IMAGING for PLASTIC SURGERY

IMAGING for PLASTIC SURGERY

Edited by
Luca Saba
Warren M. Rozen
Alberto Alonso-Burgos
Diego Ribuffo

CRC Press
Taylor & Francis Group
Boca Raton London New York

CRC Press is an imprint of the
Taylor & Francis Group, an **informa** business

CRC Press
Taylor & Francis Group
6000 Broken Sound Parkway NW, Suite 300
Boca Raton, FL 33487-2742

First issued in paperback 2018

ISBN 13: 978-1-138-74754-8 (pbk)
ISBN 13: 978-1-4665-5111-4 (hbk)

Visit the Taylor & Francis Web site at
http://www.taylorandfrancis.com

and the CRC Press Web site at
http://www.crcpress.com

Luca Saba dedicates this book to his parents,
Giovanni Saba and Raffaela Polla, for their love.

Diego Ribuffo dedicates this book to his wife, Stella, and to his wonderful girls, Chiara and Lavinia, for their continuous support during the years in Cagliari.

Warren M. Rozen dedicates this book and the time that has gone into it to his wife, Genia, and daughters, Rebecca and Hayley, to whom he will repay that time in full.

Alberto Alonso-Burgos dedicates this book to the real engine of his life, his wife Arantxa and sons Pilar and Miguel and to the memory of his father, José.

Contents

Foreword

It is not strange that a few years after the discovery by Röntgen of the x-rays, several researchers were trying to depict, by using the new and revolutionary *light*, the anatomy of the vessels. The morphology of arteries and veins was some kind of mystery, only available by anatomical dissections and by casts obtained after its extraction. Once liquid intravascular contrasts were developed, many groups worldwide produced, by using rudimentary but at the same time very imaginative techniques, new images of the flow within the vessel lumen.

Since that time, this effort has never decreased, and there is still a maintained interest in actualizing the imaging of the vessel walls and the study of all the intrinsic peculiarities of the vascular flow. Sectional imaging methods have replaced the conventional angiographic techniques in which a catheter is placed within the lumen by percutaneous approach. Such classic procedures are now used exclusively for therapeutic purposes like angioplasty or embolization.

The new methods for vascular diagnosis must include several concepts such as a meticulous analysis of its morphology, branching, and relation with other structures. Also, a careful evaluation of the vessel wall layers with precise knowledge of its characteristics, thickness, pathology, and also its flow, in terms of amount, velocity, or direction of the main stream, which may have great influence on the performance of any endovascular procedure as well as on the consequences that any endovascular therapy may have in the future must be done.

Vascular diagnosis should then contemplate not only morphology but also function and should be associated with the study of biomarkers that may allow the early detection and subsequent quantification of the consequences that any flow change (e.g., insufficiency or turbulence) may have in the targeted viscera or organ.

Imaging techniques allow, at this moment, the evaluation of the morphology of the vessels in such a way that many outstanding anatomists could never imagine just before Röntgen introduced the *light to see in depth*. This book is an outstanding example.

José I. Bilbao, MD
Head of Vascular and Interventional Unit
University of Navarra Clinic
Pamplona, Spain

Over the past years, we have seen continuous and increasingly rapid development of accessible imaging techniques. Imaging procedures allow integrating the information strictly anatomical, with submillimeter resolution, with that of a functional nature related to molecular imaging. All detailed derived information allows plastic surgeons to have precise preoperative data strictly related to the real clinical status of the patient. This book comes at the right time. The accurate presentation, to the interested reader, of the most recent and relevant imaging methodologies, from innovative ultrasound procedures to CT and from MRI to numerous and sophisticated surveys of nuclear medicine, helps to make valuable contributions of knowledge to a competent user who is here the modern plastic surgeon. Its success is largely due to Dr. Saba's and coeditors' broad experience and enthusiasm and their special talent of involving skilled colleagues in relation to their specific competence.

Mario Piga, MD
Professor of Nuclear Medicine
and
Chief of Radiology and Nuclear Medicine Department
University Hospital, Cagliari, Italy

New modalities for instrumental evaluation are getting more and more reliable and are now able to show fine vascular structures even in the skin and soft tissues. This possibility allows plastic surgeons to plan flaps (in particular, microsurgical flaps, but also propeller and fasciocutaneous flaps) in a refined and precise way, thus selecting the best option for the patient. Nowadays, after the era of anatomically predefined flaps, we are getting back to planning based on the single vessel and its newly discovered territory (angiosome). This reality induces us to use preoperative imaging as a routine and finalized method, not only to study the recipient area and vessels (as we used to do in the past years) but also to ascertain which is the best surgical indication with minimal morbidity. This book, to which our group has made an important contribution, provides the reader with a precise and reliable state of the art in modern plastic surgery.

Nicolò Scuderi, MD
Professor of Plastic Surgery
and
Chief of Plastic Surgery Unit
Sapienza University Hospital, Rome, Italy

Preface

Over the past five years, preoperative imaging has become increasingly adopted for preoperative planning in plastic surgery, with particular applications in perforator flap surgery and 3-D facial reconstruction at the forefront. Accurate preoperative analysis can reduce the length of operations and maximise surgical design and dissection techniques. This is the first collection to be published dedicated to the application of advanced imaging technologies in plastic and reconstructive surgery.

New imaging modalities have advanced to previously inconceived heights, with high-resolution, 3-D analysis of vascular anatomy and perfusion now attainable. Computed tomography (CT) and magnetic resonance imaging (MRI) have recently emerged as outstanding non-invasive techniques for the study of the vascular and non-vascular systems. In particular, CT angiography has probably now imposed itself as the *state-of-the-art* technique to explore the vascular system, with evolving MR angiography (MRA) sequences and greater magnetic fields (3 T or more) with the potential to become a matching modality in the future.

This project arises from the cooperation and friendship between the groups of radiology and plastic surgery of the European and Australian universities that shared an extensive experience in these topics in the last 10 years. The authors are world-renowned scientists who have dedicated most of their work to this exciting field. This book is the concrete example of how multidisciplinary cooperation and friendship can lead to excellent results.

The scientific purpose of this book is to comprehensively present all of the imaging techniques, potentialities, and present and future applications as applied to plastic and reconstructive surgery.

Luca Saba
Warren M. Rozen
Alberto Alonso Burgos
Diego Ribuffo

Acknowledgements

It is not possible to overstate the gratitude to the many individuals who helped to produce this book. In particular, the editors thank Matteo Atzeni for his help.

Dr. Luca Saba acknowledges the patience and understanding displayed by Tiziana throughout his work. Without her continuous encouragement, this book would not have been completed.

Diego Ribuffo thanks all the contributors from his home university for their enthusiasm and collaboration.

Warren M. Rozen thanks the contributors and coauthors with whom he has collaborated in this volume and the ongoing institutional support for his research interests and advances.

Alberto Alonso-Burgos thanks all the colleges involved in this book for their enthusiasm and collaboration and the support from the University of Navarra Clinic then and the University Hospital Fundación Jiménez Díaz now.

The editors have received considerable support and cooperation from individuals at CRC Press/ Taylor & Francis Group, particularly Michael Slaughter, Jessica Vakili, Joette Lynch, and Michele Smith, and from Dennis Troutman at diacriTech, each of whom helped to minimize the obstacles editors encountered.

Acknowledgements

It is not possible to enumerate the gratitude to the many individuals who helped to produce this book. In particular, the editors thank Martin Sexton for his help.

Dr. Luca Saba acknowledges the patience and understanding displayed by Lysanna throughout the work; without her continuous encouragement, this book would not have been completed.

Diego Ribuffo thanks all the contributors from his home University for their enthusiasm and collaboration.

Warren M. Rozen thanks the contributors and coauthors with whom he has collaborated in this volume and the ongoing institutional support for his research interests and endeavors.

Alberto Alonso-Burgos thanks all the colleagues involved in this book for their enthusiasm and collaboration and the support from the University of Navarra Clinic and the University Hospital Fundación Jiménez Díaz.

The editors have received considerable support and cooperation from individuals at CRC Press, Taylor & Francis Group, particularly Michael Slaughter, Jessica Vakili, Jennifer Lynch, and Michele Smith, and from Dennis Troutman at diacriTech, each of whom helped to minimize the obstacles the editors encountered.

Editors

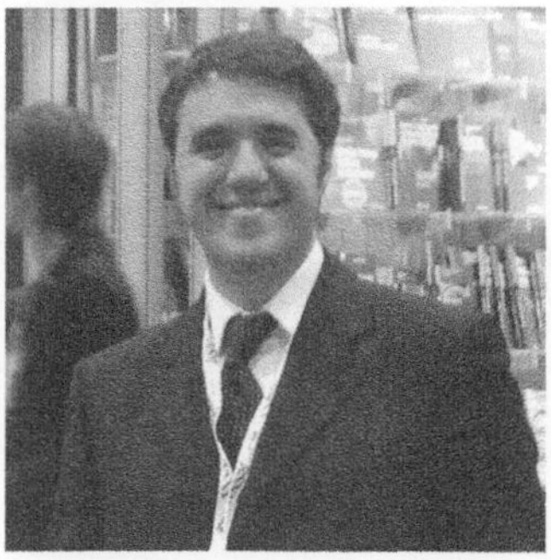

Luca Saba received his MD from the University of Cagliari, Italy, in 2002. Today he works in the AOU (Azienda Ospedaliero Universitaria) of Cagliari. Dr. Saba's research focuses on multi-detector-row computed tomography, magnetic resonance, ultrasound, neuroradiology, and diagnostics in vascular sciences.

His works as lead author include more than 130 high-impact-factor, peer-reviewed journals such as the *American Journal of Neuroradiology, Atherosclerosis, European Radiology, European Journal of Radiology, Acta Radiologica, CardioVascular and Interventional Radiology, Journal of Computer Assisted Tomography, American Journal of Roentgenology, Neuroradiology, Clinical Radiology, Journal of Cardiovascular Surgery, Cerebrovascular Diseases, Brain Pathology, and Medical Physics.*

He is a well-known speaker and has given more than 45 speeches at the national and international levels.

Dr. Saba has won 15 scientific and extracurricular awards during his career. He has presented more than 450 papers and posters in national and international congresses (RSNA, ESGAR, ECR, ISR, AOCR, AINR, JRS, SIRM, AINR). He has written 18 book chapters and is editor of 7 books in the fields of computed tomography, cardiovascular, plastic surgery, gynaecological imaging, and neurodegenerative imaging.

He is member of the Italian Society of Radiology (SIRM), the European Society of Radiology (ESR), the Radiological Society of North America (RSNA), the American Roentgen Ray Society (ARRS), the and European Society of Neuroradiology (ESNR) and serves as reviewer of more 30 scientific journals.

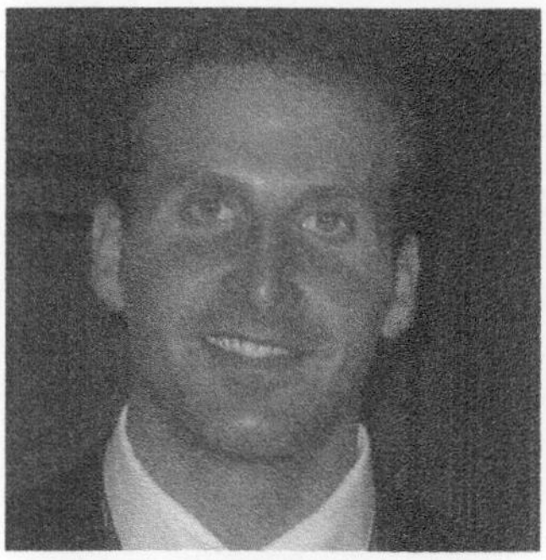

Warren M. Rozen is a consultant plastic and reconstructive surgeon in Melbourne, Australia. He combines clinical practice in plastic and reconstructive surgery with translational research at Monash University and James Cook University, following completion of postgraduate studies in surgical anatomy through an MD and a PhD. He has contributed to more than 400 publications, has given more than 100 national and international research presentations, and is on the editorial board of 9 international journals including the *Annals of Plastic Surgery and Microsurgery.* His academic interests include reconstructive flap design and preoperative flap planning.

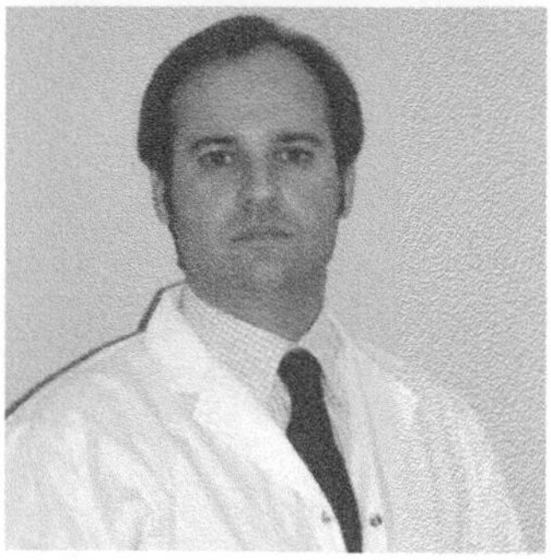

Alberto Alonso-Burgos MD, PhD, is a consultant radiologist in the Vascular and Interventional Radiology Unit at the University Hospital Fundación Jiménez Díaz (Madrid, Spain). He completed all his medical training (MD, 2003; PhD, 2009; and diagnostic radiology residency, 2008) at the University of Navarra and Clinic University of Navarra (Pamplona, Spain). His main interest and research have been focused on CT and MRI angiography for reconstructive surgery and preoperative 3D planning as well as oncologic interventional radiology. He has published more than 25 papers and 10 chapters and has been the editor of textbooks, including the first general imaging text for reconstructive plastic surgery.

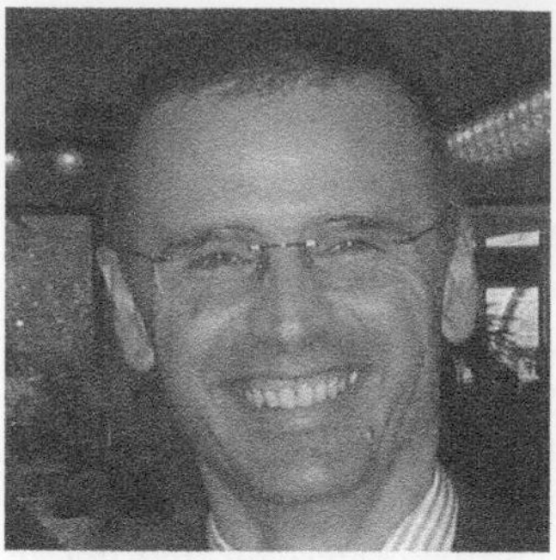

Diego Ribuffo MD, PhD is a European Board–certified plastic surgeon. He combines clinical practice with teaching and research at Sapienza University in Rome, Italy. His main clinical interests are reconstructive microsurgery and breast surgery. He has authored over 200 publications and 2 books and has given over 100 presentations at national and international meetings. He has won several scientific prizes and is on the editorial board of two international journals.

After completing two fellowships in Atlanta and Melbourne, and being associate professor for eight years at Cagliari University, Professor Diego Ribuffo is now back at his home university, where he currently serves as associate professor of plastic surgery in the Department of Surgery, Pietro Valdoni at Sapienza University of Rome.

Contributors

Robert J. Allen
The Center for the Advancement of Breast Reconstruction at New York
New York Eye and Ear Infirmary
and
New York University Medical Center
New York

and

Medical University of South Carolina
Charleston, South Carolina

and

Louisiana State University Health Sciences Center
New Orleans, Louisiana

Xavier Alomar
Department of Radiology
Creu Blanca Clinic
Barcelona, Spain

Alberto Alonso-Burgos
Department of Radiology
University Hospital Fundación Jiménez Díaz
Autonomous University of Madrid
Madrid, Spain

Anuja K. Antony
Division of Plastic and Reconstructive Surgery
Department of Surgery
University of Illinois at Chicago
Chicago, Illinois

Michele Anzidei
Department of Radiology
Policlinico Umberto I
Sapienza University of Rome
Rome, Italy

Mark W. Ashton
Department of Plastic and Reconstructive Surgery
Royal Melbourne Hospital
Parkville, Victoria, Australia

Matteo Atzeni
Section of Plastic Surgery
Department of Surgery
Cagliari University Hospital
Cagliari, Italy

Alberto Benito
Department of Radiology
Clínica Universidad de Navarra
Pamplona, Spain

Barbara Cagli
Division of Plastic and Reconstructive Surgery
Campus Bio-Medico of Rome University
Rome, Italy

Pietro Giorgio Calò
Department of Surgical Sciences
University of Cagliari
Cagliari, Italy

David Cano
Department of Radiology
Clínica Universidad de Navarra
Pamplona, Spain

Jon Etxano Cantera
Department of Radiology
Clínica Universidad de Navarra
Pamplona, Spain

Bruno Carlesimo
Unit of Plastic and Reconstructive Surgery
Policlinico Umberto I
Sapienza University of Rome
Rome, Italy

Carlo Catalano
Department of Radiology
Policlinico Umberto I
Sapienza University of Rome
Rome, Italy

Can Çevikol
Department of Radiology
School of Medicine
Akdeniz University
Antalya, Turkey

Michael P. Chae
Department of Surgery
Monash Plastic Surgery Research Unit
Monash University
Clayton, Victoria, Australia

Hung-Chi Chen
Plastic and Reconstructive Surgery Department
Superintendent of International Medical Center
China Medical University
Taichung, Taiwan

Wei F. Chen
Division of Plastic and Reconstructive Surgery
Department of Surgery
University of Iowa Hospitals and Clinics
Iowa City, Iowa

Sotirios Chondrogiannis
PET Unit
Department of Nuclear Medicine
Santa Maria della Misericordia Hospital
Rovigo, Italy

Emanuele Cigna
Unit of Plastic Surgeon
Department of Surgery
Sapienza University of Rome
Rome, Italy

Federica Ciolina
Policlinico Umberto I
Department of Radiology
Sapienza University of Rome
Rome, Italy

Riccardo Cipriani
Division of Plastic Surgery
S. Orsola-Malpighi University Hospital
Bologna, Italy

Juan Angel Clavero
Department of Radiology
Creu Blanca Clinic
Barcelona, Spain

Andrea Conversi
Unit of Plastic and Reconstructive Surgery
Department of Surgery
Sapienza University of Rome
Rome, Italy

Francesco Stagno d'Alcontres
Plastic Surgery Unit
Policlinico "G. Martino" University Hospital
Messina, Italy

Gabriele Delia
Plastic Surgery Unit
Policlinico "G. Martino" University Hospital
Messina, Italy

Carlo De Masi
Department of Radiology
S.M. Goretti Hospital
Latina, Italy

Luca Andrea Dessy
Unit of Plastic Surgery
Department of Surgery
Sapienza University of Rome
Rome, Italy

Valerio Duce
Regional Center of Nuclear Medicine
Department of Translational Research and Advanced Technologies in Medicine and Surgery
University of Pisa
Pisa, Italy

Joan Duch
Department of Nuclear Medicine
Santa Creu i Sant Pau Hospital
Autonomous University of Barcelona (UAB)
Barcelona, Spain

Ahmet Duymaz
Department of Plastic and Reconstructive Surgery
School of Medicine
Akdeniz University
Antalya, Turkey

Zdeněk Dvořák
Medical Faculty of Masaryk University Brno
Clinic of Plastic and Aesthetic Surgery
St. Anna's University Hospital
Brno, Czech Republic

Edmund W. Ek
Department of Surgery
and
Melbourne Institute of Plastic Surgery
University of Melbourne
Parkville, Victoria, Australia

Arlette Elizalde
Department of Radiology
Clínica Universidad de Navarra
Pamplona, Spain

Mariana Elorz
Department of Radiology
Clínica Universidad de Navarra
Pamplona, Spain

Paola A. Erba
Regional Center of Nuclear Medicine
Department of Translational Research and Advanced Technologies in Medicine and Surgery
University of Pisa
Pisa, Italy

Piergiorgio Falappa
Institute of Rome Italy
Bambino Gesù Children's Hospital—I.R.C.C.S.
Rome, Italy

Nefer Fallico
Department of Plastic and Reconstructive Surgery
Sapienza University of Rome
Rome, Italy

Gloria Pasqua Fanelli
Department of Radiology
S.M. Goretti Hospital
Latina, Italy

Emilio García-Tutor
Plastic and Reconstructive Surgery Department
Guadalajara General Hospital
Guadalajara, Spain

Andrea Ghezzi
Director of Hand Surgery Department
St. Joseph Hospital MultiMedica Group
and
Plastic Surgery School
University of Milan
Milan, Italy

Francesca Granata
Neuroradiology Unit
Policlinico "G. Martino" University Hospital
Messina, Italy

Manfredi Greco
Unit of Plastic and Reconstructive Surgery
Department of Surgery
University of Catanzaro
Catanzaro, Italy

Maristella Guerra
Unit of Plastic Surgery
San Gallicano-IFO Hospital
Rome, Italy

Luis Pina Insauti
Department of Radiology
Clínica Universidad de Navarra
Pamplona, Spain

Kamil Karaali
Department Radiology
School of Medicine
Akdeniz University
Antalya, Turkey

Tara Karnezis
The Taylor Lab
Department of Anatomy and Neurosciences
University of Melbourne
Parkville, Victoria, Australia

Nolan Karp
Department of Plastic Surgery
New York University School of Medicine
New York, New York

Cara Michelle Le Roux
The Taylor Lab
Department of Anatomy and Neurosciences
University of Melbourne
Parkville, Victoria, Australia

Steven Lo
Canniesburn Plastic Surgery Unit
Glasgow, United Kingdom

Luisa Locantore
Regional Center of Nuclear Medicine
Department of Translational Research and Advanced Technologies in Medicine and Surgery
University of Pisa
Pisa, Italy

Marcello Longo
Neuroradiology Unit
Policlinico "G. Martino" University Hospital
Messina, Italy

Ángeles Franco López
Cardiac Imaging Unit
Department of Radiology
University Hospital Fundación Jiménez Díaz
Madrid, Spain

Maria M. Lotempio
Center for the Advancement of Breast Reconstruction at New York
New York Eye and Ear Infirmary
New York, New York
and
Medical University of South Carolina
Charleston, South Carolina

Federico Lo Torto
Unit of Plastic and Reconstructive Surgery
Policlinico Umberto I
Sapienza University of Rome
Rome, Italy

Flavia Lupo
Plastic Surgery Unit
Policlinico "G. Martino" University Hospital
Messina, Italy

Anna Margherita Maffione
PET Unit
Department of Nuclear Medicine
Santa Maria della Misericordia Hospital
Rovigo, Italy

Marta Tomás Mallebrera
Cardiac Imaging Unit
Department of Radiology
University Hospital Fundación Jiménez Díaz
Madrid, Spain

Carlo Augusto Mallio
Division of Radiology
Campus Bio-Medico of Rome University
Rome, Italy

Gianpiero Manca
Regional Center of Nuclear Medicine
Department of Translational Research and Advanced Technologies in Medicine and Surgery
University of Pisa
Pisa, Italy

Marco Marcasciano
Unit of Plastic and Reconstructive Surgery
Policlinico Umberto I
Sapienza University of Rome
Rome, Italy

Claudio Marchetti
Division of Oral and Maxillo-Facial Surgery
S. Orsola-Malpighi University Hospital
Bologna, Italy

Adriano Marcolongo
Santa Maria della Misericordia Hospital
Rovigo, Italy

Giuliano Mariani
Regional Center of Nuclear Medicine
Department of Translational Research and Advanced Technologies in Medicine and Surgery
University of Pisa
Pisa, Italy

Michele Maruccia
Unit of Plastic Surgery
Department of Surgery
Sapienza University of Rome
Rome, Italy

Jaume Masia
Department of Plastic Surgery
Santa Creu i Sant Pau Hospital
Autonomous University of Barcelona (UAB)
Barcelona, Spain

Sara Mazzarri
Regional Center of Nuclear Medicine
Department of Translational Research and Advanced Technologies in Medicine and Surgery
University of Pisa
Pisa, Italy

Fabio Medas
Department of Surgical Sciences
University of Cagliari
Cagliari, Italy

Arianna Milia
Unit of Plastic and Reconstructive Surgery
Department of Surgical, Oncological and Stomatological Sciences
University of Palermo
Palermo, Italy

Alessandro Napoli
Department of Radiology
Policlinico Umberto I
Sapienza University of Rome
Rome, Italy

Maria Luisa Nardulli
Department of Plastic Surgery
Santa Creu i Sant Pau Hospital
Autonomous University of Barcelona (UAB)
Barcelona, Spain

Luca Negosanti
Division of Plastic Surgery
S. Orsola-Malpighi University Hospital
Bologna, Italy

Jeremy Nickfarjam
Division of Plastic Surgery
Albert Einstein School of Medicine
Bronx, New York

Angelo Nicolosi
Department of Surgical Sciences
University of Cagliari
Cagliari, Italy

Vachara Niumsawatt
Department of Surgery
Monash Medical Centre
Clayton, Victoria, Australia

Federica Orsini
Regional Center of Nuclear Medicine
Department of Translational Research and Advanced Technologies in Medicine and Surgery
University of Pisa
Pisa, Italy

Ömer Özkan
Department of Plastic and Reconstructive Surgery
School of Medicine
Akdeniz University
Antalya, Turkey

Özlenen Özkan
Department of Plastic and Reconstructive Surgery
School of Medicine
Akdeniz University
Antalya, Turkey

Giorgio Pajardi
Director of Hand Surgery Department
St. Joseph Hospital MultiMedica Group
and
Plastic Surgery School
University of Milan
Milan, Italy

Tiziano Pallara
Division of Plastic and Reconstructive Surgery
Campus Bio-Medico of Rome University
Rome, Italy

Paola Parisi
Department of Surgery
Monash Plastic Surgery Research Unit
Monash University
Clayton, Victoria, Australia

Emilia Pascali
Division of Radiology
S. Orsola-Malpighi University Hospital
Bologna, Italy

Philippe Pelissier
Department of Plastic Reconstructive and Aesthetic Surgery
Centre of F. Michelet
University Hospital of Bordeaux
Bordeaux, France

Paolo Persichetti
Division of Plastic and Reconstructive Surgery
Campus Bio-Medico of Rome University
Rome, Italy

Mario Piga
Department of Nuclear Medicine
Nuclear Medicine Center
University of Cagliari
Cagliari, Italy

Giuseppe Pisano
Department of Surgical Sciences
University of Cagliari
Cagliari, Italy

Gemma Pons
Department of Plastic Surgery
Santa Creu i Sant Pau Hospital
Autonomous University of Barcelona (UAB)
Barcelona, Spain

Hayley Reynolds
The Taylor Lab
Department of Anatomy and Neurosciences
University of Melbourne
Parkville, Victoria, Australia

Diego Ribuffo
Department of Surgery
Sapienza University
Rome, Italy

and

Department of Surgery
University of Cagliari
Cagliari, Italy

Warren M. Rozen
Department of Surgery
Monash Plastic Surgery Research Unit
Monash University
Clayton, Victoria, Australia

Domenico Rubello
PET Unit
Department of Nuclear Medicine
Santa Maria della Misericordia Hospital
Rovigo, Italy

Marco Ruggiero
Unit of Plastic and Reconstructive Surgery
Policlinico Umberto I
Sapienza University of Rome
Rome, Italy

Luca Saba
Unit of Radiology
Department of Medical Sciences Mario Aresu
and
Department of Radiology
University of Cagliari
Cagliari, Italy

Michel Saint-Cyr
Southwestern Medical Center
University of Texas
Dallas, Texas

Luigino Santecchia
Department of Surgery
Institute of Rome
Bambino Gesù Children's Hospital—I.R.C.C.S.
Rome, Italy

Mark Schaverien
Department of Plastic Surgery
Ninewells Hospital
Dundee, United Kingdom

Nicolò Scuderi
Department of Plastic and Reconstructive Surgery
Sapienza University of Rome
Rome, Italy

Alessandra Serra
Department of Nuclear Medicine
Nuclear Medicine Center
University of Cagliari
Cagliari, Italy

Francesco Serratore
Department of Plastic and Reconstructive Surgery
Sapienza University of Rome
Rome, Italy

Rossella Sgarzani
Division of Plastic Surgery
S. Orsola-Malpighi University Hospital
Bologna, Italy

Ramin Shayan
The Taylor Lab
Department of Anatomy and Neurosciences
University of Melbourne
Parkville, Victoria, Australia

Pedro Slon
Department of Radiology
Clínica Universidad de Navarra
Pamplona, Spain

David J. Hunter-Smith
Department of Surgery
Monash Plastic Surgery Research Unit
Monash University
Clayton, Victoria, Australia

Gary Xia Vern Tan
Department of Surgery
Monash Medical Centre
Clayton, Victoria, Australia

Elisa Tardelli
Regional Center of Nuclear Medicine
Department of Translational Research and Advanced Technologies in Medicine and Surgery
University of Pisa
Pisa, Italy

Achille Tarsitano
Division of Oral and Maxillo-Facial Surgery
S. Orsola-Malpighi University Hospital
Bologna, Italy

Oren Tepper
Division of Plastic Surgery
Albert Einstein School of Medicine
Bronx, New York

Jeannette W. Ting
Department of Surgery
Monash Medical Centre
Clayton, Victoria, Australia

Manuel Tredici
Regional Center of Nuclear Medicine
Department of Translational Research and Advanced Technologies in Medicine and Surgery
University of Pisa
Pisa, Italy

Donata Maria Antonia Assunta Vaccaro
Division of Radiology
Campus Bio-Medico of Rome University
Rome, Italy

Julie Vasile
Northern Westchester Hospital
Mt. Kisco, New York

Jiří Veselý
Medical Faculty of Masaryk University Brno
Clinic of Plastic and Aesthetic Surgery
St. Anna's University Hospital
Brno, Czech Republic

Fu Chan Wei
Department of Plastic Surgery
College of Medicine
Chang Gung Memorial Hospital
Chang Gung University
Linkou, Taiwan, Republic of China

Iain S. Whitaker
Chair of Plastic and Reconstructive Surgery
The Welsh Centre for Burns and Plastic Surgery
Morriston Hospital
Swansea, Wales

Takumi Yamamoto
Department of Plastic and Reconstructive Surgery
Graduate School of Medicine
The University of Tokyo
Tokyo, Japan

Hidehiko Yoshimatsu
Department of Plastic and Reconstructive Surgery
Graduate School of Medicine
The University of Tokyo
Tokyo, Japan

Fulvio Zaccagna
Department of Radiology
Policlinico Umberto I
Sapienza University of Rome
Rome, Italy

Mario Zama
Plastic and Maxillofacial Unit
Institute of Rome
Bambino Gesù Children's Hospital—I.R.C.C.S.
Rome, Italy

Bruno Beomonte Zobel
Division of Radiology
Campus Bio-Medico of Rome University
Rome, Italy

and

Northern Westchester Hospital
Mount Kisco, New York

1 Computed Tomography

Michele Anzidei, Federica Ciolina, Fulvio Zaccagna, Alessandro Napoli, and Carlo Catalano

CONTENTS

In the last few years, the use of computed tomography angiography (CTA) in the clinical workup of patients with known or suspected cardiovascular disease has grown rapidly. With the introduction of spiral CT scanning in the 1990s and the transition to multidetector row technology, and the consequent reduction in acquisition times, CTA has developed so fast that in a few years it has become an easy-to-perform and well-standardised technique. At present, CTA plays a major role in the diagnosis and follow-up of cardiovascular disease, including coronary pathologies, and can be considered as a robust alternative to invasive catheter angiography under different circumstances (e.g. diagnosis of complex vascular and skeletal anomalies, traumatic injuries and their preoperative evaluation). In parallel to these applications, CTA was recently used for vascular mapping in patients undergoing plastic surgery interventions.

1.1 EXAMINATION TECHNIQUE

Computed tomography (CT) is a tomographic technique that uses x-ray to produce images. One or, more recently, two x-ray sources rotate around the patient, and the x-ray beams produced by these sources are detected by a panel of detectors on the other side of the gantry. After the acquisition of x-ray attenuation data, a mathematical image reconstruction (inverse Radon transformation) approach is used to calculate the local attenuation of each point of acquisition volume, and hence, CT images were produced in greyscale to represent the attenuation data.

The introduction of helical acquisition yields a reduction in acquisition time as mentioned earlier, but it also permits performing a volumetric acquisition that is mandatory to obtain CTA images of adequate quality. Moreover, the use of contrast medium (CM) and proper timing is mandatory to obtain a good-quality CTA acquisition.

1.2 VOLUMETRIC ACQUISITION AND QUALITY ASSESSMENT OF CTA

Volumetric acquisition is a continuous acquisition that occurs during the constant movement of table along the *z*-axis using a spiral pattern around the patient in a single apnoea. This type of acquisition begins efficiently with the introduction of a multidetector system that rotates integrally with the x-ray source around the patient during the scanning (third-generation technology of CT scan) (Figure 1.1).

The introduction of volumetric acquisition yields the following advantages: lower acquisition time, the possibility to examine large volumes at thin layer, and the possibility to obtain isotropic voxel (mandatory for high-quality reconstructions). With these advantages, it is clear that this type of acquisition has radically changed the feasibility of CTA, revolutionising its application fields.

To evaluate vessels, particularly those of small dimensions such as coronary arteries or perforating arteries, it is mandatory to use the maximum achievable spatial resolution with an adequate layer thickness. Sometimes, the use of maximum spatial resolution is not allowed due to signal-to-noise ratio (which is defined as 'a numerical size which correlates the power of the useful signal with the noise in any system of acquisition, processing or transmission of the information'), so acquisition parameters need to be optimised to obtain the best compromise between spatial and temporal resolution and image quality (represented by the SNR). In particular, with the new generation multidetector CT (MDCT) scans, above 64 slices, it is now possible to acquire slices under 1 mm, but this increase in spatial resolution induces a reduction of the SNR.

Considering how important it is to obtain adequate quality images, handling both acquisition and reconstruction parameters is essential.

The most important acquisition parameters are the number of active detectors and detector collimation, pitch, tube load, and tube voltage. Meanwhile, the most important reconstruction parameters are section thickness, reconstruction increment or interval, field of view, reconstruction matrix size, and reconstruction filter or algorithm.

1.3 ACQUISITION PARAMETERS

The number of active detectors is the number of sections that are acquired simultaneously, and it could be as high as the detector rows of the CT scan but could also be less than the maximum achievable.

Detector collimation is determined by the opening degree of detectors, and it varies the amplitude of the photon beam used to detect the attenuation profiles of the object under examination.

Pitch factor is the relation between the table feed and the total width of the acquired volume. Pitch factor is obtained by the following relation: $P = TF/(N \times C)$, where TF is the table feed, N is the detector number, and C is the beam collimation.

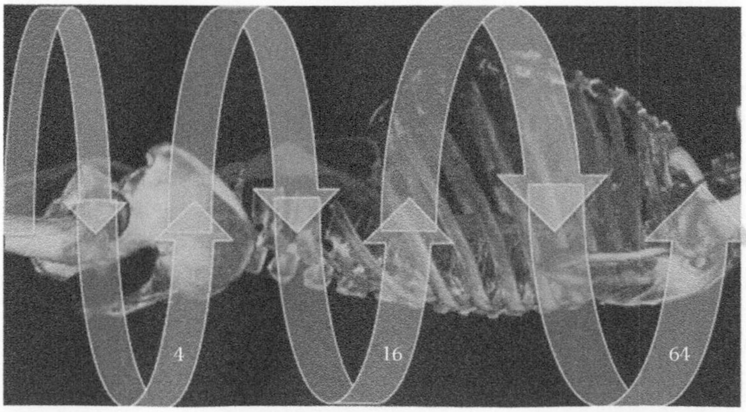

FIGURE 1.1 Volumetric spiral scan: the highest detectors number, the greatest volume acquired.

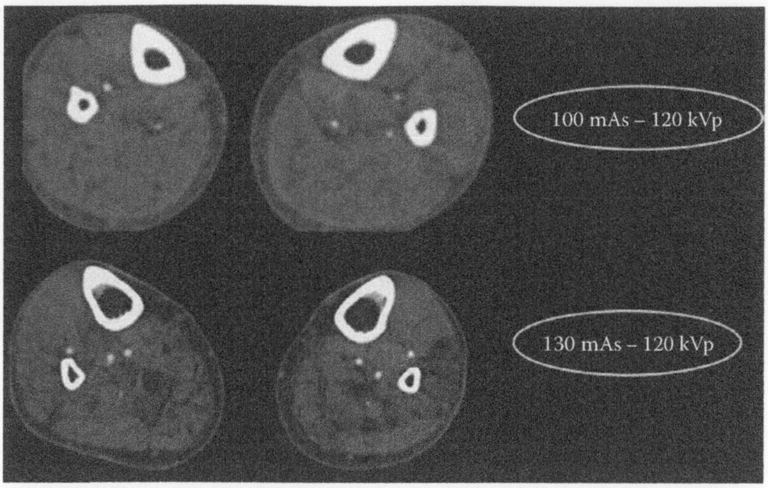

FIGURE 1.2 Study of the peripheral system in two patients with a similar body mass, evaluated both at 120 kVp but with 100 mAs and 130 mAs, respectively. The use of a greater amount of mAs produces an image with less noise and a greater contrast resolution.

Tube load (mAs) determines the number of photons produced by the x-ray tube and is proportional to the radiation dose. Tube voltage (kVp) is the potential difference between the two extremities of the x-ray tube, and it determines the energy of the x-ray beam. These two parameters are the most important to limit radiation exposure. In fact, the dose increased linearly with an increase of mAs and with an exponential relationship with an increase of kVp. It is mandatory to know that with a decrease of the kVp, the photon energy lessens and the tissue attenuation (CM included) increases, with a consequent greater contrast resolution (Figure 1.2). With this rule, in cases in which a lesser volume of CM is required (e.g. in patients with cardiac or renal failure or in paediatric patients), using a lower kVp value could balance the lower enhancement due to the lower CM volume and achieve a good contrast resolution.

1.4 RECONSTRUCTION PARAMETERS

Section thickness is the width of the contiguous layer in the final images, and it refers to the images obtained in all the three reconstruction planes. It can be equal to or greater than the value of the collimation, but not less than it. Using a section thickness greater than collimation, we can have a lower noise in the final data set.

Reconstruction interval represents the overlap between two contiguous layers. It could be higher, equal to, or lesser than the layer thickness, resulting, respectively, in layers which are spaced, adjacent, or overlapped.

Field of view (FoV) represents the size of the planar images on the transverse plane. Using a small FoV generates higher-resolution images but with a higher noise (Figures 1.3 and 1.4).

Reconstruction matrix is the number of pixels that constitute the image. It is normally of fixed size (512 × 512), but new CT scanners can have a bigger matrix to increase spatial resolution.

Reconstruction algorithms (or convolution filters) are used to reconstruct images from the raw data. Information on the attenuation profiles of the object under examination is reworked by means of mathematical algorithms which apply appropriate correction functions of the data before the production of the final image. By using this, we can obtain the highest influence on the quality of the planar reconstructed image (Figure 1.5).

The use of high-definition filters (sharp) increases the spatial resolution, but also the image noise; the use of soft filters (smooth) reduces the definition, but also the noise level.

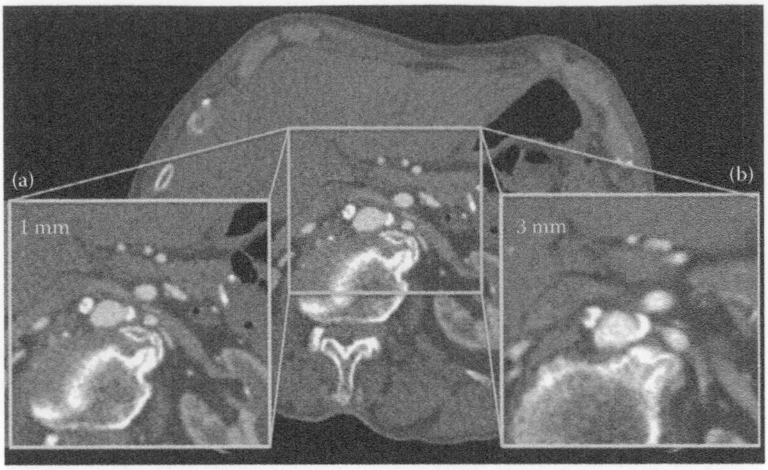

FIGURE 1.3 Particular of the abdomen reconstructed using a slice thickness of 1 mm (a) and 3 mm (b).

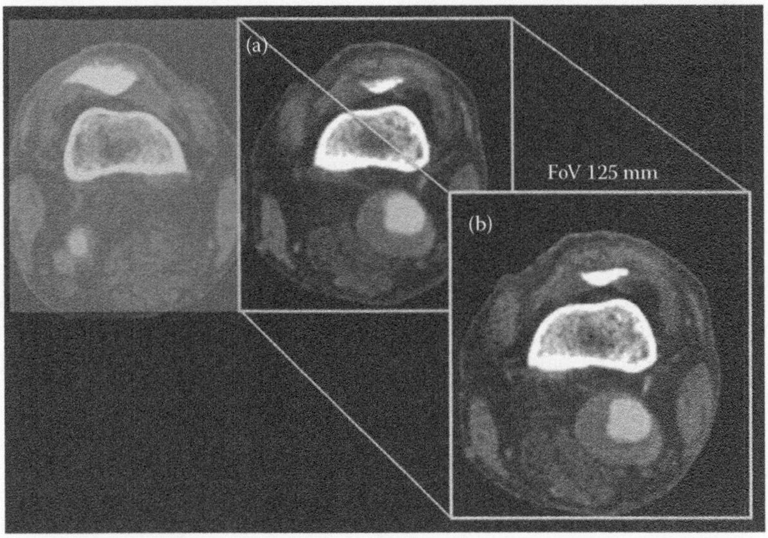

FIGURE 1.4 Patient with aneurism of the popliteal artery of the left inferior limb: FoV reconstruction of 350 mm (including both legs) (a) and limited to one leg (b).

1.5 CONTRAST MEDIUM ADMINISTRATION

The use of CM in CTA is mandatory to achieve opacification of vascular structure. The CMs used in CT are water-soluble derivatives of symmetrically iodinated benzene (triiodobenzene) with a high atomic number able to determine x-ray attenuation. The goal of CM administration is to achieve the maximum achievable opacification of vascular structure, and as it seems obvious that for the same administration (total dose of CM and infusion speed expressed in mL/s) and scanning parameters (mAs and kVp), the higher the iodine concentration is (expressed in mgI/mL), the greater will be the enhancement, hence, it is mandatory to know the principle of CM administration well to adapt it to the patient and the CT scanner.

At present, different CMs are available on the market that have different iodine concentrations and other chemical–physical characteristics. But they are used only for their ability to determine the x-ray attenuation, and hence, all pharmacological effects are generally undesired. Ionic CMs are no longer available on the market due to adverse effects, and hence, all the CMs available now are non-ionic.

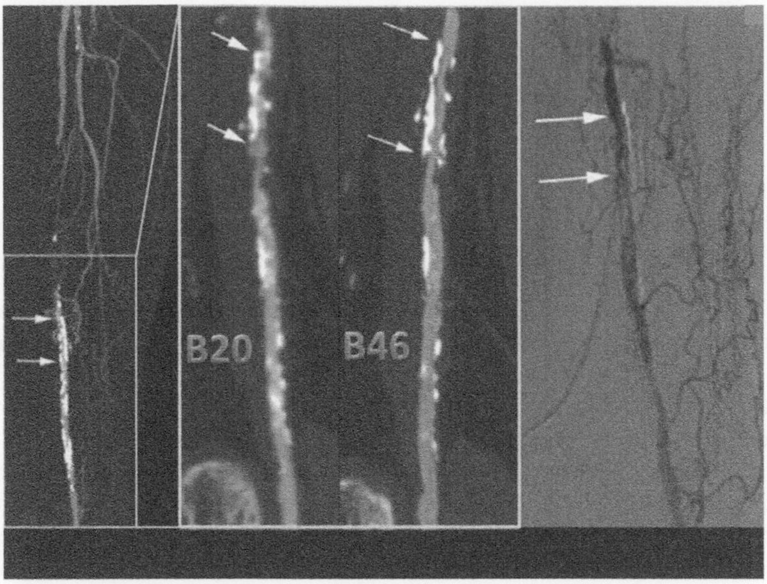

FIGURE 1.5 Use of different kernel reconstruction to obtain better image quality.

These contrast agents are molecules with an interstitial-type bio-distribution; once administered intravenously, they undergo an initial phase of vascular distribution, followed by an interstitial distribution.

1.6 CONTRAINDICATIONS TO THE CM USE IN CTA EXAMINATIONS

Contraindications to the use of iodinated contrast agents include the following:

- History of previous allergic events related to CM or atopy. In these cases, an appropriate prophylaxis must be applied (ESUR guidelines: prednisolone 30 mg 12 h and 2 h before the examination).
- Renal failure (GFR <30 mL/min): It requires both proper hydration (before and after the examination) and reduction of the total amount of administered contrast agent. In the cases of advanced renal failure, a dialysis treatment will be necessary.
- Heart failure: The danger is related to a cardiovascular failure due to a circulatory overload. In this patient, it is mandatory to minimise the total amount of contrast agent administered.
- Pregnancy and nursing: Although there is no definitive information, it is possible that a portion of the CM can be temporarily secreted in mother's milk. Breastfeeding should be discontinued for approximately 24 h after the examination.
- Multiple myeloma and Waldenström's macroglobulinemia.
- Patients treated with nephrotoxic drugs (NSAIDs or especially metformin): Therapy should be discontinued at least 48 h before the examination and should be resumed 48 h after.

These contraindications can increase the risk of adverse effects and also the risk of contrast-induced nephropathy (CIN). In particular, CIN is a clinical entity characterised by acute deterioration of renal function that occurs 48–72 h after CM administration in the absence of other possible causes.

According to the severity of the clinical manifestations, allergic reactions that may occur following CM administration can be classified as

- Side effects (nausea, emesis, altered taste, sweating, etc.)
- Mild side effects (itching, hives, coughing, sneezing, etc.)

- Moderate side effects (dyspnoea, bronchospasm, hypotension, etc.)
- Severe side effects (loss of consciousness, seizures, arrhythmias, cardiac arrest)

According to the time of onset, allergic reactions can also be classified as

- Early effects
- Late effects (1–7 days after administration of CM)

1.7 CM ADMINISTRATION STRATEGY

To obtain a good opacification of vascular structure, administration strategy of CM is the key. The goal of CM administration is to maintain a constant and complete opacification in the arterial lumen during the entire scan duration, without overlapping opacification of venous vessels (Figure 1.6).

However, this constant opacification is already impossible in vivo because CM distribution tends to be a parabolic curve that is different from patient to patient.

Moreover, CM, after the first arterial phase, will distribute into the parenchymal interstitial space (parenchymal enhancement), and a small amount will enter a phase of 'recycling' going back to the vascular space. In relation to these physiological data, it is therefore possible to consider a single bolus of CM as the set of multiple fractions of volume, subjected to the recirculation phenomena, each of which contribute to a greater and longer-lasting enhancement ('additive model', Figure 1.7).

1.8 CM VOLUME AND IODINE DELIVERY RATE

The choice of CM volume is linked to the speed of injection and iodine concentration. For CTA, it is necessary to use high-speed injection rates in order to avoid bolus dilution within the vascular site and to obtain an intense and lasting enhancement through the acquisition time. By using high-speed injection rates, the intensity of vascular enhancement will be greater but its duration will be reduced.

For CT scanner under 16-channel, the CM was injected for a time equal to the scan time and so the CM quantity is directly obtained from scan duration and speed of injection. In this manner, opacification of vascular structure was constant during the entire scan, but sometimes it requires a lot of CM.

The last generation MDCT scan with a high number of detectors (64–128–320 MDCT) and the consequent reduction in acquisition time have made this approach obsolete (Figure 1.8).

For example, if we consider a carotid artery acquisition with a >16 MDCT scan, the duration of acquisition will be 6 s, and therefore, considering an injection speed of 4 mL/s, the suggested dose is only 24 mL of CM, too less to achieve a good opacification.

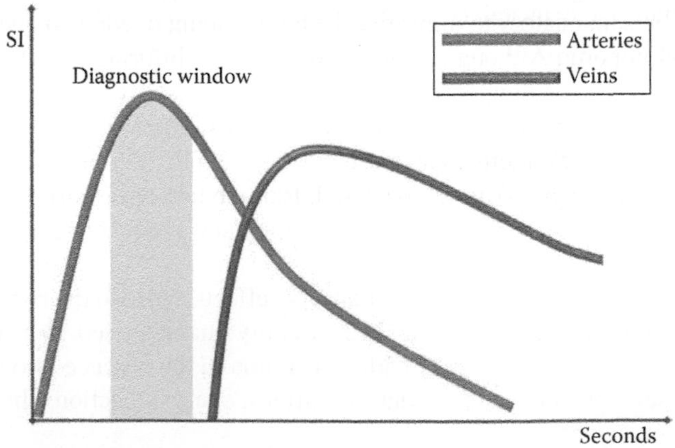

FIGURE 1.6 In vascular study the perfect diagnostic window is during the arterial peak phase; acquisition during the venous phase results in parenchimal study.

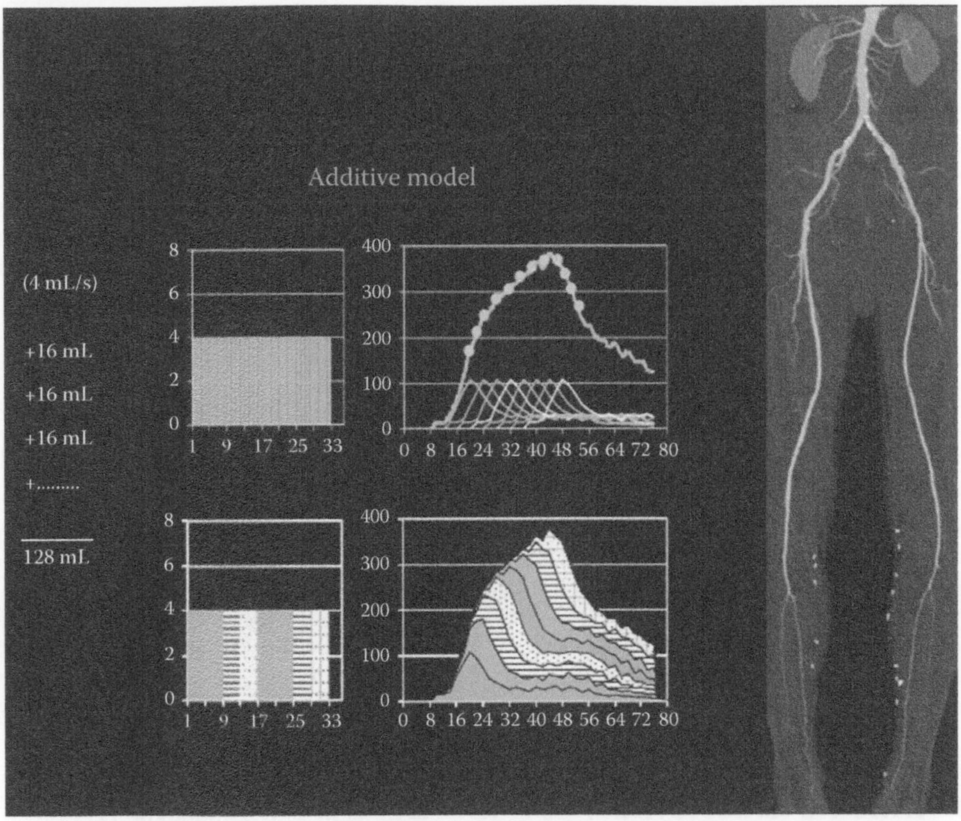

FIGURE 1.7 Continuous administration of 128 mL of contrast agent may be considered as a subsequent injection of multiple little bolus of 16 mL. The effective vascular enhancement results in the bell curve of contrast media. (Fleischmann et al. Eur Radiol 2002; 12: S11–16).

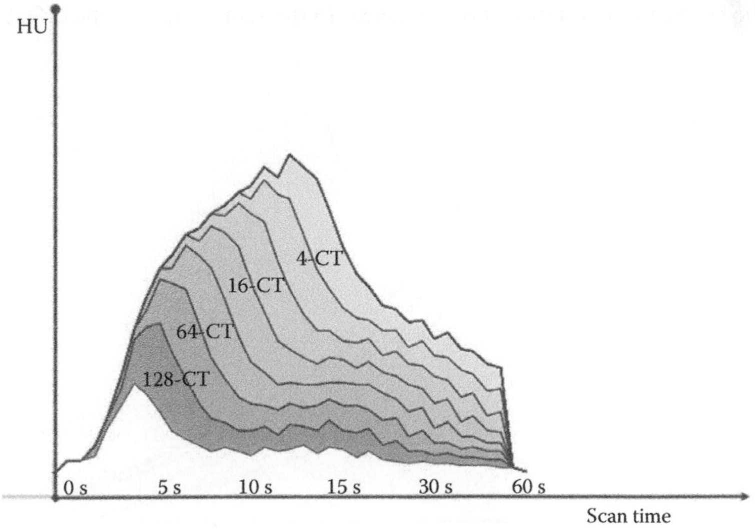

FIGURE 1.8 The greatest is the number of detectors the lowest is the scan time and the earliest peak enhancement.

For this reason, the old approach was abandoned on >16 MDCT and a new approach was proposed. Considering that in a vascular study the vascular enhancement depends on iodine administration per time unit (iodine flow expressed in mgI/s) and blood volume per time unit (cardiac output, expressed in L/min), a new technique based on the iodine delivery rate (IDR) was proposed. The IDR describes the total amount of iodine molecules released in a fluid volume in the unit of time, and obviously the greater it will be, the greater will be the vascular opacification.

Moreover, IDR also depends on iodine concentration of CM. Therefore, a higher iodine concentration corresponds to a higher IDR at the same speed injection and so a higher enhancement peak.

Considering this fact, for CTA of good quality, it is suggested that we use a high iodine concentration CM (350–400 mgI/mL).

These strategies however need to be modified case by case. The use of higher volumes of CM determines a vascular enhancement of greater intensity and duration, but with a slower onset, while a reduced volume of CM produces faster enhancement but of less intensity and duration. So higher volumes of CM could be used for large vascular segments (peripheral circulation, thoracic and abdominal aorta, or whole-body examination), while smaller volumes of CM could be used for smaller regions (neck vessels or coronary circulation).

1.9 SALINE FLUSH

The use of a saline bolus of 40–50 mL injected at a high flow (3.5–4 mL/s, usually 0.5 mL/s higher than the CM considering the different viscosity of the two solutions) immediately after the administration of CM to flush the venous system could improve the quality of CTA. This high-speed bolus helps the progression of the contrast agent avoiding its presence in the venous site, consolidates the CM bolus, and moreover brings to a reduction the total amount of CM administered.

1.10 PATIENTS' CHARACTERISTICS AND VASCULAR ENHANCEMENT

Vascular opacification is due to many factors, some related to acquisition technique as stated earlier and others due to patients' characteristics such as cardiac output or body mass.

The cardiac ejection fraction directly influences the distribution speed of the contrast agent through the vascular site, with a particular effect on the arterial concentration during the first pass. In patients with a history of heart failure, the circulation speed of the contrast agent is reduced and its arrival in the target vascular territories is delayed. In the same way also the effect of the venous

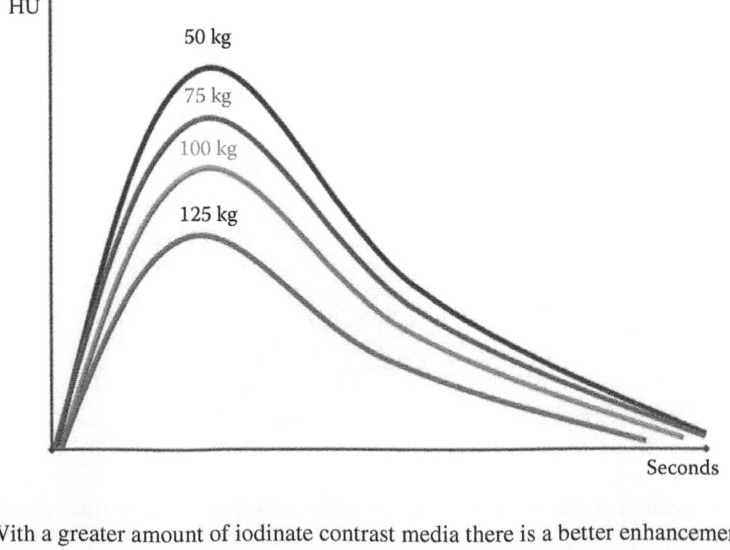

FIGURE 1.9 With a greater amount of iodinate contrast media there is a better enhancement.

washout is delayed by the reduced cardiac function. The final result of these phenomena is therefore a delayed peak of enhancement but more intense than the one that we have in the case of a normal cardiac function; the effect is more apparent to progressively reduced ejection fraction.

Patients' body mass influences the distribution volume of CM as well as its pharmacodynamics and pharmacokinetics (Figure 1.9). So it is necessary to adjust the amount of CM in relation to body weight. In subjects with a high body mass, the CM is mainly diluted in the blood, resulting in a lower iodine concentration and a lower enhancement. Correction of the CM volume for the body mass is necessary for subjects with a weight less than 60 kg or greater than 90 kg (reducing or increasing, respectively, 20% of the standard volume of CM and varying the same percentage of the administration rate).

1.11 TIMING OF CTA ACQUISITION

The right scan timing (or scan synchronisation) is mandatory to obtain a good-quality CTA examination. The following are the techniques used to synchronise CM administration and CTA acquisition:

- Fixed delay (now considered obsolete): It is based on the use of fixed delay between CM administration and the beginning of the scan.
- Test bolus: It is based on the administration of a small amount of CM (15–20 mL) used to determine the time needed to reach peak enhancement to set delay of CTA acquisition (Figure 1.10). It is a technically valid method but is now replaced by the more simple and rapid technique of bolus tracking.
- Bolus tracking: It is based on a real-time monitoring of the enhancement in a vessel in which attenuation is continuously measured (Figure 1.11). When attenuation reaches a selected threshold value (expressed in HU), CTA scan will start automatically after a delay that is settled as lower as possible (usually 6–8 s). Threshold attenuation value (expressed in HU) is variable according to vascular region (70–90 HU for the carotid arteries, 150–200 HU for the aorta, and 50–60 HU for pulmonary arteries) and to the speed of acquisition (with faster scanners it should be set at higher threshold values in order to avoid the bolus overcome and a subsequent too early inadequate acquisition).

To summarise, among latest CT scans, the bolus tracking technique is the technique of choice; however, the test bolus could be a good alternative among older-generation CT scans.

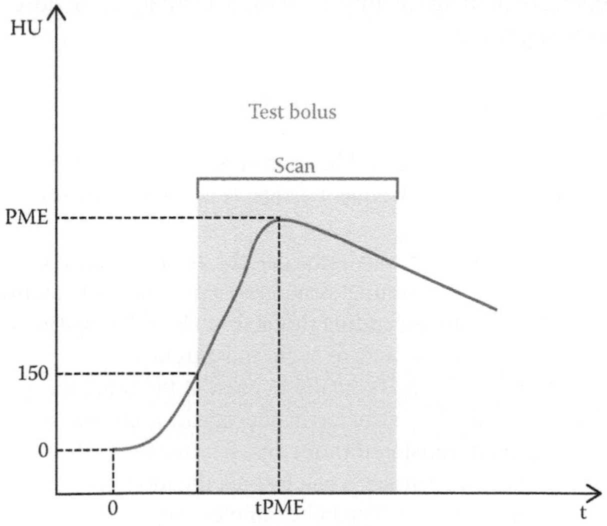

FIGURE 1.10 Test bolus.

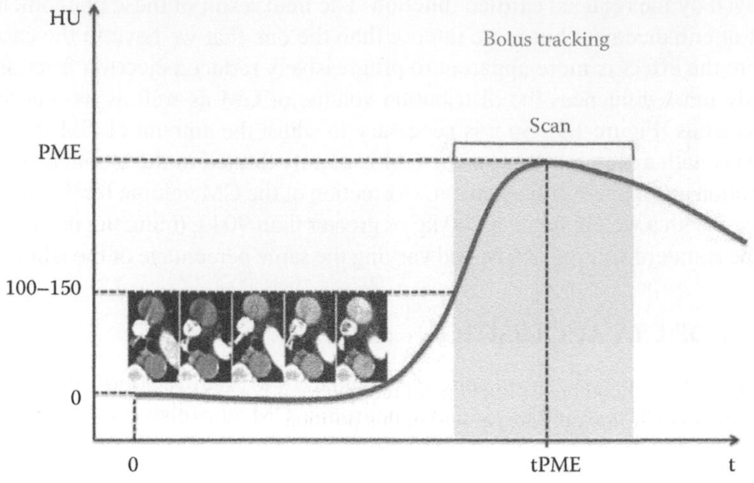

FIGURE 1.11 Bolus tracking.

1.12 RADIATION DOSE CONSIDERATIONS

Radiation dose in CT depends on mAs and kV, layer collimation, and acquisition time. The administered radiation dose is measured as CTDIvol, which is the average exposure dose in a given volume, and is expressed in milligray (mGy). CTDIvol is automatically calculated based on the pitch, mAs, kVp, and on some specific scanner parameters.

In patients with a mean BMI, the recommended maximum CTDIvol for a CTA examination of the thoracic and abdominal vessels is, respectively, 5–6 mGy and 8–15 mGy. In overweight patients, it is necessary to use higher doses to maintain an acceptable image quality. As stated previously, it is important to remember that the use of low kVp (80–100), in patients with mean BMI, can increase the iodine attenuation. Moreover, a variation in acquisition parameters influences both radiation dose and image quality, so it is important to balance dose exposure and quality of the acquired images.

Recently, new techniques based on a real-time modulation of the x-ray tube load (mAs) along the *z*-axis considering the different body thickness determine an exposure dose reduction up to 20%–30% without a decrease in image quality. So if these techniques of dose modulation are available, their use is strongly suggested.

1.13 ARTEFACTS

As for every CT scan, artefacts in CTA could be caused by patients' movements or by the technical performances. The most important and frequent artefacts are the following:

- Heartbeat and respiration: Pulse movement of the heart creates a change in diameter, shape, and position of adjacent vascular structures; this artefact is manifested as a 'double contour' of the vessel (typically ascending thoracic aorta). ECG-gating techniques are useful to reduce the pulsation effects, and so avoid this artefact.
- Contrast agent over-concentration: Typically evident at the brachiocephalic venous trunk. It determines a beam-hardening artefact in the aortic arch and epiaortic vessels. It is reduced by a saline flush administered immediately after the CM.
- Turbulent and slow flow: It determines a patchy opacification of a vessel caused by low and inhomogeneous CM concentration. Typical examples are represented by the patchy effect induced by the flow turbulence in the aneurysmal sacs or by the asymmetrical enhancement of the leg distal vessels in patients with a slow circulation time.

- Calcifications, stent devices, embolic materials, and other metallic implants: Even if the CTA capability to identify the wall calcifications is an undeniable advantage, it may also constitute a limitation of the study because it hinds proper evaluation of vessel lumen due to 'blooming artefact' owing to beam hardening. Similar alterations are observed in the presence of metallic materials (implants, stent devices, and embolic agents). The effect of these artefacts can be reduced with the use of high-spatial resolution reconstruction techniques and the application of high-definition convolution filters.

1.14 CT APPLICATIONS IN PLASTIC SURGERY

In plastic surgery, it is often mandatory to assess vascular and skeletal anatomy before surgical repair of congenital diseases and post-traumatic injuries (Figure 1.12).

Moreover, CTA has a central role in surgical reconstruction in patients that underwent demolitive surgery for tumours, such as breast reconstruction: it is considered safe and reliable in the assessment of vascular anatomy during perforator flap reconstruction (using the deep inferior epigastric artery, the superficial inferior epigastric artery, or the gluteal arteries), and may prevent the number of post-operative complications. It enables flap selection (based on size, location, course, and length), target donor vessel, level and type of anastomosis through the use of multiplanar reformations (MPRs), volume rendering (VR), and maximum intensity projection (MIP) reconstructions in different planes.

In addition, the use of dedicated software with a scale grid superimposed on the image may show the relations of the little vessels to other anatomical structures, guiding the surgeon during the intervention and resulting in a decreased mean operating time, a lower rate of complications related to flap viability, and a significant reduction in donor site morbidity.

CT reconstructions frequently used are as follows:

- MPR are two-dimensional reformatted images that are reconstructed secondarily in different planes (coronal or sagittal) from the stack of axial image data. Particular applications of MPR imaging are the curved-planar reformations (CPR) that are generally needed to depict structures that pass through multiple axial planes of section (e.g. vessels).
- MIP images are volume-rendering techniques in which suitable editing methods are used to define the volume of interest (VOI). Images are generated by projecting the volume of interest into a viewing plane and displaying the maximum CT numbers that are encountered along the direction of the projection (the viewing angle). MIP are generally used to assess vessels in CT angiography (Figures 1.13 and 1.14).

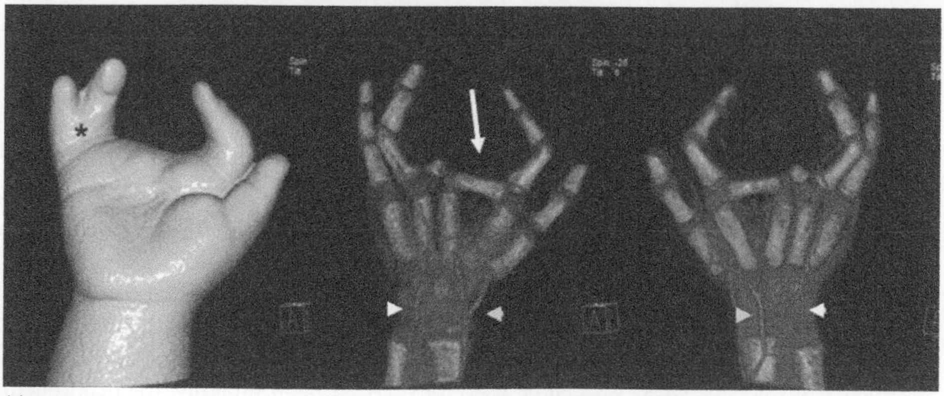

(a) (b) (c)

FIGURE 1.12 Right hand of patient affected by syndactytilies: VR reconstructions (a,b,c) show the fusion of the IV and V finger, absence of the III and fusion of the proximal phalange with the second interphalang (white arrow). Ulnar (white arrow head) and radial arteries (yellow arrow head).

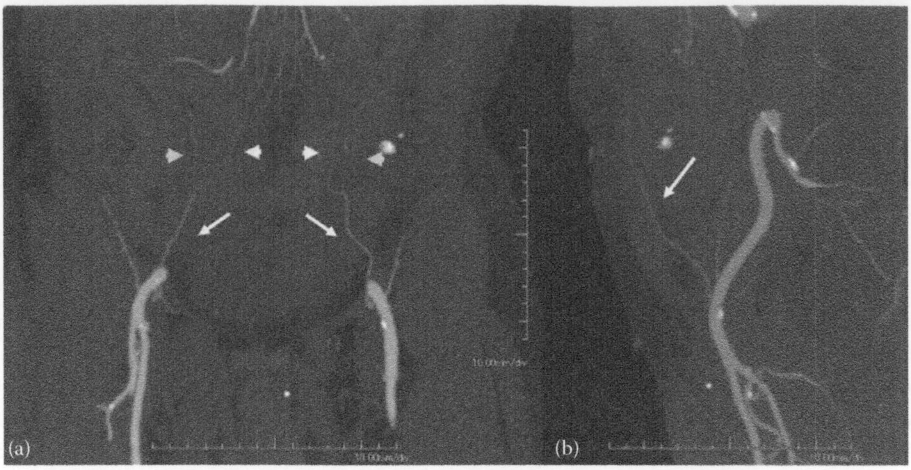

FIGURE 1.13 MIP coronal (a) and sagittal (b) images show deep inferior epigastric artery (white arrow) and its bifurcation in medial (white arrow head) and lateral (yellow arrow head) branches.

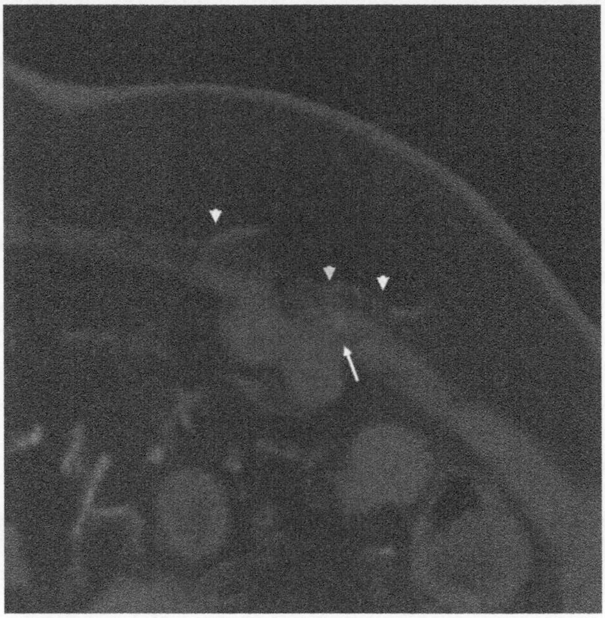

FIGURE 1.14 Axial MIP image shows intramuscular (white arrow), subfascial (yellow arrow head) and subcutaneous (white arrow head) segments of the left deep inferior epigastric perforating artery.

- VR assigns a range of opacity values to CT numbers, giving a better definition of object contours or semi-transparent displays. In this process, all CT numbers belonging to the 3D object (in the chosen threshold range) have maximum opacity, while all CT numbers outside the range have zero opacity and do not contribute to the image. Since all the voxels within the CT range have maximum opacity, only the surface of the object is depicted in the shaded surface displays. VR can be used for CTA, skeletal imaging, tracheobronchial imaging, colon and abdominal organ as a primary tool for image analysis. In particular, in CTA, it is very useful because it shows vessel lumen and calcifications in separate colours and makes it easy to localise calcified plaques and differentiates arterial and venous vessels and organs with different contrast enhancement (Figures 1.15 and 1.16).

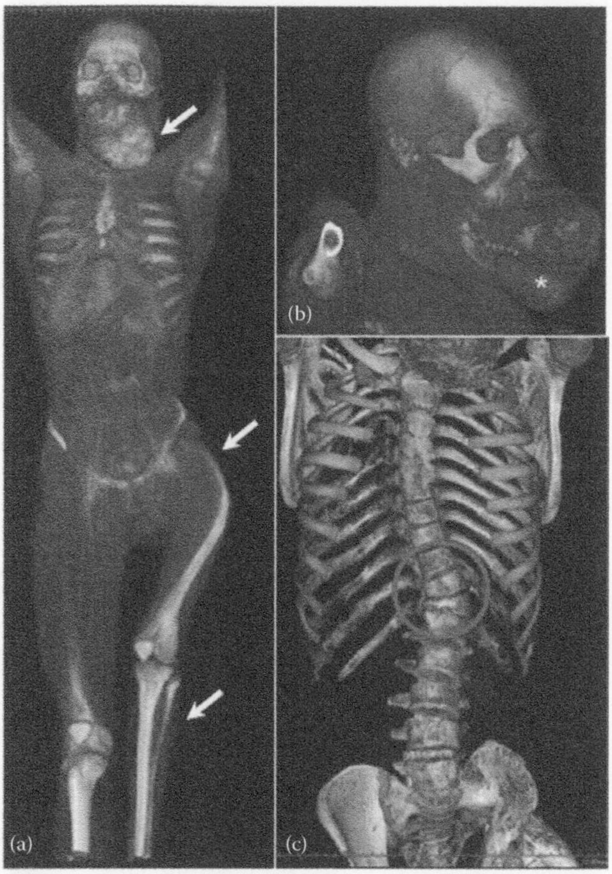

FIGURE 1.15 VR image of a patient affected by fibrous dysplasia with multiple bone deformities (a) (white arrows). (b) Mandibular localization (*); (c) vertebral fracture (red circle).

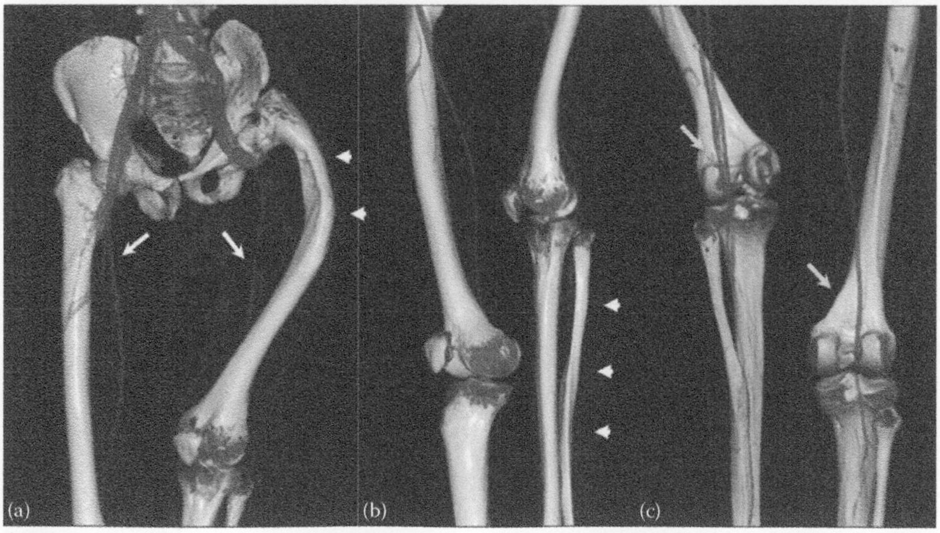

FIGURE 1.16 VR images of the same patient depict femural deformity (arrow head) and superficial femural artery (white arrow) in (a), fibular deformity in (b) and popliteal vessels in (c).

2 MRI Physics Principles

Marta Tomás Mallebrera and Ángeles Franco López

CONTENTS

2.1 SUMMARY: BASIC PRINCIPLES OF MRI

Magnetic resonance imaging (MRI) uses the hydrogen atoms in the body to generate an image. When hydrogen atoms are introduced into a magnetic field, they align in the direction of the magnetic field (Bo). A radio-frequency (RF) pulse is then applied, which provides energy to the atoms and causes some to be aligned in different directions. When the RF pulse ceases, the atoms return to their rest position, releasing energy and emitting a signal. This signal is picked up and converted into an image.

2.2 ORIGIN OF MRI SIGNAL

The primary origin of the MR signal is the hydrogen nuclei (consisting of a single proton) of water and fat molecules in the patient's tissue. These protons have the nuclear property of spin which causes them to act like tiny magnets with a north and a south pole. When they are introduced in an external magnetic field, they tend to align either toward or against the magnetic field (Bo), quickly reaching an equilibrium state where there are a greater number of protons that align with the magnetic field direction (more energetically favourable direction) and form a net magnetic field or net magnetisation (Mo). As well as aligning with the field, the protons rotate (precess) around their own axis and around the magnetic field. The frequency with which spins precess is proportional to the size of the magnetic field and is known as the Larmor frequency: $\omega = \gamma \times Bo$.

The scheme can be represented by two cones, one aligned with the magnetic field and one aligned against it (Figure 2.1).

An RF pulse can perturb this alignment and the net magnetisation moves away from its alignment with Bo and rotates perpendicularly about the magnetic field (excitation). The angle of this rotation will depend on the amplitude and duration of RF pulse (Figure 2.2). The frequency of the RF pulse must be the same as the Larmor frequency; this is the resonance condition of MR.

When the RF pulse ceases, the hydrogen atoms tend to return to the equilibrium state (what is known as relaxation), and they release energy which is emitted as a small signal. After an amplification and transformation process, the signal is used for imaging.

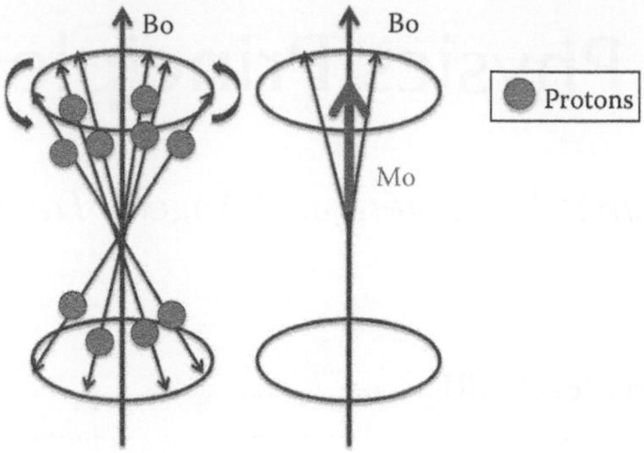

FIGURE 2.1 The precession of spins forms two cones. The cancellation of opposing spins leaves a small number of *unpaired* spins, which creates a net magnetisation vector (Mo) aligned with the magnetic field (Bo).

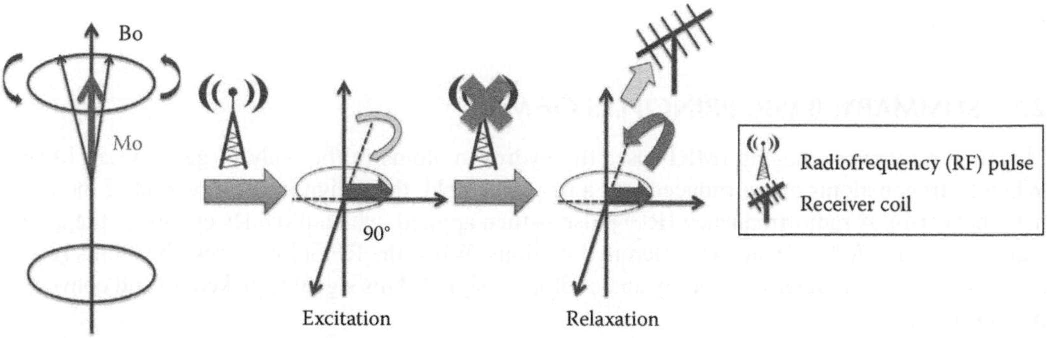

FIGURE 2.2 Effect of RF pulse.

2.3 MR SIGNAL CHARACTERISTICS: T1, T2, AND T2* RELAXATION

The signal to return to the equilibrium state oscillates at the Larmor frequency and decreases in a characteristic time known as *transverse relaxation time or* T2. The signal can drop faster when the field is not homogeneous. This faster decrease is called T2* and may be elongated improving the homogeneity of the magnetic field (a process called shimming). The recovery of the magnetisation vector back to its initial position occurs in a characteristic time which is called the *longitudinal relaxation time* T1 (the time which it takes to return to its equilibrium state).

T1 and T2 are characteristic properties of each tissue and are responsible for one of the major advantages of MRI over other techniques: the ability to generate tissue contrast. Different types of tissue show different T1 and T2 relaxation times. This is key to the sharp image contrast obtained with MR.

2.4 MR SCANNER COMPONENTS

To obtain magnetic field strengths high enough for MR, a superconducting magnet is needed, which need to be cooled to extremely low temperatures (for that, helium is used). To ensure that the helium remains cold and in a liquid form, a compressor is used which makes the characteristic noise of an MR scanner. Once in service, the magnet is always on even when the console is turned off.

The gradient system is necessary to spatial differentiation. It generates a magnetic field in the same direction as Bo but with a strength that varies with position along the x, y, z. It is the origin of the noise and vibration of the equipment.

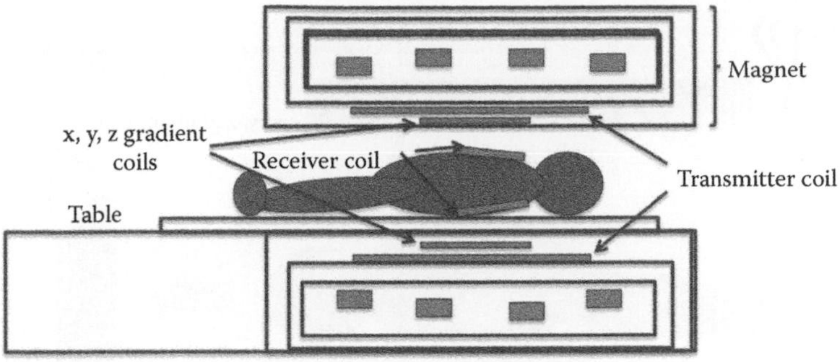

FIGURE 2.3 Components of an MR scanner.

RF system is composed of an RF transmit coil, an RF amplifier, and an RF receiver coil. An RF transmit coil is used to excite the protons. An RF amplifier is sited in the scanner and drives the RF transmit coil. RF receiver coils are critical to the quality of the image. As shown in Figure 2.3, they must be near the area studied. Coil selection is also crucial to obtain a good image. A too big coil will have too much noise and a too small coil will not permit to see very far into the patient. The table allows the patient to be positioned in the centre of the system. It moves the region of interest exactly in the centre of the field to get a better picture quality.

2.5 MR IMAGE GENERATION

The basis for an MR image is the spatial location of individual MR signals. It is necessary to identify each point inside the image. If all hydrogen atoms in the body were excited at the same time, the generated signal would be impossible to locate in an area. So we need to excite only a slice at a time. The method that spatially differentiates MR signals is the gradient coils. The gradient coils create magnetic field gradients which are superimposed on the main magnetic field and change the main magnetic field strength in different positions. The magnetic field gradients are applied simultaneously with the RF pulse.

The RF pulse is designed to contain only a small range of frequencies (bandwidth), and only protons that precess to those certain frequencies (proportional to the magnetic field strength by the Larmor equation) will excite. Outside the image slice, spins are not affected by the RF pulse (Figure 2.4).

Following the excitation of spins, several steps are required to identify the position of their signal within the slice. To localise the signal of each spin, a phase-encoding gradient and frequency-encoding gradient are switched. This means that each signal emitted has a frequency and phase which enables their location.

Through a complex mathematical model, the received signals with different frequencies and phases are transformed into an image. This process is called *Fourier transformation*.

2.6 K-SPACE

The collected data (with many frequencies and phases) are put into a matrix, known as K-space. The ways in which K-space can be filled are almost infinite and determine the image properties. The data in the centre of the K-space generate the image contrast: If only the centre of the image is acquired, we will have an image high in signal but of low in resolution. The data obtained from the periphery of the K-space generate the structure and edges of the image: If only the data from the periphery of K-space are acquired, the image is low in signal but fine in details (Figure 2.5).

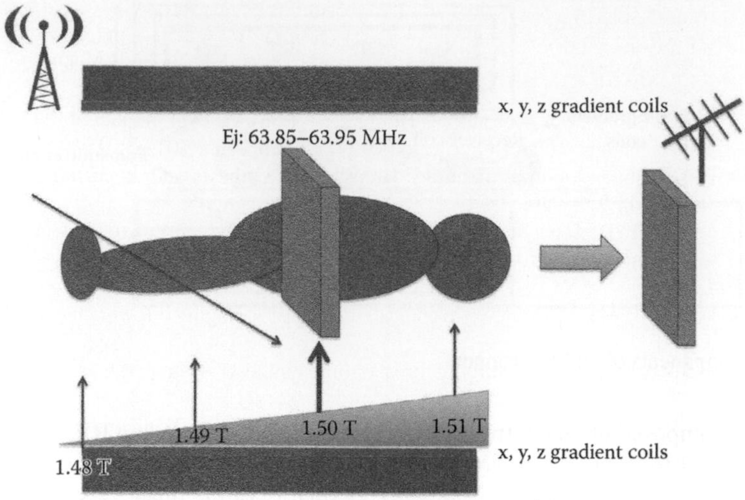

FIGURE 2.4 The gradient coils create a change in the magnetic field in a specific direction. Only spins inside the selected slice will resonate. Outside the slice, spins are not affected by RF pulse.

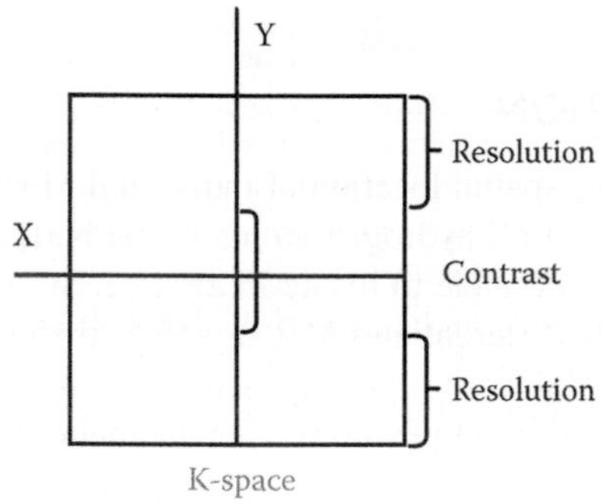

FIGURE 2.5 Scheme for basic understanding K-space.

2.7 PULSE SEQUENCES AND IMAGE CONTRAST

All the steps we have discussed are repeated multiple times with different gradients to generate a series of signals that form the complete anatomical image. The time between successive excitations is called the repetition time or TR. The time between the excitation of the protons and acquisition of data is called the echo time or TE (Figure 2.6).

As previously described, one of the most important advantages of MRI over other imaging modalities is its ability to generate contrast of different tissue types. This is because different tissues

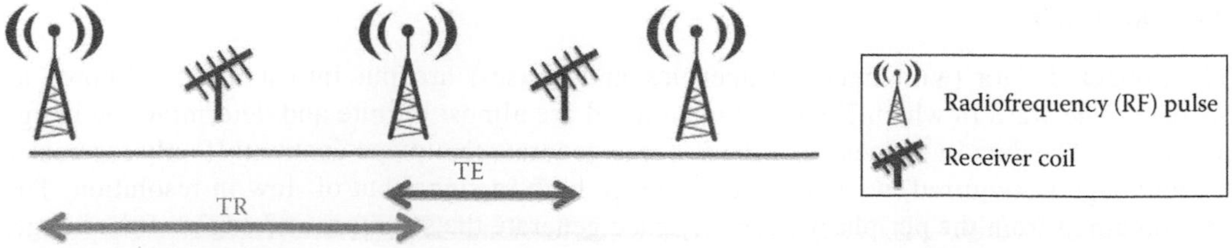

FIGURE 2.6 Squeme for basic understanding TR and TE concepts.

have different characteristic T1 and T2 relaxation times. TR and TE are the most important parameters for controlling the image contrast, because they determine the enhancement of a contrast type or weighting. For a T1 contrast, the image must be acquired with a short TR and short TE. When using a short TR, tissues with a short T1 (i.e. fat) have greater longitudinal relaxation component and their signal will be high. For a T2 contrast, the image must be acquired with a long TR and long TE. When the image is acquired with a long TR and short TE, the image is weighted with proton density contrast.

There are many possible ways of controlling the previously mentioned sequence of events, with different timings, RF pulses, and gradients, to generate different types of image. The combination of these aspects is programmed into the computer scanner and is termed a *sequence*. A typical image session may use several different sequences, depending on the type of images required.

BIBLIOGRAPHY

Balaban RS, Peters DC. Basic principles of cardiovascular magnetic resonance. In Manning WJ, Pennell DJ (eds.), *Cardiovascular Magnetic Resonance*, 2nd edn. Philadelphia, PA: Saunders; 2010, pp. 3–18.

Bitar R, Leung G, Perng R, Tadros S, Moody AR, Sarrazin J, McGregor C et al. MR pulse sequences: What every radiologist wants to know but is afraid to ask. *Radiographics* 2006;26(2):513–537. Review.

Finn PJ (ed.). *Physics of MR Imaging* (Magnetic Resonance Imaging Clinics of North America). Philadelphia, PA: W.B. Saunders; 1999, pp. 607–808.

Myerson SG, Francis J, Neubauer S (eds.). *Cardiovascular Magnetic Resonance* (Oxford Specialist Handbooks in Cardiology). Oxford, U.K.: Oxford University Press, 2010.

Ridgway JP. Cardiovascular magnetic resonance physics for clinicians: Part I. *Journal of Cardiovascular Magnetic Resonance* 2010;12:71.

3 Diagnostic Ultrasound

Alberto Benito, David Cano, Mariana Elorz, and Pedro Slon

CONTENTS

3.1 INTRODUCTION

Since their first reports in 1994, free deep inferior epigastric perforator (DIEP) flaps have been rapidly rising in popularity and have become the standard surgery procedure in breast reconstruction. Imaging techniques currently available allow preoperative location of the individual perforator of choice in order to design the kind and the volume of the flap. These will make the surgical procedure much easier and also would decrease patient morbidity preventing unnecessary perforator dissections, proceeding in a faster and safer way.

Preoperative imaging to give accurate information about the location, origin, course, calibre, and anatomical variations of perforator arteries before perforator-based free flaps surgery is mandatory to reduce flap failures or partial necrosis due to individual variations in perforator anatomy.

Different non-invasive diagnostic techniques have been purposed. Although some classic studies reported a very high proportion of false positives for preoperative ultrasound (US), many have recommended its use in addition with pulsed Doppler and colour Doppler to find perforating arteries coming from the deep epigastric vessels for DIEP flaps. In this chapter, the basics and the role of US and Doppler in the study of perforating vessels will be discussed.

3.2 BASICS OF ULTRASOUND

US is one of the most widely used imaging techniques in medicine. It has great advantages such as the relative low cost, absence of ionising radiation, and its portable and non-invasive nature. Another important characteristic is that images can be acquired in real time and in different views, offering a dynamic and cross-sectional view of anatomical structures.

3.3 B-MODE ULTRASOUND

A basic understanding of the physical principles involved in US image generation is essential. Modern medical US is performed primarily using a pulse-echo approach with a brightness-mode (B-mode) display. This involves transmitting small pulses of US echo from a transducer into the body.

US transducers (or probes) contain multiple piezoelectric crystals that vibrate in response to an applied electric current, a phenomenon called the piezoelectric effect, originally described by the Curie brothers in 1880. These vibrating mechanical sound waves create alternating areas

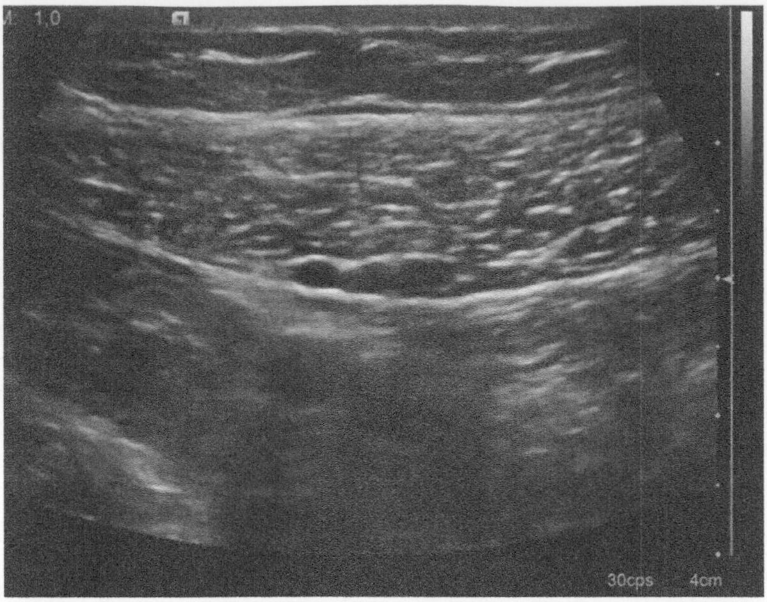

FIGURE 3.1 Deep epigastric vessels behind the rectus abdominis muscle (greyscale US).

of compression and rarefaction when propagating through body tissues. As the US waves penetrate body tissues of different acoustic impedances, some are reflected back to the transducer and some continue to penetrate deeper. The different densities of tissues in the body absorb different amounts of energy and these differences are expressed as different shades of grey in the US image (Figure 3.1).

Medical US devices use sound waves that have frequencies that exceed the upper limit for audible human hearing, using sound waves ranging from 1 to 20 MHz. Proper selection of transducer

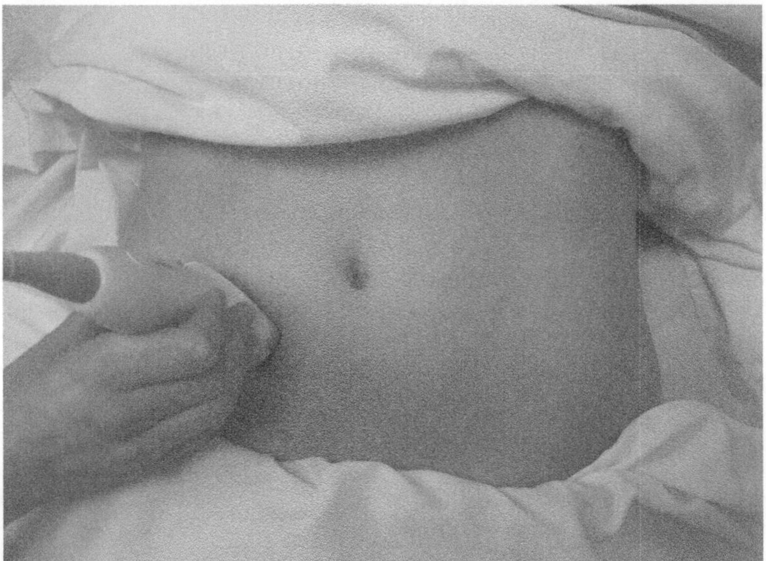

FIGURE 3.2 US study using a linear transducer in the infraumbilical area.

frequency is an important concept for providing optimal image resolution in diagnostic and procedural US. Low-frequency waves offer images of lower resolution but can penetrate to deeper structures due to a lower degree of attenuation. High-frequency US waves generate images of high resolution. However, they are more attenuated; thus, they are suitable for imaging mainly superficial structures. For this reason, it is best to use high-frequency transducers to image superficial structures and low-frequency transducers for imaging deep structures.

There are different kinds of transducers. The linear array transducer emits sound waves parallel to each other and produces a rectangular image. They are primarily used with high frequencies (5.0–10.0 MHz) for evaluating soft tissues and superficial structures. The sector transducer produces a fan-like image that is narrow near the transducer and increases in width with deeper penetration. This array is usually used in cardiology. Finally, the curved or convex array transducers are predominantly used in abdominal sonography with frequencies from 2.5 to 5.0 MHz (Figure 3.2).

3.4 PULSED AND COLOUR DOPPLER

Doppler US has been available for clinical use for more than 40 years. The Doppler effect (or Doppler shift), discovered by Christian Andreas Doppler (1803–1853), is a change in frequency that occurs when sound is emitted from a moving object. This phenomenon enables US to be used to detect the motion of blood and to measure the velocity of blood flow. When a moving target (i.e. blood cells) reflects a sound, the frequency of the reflected sound wave is altered. The frequency is shifted up by an approaching target and shifted down by a receding target. The amount of the shifted frequency is proportional to the velocity of the moving object. When properly performed, Doppler US provides rapid, comprehensive, and accurate evaluation of the vasculature.

There are two main display modes used in modern Doppler systems, 2D colour flow imaging and spectral Doppler. Colour flow Doppler superimposes a colour image representing motion into a B-mode image to illustrate motion of blood flow. A unique colour (or brightness) is assigned to an individual frequency. Typically, a greater frequency shift (corresponding to a higher velocity) is assigned a brighter colour. Analysis of the colour flow image gives a graphic illustration of the direction and speed of blood flow within soft tissue. The colour-coded flow information is usually displayed in a limited region of interest called the colour box within the displayed B-mode image. Conventionally, the flow towards the probe is coded with red colour and the flow away from the probe is coded with blue. The brightness of the colour determines the flow velocity (Figure 3.3). Power Doppler mode is a variation on colour flow imaging in which the displayed intensity is not based on the intensity of the Doppler frequency signal. This mode does not provide blood velocity information, but rather information about the total number of moving red blood cells, usually used to display the flow in small vessels.

Spectral Doppler is used to detect the blood velocity information from a single location within the blood vessel. The velocity information is displayed in the form of a Doppler spectrum. Doppler spectrum displays time along the horizontal axis and the measured Doppler frequency shift of calculated velocity along the vertical axis. Conventionally, positive Doppler frequencies and velocities (blood flowing towards the probe) are plotted above the baseline and negative Doppler frequencies and velocities (blood flowing away from the probe or reverse flow) below the baseline (Figure 3.4).

Doppler systems for spectral Doppler measurements can be divided into two groups, continuous-wave systems and pulsed wave systems:

- Continuous-wave Doppler uses two piezoelectric crystals, one for the continuous transmission of US pulses (continuous wave) and one for the reception of reflected US signals. The frequency spectra of returning echoes are displayed acoustically and also visually if desired. The frequency shifts can be used to calculate the direction and velocity of blood flow.

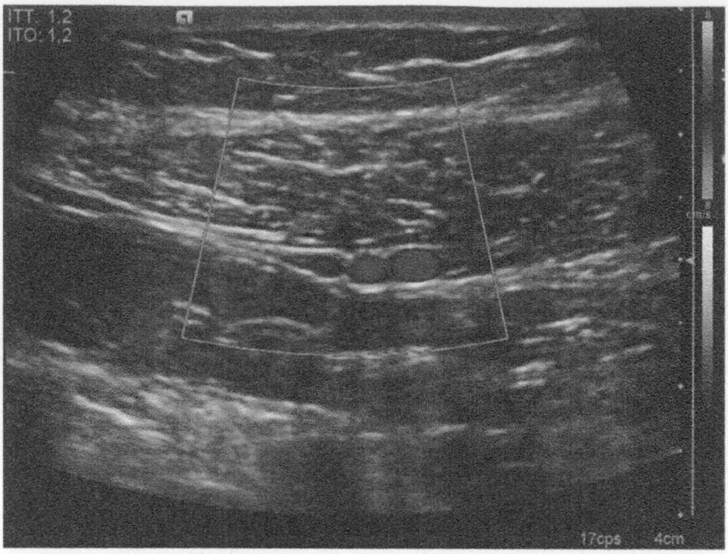

FIGURE 3.3 Deep epigastric vessels behind the rectus abdominis muscle (colour Doppler US). The artery appears in the middle between the two veins.

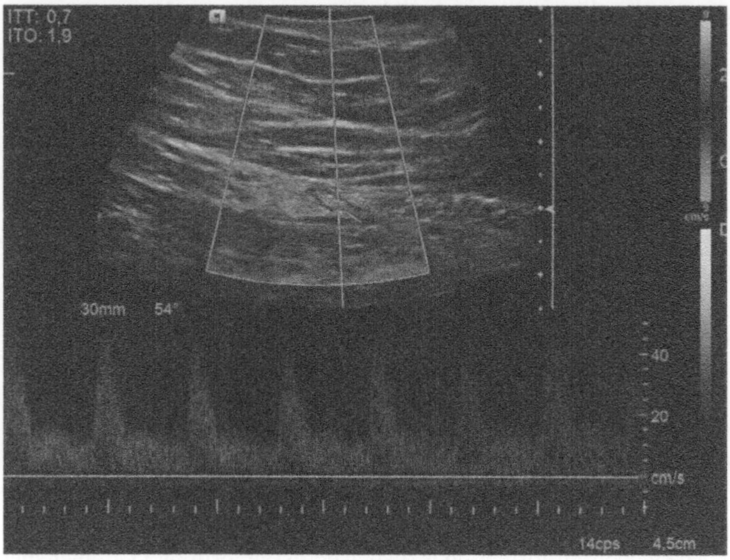

FIGURE 3.4 Pulsed-Doppler mode epigastric artery showing arterial pattern.

This technique does not, however, provide information on the depth or range of the echo source so it is not very useful in the identification of perforating branches from the deep epigastric artery.

- Pulsed Doppler employs one piezoelectric crystal that functions alternately as a transmitter and receiver (pulse wave). Echo signals are recorded from a designated sample volume during the receiving phase of the scan. This makes it possible to determine the depth and width of the sample volume and investigate blood flow within a circumscribed area.

Today, pulsed-Doppler systems for spectral Doppler measurements are usually used in conjunction with US B-mode imaging, known as duplex US.

3.5 BASIS OF SIGNAL PROCESSING AND SETTINGS

When a Doppler US is performed, there are a variety of operator-dependent technical parameters that must be optimised. Changes in these parameters independently influence both the colour and spectral components of the Doppler US examination, and parameters should be optimised separately for each patient. It will be very important to manage properly the equipment (Figure 3.5). The most important of those parameters are the following:

- *Transmit power*: It determines the amplitude of the US transmitted into the tissue. An increase of the output power will increase the amplitude of returning Doppler-shifted signal, but it will also increase the exposure to US.
- *Gain*: The spectral gain increases the brightness of the spectrum on the screen.
- *Frequency*: High-frequency sound waves provide high-resolution images but are more attenuated than the low-frequency ones. The appropriate Doppler transmit frequency will need to be selected to ensure adequate penetration of US.
- *Pulse repetition frequency (PRF)*: The PRF indicates the rate (frequency) at which data are sampled. This variable is directly related to the velocity range because higher flow velocities will require more rapid sampling to obtain accurate measurements.
- *Baseline*: The baseline represents the zero Doppler frequency shift. The position of the baseline can be changed to optimise the spectral display, depending on the relative size of the forward and reverse flow velocities.
- *Inversion of the spectrum*: This control enables to display positive velocities below the baseline and negative velocities above the baseline.
- *Wall filter*: Wall filters selectively filter out all acquired information below an operator-defined frequency threshold. Filters eliminate the typically low-frequency–high-intensity noise that may arise from vessel wall motion.
- *Angle correction*: Angle correction refers to adjustment of the Doppler angle and is used to calibrate the velocity scale for the angle between the US beam and the blood flow

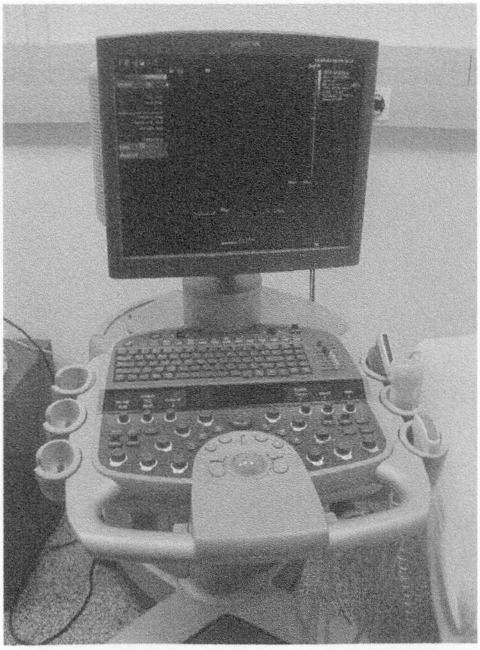

FIGURE 3.5 High-resolution US equipment.

being measured. Errors in the alignment of the angle correction cursor can lead to significant errors in velocity measurements.
- *Focal depth*: It is used to focus the Doppler beam to the sample volume.
- *Gate size and position*: To maximise depiction of flow, the gate should be positioned over the central part of the vessel being studied.

3.6 DOPPLER US FOR DIEP FLAPS

Doppler US is inexpensive, portable, ready to use, and available in all hospitals. When applied to the skin with an interface layer of gel to facilitate transmission, it emits audible or visible signals when over blood vessels (the Doppler effect).

Old blind devices have been used several years ago as early as 1975 and it has been a common practice since 1990 for planning microvascular free flaps. These handheld Doppler equipments have been mainly described for assisting in identifying donor vessels before surgery. Although studies showed the Doppler probe to have reasonable accuracy in identifying perforators in preparation for various free-flap operations, some reports present worrying inaccuracies when compared with operative findings or with newer imaging modalities. In addition, it is a relatively time-consuming technique with low accuracy and high interobserver variability. For these old reasons, Doppler US has not been widely considered enough for perforator mapping and cannot achieve the sensitivity and breadth of information provided with CT or MR angiography (MRA). However, some authors consider that the new Doppler US technology is a suitable preoperative imaging modality alone, although skilled radiologists would be usually desirable.

For DIEP flap planning, US can be performed the day before or the same day of the intervention. The patient is placed in a supine position (as in the surgery room), and to obtain the best possible Doppler US signal, the probe was held perpendicular to the skin outline. Each side of the abdomen must be explored from 5 cm above the umbilicus to the inguinal ligament scanning at both axial and longitudinal projections covering both 10 cm sides to the right and to the left (Figure 3.2). High-frequency probes (5–17 MHz) are needed in order to acquire high-resolution images.

The study must begin with the identification of the deep epigastric vessels behind the abdominal rectus muscles that is usually easy using colour Doppler (Figure 3.3), but their origin from the iliac artery or vein in the groin area can be useful or sometimes necessary in order to identify the epigastric vessels (Figures 3.6 and 3.7). The deep epigastric artery and veins can be identified by the different flow directions assessed by using colour (Figure 3.3) or pulsed Doppler (Figure 3.4).

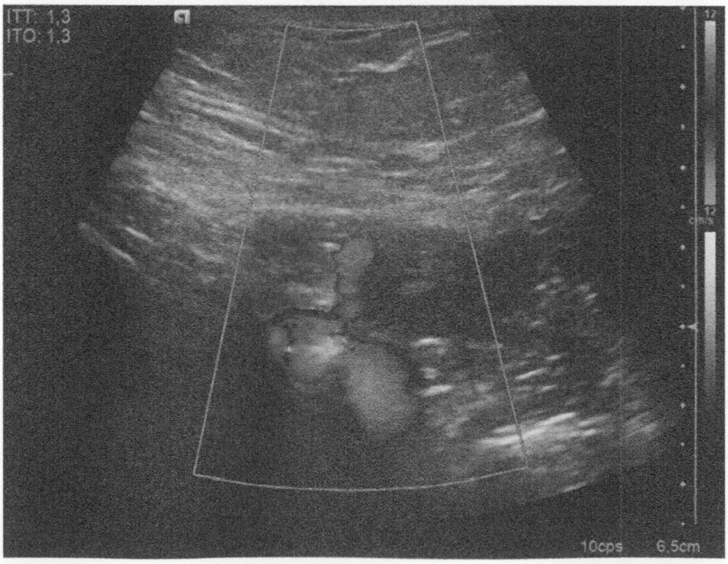

FIGURE 3.6 Deep epigastric artery arising from the iliac artery.

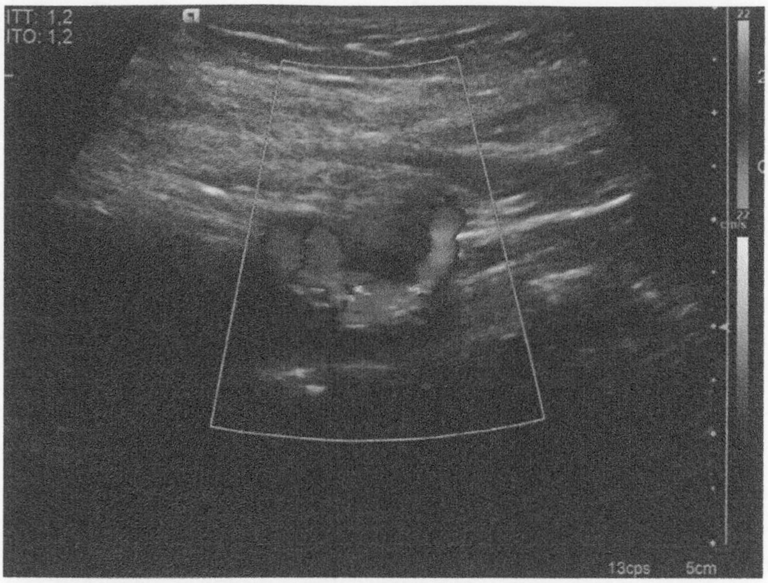

FIGURE 3.7 Deep epigastric vein draining to the iliac–femoral vein.

The perforating branches from deep epigastric vessels are included in the area between the umbilicus and the groin. The study is traced superiorly until the first perforator is detected. The exact location of the penetrating points of the perforators through the superficial fascia of the rectus abdominis is mandatory for successful intra-operative dissection. These pedicles (arteries and veins) will be identified as pulsatile vessels, visualised as either red or blue streaks on the colour Doppler map depending on the beam orientation (Figure 3.8).

The corresponding points are therefore accurately marked with a felt-tip point pen and the position of their outflow from the deep fascia can and must be marked on the overlying skin (Figure 3.9).

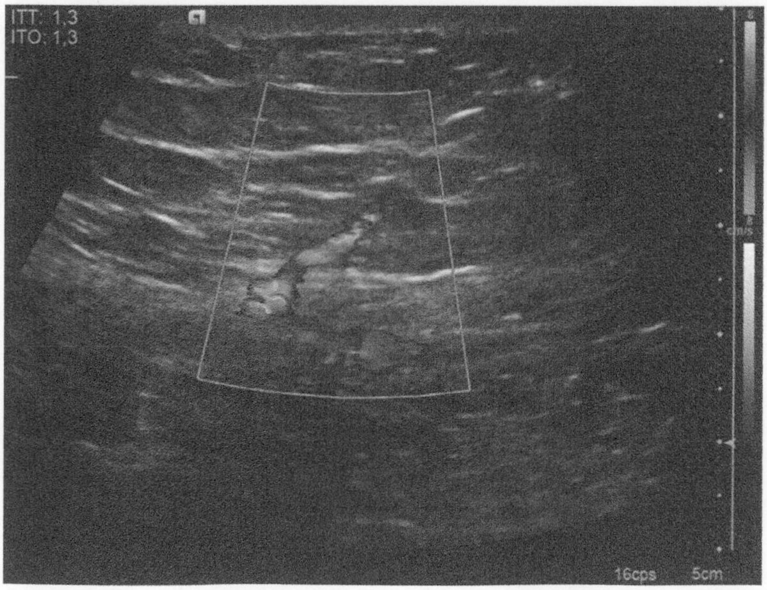

FIGURE 3.8 Identification of the perforation point on the muscular fascia.

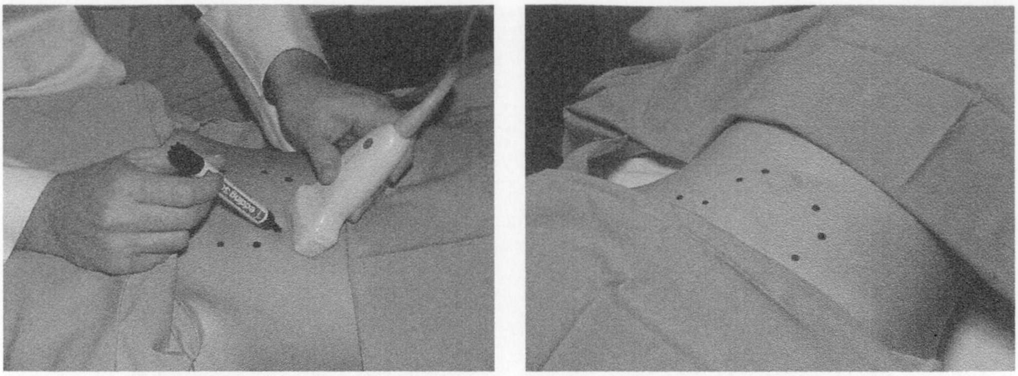

(a) (b)

FIGURE 3.9 Marks done with a felt-tip pen in the position of the outflow of perforators from the deep fascia marked on the overlying skin (a: marking; b: final result).

Special attention should be paid to the best and largest perforator, although the calibre can also be measured. If possible, the intramuscular and different courses of the perforating vessels will be described as short, long, straight, or tortuous (Figures 3.10 through 3.12). Conventional anatomy can be identified, but variants or congenital alterations can also be reported.

Subcutaneous fat must be explored to identify branches of the superficial inferior epigastric veins that link across the midline.

Duplex US, as handheld colour US, is a non-invasive imaging technique that relies in the same physical principle as handheld colour US. Blood flow is detected by the physical principle of a direct relationship between the recorded Doppler frequency shift and the blood-flow velocity. In addition, different velocities and directions of moving blood stream can be displayed on a screen (Figure 3.4). Colour Doppler has also been found to be of value in cases in which the perforating vessels might have been damaged as it offers information about the amount of flow in vessels.

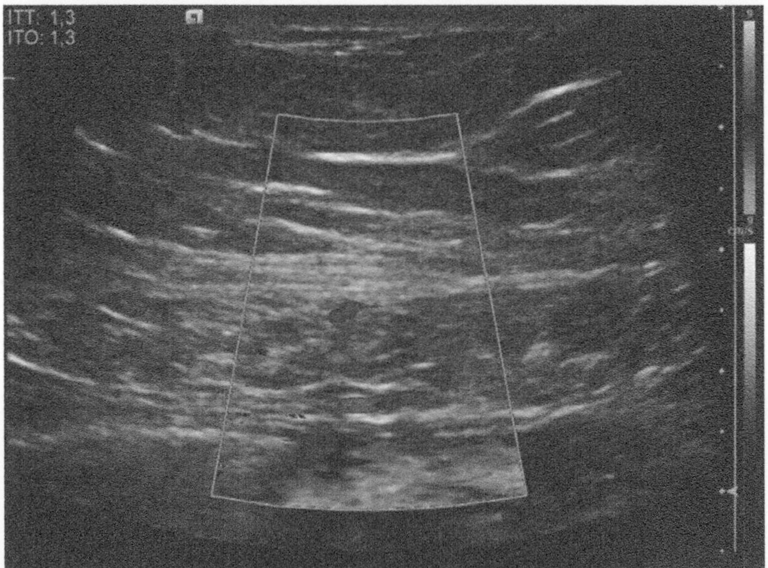

FIGURE 3.10 Short and perpendicular intramuscular perforator tract.

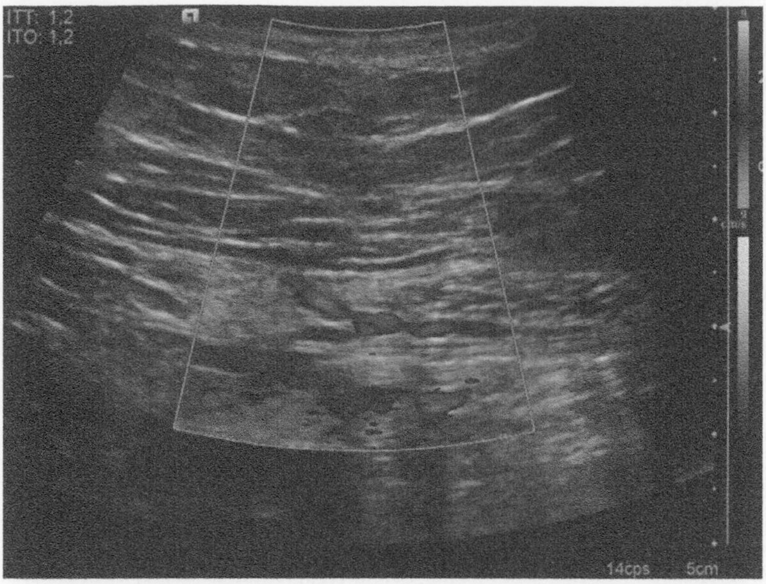

FIGURE 3.11 Long and oblique intramuscular tract and the outflow to the subcutaneous fat.

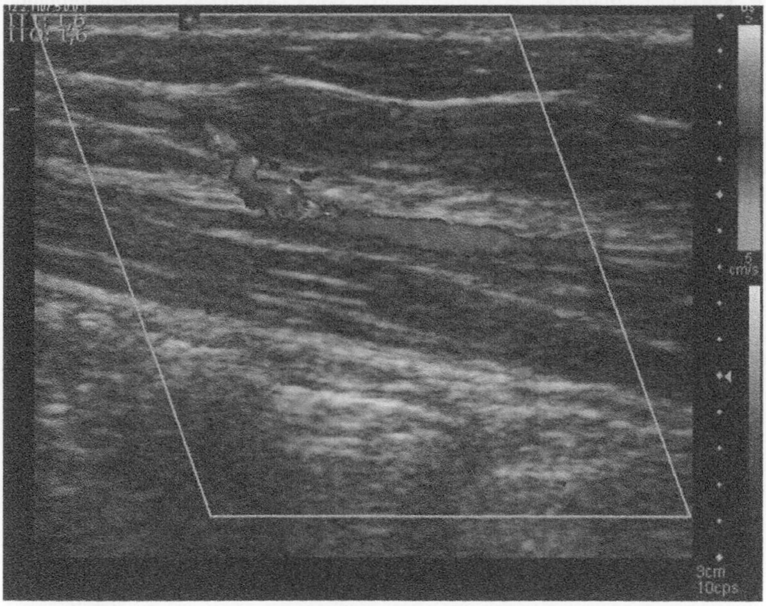

FIGURE 3.12 Long subfascial perforating pedicle before its outflow to the subcutaneous fat.

In cases of overweight patients, the sensitivity significantly drops due to the depth of the interrogated vessels and the major pressure on the abdominal wall needed.

The major disadvantage of Doppler US is the need of skillness with knowledge about free-flap anatomy and Doppler technology. Doppler US usually takes between 30 and 50 min depending on the size of the patient and the individual anatomical variants. Another disadvantage in comparison to CTA or MRA is that Doppler does not reproduce a 2D or 3D map of the complete vascular anatomy which can be used by the surgeon in the flap design or in the surgery room. However, Doppler US does not require radiation exposure.

In summary, although CTA may be considered the gold standard in the evaluation of perforator vessels, colour Doppler US can be enough and is able to identify the course of deep inferior epigastric vessels, main branching, and perforator pattern especially when other complex techniques are not available.

REFERENCES

1. Boote E. AAPM/RSNA physics tutorial for residents: Topics in US. Doppler US techniques: Concepts of blood flow detection and flow dynamics. *Radiographics* 2003;23: 1315–1327.
2. Hangiandreou N. AAPM/RSNA physics tutorial for residents: Topics in US. B-mode US basic concepts and new technology. *Radiographics* 2003;23: 1019–1033.
3. Middleton W, Kurtz A, Herzberg B. Practical physics. In: *Ultrasound, the Requisites*, 2nd edn. St Louis, MO: Mosby Inc., 2004, pp. 3–27.
4. Kruskal J, Newman P, Sammons L, Kane R. Optimizing Doppler and color flow US: Application to hepatic sonography. *Radiographics* 2004;24: 657–675.
5. Merritt CRB. Physics of ultrasound. In: Rumack C (ed.), *Diagnostic Ultrasound*, 4th edn. Philadelphia, PA: Elsevier-Mosby, 2011, pp. 2–33.
6. Taylor GI, Doyle M, McCarten G et al. The Doppler probe for planning flaps: Anatomical study and clinical applications. *Br J Plast Surg* 1990;43: 1–16.
7. Ogawa R, Hyakusoku H, Murakami M et al. Colour Doppler ultrasonography in the planning of microvascular augmented "super-thin" flaps. *Plast Reconstr Surg* 2003;112: 822–828.
8. Hallock GG. Doppler sonography and colour duplex imaging for planning a perforator flap. *Clin Plast Surg* 2003;30: 347–357.
9. Tsukino A, Kurachi K, Inamiya T et al. Preoperative color Doppler assessment in planning of anterolateral thigh flaps. *Plast Reconstr Surg* 2004;113: 241–246.
10. De Frene B, Van Landuyt K, Hamdi M et al. Free DIEAP and SGAP flap breast reconstruction after abdominal/gluteal liposuction. *J Plast Reconstr Aesthet Surg* 2006;59: 1031–1036.
11. Yu P, Youssef A. Efficacy of the handheld Doppler in preoperative identification of the cutaneous perforators in the anterolateral thigh flap. *Plast Reconstr Surg* 2006;118: 928–933.
12. Rozen WM, Phillips TJ, Ashton MW et al. Preoperative imaging for DIEA perforator flaps: A comparative study of computed tomographic angiography and Doppler ultrasound. *Plast Reconstr Surg* 2008;121: 9–16.
13. Rozen WM, Garcia-Tutor E, Alonso-Burgos A et al. Planning and optimising DIEP flaps with virtual surgery: The Navarra experience. *J Plast Reconstr Aesthet Surg* 2010;63: 289–297.
14. Smit JM, Klein S, Werker PM. An overview of methods for vascular mapping in the planning of free flaps. *J Plast Reconstr Aesthet Surg* 2010;63: 674–682.
15. Cina A, Salgarello M, Barone-Adesi L et al. Planning breast reconstruction with deep inferior epigastric artery perforating vessels: Multidetector CT angiography versus color Doppler US. *Radiology* 2010;255: 979–987.

4 Nuclear Medicine

Alessandra Serra and Mario Piga

CONTENTS

4.1 INTRODUCTION

The nuclear medicine imaging is based on the assessment of radiotracer distribution in the organs after in vivo administration of a molecule containing radioactive atoms (radiopharmaceuticals) to distinguish between physiological and pathophysiological functions of the examined tissues.

The diagnostic information obtained from radiopharmaceutical distribution is fundamentally functional – differing from other imaging procedures, which display primarily anatomical data. More specifically, nuclear medicine is a part of molecular imaging because it produces images that reflect biological processes that take place at the cellular and subcellular levels. We can distinguish two types of radionuclide imaging techniques: scintigraphy and positron emission tomography (PET). Scintigraphic technique, which uses radioisotopes that emit a single γ-photon, provides both planar and single-photon emission computed tomography (SPECT) imaging. A wide selection of radiopharmaceuticals is available for single-photon imaging designed to study numerous physiological processes within the body. The PET uses biologically active tracers labelled with a positron-emitting isotope. Following the decay of the radioisotope, the positron annihilates with a nearby electron emitting two γ-rays. Dual-photon imaging is the principle underlying PET and is fundamentally tomographic. PET has expanded rapidly due to the clinical impact of the radiopharmaceutical ^{18}F-fluorodeoxyglucose (FDG), a glucose analogue particularly used for imaging of malignancy. A combined structure–function approach utilising a fusion device permits an anatomical localisation of the uptake areas representing the major innovation of recent times in the area of medical imaging. Clinically, the best example of multimodality imaging is seen in the rapid evolution of hybrid PET/computed tomography (CT) and SPECT/CT scanners. Hybrid imaging has been successfully applied in oncology, orthopaedic surgery, and the other areas including the evaluation of benign diseases.

4.1.1 Physical Basic of Nuclear Medicine

Nuclear medicine is a branch of medicine which utilises molecules containing radioactive atoms (radionuclides) for the diagnosis and treatment of diseases. A radionuclide (also referred to as a radioisotope) is an atom with an unstable nucleus characterised by excess of energy. In general, radioactive elements are those which have an excess of protons or neutrons. Eventually, the imbalance is corrected by the release of excess neutrons or protons by spontaneously emitting particles and/or photons. This process is referred to as radioactive decay.

In order to reach a stable state, a radionuclide may decay in different modes by emitting different types of ionising radiation: α-emission, β– emission, positron (β+) emission, isomeric transition (γ-emission), internal conversion (IC), electron capture (EC), and nuclear fission. For diagnostic nuclear medicine purposes, the α-emission and nuclear fission are of relatively little importance. The other modes are briefly described.

Beta minus (β–) decay particles are negatively charged electrons emitted from radionuclides that have an excess number of neutrons compared to the number of protons. A neutron in this nuclide is converted into a proton with the ejection of an electron (β–) from the nucleus. Often, during the β– decay, the daughter radionuclide is formed in an excited state that transits nearly instantaneously to a stable state with emission γ-rays. As the nuclear states have well-defined energies, the gamma ray energy emitted in the transition from state to state is also well defined.

For example, an important radionuclide used in nuclear medicine for both diagnostic and therapeutic purposes is the iodine-131 (^{131}I) that decays with the emission of β- and γ-rays. In nuclear medicine, important types of radioactive decay are by isomeric transition. Often, during radioactive decay, a daughter is formed in an excited state. Most excited states transit nearly instantaneously to lower energy states with the emission of γ-rays. Some nuclides can exist in excited states for extended periods of time, before releasing the excess energy in the form of gamma radiation, but without altering the composition of the nuclide. These excited states that are called metastable or isomeric states (denoted by the letter m after the mass number) are very important for nuclear medicine as they represent nuclides capable of delivering only gamma rays without any contribution from the particle. Technetium-99m (^{99m}Tc), which is the most commonly used radionuclide in nuclear medicine imaging (half-life 6 h), is a metastable daughter product of molybdenum-99 (^{99}Mo) (half-life of 66 h) that decays by isomeric transition to ^{99}Tc by emitting a gamma photon of 140 keV.

Positron decay (β+) occurs with neutron-poor radionuclides. A proton is converted into a neutron with the simultaneous ejection of a positron (β+). The positron is the antimatter conjugate of the electron emitted in β– decay (β+ and β– have the same physical characteristics, with the exception of electric polarity). After ejection from the nucleus, a positron loses its kinetic energy in collisions with atoms of the surrounding matter and comes to rest within approximately 10^{-9} s. The positron then combines with an ordinary electron in an annihilation reaction, in which the entire rest mass of both particles is instantaneously converted to energy and emitted as two oppositely directed 511 keV γ-ray photons. PET is a nuclear medicine technique which produces the images of positron-emitting radionuclides measuring the annihilated γ-rays. Radionuclides used in PET are short-lived radionuclides (Table 4.1), and most are produced on site by cyclotron. They represent the main constituents of most biological molecules.

TABLE 4.1
Common PET Radioisotopes

Radioisotope	Half-Life	Decay%
Carbon (^{11}C)	20.3 min	β^+ 99.8, EC 0.2
Nitrogen (^{13}N)	9.96 min	β^+ 100
Oxygen (^{15}O)	122 s	β^+ 99.9, EC 0.1
Fluorine (^{18}F)	109.8 min	β^+ 96.9, EC 3.1
Rubidium (^{82}Rb) (gen.)	75 s	β^+ 96, EC 4
Iodine (^{124}I)	4.15 days	β^+ 25, EC 075

TABLE 4.2
Common SPECT Radioisotopes

Radionuclides	Physical Half-Life	Modes of Decay	Principle Gamma Photon Radiation Emission(s) (keV)
Technetium (^{99m}Tc)	6.04 h	Isomeric transition	140
Indium (^{111}In)	67.4 h (2.81 days)	EC	171, 245
Galium (^{67}Ga)	78.3 h (3.26 days)	EC	93, 184, 300
Iodine (^{123}I)	13.2 h	EC	159
Iodine (^{131}I)	193.0 h (8.04 days)	β- and γ-rays	284, 364, 637
Thallium (^{201}Tl)	73.0 h (3.04 days)	EC	72, 135, 167

EC is an alternative way for positron decay involving neutron-poor radionuclides. In this mode, an unstable nucleus captures an orbital electron, with the conversion of a proton into a neutron. Additional characteristic x-rays are generated when the vacancy in the electron shell created by EC is filled by an electron from a higher-energy shell. The EC decay frequently results in a daughter nucleus that is in an excited state. Thus, γ-rays (or conversion electrons) may also be emitted. Examples of EC radionuclides are gallium-67 (^{67}Ga), indium-111 (^{111}In), iodine-123 (^{123}I), and thallium-201 (^{201}Tl) (Table 4.2).

4.2 RADIOACTIVE DECAY

The exact moment at which an atom will decay cannot be predicted. Radioactive decay was found to follow a statistical law, that is, it is impossible to predict when any given atom will disintegrate, but the decay rate itself over a long period of time is constant. So if we have N radioactive atoms at time t_0, we expect to have a decrease dN after an interval of time dt of $dN = -\lambda dt$ where λ is called the decay constant that is characteristic of each radionuclide. The rate at which a radioactive substance N decays is given by $dN/dt = -\lambda N$, which represents the probability per unit time for one atom to decay. Integration over time yields $N_{dt} = N_{t0}e^{-\lambda(dt)}$.

Physical half-life (T½) is a useful parameter related to the decay constant defined as the time required for the number of radioactive atoms in a sample to decrease by one-half. The decay constant and physical half-life are inversely related and unique for each radionuclide and have the following relationship: $T½ = \ln(2)/\lambda = 0.693/\lambda$.

The amount of a radioactive substance is quantified by the *activity* (A). The activity of radioactive material is defined as the number of radioactive atoms undergoing radioactive decay per unit time (t). Therefore, the activity is equal to the change (dN) in the total number of radioactive atoms (N) in a given period (dt): $A = -dN/dt$.

The SI unit of activity is becquerel (Bq), which is named after Henri Becquerel, who discovered radioactivity in 1896. One Bq is defined as one disintegration per second (dps). Because a Bq is a very tiny amount of activity, the curie (Ci; the historical unit of activity) is more frequently used in nuclear medicine. One curie is the activity of 1 g of pure 226 Ra. Ci and Bq have the following relationship: $1\ Ci = 3.7 \times 10^{10}\ Bq$; 1 mCi = 37 MBq.

Interaction of radiation with matter: When a photon passes through a thickness of absorber material, the probability that it will have an interaction depends on its energy and on the composition and thickness of the absorber. In the body, attenuation is very undesirable but, unfortunately, unavoidable. The intensity of gamma rays travelling through material is gradually reduced by absorption or scattering. The attenuation of a photon beam through a thickness of an absorber material is mainly caused by four types of interactions: coherent scattering, photoelectric effect, Compton effect and pair production. Thus each of these processes can be represented by its own coefficient of attenuation that varies according to the incident photon energy and atomic number of absorbed material.

Over the range of gamma ray energies used in radionuclide imaging (Table 4.2), the two primary interactions that contribute to the attenuation coefficient are photoelectric absorption and Compton scattering.

Photoelectric absorption refers to the total absorption of the gamma ray by an inner-shell atomic electron. In photoelectric interactions, an incident (incoming) photon with slightly more energy than the binding energy of a k-shell electron encounters one of these electrons and ejects it from its orbit; because all its energy is imparted to the orbital electron, the photon disappears in the vicinity of the nucleus. The ejected photoelectron possesses kinetic energy equal to the energy from the incident photon minus the energy required to eject the electron from its orbit. The resultant vacancy in the k-shell is filled by a shell electron, which gives up energy in the form of an x-ray photon. The energy of radiation produced by the movement of electrons within an atom is a characteristic of each element and is therefore called characteristic radiation. It is the primary interaction in high-Z materials such as sodium iodide (the detector material used in the scintillation camera) and lead. In low-Z materials such as body tissues, its contribution to attenuation is relatively small.

Compton scattering results from a collision between a high-energy incident photon and a loosely held outer-shell electron. The incident photon transfers some of its energy to the electron, which is ejected from its orbit by the collision. Because incident photons cannot transfer all their energy to the orbiting electron, Compton scattering always produces an ion pair, a positive ion and the ejected negative electron (called a recoil electron), and always results in the formation of a scatter photon. The amount of energy lost in the event depends on the angle between the gamma ray and scattered photons. Compton scattering is the dominant interaction in body tissues.

4.2.1 Radiopharmaceuticals

A radiopharmaceutical is a molecule that incorporates one or more radionuclides (radioactive isotopes). Radiopharmaceuticals usually have no pharmacologic effects, as they are used in tracer quantities for diagnosis or therapeutic treatment. There is no dose–response relationship in this case, which thus differs significantly from conventional drugs. Radiation is an inherent characteristic of all radiopharmaceuticals which contain at least two major components:

1. *A radionuclide* that must emit gamma rays of sufficient energy to escape from the body and must have a half-life short enough for it to decay away soon after study is completed
2. *A chemical compound* with structural or chemical properties that determine the in vivo distribution and physiological behaviour of the radiopharmaceutical

The radionuclides used in diagnostic are chosen for their particular radioactive properties such as half-life, type of radiation emitted, photon energy, cost, and availability. Diagnostic radiopharmaceuticals should be a pure gamma ray emitter, decaying by either EC or isomeric transition. Furthermore, modern imaging equipment has been tailored to function in energy range 100–250 keV. Thus, the classical example of ideal radionuclide is ^{99m}Tc (used in more than 80% of nuclear medicine studies). The short half-life and the absence of particulate emission result in a low radiation dose to the patient. Its logistics also favour its use. Technetium generators, a lead pot enclosing a glass tube containing the radioisotope, are supplied to hospitals from the nuclear reactor where the isotopes are made. The ^{99m}Tc is washed out of the lead pot by saline solution when it is required.

Technetium generator contains molybdenum-99 (^{99}Mo), with a half-life of 66 h, which progressively decays by the emission of a 140 KeV gamma ray to ^{99m}Tc. The chemistry of technetium is so versatile it can form tracers by being incorporated into a range of biologically active substances to ensure that it concentrates in the tissue or organ of interest. According to the physiological process that is being targeted, there are different pharmaceuticals available.

For example, ^{123}I or ^{131}I can be substituted for stable (nonradioactive) ^{127}I within sodium iodide (NaI), which is still taken up by the thyroid gland in a manner identical to the nonradioactive substrate. More commonly, because of limitations in available radionuclides and their imaging properties, an analogue of the molecule of interest is created which shares critical biochemical features, although its chemical structure differs and its biological fate is not identical to that of the original compound. ^{18}F-FDG, the most frequently used PET tracer, represents a radiopharmaceutical which shares some, but not all, features of glucose yet is of important clinical utility.

A radiopharmaceutical can be as simple as a radioactive element such as ^{133}Xe, a simple salt such as ^{131}I-NaI, or a labelled compound such as ^{131}I-iodinated proteins and ^{99m}Tc-labelled compounds. Typically, the radiopharmaceutical is injected intravenously, but some studies require inhalation (as a radioactive gas) or ingestion. Unlike radiographic procedures, which depend almost entirely upon tissue density differences, external imaging of radiopharmaceuticals is essentially independent of the density of the target organ. The mechanism of localisation of a radiopharmaceutical in a particular target organ depends on different processes as antigen–antibody reactions, physicochemical adsorption or chemisorption, receptor site binding, and transport of a chemical species across a cell membrane and into the cell. The biological functions can be displayed as images, numerical data, or time–activity curves.

The different uptake of the radiopharmaceutical can reveal the normal or altered state of tissue metabolism or specific function of an organ system. Another important use is to predict the effects of surgery and assess changes since treatment.

4.2.2 Nuclear Medicine Instrumentation

4.2.2.1 Gamma Camera Detector

4.2.2.1.1 Introduction

The purpose of nuclear medicine imaging is to obtain a picture of the distribution of a radiopharmaceutical within the body after the administration and its metabolism in the patient. In order to get images, it is necessary to detect the radiation emitted by the radionuclide. Alpha particles and electrons ($\beta\pm$ particles, auger and conversion electrons) are not used for imaging because they cannot penetrate more than a few millimetres of tissue. Gamma (γ) radiation is non-particulate and penetrating, making it useful for diagnostic imaging purposes. Gamma ray in the approximate energy range of 60–600 keV (or annihilation photons, 511 keV in PET) is sufficiently penetrating in body tissues to be detected by an external radiation detector used in diagnostic nuclear medicine.

There are two types of nuclear imaging methods: single-photon imaging and PET. The distinction between these two imaging modalities is based on the physical properties of the radioisotopes used for imaging. Radioisotopes emitting single γ-ray are used to obtaine single-photon imaging (Table 4.2). The most widely used single-photon emitters include ^{99m}Tc, ^{201}Tl, and ^{123}I. In contrast to single-photon imaging, PET uses the radioisotopes that finally emit two γ-ray photons simultaneously. A single-photon imaging device is the gamma camera. It is also called the Anger camera in honour of Hal O. Anger, who developed the first one in the late 1950s [1]. Various designs of gamma cameras have been proposed and made available, but the Anger camera with a single crystal is by far the most widely used.

4.2.2.2 Component of Gamma Camera

The Anger type of a modern gamma camera consists of a camera head, a gantry, an electronic processing unit for position and energy determination, and a computer for data acquisition and image reconstruction.

The camera head contains the detector assembly, consisting of a gamma ray–sensitive element, a scintillation crystal, photomultiplier tubes (PMTs) and light guides, and a collimator, shielded with lead to reduce the detection of background radiation of the crystal (Figure 4.1).

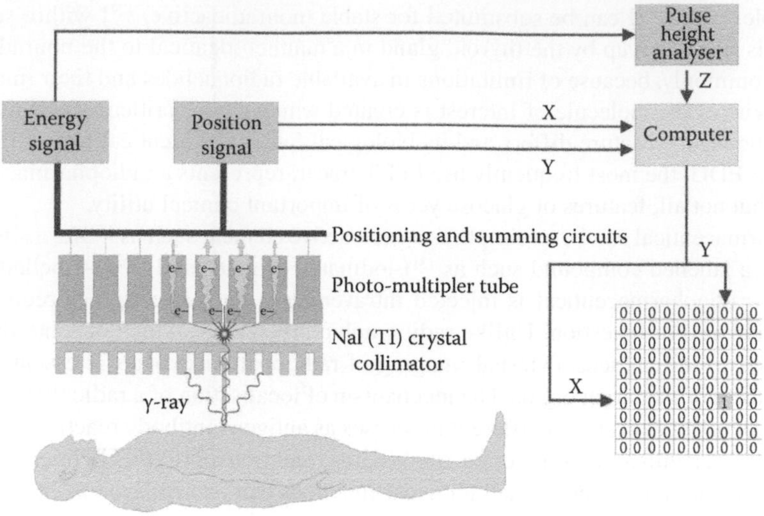

FIGURE 4.1 Basic components and principles of the gamma camera: radiopharmaceutical within the patient's body emits γ-photons in an isotropic manner. Only the photons travelling in a direction of collimator holes strike and are absorbed by the Na(I) crystal. The energy of the photon is transformed to visible light emitted within the crystal. The light signal is simultaneously detected by an array of PMTs that convert the light signal to an electronic pulse which is amplified and then analysed by the positioning and summing circuits to determine the location (x, y) and energy (z) of a scintillation event. If a scintillation event falls within the selected energy range, the transfer of X- and Y-position signals to the computer is enabled.

In clinical systems, scintillation crystals of sodium iodide, purposely contaminated or *doped* with thallium ions [NaI(Tl)], are commonly used. NaI(Tl) converts gamma ray energy into visible light. The scintillation stops the photon via photoelectric absorption or via multiple scattering events. The resulting photoelectron travels through the crystal, distributing its kinetic energy over a few thousand other electrons in multiple collisions. After a short time, these electrons will release their energy in the form of a photon of a few eV.

These photons contain just the right amount of energy to drive an electron from a lower level to the higher one. In pure NaI, the photons are reabsorbed and the scintillation light never leaves the crystal. To avoid this, the NaI crystal is doped with a bit of Tl (thallium). This disturbs the lattice and creates additional energy levels. Electrons returning to the ground state via these levels emit photons (which are not reabsorbed) in the form of light, hence the term scintillation detector. It is the detector of choice due to this crystal's optimal detection efficiency for the gamma ray energies of radionuclide emission common in nuclear medicine. Most current cameras incorporate large (40 cm × 50 cm) rectangular crystal, which results in increased efficiency. The features that make this crystal desirable include high mass density and atomic number (Z), thereby effectively stopping γ-photons, and high efficiency of light output. The choice of thickness of the crystal is a trade-off between its detection efficiency (which increases with increasing thickness) and its intrinsic spatial resolution (which deteriorates with increasing thickness). Due to the fact that most gamma cameras are designed for imaging ^{99m}Tc-labelled pharmaceuticals with 140 keV low-energy γ-photon emissions, a crystal thickness of 9–12 mm provides the best compromise between resolution and efficiency. Thus, the energy of the γ-ray is absorbed by the scintillation crystal and part of this energy is converted into visible light. The amount of light produced following the interactions of a single particle is proportional to the energy deposited by the incident radiation in the scintillator. Converting the gamma ray energy to visible light is only the first step. In order for the information from the scintillation to be useful, it has to be converted into an electronic signal. All this is usually obtained with PMTs, in which the visible light photons are converted into an electrical signal that is amplified to detectable levels.

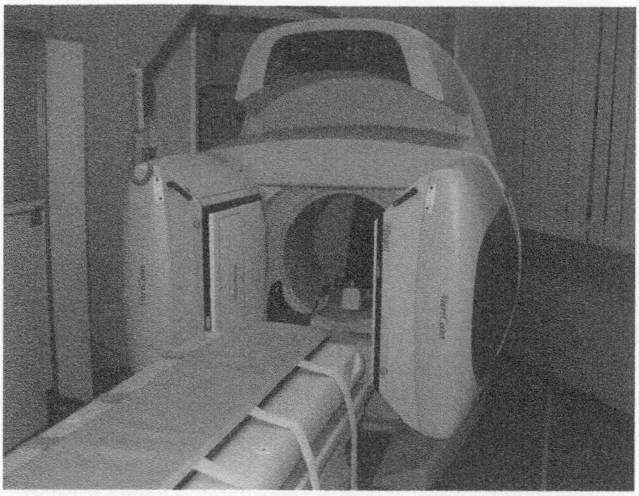

FIGURE 4.2 Gamma camera (VariCam, General Electric Medical System). Two gamma camera heads are mounted onto a rotating gantry for SPECT and a moving bed is incorporated to permit imaging of the whole body.

In the Anger camera design, the NaI(Tl) crystal is optically coupled to an array of PMTs which is packed to the back face of the crystal and arranged in a hexagonal pattern to maximise the area of the scintillation crystal. It is usually necessary to provide a light guide to interface the scintillation crystal to the photomultipliers. The light guide helps to minimise the light losses in the transfer of light from the scintillation crystal to the photomultiplier.

A typical gamma camera has between 30 and 100 PMTs. The number of PMTs affects the intrinsic resolution of the camera. The PMT consists of multiple dynodes (about 10), the first of which (the photocathode) is in optical contact with the crystal and an anode (Figure 4.2). The principle of operation of these devices is that when incident light reaches the entrance window, which is coated with a photocathode, electrons are ejected and focused towards a dynode. The dynode is maintained at a positive voltage relative to the photocathode attracting the electrons to it. The dynodes are coated with a material having relatively high secondary emission characteristics. A high-speed photoelectron striking the first dynode surface ejects several secondary electrons secondary attracted to the next dynode which is maintained at 50–150 V higher potential than the first one; here, the electrons are again ejected to the next dynode and so on. Finally, after about 10 dynode steps, the number of electrons has been multiplied by a factor ~10^6. Finally, the anode collects all the electrons produced from the final dynode and emits an output voltage signal. Each γ-photon originally absorbed in the crystal results in a discrete pulse of current exiting from the PMT; the amplitude of this pulse is proportional to the incident photon energy. This measurable voltage from the PMT outputs is digitised with an analogue-to-digital converter (ADC) to deduce for each scintillation event the position and the energy (~amount of scintillation photons). The output of each PMT is used to define the X,Y coordinates of the point of interaction of the γ-ray in the detector by the use of an X-, Y-positioning circuit (the position of the event is determined by summing weighted outputs from each PMT) and also is summed up by a summing circuit to form a pulse known as the Z pulse that indicates its energy (based on the linear relationship between gamma ray energy and the number of scintillation photons produced) (2). The Z pulses are then subjected to pulse-height analysis (PHA) amplitude and are accepted only if they fall within the range of desired energy (Figure 4.1). PHA is necessary in avoiding distorted signals. In modern gamma cameras, two or three PHAs are used to select simultaneously two or three γ-rays of different energies. These types of cameras are useful in imaging with ^{111}In and ^{67}Ga that possess two or three predominant γ-rays. In the initial designs, positioning circuit in the gamma camera was analogue in nature, and literally all the PMTs participated in the energy and position signal summations. It is subsequently found that the signal from PMTs located far from the event contributed mostly noise. A commonly used tactic that is employed in both digital and analogue cameras to improve the positioning accuracy is to include in the position calculation only PMTs with signals above a certain threshold. When an event falls within the selected energy window, the transfer of X- and Y-position signals to the computer is enabled. This has two important benefits. First, by using the signal only from those PMTs that produce a significant pulse amplitude, the noise from the PMTs that have negligible pulse amplitude (and that therefore contribute no position information) is not included into the position calculation means to discriminate against γ-rays that have scattered in the body and therefore lost their positional information. Second, with signal thresholding, only a small number of PMTs surrounding the interaction location are used for position determination. This allows a gamma camera to detect multiple events simultaneously when they occur in different portions of the gamma camera and their light cones (the projection of the scintillation light on the PMT array) do not significantly overlap. This improves the count rate performance of the gamma camera, reducing dead time losses.

The precision of locating gamma ray events by a scintillation camera is referred to as *intrinsic spatial resolution*. With the improvement in electronics and pulse-processing methods, the intrinsic spatial resolution of the scintillation camera has improved steadily, approaching 3 mm in modern systems.

4.2.2.3 Collimators

The interaction of a gamma ray with the crystal results in a burst of isotropically emitted scintillation photons. In order to form images with a gamma camera, a collimator must be placed in front of the scintillation crystal. The purpose of collimation in gamma camera is to allow a geometric correspondence or mapping between gamma rays emitted within the patient and the location of their interaction in the scintillation crystal. A mechanical collimator is made of lead or tungsten and is crossed by a distributed set of holes with different geometric patterns. The lead bricks between the holes are called septa. This collimator projects an image of the source distribution onto the detector by allowing only those γ-rays travelling along certain directions to reach the detector. Gamma rays not travelling in the proper direction are absorbed by the collimator before they reach the detector. Photons that pass through the collimator have momenta that are restricted to a small solid angle. In the absence of scattering within the patient, the photons propagate in a straight line from the point of emission to the point of detection in the gamma camera. Consequently, the collimator imposes a strong correlation between the position in the image and the point of origin. Because the collimator restricts the photon momenta to such a small solid angle, most of the photons are absorbed in the collimator material. This is one of the underlying reasons for the relatively poor quality of radionuclide images.

The mechanical collimator has a dominating effect on the resolution and sensitivity of the gamma camera. Unfortunately, these two factors are inversely related in that the use of a collimator which produces images of good spatial resolution generally implies that the instrument is not very sensitive to radiation. To improve the count sensitivity, the collimator hole size could be increased and the hole length shortened, but these changes degrade the spatial resolution and vice versa. Collimator geometry is another fundamental design and it requires the specification of the orientation of the hole axes. The orientation of the hole axes has the greatest effect on the imaging properties of the collimator. Parallel-hole collimators that have hole axes oriented perpendicular to the collimator face are the most frequent in nuclear medicine. This one only permits passage of γ-photons normal to the crystal face. The projected image is the same size as the source distribution onto the detector.

One very important property to remember about collimators is that the spatial resolution gets worse as the source-to-collimator distance increases. In the absence of scattering within the patient, the photons propagate in a straight line from the point of emission to the point of detection in the gamma camera. Consequently, the collimator imposes a strong correlation between the position in the image and the point of origin of the photon. To obtain the best-quality images with parallel-hole collimator, spatial resolution comes at the price of count sensitivity; therefore, it is crucial to keep the collimator as close to the patient as possible. The spatial resolution of the collimator is constrained by the geometry of the holes and is typically in the range of 6–8 mm to 10 mm when used with ^{99m}Tc.

Many modern gamma cameras are completely digital, in the sense that the output of each PMT is directly digitised by an ADC. The calculation of X-, Y-position and pulse height is performed by using a software based on the digitised PMT signals, and the errors in energy and positioning due to noise and pulse distortions caused by the positioning circuitry are eliminated. In a digital image, the X- and Y-values corresponding to the event position are limited to certain discrete values. The requirement for discrete values leads to a grid-like arrangement called an imaging matrix. Each possible position in the grid is called a picture element or pixel. The analogue X- and Y-signals coming from an event registered by the gamma camera are converted to digital X- and Y-values that in turn locate the event in one of the pixels of the image matrix; the computer increments the count of that pixel by 1 (Figure 4.1). In a complete image, three numbers specify each: its X- and Y-coordinates and the number of counts registered in it. The latter value is most commonly correlated to a grey or colour scale. The resultant image can be manipulated and analysed after acquisition and stored in digital media.

4.2.2.4 Nuclear Medicine Imaging Characteristics

To produce nuclear images of the best quality, two conditions are essential:

1. The body must absorb very little radiation.
2. The detector must absorb as much radiation as possible.

In radionuclide imaging, the flux of gamma rays available is in orders of magnitude less than that used in x-ray radiography or x-ray CT. As a result, the images produced in nuclear medicine studies are usually noisier and of less spatial resolution than an x-ray image.

The decay of radioactive nuclei is *random*, which means that the activity within a subject produces a random distribution of counts. This randomness is known as noise when it appears in an image. Image noise is most apparent in images that have a small number of counts. As the number of counts increases, randomness averages out, and noise will decrease. Images that have a large number of counts show improved contrast and resolution. These parameters will improve up to the imaging limitations of the gamma camera itself.

A scattered ray that loses a small amount of energy will deviate from its original path by a small amount; if it passes through the collimator holes, it will appear to have come from a tissue near the original source. The scatter acts as increased background on which sources of activity are superimposed and results in loss of image contrast.

However, several factors will degrade the image quality, some of which are due to inherent properties of the imaging device such as spatial resolution, energy resolution, non-uniformity, or distortions. Other degrading factors are dependent on the patient and organ localisation. A large patient will increase the influence of scattered photons. An organ deep in the body will be overlapped by other tissues, which will increase the background registrations. Patient and organ movements will also degrade the image quality. Finally, some important factors are due to the operation of the imaging device and can be optimised by the user. These include spatial resolution by keeping the distance between the detector and the patient as short as possible and noise reduction by selecting an optimum examination time and matrix size. Scattered radiation can be reduced by a proper setting of the pulse-height analyser.

4.2.2.5 SPECT Instrumentation

Common types of gamma camera are the single- or dual-head gamma cameras. In these systems, one or two gamma camera heads are mounted onto a gantry that allows the camera heads to be positioned in a flexible way over different regions of the patient's body, and a moving bed is incorporated to permit imaging studies of the whole body (Figure 4.2). In addition, its rotating gantry allows to produce tomographic images. An obvious advantage of a dual-head system is that the acquisition time is reduced by a factor of 2 over a single detector. Triple-head systems exist primarily for tomographic studies. Multihead camera offers more optimal spatial resolution and sensitivity characteristics than are available with a single-head system.

Planar imaging produces a 2D image of a 3D object. As a result, images contain no depth information and some details can be superimposed on top of each other and partially obscured as a result. Images of higher contrast and better localisation can be obtained by SPECT. This type of acquisition produces tomographic images of the distribution of an administered radiotracer within an organ. SPECT studies are usually acquired over a full 360° arc on a matrix of 64 × 64 or 128 × 128 pixels. The acquisitions are performed with the scintillation camera located at preselected angular locations (step-and-shoot mode) or in a continuous rotation mode (Figure 4.3). In a dual-head system, two 180° opposed camera heads are used. During the rotation procedure, multiple 2D projections of the 3D radiopharmaceutical distribution can be acquired to provide an estimate of 3D distribution of the radiotracer using image reconstruction from multiple projections. In standard SPECT examination, the projection images are acquired every 3°–6° around the object with a total of 60–120 images. Total scan time requires about 20–30 min. The 2D projection images are the first corrected for non-uniformities, and then mathematical algorithms are used to reconstruct 3D matrices of selected planes from the 2D projection data (Figure 4.3). There are two methods to reconstruct SPECT images, either iteratively or by filtered back projection (FBP) technique [3]. The quality of the final tomographic image is limited by several factors. Some of these are the attenuation and scatter of gamma ray photons, the detection efficiency, and the spatial resolution of the collimator–detector system [4]. The main advantage of SPECT imaging is that overlaying and underlying activity is eliminated from the image. Although SPECT data, in general, have proved superior to those of planar imaging, SPECT images contain occasionally little or no anatomical landmarks that can be correlated with anatomical reference points as a result of an inability to provide accurate anatomical localisation of an identified abnormality.

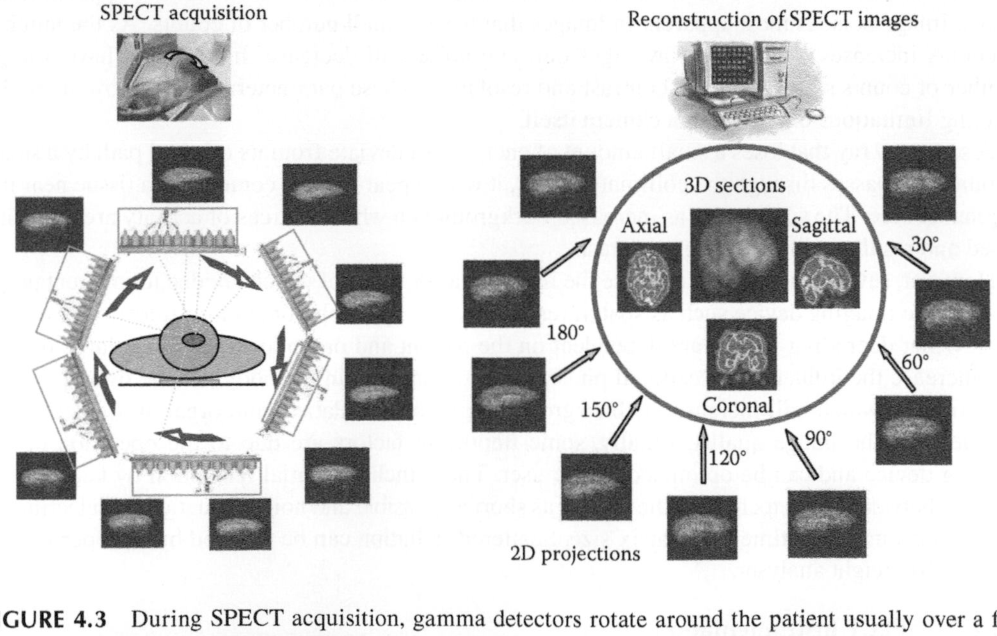

FIGURE 4.3 During SPECT acquisition, gamma detectors rotate around the patient usually over a full 360 arc, and projections from different views around the patient are acquired at selected angles (typically every 3°–6°). These projection images are then processed to generate cross-sectional images (transaxial, sagittal, and coronal).

4.2.2.6 Hybrid System SPECT/CT

Nuclear medicine imaging is based on the bio-distribution of a radioactive agent over time and space, thus visualising dynamic physiological and pathophysiological processes that define the functional characteristics of disease. Due to inherent characteristics of nuclear medicine images, it is difficult to define the precise location of diseases, making often the interpretation of studies very difficult. SPECT provides several clinically important advantages over planar imaging. The main advantage of SPECT is accurate localisation which improves the specificity of the scan. It is beneficial in the evaluation of lesions in areas where the complexity of the structures can result in false-positive/false-negative finding on planar images. The 3D image reconstruction of SPECT allows separation of the overlying tracer accumulation from areas of interest and, thus, also may be able to differentiate pathological from physiological tracer distribution. However, the visual quality and quantitative accuracy of radionuclide imaging SPECT is limited by some other important physical characteristics such as lack of anatomical landmarks that are needed to precisely localise the disease. This is particularly important in SPECT studies with low count density due to unfavourable physical properties of some radionuclides (^{131}I, ^{67}Ga, ^{201}Tl, etc.) or with highly specific radiopharmaceutical accumulation because there are a few reference points for localisation. In contrast, imaging modalities such as CT and MRI are based on morphologic criteria providing information regarding changes in organ size and tissue density as well as their precise spatial localisation and topographic landmarks. To overcome nuclear medicine imaging limitation, the molecular and functional imaging provided by PET and SPECT and the anatomical imaging provided by CT and more recently by MRI have been merged into *hybrid imaging* using combined scanners such as SPECT/CT or PET/CT. Hybrid imaging technology SPECT/CT allows to acquire and co-record both structural and functional tomographic images that determine the geometric relationship between two different modality imaging studies [5]. The imaging study is performed with the patient remaining on the patient table, which is translated from the CT scanner to the PET or SPECT system to acquire the correlated x-ray and radionuclide image data. The resulting dual-modality image data then can be transferred electronically to a common computer for data correction, reconstruction, display, integration, and analysis. In addition, the transmission data of TC are reconstructed to generate a patient-specific map of attenuation coefficients for attenuation correction of the radionuclide image to improve both the visual quality (improved sensitivity) and the quantitative accuracy of the radionuclide images. SPECT attenuation correction data helps to remove artefacts associated with attenuated photons, particularly important for deeper structures.

While image fusion techniques have been in clinical use for many years, the first commercial SPECT/CT system was only introduced in 1999. This hybrid system combined a low-power x-ray tube opposite gamma ray detectors mounted on the same slip ring gantry (Figure 4.4). The x-ray system operated at 140 kV with a tube current of only 2.5 mA to provide a high-quality attenuation map and fair anatomical images with a significantly lower patient dose than that received during a conventional CT imaging procedure (by a factor of 4–5), but the quality of the CT images was inferior to state-of-the-art CT. This system has recently been equipped with a 4-slice low-dose CT scanner yielding an axial slice thickness of 5 mm with each rotation instead of one 10 mm slice. Thus, in an effort to further improve imaging quality and reduce acquisition time, new hybrid systems employing a variety of multi-slice CT scanners and the state-of-the-art spiral CT scanners have been developed (Figure 4.5). These systems combine dual-head gamma cameras with full diagnostic, up to 16-slice CT scanners that allow variation of CT slice thickness from 0.6 mm up to 10 mm, yielding diagnostic-quality CT images with a scan speed shorter than 30 s for a 40 cm axial field of view [6,7].

Improving qualitative and quantitative radionuclide assessments by SPECT/CT and PET/CT would be particularly important in oncology. The combined presence or absence of pathological changes observed on the CT in conjunction with the radiotracer uptake observed in SPECT or

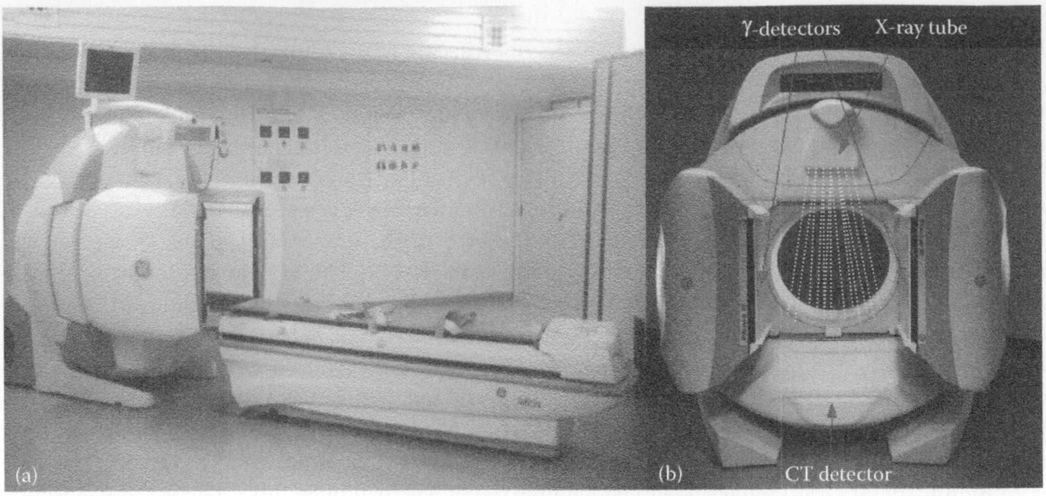

FIGURE 4.4 (a) Hybrid dual-head gamma camera CT (Infinia Hawkeye, GE Healthcare). Frontal view of a dual-head gamma camera with an integrated low-dose CT scanner built onto the same rotating gantry (b). CT source and CT detectors are oriented perpendicular to the two gamma camera heads and rotate on the same gantry.

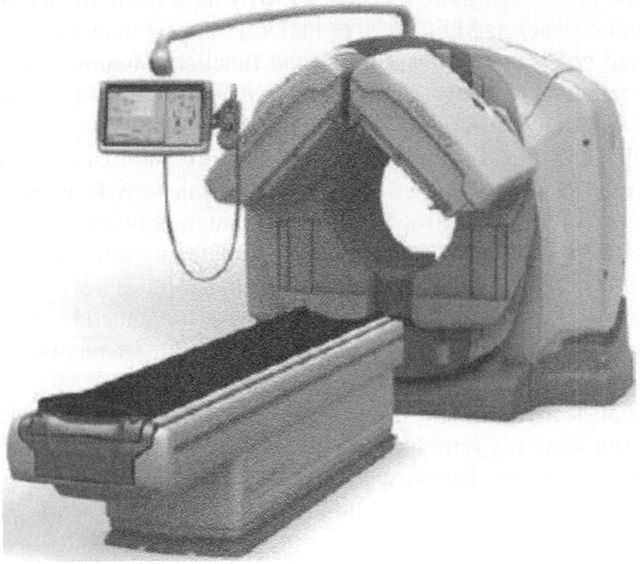

FIGURE 4.5 Two gamma detectors suspended to a moving arm combined with a 16-slice CT component. (Courtesy of GE Healthcare.)

PET can improve the diagnostic accuracy of the procedure. In oncology, hybrid systems can allow more accurate tumour localisation such as evaluating therapeutic response to surgery, radiation treatment, or chemotherapy. In addition, dosimetry has made great progress recently with the widespread availability of SPECT and/or SPECT/CT that allows a 3D radionuclide distribution, as well as volume measurements of tumours and normal organs for treatment planning and monitoring [8,9]. Clinical utility of SPECT/CT has been also demonstrated in cardiology, musculoskeletal applications, infection, neurology, and general nuclear medicine [10]. Finally, SPECT/CT can also aid in guiding interventional procedures where it is especially suited to support the minimally invasive surgery.

REFERENCES

1. Anger HO. Scintillation camera. *Rev. Sci. Instrum.* 29:27–33, 1958.
2. Cherry SR, Sorenson JA, Phelps ME. *Physics in Nuclear Medicine*, 3rd edn. Saunders, Philadelphia, PA, 2003.
3. Groch MW, Erwin WD. SPECT in the year 2000: Basic principles. *J. Nucl. Med. Technol.* 28(4):233–244, 2000.
4. Madsen MT. Recent advances in SPECT imaging. *J. Nucl. Med.* 48:661–673, 2007.
5. Hasegawa BH, Iwata K, Wong KH et al. Dual-modality imaging of function and physiology. *Acad. Radiol.* 9:1305, 2002.
6. Patton JA, Turkington TG. SPECT/CT physical principles and attenuation correction. *J. Nucl. Med. Technol.* 36(1):1–10, 2008.
7. O'Connor MK, Kemp BJ. Single-photon emission computed tomography/computed tomography: Basic instrumentation and innovations. *Semin. Nucl. Med.* 36:258–266, 2006.
8. Mansberg R, Sorensen N, Mansberg V et al. Yttrium 90 Bremsstrahlung SPECT/CT scan demonstrating areas of tracer/tumour uptake. *Eur. J. Nucl. Med. Mol. Imaging* 34(11):1887, 2007.
9. Boucek JA, Turner JH. Validation of prospective whole-body bone marrow dosimetry by SPECT-CT multimodality imaging in ^{131}I-anti-CD20 rituximab radioimmunotherapy of non-Hodgkin's lymphoma. *Eur. J Nucl. Med. Mol. Imaging* 32:458–469, 2005.
10. Mariani G, Bruselli L, Kuwert T, Kim EE, Flotats A, Israel O, Dondi M, Watanabe N. A review on the clinical uses of SPECT/CT. *Eur. J. Nucl. Med. Mol. Imaging* 37:1959–1985, 2010.

5 Mammography

Luis Pina Insauti, Jon Etxano Cantera, Pedro Slon, and Arlette Elizalde

CONTENTS

5.1 INTRODUCTION

Breast cancer is nowadays the most common malignancy among women in developed countries [1], being the third most common cancer in Europe after lung and colorectal cancers. The high prevalence of breast cancer (out of every 10 women, 1 will develop a breast malignancy during her life) promotes that an important number of women suffer the consequences of this disease, which vary from breast surgery to death. More than 15,000 cases of breast cancer are diagnosed each year in Spain. In 2012, this disease caused around 6,000 deaths [2].

The treatment of breast cancer has completely changed in the last years. Nowadays, breast-conserving surgery is the first choice for most cases. The revolution produced by new oncoplastic surgeries has changed the concept of breast surgery, avoiding mastectomy for many cases. In recent years, there has also been a general decrease in mortality from breast cancer [3]. This fat can be explained by several reasons. The development of new protocols of adjuvant systemic chemotherapy and the inclusion of local radiotherapy have improved the prognosis of patients with breast cancer. The development of these new treatments has been of quite relevance, but it has been the introduction and consolidation of breast cancer detection programmes the principal factor which has made possible to achieve a reduction in the mortality of this disease.

The first breast cancer detection trials based on mammography were the Health Insurance Plan (HIP) trial and the Swedish two-county study [4,5]. Both studies were based on mammography, which is still today the first imaging technique for the detection of breast cancer.

Many other breast cancer screening studies have been launched after them. Nowadays, all the poblational screening programmes are based on mammography, and the literature confirms the results of the first screening programmes, as they can reduce mortality up to 20%–30% [6].

Nevertheless, breast screening programmes are not perfect, because all cancers cannot be detected on mammography. It is well documented that 20%–30% of all cancers are missed on screening. Several factors contribute to the difficulty in detecting malignant breast lesions on mammography. Breast density is one of the most important related to the decrease of mammographic sensitivity [7]. This is one of the reasons why the actual trend is to complete the mammographic study of patients with dense breasts with complementary digital breast tomosynthesis (DBT) or ultrasound.

In this chapter, we are going to describe the mammographic imaging technique, the semiology of breast lesions, and recent advances on mammography.

5.2 MAMMOGRAPHY AND PHYSICS

Mammograph is the equipment capable of performing images of the breast using x-rays. The features of the breast and the breast lesions make a mammograph be a quite specific machine, different of other x-ray equipment.

The breast is a good example of what is called *soft tissue*, with low absorption of radiation and low contrast between the different fat and glandular tissue that compose it. In other words, it is difficult to detect a breast lesion using a conventional x-ray technique.

Moreover, some breast cancers produce microcalcifications. These are very tiny particles of calcium, measuring as little as 100 μm or less, so a high spatial resolution is crucial.

To accomplish both purposes (high contrast and high spatial resolution), a low energy radiation beam is used, usually between 17 and 22 kV, generated by a very small focus (anode). The anode is the component of the tube that generates the radiation beam, and it is often made of molybdenum. This metal generates a characteristic radiation beam of the previous energy. Rhodium is another metal used in anodes, whose radiation is more energetic, being useful for dense breasts [8].

One of the typical components of a mammograph is the compressor paddle, which is responsible for the complaints and pain of many patients after a mammographic examination. The applied compression is about 10–15 kg for most breasts, although it can be adjusted for every patient. The reasons for such a strong compression are the following:

- Superposition of different structures is avoided. The breast is a tridimensional structure that is represented in a bidimensional image (mammography), so different structures are superimposed, and they potentially can produce a false image. These images can be interpreted as a lesion (false-positive result). A gentle compression can reduce this superposition.
- The breast thickness is smaller, so a significant decrease of both the radiation dose for the patient as well as the scattered radiation can be obtained.
- The fibroglandular tissue is dispersed, so lesions can be easily detected.

Most mammographs contain a grid made of plumb which is responsible for the elimination of the scattered radiation. This grid is also known as *bucky*.

TABLE 5.1
Desirable and Acceptable Radiation Dose Values according to Thickness

Thickness (cm)	Desirable Value (mGy)	Acceptable Value (mGy)
2.1	<0.6	<1.0
3.2	<1	<1.5
4.5	<1.6	<2.0
5.3	<2.0	<2.5
6	<2.4	<3.0
7.5	<3.6	<4.5
9	<5.1	<6.5

All mammographs include an automatic system to adjust the parameters of the tube to the composition of each breast. This system is called automatic exposure.

Nowadays, most mammographs are digital and use flat panels as receptors to produce the image. Originally, the receptor was analogue, using a combination of a film and a screen inside a cassette. Once this cassette was used, the film was introduced in a processor where, after a chemical procedure, the mammogram was obtained. This procedure was unstable and required a strict control of temperature and other parameters. The chemical liquids (revelator and fixer) were highly contaminants for the environment. Despite all of these problems, conventional mammography was a successful technique capable to produce high-quality images at a very low cost.

As an evolution of the conventional mammography, the computed radiography systems were introduced to replace conventional mammographs with lower cost. A cassette, similar to the analogic one, was used. However, this cassette had a photostimulable screen made of phosphor. This screen was able to store a latent image after stimulation. A laser processor was used to read the latent image, to digitise it, and to erase the screen, allowing a quick use of the cassette again and again.

Definitively, flat panels have become the final stage of the receptor technology. The flat panels can be made of amorphous selenium or cesium iodide with silicium, depending on the manufacturers. Anyway, flat panels join a high spatial resolution and high contrast. The size of the receptor pixels can vary from 50 to 100 μm. The advantages of flat panels are obvious: The image is formed in a few seconds, no additional manipulation with a cassette or processor is needed, the productivity increases, the image formation is very stable and reproducible, the digital image can be postprocessed and stored, and the received radiation dose is reduced. Probably, the main disadvantage is the high cost of the technology.

The radiation dose depends on several factors: composition and thickness of the compressed breast, characteristics of the mammograph, technical parameters used to form the image (kilovolts, milliamperes, time of exposure), and optical density of the image. The recommended radiation doses are shown in Table 5.1 [9,10].

5.3 QUALITY CONTROL

Mammography should be a high-quality exploration of breasts able to detect small cancers. It is very important to test the quality in order to prevent low-quality images that can misdiagnose a breast cancer.

The next items should be taken into account:

- Positioning: An adequate positioning of the breast is extremely important, because if it is not correct, a breast cancer can be omitted. The standard views of a mammographic study comprises both the mediolateral oblique (45° MLO) and the craniocaudal (CC)

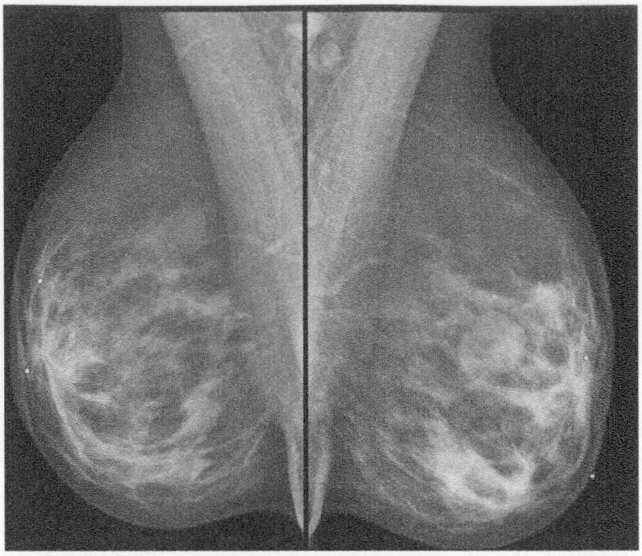

FIGURE 5.1 45° MLO views of both breasts. Note that the pectoralis muscle is seen below the level of the nipples.

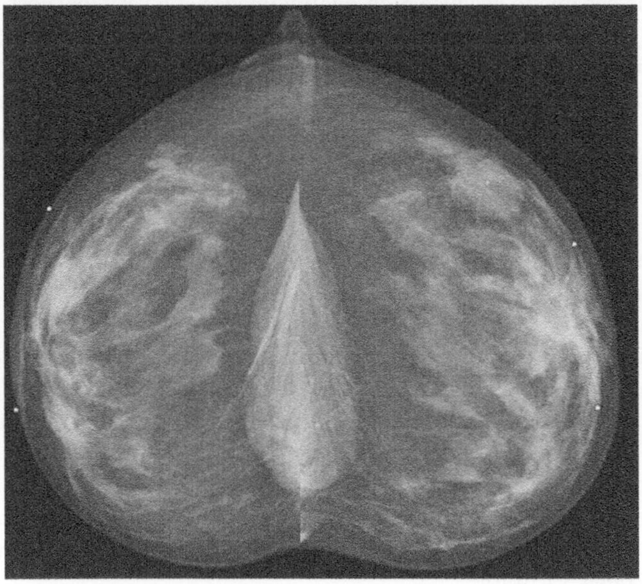

FIGURE 5.2 CC views of both breasts. Up to 30% of cases, the pectoralis muscle can be seen.

views (Figures 5.1 and 5.2). The MLO view shows the maximum quantity of fibroglandular tissue. The major pectoralis muscle is gently represented until the nipple level in this view, and the inframammary angle should be opened. In the CC view, the nipple should be seen tangential to the breast, and the retromammary fat should be detected. The major pectoralis can be seen in up to 30% of cases.

Moreover, there are additional views that can be used for specific situations. Lateromedial views, magnification views, and spot views are included among them.

- Compression: A deficiency of compression can generate false images and distortions, and calcifications cannot be properly detected.

- Exposition: Both a subexposition and superexposition can influence the quality of the image. These factors were very important using screen–film technology. Nowadays, most equipments are digital and image postprocessing can correct both.
- Spatial resolution: The image receptor has a specific spatial resolution. However, the movement of the breast during the exposure or a lack of compression can decrease the resolution.
- Contrast: For a good contrast between fat and fibroglandular tissue, a low voltage should be used.
- Noise: It usually increases in subexposed mammograms. The noise can hide or mimic microcalcifications and can make it difficult to evaluate the margins of a mass.
- Artefacts: Artefacts are false images, usually due to dust and dirty or electrostatic charges on conventional mammography and due to problematic pixels on digital mammography. The introduction of digital mammography has decreased dramatically the number of artefacts, and this is a great advantage of this technology.

5.4 INDICATIONS

The indications for performing mammography can vary, depending on the patient.

Several scenarios should be taken in mind: the asymptomatic woman, the symptomatic one, and mammography in men [11].

- Asymptomatic women: The role of mammography is the detection of an early breast cancer, so that mortality due to breast cancer should decrease in the screened population. There is a controversy among several Scientific Societies about the age to start the screening and the intervals between examinations. Most Scientific Societies in the United States recommend starting at 40 years old with periodic examinations every year. Population screening programmes in Europe are variable, but most of them start later (50 years old) and the periodic examinations every 2 years.
- Women with family antecedents of breast cancer (mother, sister, grandmother) or other risk factors should start earlier (35 years old).
- Symptomatic women: Mammography can be performed for women older than 30 years old if breast cancer cannot be ruled out due to symptoms (breast lump, nipple discharge, etc.) or if other examinations are inconclusive.
- Mammography should be performed for all women with a diagnosis of breast cancer, prior to surgery and during posterior follow-up.
- Mammography in male: Males can suffer from breast cancer, although this entity is very rare. The most common pathologies in males are lipomastia and gynaecomastia, both benign entities. Most of these are typically diagnosed by palpation, with no need for additional explorations.

Only 1 in 100 of breast cancers occurs in male patients. Most of these are symptomatic, breast lump or nipple discharge being the most common findings. When the clinical exploration is inconclusive, mammography is indicated.

5.5 MAMMOGRAPHIC READING

Several years ago, all mammograms were read on negatoscopes. These had to be specifically dedicated to mammography, with a very intense light (3500 cd/m^2) and appropriate collimation to avoid glare. Today, all new mammographs are digital, so images are viewed on dedicated high-resolution monitors (5 megapixel). The ambient conditions required include a pale light to avoid reflected light on the monitors. Also a quiet ambience is needed to concentrate in reading, avoiding noises (and telephones!) that can reduce attention.

Systematic reading of mammography comprises several steps [11]:

1. Clinical information about the patient. This information is really important, because some cancers can be clinically detected but not on mammography. Unfortunately, this information is not always available, especially in a screening setting. However, the radiographers can play an important role asking the patient about breast symptoms while they are performing the exploration and about family history of breast cancer.
2. Evaluation of the image quality: if it is not acceptable, mammography should be repeated (Figure 5.3).
3. Is the study normal or not? All the fields of the mammogram should be carefully evaluated, searching for masses, microcalcifications, architectural distortions, asymmetries, and other lesions. If there are no lesions, the examination can be considered normal. We should not forget that breast cancer can also present atypical mammographic findings that should be considered too, such as skin thickening or retraction and axillary lymph nodes. If clinical symptoms are presented, additional imaging techniques should be added.
4. Is the lesion real or is it a false image? Some lesions are very clearly seen on mammography, but others are not. And superposition of fibroglandular tissue can create a false image that can mimic a lesion. So additional views (tomosynthesis, spot compressions, magnification views, etc.) are needed to give additional information.
5. If the lesion is real, what is the concern? In other words, we need to classify the lesion according to different suspicion levels, so that an appropriate management of the patient can be performed. See the Breast Imaging Reporting and Data System (BI-RADS) categories later.

Modern workstations are equipped with computer-aided diagnosis (CAD) systems. These systems analyse the mammograms using mathematical algorithms and detect mass and calcifications. The sensitivity of these systems is quite high, and they can play a role as a second reader, but specificity is really bad.

Another advantage of digital mammography is telemedicine. The images can be sent to other readers worldwide.

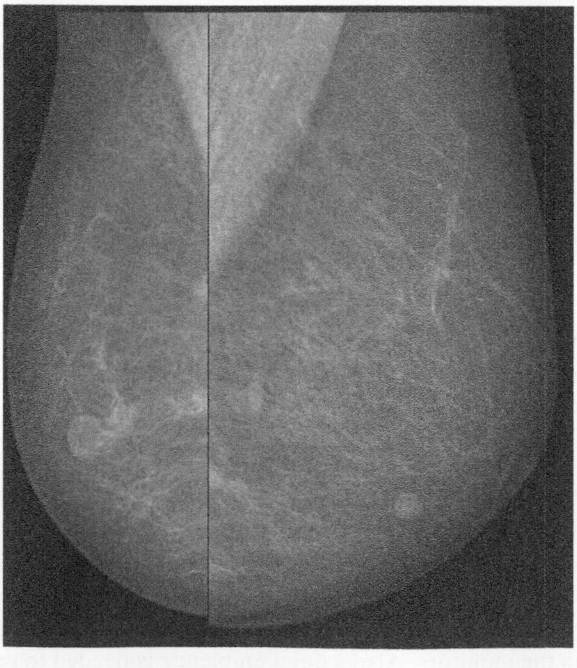

FIGURE 5.3 45° MLO views with incorrect positioning of both breasts.

5.6 BI-RADS SYSTEM

The BI-RADS was edited by the American College of Radiology as an atlas and a document with three aims [12]:

1. To standardise the mammographic reports
2. To reduce the interpretations of ambiguous reports
3. To improve the management of patients

The most important contributions of the BI-RADS have been the creation of a *lexicon* and the classification in different *categories*, regarding the suspicion.

5.6.1 BI-RADS Lexicon

1. Masses: Three descriptors should be used.
   1.1 Morphology: A mass can be rounded, oval, lobulated, or irregular (Figures 5.4 through 5.6).
   1.2 Margins: Circumscribed, microlobulated, occult, indistinct, and spiculated (Figure 5.7).
   1.3 Density: Regarding the fat tissue, it can be hyperdense, isodense, or hypodense (Figure 5.8).
2. Calcifications:
   2.1 Typically benign:
      2.1.1 Skin calcifications
      2.1.2 Vascular calcifications (Figure 5.9)
      2.1.3 Radiolucent calcifications (Figure 5.10)
      2.1.4 Rod-like calcifications (Figure 5.11)
      2.1.5 Popcorn calcifications (Figure 5.12)

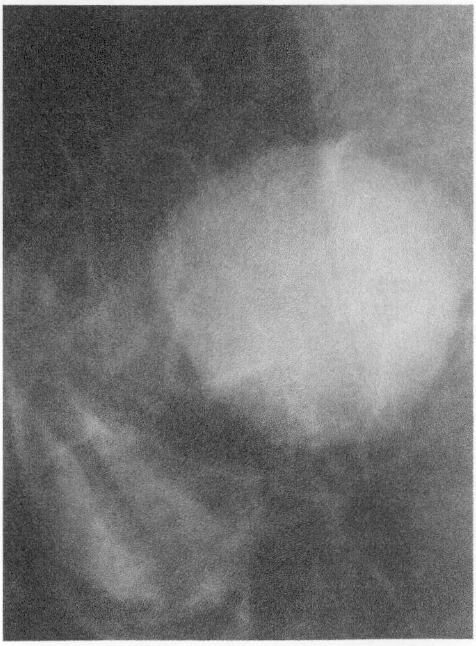

FIGURE 5.4 Well-defined round mass.

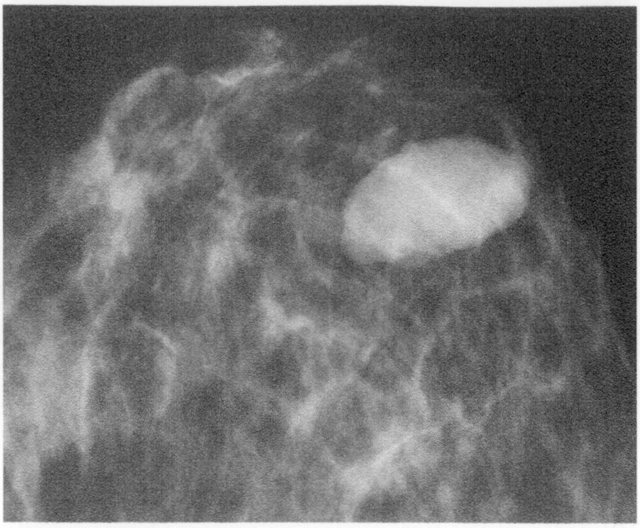

FIGURE 5.5 Well-defined oval mass.

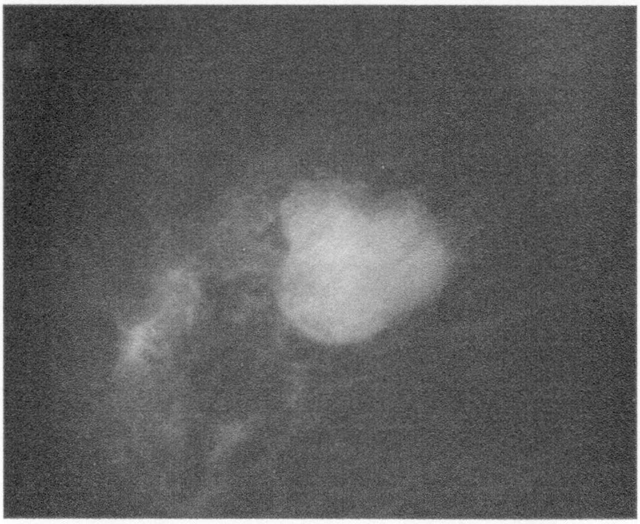

FIGURE 5.6 Well-delimited lobulated mass.

- 2.1.6 Rounded and punctate calcifications
- 2.1.7 Eggshell calcifications
- 2.1.8 Milk of calcium (Figure 5.13)
- 2.1.9 Calcifies sutures
- 2.1.10 Dystrophic calcifications

2.2 Intermediate concern:

- 2.2.1 Amorphous calcifications
- 2.2.2 Gross heterogeneous calcifications

2.3 Suspicious calcifications:

- 2.3.1 Fine pleomorphic calcifications (Figure 5.14)
- 2.3.2 Fine linear or branching calcifications (Figure 5.15)

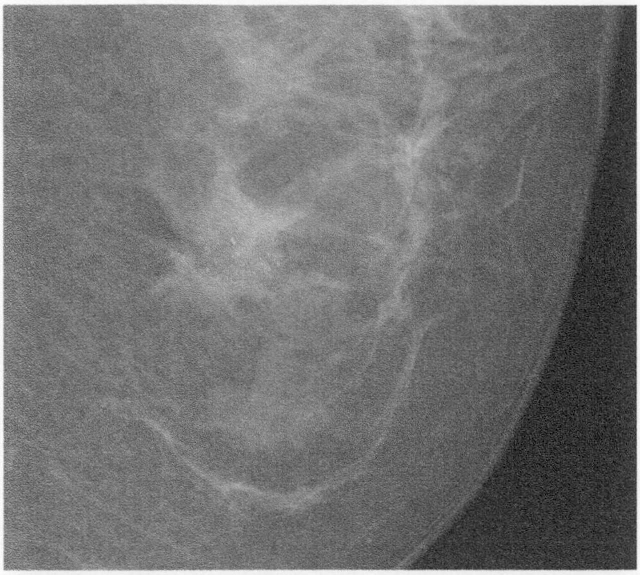

FIGURE 5.7 Irregular, spiculated mass with associated suspicious microcalcifications. Pathology: invasive ductal carcinoma.

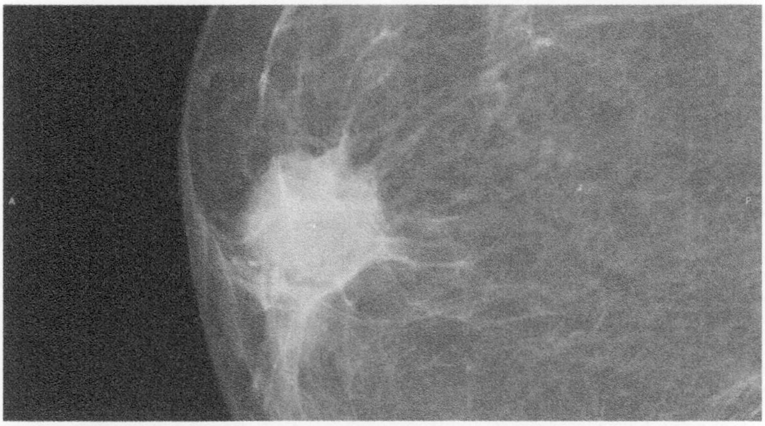

FIGURE 5.8 Irregular, spiculated mass. Note the high density of the lesion. Pathology: invasive ductal carcinoma.

- 2.4 Distribution pattern:
  - 2.4.1 Diffuse
  - 2.4.2 Regional
  - 2.4.3 Clustered
  - 2.4.4 Lineal
  - 2.4.5 Segmental

3. Architectural distortion: The normal architecture of the breast is altered (Figure 5.16).
4. Special cases:
   - 4.1 Asymmetric tubular structure
   - 4.2 Intramammary lymph node (Figure 5.17)
   - 4.3 Global asymmetry
   - 4.4 Focal asymmetry

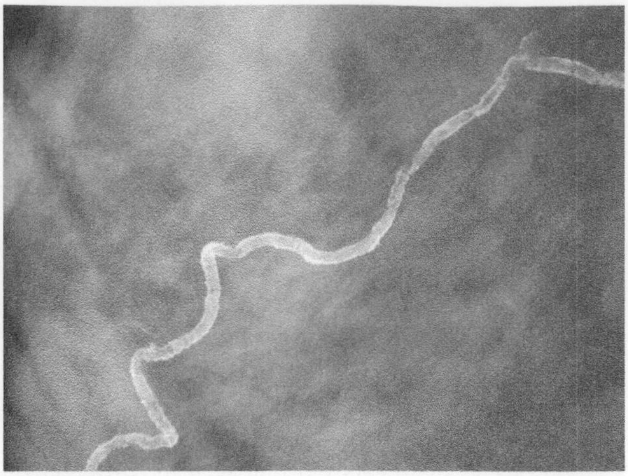

FIGURE 5.9 Vascular arterial calcifications.

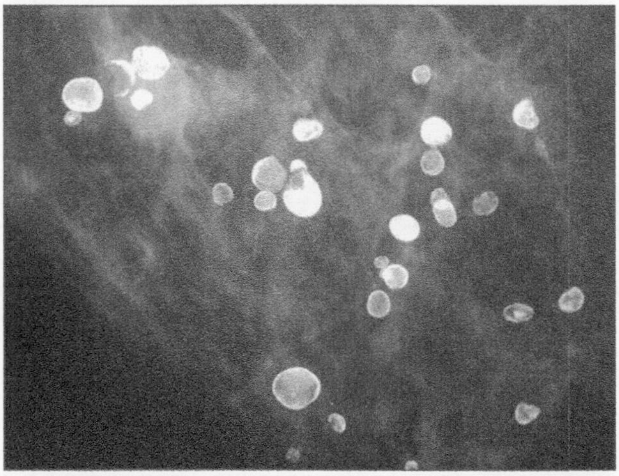

FIGURE 5.10 Radiolucent calcifications with typical benign radiological appearance related to fat necrosis.

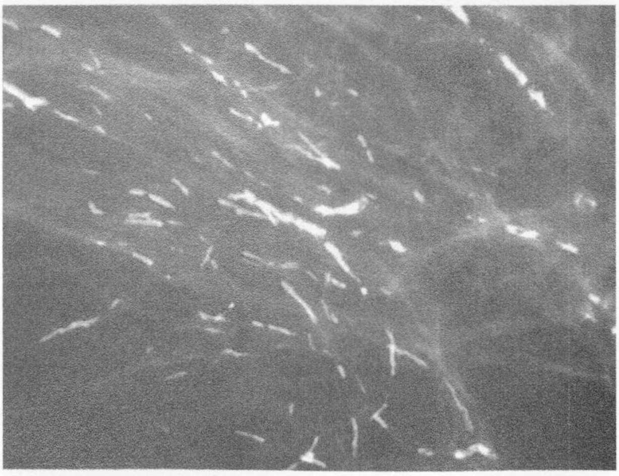

FIGURE 5.11 Rod-like calcifications represent ductal calcifications due to inflammatory benign conditions (secretory disease).

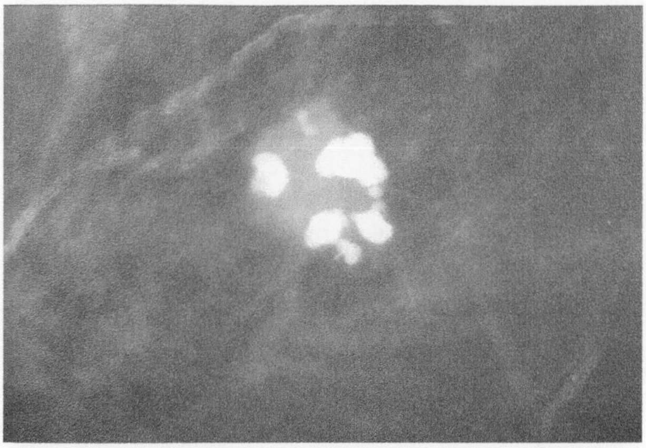

FIGURE 5.12 Well-delimited mass with gross, heterogeneous calcifications resembling a popcorn. Pathology: calcified fibroadenoma.

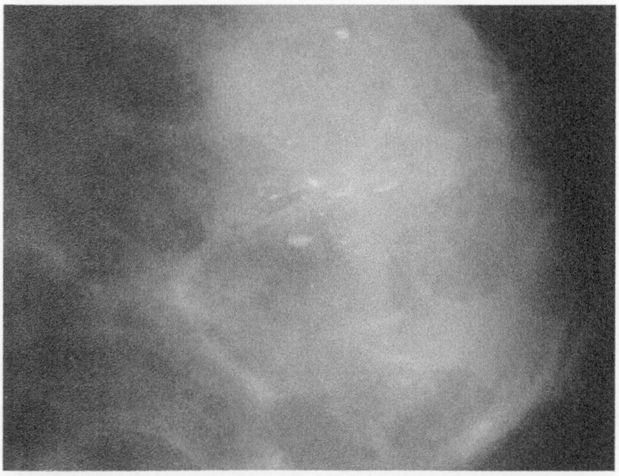

FIGURE 5.13 Milk of calcium of teacup calcifications. Note the horizontal distribution on 90° lateral view.

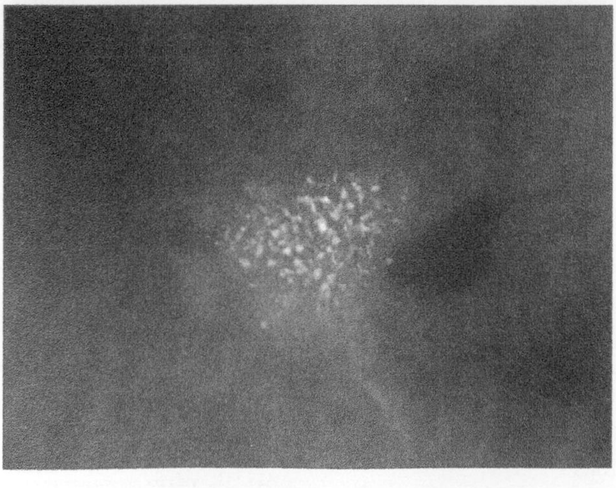

FIGURE 5.14 Fine, pleomorphic clustered calcifications highly suspicious of malignancy. Pathology: ductal carcinoma in situ.

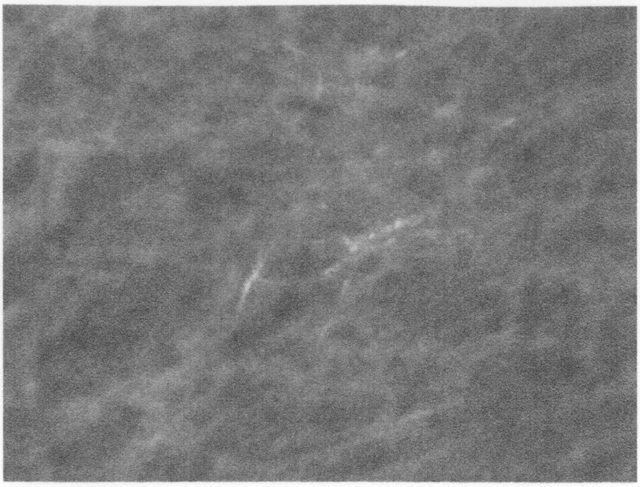

FIGURE 5.15 Fine, linear, and branching clustered calcifications highly suspicious of malignancy. Pathology: ductal carcinoma in situ.

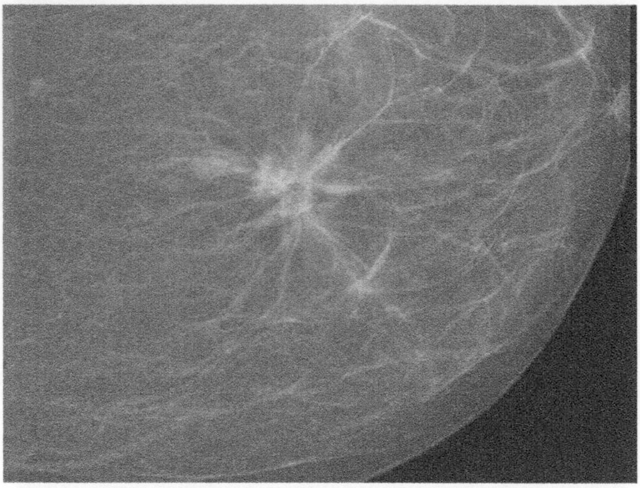

FIGURE 5.16 Architectural distortion with radiolucent core. Pathology: radial scar.

5. Associated findings:
   - 5.1 Skin retraction
   - 5.2 Nipple retraction
   - 5.3 Skin thickening
   - 5.4 Trabecular thickening (Figure 5.18)
   - 5.5 Skin lesion
   - 5.6 Axillary nodes
   - 5.7 Architectural distortion
   - 5.8 Calcifications

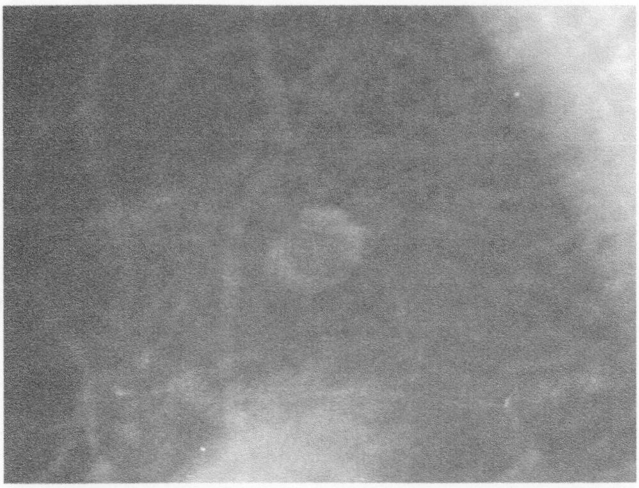

FIGURE 5.17 Intramammary lymph node. Note the presence of fatty hilar notch.

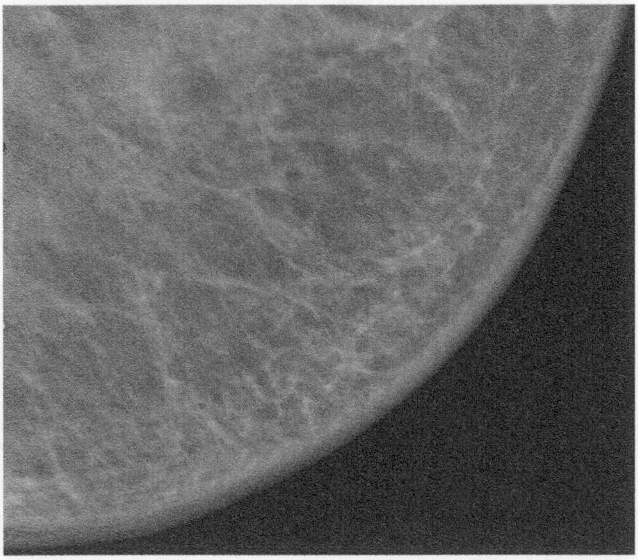

FIGURE 5.18 Skin and trabecular thickening can be seen in this inflammatory carcinoma.

5.6.2 BI-RADS Categories

The final categories are an important contribution too, because the classification itself implies the management for the radiologist and the clinician [12]. It is not a mere description of lesions or the likelihood of malignancy, but an active recommendation about the management of the case.

Seven categories are proposed:

- Category 0: Additional views or other techniques are needed. The examination itself cannot be classified in the remaining categories.
- Category 1: Negative. No lesions are detected. Routine follow-up is recommended.

- Category 2: Benign findings. The mammographic study is normal, but there are some benign lesions that are referred in the report. Typical benign lesions are calcified fibroadenomas, lipomas, etc.
- Category 3: Probably benign finding. Short-term follow-up is recommended. The positive predictive value is lower than 2%. Typical included lesions are solid well-delimited masses, non-palpable focal asymmetries, and clustered punctate calcifications. Although follow-up is the most accepted management, a percutaneous biopsy can be considered in some specific situations.
- Category 4: Suspicious finding. A biopsy should be recommended. The likelihood of malignancy is variable, showing a wide range (from 3% to 94%). In fact, three subcategories have been proposed: 4A (low probability of cancer), 4B (intermediate probability of cancer), and 4C (high probability of cancer).
- Category 5: Highly suspicious findings. The positive predictive value for this category is greater than 95%.
- Category 6: Malignancy is histologically proven. Typically, this category is used before the treatment or during the monitorisation of neoadjuvant chemotherapy.

Furthermore, the composition of the breast can be classified in a 4-level density scale (Figure 5.19):

- ACR (American College of Radiology) density pattern 1: Almost entirely fat. Fibroglandular tissue is less than 25%.
- ACR density pattern 2: Scattered areas of fibroglandular tissue (26%–50%).
- ACR density pattern 3: Heterogeneously dense breasts (51%–75%).
- ACR density pattern 4: Extremely dense. More than 75% is occupied by fibroglandular tissue.

This classification regarding the composition is very important, because it is well known that the sensitivity of mammography drops dramatically in dense patterns. In fact, sensitivity can be as

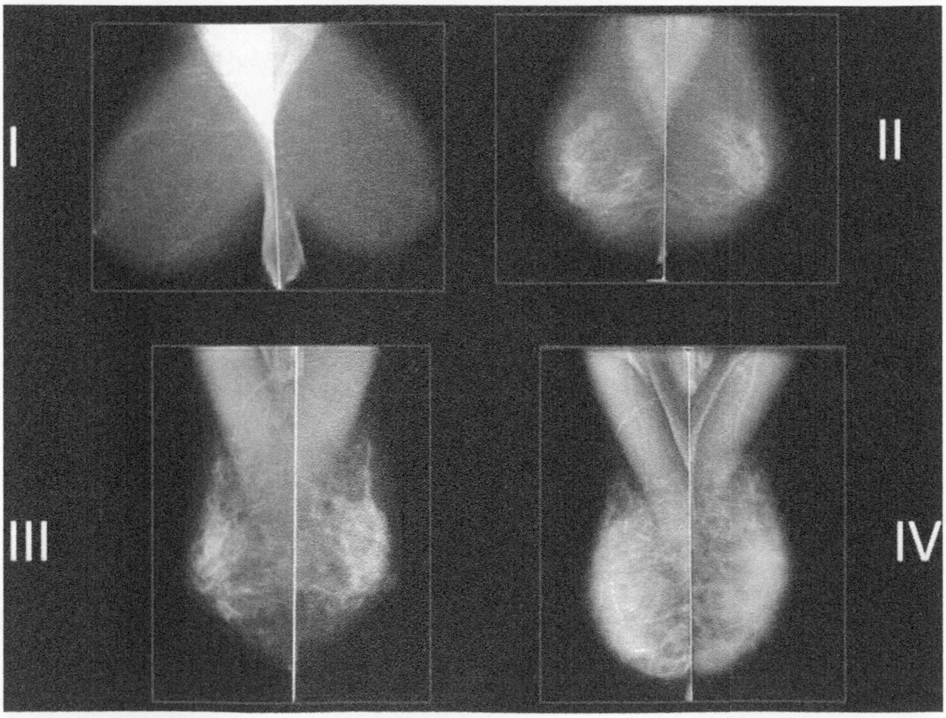

FIGURE 5.19 Representative of ACR density patterns I–IV.

low as 50% for dense patterns. Breast density can be genetically determined, but also it can be influenced by changes in body weight and by age. The younger the women are, the denser the breasts show on mammography. This is one of the reasons why mammography has started in many screening programmes for women older than 50 years old: these women, mostly postmenopausal, have fatty breasts.

5.6.3 Report Organisation

The following approach is recommended [12]:

1. Describe the indication for the study.
2. Describe the breast composition.
3. Describe any significant finding.
4. Compare to previous studies.
5. Conclude to a final assessment category.
6. Give management recommendations.

5.7 PLASTIC SURGERY AND MAMMOGRAPHY

5.7.1 Augmented Breast

Several types of breast implants have been used in the past decades for breast augmentation. Regarding the breast density of the implants on mammography, three major categories can be observed:

- Fat density implants: These implants are filled with soy oil and are radiolucent on mammography. They are no longer in use.
- Water density implants: These implants are filled with saline and its density is similar to that of water (Figure 5.20).
- High density or radio-opaque implants: These are the commonly used silicon implants, including single- and double-lumen implants.

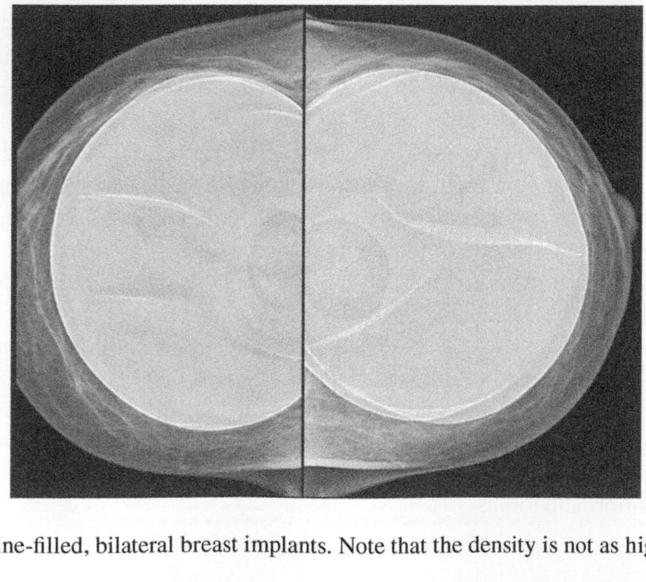

FIGURE 5.20 Saline-filled, bilateral breast implants. Note that the density is not as high as in silicon-filled breast implants.

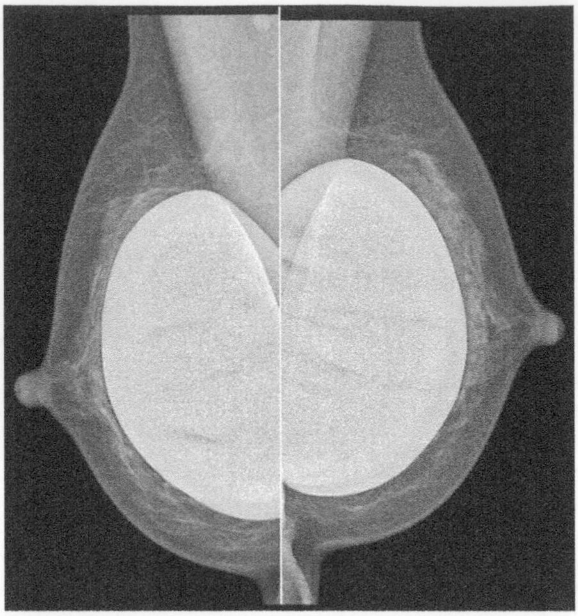

FIGURE 5.21 Bilateral, silicon breast implants in subglandular position.

Nowadays, all implants are composed of silicon, and they can make the detection of a breast cancer difficult, because the presence of a breast implant can hide a breast cancer.

The position of the implant may be variable, with some implications for diagnosing:

- Subglandular implants usually mask breast lesions, especially those that are located at the periphery (Figure 5.21).
- Implants located behind the pectoralis muscle: In these cases, most of the fibroglandular tissue is properly evaluated on mammography (Figure 5.22).

The mammographic technique has to be adapted to breast implants [13]. Modern mammographs and workstations have special postprocessing algorithms to correct the high difference between the density of the implant and that of the fibroglandular tissue. But positioning can be different too: most implants can be displaced posteriorly out of the field of view of mammography, so the fibroglandular tissue can be correctly compressed. This is known as Eklund's view.

Mammography is not a good technique to detect implant ruptures. Ultrasound or MRI is capable to evaluate more accurately the structure of the implant. Nevertheless, mammography can detect extracapsular ruptures, showing free silicon out of the implant, and can also suggest a rupture when a deformity or a change on the shape of the implant is seen.

Gross calcifications can be detected surrounding the implants when they are contractured (Figure 5.23). Moreover, folds can be detected when capsular retraction occurs.

Although mammography applies compression to the implant, it is unlikely that it can damage the implant. Radiographers are aware of implants and take care of them.

Other techniques for breast augmentation consist on the injection of biocompatible materials, such as autologous fat or hyaluronic acid. Lipofilling is now being used in the breast, and it induces the formation of multiple oil cysts. Hyaluronic acid forms dense well-delimited nodules, resembling cysts or fibroadenomas.

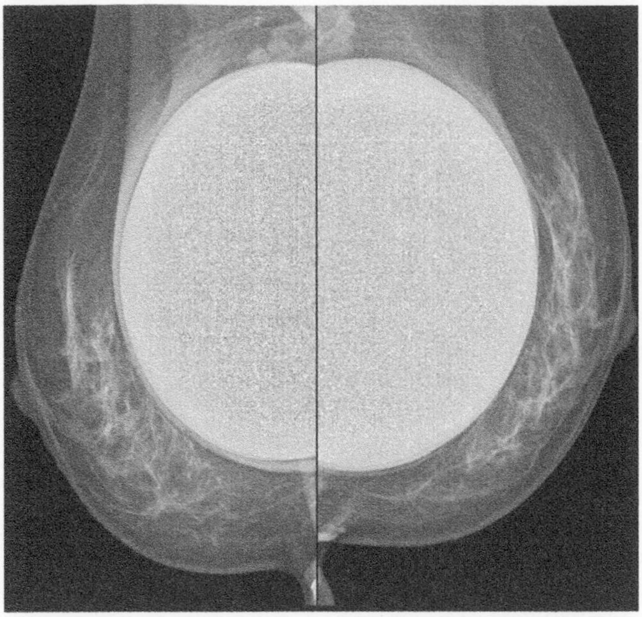

FIGURE 5.22 Bilateral, silicon breast implants in retropectoral position. Note that glandular tissue can be better evaluated when breast implants are located in this position.

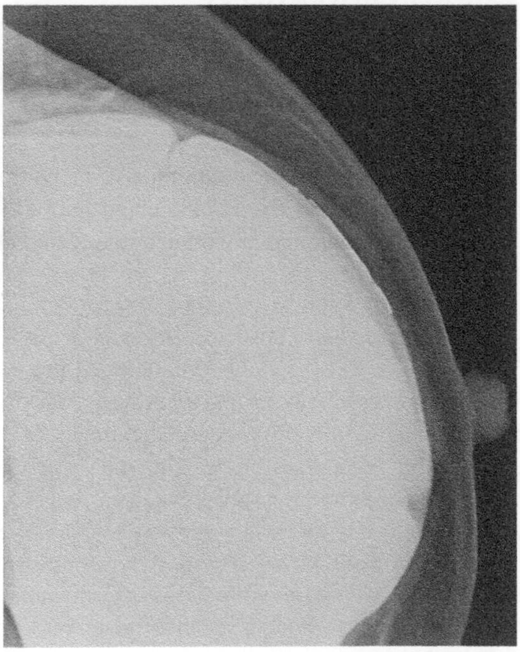

FIGURE 5.23 Contractured, silicon breast implant. Note the foldings and peripheral, gross calcifications.

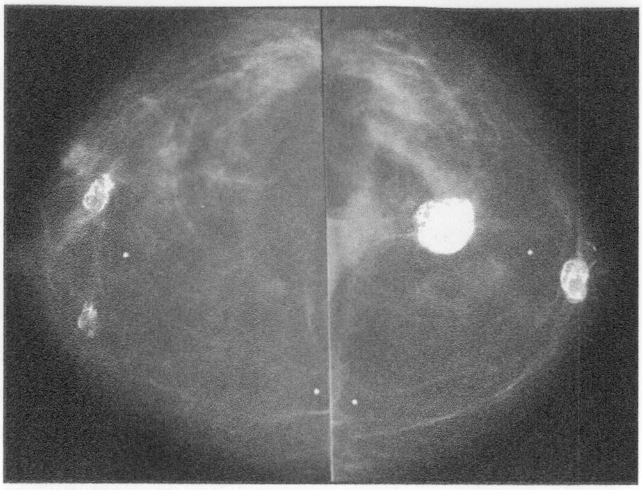

FIGURE 5.24 Bilateral breast reduction. 45° MLO mammograms show typical calcified lipid cysts and scars secondary to surgery.

5.7.2 Reduced Breast

All the surgical interventions of the breast can produce changes that are detected on mammography [13]. Breast reduction surgery typically induces the formation of fat necrosis, which usually produces oil cysts and gross calcifications. Large scars are also visible (Figure 5.24).

5.7.3 Reconstruction after Mastectomy

Several techniques can be used for reconstruction after mastectomy [13]:

- Breast implant: The implant is located behind the pectoralis muscle. The utility of mammography to detect a recurrence is low, because most of the volume of the breast is due to the implant.
- Autologous tissue: Both DIEP and TRAM techniques can be used (Figures 5.25 and 5.26). Mammography is useful because the reconstructed breast is entirely composed of fat. Typical complications are haematomas and fat necrosis. Mammographically, oil cysts and gross calcification are detected.

5.7.4 Screening Programmes Based on Mammography

The main objective of a breast cancer screening programme is the reduction of mortality due to breast cancer. The HIP trial started in New York in December 1963, and it included women from 40 to 64 years old. All the participants were randomised in two groups: The first one was explored by palpation and received a mammography every year, while the second group did not receive any explorations. The reduction of mortality was about 30% 10 years before the beginning of the trial, and other trials, like the Swedish two-county trial, found similar results [4,5]. Three decades later, this last trial continues showing similar results. Nowadays, poblational screening programmes are widely used in Europe. Recent articles have found a reduction of mortality ranging from 26% to 36% [6].

To achieve this ambitious objective, it is necessary to have high-quality criteria in all the steps of the screening. Table 5.2 shows some of the most important quality criteria that all screening programmes should fulfil [14].

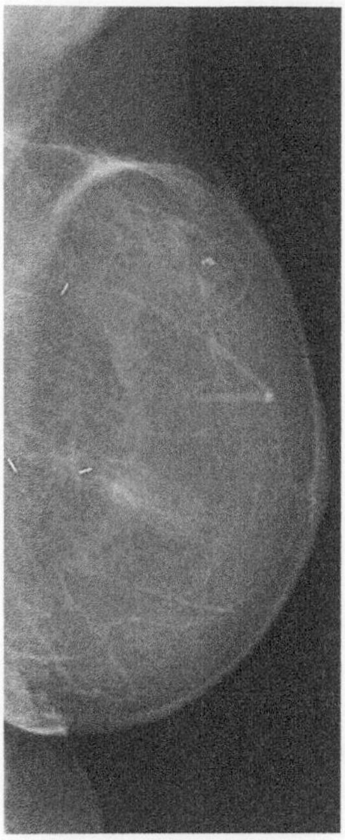

FIGURE 5.25 45° MLO view of the left breast after mastectomy and DIEP reconstruction. Note that the entire reconstruction is composed of fat tissue.

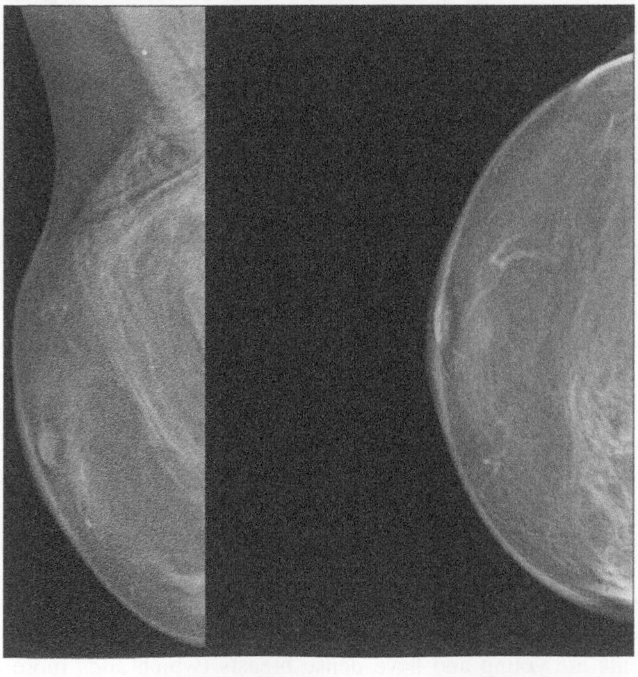

FIGURE 5.26 45° MLO and CC views of the right breast after mastectomy and TRAM reconstruction. Note that mixed composition of the flap showing fat and a piece of the rectus abdominis muscle.

TABLE 5.2
Summary of Mammographic Performance

Indicator	Minimum Standard	Desirable Standard
Participation rate	>70%	>75%
Technical repeat rate	<3%	<1%
Detection rate in women at initial examination/expected incidence rate	3	>3
Detection rate in women at subsequent examination/expected incidence rate	1.5	>1.5
Recall rate in initial screening	<7%	<5%
Recall rate in subsequent-regular screening	<5%	<3%
Benign-to-malignant biopsy ratio in women at initial examination	<1:1	<0.5:1
Benign-to-malignant biopsy ratio in women at subsequent-regular screening	<1:1	<0.2:1
Proportion of screen-detected breast cancer with a preoperative diagnosis of malignancy	>70%	>90%
Proportion of image-guided biopsies with an insufficient result	<20%	<10%
Proportion of invasive cancers detected at initial screening	>20%	>25%
Proportion of invasive cancers detected at subsequent screening	>25%	>30%
DCIS as a proportion of all screen-detected cancers	10%	>15%
N0 cancers/total of invasive cancers	75%	>75%
Rate of interval cancers/incidence rate 0–11 months	30%	<30%
Rate of interval cancers/incidence rate 12–23 months	50%	<50%

Despite the fact that screening programmes are widely spread throughout Europe and the United States, there are some discordant and controversial opinions. These are the topics of discordance [15–21]:

- Reduction of mortality: Some authors found a lower decrease in mortality than the most accepted data, with no more than 12% in reduction. The arguments for such a discrepancy were as follows [14]:
  - The randomisation in the clinical trials was not correctly performed.
  - The screening programmes have not decreased the rate of locally advanced tumours.
  - The actual adjuvant treatments are very effective and can influence in the mortality reduction.
- False-positive cases: The likelihood of a false-positive result for one patient participating in a screening programme during 10 consecutive rounds ranges from 8% to 21%. And the likelihood of a biopsy with a benign result is about 1.8%–6.3%. These false-positive results can produce anxiety to the patient, who can even give up the programme.
- Overdiagnosis and overtreatment: Not all diagnosed cancers are capable to cause the death of the patient, even in the absence of any treatments. So perhaps, there is not a real benefit diagnosing and treating some cancers. The problem is that we do not have specific tests to rule out these cancers. During many years, it was postulated that the increase of DCIS was a great benefit of screening. However, nowadays, some of these DCIS can be considered as overdiagnoses. Moreover, overdiagnosis implies overtreatment too, with aggressive treatments and side effects. It is estimated that up to 10% of all diagnosed breast cancers are in fact overdiagnoses.
- High-risk patients: Patients having mutations in BRCA 1/2 genes are at a high-risk situation of developing a breast cancer (more than 25% through their lives). It is well known that these patients are more sensitive to the carcinogenic effect of radiation. Moreover, most of these patients are young and have dense breasts (which adds more difficulty to the detection), and the appearance of malignant tumours on mammography does not show the typical features of malignancy.

- Dense breasts: The denser the breast is, the lower the sensitivity will be. In extremely dense breasts, the sensitivity can be as low as 50%, which is really unacceptable for screening. Women with breast implants can show this decrease of sensitivity too.
- The false security caused by screening: It is not infrequent to find patients and even physicians who think that a normal mammographic examination excludes the possibility of having a breast cancer. Some women will underestimate a breast lump as suspicious if a recently performed mammography is normal.

Keeping in mind all these arguments, it is obvious that some changes should be considered for improving the results of the screening programmes. These changes could be performed in two lines: a better classification of patients according to their risk of developing breast cancer and introducing complementary techniques to improve the sensitivity, such as DBT or ultrasound.

5.8 RECENT ADVANCES IN MAMMOGRAPHY

In the last two decades, the world of breast screening with mammography underwent a revolution with the development of new materials to design better detectors of radiation and the replacement of conventional film–screen mammography by digital mammography. These technical advances improved the contrast of mammography and decreased the radiation dose given with every exploration. With these new advantages, mammography was able to perform more detailed characterisation of breast lesions (especially for microcalcifications) [22]. However, these technical advances did not resolve one of the most important limitations of mammography, which is breast glandular tissue overlapping. As a bidimensional imaging technique, mammography has problems to detect and characterise breast malignancies without calcifications in patients with dense breasts. The sensitivity of digital mammography drops in the examination of dense breasts, ranging around 50% [7]. This is a significant problem to be considered, because it may significantly increase the number of non-detected malignant breast lesions and the generation of false suspicious breast lesions. This fact can produce a delay in breast cancer diagnosis and lead to an increased number of recalls or to the performance of unnecessary biopsies.

5.8.1 Digital Breast Tomosynthesis

Recently, an emerging new breast imaging technique has been developed to try to avoid these problems: DBT. This 3D imaging technique has the capability to obtain a series of consecutive thin and low-radiation slice images, which result in a reduction of the overlapping of tissues and a decrease of the anatomical noise.

5.8.2 Technical Aspects of Digital Breast Tomosynthesis

5.8.2.1 Generation of the Images

In DBT studies, the x-ray tube moves making a variable amplitude arch (depending on the manufacturer, it can range from 11° to 60°), while it sends multiple exposures of low radiation. As in digital mammograms, all the equipments include an automatic system to adjust the parameters of the tube to the composition of every breast. However, the number, energy, and distribution of the emitted x-ray pulses vary among different equipment of DBT. Some of them send pulses regularly every 1° or 2°, whereas others focus the emission of a higher number of x-ray exposures in the centre of the arch. This discrepancy in x-ray emission technique is responsible for the differences in DBT images observed in the different commercial equipment.

After the emission of the x-ray pulses, the radiation crosses the different tissues that constitute the breast. All the radiation collected by the receptors is codified and transformed into electronic signal, and with this information, the raw data of the DBT are generated.

As in the other 3D imaging techniques, the raw data of DBT are processed and reconstructed into 1 mm thick slices using different reconstruction algorithms. And these are the slices that finally compound the series of sequential images of DBT.

5.8.2.2 Radiation Dose of Digital Breast Tomosynthesis

DBT is formed by a variable number of low radiation x-ray exposures. As it has been explained before, different combinations of a number and energy of x-ray are currently used. Although this variety in acquisition protocols exists, all of them have agreed by consensus a maximum radiation dose per exploration, which never has to exceed 3 mGy for a breast thickness of 5 cm [23]. Therefore, the average dose emitted with each DBT is similar to that given when a conventional digital mammography is performed (2.5 mGy) for the most common breast thickness (about 5 cm) [24–26].

This similitude in the radiation dose between both imaging techniques is not always true. There are many factors that we must consider when we want to estimate the real dose that each patient is going to receive in the acquisition of a projection of DBT. The most important are breast thickness and breast glandular density. When either increases, the radiation required to obtain a standard DBT significantly rises up, reaching almost twice the radiation used in conventional digital mammography. Nevertheless, the radiation dose used in these cases is always within the limits allowed by the FDA to perform breast imaging studies [27].

5.8.3 Utility of Digital Breast Tomosynthesis

When DBT was developed, a great effort was put to learn about what could be the role of this innovating imaging technique in the detection of breast cancer. At the beginning, many studies were performed to identify its advantages and strengths. As we know, DBT is based on x-ray technology, and it has many similarities to digital mammography. Many studies have made comparison between the diagnostic accuracy of DBT and digital mammography in different modalities and combinations on both techniques. The following are the main conclusions of the most important studies:

- Increased rate of detection of breast cancer with the combination of DBT and digital mammography

  There is more and more evidence in the literature about the improvement in breast cancer detection rate with the combined use of both techniques compared to the isolated use of mammography [28–30].

  These results were first found in small cohorts of patients and in clinical setting. But latest studies have confirmed the idea that DBT and digital mammography could be excellent complementary imaging techniques for the detection of breast cancer in both clinical and screening scenarios.
- Decreased number of unnecessary recalls

  DBT has been proven as a useful complementary imaging technique to digital mammography to solve cases in which conventional projections have found dubious or suspicious breast lesions. With the addition of DBT, an important decrease in the recall rate (up to 70%) compared with the isolate use of conventional projections of digital mammography has been found. Other studies have investigated about the differences in the recall rate using a combination of DBT and digital mammography versus conventional digital mammography projections (MLO and CC) plus additional views. Almost all studies have found a significant decrease in the recall rate [31] using both techniques. It is an important data to consider for a possible future establishment of DBT as a complementary imaging technique to digital mammography on screening programmes, because the number of unnecessary recalled patients has a great impact on the screening programmes workflow. Moreover, it should also decrease the anxiety and inconveniences that these false-positive and inconclusive explorations generate in recalled women, which is also very important.

Nevertheless, a recent article has been published about the impact of the addition of DBT in a screening programme in progress [32]. It has thrown different results, with higher recall rate when both DBT and digital mammography were used for screening. Further investigation and more experience are needed to assess if there is a real reduction in recall rate when DBT is added in large screening programmes.

- Features of additional breast lesions detected by DBT
  DBT is able to perform a better evaluation of the margins of breast nodules than digital mammography. It allows to identify poorly defined or spiculated suspicious margins that conventional mammography may ignore. DBT is also very sensitive in the detection of architectural distortions (sclerosing lesions, radial scars), because it can differentiate the spikes that are characteristics of these lesions [33,34]. These features explain why DBT is more useful in the detection of invasive cancers, because most common radiological presentations are nodules and architectural distortions.

  There is plenty of evidence in the literature about the superiority of the combination of DBT and digital mammography in the detection and characterisation of soft tissue breast lesions. However, there is no such agreement about the utility of the combination of both imaging techniques in the detection of microcalcifications [35,36]. Additional DBT can be of great use to improve the characterisation and localisation of microcalcifications which with conventional mammographic studies result inconclusive (teacup microcalcification, skin microcalcifications, or uncertain microcalcifications in which DBT may discover an associated malignant nodule missed on digital mammography).

5.8.4 Establishment of Digital Breast Tomosynthesis in Our Daily Work

After the verification of DBT as an excellent technique for the detection of breast cancer, a great effort should be done to establish what could be the most appropriate role of this imaging technique.

We do not only have to evaluate which patients may benefit from the use of DBT. We also have to take into account other important factors as the additional radiation dose or the reading time increase that involves the performance of an additional x-ray-based imaging technique.

Two different settings can be considered.

5.8.4.1 Clinical Setting

In breast imaging areas, the improvement of breast detection rate is one of the most important factors to be considered. The number of patients that a doctor deals with per day in this setting is smaller, so is not a big problem to handle an additional imaging exploration which is not long time-consuming (reading a DBT in combination and digital mammography consumes double time than reading digital mammography alone). The percentage of symptomatic women and prevalence of cancer are higher in this setting. The combination of both techniques has several advantages, because they significantly improve breast cancer detection rate and they could avoid the performance of unnecessary biopsies.

The recall rate in clinical setting is not so crucial than in screening programmes. To recall patients is less problematic in these settings, because, as they cover a smaller population, it has less impact on their workflow. However, the anxiety and worry that produces recalls in women must be also considered.

5.8.4.2 Screening Setting

This setting has many different aspects to be considered. First of all, the screening programmes include a huge number of women which are mostly asymptomatic. The improvement of the sensitivity and specificity in breast cancer detection is also very important, but the recall rate and reading time have a greater impact in this setting. The introduction of an additional imaging technique can significantly affect the workflow. So these two facts must carefully be studied before the establishment of DBT in screening programmes.

Other two important problems to analyse are the economic issue and the additional radiation dose that means the addition of DBT in this setting. Whereas the first one is a problem for the administration, many efforts are being done to reduce the second one (e.g., the development of synthetic images or post-procedure software to erase scattered radiation).

5.9 CONCLUSION

DBT represents a promising imaging technique which has demonstrated a high accuracy in the detection of breast cancer. It has been proved as an excellent complementary imaging technique to digital mammography, although more research must be done to find out which patients and settings could have more benefits from its use.

REFERENCES

1. Smith RA, Duffy SW, Tabár L. Breast cancer screening: The evolving evidence. *Oncology (Williston Park)* 2012;26:471–475, 479–481, 485–486.
2. Sánchez MJ, Payer T, De Angelis R, Larrañaga N, Capocaccia R, Martinez C, CIBERESP Working Group. Cancer incidence and mortality in Spain: Estimates and projections for the period 1981–2012. *Ann Oncol* 2010;21:30–36.
3. Álvaro-Meca A, Debón A, Gil Prieto R, Gil de Miguel Á. Breast cancer mortality in Spain: Has it really declined for all age groups? *Public Health* 2012;126:891–895.
4. Strax P. Results of mass screening for breast cancer in 50,000 examinations. *Cancer* 1976;37:30–35.
5. Tabár L, Fagerberg CJ, Gad A, Baldetorp L, Holmberg LH, Gröntoft O et al. Reduction in mortality from breast cancer after mass screening with mammography: Randomised trial from the Breast Cancer Screening Working Group of the Swedish National Board of Health and Welfare. *Lancet* 1985;1:829–832.
6. Moss SM, Nyström L, Jonsson H, Paci E, Lynge E, Njor S et al. The impact of mammographic screening on breast cancer mortality in Europe: A review of trend studies. *J Med Screen* 2012;19:26–32.
7. Pisano ED, Gatsonis C, Hendrick E, Yaffe M, Baum JK, Acharyya S et al. Digital Mammographic Imaging Screening Trial (DMIST) Investigators Group. Diagnostic performance of digital versus film mammography for breast-cancer screening. *N Engl J Med* 2005;353:1773–1783.
8. Van Woudenberg S, Thijssen M, Young K. European protocol for the quality control of the physical and technical aspects of mammography screening. In: Perry N, Broeders M, de Wolf C, Törnberg S, Holland R, von Karsa L (eds.), *European Guidelines for Quality Assurance in Breast Cancer Screening and Diagnosis*, 4th edn. Luxembourg: Office for Official Publications of the European Communities; 2006, pp. 69–128.
9. Regs E, Foster PK. Quality control and radiation protection of the patient in diagnostic radiology and nuclear medicine. *Rad. Prot. Dosimetry* 1995;57(1–4); CEC-Report EUR 15257.
10. Young KC, Ramsdale ML, Rust A. Mammography dose and image quality in the UK breast screening programme. NHSBSP Report 35, 1998.
11. Heywang-Köbrunner SH, Dershaw DD, Schreer I. Mammography. In: Heywang-Köbrunner SH, Dershaw DD, Schreer II (eds.), *Diagnostic Breast Imaging*, 2nd edn. Stuttgart, Germany: Thieme, pp. 14–86.
12. American College of Radiology. *Breast Imaging Reporting and Data System® (BI-RADS®) 4*. Reston, VA: American College of Radiology; 2003.
13. Heywang-Köbrunner SH, Dershaw DD, Schreer I. Post-traumatic, post-surgical and post-therapeutic changes. In: Heywang-Köbrunner SH, Dershaw DD, Schreer II (eds.), *Diagnostic Breast Imaging*, 2nd edn. Stuttgart, Germany: Thieme, pp. 339–374.
14. Rosselli del Turco M, Hendriks J, Perry N, Azavedo E, Skaane P. Radiological guidelines. In: Perry N, Broeders M, de Wolf C, Törnberg S, Holland R, von Karsa L (eds.), *European Guidelines for Quality Assurance in Breast Cancer Screening and Diagnosis*, 4th edn. Luxembourg: Office for Official Publications of the European Communities; 2006, pp. 181–195.
15. Gøtzsche PC, Olsen O. Is screening for breast cancer with mammography justifiable? *Lancet* 2000;355:129–134.

16. Jørgensen KJ, Keen JD, Gøtzsche PC. Is mammographic screening justifiable considering its substantial overdiagnosis rate and minor effect on mortality? *Radiology* 2011;260:621–627.
17. Gøtzsche PC. Time to stop screening? *CMAG* 2011;183:1957–1958.
18. Gøtzsche PC, Jorgensen KJ, Zahl PH, Maehlen J. Why mammography screening has not lived up to expectations from the randomized trials? *Cancer Causes Control* 2012;23:15–21.
19. Hofvin S, Ponti A, Patnick J, Ascunce N, Njor S, Broeders M et al. False-positive results in mammographic screening for breast cancer in Europe: A literature review and survey of service screening programs. *J Med Screen* 2012;19:57–66.
20. Puliti D, Duffy SW, Miccinesi G, de Koenig H, Lynge E, Zappa M et al. Overdiagnosis in mammographic screening for breast cancer in Europe: A literature review. *J Med Screen* 2012;19:42–56.
21. Berg WA, Blume JD, Cormack JB, Mendelson EB, Lehrer D, Böhm-Vélez M et al. Combined screening with ultrasound and mammography vs mammography alone in women at elevated risk of breast cancer. *JAMA* 2008;299:2151–2163.
22. Mellado M, Osa AM, Murillo A, Bermejo R, Burguete A, Pons MJ et al. Impact of digital mammography in the detection and management of microcalcifications. *Radiologia* 2013;55:142–147.
23. Helvie MA. Digital mammography imaging: Breast tomosynthesis and advanced applications. *Radiol Clin North Am* 2010;48:917–929.
24. Tagliafico A, Astengo D, Cavagnetto F, Rosasco R, Rescinito G, Monetti F, Calabrese M. One-to-one comparison between digital spot compression view and digital breast tomosynthesis. *Eur Radiol* 2012;22:539–544.
25. Kilburn-Toppin F, Barter SJ. New horizons in breast imaging. *Clin Oncol (R Coll Radiol)* 2013;25(2):93–100.
26. Feng SS, Sechopoulos I. Clinical digital breast tomosynthesis system: Dosimetric characterization. *Radiology* 2012;263:35–42.
27. Mammography Quality Standards Act of 1992. Public Law 102-539. As amended by the Mammography Quality Standards Reauthorization Act of 1998. Pub. L. No. 105-248. Title 42 Subcharter II Part F Subpart 3, § 354 (42 USC 263b), certification of mammography facilities.
28. Michell MJ, Iqbal A, Wasan RK, Evans DR, Peacock C, Lawinski CP et al. A comparison of the accuracy of film-screen mammography, full-field digital mammography, and digital breast tomosynthesis. *Clin Radiol* 2012;67:976–981.
29. Gur D, Bandos AI, Rockette HE, Zuley ML, Sumkin JH, Chough DM et al. Localized detection and classification of abnormalities on FFDM and tomosynthesis examinations rated under an FROC paradigm. *AJR Am J Roentgenol* 2011;196:737–741.
30. Waldherr C, Cerny P, Altermatt HJ, Berclaz G, Ciriolo M, Buser K et al. Value of one-view breast tomosynthesis versus two-view mammography in diagnostic workup of women with clinical signs and symptoms and in women recalled from screening. *AJR Am J Roentgenol* 2013;200:226–231.
31. Skaane P, Bandos AI, Gullien R, Eben EB, Ekseth U, Haakenaasen U et al. Comparison of digital mammography alone and digital mammography plus tomosynthesis in a population-based screening program. *Radiology* 2013;267(1):47–56.
32. Skaane P, Bandos AI, Gullien R, Eben EB, Ekseth U, Haakenaasen U et al. Prospective trial comparing full-field digital mammography (FFDM) versus combined FFDM and tomosynthesis in population-based screening programme using independent double reading with arbitration. *Eur Radiol* 2013;23(8):2061–2071.
33. Skaane P, Gullien R, Bjørndal H, Eben EB, Ekseth U, Haakenaasen U et al. Digital breast tomosynthesis (DBT): Initial experience in a clinical setting. *Acta Radiol* 2012;53:524–529.
34. Zuley ML, Bandos AI, Ganott MA, Sumkin JH, Kelly AE, Catullo VJ et al. Digital breast tomosynthesis versus supplemental diagnostic mammographic views for evaluation of noncalcified breast lesions. *Radiology* 2013;266:89–95.
35. Kopans D, Gavenonis S, Halpern E, Moore R. Calcifications in the breast and digital breast tomosynthesis. *Breast J* 2011;17:638–644.
36. Timberg P, Baath M, Andersson I, Mattsson S, Tingberg A, Ruschin M. Visibility of microcalcification clusters and masses in breast tomosynthesis image volumes and digital mammography: A 4AFC human observer study. *Med Phys* 2012;39:2431–2437.

6 PET-CT in Oncology

Anna Margherita Maffione, Sotirios Chondrogiannis, Adriano Marcolongo, and Domenico Rubello

CONTENTS

6.1 INTRODUCTION

Industrial and scientific developments in the latter decades have made achievable to visualise metabolic processes within the human body. These imaging modalities, such as positron emission tomography (PET), allow in vivo evaluation of radiolabelled compounds, by recognition of emitted radiation from the patient. Pharmaceuticals, indeed, interact with the tissue through a metabolic process and the isotopes allow to track, map, and measure it.

Diagnostic morphological techniques, despite their precision and accuracy, are often notably limited in revealing and interpreting lesions for an accurate staging.

The accessibility of a variety of radiotracers labelled with positron emitters currently enables the assessment (and also the quantification) of not only the glycolytic metabolism but also the amount of protein expression, the presence and degree of receptor density, the neurotransmitter activity, angiogenesis, blood flow, and tissue hypoxia. This enables to visualise early molecular modifications that often occur during the time before comprehensible structural changes. The ability to exhibit molecular alterations opens up interesting possibilities for characterising lesions, determining their real extension, making an early evaluation of the response to therapy, and identifying the sites of possible relapse.

6.2 TECHNICAL ASPECTS

PET imaging is based on coincidence detection of two simultaneously emitted gamma photons, which occurs when a positron annihilates after combination with an electron. Positron emitting isotopes, produced in a cyclotron or, in the few cases like gallium-68 or rubidium-82, by a generator, can be chemically linked to a probe molecule and then i.v. injected into the patient. Once within the body, the two positrons combine with as many electrons, with all the mass being converted into photons. In order to conserve energy and linear momentum, the electromagnetic radiation appears in the form of two gamma rays of equal energy (511 keV), which are emitted at opposite directions. The emitted photons are detected by a technique known as coincidence detection, whereby a coincident signal is transmitted when two opposite detectors are stimulated simultaneously. Semi-quantitative methods such as standardised uptake values (SUV) can measure the amount of radiotracer uptake into a specific region of interest (ROI) at a certain time point after injection.

The physics of positron emission imposes definite boundaries on the temporal, spatial, and contrast resolution that can be obtained in a PET scan. Nowadays, the spatial resolution of a PET exam in a typical clinical circumstance is about 6 mm [1].

At the present time, fluorine-18 radiolabelled fluorodeoxyglucose (FDG) is the most employed compound in the clinical practice because cancer cells are known to have increased anaerobial glycolytic activity and higher expression of glucose transporters. FDG PET allows to study in vivo tissue metabolism and thus to demonstrate malignant tumours as hypermetabolic lesions, showing an increase of tracer uptake.

FDG is initially carried into the cell by glucose transporters, exactly as the normal glucose, and then is rapidly phosphorylated and trapped in the cells. Physiological sites of FDG accumulation

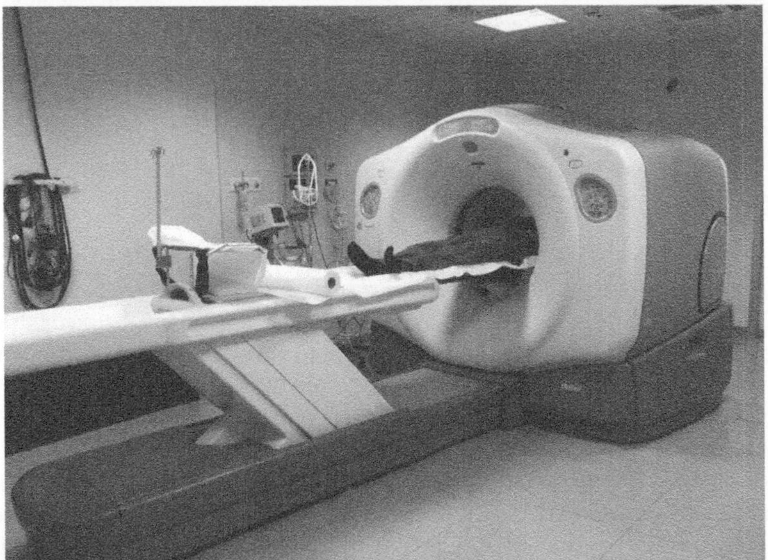

FIGURE 6.1 PET-CT scanner 16 slices, GE discovery STE.

are the grey matter of the brain, myocardium (according as the insulinemic level), and, but fewer, spinal marrow, liver, and spleen. Also all the FDG elimination ways are noticeable: kidneys, ureters, bladder, and variably the gastrointestinal system.

Since pure PET images lack anatomical data (a serious disadvantage in regions of particular anatomical complexity as head and neck), the introduction on clinical practice of hybrid scanner systems (PET and computed tomography [CT] hardware fusion – PET-CT [Figure 6.1]) has permitted both morphological and metabolic imaging to be performed in a single session, reducing false-positive findings and inconclusive studies, thus increasing diagnostic accuracy [2]. PET-CT scanner is a typical example of an evolution in imaging technology whereby the fusion of two established modalities becomes greater than the sum of the individual parts.

Rather than oncology, the other fields where PET is employed are cardiology, neurology, vasculitis, sarcoidosis, pyrexia of unknown origin and infection disease, even if in a less amount.

6.3 PET-CT ONCOLOGIC APPLICATIONS

Many international papers have demonstrated PET appropriate indications for each neoplastic disease, in terms of improving diagnostic performance (compared with other current techniques) and influence of patient's outcome either through adoption of more effective therapeutic strategies or through non-adoption of ineffective or harmful practices.

Currently, PET-CT imaging is employed in almost all oncologic diseases thanks to the development of many radiopharmaceuticals able to trace different metabolic pathways.

The analysis of main indications for PET-CT scanning is examined in the following.

6.3.1 Diagnosis

6.3.1.1 Characterisation of Mass Lesion

Actually the main use of PET in the field of diagnosis is focused on the characterisation of the solitary pulmonary nodule (SPN). Most lung nodules are discovered incidentally on chest radiographs, and a variable percentage of them are malignant (15%–75%, depending on the population studied).

CT represents the first step for localising and characterising the lesion (e.g., CT features as calcification or speculation are indicative for benign cause or malignancy, respectively) but it could represent a diagnostic challenge, especially if biopsy may be dangerous.

Otherwise, FDG PET identifies malignant lesions on the basis of their glucidic metabolism.

FDG PET is a non-invasive method to differentiate malignant from benign SPN, with a high specificity [3] (82% in lesions 1 cm in diameter or larger) and therefore high negative predictive value. SPN with high FDG uptake should be considered malignant (Figure 6.2), whereas lesions with low uptake are likely to be benign or slowly growing malignancies such as broncho-alveolar carcinoma (BAC) and may be considered for surveillance using CT scanning. The use of PET for diagnostic characterisation of SPN is cost effective.

Another application is the characterisation of pancreatic lesion in case of indeterminate CT report: the major limitation of morphological imaging techniques is their incapability to confidently characterise small as well as cystic lesions. PET/CT may be helpful, with high sensitivity (85%–100%) and moderate specificity (67%–90%) [4] in evaluating lesions without the need for biopsy or surgery, which may increase morbidity [5].

Concerning cholangio- and gallbladder carcinomas, the use of PET may be appropriate in discriminating benign from malignant strictures of the biliary tract [6].

Furthermore, regarding the primary tumours of central nervous system (CNS), there is a good correlation between FDG uptake and tumour grade, although the high background in normal grey matter could limit the ability to detect lesions. It has to be underlined that FDG PET is not helpful neither for exact tumour delineation nor for monitoring response to radiosurgery [7], a role accomplished by aminoacidic radiopharmaceuticals (see non-FDG chapter).

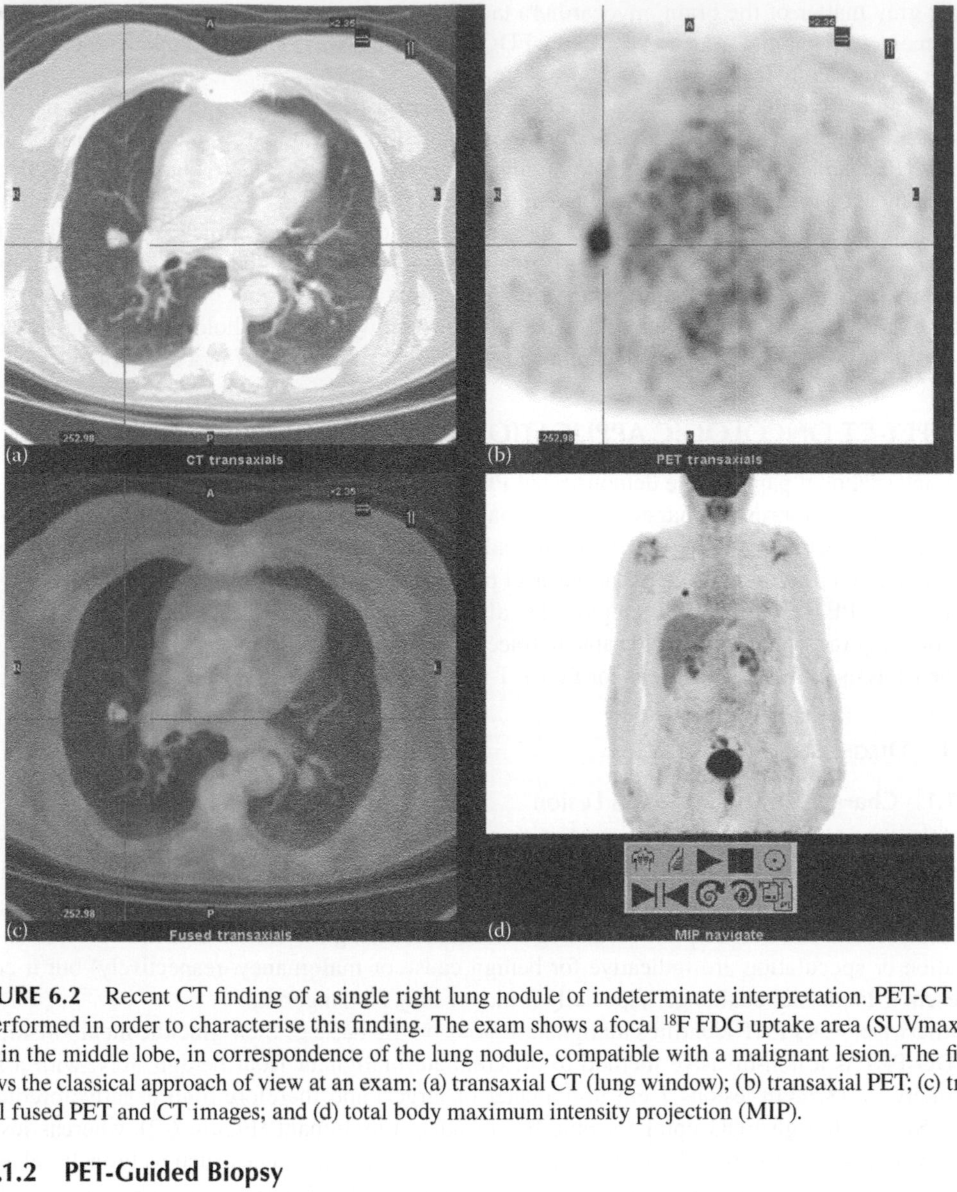

FIGURE 6.2 Recent CT finding of a single right lung nodule of indeterminate interpretation. PET-CT scan is performed in order to characterise this finding. The exam shows a focal ^{18}F FDG uptake area (SUVmax 8.7) within the middle lobe, in correspondence of the lung nodule, compatible with a malignant lesion. The figure shows the classical approach of view at an exam: (a) transaxial CT (lung window); (b) transaxial PET; (c) transaxial fused PET and CT images; and (d) total body maximum intensity projection (MIP).

6.3.1.2 PET-Guided Biopsy

PET scan may support in guiding biopsy to the region of a tumour with the highest metabolic activity, identified by the area(s) of highest radiopharmaceutical uptake.

The use of PET to identify the optimal biopsy site has a strong rationale, as in sarcoma tumours or in primary tumours of CNS [8], when treatment may change according to the tumour grade.

Another possibility of PET application is the selected group of patients with high suspicion of prostate cancer but negative ultrasound (US)-guided biopsy.

6.3.1.3 Detection of Occult Primary Cancer

Unknown primary cancer (UPC) is defined as a biopsy-proven secondary lesion with no detectable primary tumour after physical examination and conventional imaging tests. Whole-body FDG PET-CT has been successfully used for identifying UPC of the most common histologies, that is, adenocarcinomas, squamous cell carcinoma, and poorly differentiated carcinoma with a sensitivity of 36%, not so low if compared with the CT ones (15%) [9].

It is well known that ^{18}F-FDG is of limited value in tumours that usually do not show enhanced glycolytic metabolism, and for this reason, alternative PET tracers have been proposed in the detection of primary tumours (see non-FDG chapter).

6.3.1.4 Incidentaloma

A special role of PET is concerning incidentalomas: an incidentaloma is a lesion found by coincidence without clinical symptoms or suspicion.

One of the most common incidental FDG uptake findings is a lesion within the thyroid, with a prevalence of 3.8% and a further malignancy detection of 64% in lesions with focal uptake [10].

Another recurrent incidental finding in PET, as well in CT scan, is an adrenal mass. PET/CT is a highly accurate method for differentiating benign from malignant adrenal masses, particularly when using qualitative, rather than quantitative, PET data [11].

Colorectal FDG uptake findings are, in addiction, quite common: there are numerous cases where unsuspected and asymptomatic colorectal cancers have been detected on FDG PET scans performed for other purposes.

6.3.1.5 Raised Tumour Markers

PET/CT may not be routinely recommended in patients with a suspicion of cancer on the mere detection of increased blood tumour markers.

6.3.2 Staging

While T staging is often better defined by conventional imaging (CT, US, or magnetic resonance imaging [MRI]), at present, the use of PET imaging for N and M staging is validated by literature for many tumours: non–small-cell lung cancer (NSCLC), lymphoma, melanoma, uterine and cervical cancer, colorectal cancer, oesophageal and gastric carcinoma, nasopharyngeal carcinoma, and GIST.

The definition of NSCLC staging often requires invasive procedures and multiple tests. Whole-body PET may simplify and improve the evaluation of patients affected by this tumour. PET represents the standard of care for staging NSCLC in many countries, with meta-analysis indicating a higher sensitivity and specificity for PET than for CT scanning. This is especially important for mediastinal lymph nodes close to normal size (mediastinoscopy is still the gold standard for staging, even if invasive and not all mediastinal lymph nodes can be easily accessed) [12].

The use of PET modifies also the staging (down or up) of about 50% of patients and thus has an incontestable positive effect on treatment (Figure 6.3a,b).

Due to its superior sensitivity and specificity for most types of lymphoma, FDG PET is appropriate for staging both Hodgkin's disease (HD) and aggressive non–Hodgkin's lymphomas (NHL), but not for low-grade ones. As spread bone marrow involvement and small localisation may be missed, FDG PET should not replace bone marrow biopsy at initial staging. A baseline FDG PET scan is also recommended when succeeding evaluation of response to treatment with PET is considered.

Regarding melanoma, PET staging is improper for stages I and II and low pretest probability of metastases because less sensitive than sentinel node biopsy. In case of high pretest probability of metastases (melanoma of the head, neck, and trunk, Breslow index >4 mm, ulceration, high mitotic rate), or stage III, FDG PET is appropriate for detecting potentially operable metastases.

Concerning the uterine and cervical cancer, PET changes the patient's management in 14.1% and in 9.1%, respectively.

T staging of oesophageal cancer is usually made at endoscopic biopsy, and CT or MRI is used to demonstrate infiltration of adjacent structures and local adenopathy. FDG PET-reported sensitivity in detecting metastatic disease varies, but it is always superior to that of CT. This feature is important, as upstaging usually indicates that surgery with radical intent is unsuitable.

The capability of entire body scanning with a single examination at one time is evidently an advantage of FDG PET, compared with the other imaging modalities. A positive PET scan for

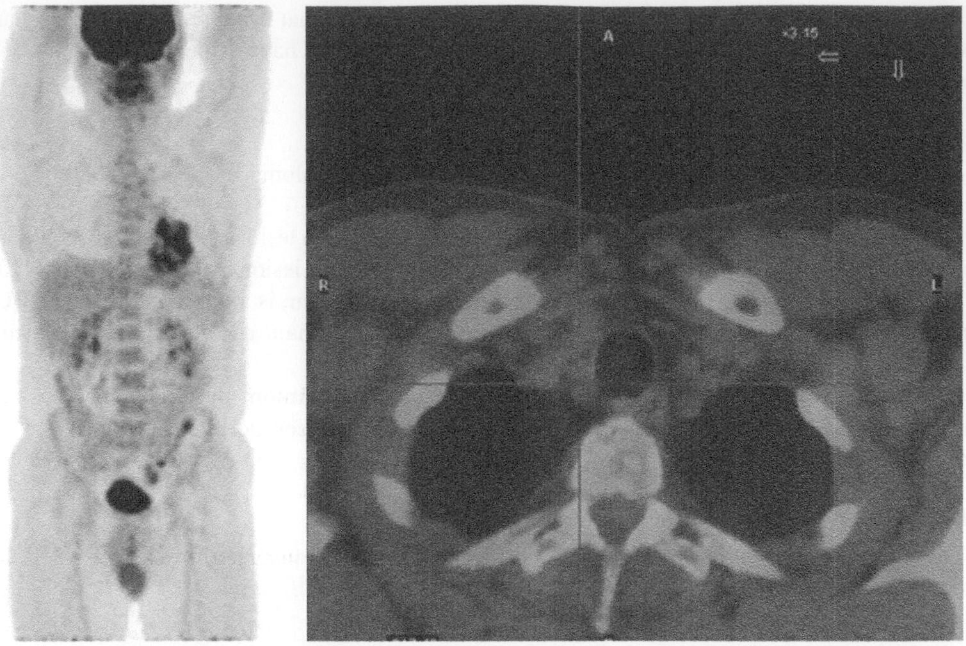

(a) (b)

FIGURE 6.3 (a) Left lung cancer staging. The MIP image shows the large mass within the inferior left lung lobe (SUVmax 10.9). Two FDG avid mediastinal lymph nodes (SUVmax 3.0), subaortic and subcarinal stations, are noted, consistent with lymphatic metastasis. (b) Transaxial CT and PET fused image shows two more hypermetabolic (SUVmax 3.2) upper paratracheal slightly enlarged lymph nodes on the right side (therefore contralateral to the primary tumour). These findings are highly suspected to represent other metastatic sites, upstaging the tumour (N3 and therefore IIIB stage).

distant metastatic disease would lead to the decision to avoid useless surgery with radical intent reducing costs and morbidity. PET staging, but with regard only for distant metastasis detection, is particularly appropriate for breast cancer, head and neck cancer, and pancreatic cancer.

With regard to breast cancer, FDG PET allows detection of extra-axillary nodes (axillary nodes are better staged by sentinel node biopsy able to detect also micrometastasis) and distant metastases with higher sensitivity than other diagnostic imaging methods, with exception of brain metastases, better staged by MRI.

Head and neck carcinoma staging is very complex. This is confirmed by the huge discordance in the published literature. Clinical N0 is the most critical situation: CT, PET-CT, and US show various accuracy values [13]. Although diagnostic tools have developed significantly, there are no effective procedures available to identify hidden metastatic disease in the cervical lymph nodes of patients with oral cancer. Since the incidence of cervical adenopathy is around 30%, the use of elective neck dissection is the common practice in the staging of regional disease in oral cancer. On the contrary, PET-CT is highly recommended for the detection of hematogenous metastasis (sensitivity 100% and specificity 90%), and patients with advance node disease (N3) would benefit the most [14] avoiding useless and aggressive surgery.

6.3.3 Response Evaluation

Commonly, structural variations in tumour volume are interpreted as a prospective endpoint to assess drug action as a substitute for other measures of clinical benefit such as disease-free and overall survival. Moreover, in routine practice, clinicians use volume changes to modify the treatment management.

Since tissue metabolism varies more quickly than morphology, changes in tumour FDG uptake may predate volume alteration. This is emblematic in malignant lymphomas, where anatomical imaging after therapy completion often reveals residual masses that could represent either persistent disease or fibrotic tissue [15]. Identification of residual disease after radio- or chemotherapy is clearly influencing prognosis and further treatment options. Positive FDG PET findings after the end of therapy in patients affected by HD is a strong predictor of relapse, while a negative PET study is also an excellent predictor of good prognosis (positive predictive value of PET = 100% vs. CT = 42%). However, a negative PET scan does not exclude the presence of minimal residual disease, under the spatial resolution, that could lead to a later relapse [16]. Nowadays, PET-CT is the technique of choice for the assessment of response to therapy in HD and NHL with baseline FDG avidity lesions, being superior to the CT evaluation based on International Workshop Criteria.

Patients affected by NSCLC with stages III and IV are usually treated with chemotherapy or chemoradiotherapy. Therefore, there is the need for therapy response monitoring, but conventional imaging cannot reliably distinguish necrotic tumour or fibrotic scar from residual tumour tissue. Response evaluation with these morphological imaging methods does not well correlate with pathologic response nor with changes at the cellular level or with tumour viability. Instead, metabolic imaging provided by FDG PET can detect cell behaviour determining potential residual tumour disease. Therefore, PET can determine response soon after radical radiotherapy or chemoradiotherapy and is significantly associated with overall survival compared with CT scan [17].

Management of locally advanced rectal cancer included a treatment with chemoradiotherapy before surgery. Several works in literature underline the higher accuracy of FDG PET, compared with CT or MRI, in assessing neo-adjuvant chemoradiotherapy response due to its intrinsic capacity to identify precociously changes in tumour behaviour [18].

The PET response following neo-adjuvant chemotherapy can be used to select the patients who shift from inoperable condition to candidate to surgical resection. For example, in the case of stage III of NSCLC, if metastatic mediastinal lymph nodes show good response to chemotherapy, debulking or curative surgery may be considered. On the contrary, if there is poor PET response in mediastinal nodes, survival is very poor and patients probably should not undergo surgery.

The assessment of therapy response with PET is also valid for other tumours, such as ovarian, head and neck, germinal, gastric, neuroendocrine, prostate, oesophageal, cervical, and pancreatic tumours, sarcomas, primary tumour of the CNS, gastrointestinal stromal tumours (GIST), and multiple myeloma.

6.3.3.1 Early Response Assessment

Chemotherapy is currently the treatment of choice for many high-risk metastatic tumours, but the response assessment by conventional imaging after several cycles of chemotherapy by changes in tumour size requires a lot of time. Furthermore, response evaluation with morphological imaging methods does not correlate well with pathologic response, with changes at the cellular level or with tumour viability. In contrast, FDG PET is able to detect cell behaviour and thus to identify potential residual tumour disease.

Several studies have considered the utility of PET-CT for response evaluation *ad interim*. Early identification of non-responding patients provides a basis for substitute treatment strategy choice, reducing the costs and side effects of a worthless therapy.

For example, FDG PET can predict the response soon after a few cycles of chemotherapy for metastatic breast cancer. The use of FDG PET as a surrogate endpoint for monitoring therapy response offers improved and personalised patient care by individualising treatment and avoiding ineffective chemotherapy [19]. Furthermore, FDG PET is a valid tool for prognostic stratification in patients with metastatic breast cancer treated with high-dose chemotherapy [20].

In addition, in comparison with CT scan findings, FDG PET results show a significantly closer association with overall survival.

It has to be underlined that if a PET scan is performed early after radiotherapy (less than 6 weeks), false-positive results due to inflammatory post-actinic changes are possible, although there is no consensus in international literature about the minimal time that has to be waited prior to performing a post radiotherapy PET scan [21].

6.3.3.2 Response to Targeted Therapies Assessment

One of the principal pathways of communication between cells is the binding of polypeptide ligands to cell surface receptors with tyrosine kinase (TK) activity. Alteration of TK signalling can lead also to malignant transformation. During the last few decades, these networks have been examined in detail and drugs targeted at key molecules produced. Though many agents have failed, either humanised monoclonal antibody as bevacizumab, trastuzumab, and cetuximab or epidermal growth factor receptor (EGFR) inhibitors like gefitinib and erlotinib have already become part of the standard care for widespread tumours like breast, colorectal, ovarian, lung, and head and neck cancers. Additionally, imatinib, a receptor TK inhibitor, has revealed unsurpassed efficacy in GIST and chronic myeloid leukaemia. The clinical success of these drugs is funded on the increasing awareness of the molecular networks that govern the growth of a cancer phenotype [22].

The selection of patients who are likely to benefit from TK inhibitors is mandatory not only for clinical but also for economic reasons, since receptor-targeted therapies are very expensive. This scenario requires a revaluation of the standard criteria to assess treatment response (response evaluation criteria in solid tumours – RECIST), and PET-CT may play a relevant role in the molecular insight of the tumour.

Regarding GIST patients (Figure 6.4a,b), the use of FDG PET has been judged appropriate in assessing treatment response to TK inhibitor therapy [23]. Moreover, ^{18}F-FDG PET allows an early assessment of treatment response and is a strong predictor of clinical outcome [24].

6.3.4 Suspected Recurrence

Routine oncologic follow-up includes clinical evaluation, laboratory tests, tumour markers, and diagnostic imaging. In some cases, cancer relapse is suggested by rising tumour markers, while morphological imaging modalities may remain negative for a long time: this is the case of ovarian, prostate, testicular, and thyroid cancer. In these diseases, most studies [25–27] showed the diagnostic accuracy of PET-CT to be superior to that of other imaging methods, in particular contrast-enhanced CT: PET scan can found little areas of locoregional relapse (e.g., non-enlarged but hypermetabolic lymph nodes) or distant metastasis, changing the clinical management in a wide portion of patients.

Furthermore, FDG PET could also exclude or set the presence of recurrence in cases of indeterminate findings by other imaging modalities. In fact, NSCLC [28], melanoma [29], head and neck, breast [30], pancreas [31], oesophagus [32], stomach, and colorectal cancer [33] are frequently evaluated prior to radiological procedures (mostly CT scan), and in case of a discordance between methods or the presence of an inconclusive report, FDG PET has to be proposed for identifying early recurrent cancer.

6.3.5 Treatment Planning

Such as other imaging procedures, PET influences further therapeutic decisions, that is, if it is advisable to operate or not, which approach is the most appropriate, or the feasibility of advanced therapies (as autologous bone marrow transplantation in lymphoma).

There are therapies that take advantage of PET to improve the results and reduce adverse reactions: the use of intensity-modulated radiotherapy (IMRT) allows individualised dose delivery while sparing the surrounding normal and radiosensitive tissue (a daily challenge in head and neck or in pelvic region). This method carries the potential benefit of increasing the therapeutic ratio by limiting the amount of normal tissues receiving radiation and maximising coverage of tumour volumes. Although CT remains the gold standard of anatomic image acquisition for the purpose of

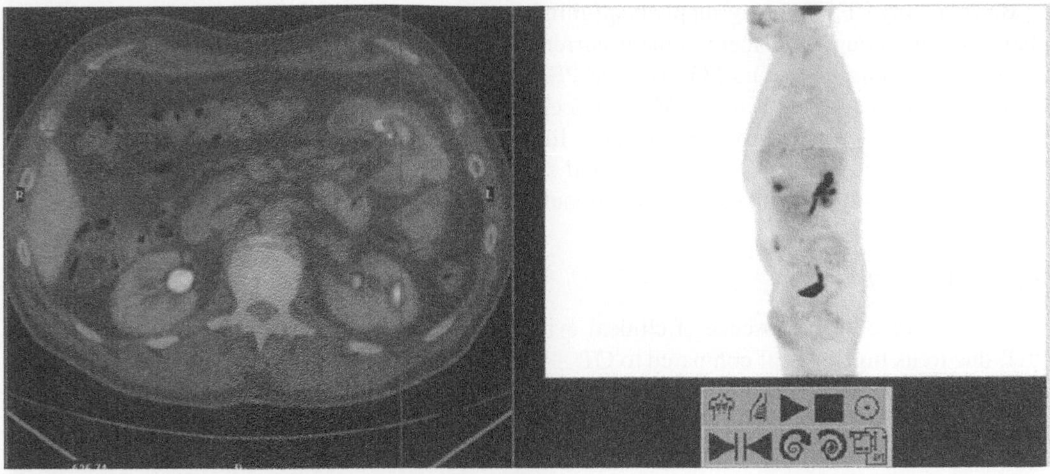

(a)

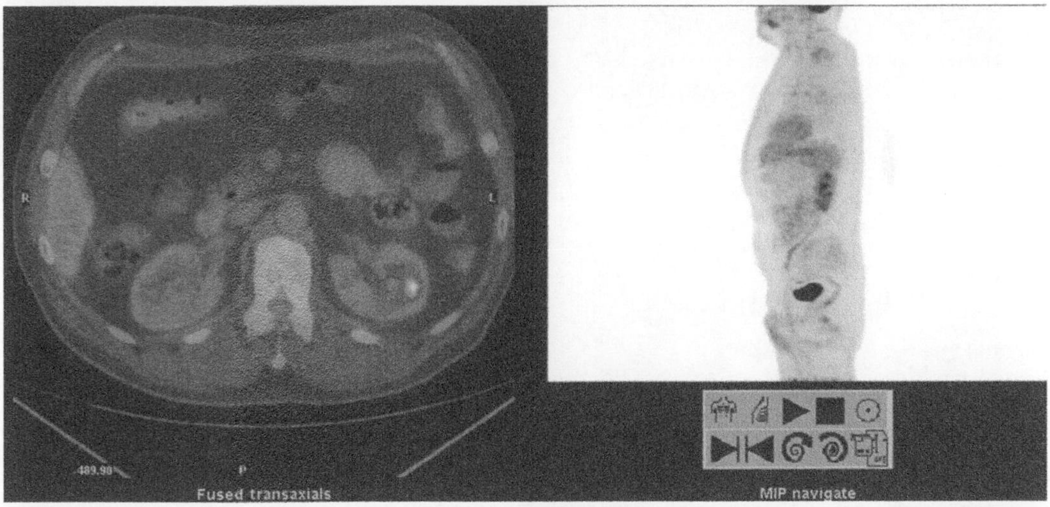

(b)

FIGURE 6.4 (a) GIST restaging after surgical resection of a jejunal GIST mass. Transaxial CT and PET fused and MIP images show a left hypochondrial area of FDG pathological uptake (SUVmax 7.1), consistent with local residual disease mass. (b) GIST restaging after 3 months of therapy with imatinib. Transaxial PET-CT fused and MIP images show the normalisation of FDG uptake within the intestinal loops in the left hypochondrium, refers to a complete metabolic response.

target volume definition and dose calculation in radiotherapy treatment planning, CT has several limitations. Anatomic details may be compromised by metal artefacts, and gross tumour volume (GTV) definition may be affected by insufficient contrast between soft tissue and tumour.

Functional imaging with PET can provide information that can influence RT planning in many ways: PET can improve staging revealing targets, even far from the primary tumour, that are not well visualised by CT or MRI or excluding non-pathological areas as reactive lymphadenopathy or atelectatic regions of a lung. Furthermore, the imaging of biologic heterogeneity within sub-volumes of the tumour may offer the possibility to adapt doses to local differences in radiosensitivity (known as dose painting). Additionally, PET can be useful for the evaluation of residual masses after chemotherapy, helping to determine which regions, if any, require radiation therapy and helping to choose between a lower dose for presumed microscopic residual disease or a higher dose for gross residual disease [34].

But, not only ^{18}F FDG may supply helpful information which may influence radiation treatment planning, for example, ^{11}C-methionine is currently one of the best available PET tracers for delineating brain tumour contours [35], choline PET is widely used for prostatic cancer [36], and ^{18}F FMISO, ^{18}F FAZA, and ^{64}Cu ATSM are tracers allowing non-invasive determination of hypoxia that gives radioresistancy to tumour cells, limiting locoregional control by radiotherapy [37]. ^{18}F-Fluorothymidine [38] is a nucleoside and surrogate for proliferation activity, which may also add information to adequate radiation treatment planning.

6.3.6 Follow-Up

The surveillance in the absence of clinical evidence of recurrence is not routinely performed by PET, due to its high costs if compared to CT.

Nevertheless, PET is commonly performed in the case of tumours at high risk of recurrence because of its better sensitivity to identify active disease (Figure 6.5).

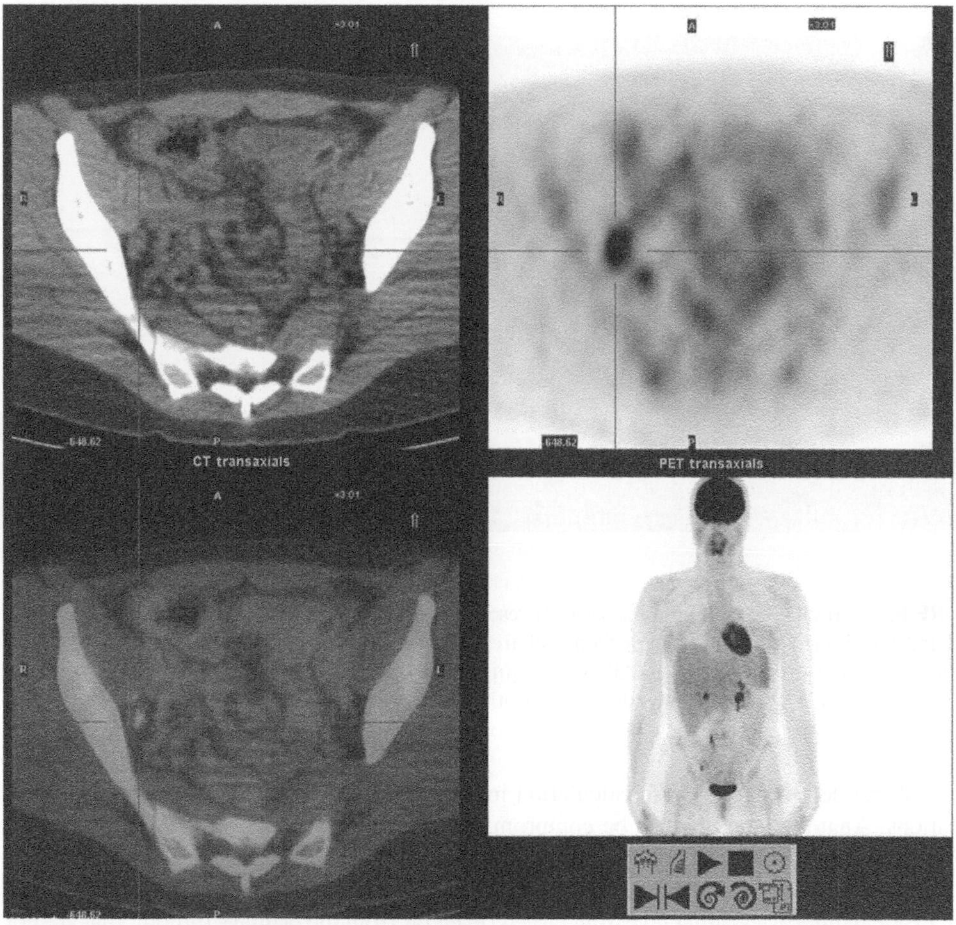

FIGURE 6.5 Hodgkin's lymphoma (subdiaphragmatic disease localisation), treated by chemotherapy 18 months before with complete response. The patient is referred to a follow-up PET-CT scan. The figure is composed by the transaxial CT, PET, fused PET-CT images, plus total body MIP. A single FDG avid lymph node below the bifurcation of the right common iliac artery is noted (SUVmax 6.7; maximum axial diameter 1.6 cm), suspected for a disease relapse.

Moreover, FDG PET may be useful for detecting recurrence at an early stage, when salvage therapy may be possible, more effective, or less mutilating. This is particularly indicated for colorectal cancer, sarcomas, GIST, and lymphoma. For primary tumour of the CNS, PET has to be used for routine surveillance of untreated low-grade gliomas to assess transformation to high-grade lesions.

6.4 CHANGES IN PATIENT MANAGEMENT

Like other imaging tests, PET is used to update decision-making, that is, whether a surgical approach is worthwhile, which intervention will be most fitting, and if advanced therapies are practicable. Moreover, molecular imaging could be employed to personalise therapy by guiding radiation therapy planning (the most significant example is IMRT) and improving definition of tumour target volumes.

To be cost effective, the information from PET must alter management appropriately. The average management change across all applications was estimated to be 30% on studies only with PET alone [39]. More recently, studies on hybrid PET-CT show different percentage of modification in therapeutic decision, on the basis of the different diseases (i.e., 51% in suspected recurrence breast cancer or 15% in stage III melanoma [40]).

Commonly, PET-CT scan brings upstaging of the patient depicting more regional lymph nodes or distant metastases which led to the use of primary systemic therapy as opposed to radical surgery.

6.5 NON-FDG RADIOPHARMACEUTICALS

FDG PET has a well-established role in the management of a range of cancers, as just described. Nevertheless, FDG is not a perfect tumour-specific tracer and its specificity may be reduced by increased uptake in sites of inflammation or by physiological FDG uptake region (brain, bladder, and urinary tract) interfering with interpretation. These limitations explain the strong and continued research for development of other PET tracers. A variety of biological substances can be labelled with positron emitters such as ^{11}C, ^{15}O, ^{13}N (due to their very short half-life, only used at the production centres equipped with a cyclotron), and ^{18}F to the study of many metabolisms: cellular proliferation, receptor activity, protein or membrane phospholipids metabolism, hypoxia, apoptosis, and angiogenesis, for example. Tumours showing alteration of these kinds of metabolism will concentrate PET radiotracers more intensively than healthy tissue with a high tumour-to-background rate.

6.5.1 Choline

Given the poor results of FDG as a tracer for prostate cancer, efforts have been directed to alternative radiopharmaceuticals, and choline is probably the most studied at the moment. Principles of choline accumulation are related to the synthesis of phospholipids in cell membranes, whose major is phosphatidylcholine.

Choline can be labelled both with ^{11}C (20 min of half-life) and ^{18}F (110 min of half-life): the former being preferable due to lower urinary excretion and patient's exposure while the latter is the only option for centres lacking on-site cyclotron.

The usefulness and accuracy of choline PET in prostate cancer patients has been described in many original papers, mostly in the setting of relapse identification but also for biopsy guiding in patients with high prostate-specific antigen (PSA) rising but negative US-guided biopsy (Figure 6.6a,b).

In patients radically treated for prostate cancer with PSA serum level increased and negative conventional diagnostic flow chart, choline PET seems to have very high accuracy in the detection of early metastatic lymph node and little scheletric lesions (also if compared with bone scintigraphy). Choline PET is also useful in local recurrence detection, however, with a lower sensitivity [41,42].

6.5.2 Methionine and Tyrosine

Methionine uptake, as well as tyrosine uptake, is associated with increased amino acid transport and protein synthesis. Thanks to its low uptake in the normal brain, it has advantages over FDG in the evaluation of brain lesions.

Although MRI is the most appropriate imaging tool to assess cerebral tumours, it is not accurate enough in evaluating grading and in distinguishing tumour recurrence from post-surgical fibrosis, radionecrosis, or oedema. The main limitation of methionine use is related to ^{11}C labelling, which implies the availability of on-site cyclotron, and therefore ^{18}F-labelled tyrosine has been suggested as an alternative.

One of the principal applications of these amino acid PET tracers is the detection of residual or relapsed cerebral glioblastomas, astrocytomas, oligodendrogliomas, and meningiomas following surgery or radiotherapy. In these cases, PET significantly shortens the time of diagnosis, allowing a quick second line treatment. ^{11}C-methionine PET has also been used both to better define the radiotherapy field and localise the most metabolic area inside a brain mass to guide the biopsy [43].

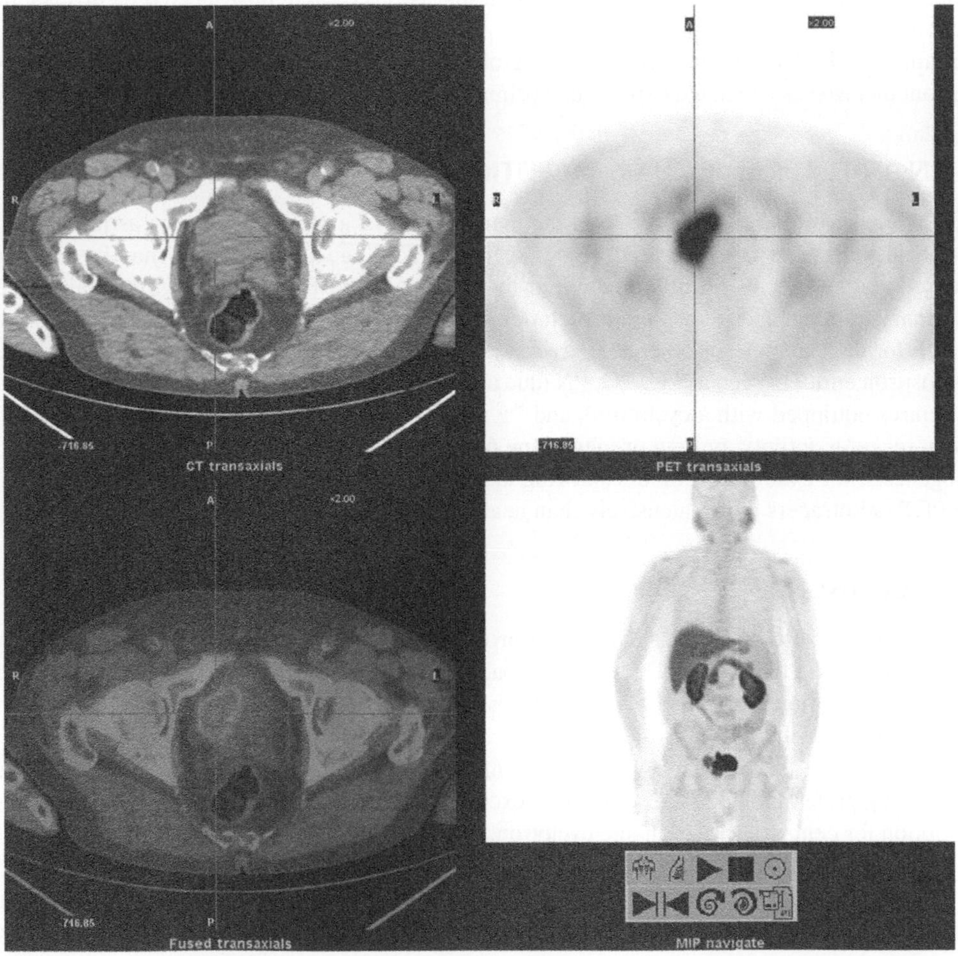

(a)

FIGURE 6.6 (a) Suspected prostate cancer on the basis of PSA rising (113 ng/mL). Two transrectal US-guided prostate biopsies were negative. The figures, composed by the transaxial CT, PET, fused PET-CT images, and total body MIP, show a detection PET-CT with ^{18}F-choline. The image shows high choline uptake within the right prostatic lobe (SUVmax 9.9) which refers to a malignant lesion. *(Continued)*

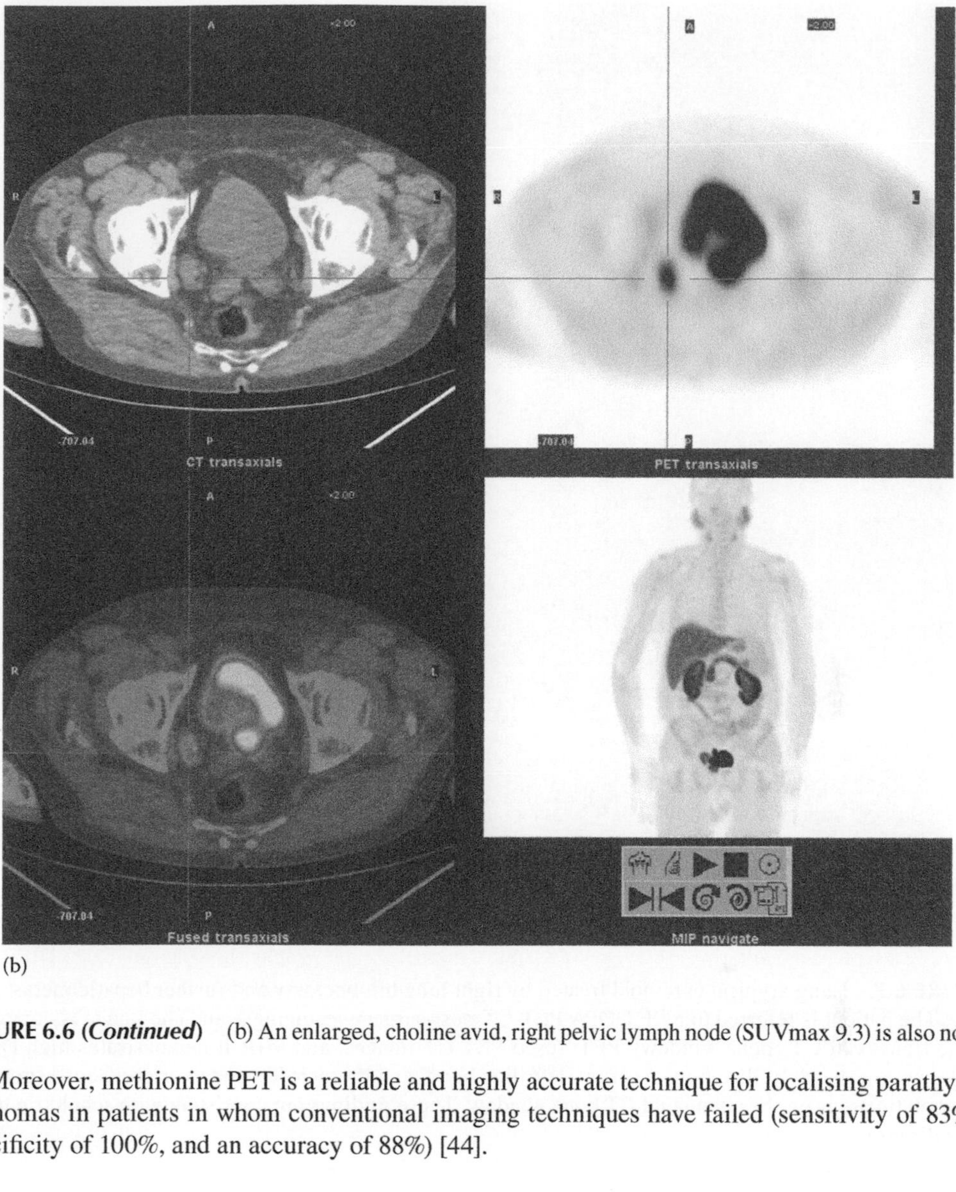

(b)

FIGURE 6.6 (*Continued*) (b) An enlarged, choline avid, right pelvic lymph node (SUVmax 9.3) is also noted.

Moreover, methionine PET is a reliable and highly accurate technique for localising parathyroid adenomas in patients in whom conventional imaging techniques have failed (sensitivity of 83%, a specificity of 100%, and an accuracy of 88%) [44].

6.5.3 DOPA

Neuroendocrine tumours (NET) show increased metabolism of amino acids like dihydroxyphenylalanine (DOPA) which are therefore used, labelled with ^{18}F, as tracer to detect primary and metastatic neoplastic diseases like carcinoids (Figure 6.7), medullary thyroid cancer, neuroblastoma, small cell lung cancer, and pheochromocytoma [45]. Moreover, ^{18}F-DOPA PET-CT scan is feasible for studying NET of unknown origin. However, the difficulties and high costs of its synthesis process have confined its extensive use in the clinic [46].

6.5.4 DOTA-Somatostatin Receptor Analogues

Somatostatin receptors (SSTRs) are overexpressed in many tumours (NET, melanoma, lung, and breast tumours), with different subtype specificity. Until now, five receptor subtypes of somatostatin have been identified.

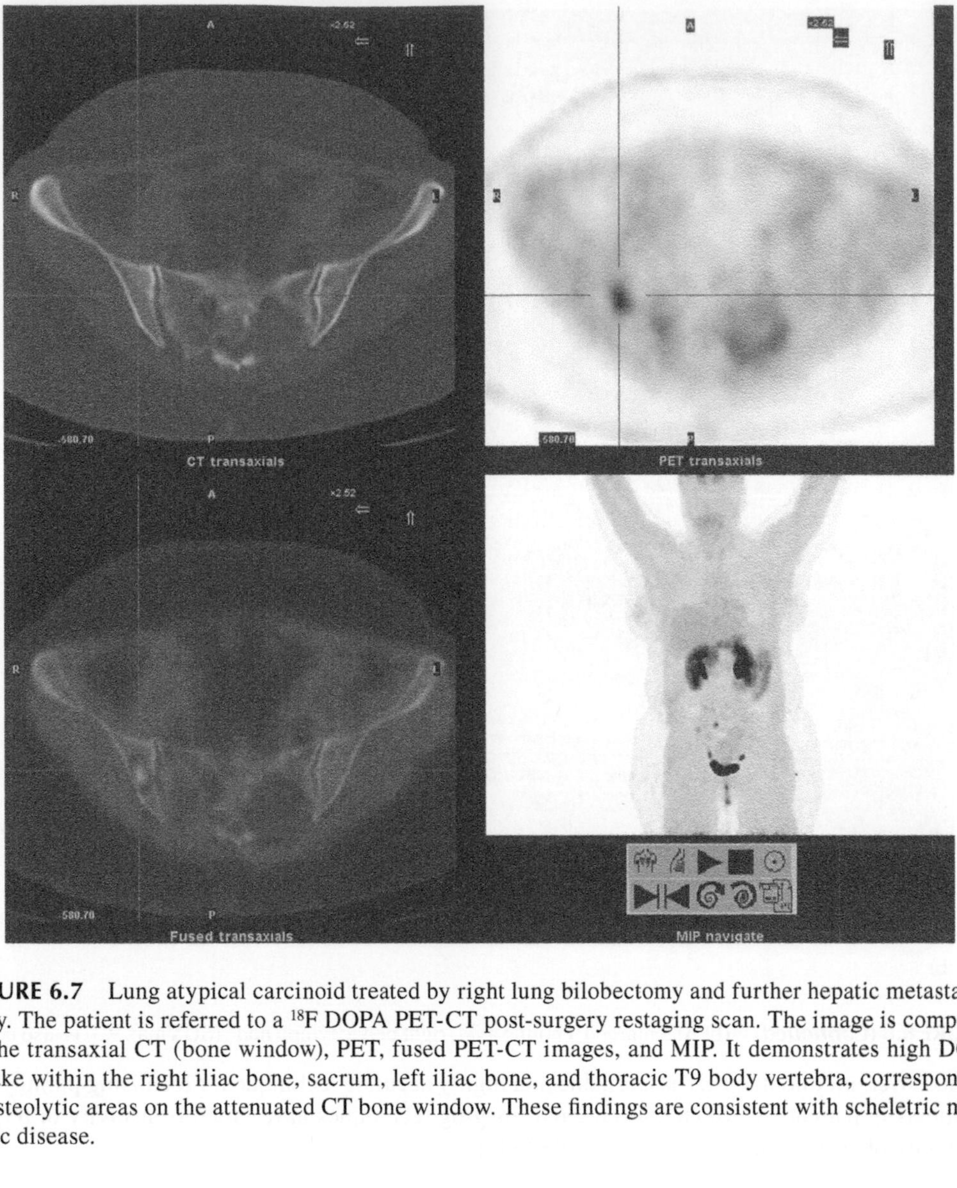

FIGURE 6.7 Lung atypical carcinoid treated by right lung bilobectomy and further hepatic metastasectomy. The patient is referred to a ^{18}F DOPA PET-CT post-surgery restaging scan. The image is composed by the transaxial CT (bone window), PET, fused PET-CT images, and MIP. It demonstrates high DOPA uptake within the right iliac bone, sacrum, left iliac bone, and thoracic T9 body vertebra, corresponding to osteolytic areas on the attenuated CT bone window. These findings are consistent with scheletric metastatic disease.

Different SSTR imaging agents, such as TATE (octreotate, a SSTR2-selective ligand), TOC (octreotide), and NOC (1-NaI3-octreotide, with SSTR 2, 3, and 5 affinity), have been developed and labelled with the isotope gallium-68, produced by a generator and therefore independently from an on-site cyclotron.

Since most NETs show low FDG uptake, ^{68}Ga DOTA-octreotide analogues offer excellent diagnostic accuracy for NET management with a very high tumour-to-background ratio, compared with conventional SSTR scintigraphy and diagnostic CT [47]. In recent years, radionuclide treatments using SSTR agents have resulted in improved quality of life, and survival for patients with NETs and SSTR imaging helps to select and manage patients for radionuclide therapy [48].

Moreover, the use of ^{68}Ga-DOTA-NOC PET-CT seems to be valuable to reveal unknown primary tumour of neuroendocrine nature.

6.5.5 Acetate

This PET tracer can be considered an intermediate molecule both in the glucose catabolism pathways and in membrane metabolism. Acetate, labelled with ^{11}C, was first used like choline for the detection of prostate cancer, showing a similar sensitivity and specificity [49]. Another field of acetate use, in association with FDG, is for the evaluation of liver masses: ^{11}C acetate has good sensitivity for low-grade hepatocellular carcinoma, while FDG shows good accuracy for high-grade ones [50].

6.5.6 Other Non-FDG Tracers

^{18}F-FLT (fluoro-levo-thymidine) is one of the most promising radiotracers synthesised for PET oncological studies as a specific marker of cell proliferation.

Since it does not accumulate into inflammation processes can theoretically be an optimal marker of therapy response. Nowadays, its clinical indication is for therapy monitoring, especially for early detection of anti-proliferative effects of chemoradiotherapy, in lymphoma, breast cancer, and glioma [51–53].

Other interesting molecules are the markers of hypoxia: these compounds (the most important are ^{18}F-MISO and ^{64}Cu-ATSM) which highlight the presence of hypoxic areas are useful for patients who must be treated with radiotherapy. In fact, it is well known that hypoxia is one of the strongest radioresistance factors and should be over-treated compared to non-hypoxic malignant tissues [54].

REFERENCES

1. Valk PE, Delbeke D, Bailey DL et al. *Positron Emission Tomography: Clinical Practice*. London, U.K.: Springer-Verlag London Ltd. 2006, p. 4.
2. Freudenberg LS, Antoch G, Schutt P et al. FDG-PET/CT in re-staging of patients with lymphoma. *Eur J Nucl Med Mol Imaging* 2004;31(3):325–329.
3. Fletcher JW, Kymes SM, Gould M et al. A comparison of the diagnostic accuracy of 18F-FDG PET and CT in the characterization of solitary pulmonary nodules, VA SNAP Cooperative Studies Group. *J Nucl Med* 2008;49(2):179–185.
4. Heinrich S, Goerres GW, Schäfer M et al. Positron emission tomography/computed tomography influences on the management of resectable pancreatic cancer and its cost-effectiveness. *Ann Surg* 2005;242(2):235–243.
5. Fletcher JW, Djulbegovic B, Soares HP et al. Recommendations on the use of 18F-FDG PET in oncology. *J Nucl Med* 2008;49(3):480–508.
6. Nishiyama, Y, Yamamoto Y, Kimura N et al. Comparison of early and delayed FDG PET for evaluation of biliary stricture. *Nucl Med Commun* 2007;28(12):914–919.
7. Liu RS, Chang CP, Guo WY et al. 1-11C-acetate versus 18F-FDG PET in detection of meningioma and monitoring the effect of gamma-knife radiosurgery. *J Nucl Med* 2010;51(6):883–891.
8. Fischman AJ. PET imaging of brain tumors. *Cancer Treat Res* 2008;143:67–92.
9. Kwee TC, Kwee RM. Combined FDG-PET/CT for the detection of unknown primary tumors: Systematic review and meta-analysis. *Eur Radiol* 2009;19(3):731–744.
10. Chen W, Parsons M, Torigian DA et al. Evaluation of thyroid FDG uptake incidentally identified on FDG-PET/CT imaging. *Nucl Med Commun* 2009;30(3):240–244.
11. Boland GW, Blake MA, Holalkere NS et al. PET/CT for the characterization of adrenal masses in patients with cancer: Qualitative versus quantitative accuracy in 150 consecutive patients. *AJR Am J Roentgenol* 2009;192(4):956–962.
12. MacManus M., Hicks RJ. The use of positron emission tomography (PET) in the staging/evaluation, treatment, and follow-up of patients with lung cancer: A critical review. *Int J Radiat Oncol Biol Phys* 2008;72(5):1298–1306.
13. Stoeckli SJ, Steinert H, Pfaltz M, Schmid S. Is there a role for positron emission tomography with 18F-fluorodeoxyglucose in the initial staging of nodal negative oral and oropharyngeal squamous cell carcinoma. *Head Neck* 2002;24(4):345–349.
14. Yen TC, Chang JT, Ng SH et al. The value of 18F-FDG PET in the detection of stage M0 carcinoma of the nasopharynx. *J Nucl Med* 2005;46(3):405–410.

15. Juweid ME, Stroobants S, Hoekstra OS et al. Use of positron emission tomography for response assessment of lymphoma: Consensus of the Imaging Subcommittee of International Harmonization Project in Lymphoma. *J Clin Oncol* 2007;25(5):571–578.
16. Zinzani PL, Fanti S, Battista G et al. Predictive role of positron emission tomography (PET) in the outcome of lymphoma patients. *Br J Cancer* 2004;91(5):850–854.
17. De Geus-Oei LF, van der Heijden HF, Corstens FH, Oyen WJ. Predictive and prognostic value of FDG-PET in nonsmall-cell lung cancer: A systematic review. *Cancer* 2007;110(8):1654–1664.
18. Denecke T, Rau B, Hoffmann KT et al. Comparison of CT, MRI and FDG-PET in response prediction of patients with locally advanced rectal cancer after multimodal preoperative therapy: Is there a benefit in using functional imaging? *Eur Radiol* 2005;15(8):1658–1666.
19. Yang DH, Min JJ, Song HC et al. Prognostic significance of interim ^{18}F-FDG PET/CT after three or four cycles of R-CHOP chemotherapy in the treatment of diffuse large B-cell lymphoma. *Eur J Cancer* 2011;47(9):1312–1318.
20. Dose Schwarz J, Bader M, Jenicke L, Hemminger G, Janicke F, Avril N. Early prediction of response to chemotherapy in metastatic breast cancer using sequential 18F-FDG PET. *J Nucl Med* 2005;46(7):1144–1150.
21. Castellucci P, Zinzani P, Nanni C et al. 18F-FDG PET early after radiotherapy in lymphoma patients. *Cancer Biother Radiopharm* 2004;19(5):606–612.
22. Erman M. Molecular mechanisms of signal transduction: Epidermal growth factor receptor family, vascular endothelial growth factor family, Kit, platelet-derived growth factor receptor, Ras. *J BUON* 2007;12(Suppl. 1):S83–S94.
23. Appropriate use of FDG-PET for the management of cancer patients. Vienna, Austria: International Atomic Energy Agency, 2010.
24. Treglia G, Mirk P, Stefanelli A, Rufini V, Giordano A, Bonomo L. 18F-Fluorodeoxyglucose positron emission tomography in evaluating treatment response to imatinib or other drugs in gastrointestinal stromal tumors: A systematic review. *Clin Imaging* 2012;36(3):167–175. Review.
25. Nanni C, Rubello D, Farsad M et al. (18)F-FDG PET/CT in the evaluation of recurrent ovarian cancer: A prospective study on forty-one patients. *Eur J Surg Oncol* 2005;31(7):792–797.
26. Sanchez D, Zudaire JJ, Fernandez JM et al. 18F-fluoro-2-deoxyglucose-positron emission tomography in the evaluation of nonseminomatous germ cell tumours at relapse. *BJU Int* 2002;89(9):912–916.
27. Scattoni V, Picchio M, Suardi N et al. Detection of lymph-node metastases with integrated [11C]choline PET/CT in patients with PSA failure after radical retropubic prostatectomy: Results confirmed by open pelvic-retroperitoneal lymphadenectomy. *Eur Urol* 2007;52(2):423–429.
28. Hicks RJ, Kalff V, MacManus MP et al. The utility of (18)F-FDG PET for suspected recurrent non-small cell lung cancer after potentially curative therapy: Impact on management and prognostic stratification. *J Nucl Med* 2001;42(11):1605–1613.
29. Stas M, Stroobants S, Dupont P et al. 18-FDG PET scan in the staging of recurrent melanoma: Additional value and therapeutic impact. *Melanoma Res* 2002;12(5):479–490.
30. Radan L, Ben-Haim S, Bar-Shalom R, Guralnk L, Israel O. The role of FDG-PET/CT in suspected recurrence of breast cancer. *Cancer* 2006; 107(11):2545–2551.
31. Ruf J, Lopez Hanninen E, Oettle H et al. Detection of recurrent pancreatic cancer: Comparison of FDG-PET with CT/MRI. *Pancreatology* 2005;5(2–3):266–272.
32. Guo H, Zhu H, Xi Y et al. Diagnostic and prognostic value of 18F-FDG PET/CT for patients with suspected recurrence from squamous cell carcinoma of the esophagus. *J Nucl Med* 2007;48(8):1251–1258.
33. Kalff V, Hicks RJ, Ware RE, Hogg A, Binns D, McKenzie AF. The clinical impact of (18)F-FDG PET in patients with suspected or confirmed recurrence of colorectal cancer: A prospective study. *J Nucl Med* 2002;43(4):492–499.
34. The role of PET/CT in radiation treatment planning for cancer patient treatment. Vienna, Austria: IAEA, 2008.
35. Geets X, Daisne JF, Gregoire V, Hamoir M, Lonneux M. Role of 11-C-methionine positron emission tomography for the delineation of the tumor volume in pharyngo-laryngeal squamous cell carcinoma: Comparison with FDG-PET and CT. *Radiother Oncol* 2004;71:267–273.
36. Picchio M, Crivellaro C, Giovacchini G, Gianolli L, Messa C. PET-CT for treatment planning in prostate cancer. *Q J Nucl Med Mol Imaging* 2009;53:245–268.
37. Lee NY, Mechalakos JG, Nehmeh S et al. Fluorine-18-labeled fluoromisonidazole positron emission and computed tomography-guided intensity-modulated radiotherapy for head and neck cancer: A feasibility study. *Int J Radiat Oncol Biol Phys* 2008;70(1):2–13.
38. Bading JR, Shields AF. Imaging of cell proliferation: Status and prospects. *J Nucl Med* 2008;49:64S–80S.

39. Gambhir SS, Czernin J, Schwimmer J, Silverman DH, Coleman RE, Phelps ME. A tabulated summary of the FDG PET literature. *J Nucl Med* 2001;42(5 Suppl):1S–93S.
40. Visioni A, Kim J. Positron emission tomography (PET) for benign and malignant disease. *Surg Clin North Am* 2011;91(1):249–266.
41. Picchio M, Landoni C, Messa C et al. Positive [11C]choline and negative [18F]FDG with positron emission tomography in recurrence of prostate cancer. *AJR Am J Roentgenol* 2002;179:482–484.
42. de Jong IJ, Pruim J, Elsinga PH, Vaalburg W, Mensink HJ. 11C-choline positron emission tomography for the evaluation after treatment of localized prostate cancer. *Eur Urol* 2003;44:32–38.
43. Pirotte B, Goldman S, Massager N et al. Comparison of 18F-FDG and 11C-methionine for PET-guided stereotactic brain biopsy of gliomas. *J Nucl Med* 2004;45:1293–1298.
44. Beggs AD, Hain SF. Localization of parathyroid adenomas using 11C-methionine positron emission tomography. *Nucl Med Commun* 2005;26:133–136.
45. Hoegerle S, Altehoefer C, Ghanem N et al. Whole-body 18F DOPA PET for detection of gastrointestinal carcinoid tumors. *Radiology* 2001;220:373–380.
46. Nanni C, Fanti S, Rubello D. 18F-DOPA PET and PET/CT. *J Nucl Med* 2007;48(10):1577–1579.
47. Gabriel M, Decristoforo C, Kendler D et al. 68Ga-DOTA-Tyr3-octreotide PET in neuroendocrine tumors: Comparison with somatostatin receptor scintigraphy and CT. *J Nucl Med* 2007;48(4):508–518.
48. Ambrosini V, Campana D, Bodei L et al. 68Ga-DOTANOC PET/CT clinical impact in patients with neuroendocrine tumors. *J Nucl Med* 2010;51(5):669–673.
49. Dimitrakopoulou-Strauss A, Strauss LG. PET imaging of prostate cancer with 11C-acetate. *J Nucl Med* 2003;44:549–555.
50. Delbeke D, Pinson CW. 11C-Acetate: A new tracer for the evaluation of hepatocellular carcinoma. *J Nucl Med* 2003;44:222–223.
51. Kasper B, Egerer G, Gronkowski M et al. Functional diagnosis of residual lymphomas after radiochemotherapy with positron emission tomography comparing FDG- and FLT-PET. *Leuk Lymphoma* 2007;48(4):746–753.
52. Chen W, Delaloye S, Silverman DH et al. Predicting treatment response of malignant gliomas to bevacizumab and irinotecan by imaging proliferation with [18F] fluorothymidine positron emission tomography: A pilot study. *J Clin Oncol* 2007;25(30):4714–4721.
53. Kenny L, Coombes RC, Vigushin DM, Al-Nahhas A, Shousha S, Aboagye EO. Imaging early changes in proliferation at 1 week post chemotherapy: A pilot study in breast cancer patients with 3′-deoxy-3′-[18F] fluorothymidine positron emission tomography. *Eur J Nucl Med Mol Imaging* 2007;34(9):1339–1347.
54. Lewis JS, Welch MJ. PET imaging of hypoxia. *Q J Nucl Med* 2001;45:183–188.

7 Sentinel Node Biopsy

An Evolution of the Science and Surgical Principles

Ramin Shayan, Hayley Reynolds,
Cara Michelle Le Roux, and Tara Karnezis

CONTENTS

7.1 INTRODUCTION TO THE LYMPHATIC SYSTEM AND THE SCIENCE OF SENTINEL LYMPH NODE BIOPSY

Lymphatic vessels were first referred to as *vasa chylifera* or the *lacteals* by Greek physicians Herophilus and Erasistratus in human and goat dissections, around 300 BC (Robinson, 1907). Hippocrates had referred to lymph as *white blood* (Rusznyak et al., 1960), and in 1622, Italian anatomist/surgeon Aselli was fascinated by *milky vessels*, describing *lacteals* at canine vivisection. The existence of *lacteals* was supported in humans by de Peiresc, who repeated Aselli's experiment on a prisoner shortly pre-execution (Dunglison, 1841). Later, Joylife (1652) and Rudbeck (1651) independently described lymphatic drainage from all parts of the body, recognising the coalescence of individual lymphatic pathways into an organised system (Robinson, 1907; Skobe and Detmar, 2000). That same year, Pecquet (1651) would elucidate the lymph passage from the thoracic duct into the central venous system. It was Bartholin, a Danish anatomist also working on lymphatics around this period, who coined the term *vasa lymphatic* or lymph vessels (Robinson, 1907; Skobe and Detmar, 2000). The question of how lymph entered the lymphatic system, partly addressed by Hunter (1746) – who observed that the lymphatic capillaries were engaged in absorption (Skobe and Detmar, 2000) – was further clarified by von Recklinghuasen, who established the concept of *blind-ended* lymphatic capillaries, in contrast to characteristic arteriovenous *loops* of blood vessel capillary beds (Skobe and Detmar, 2000). From the earliest origins of lymphatic research, injection studies were fundamental to our understanding of the lymphatic system, including Sappey's pioneering use of mercury injections to map cadaveric collecting lymphatic's (Sappey, 1874) – diagrams of which still form the basis of many current anatomical reference texts (Last, 1998). Unfortunately, Sappey's work was never repeated due to the hazards of mercury use, and the limitations of this body of work have now begun to emerge, for example, regarding the centrifugal drainage pattern of the female breast, emanating radially from the nipple (Sappey, 1874; Uren et al., 1998b).

It would be a further 100 years before Sabin's India ink injection studies of pig embryos would shed light on lymphatic development. After a further lull in lymphatic research, the study of lymphatic physiology regained popularity from the 1940s due to works by Yoffey and Drinker (1939) and by Australian physiologist FC Courtice who further refined the cannulation of collecting lymphatic vessels and adapted it to the cannulation of the capillary (now known as *initial*) lymphatics (Courtice, 1951; Yoffey and Courtice, 1970). This interest in lymphatic function was, however, relatively short-lived, and another stagnation in large-scale lymphatic research ensued between the 1970s and the late 1990s, when breakthroughs in molecular science enabled researchers to both revisit and verify some of the findings espoused by earlier pioneers (Shayan et al., 2006). In particular, this era saw the advent of several key molecular biology techniques in scientific interrogation of the lymphatic system (lymphatic-specific immunohistochemical markers, e.g. LYVE-1 and podoplanin [Banerji et al., 1999], and the discovery of lymphangiogenic growth factors VEGF-C [Joukov et al., 1996] and VEGF-D [Achen et al., 1998]). These advances have enabled researchers to create animal models for lymphangiogenesis and cancer metastasis and to study the role of growth factors in human disease. The advent of these key tools in the study of lymphatics led to the realisation that lymphatic vessels are fundamental to cancer metastasis and many other pathological processes and have led to intense clinical and scientific interest in the lymphatic vasculature as a potentially valuable therapeutic target in these conditions (Stacker et al., 2004). In parallel with these important developments in clinical lymph node tracing, sentinel lymph node biopsy (SLNB) has also become a commonly used tool in the detection of lymph node metastasis (see below).

7.2 CANCER METASTASIS

Tumour metastasis is defined as the movement of cancer cells from the primary tumour to spread systemically, thus implanting in distant anatomical locations. These metastatic colonies may eventually become the survival-limiting factor for patients (DeVita et al., 2001; Robbins, 1999). Tumour cell sub-colonies are more likely to metastasise if equipped with properties such as expressing a range of protease enzymes enabling detachment from the primary tumour, movement through the extracellular matrix, induction and invasion of blood vessels and lymphatics, and subsequent extravasation *downstream* into distant organs (DeVita et al., 2001; Haagensen et al., 1972; Robbins, 1999). Initial spread of cancer cells is seen histologically as tumour escape beyond a defined boundary and may include local lymphatic invasion (Robbins, 1999). Further spread to regional lymph nodes represents an early metastatic extension of tumour cells beyond the primary tumour location and is itself a key diagnostic step and the most important prognostic indicator (Bilchik et al., 1998) in the disease process of many solid human cancers such as melanoma, head and neck squamous cell carcinoma, breast cancer, and many more varieties of epithelial tumours (Dadras et al., 2004; Ferris et al., 2005; Shayan et al., 2012).

Micrometastasis to lymph nodes, thought to occur prior to clinical detection of many primary tumours, may herald distant organ metastasis at the time of diagnosis or after some period of delay (Fidler, 2003). Hence, lymph node staging may alter the type and timing of treatment offered to the patient, and it is critical that all lymph nodes that may potentially harbour metastatic tumour cells are identified and removed for histological analysis (Fidler, 2003). Whether tumour cells become disseminated to distant organs from this point or whether they metastasise directly to sites such as bone, lung, liver, or brain directly remains a topic of contention (Achen and Stacker, 2008; Adams and Alitalo, 2007; Alitalo and Carmeliet, 2002; Alitalo et al., 2005; Baldwin et al., 2002; Karkkainen et al., 2002; Stacker et al., 2002a,b).

It is becoming increasingly recognised that the metastatic characteristics and propensity of individual tumours may be evident earlier in the disease process than previously thought (Ramaswamy et al., 2003) and that genetic susceptibility may play a significant role in the propensity for metastasis (Threadgill, 2005). An improved understanding of the steps controlling lymph node metastasis therefore also offers potential therapeutic options to contain metastasis (Karnezis et al., 2012). Whether or not this aim may be achieved by SLNB is still under investigation (see below).

In addition to this objective, there is an increasing emphasis on sparing patients the morbidity of undergoing unnecessary dissections and removal of the entire lymph node basin unless absolutely necessary (Shayan et al., 2012) – for example, patients in whom the presence of metastatic cells in that lymph node group has already been verified histologically (Shayan et al., 2012). Despite much research into alternative radiological evaluation techniques, however, this type of histological examination of draining regional nodes remains the gold standard in identifying even small metastatic cancer cell deposits within the lymph node (Scolyer et al., 2004). The misdiagnosis and failure to remove such affected nodes can result in dire consequences, with inadequate clearance often resulting in bulky, unresectable disease (Ferris et al., 2005). Techniques that may aid in the identification of tumours that are likely to metastasise from primary tumour characteristics are under investigation (Shayan et al., 2012).

Regarding patients in whom metastasis occurs when clinical indicators suggested that metastasis was unlikely, there are several potential explanations. Failure to detect occult metastasis may be responsible for around one-third of early-stage colorectal cancer patients, who were originally classified as histologically *lymph node negative* but later developed systemic disease (Bilchik et al., 2001, 2002). Despite our knowledge of the prognostic significance of the histological presence of metastatic cells in draining lymph nodes, the precise mechanisms by which tumour cells move preferentially towards particular lymph nodes remain poorly defined (Karnezis et al., 2012). It was originally envisaged that lymphatic invasion took place as an advancing tumour front eroding the walls of any vessels in its path and that metastasis occurred by passive drainage (Pepper, 2001). However, recent evidence indicates that a more complex interaction may take place between tumour cells and the lymphatic endothelial cells (LECs) (Qian et al., 2001). The availability of markers with specificity for LECs has enabled the identification and quantification of previously undiscernible lymphatic vessels in human cancer (Beasley et al., 2002) and other pathological states (Jeltsch et al., 1997; Karkkainen et al., 2000). Further, experimental and clinico-pathological studies indicate that lymphangiogenesis can contribute to the formation of these lymphatic vessels (Mandriota et al., 2001; Skobe et al., 2001; Stacker et al., 2001; Williams, 2003). Downstream from this lymphatic neo-vascularisation, there are likely to be pro-metastatic effects of lymphangiogenic growth factors on the collecting lymphatic vessel conduits, mediated by intermediary molecular mechanisms such as the prostaglandin pathway (Karnezis et al., 2012a,b). Finally, in the sentinel lymph node (SLN) itself, molecular signals from the primary tumour are likely to pre-induce a fertile niche for the metastasis and establishment of metastatic cell deposits (Farnsworth et al., 2011; Hirakawa et al., 2009).

Overall, an understanding of the molecular control of signalling pathways governing SLN spread may provide target molecules that may be exploited therapeutically to restrict cancer spread (Stacker et al., 2004). Thus, despite potentially significant side effects that may result from the disruption of lymphatic channels during regional lymph node clearance, this procedure remains critical in surgical oncological treatment and staging (Ferris et al., 2005). Ultimately however, the goal of clinicians would be to discover a feature of the primary tumour that would enable the prediction with greater certainty, which patients require completion of axillary lymph node clearance and which may safely be monitored without lymph node sampling or subsequent surgery (Shayan et al., 2012, 2013).

7.3 METASTASIS VIA THE LYMPHATIC SYSTEM AND SURGICAL PRINCIPLES OF SLNB

French surgeon LeDran first noted in the sixteenth century that patients in whom breast cancers spread to axillary lymph nodes had significantly worse survival outcomes than those in whom the cancers remained localised to the breast (LeDran et al., 1752). Some 200 years later, Halsted began performing radical excisions of both the primary breast cancer and the metastatic axillary lymph nodes lesions (Baum et al., 2005; Halsted, 1894). The next major clinical development regarding the lymphatics in cancer occurred in the 1950s when clinicians began to use radioisotope injections to better understand the regional lymph node groups that drained different regions of the body (Sherman and Ter-Pogossian, 1953). This work provided essential information for the identification of potential routes of cancer metastasis via the lymphatic vasculature. It was not until the 1950s that Turner-Warwick and Kinmonth adapted the idea of lymphatic injection for radiographic imaging in live patients (Kinmonth, 1972; Turner-Warwick, 1955). From this point onwards, imaging would become integral to the study of the lymphatic system. Using radioactive gold lymphoscintigraphy and radio-opaque dye, they imaged the lymphatic vasculature of living humans (Kinmonth, 1972; Turner-Warwick, 1955). Kinmonth demonstrated the collecting lymphatic vessel pathways in normal and diseased individuals, particularly in the upper and lower limbs. This methodology would come to form the basis of modern lymphoscintigraphy and SLNB. This important advance in clinical diagnostics was made initially in the 1970s, when the *SLN* theory was articulated by Cabanas for use in patients suffering squamous cell carcinoma of the penis (Cabanas, 1977). The technique was popularised for use in melanoma by Morton and Cochran (Cochran et al., 1992; Morton et al., 1992), as one method of sampling reliably those lymph nodes to which tumour cells had metastasised (Morton et al., 1992). The SLNB method has since been adapted for application to several other malignancies (Bilchik et al., 1998; Ferris et al., 2005; Shayan et al., 2006), in particular, squamous cell carcinoma of the skin (Doubrovsky et al., 2004; Thompson and Uren, 2001; Uren et al., 2001), carcinoma of the breast (Park et al., 2005), and carcinomas of the gastrointestinal tract (Wood et al., 2001).

The development of the SLNB technique (see Figure 7.1), which applied the combination of earlier lymphatic injection techniques with dynamic studies of existing drainage patterns, represented the latest in a long line of refinements to oncological surgery (Shayan et al., 2012). The use of lymphatic mapping techniques to predict each individual patient's lymphatic drainage from a specific tumour was a further step in the evolution of minimising the impact of surgical intervention in particular. The ability to identify the SLN – the first lymph node(s) draining the area of tissue in which the primary tumour occurs – enabled clinicians to select only those patients with demonstrated metastatic nodal disease for clearance of the nodal drainage basin (Cochran et al., 1992). Surgical excision of the SLN(s) is aimed at targeting the node(s) most likely to harbour metastatic

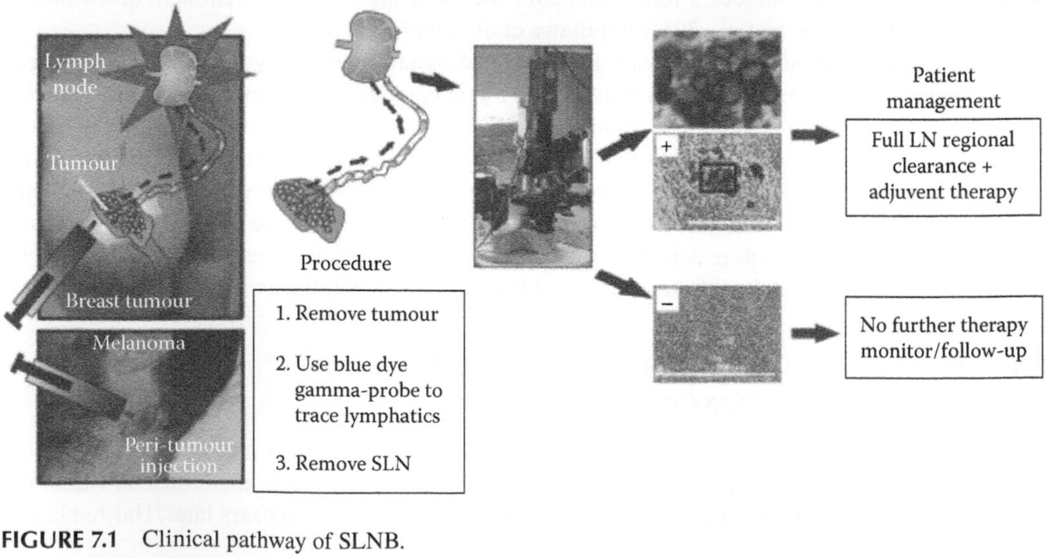

FIGURE 7.1 Clinical pathway of SLNB.

cancer cells (Cochran et al., 1992; Morton et al., 1992) and provides the node for histological examination by the pathologist. The presence or absence of metastatic cells on subsequent histological examination then determines further patient management (Sun and Haller, 2005). One of the greatest benefits that this technique offers patients is that by minimising unnecessary lymph node clearance in patients in whom detailed histological analysis reveals the SLN(s) to be free of metastasis – so-called 'SLN-negative' patients – this cohort, who would previously have been recommended to automatically undergo lymph node clearance, may be spared from this potentially morbid procedure (Wu et al., 2003). It is estimated that 80% of patients who are eligible for SLNB are negative on histological examination and that a comparatively small 20% demonstrate cells within their sampled nodes, indicating that the managing surgeon should proceed to completion lymphadenectomy in that patient.

A negative SLN finding indicates that the patient is not usually required to undergo treatment for systemic cancer dissemination (Leong, 2004), as the absence of metastatic cancer cells within the sentinel node is taken to indicate disease-free status in the remaining lymph nodes in the nodal group (Thompson et al., 2004). Sparing the morbidity of further lymphablation surgery, which can lead to undesirable side effects such as lymphoedema (Starritt et al., 2004). Avoiding lymphablation also means that the majority of the lymph nodes within the basin are intact to perform their intended role of immune surveillance and filtering of pathogens. In contrast, histologically positive SLNs may predate overt clinically detectable metastatic disease or at least provide a clue that the tumour has metastatic propensity and may have seeded distant metastasis. In either case, it does indicate a poor prognosis (Cochran et al., 1992; Morton et al., 1992; Sun and Haller, 2005), even if they occur outside the area to which the tissue surrounding a tumour is expected to drain (Thelmo et al., 2001; Uren et al., 2003). Detection of positive SLN(s) results in reclassification of a patient to a group with higher risk of recurrence, which may render the patient eligible for systemic adjuvant treatment (Sun and Haller, 2005) and thus potentially result in improved survival (Bilchik, 2001; Scolyer et al., 2004; Takeuchi, 2004; Wolmark et al., 2001). Histological examination revealing a positive SLN identifies candidates in whom comprehensive or completion surgical lymph node dissection or clearance of the regional lymph node basin from which a *positive* SLN was sampled is indicated. Patients are recommended to undergo this procedure not only for focal disease control but also for prognostication and treatment-planning purposes (Leong et al., 2005). However, whether SLNB also provides a survival benefit is undecided and still the subject of large multicentre international trials (first, the Multicenter Selective Lymphadenectomy Trial [MSLT-I] [Morton et al., 2006] and, second, the Multicenter Selective Lymphadenectomy Trial [MSLT-II] [Morton, 2012]). MSLT-I, the first of these two trials, was intended to examine for a putative survival difference, once appropriate wide local excision has been performed, between patients randomised to the biopsy arm (patients undergoing SLNB and early completion lymphadenectomy when metastatic disease was identified) and the observation arm (observation alone and delayed completion lymphadenectomy only when lymphadenopathy became clinically palpable). However, during the course of the MSLT-I, it was stated that a subset of patients enrolled in the observation arm underwent screening with high-resolution ultrasound, facilitating detection prior to nodal metastasis becoming clinically detectable, thus confounding this arm of the study (Thomas, 2009). MSLT-II patients with histopathology or RT-PCR-proven tumour in the SLN were randomly assigned to receive completion lymph node dissection (CLND) or observation using serial ultrasound scans of the nodal basin in which the SLN was detected (Amersi and Morton, 2007). Patients who developed clinically detectable lymph node metastasis then underwent CLND (Amersi and Morton, 2007).

SLN biopsy facilitates the mapping of lymphatic pathways that drain a particular area of tissue, and it identifies the lymph nodes into which they drain (Leong, 2004). The more widespread use of SLNB has also resulted in the detection and location of potentially metastatic draining lymph nodes in unexpected sites (Thompson and Uren, 2001; Uren et al., 1995, 1998b). The use of a preoperative map of lymph node(s) draining a primary cancer is obtained by injection of a radiolabelled colloid (Nieweg et al., 2001) and a gamma camera that documents the lymphatic drainage over a time sequence. In addition, the intra-operative handheld gamma probe (Leong, 2003), combined with on-table injection of lymphatic-specific Patent Blue V dye (Thompson et al., 1999), enables the reliable detection, identification, and excisional biopsy of the SLN intra-operatively (Leong, 2004). When injections are located in or around a primary tumour, the performance of SLN sampling followed by detailed histological examination of the SLN(s) is considered to give an accurate prediction of the degree of cancer metastasis (detecting greater than 95% of SLNs [Carlson et al., 2002; Leong, 2004]). This detection rate represents a significant improvement on the detection rates utilising either radiolabelled colloid (Nieweg et al., 2001) or Patent Blue V dye (Thompson et al., 1999) alone. Nuclear medicine scans involve a technetium-labelled colloid tracer (technetium-99m or ^{99m}Tc) that is injected around the primary tumour in question, and a series of images are taken: one at the time of injection and then images at incremental time points for a set time thereafter. The injection of radiolabelled colloid is usually performed in the morning prior to an afternoon operating list or in the night before a morning operating list. In addition to these LS images obtained using nuclear imaging, handheld intra-operative gamma probes emitting gamma irradiation readings and audible tone as it approaches areas of higher concentration of radiolabelled colloid were also added to the standard technique of SLNB. A comparison of blue dye alone (69.5% accuracy in identifying lymph nodes) and ^{99m}Tc sulphur colloid (83.5% accuracy in identifying lymph nodes) conducted by Albertini and colleagues demonstrated improved detection rates of true SLNs for a particular injection site to 96% (Albertini et al., 1996; Carlson et al., 2002; Leong, 2004).

Amongst the foremost proponents of the SLNB techniques, the Sydney Melanoma Unit led by Thompson and Uren was amongst the most well respected and prolific. Their early work on melanoma LS studies demonstrated that although most cases exhibited typical ipsilateral drainage patterns, certain cases exhibited more unexpected contralateral drainage that contradicted Sappey's drawings (Uren et al., 1998a). As experience with SLNB improved, so too did the confidence with which observed patterns of lymphatic drainage were seen to contradict predictions of where lymphatics draining different locations should drain, according to the original Sappey model (Leong, 2006). Sappey's mercury injection studies show an ordered pattern of predictable and almost exclusive drainage to the major lymph node basins. Another recent example of this phenomenon of observed patterns of lymphatic drainage contradicting predictions of where tumours in different locations should spread to according to the original patterns described by Sappey was melanoma metastasis from a primary tumour located on the lower posterior truncal region, through deep para-aortic lymph nodes located deep within the retroperitoneal (Uren et al., 1998) or thoracic cavity (Uren et al., 1999). This drainage pattern bypasses the inguinal lymph nodes, to which this area of skin is expected to drain, and suggests that there may be previously unknown direct communications between the lower back and intra-thoracic/abdominal lymph nodes (Uren et al., 1998a). Other examples were of forearm lesions draining to the supraclavicular lymph nodes (Uren et al., 1996), central inter-scapular primary lesions, or lesions on one or other side of the midline draining across the traditional watershed areas to the contralateral or bilateral axillary lymph node basins (Uren et al., 2003).

In performing LS, there are a number of variable factors to consider, which may be responsible for any observed variations. These include the tracer radioisotope and dosage used, the location(s) chosen to inject the tracer, and the imaging protocol(s) implemented. In most centres, ^{99m}Tc-labelled colloids for the mainstay for SLNB mapping (Uren et al., 2003).

Colloidal particle size is an important characteristic when considering which radiopharmaceutical should be used for mapping SLN in LS. Tsopelas demonstrated that the particle size of ^{99m}Tc-labelled colloids was (in 96% of particles) under 100 nm diameter (Tsopelas, 2001). SLN biopsy facilitates the mapping of lymphatic pathways that drain a particular area of tissue, and it identifies the lymph nodes into which they drain (Leong, 2004). The detection and location of potentially metastatic draining lymph nodes in unexpected sites (Thompson and Uren, 2001; Uren et al., 1998b, 1995) occur at a rate of up to 30% (Uren et al., 2006). Regardless of whether the draining nodal basin is expected (largely defined in anatomical texts by Sappey's original studies) or in an unusual location, any clinical benefits to the patient lie in the accurate detection and sampling of the true draining SLN (Uren et al., 2006).

Clinical observations of unpredictable metastatic patterns such as those outlined earlier have led to the teaching that melanoma metastasis is particularly unpredictable according to the traditional understanding of lymphatic drainage patterns. However, such phenomena may simply be due to metastatic lymphatic pathways that were not originally identified by Sappey's mercury injections over a century ago. Overall, the targeted approach employed in SLNB has seen a drastic reduction in the number of radical axillary lymph node dissections that are performed; this has decreased potential complications such as lymphoedema, which in turn increases the risk of infection and limb discomfort (Wu et al., 2003). Nevertheless, a 5%–10% complication rate is still quoted for lymphoedema. Similarly, whilst not well documented in the literature, there are definitely risks of injury in particular to cutaneous nerves in and around the major lymph node basins. A worldwide web-based survey was conducted amongst melanoma surgeons to investigate opinions about CLND in patients with positive SLNs. The questionnaire was designed by a group of melanoma surgeons (30.1% in a dedicated melanoma unit, 44.6% in a surgical oncology unit) identified through a systematic review of the SLNB and CLND literature and invited by e-mail. Of 193 surgeons (from 25 countries), 91.8% of surgeons responded that they would recommend that patients with a positive SLNB undergo CLND. For patients requiring CLND in the neck, 62% base the extent of dissection on primary site and lymphatic mapping patterns, whereas empirical level 1–5 dissections were recommended by 35% of responders. Most surgeons (81%) perform full axillary dissections in positive SN cases. Enrolment in the MSLT-II was recommended to patients by only 71 (37%) responders, with 64 of the 71 suggesting entering patients into trials to majority of patients.

7.4 NEW FRONTIERS IN SLNB

Whilst it is currently the gold standard in patient prognostication, lymph node sampling is not without potentially significant adverse effects. Researchers have continually been trying to refine the process and reduce the surgical risk to patients and to be able to more accurately predict which patients will derive potential benefit from lymph node clearance surgery. To this end, Reynolds et al. developed computational models to provide improved visualisation and analysis of the functional lymphatic anatomy of the skin and to assess historical assumptions about lymphatic anatomy (Reynolds et al., 2007, 2009). In their studies, accumulated 2D melanoma LS data were used from over 5000 patients with cutaneous melanoma treated at the Sydney Melanoma Unit, Australia. The 2D LS data were mapped onto an anatomically based 3D computer model of the skin and lymph nodes. Spatial analysis was then carried out to visualise the relationship between primary melanoma sites and the locations of draining SLNs, which collectively showed patterns of skin lymphatic drainage.

Probability diagrams known as *heat maps* were generated to represent the data and to enable visualisation of the patterns of drainage from the skin to each node field, highlighting the inter-patient variability in skin lymphatic drainage and showing the skin regions in which the most highly variable drainage would occur. Results from these studies indicated that the most variable drainage patterns included skin on the torso close to Sappey's lines (Reynolds et al., 2007) and skin on the head and neck[3] and that, overall, the commonly used concept of Sappey's lines were not effective in predicting lymphatic drainage. Results also showed that although lymphatic drainage of the head and neck is highly complex and clinically unpredictable, there were still clear patterns of drainage shown. Some nodal fields drained relatively circumscribed areas of skin, particularly the pre-auricular and occipital node fields, which drained large regions of the head and neck. Overall, the 3D models developed by Reynolds et al. quantitatively updated the knowledge of lymphatic drainage of the skin, demonstrating how they differed from traditional anatomical descriptions and are available to view online at www.bioeng.auckland.ac.nz/melanoma and www.bioeng.auckland.ac.nz/head.

Further, Reynolds et al. conducted a thorough statistical analysis to move towards a purely data-driven approach (Reynolds et al., 2010). Results indicated that most skin regions showed symmetric lymphatic drainage about the coronal midline of the body. Subsequent cluster analysis showed a clear anatomical division of the skin into nine separate clusters, primarily grouping regions of skin according to the dominant draining node fields: the axilla, groin, cervical level II, and pre-auricular node fields. Interestingly, the clusters draining primarily to axillary and groin node fields divided the trunk into regions comparable to Sappey's lines. Even though there was variability of lymphatic drainage on the torso between individuals, Sappey's lines appeared to conform to the most likely drainage behaviour of these data.

LS imaging has also been used to determine SLN locations in patients with breast cancer, demonstrating lymphatic drainage patterns of the breast. In 2011, Blumgart et al. conducted studies into lymphatic drainage of the breast using aggregated LS data from 2304 patients from the Royal Prince Alfred Hospital, Sydney, Australia (Blumgart et al., 2011a). Their study aimed to test commonly held assumptions of breast lymphatic anatomy, where results confirmed the left and right breasts are likely to have symmetric drainage patterns and that there is likely no statistically significant difference between the draining breast lymphatics of males and females. Furthermore, results showed that direct lymphatic drainage of the breasts is likely to be independent between node fields.

These breast LS data were also modelled and mapped onto a 3D computational model of the breast and sentinel node field locations (Blumgart et al., 2011b). The likelihood of drainage to each node field from the whole breast and from each breast region was calculated using Bayesian inferential techniques. Patterns were observed in the drainage where regions anatomically close to each node field showed an increased drainage to that node field. In addition, as expected, the breast almost always drained to the axillary node field (98.2%) and frequently to the internal mammary node field (35.3%). Additional draining node fields included the infraclavicular, supraclavicular, and interpectoral node fields with 1.7%, 3.1%, and 0.7% patients, respectively. These results are available to visualise online at www.abi.auckland.ac.nz/breast-cancer.

7.5 PRIMARY TUMOUR CHARACTERISTICS AS MARKERS OF SENTINEL LYMPH NODE STATUS

The recent advent of markers with affinity for lymphatics has allowed the identification and quantification of lymphatic vessels in tissue (Shayan et al., 2006), and some studies suggest that the amount of lymphangiogenesis within the tumours (as shown by lymphatic vessel density [LVD]) could predict which of the regional lymph nodes harbour tumour cells and therefore may also provide a valuable prognostic indicator (Shayan et al., 2012). It is unclear, however, whether the presence, density, distribution, or patency of lymphatics in different regions of the primary tumour (e.g. intra-tumoural vs. peri-tumoural areas) is the most important in predicting the risk of metastasis (Shayan et al., 2012) or whether collecting vessels between the primary tumour and lymph node(s) could also be a contributing factor (Karnezis et al., 2012). If significant differences between LVDs in metastasising tumours and non-metastasising tumours were present, the LVD could be used to assist in disease staging, prognostication, and clinical decision-making, in addition to selecting patients who could benefit from therapeutic trials. The ultimate aim would be to use the LVD analysis of the primary tumour to obviate the need for SLNB, altogether.

To directly address whether lymphatic vessel nature or location influenced the metastatic potential melanomas, Shayan et al. identified and compared the number (LVD) and morphology of lymphatic vessels in two groups of primary cutaneous melanomas, which had been matched for key established prognostic factors. These factors included tumour thickness, mitotic rate, and whether or not the tumours were ulcerated, and tumours that had been shown to result in a positive SLN were matched with identical tumours that were non-metastatic. The sample groups, obtained from the Sydney Melanoma Unit database, consisted of 11 metastasising and 11 non-metastasising primary melanoma samples that were analysed using antibody to podoplanin. Significant differences were identified between the LVDs in the peripheral (5.73 ± 0.68) and central regions (1.79 ± 0.42) of the metastasising tumour group ($P < .001$) and between the LVDs in the peripheral areas of metastasising (5.73 ± 0.68) and non-metastasising tumours (4.21 ± 0.37) ($P < .01$). Conversely, no overall difference was found between the total average LVDs in the two tumour groups nor between their vessel morphologies. Overall, the results of this study show that LVD is associated with the risk of lymph node metastasis and, furthermore, that the ratio of central LVD to peripheral LVD may prove to be a useful marker of primary melanomas that are likely to metastasise to the lymph node. This and other patterns or features that could differentiate between patients likely to harbour a metastatic deposit in a draining lymph node basin could serve as an indicator of which patients should proceed to a lymphatic mapping procedure or a regional lymph node clearance operation.

7.6 SPECT/CT IMAGING

Gamma cameras have been used traditionally during LS imaging; however, recent advances have been made in locating SLNs using SPECT/CT imaging. This hybrid imaging technology allows the nuclear medicine physician to determine the exact anatomical position of the SLN during preoperative LS in patients.

Due to the precise anatomical detail available in SPECT/CT, knowledge of the lymphatic anatomy can be further refined. For example, in a study by Uren et al., the anatomy of the axillary node field draining the breast has been reassessed using such images (Uren et al., 2012). Historically, it has been suggested that the lymphatic drainage of the breast was to lymph nodes lying in the antero-pectoral group of nodes in the axilla, just lateral to the pectoral muscles. Uren et al. were able to use LS performed using the SPECT/CT modalities to show that the breast does not always drain to the anterior group of level I lymph nodes in the axilla but may drain to the mid-axilla and/or posterior group in about 50% of patients with breast cancer, regardless of the location of the cancer within the breast itself. Further refinement of lymphatic anatomy should be possible using such imaging techniques and comparing them with current anatomical descriptions of the lymphatic network.

Preoperative injections of radioisotope tracer and Patent Blue V dye allow intra-operative identification of the SLN or SLNs. These are the lymph nodes deemed to be the primary draining lymph node or nodes on preoperative imaging and/or intra-operative detection by visualisation of a blue dye and/or detection of a radioactive count using a handheld gamma camera. The detected lymph node(s) is removed, fixed, and sectioned for review by a trained pathologist who identifies whether metastatic cells are present (meaning that, on the basis of evidence from large population-based studies, adjuvant treatment using chemo-/radiotherapy may be warranted) or absent (indicating that only careful monitoring and follow-up is sufficient to detect any unexpected recurrence or spread of disease in these patients).

Printed with permission: Ramin Shayan, Characterizing lymphatic vessel subtypes and their role in cancer metastasis (2009). PhD thesis, The University of Melbourne.

REFERENCES

Achen, M.G., Jeltsch, M., Kukk, E., Makinen, T., Vitali, A., Wilks, A.F., Alitalo, K., and Stacker, S.A. (1998). Vascular endothelial growth factor D (VEGF-D) is a ligand for the tyrosine kinases VEGF receptor 2 (Flk1) and VEGF receptor 3 (Flt4). *Proc Natl Acad Sci USA* 95, 548–553.

Achen, M.G. and Stacker, S.A. (2008). Molecular control of lymphatic metastasis. *Ann NY Acad Sci* 1131, 225–234.

Adams, R.H. and Alitalo, K. (2007). Molecular regulation of angiogenesis and lymphangiogenesis. *Nat Rev Mol Cell Biol* 8, 464–478.

Albertini, J.J, Cruse, C.W., Rapaport, D., Wells, K., Ross, M., DeConti, R., Berman, C.G. et al. (1996). Intraoperative radio-lympho-scintigraphy improves sentinel lymph node identification for patient with melanoma. *Ann Surg* 223(2), 217–224.

Alitalo, K. and Carmeliet, P. (2002). Molecular mechanisms of lymphangiogenesis in health and disease. *Cancer Cell* 1, 219–227.

Alitalo, K., Tammela, T., and Petrova, T.V. (2005). Lymphangiogenesis in development and human disease. *Nature* 438, 946–953.

Amersi, F. and Morton, D.L. (2007). The role of sentinel lymph node biopsy in the management of melanoma. *Adv Surg* 41, 241–256.

Baldwin, M.E., Stacker, S.A., and Achen, M.G. (2002). Molecular control of lymphangiogenesis. *Bioessays* 24, 1030–1040.

Banerji, S., Ni, J., Wang, S.-X., Clasper, S., Su, J., Tammi, R., Jones, M., and Jackson, D.G. (1999). LYVE-1, a new homologue of the CD44 glycoprotein, is a lymph-specific receptor for hyaluronan. *J Cell Biol* 144, 789–801.

Baum, M., Demicheli, R., Hrushesky, W., and Retsky, M. (2005). Does surgery unfavourably perturb the "natural history" of early breast cancer by accelerating the appearance of distant metastases? *Eur J Cancer* 41, 508–515.

Beasley, N.J., Prevo, R., Banerji, S., Leek, R.D., Moore, J., van Trappen, P., Cox, G., Harris, A.L., and Jackson, D.G. (2002). Intratumoral lymphangiogenesis and lymph node metastasis in head and neck cancer. *Cancer Res* 62, 1315–1320.

Bilchik, A.J., Giuliano, A., Essner, R., Bostick, P., Kelemen, P., Foshag, L.J., Sostrin, S., Turner, R.R., and Morton, D.L. (1998). Universal application of intraoperative lymphatic mapping and sentinel lymphadenectomy in solid neoplasms. *Cancer J Sci Am* 4, 351–358.

Bilchik, A.J., Nora, D., Tollenaar, R.A., van de Velde, C.J., Wood, T., Turner, R., Morton, D.L., and Hoon, D.S. (2002). Ultrastaging of early colon cancer using lymphatic mapping and molecular analysis. *Eur J Cancer* 38, 977–985.

Bilchik, A.J., Saha, S., Tsioulias, G.J., Wood, T.F., and Morton, D.L. (2001). Aberrant drainage and missed micrometastases: The value of lymphatic mapping and focused analysis of sentinel lymph nodes in gastrointestinal neoplasms. *Ann Surg Oncol* 8, 82S–85S.

Blumgart, E.I., Uren, R.F., Nielsen, P.M.F., Nash, M.P., and Reynolds, H.M. (2011a). Lymphatic drainage and tumour prevalence in the breast: A statistical analysis of symmetry, gender and node field independence. *J Anat* 218, 652–659.

Blumgart, E.I., Uren, R.F., Nielsen, P.M.F., Nash, M.P., and Reynolds, H.M. (2011b). Predicting lymphatic drainage patterns and primary tumour location in patients with breast cancer. *Breast Cancer Res Treat* 130, 699–705.

Cabanas, R.M. (1977). An approach for the treatment of penile carcinoma. *Cancer Cell* 39, 456–466.

Carlson, G.W., Murray, D.R., Thourani, V., Hestley, A., and Cohen, C. (2002). The definition of the sentinel lymph node in melanoma based on radioactive counts. *Ann Surg Oncol* 9, 929–933.

Cochran, A.J., Wen, D.R., and Morton, D.L. (1992). Management of the regional lymph nodes in patients with cutaneous malignant melanoma. *World J Surg* 16, 214–221.

Courtice, F.C. (1951). Extravascular protein and the lymphatics. *Med J Aust* 2, 169–170.

Dadras, S.S., Bertoncini, P.T., Brown, L.F., Muzikansky, A., Jackson, D.G., Ellwanger, U., Garbe, C., Mihm, M.C., and Detmar, M. (2004). Tumor lymphangiogenesis: A novel prognostic indicator for cutaneous melanoma metastasis and survival. *Am J Pathol* 162, 1951–1960.

DeVita, V.T., Hellman, S., and Rosenberg, A. (2001). *Cancer, Principles and Practice of Oncology*, 6th edn. Philadelphia, PA: Lippincott, Williams and Wilkins.

Doubrovsky, A., De Wilt, J.H., Scolyer, R.A., McCarthy, W.H., and Thompson, J.F. (2004). Sentinel node biopsy provides more accurate staging than elective lymph node dissection in patients with cutaneous melanoma. *Ann Surg Oncol* 11, 829–836.

Dunglison, R. (1841). *Human Physiology*, Vol. 2. Philadelphia, PA: Lea and Blanchard.

Farnsworth, R., Karnezis, T., Shayan, R., Matsumoto, M., Nowell, C., Achen, M., and Stacker S. (2011). A role for bone morphogenetic protein-4 in lymph node vascular remodeling and primary tumor growth. *Cancer Res* 71, 6547–6557.

Ferris, R.L., Xi, L., Raja, S., Hunt, J.L., Wang, J., Gooding, W.E., Kelly, L., Ching, J., Luketich, J.D., and Godfrey, T.E. (2005). Molecular staging of cervical lymph nodes in squamous cell carcinoma of the head and neck. *Cancer Res* 65, 2147–2156.

Fidler, I.J. (2003). The pathogenesis of cancer metastasis: The 'seed and soil' hypothesis revisited. *Nat Rev Cancer* 3, 453–458.

Haagensen, C.D., Feind, C.R., Herter, F.P., Slanetz, C.A., and Weinberg, J.A. (1972). *The Lymphatics in Cancer*, 1st edn. Philadelphia, PA: W.B. Saunders.

Halsted, W. (1894). The results of operations for the cure of cancer of the breast. *Johns Hopkins Hosp Rep* 4, 297–350.

Hirakawa, S., Kodama, S., Kunstfeld, R., Kajiya, K., Brown, L.F., and Detmar, M. (2005). VEGF-A induces tumor and sentinel lymph node lymphangiogenesis and promotes lymphatic metastasis. *J Exp Med* 201, 1089–1099.

Jeltsch, M., Kaipainen, A., Joukov, V., Meng, X., Lakso, M., Rauvala, H., Swartz, M., Fukumura, D., Jain, R.K., and Alitalo, K. (1997). Hyperplasia of lymphatic vessels in VEGF-C transgenic mice. *Science* 276, 1423–1425.

Joukov, V., Pajusola, K., Kaipainen, A., Chilov, D., Lahtinen, I., Kukk, E., Saksela, O., Kalkkinen, N., and Alitalo, K. (1996). A novel vascular endothelial growth factor, VEGF-C, is a ligand for the Flt-4 (VEGFR-3) and KDR (VEGFR-2) receptor tyrosine kinases. *EMBO J* 15, 290–298.

Karkkainen, M.J., Ferrell, R.E., Lawrence, E.C., Kimak, M.A., Levinson, K.L., McTigue, M.A., Alitalo, K., and Finegold, D.N. (2000). Missense mutations interfere with VEGFR-3 signalling in primary lymphoedema. *Nat Genet* 25, 153–159.

Karkkainen, M.J., Mäkinen, T., and Alitalo, K. (2002). Lymphatic endothelium: A new frontier of metastasis research. *Nat Cell Biol* 4, E2–E5.

Karnezis, T., Shayan, R., Caesar, C., Roufail, S., Ardipradja, K., Harris, N.C., Farnsworth, R.H. et al. (2012a). VEGF-D promotes tumor metastasis by regulating prostaglandins produced by the collecting lymphatic endothelium. *Cancer Cell* 21, 181–195.

Karnezis, T., Shayan, R., Fox, S., Achen, M.G., and Stacker, S.A. (2012b). The connection between lymphangiogenic signaling and prostaglandin biology: A missing link in the metastatic pathway. *Oncotarget* 3(8), 890–903. Epub 2012 Aug 19.

Kinmonth, J.B. (1972). *The Lymphatics: Diseases, Lymphography, and Surgery*, 1st edn. London, U.K.: Edward Arnold.

Last, R.J. (1998). *Last's Anatomy: Regional and Applied*, 9th edn. Edinburgh, U.K.: Churchill Livingstone.

LeDran, H., Gataker, T., and Chelsden, W. (1752). *Traite des operations de chirurgie* [English tanslation Gataker], 2nd edn. London, U.K.: C Hitch, R Dosley.

Leong, S.P. (2003). Selective sentinel lymphadenectomy for malignant melanoma. *Surg Clin North Am* 83, 157–185, vii.

Leong, S.P. (2004). Sentinel lymph node mapping and selective lymphadenectomy: The standard of care for melanoma. *Curr Treat Options Oncol* 5, 185–194.

Leong, S.P., Morita, E.T., Sudmeyer, M., Chang, J., Shen, D., Achtem, T.A., Allen, R.E., Jr., and Kashani-Sabet, M. (2005). Heterogeneous patterns of lymphatic drainage to sentinel lymph nodes by primary melanoma from different anatomic sites. *Clin Nucl Med* 30, 150–158.

Mandriota, S.J., Jussila, L., Jeltsch, M., Compagni, A., Baetens, D., Prevo, R., Banerji, S. et al. (2001). Vascular endothelial growth factor-C-mediated lymphangiogenesis promotes tumour metastasis. *EMBO J* 20, 672–682.

Morton, D.L. (2012). Overview and update of the phase III Multicenter Selective Lymphadenectomy Trials (MSLT-I and MSLT-II) in melanoma. *Clin Exp Metastasis* 29(7), 699–706. doi: 10.1007/s10585-012-9503-3. Epub 2012 June 24.

Morton, D.L., Thompson, J.F., Cochran, A.J., Mozzillo, N., Elashoff, R., Essner, R., Nieweg, O.E. et al. (2006). Sentinel-node biopsy or nodal observation in melanoma. *N Engl J Med* 355, 1307–1317. doi: 10.1056/NEJMoa060992.

Morton, D.L., Wen, D.R., Wong, J.H., Economou, J.S., Cagle, L.A., Storm, F.K., Foshag, L.J., and Cochran, A.J. (1992). Technical details of intraoperative lymphatic mapping for early stage melanoma. *Arch Surg* 127, 392–399.

Nieweg, O.E., Tanis, P.J., and Kroon, B.B. (2001). The definition of a sentinel node. *Ann Surg Oncol* 8, 538–541.

Park, C., Seid, P., Morita, E., Iwanaga, K., Weinberg, V., Quivey, J., Hwang, E.S., Esserman, L.J., and Leong, S.P. (2005). Internal mammary sentinel lymph node mapping for invasive breast cancer: Implications for staging and treatment. *Breast J* 11, 29–33.

Pepper, M.S. and Skobe, M. (2003). Lymphatic endothelium: Morphological, molecular and functional properties. *J Cell Biol* 163, 209–213.

Qian, F., Hanahan, D., and Weissman, I.L. (2001). L-selectin can facilitate metastasis to lymph nodes in a transgenic mouse model of carcinogenesis. *Proc Natl Acad Sci USA* 98, 3976–3981.

Ramaswamy, S., Ross, K.N., Lander, E.S., and Golub, T.R. (2003). A molecular signature of metastasis in primary solid tumors. *Nat Genet* 33, 49–54.

Reynolds, H.M., Dunbar, P.R., Uren, R.F., Thompson, J.F., and Smith, N.P. (2007). Three-dimensional visualisation of lymphatic drainage patterns in patients with cutaneous melanoma. *Lancet Oncol* 8, 806–812.

Reynolds, H.M., Smith, N.P., Uren, R.F., Thompson, J.F., and Dunbar, P.R. (2009). Three-dimensional visualization of skin lymphatic drainage patterns of the head and neck. *Head & Neck* 31, 1316–1325.

Reynolds, H.M., Walker, C.G., Dunbar, P.R., O'Sullivan, M.J., Uren, R., Thompson, J.F., and Smith, N.P. (2010). Functional anatomy of the lymphatics draining the skin: A detailed statistical analysis. *J Anat* 216, 344–355.

Robbins, S. (1999). *Pathologic Basis of Disease*, 6th edn. Philadelphia, PA: W.B. Saunders Company.

Robinson, B. (1907). Chapter XXXVIII: The pathologic physiology of (I.) tractus lymphaticus, (II.) lymph. In *The Abdominal and Pelvic Brain*.

Rusznyak, I., Foldi, M., and Szabo, G., eds. (1960). *Lymphatics and Lymph Circulation*. New York: Pergamon Press.

Sappy, P.C. (1874). *Anatomie, physiologie, pathologie des vaisseaux lymphatiques: considérés chez l'homme et les vertébrés* [Anatomy, Physiology and Pathology of Lymphatic Vessels in Man and Vertebrates]. Paris, France: DeLahaye, A & Lacrosnier, E Eds.

Scolyer, R.A., Thompson, J.F., Li, L.X., Beavis, A., Dawson, M., Doble, P., Ka, V.S. et al. (2004). Failure to remove true sentinel nodes can cause failure of the sentinel node biopsy technique: Evidence from antimony concentrations in false-negative sentinel nodes from melanoma patients. *Ann Surg Oncol* 11, 174S–178S.

Shayan, R., Achen, M.G., and Stacker, S.A. (2006). Lymphatic vessels in cancer metastasis: Bridging the gaps. *Carcinogenesis* 27, 1729–1738.

Shayan, R., Inder, R., Karnezis, T., Caesar, C., Paavonen, K., Ashton, M.W., Mann, G.B., Taylor, G.I., Achen, M.G., and Stacker, S.A. (2013). Tumor location and nature of lymphatic vessels are key determinants of the metastatic spread of cancer. *Clin Exp Metastasis* 30(3), 345–356. doi: 10.1007/s10585-012-9541-x.

Shayan, R., Karnezis, T., Murali, R., Wilmott, J., Ashton, M.W., Taylor, G.I., Thompson, J.F. et al. (2012). Lymphatic vessel density in primary melanomas predicts sentinel lymph node status and risk of metastasis. *Histopathology* 61, 702–710. doi: 10.1111/j.1365-2559.2012.04310.x.

Sherman, A.I. and Ter-Pogossian, M. (1953). Lymph-node concentration of radioactive colloidal gold following interstitial injection. *Cancer* 6, 1238–1240.

Skobe, M. and Detmar, M. (2000). Structure, function, and molecular control of the skin lymphatic system. *J Invest Dermatol Symp Proc* 5, 14–19.

Skobe, M., Hawighorst, T., Jackson, D.G., Prevo, R., Janes, L., Velasco, P., Riccardi, L., Alitalo, K., Claffey, K., and Detmar, M. (2001). Induction of tumor lymphangiogenesis by VEGF-C promotes breast cancer metastasis. *Nat Med* 7, 192–198.

Stacker, S.A., Achen, M.G., Jussila, L., Baldwin, M.E., and Alitalo, K. (2002a). Lymphangiogenesis and cancer metastasis. *Nat Rev Cancer* 2, 573–583.

Stacker, S.A., Baldwin, M.E., and Achen, M.G. (2002b). The role of tumor lymphangiogenesis in metastatic spread. *FASEB J* 16, 922–934.

Stacker, S.A., Caesar, C., Baldwin, M.E., Thornton, G.E., Williams, R.A., Prevo, R., Jackson, D.G., Nishikawa, S., Kubo, H., and Achen, M.G. (2001). VEGF-D promotes the metastatic spread of tumor cells via the lymphatics. *Nat Med* 7, 186–191.

Stacker, S.A., Hughes, R.A., and Achen, M.G. (2004). Molecular targeting of lymphatics for therapy. *Curr Pharm Des* 10, 65–74.

Starritt, E.C., Joseph, D., McKinnon, J.G., Lo, S.K., de Wilt, J.H., and Thompson, J.F. (2004). Lymphedema after complete axillary node dissection for melanoma: Assessment using a new, objective definition. *Ann Surg* 240, 866–874.

Sun, W. and Haller, D.G. (2005). Adjuvant therapy of colon cancer. *Semin Oncol* 32, 95–102.

Thelmo, M.C., Morita, E.T., Treseler, P.A., Nguyen, L.H., Allen, R.E., Jr., Sagebiel, R.W., Kashani-Sabet, M., and Leong, S.P. (2001). Micrometastasis to in-transit lymph nodes from extremity and truncal malignant melanoma. *Ann Surg Oncol* 8, 444–448.

Thompson, J.F., Stretch, J.R., Uren, R.F., Ka, V.S., and Scolyer, R.A. (2004). Sentinel node biopsy for melanoma: Where have we been and where are we going? *Ann Surg Oncol* 11, 147S–151S.

Thompson, J.F. and Uren, R.F. (2001). Anomalous lymphatic drainage patterns in patients with cutaneous melanoma. *Tumori* 87, S54–S56.

Thompson, J.F., Uren, R.F., Shaw, H.M., McCarthy, W.H., Quinn, M.J., O'Brien, C.J., and Howman-Giles, R.B. (1999). Location of sentinel lymph nodes in patients with cutaneous melanoma: New insights into lymphatic anatomy. *J Am Coll Surg* 189, 195–204.

Threadgill, D.W. (2005). Metastatic potential as a heritable trait. *Nat Genet* 37, 1026–1027.

Tsopelas C. (2001). Particle size analysis of (99m)Tc-labeled and unlabeled antimony trisulfide and rhenium sulfide colloids intended for lymphoscintigraphic application. *J Nucl Med* 42(3), 460–466.

Turner-Warwick, R.Y. (1955). The demonstration of lymphatic vessels. *Lancet* 2, 1371.

Uren, R.F., Howman-Giles, R., Chung, D., Spillane, A., Noushi, F., Gillett, D., Gluch, L. et al. (2012). SPECT/CT scans allow precise anatomical location of sentinel lymph nodes in breast cancer and redefine lymphatic drainage from the breast to the axilla. *Breast* 21, 480–486.

Uren, R.F., Howman-Giles, R., Renwick, S.B., and Gillett, D. (2001). Lymphatic mapping of the breast: Locating the sentinel lymph nodes. *World J Surg* 25, 789–793.

Uren, R.F., Howman-Giles, R., and Thompson, J.F. (1998a). Lymphatic drainage from the skin of the back to retroperitoneal and paravertebral lymph nodes in melanoma patients. *Ann Surg Oncol* 5, 384–387.

Uren, R.F., Howman-Giles, R., and Thompson, J.F. (1999). Direct lymphatic drainage from a melanoma on the back to paravertebral lymph nodes in the thorax. *Clin Nucl Med* 24, 388–389.

Uren, R.F., Howman-Giles, R., and Thompson, J.F. (2003). Patterns of lymphatic drainage from the skin in patients with melanoma. *J Nucl Med* 44, 570–582.

Uren, R.F., Howman-Giles, R., Thompson, J.F., and Quinn, M.J. (1996). Direct lymphatic drainage from the skin of the forearm to a supraclavicular node. *Clin Nucl Med* 21, 387–389.

Uren, R.F., Howman-Giles, R.B., Thompson, J.F., Roberts, J., and Bernard, E. (1998b). Variability of cutaneous lymphatic flow rates in melanoma patients. *Melanoma Res* 8, 279–282.

Uren, R.F., Howman-Giles, R.B., Thompson, J.F., Shaw, H.M., and McCarthy, W.H. (1995). Lymphatic drainage from peri-umbilical skin to internal mammary nodes. *Clin Nucl Med* 20, 254–255.

Uren, R.F., Thompson, J.F., Howman-Giles, R., and Chung, D.K. (2006). The role of lymphoscintigraphy in the detection of lymph node drainage in melanoma. *Surg Oncol Clin N Am* 15(2), 285–300.

Wolmark, N., Wang, J., Mamounas, E., Bryant, J., and Fisher, B. (2001). Preoperative chemotherapy in patients with operable breast cancer: Nine-year results from National Surgical Adjuvant Breast and Bowel Project B-18. *J Natl Cancer Inst Monogr* 96–102.

Wood, T.F., Spirt, M., Rangel, D., Shen, P., Tsioulias, G.J., Morton, D.L., and Bilchik, A.J. (2001). Lymphatic mapping improves staging during laparoscopic colectomy for cancer. *Surg Endosc* 15, 715–719.

Wu, C.T., Morita, E.T., Treseler, P.A., Esserman, L.J., Hwang, E.S., Kuerer, H.M., Santos, C.L., and Leong, S.P. (2003). Failure to harvest sentinel lymph nodes identified by preoperative lymphoscintigraphy in breast cancer patients. *Breast J* 9, 86–90.

Yoffey, J.M. and Courtice, F.C. (1970). *Lymphatics, Lymph and the Lymphomyeloid Complex.* London, U.K.: Academic Press.

Yoffey, J.M. and Drinker, C.K. (1939). Some observations on the lymphatics of the nasal mucous membrane in the cat and monkey. *J Anat* 74, 45–52.

8 Free Flap Revascularisation Process

Emanuele Cigna, Federico Lo Torto, Alessandro Napoli, Jiří Veselý, and Diego Ribuffo

CONTENTS

8.1 HISTORY

Between the end of the sixteenth and the beginning of the twentieth century, surgeons began to approximate the vessels.[1,2]

First in 1902, Alexis Carrel reported the triangulation method of end-to-end anastomosis, which is still routinely used today and for which he was awarded the Nobel Prize in 1912. At the same time, he suggested to use the latero-terminal (LT) technique for the anastomosis of vessels of different size.[3] Finally, the innovation that led to the foundation of modern microvascular surgery was the introduction of the operating microscope by Nylen.[4]

Subsequently, in 1958, Onji and Tamai attempted to revascularise an incompletely amputated thigh on a 12-year-old girl at the Nara Medical University Hospital in Japan, but the extremity was lost 4 weeks after the revascularisation because of overwhelming infection and thrombosis.[5]

Following this first report, in 1962, Malt and McKhann performed the first replantation of a completely amputated arm in a 12-year-old boy in Boston. Two years later, Kleinert and Kasdan successfully revascularised an incompletely amputated thumb.

However, the first reported successful transfer of the greater omentum for scalp reconstruction in a patient was performed by McLean and Buncke.[6]

Daniel and Taylor performed a free-tissue transfer of groin flap for scalp reconstruction in 1973; so it represents the world's first clinical free skin flap transfer.[7]

During this period, new tissue donor sites and flap variations were described and research on limb–digit replantation and free-tissue transfer went along worldwide.[8]

Furthermore, Taylor and Palmer mapped the vascular anatomy of the skin, identifying an average of 374 dominant cutaneous vessels of 0.5 mm or greater in diameter and introduced the angiosome concept.[9–11]

Nowadays different microvascular flaps are available varying in size, volume, tissue, texture, and blood supply.

The advent of reconstructive microsurgery has allowed both the coverage of complex defects and the reduction of instances of inoperability. However, although the use of free flaps has become a routine practice with a success rate of 95%–100%,[12–17] the pathophysiology of these autologous transplantations is not yet clear.

However, radiological techniques have allowed to study the revascularisation process of free flaps and to evaluate their vascular changes over time.

Various techniques and measurements are described in literature for the postoperative monitoring of free flaps.[18–22] Several retrospective clinical studies have been performed to highlight the causes of the complications of free flap as bruising, bleeding,[23,24] postoperative thrombosis,[25–27] and necrosis or free flap failure.[28–31] However, few studies have investigated the postoperative haemodynamic changes charged to the free flap and the recipient area. Few studies have tried to investigate clinical cases, in which a free flap survived after a total thrombosis of its pedicle[32–38] or cases where the transplant developed total necrosis a few years after its transfer.[39]

8.2 FASCIOCUTANEOUS FREE FLAPS

Free cutaneous, fasciocutaneous, and fascial flaps are characterised by a low metabolic rate, reflecting in a long ischaemia time. Their versatility can afford coverage or reconstruction of defects of any region of the body from the head and neck to the lower limbs (LLs).[40–47] For this reason, they are probably the most used in microsurgery.

O'Brien reported one of the first experimental studies on animals in 1978[46] noting that, in all cases, the free flap survived to the section of its pedicle after the eighth postoperative day. However, the survival of the flap was considered unpredictable when the section occurred previously. Interestingly, in 1982, Fried[47] performed a study investigating three different aspects of free flap revascularisation:

1. The role of the pedicle
2. The role of the recipient site
3. The role of the contact surface between the flap and recipient site

The outcomes showed that the most important factor was the pedicle. In fact, the section led to flap necrosis in 90% of cases.

In 1988, Oswald evaluated free flap survival after ligation of its pedicle in an experimental model. When performed in the second postoperative day, it led to necrosis in all of the reported cases, while the binding in the second to the fourth day had controversial results. However, the study demonstrated the absence of necrosis in case of ligation of the pedicle after the fifth post operative days (POD). The authors also suggested that the venous connection was formed earlier than the arterial around the fourth postoperative day.[48]

The first clinical case described in literature of free flap survival after ligation of the pedicle was reported by Gilbert in 1976. He described a flap survived after occlusion of its pedicle in the 14th POD.[49] Similar cases were reported by Acland[50] and Ribuffo,[38] respectively, in 1983 and 2004.

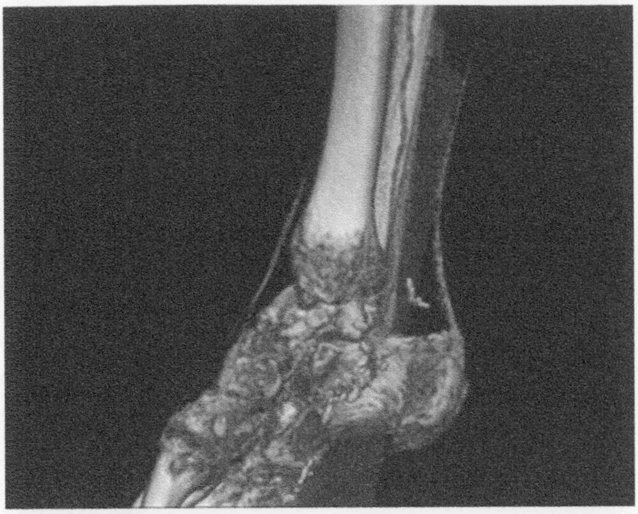

FIGURE 8.1 Angio-TC: no signal pedicle of an anterolater thigh free flap for foot reconstruction.

Recently, Mucke et al. published an interesting study on revascularisation of flaps inserted into the oral cavity. This study revealed that free flaps were able to autonomise over time according to the clinical situation of each patient: preoperative radiation, tumour site, and type of free flap reconstruction. Values were found to be significantly different at the different sites of reconstruction, revealing the influence of the recipient area.[51]

He demonstrated that revascularisation was reached at 4 weeks depending on the flap type, the area of reconstruction, and the recipient bed. Even after 12 weeks, some flaps at the hard or soft palate were still dependent on their axial blood supply.

Moreover, remarkable is the case reported by Dr. Sean R. Wise. An anterolateral thigh free flap was transferred for reconstruction of a tongue base defect, with the flap surviving despite loss of its arterial and venous pedicle on postoperative day 9 (Figure 8.1).[52] The imagine 8.1 is an example and does not refer to a specific case.

8.3 MUSCULOCUTANEOUS AND MUSCLE FREE FLAP

Musculocutaneous and muscle free flaps are characterised by a high metabolic rate.

Salmi et al. demonstrated that muscle free flaps tended to maintain the vascular pedicle more active when used for reconstruction of the LLs (91%) rather than for other districts.[53]

In 1988, Machens reported an interesting study on the vascular pedicle of the latissimus dorsi (LAT D). He noted that, in 100% of cases in study,[54] the pedicles were pervious and active 10 years after the transfer; he also studied how this result varied according to the number of complications encountered in the early postoperative period.[55] In fact, two groups of patients with 8–10 years of follow-up were compared: the first group had no perioperative complications, while the second group was composed by patients who underwent to a revision surgery for several reasons with clinical success.[55]

The study showed that in the first group, 100% of the flaps were dependent by the pedicle, while in the second group only a 50% of cases.

As in the previous case, another study reported a 100% patency of the pedicle of muscle free flaps examined. The same result was obtained in different free muscle flaps as LAT D, Transverse Rectus Abdominis Musculocutaneous (TRAM), or gracilis muscle flap.[56] The role of pedicle was confirmed also in patients with arterial bypass used for blood supply of LLs and free flaps.[57–59] In 1982, Khoo reported his experience with three cases of failure in the 17th and 14th postoperative day of muscle free flaps for reconstruction of the LLs.[60]

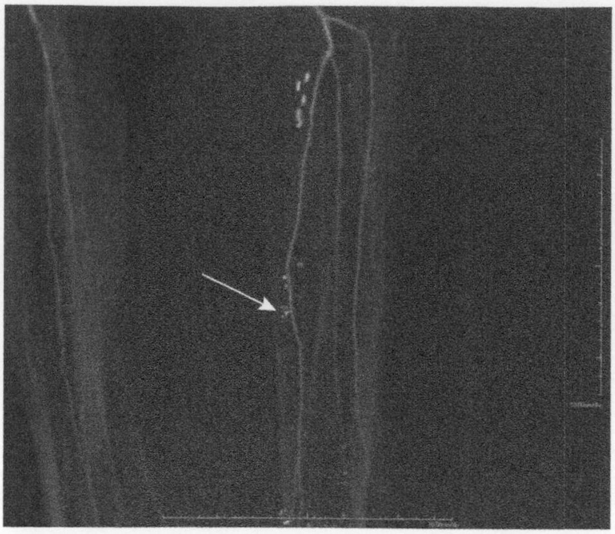

FIGURE 8.2 Angio CT scan showing the pedicle of a gracilis free flap for tibial osteomyelitis.

One case of rectus abdominis flap was recently reported by Lau,[61] used to reconstruct two amputated limbs. At the sixth postoperative week, the flap was divided and no necrosis occurred in the revascularised side (Figure 8.2). The imagine 8.2 is an example and does not refer to a specific case.

8.4 PERFORATOR FREE FLAPS

Perforator free flaps seem to behave in an intermediate manner between the fasciocutaneous flaps and the muscle flaps, resembling to the one or to the other depending on the volume of tissue transferred. In fact, in 2005, Moolenburgh reported some Deep Inferior Epigastric Perforator (DIEP) failures 3 years after its transfer.[39]

8.5 BONE FREE FLAP

The bone free flaps are characterised by a low metabolic rate. In addition, venous anastomosis is not essential because venous drainage can be performed by the bone marrow.[62] Furthermore, the osteocutaneous free flaps (e.g. fibula free flap) can be compared to the fasciocutaneous flaps. In fact, Salgado reported the survival of five osteocutaneous free flaps despite vascular occlusion of the pedicle, occurred from the 8th to the 20th postoperative day. Just one failure was described in the 42 postoperative day, in a case where irradiation of the recipient site (7200 cGy)[36] was performed before the tissue transfer.

8.6 INTESTINAL FREE FLAP/JEJUNAL FREE FLAP

Intestinal free flaps are mainly used in the reconstruction of the cervical oesophagus and pharynx, where perfusion pressure is high and allows to perform random flaps with a length/width of the flap ratio that has no equal in other human regions.[63] Concerning that, an interesting study on experimental animal models[6] showed that jejunal free flaps used for neck reconstructions had success rates of 100%, 83%, 60%, and 0%, after the section of pedicle, respectively, at fourth, third, second, and first week after transfer.[63] Clinically, Chen HC et al. reported three cases of vascular occlusion occurred in jejunal free flaps. In the first two cases, free flap thrombosis occurred in the seventh postoperative day with both free flap ischaemia (failure of one case and salvage with re-anastomosis of the second case). In the third case, the free flap thrombosis occurred in the 17th postoperative day without causing flap ischaemia and its failure. Chen HC et al. demonstrated that the flap survived through the revascularisation obtained from the recipient bed.[34] A similar case was later reported by Dr. Urken, describing a vascular occlusion in the 20th postoperative day.[64] Recently, Dr. Hirano reported the survival of a free jejunal flap, despite venous occlusion, at 5 weeks after the procedure.[65]

8.7 RADIOTHERAPY

The effects of radiotherapy on tissues have been known for decades. Their effect appears closely related to the interval of administrations. Only in a relatively recent period, its effects on revascularisation in rats have been studied by Clarke.[66,67] Microvascular flaps were transferred to an irradiated recipient bed. After the ligation of the pedicle, the area of flap necrosis was higher in irradiated cases, than in healthy controls. However, after the sixth postoperative day, the difference between the two groups became not as significant to demonstrate that the neovascularisation occurs even in irradiated sites, but it requires a longer period.[66]

Doyle investigated the effects of radiation on revascularisation and showed that, at low doses (300–600 cGy), alterations did not occur, compared to control cases. However, increasing the dose (>900 cGy), the effects on the tissues were higher. Doyle also showed that revascularisation was less influenced by preoperative radiotherapy, compared to the postoperative one.[67]

Very interesting was the review reported by Salgado about effects of late loss of arterial inflow on free flap survival.[36] He focused his attention on the receiving site and concluded that the fibrous barrier (caused by previous surgery or radiotherapy) had prevented revascularisation. In fact, multifactorial mechanisms have a greater influence in LL reconstruction compared to other districts, such as the head–neck (H&N) where the high flow appears to be sufficient to revascularise every free flap.

8.8 SMOKING

The effect of cigarette smoking on the survival of free and pedicled flaps was demonstrated by van Adrichem et al. They showed that smoking reduced survival of both flaps, in particular of free-tissue transfers.[68] Van Adrichem et al. also demonstrated how the rats exposed to preoperative smoking had fewer complications, compared with rats exposed to both preoperative and postoperative smoking.[68]

8.9 RECEIVING SITE

The receiving site influences significantly the process of revascularisation of a free flap. In particular, the type of flow plays an important role as in wound healing. Therefore, based on blood flow perfusion, areas of the body can be divided into five categories:

1. H&N high flow area
2. Upper limb (UL) high/intermediate flow area
3. Trunk (T) intermediate flow area
4. Perineum (G) intermediate/low flow area
5. LL low flow area

8.10 CHRONIC ISCHAEMIA, BLOOD DISEASE, ATHEROSCLEROSIS, DIABETES, PERIOPERATIVE COMPLICATIONS, AND VASCULAR STEAL PHENOMENON

Haematologic diseases, such as atherosclerosis and diabetes, do not influence revascularisation, except from those diseases that cause thrombosis of the microcirculation as vasculitis (Churg–Strauss disease) and atherosclerotic plaques (causing the maximum peripheral vasodilation).[69–71] In patients with arterial bypass, the free flap determines an increase of blood supply, compared to a local flap.[53–55,57–59,72–79] On the other hand, the high metabolic rate of a large muscle flap, as a flap of LAT D, can also aggravate the ischaemia of the limb[80,81] by the vascular steal phenomenon.

8.11 VOLUME OF THE FLAP AND AREA OF CONTACT BETWEEN THE FREE FLAP AND THE RECEIVING SITE

The total volume of a free flap is another important parameter in the evaluation of its potential revascularisation as shown previously concerning bulky perforator flap as the DIEP flap. However, this is closely related to other parameters, such as the contact surface between the free flap and the receiving site and the type of tissue.[47] In literature are reported different cases of large flaps with high metabolic rate failed after several months after their transplantation.[60,82] Similar cases are described for large and bulky flaps with low metabolic rate as the DIEP flap, while they are not described for smaller flaps with low metabolic rate as the fascial or the fasciocutaneous flaps.[32–33,38]

8.12 ANGIOGENESIS

The angiogenesis is realised through several steps, which include the retraction of pericytes, the secretion of proteases by endothelial cells that destroy the cell–matrix interactions. In adults, the vessels are in a quiescent state, governed by a balance between activating factors and inhibiting factors of angiogenesis. When this balance is altered, vessels respond by activating the angiogenic mechanism. This is regulated by the family of Vascular Endothelial Growth Factor (VEGF). Other key molecules include mitogens, such as Fibroblast Growyh Factor (FGF-1 and FGF-2), Trasforming Growth Factor (TGF β), Platelet-derived growth Factor (PDGF), and Tumor Necrosis Factor-α (TNF-α). Hyaluronic acid, the major constituent of extracellular matrix, plays both a structural and a functional role. Its fragments (enzyme hyaluronidase) have an extraordinary angiogenic power.[83–88]

Angiogenesis can be induced at both macroscopic and molecular level. In fact, angiogenesis can be induced by the delay phenomenon. It produces hypoxia, which is a stimulus to angiogenesis.[89]

Therefore, in literature, various proangiogenesis techniques are reported, such as shockwave therapy and pulsed magnetic energy.[90,91]

On the other hand, at a molecular level, it is reported that hyperbaric oxygen also stimulates angiogenesis and increases wound healing. The impact of different drugs on angiogenesis was studied: sympatholytic agents, vasodilators, calcium channel blockers, antithrombotic agents, antioxidants, and opioids. Only a few of these substances have been shown to have a therapeutic effect. Recent studies with topical nifedipine (calcium channel antagonist) and salicylates (anti-inflammatory analgesics) showed a significant increase in free flap survival.[92,93]

Vacuum-assisted closure (VAC) therapy plays also a proangiogenic role. In fact, several studies showed that mechanical stress applied on the cells increases the expression of growth factors, such as VEGF and FGF-2, resulting in angiogenesis and cell proliferation.[94,95]

8.13 REVASCULARISATION PROCESS

Once the patient is discharged from the hospital, different events may occur that lead to failure of the surgical procedure. At more than 30 years by the pioneering interventions that made the history of microsurgery,[1,7,40,96,97] still little is known about the interaction between the vascular free flap and the receiving site, a phenomena defined *revascularisation*.

The question of how long a flap is dependent on its pedicle cannot clearly be answered from the information available in the literature. Although there are some known factors that seem to be stimulating or inhibiting this process, continues without a solution to the scientific debate, whether or not is safe to disconnect the pedicle, in part because of the limited cases of each microsurgery centre.[31–63]

Literature review and radiological techniques have allowed to study the revascularisation process of free flaps and to identify the factors that influence it.

Inhibiting Factor	Stimulating Factor
Radiotherapy	Time
Fibrosis of receiving area	Proangiogenic factors
Atrophy of receiving area	Buried flap
Vasculopathy	Delay phenomenon
Smoking	Postoperative complications
Functioning muscle	Intraoperative complications
Body Area	**Flow Rate**
Head and neck	High flow area
UL	Intermediate/high flow area
T	Intermediate flow area
G	Intermediate/low flow area
LL	Low flow area

The influence of the intra- and postoperative complications on revascularisation was brilliantly reported by Machens.[54,55] He noted that the pedicles were patent and active 10 years after the transfer in all cases[54] and how this result varied significantly according to the number of complications encountered in the early postoperative period.[55]

Supporting the activity of complications, to allow the vascular independence of free flaps, was the case reported by Salgado,[36] in which the patient received a TRAM flap for mammary reconstruction. It presented 66% of survival possibly due to a seroma, which acted as pro-revascularisation factor.

The type of flap is another variable useful in predicting the probability of survival. In fact, flaps with low metabolism (fasciocutaneous flaps) are more likely to survive to an early section of the pedicle than those with a high metabolic rate (musculocutaneous flaps), especially, in relation to the recipient area in which they are transferred. In particular, Ichinose et al. showed that[98] vascularity of the radial forearm flap increases over time up to two postoperative weeks, and then decreased slowly (Figure 8.3).

On the other hand, the venous drainage increases after the third day, but it is not proportional to the arterial flow, being 60% at the sixth postoperative month. In fact, venous return is also obtained by the recipient site starting in the period from the fourth to the seventh postoperative day.

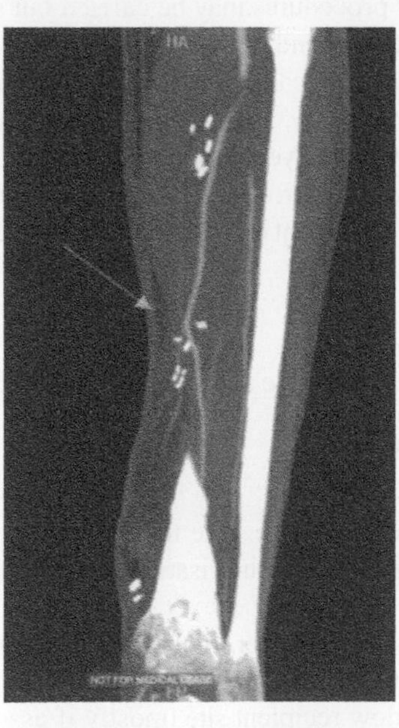

FIGURE 8.3 Angio-CT scan showing anastomosis T-L between Ascending branch of medial circumflex femoral artery and posterior tibial artery.

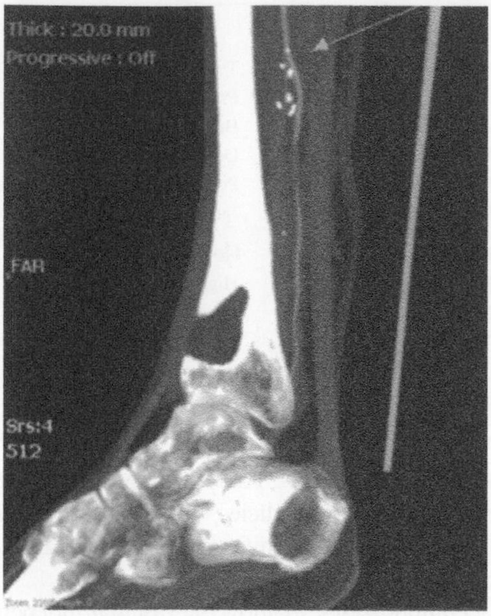

FIGURE 8.4 Lateral view of the anastomosis.

Moreover, the flow of a free flap tends to become proportional to the function of the organ or tissue that is reconstructed, regardless of the anatomic area, and is still closely related to the function. For this reason, it is clear that any muscle or musculocutaneous free flap, which has a contractile function and requires a high metabolic rate and thus blood flow tends to maintain a dependently from its pedicle.

An understanding of the timing of the revascularisation process should optimise the safety of secondary procedures involving the flap. Therefore, based on our clinical experience, we propose some suggestions to avoid free flap complications after secondary procedures. For flaps transferred to head and neck area, secondary procedures may be carried out safely because of their high blood flow. However, it should be delayed beyond 12 weeks as reported by Mucke et al.[51]

In case of trunk reconstruction, surgical revision should be carried out more carefully because the revascularisation occurs more slowly. It is confirmed by Moolenburgh et al. that reported a DIEP-flap failure after pedicle division 3 years following transfer (Figure 8.4).[39]

For flap transferred to LL, secondary procedures may be carried out only if strictly necessary. In fact, in this area, free flap remains dependent on its pedicle over time especially in case of muscle flaps.

8.14 CLASSIFICATION

The dependence of free flap from its pedicle can then be classified into three groups.

8.14.1 Type 1

The pedicle has maintained its original size. The flap generally survives after vascular occlusion only if one or more factors enhancing revascularisation are present and not inhibitory:

- Functional free flap (toe to hand transfer, functioning muscle transfer)
- High flow free flap to low/moderate flow recipient site
- High flow free flap to low flow recipient site (mostly if associated with inhibiting factors) (Figure 8.5)

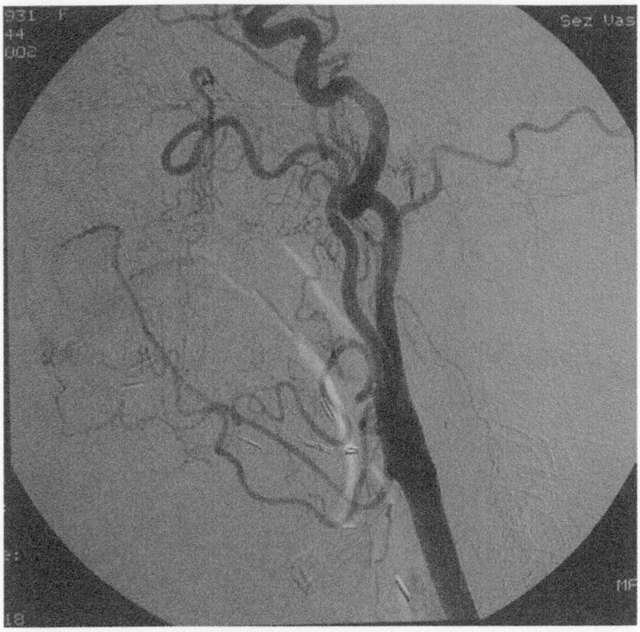

FIGURE 8.5 The pedicle has its original sizel.

8.14.2 Type 2

The pedicle is active and partial atrophic. Revascularisation is present; the flap is partially dependent on the pedicle:

- In case of multiple revision of free flap
- High flow free flap to high flow recipient site
- Low flow free flap to low/moderate flow recipient site (mostly if associated with inhibiting factors) (Figure 8.6)

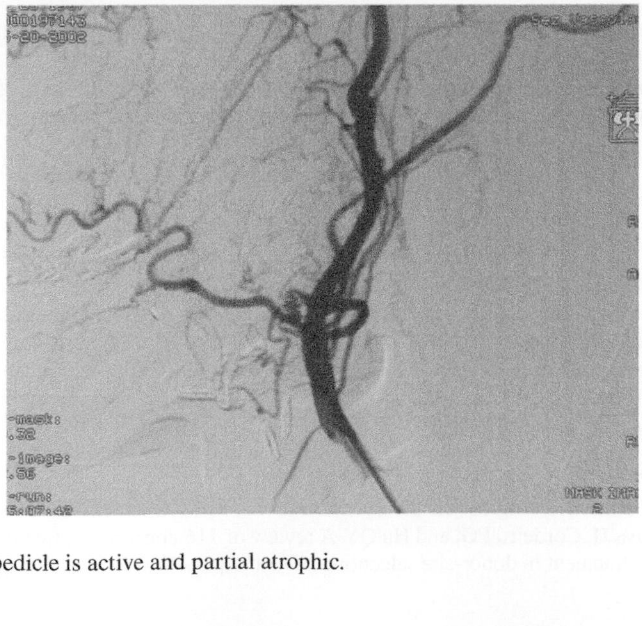

FIGURE 8.6 The pedicle is active and partial atrophic.

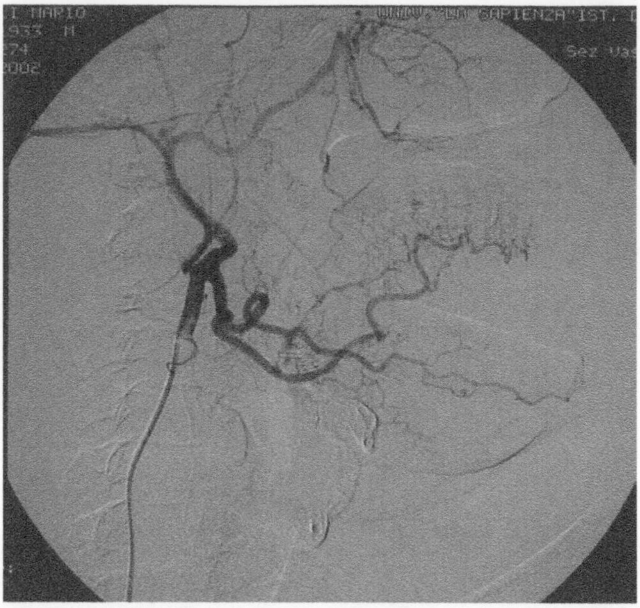

FIGURE 8.7 The pedicle is atrophic.

8.14.3 Type 3

The pedicle is atrophic, and the flap is revascularised and independent from its pedicle:

- Low flow free flap to high/moderate flow recipient site
- High flow free flap to high flow recipient site
- Low flow free flap to low flow recipient site (mostly if associated with enhancing factors) (Figure 8.7)

REFERENCES

1. Murphy JB. Resection of arteries and veins injured in continuity: End-to-end suture: Experimental and clinical research. *Med Rec* 1897;51: 73.
2. Guthrie CC. Some physiologic aspects of blood vessel surgery. *JAMA* 1908;51: 1658.
3. Carrel A. The operative technique of vascular anastomoses and the transplantation of viscera. *Med Lyon* 1902;98: 859.
4. Nylen CO. The otomicroscope and microsurgery, 1921–1971. *Acta Otolaryngol* 1972;73: 453.
5. Tamai S. History of microsurgery—From the beginning until the end of the 1970s. *Microsurgery* 1993;14: 6–13.
6. McLean D and Buncke H. Autotransplant of omentum to a large scalp defect with microsurgical revascularization. *Plast Reconstr Surg* 1972;49: 268–274.
7. Daniel R and Taylor G. Distant transfer of an island flap by microvascular anastomosis. *Plast Reconstr Surg* 1973;52: 111–117.
8. Tamai S. History of microsurgery. *Plast Reconstr Surg* 2009;124(6 Suppl): e282–e294.
9. Watterson PA, Taylor GI, and Crock JG. The venous territories of muscles: Anatomical study and clinical implications. *Br J Plast Surg* 1988;41: 569–585.
10. Taylor GI and Palmer JH. The vascular territories (angiosomes) of the body: Experimental study and clinical applications. *Br J Plast Surg* 1987;40(2): 113–141.
11. Taylor GI and Palmer JH. Angiosome theory. *Br J Plast Surg* 1992;45(4): 327–328.
12. Hidalgo DA, Disa JJ, Cordeiro PG, and Hu QY. A review of 716 consecutive free flaps for oncologic surgical defects: Refinement in donor-site selection and technique. *Plast Reconstr Surg* 1998;102: 722–732.

13. Khouri RK, Cooley BC, Kunselman AR, Landis JR, Yeramian P, Ingram D, Natarajan N, Benes CO, and Wallemark C. A prospective study of microvascular free-flap surgery and outcome. *Plast Reconstr Surg* 1998;102: 711–721.
14. Oliva A, Lineaweaver W, Buncke HJ, Siko P, Jackson RL, Samaha FJ, and Alpert BA. Salvage of wounds following failed tissue transplantation. *J Reconstr Microsurg* 1993;4: 257–263.
15. Serletti JM, Deuber MA, Guidera PM, Reading G, Herrera HR, Reale VF, Wray RC, Jr., and Bakamjian VY. Comparison of the operating microscope and loupes for free microvascular tissue transfer. *Plast Reconstr Surg* 1995;95: 270–276.
16. Singh B, Cordeiro PG, Santamaria E, Shaha AR, Pfister DG, and Shah JP. Factors associated with complications in microvascular reconstruction of head and neck defects. *Plast Reconstr Surg* 1999;103: 403–411.
17. Yuen JC and Feng Z. Monitoring free flaps using the laser Doppler flowmeter: Five-year experience. *Plast Reconstr Surg* 2000;105: 55–61.
18. Wechselberger G, Rumer A, Schoeller T, Schwabegger A, Ninkovic M, and Anderl H. Free-flap monitoring with tissue-oxygen measurement. *J Reconstr Microsurg* 1997;13: 125–130.
19. Udesen A, Lontoft E, and Kristensen SR. Monitoring of free TRAM flaps with microdialysis. *J Reconstr Microsurg* 2000;16: 101–106.
20. Yuen JC and Feng Z. Monitoring free flaps using the laser Doppler flowmeter: Five-year experience. *Plast Reconstr Surg* 2000;105: 55–61.
21. Jones NF. Intraoperative and postoperative monitoring of microsurgical free tissue transfers. *Clin Plast Surg* 1992;419: 783–797.
22. Khouri RK and Shaw WW. Monitoring of free flaps with surface temperature recordings: Is it reliable? *Plast Reconstr Surg* 1992;89: 495–499.
23. Khouri RK, Cooley BC, Kunselman AR, Landis JR, Yeramian P, Ingram D, Natarajan N, Benes CO, and Wallemark C. A prospective study of microvascular free-flap surgery and outcome. *Plast Reconstr Surg* 1998;102: 711–721.
24. Kroll SS, Miller MJ, and Reece GP. Anticoagulants and hematomas in free flap surgery. *Plast Reconstr Surg* 1995;96: 643–647.
25. Khouri RK, Cooley BC, Kunselman AR, Landis JR, Yeramian P, Ingram D, Natarajan N, Benes CO, and Wallemark C. A prospective study of microvascular free-flap surgery and outcome. *Plast Reconstr Surg* 1998;102: 711–721.
26. Komuro Y, Sekiguchi J, Nomura S, Ohmori K, Takasugi Y, and Arai C. Blood coagulation activity during microsurgery. *Ann Plast Surg* 1998;40: 53–58.
27. Thomson JG, Kim JH, Syed SA, Reid MA, Madsen J, and Restifo RJ. The effect of prolonged clamping and vascular stasis on the patency of arterial and venous microanastomoses. *Ann Plast Surg* 1998;40: 436–441.
28. al-Qattan MM. Ischaemia-reperfusion injury. Implications for the hand surgeon. *J Hand Surg* 1998;23: 570–573.
29. Kroll SS, Gherardini G, Martin JE, Reece GP, Miller MJ, Evans GR, Robb GL, and Wang BG. Fat necrosis in free and pedicled TRAM flaps. *Plast Reconstr Surg* 1998;102: 1502–1507.
30. Jones NF, Johnson JT, Shestak KC, Myers EN, and Swartz WM. Microsurgical reconstruction of the head and neck: Interdisciplinary collaboration between head and neck surgeons and plastic surgeons in 305 cases. *Ann Plast Surg* 1996;36: 37–43.
31. Suominen S and Asko-Seljavaara S. Free flap failures. *Microsurgery* 1995;16: 396–399.
32. Gilbert A and Beres J. Unusual complication of a free flap. *Ann Chir Plast* 1976;21(2): 151–155.
33. Rothaus KO and Acland RD. Free flap neo-vascularisation: Case report. *Br J Plast Surg* 1983;36(3): 348–349.
34. Chen HC, Tan BK, Cheng MH, Chang CH, and Tang YB. Behavior of free jejunal flaps after early disruption of blood supply. *Ann Thorac Surg* 2002;73(3): 987–989.
35. Keen M, Arena S, and Urken M. Survival of transferred intestine after interruption of blood supply. *Plast Reconstr Surg* 1987;80(5): 750–751.
36. Salgado CJ, Smith A, Kim S, Higgins J, Behnam A, Herrera HR, and Serletti JM. Effects of late loss of arterial inflow on free flap survival. *J Reconstr Microsurg* 2002;18(7): 579–584.
37. Rath T, Piza H, and Opitz A. Survival of a free musculocutaneous flap after early loss of arterial blood supply. *Br J Plast Surg* 1986;39(4): 530–532.
38. Ribuffo D, Chiummariello S, Cigna E, and Scuderi N. Salvage of a free flap after late total thrombosis of the flap and revascularisation. *Scand J Plast Reconstr Surg Hand Surg* 2004;38(1): 50–52.

39. Moolenburgh SE, van Huizum MA, and Hofer SO. DIEP-flap failure after pedicle division three years following transfer. *Br J Plast Surg* 2005;58(7): 1000–1003.
40. Taylor GI and Daniel RK. The free flap: Composite tissue transfer by vascular anastomosis. *Aust N Z J Surg* 1973;43(1): 1–3.
41. Cho BC, Kim M, Lee JH, Byun JS, Park JS, and Baik BS. Pharyngoesophageal reconstruction with a tubed free radial forearm flap. *J Reconstr Microsurg* 1998;14: 535–540.
42. O'Brien CJ, Lee KK, Stern HS, Traynor SJ, Bron L, Tew PJ, and Haghighi KS. Evaluation of 250 free-flap reconstructions after resection of tumours of the head and neck. *Aust N Z J Surg* 1998;68: 698–701.
43. Stark B, Nathanson A, Heden P, and Jernbeck J. Results after resection of intraoral cancer and reconstruction with the free radial forearm flap. *ORL J Otorhinolaryngol Relat Spec* 1998;60: 212–217.
44. Urbaniak JR, Koman LA, Goldner RD, Armstrong NB, and Nunley JA. The vascularized cutaneous scapular flap. *Plast Reconstr Surg* 1982;69: 772–778.
45. Weinzweig N and Davies BW. Foot and ankle reconstruction using the radial forearm flap: A review of 25 cases. *Plast Reconstr Surg* 1998;102: 1999–2005.
46. Black MJ, Chait L, O'Brien BM, Sykes PJ, and Sharzer LA. How soon may the axial vessels of a surviving free flap be safely ligated: A study in pigs. *Br J Plast Surg* 1978;31(4): 295–299.
47. Fried MP, Horowitz Z, Kelly JH, and Strome M. The importance of the pedicle for the survival of a vascularized free flap: An experimental study on rats. *Head Neck Surg* 1982;5(2): 130–133.
48. Oswald P, Tilgner A, and Schumann D. The influence of postoperative vessel occlusion on the viability of free micro vascular skin-fat flap sand island flaps in rats. *J Reconstr Microsurg* 1988;4(5): 403–407.
49. Gilbert A and Beres J. Unusual complication of a free flap. *Ann Chir Plast* 1976;21(2): 151–155.
50. Rothaus KO and Acland RD. Free flap neo-vascularisation: Case report. *Br J Plast Surg* 1983;36(3): 348–349.
51. Mücke T, Wolff KD, Rau A, Kehl V, Mitchell DA, and Steiner T. Autonomization of free flaps in the oral cavity: A prospective clinical study. *Microsurgery* 2012;32(3): 201–206.
52. Wise SR, Harsha WJ, Kim N, and Hayden RE. Free flap survival despite early loss of the vascular pedicle. *Head Neck* 2011;33(7): 1068–1071.
53. Salmi A, Ahovuo J, Tukiainen E, Harma M, and Asko-Seljavaara S. Use of ultrasonography to evaluate muscle thickness and blood flow in free flaps. *Microsurgery* 1995;16: 601–605.
54. Machens HG, Pallua N, Pasel J, Mailaender P, Liebau J, and Berger A. Persistence of pedicle blood flow up to 10 years after free musculocutaneous tissue transfer. *Plast Reconstr Surg* 1998;101: 719–726.
55. Machens HG, Mailander P, Pasel J, Lutz BS, Funke M, Siemers F, and Berger AC. Flap perfusion after free musculocutaneous tissue transfer: The impact of postoperative complications. *Plast Reconstr Surg* 2000;105: 2395–2399.
56. Kumar K, Jaffe W, London NJ, and Varma SK. Free flap neovascularization: Myth or reality? *J Reconstr Microsurg* 2004;20(1): 31–34.
57. Gooden MA, Gentile AT, Mills JL, Berman SS, Demas CP, Reinke KR, Hunter GC, Westerband A, and Greenwald D. Free tissue transfer to extend the limits of limb salvage for lower extremity tissue loss. *Am J Surg* 1997;174: 644–648.
58. Lepäntalo M and Tukiainen E. Combined vascular reconstruction and microvascular muscle flap transfer for salvage of ischaemic legs with major tissue loss and wound complications. *Eur J Vasc Endovasc Surg* 1996;12: 65–69.
59. Serletti JM, Hurwitz SR, Jones JA, Herrera HR, Reading GP, Ouriel K, and Green RM. Extension of limb salvage by combined vascular reconstruction and adjunctive free-tissue transfer. *J Vasc Surg* 1993;18: 972–978.
60. Khoo CT and Bailey BN. The behaviour o free muscle and musculocutaneous flaps after early loss of axial blood supply. *Br J Plast Surg* 1982;35(1): 43–46.
61. Lau KN, Park D, Dagum AB, and Bui DT. Two for one: Salvage of bilateral lower extremities with a single free flap. *Ann Plast Surg* 2008;60(5): 498–501.
62. el Danaf A, Abou Elseoud A, Alhussein T, and Fansa M. Venous drainage through marrow coaptation in free bone transfer: Two case reports. *J Reconstr Microsurg* 1986;2(3): 165–167, 169.
63. Cordeiro PG, Santamaria E, Hu QY, DiResta GR, and Reuter VE. The timing and nature of neovascularization of jejunal free Flaps: An experimental study in a large animal model. *Plast Reconstr Surg* 1999;103(7): 1893–1901.
64. Keen M, Arena S, and Urken M. Survival of transferred intestine after interruption of blood supply. *Plast Reconstr Surg* 1987;80(5): 750–751.
65. Hirano T, Fujita K, Kodama S, Takeno S, and Suzuki M. Survival of a free jejunal flap with venous occlusion. *Ann Thorac Surg* 2010;89(5): 1656–1659.

66. Clarke HM, Howard CR, Pynn BR, and McKee NH. Delayed neovascularization in free skin flap transfer to irradiated beds in rats. *Plast Reconstr Surg* 1985;75(4): 560–564.
67. Doyle JW, Li YQ, Salloum A, FitzGerald TJ, and Walton RL. The effects of radiation on neovascularization in a rat model. *Plast Reconstr Surg* 1996;98(1): 129–135; discussion 136–139.
68. van Adrichem LN, Hoegen R, Hovius SE, Kort WJ, van Strik R, Vuzevski VD, and van der Meulen JC. The effect of cigarette smoking on the survival of free vascularized and pedicled epigastric flaps in the rat. *Plast Reconstr Surg* 1996;97(1): 86–96.
69. Chen HC, Coskunfirat OK, Ozkan O, Mardini S, Cigna E, Salgado CJ, and Spanio S. Guidelines for the optimization of microsurgery in atherosclerotic patients. *Microsurgery* 2006;26(5): 356–362.
70. Ozkan O, Chen HC, Mardini S, Cigna E, Hao SP, Hung KF, and Chen HS. Microvascular free Tissue transfer in patients with hematological disorders. *Plast Reconstr Surg* 2006;118(4): 936–944.
71. Ozkan O, Chen HC, Mardini S, Cigna E, Feng GM, and Chu YM. Principles for the management of toe-to-hand transfer in reexploration: Toe salvage with a tubed groin flap in the last step. *Microsurgery* 2006;26(2): 100–105.
72. Salmi A, Lamminen A, Tukiainen E, and Asko-Seljavaara S. Magnetic resonance imaging of free muscle flaps. *Eur J Plat Surg* 1996;19: 21–25.
73. Salmi A, Tukiainen E, Harma M, and Asko-Seljavaara S. A prospective study of changes in muscle dimensions following free-muscle transfer measured by ultrasound and CT scanning. *Plast Reconstr Surg* 1996;97: 1443–1450.
74. Chen LE, Seaber AV, Bossen E, and Urbaniak JR. The effect of acute denervation on the microcirculation of skeletal muscle: Rat cremaster model. *J Orthop Res* 1991;9: 266–274.
75. Chen LE, Seaber AV, and Urbaniak JR. Combined effect of acute denervation and ischemia on the microcirculation of skeletal muscle. *J Orthop Res* 1992;10: 112–120.
76. Siemionow M, Andreasen T, Chick L, and Lister G. Effect of muscle flap denervation on flow hemodynamics: A new model for chronic in vivo studies. *Microsurgery* 1994;15: 891–894.
77. Wang WZ, Anderson G, and Firrell JC. Arteriole constriction following ischemia in denervated skeletal muscle. *J Reconstr Microsurg* 1995;11: 99–106.
78. Mätzke S, Tukiainen EJ, and Lepantalo MJ. Survival of a microvascular muscle flap despite the late occlusion of the inflow artery in a neuroischaemic diabetic foot. *Scand J Plast Reconstr Surg Hand Surg* 1997;31: 71–75.
79. McDaniel MD, Zwolak RM, Schneider JR, Cvonenwett JL, Walsh DB, Reus WF, and Colen LB. Indirect revascularization of the lower extremity by means of microvascular free-muscle flap—A preliminary report. *J Vasc Surg* 1991;14: 829–830.
80. Musser DJ, Berger A, and Hallock GG. Free flap "steal" hastening amputation of a revascularized lower limb. *Eur J Plast Surg* 1995;18: 311–313.
81. Sonntag BV, Murphy RX Jr., Chernofsky MA, and Chowdary RP. Microvascular steal phenomenon in lower extremity reconstruction. *Ann Plast Surg* 1995;34: 336–339.
82. Fisher J and Wood MB. Late necrosis of a latissimus dorsi free flap. *Plast Reconstr Surg* 1984;74(2): 274–281.
83. Matthews W, Jordan CT, Gavin M et al. A receptor tyrosine kinase cDNA isolated from a population of enriched primitive hematopoietic cells and exhibiting close genetic linkage to ckit. *Proc Natl Acad Sci USA* 1991;88: 9026e30.
84. Yamaguchi TP, Dumont DJ, Conlon RA et al. Flk-1, an flt-related receptor tyrosine kinase is an early marker for endothelial cell precursors. *Development* 1993;118: 489e98.
85. Ferrara N, Gerber HP, and LeCouter J. The biology of VEGF and it receptors. *Nat Med* 2003;9: 669e76.
86. Neufeld G, Cohen T, Gengrinovitch S et al. Vascular endothelial growth factor (VEGF) and its receptors. *FASEB J* 1999;13: 9e22.
87. Weige P. Chemistry and biology of hyaluronan. In: *The Hyaluronan Synthases*, Garg H and Hales CA (eds.), Chapter 25, page 553–564. Amsterdam. Elsevier, 2004.
88. Gerecht S, Brudick JA, and Vunjak-Novakovic G. Hyaluronic acid hydrogel for controlled self-renewal and differentiation of human embryonic stem cells. *PNAS* 2005;104: 11298e303.
89. McFarlane RM, Heagy FC, Radin S et al. A study of the delay phenomenon in experimental pedicle flaps. *Plast Reconstr Surg* 1965;35: 245e62.
90. Weber RV, Navarro A, Wu JK et al. Pulsed magnetic fields applied to a transferred arterial loop support the rat groin composite flap. *Plast Reconstr Surg* 2004;114: 1185e9.
91. Noma M, Tomoike H, Ando H et al. Collateral development induced by repetitive brief coronary occlusion relates to the functional state of pre-existing collaterals. *Jpn Circ J* 1994;58: 269e77.

92. Kerrigan CL and Daniel RK. Pharmacologic treatment of the failing skin flap. *Plast Reconstr Surg* 1982;70: 541e9.
93. Zhang F, Waller W, and Lineaweaver WC. Growth factors and flap survival. *Microsurgery* 2004;24: 162e7.
94. Kryger Z, Dogan T, Zhang F et al. Effects of VEGF administration following ischemia on survival of the gracilis muscle flap in the rat. *Ann Plast Surg* 1999;43: 172e8.
95. Urschel JD, Scott PG, and Williams HT. The effect of mechanical stress on soft and hard tissue repair; a review. *Br J Plast Surg* 1988;41: 182e6.
96. Taylor GI and Daniel RK. The anatomy of several free flap donor sites. *Plast Reconstr Surg* 1975;56: 243–253.
97. Taylor GI, Townsend P, and Corlett R. Superiority of the deep circumflex iliac vessels as the supply for free groin flaps. *Plast Reconstr Surg* 1979;64: 595–604.
98. Ichinose A, Tahara S, Terashi H, and Yokoo S. Reestablished circulation after free radial forearm flap transfer. *J Reconstr Microsurg* 2004;20(3): 207–213.

9 Application of Virtual 3D Plastic Surgery

Alberto Alonso-Burgos, Vachara Niumsawatt, and Warren M. Rozen

CONTENTS

9.1 OVERVIEW

Virtual three-dimensional (3D) imaging has been used in surgery as a tool to allow 3D analysis of images in a way that is meaningful to reconstructive surgeons, achieving increased insight and understanding of patients' anatomy. It is a way to see more than one plane at the same time within the same image, thus allowing the viewing of the image data from various points in space. The characteristics of anatomical structure such as the anatomical construct, contour, and relationship to other structures are easier to view and interpret than that of a flat single plane. Advances in imaging techniques have expended the capability of computer tomography (CT), magnetic resonance imaging (MRI), and ultrasound scanning (US) software to produce 3D images.[1,2] Traditionally, CT and MRI scans produced 2D static outputs on film slices. A virtual 3D image reconstruction is made by combining a series of 2D film slice scans. The computer software then produced a digital 3D model, which can then be manipulated to enhance the visual information. Application of visual 3D images has been utilized in medicine in various fields including plastic and reconstructive surgery, and applications within these specialities as well as into other specialities continue to evolve (see Tables 9.1 and 9.2). Its use in pre-operative planning has been proven to improve accuracy, reduce operative time, and decrease morbidity. The method is reproducible and easier to visualize than in conventional imaging such as x-ray, CT, MRI, and US and has thus been allowed to be used as an educational tool for both junior doctors and patients.

TABLE 9.1
3D Surface Imaging Systems

Surface Imaging Device	Principle
Laser imaging technology	A laser beam (spot or strip) is scanned across a target object to determine the surface coordinates.
Structured light technology	Similar to laser imaging, but an organized pattern of white light is used in the forms of grids, dots, or strips.
Stereophotogrammetric technology	Two pictures of the object are taken o recorded pattern on the surface. The stereoalgorithms then produce an image that includes depth perception. These can be divided into active or passive.
Active stereophotogrammetric technology	It deploys the projection of a focused random unstructured light pattern on the actual surface of the target object to generate a quality 3D geometry. No special external lighting conditions are needed for this technique, and it is resilient to the effects of ambient lighting.
Passive stereophotogrammetric technology	In contrast to active stereophotogrammertic, it generates 3D geometry solely based on the natural patterns of the target object's surface with the use of high-resolution cameras to allow for enough surface detail. Care is needed to avoid distortion by ambient light.

TABLE 9.2
Commercially Available 3D Imaging Software

Software Program	Cost (Estimates May Vary)
Amira (Visage Imaging GmbH, Germany)	$4,800 (base package)
Alma3D (Alma IT Systems, Spain)	NA
Analyze (AnalyzeDirect, Inc., Kansas)	$5,000
ImageJ (National Institutes of Health, USA)	Free (http://rsbweb.nih.gov/ij/)
iNtellect Cranial Navigation System (Stryker, Germany)	NA
iPlan (BrainLab, USA)	$30,000 (planning station and software)
Maxilim (Medicim, Belgium)	NA
Mimics (Materialise, Belgium)	NA
Osirix (Osirix, Switzerland)	Free (http://www.osirix-viewer.com)
SurgiCase CMF (Materialise, Belgium)	$650,000
SimPlant OMS (Materialise Dental, Belgium)	NA
Voxim (IVS Solutions, Germany)	$20,000 (Voxim basics)
3dMD (Atlanta, USA)	NA

9.2 HISTORY OF VIRTUAL 3D IN MEDICINE

Radiographic imaging has been used to assist health professionals in diagnosing and managing patients who suffer from various conditions (see Figure 9.1). The radiographic image is the sum of shadows of all the objects located between the radiation tube and the photographic film. The resultant image is thus a bidimensional projection of a tridimensional volume. Interpretation of a bidimensional image or 2D images can be extremely difficult, as the level at which the shadows are located cannot be determined. Radiologists and radiation physicians have attempted to overcome this issue using profile image or use of fluoroscopy while mobilizing the patient. However, these methods lacked accuracy, which resulted in distortion of images. It was clear that other means to obtain and view images in a third dimension are required.

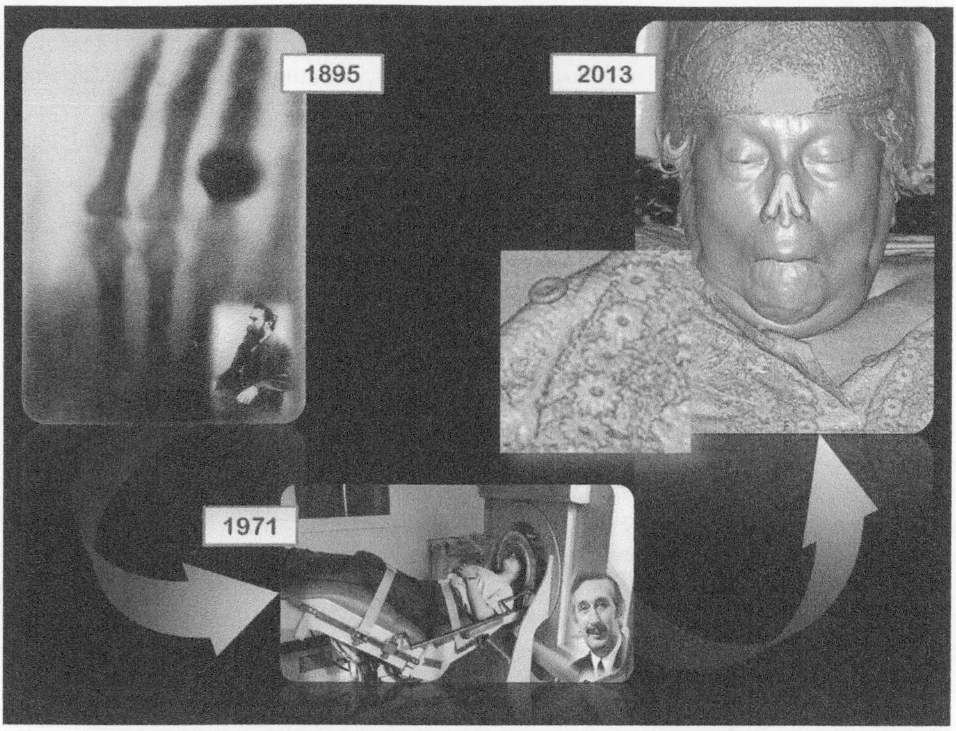

FIGURE 9.1 Evolution of imaging. From past times where x-ray plain films revealed hidden anatomy, Sir Hounsfield and his 'computerized assisted tomography' facilitated a crucial step in the development of 3D images. Note the detail obtained from a volume-rendered reconstruction of a woman and her ancient clothes in a past cranial computed tomography (CT) study.

9.2.1 Radiostereoscopy

The original concept of 3D reconstruction of radiographic images was based on the principles of stereoscopy by Sir Wheatstone, a professor in experimental philosophy at King's college in London. In 1838, he showed that our impression of solidity is gained by the combination of two separate pictures of an object taken by both of our eyes from different points of view in our mind, thus, it is the creation of stereoscope concept by using two photographs of the same object taken from different points. These is image is view through lens or reflection of mirrors with the images is combined as to make the object stand out with a solid aspect. From this basis, he developed an instrument that produced a 3D image from two flat plane images.[3] The produced images provide more realistic depth perception to the viewer than conventional 2D images. The idea was adopted by Brewster, a Scottish physicist who invented a refracting stereoscope device called the lenticular stereoscope, which consisted of a closed box with an opening for the introduction of light into the box and two lenticular lenses. This enables the viewer to see a 3D image on the floor of the closed box.

The first use of radiostereoscopy in experimental medicine developed with the combination of the stereoscopic concepts and x-ray in 1895 by Sir Thomson[4] and later utilized in clinical work by Davidson in 1898.[5,6] Based on Wheatstone concept, two x-ray images taken from different views were placed on a platform with their reflection superimposed on one another. However, it was difficult to align the films precisely. Therefore, the radiologists often experienced discomfort and eye strain when using the device. Nevertheless, the growing interests for stereoscopic x-ray devices that can produce a more realistic image of tissue morphology and anatomy gradually increase. Stereography remained in use until the end of the twentieth century, until the discovery of slice radiography or tomography. The concept was only recently resurrected to improve depth perception when optical device is used intra-operatively. This led to the development of stereoscopic endoscope, stereoscopic microscope, and robotic surgery such as a Da Vinci surgical root system, which are commonly used by urologists and abdomen, colorectal, and vascular surgeons.[7,8] Moreover, with the improvement in laser technology, the device has gained interest in surface imagery, which has been used in aesthetic surgery.

9.2.2 3D Imaging: Computed Tomography and Magnetic Resonance Imaging

The revolution of digital 3D image reconstruction started with the development of computed tomography (CT). Sir Godfrey Hounsfield, a British electrical engineer, recognized the limitations inherent in conventional x-ray images and devised a method for creating an image, in great detail, of a narrow cross section of a portion of the body. The instrument delivered hundreds of narrow x-ray beams at various angles through a specific part of the anatomy. The collected information was then analysed by computer software that produced a very detailed image of the slice. He called this technology 'computerized assisted tomography' or CAT scan for short and introduced it in 1972. This technique marked the first time that computers were integrated into the process of constructing a medical image for which he later won a Nobel Prize in physiology or medicine in 1979.[9] CAT scan images can be arranged in sequence to approximate a 3D structure, which began in the early 1980s. This development came from the work of cardiologists in an attempt to ascertain the volume of cardiac chambers. Further improvement in computer software has allowed the reconstructed digital information to not only be reviewed but also be animated and manipulated. This application was used largely in neurosurgery and tissue reconstruction such as facial aesthetic, craniofacial, spine, and joint surgery (see Figure 9.2).

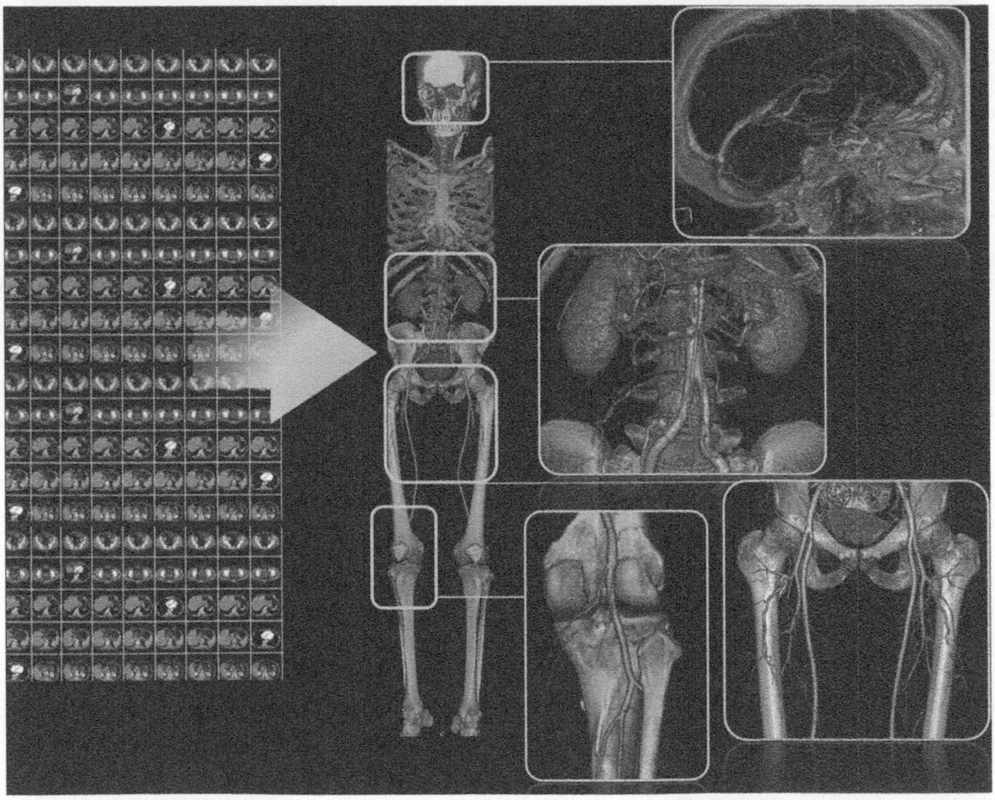

FIGURE 9.2 Post-processing tools and software have allowed the management of hundreds and even thousands of single images to form current technology in computed tomography (CT) and magnetic resonance imaging (MRI) into reformatted 3D images from anywhere in the anatomy of the body.

Similarly, MRI has been used to create a visual 3D reconstruction in a similar manner as CT. It is hypothesized that it could provide a high fidelity in distinguishing different anatomical soft-tissue density. The first 1D MRI scanner was developed by Herman Carr, an American physicist, in 1952.[10] Further development of MRI allowed a production of 2D or 3D images by Paul Lauterbur, an American chemist who received a Nobel Prize in physiology or medicine in 2003.[11] This allowed for a greater quality image showing cross sections through body parts at regular intervals. The images are so precise that radiologists are often able to get as much information from a scan as from looking at the tissue directly. MRI is the state-of-the-art radiological imaging method that has far superior soft tissue in contrast to any other radiological methods. Not surprisingly, its applications have grown rapidly in recent years (see Figure 9.3a through c).

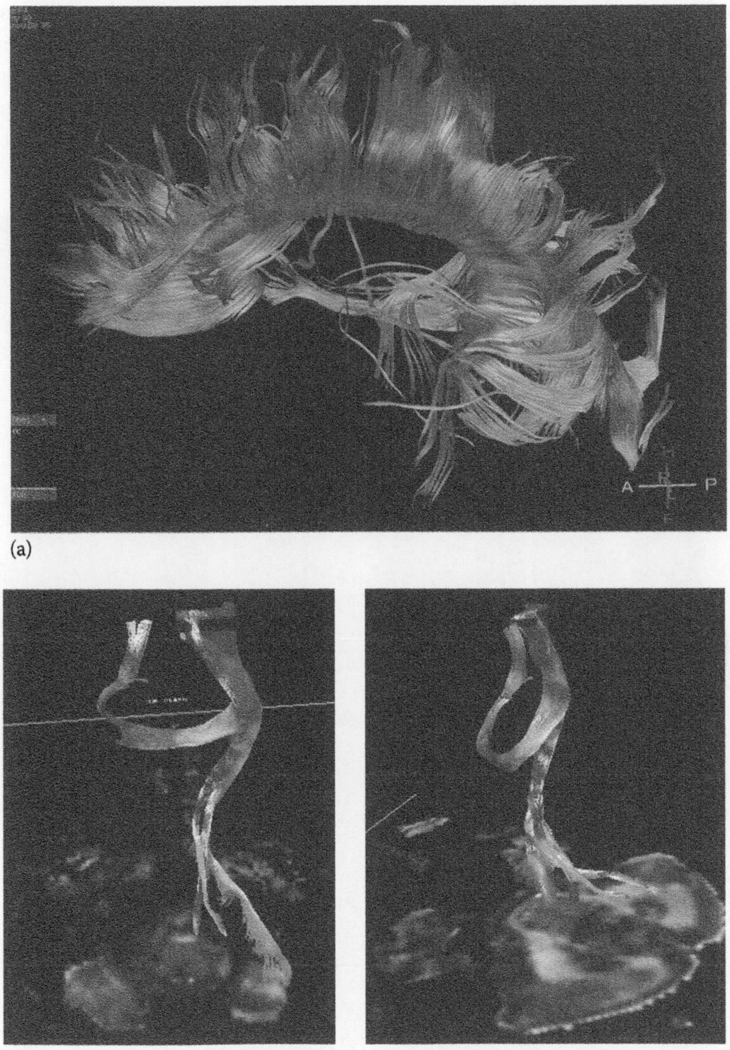

(a) (b) (c)

FIGURE 9.3 (a–c) Recent advances in MRI techniques allow performing almost any 3D evaluation in almost any tissue or structure. (a) Corpus callosum MRI 3D tractography. White matter fibres' direction is colour-encoded: red, transverse; green, anteroposterior; and blue, craniocaudal. (b and c) Corticospinal tract MRI 3D tractography in two different views. In this case, a huge number of blue fibres can be observed, due to cranio-caudal direction. Upper region in red corresponds to corpus callosum. (Imaging courtesy of Julia Montoya, M.D., Radiology Department (Neuroradiology Unit), University Hospital Fundación Jimenez Díaz, Spain.)

9.3 DEVELOPMENT OF VIRTUAL 3D IN PLASTIC SURGERY

Extension in the use of virtual 3D reconstruction in plastic surgery has expanded largely in the form of pre-operative assessment and patient education. However, the most noticeable utility of this technique is in pre-operative reconstructive planning such as flap reconstruction and surface imagery in aesthetic surgery (see Figure 9.4).

9.3.1 Stereolithography Free Fibular Flap Reconstruction

Since the introduction of free fibular flap reconstruction for mandible defect by Hidalgo,[12] contouring of the fibula has been classically performed with a freehand approach. This however can be inaccurate and subject to human error. A more aesthetically pleasing result is obtained only through the accumulation of experience and sculpture skill. Various literatures have reported the use of computer-aided surgical planning in an animated form of a virtual environment. This allowed the reconstructive surgeons to plan the angle and length for fibular osteotomy. The process is repeatable, thus allowing several mistakes and adjustments to be made without compromising

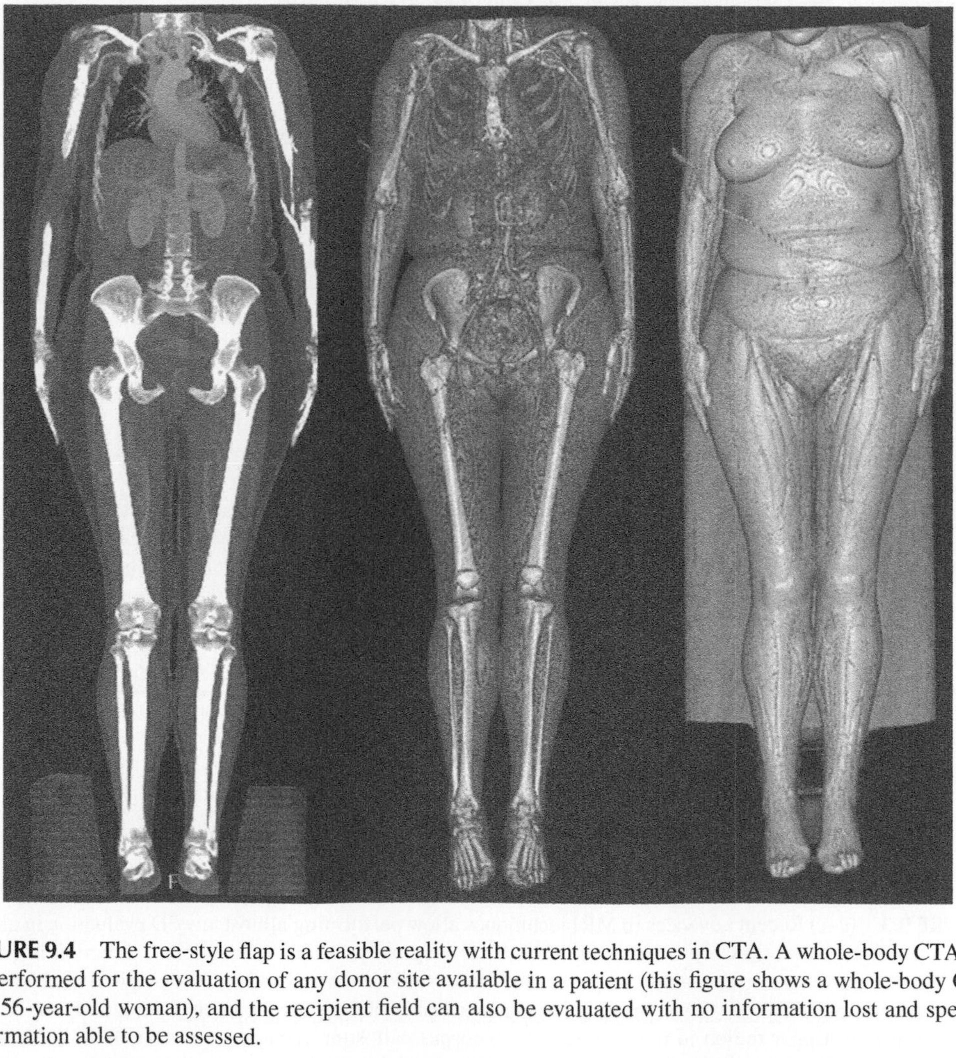

FIGURE 9.4 The free-style flap is a feasible reality with current techniques in CTA. A whole-body CTA can be performed for the evaluation of any donor site available in a patient (this figure shows a whole-body CTA in a 56-year-old woman), and the recipient field can also be evaluated with no information lost and specific information able to be assessed.

the operation. Due to the improved computer software system, an animation of the reconstructed images can be manipulated and rotated to simulate the resulting reconstruction. Anuja et al. used the virtual reconstruction to perform a pre-operative measurement of the fibular osteotomy angle to match that of the native curvature of the mandible. The computer software helps to obtain a direct angle measurement of each section of the mandible, but final decision is relied upon a trial-and-error process. With these data, stereolithographic models of the neomandible fibular cutting guides and a plate-bending template can be manufactured.[13] A reconstruction plate can be prefabricated and shaped according to the specification of the virtual reconstructed. Thus, the reconstructive surgeons see the resulting reconstruction prior to any incision made.

This method of pre-operative measurement, animation, stereolithographic models, cutting guide, and plate prefabrication has eliminated the need for an intra-operative freehand contouring by means of manual measurement, which is crude and imprecise. The pre-blended plate is more accurate in its curvature and fixation. Furthermore, several plates can be made prior to surgery and can be used as a replacement in the event of intra-operative error. A manufactured stereolithographic mandibular model allows the surgeon to perform a real-world manual measurement, practice the reconstruction, and see the result prior to the operation. The main reported advantage of this novel technology has been the reduction in operative time and improvement in accuracy. Anuja et al. and Sink et al. have both reported an average reduction of intra-operative time by 60 min.[13,14] Roser et al. have reported a high accuracy when comparing the virtual images to intra-operative finding. They found that mean percentage volumes of the actual post-operative fibula compared to the planned fibula were 90.93% ± 18.03%, and a total mean distance of the actual fibula osteotomy when compared to the virtual fibula osteotomy was 1.30 ± 0.59 mm.[15] A further benefit is that reconstructive surgeons are able to foresee potential complicating factors, improve bone-to-bone contact, and reduce morbidity, thus enabling a better functional (mastication and speech articulation) and aesthetic result.

9.3.2 Use of Virtual 3D in Perforator Flap Reconstruction

The increased use of perforator flaps has raised the need for pre-operative familiarity with an individual's particular anatomical feature of the axial arteries and their perforating branches, particularly when there is such a significant variation of the vascular anatomy. Image-guided technique played an important role in plastic and reconstructive surgery, especially in the domain of perforator flaps since pre-operative awareness of perforator location and course can permit improved flap design and reliability, decrease morbidity, and identify and protect vascular pedicle. Furthermore, it can be used to identify the most suited perforators to base the flap on, thus helping in the decision making to reduce operative time and improve flap survival.

The use of pre-operative computed tomographic angiography (CTA) imaging has gained more acceptance in perforator flap reconstruction.[15] With the advance in computer software and the need for a better description of the perforator vessels, there is a need for a virtual 3D reconstruction. These are achieved using computer software that performs multiplanar reconstructions. Volume-rendered technique (VRT) and maximum-intensity projection (MIP) reconstructions are widely used for this purpose and can be achieved with a wide variety of software programs from many software companies.[16] Both VRT and MIP help enhancing visual images by helping to distinguish different anatomical structures. VRT reconstructions assign colour to data points that display a 2D representation of the 3D dataset. MIP reconstructions are optimal for demonstrating the axial pedicles and the intramuscular course of perforators.[15,16] In the virtual 3D reality environment, anatomical structure can be viewed in different angles, and relationships to other structures are optimally appreciated. The calibre, position, and fasciocutaneous, septal, and intramuscular course can be evaluated. Several software modifications have additional features that can provide even more descriptive information. Individual structures can

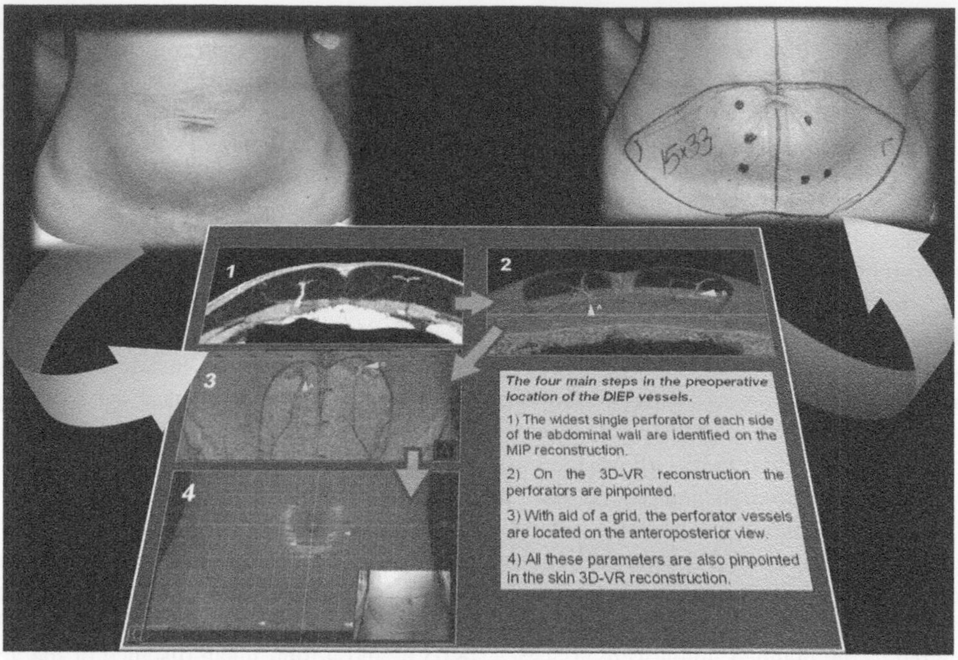
1
2
3
4
15x33
The four main steps in the preoperative location of the DIEP vessels.
1) The widest single perforator of each side of the abdominal wall are identified on the MIP reconstruction.
2) On the 3D-VR reconstruction the perforators are pinpointed.
3) With aid of a grid, the perforator vessels are located on the anteroposterior view.
4) All these parameters are also pinpointed in the skin 3D-VR reconstruction.

FIGURE 9.5 A detailed anatomical study for each flap is presented. Classic anatomical studies do not allow sufficient anatomical detail and offer inconstant information for a 'blinded' surgical approach. In 2006, CTA was established as a new gold standard and the perfect workhorse for this purpose. Perforator vessels were clearly visualized with this technique, and new flaps and surgical techniques promptly took advantage of this.

be faded in and out of view by intuitive and user-friendly interfaces built into the model. The conversion of more superficial structures into phantom images makes it possible for the viewer to grasp the 3D relationship of superficial and deeper structures. Colour representation allows for a better descriptive feature of each individual structure. The ability to rotate and eliminate irrelevant structures (crop feature) helps the reconstructive surgeon to view the anatomy, which is not possible with flat plane images or even on the actual patient. The surgeon can choose the right perforator not having to rely on clinical evaluation but on technical aspects aided by the navigation system (see Figure 9.5).

This concept has also been used in various perforator flaps such as superior gluteal artery perforator, lumbar artery musculocutaneous perforator flap, and more extensively in deep inferior epigastric perforator (DIEP).[18–22] In the DIEP flap, Gomez-Cía et al. demonstrated a high accuracy showing an average error rate of only 0.228 cm (95% CI, 0.17–0.30) compared to previous experience with conventional CTA that demonstrated an error localization margin of 0.5 cm.[22] Gacto et al. and Rozen et al. have also demonstrated a similar result in their studies.[18,19,21] All of these studies were able to describe the artery pattern prior to surgery, which allows for an identification of the most suitable perforator with a significant volume to assess flap survival. The main disadvantages of this technology are the cost and the technical expertise required to apply the data, manipulate virtual reconstruction images, and interpret the images. The fact that the examination does involve both ionizing radiation and the injection of iodinated contrast medium is also an issue. However, the risk is no different when compared to conventional CTA.

9.3.3 Facial Aesthetic Surgery

In facial aesthetic surgery of the face, the key soft-tissue anatomy is relied on a 3D relationship that is not easily appreciated by conventional means like CT and MRI. Adding a third dimension to the displayed information allows for a more realistic view assessment and prediction of the outcome. An early work by Marsh et al. and Cutting et al. has applied the use of CT data to recreate a 3D virtual model of the skeletal anatomy.[23,24] This method helps to clarify skeletal feature and assists in pre-operative planning by assessing numerous manipulation to optimize best reconstructive result. However, the use of CT and MRI does not allow for a full appreciation of the surface anatomy. Instead of CT or MRI, many devices have been developed to recreate surface anatomy, which include a third dimension. This included the work of Nkenke et al.,[25] who have used 3D surface imaging to measure orbital globes position. Ferrario et al.[26] have applied 3D surface scanning to analyse facial morphology in ectodermal dysplasia patient. Ji et al.[27] have used 3D surface scanning for the assessment of facial tissue expansion. Most of the recent developments in 3D surface imaging systems had been on the use of laser- and optical-based surface imaging technologies. They are based on the principle of structured light imaging and stereophotogrammetry. These technologies included laser imaging, structure light technology, stereophotogrammetric technologies, active stereophotogrammetric technology, and passive stereophotogrammetric technology. The description of these devices is summarized in Table 9.1.

9.4 PRACTICAL ASPECTS OF VIRTUAL 3D IN PLASTIC SURGERY

There are several devices that have been developed in an attempt to measure and reconstruct images into 3D images. These include CT, MRI, US, stereophotogrammetry, image subtraction technique, liquid crystal scanning, light luminance scanning, laser scanning, stereolithography, and video systems. From these developments, we can conclude that an ideal virtual 3D imaging should be able to fulfil several characteristics.

Characteristics of virtual 3D imaging include[28] the following:

- Imaging should be quickly acquired.
- It should be consistently repeatable.
- There is no adverse outcome to the patient.
- Imaging should yield sub-millimetre 3D data including skin surface, tone, underlying soft tissue, muscle, bone, and teeth.
- It should provide detailed contrast and colour of individual structure.
- It should capture and store the patient's images including all of their anthropometric data.
- Three-dimensional images can be viewed from any angle.
- Selected anatomical parts can be made transparent.

Another crucial aspect of virtual 3D imaging is the innovation of computer-aided design and computer-aided modelling (CAD/CAM) software.[16,29] They are initially implemented in neurosurgery and radiology procedures, and the easy acquisition and transfer of Digital Imaging and Communications in Medicine data have facilitated the development of various proprietary software programs for use in the craniomaxillofacial skeleton. Contemporary software allows surgeons to analyse patients by performing 3D measurements and to manipulate deformed or missing anatomy by mirror imaging, segmentation, or insertion of an unaltered or ideal skeletal construct. The virtual reconstruction may be transferred to the patient by using custom stereolithographic models (SLMs), implants, or cutting jig splints that are constructed using a CAD/CAM process, or through image-guided surgery in the form of intra-operative navigation (frameless stereotaxy) performed to the idealized virtual image.[16] The process of a virtual 3D reconstruction in plastic surgery can be divided into four phases:[29] (1) Data acquisition phase, in which all clinical information and measurements are obtained usually by way of image devices such as CT, MRI, or surface imagery technologies; (2) pre-operative planning phase, in which CT data are imported into a proprietary software program for the purposes of virtual planning before surgery. Surgical stimulation and manipulation of the 3D reconstruction using data derived from CT datasets can now be performed on several commercial and medical software systems as shown in Tables 9.1 and 9.2; (3) surgical phase, which is performed using CAD and CAM derived SLMs, guide stents, and/or intra-operative navigation; and (4) assessment phase, in which the accuracy of the treatment plan transfer is evaluated using intra-operative (or post-operative) CT imaging.

9.5 SUMMARY

Three-dimensional images add a third plane of depth to an otherwise conversional 2D image. The procedure involves the acquisition of scan images from CTA, MRI, or digital imagery, which can then be processed through computer software. The resulting reconstructed images can be manipulated using various technical features (see Figure 9.6). Objects can be enhanced or deleted and can be viewed from several directions, thus help improve both reconstructive surgeons and patients in understanding the anatomy and result after reconstruction. Further advance in virtual image is the application in reproducing a model of the interested area with the use of a 3D printer. This model can be used to pre-plan and prefabricate instruments thus reducing operative time with improved precision. It also served as a trial that allowed reconstructive surgeons to make as many mistakes as needed. However, the current status of virtual 3D is still in its early state, expensive, and requires

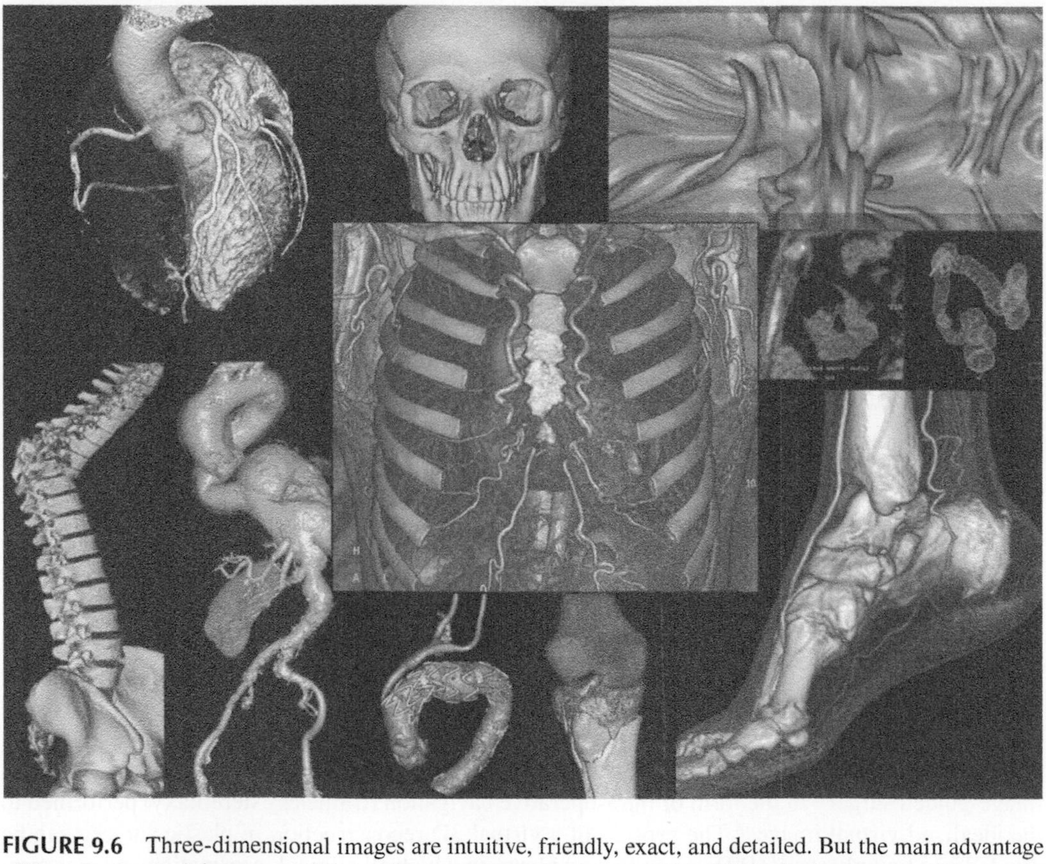

FIGURE 9.6 Three-dimensional images are intuitive, friendly, exact, and detailed. But the main advantage of these images and the reason of their wide acceptance are the capability of 'playing' with them: the user can add, remove, turn, undo, cut, colour-change, rotate – all forms of post-scan processing is possible from any anatomical site, and structure and specific reconstructive goals can be evaluated.

expertise to operate the system. With the improvement in technology and computer software, we can expect an improvement in image quality, reduction in cost, or even allow for images to be superimposed directly onto the patient for a greater accuracy.

REFERENCES

1. Smith DM, Aston SJ, Cutting CB, Oliker A, Weinzweig J. Designing a virtual reality model for aesthetic surgery. *Plast Reconstr Surg* 2005;116(3):893–897.
2. Baba K. Development of 3D ultrasound. *DSJUOG* 2010;4(3):205–215.
3. Wheatstone C. Contributions to the physiology of vision-part the first. On some remarkable, and hitherto unobserved phenomena of binocular vision. *Phil Trans R Soc London* 1838;Part I:371–394.
4. Thomson E. Stereoscopic Roentgen pictures. *Electr Eng* 1896;21:256.
5. Davidson JM. Remarks on the value of stereoscopic photography and skiagraphy: Records of clinical and pathological appearances. *Br Med J* 1898;2(1979):1669–1671.
6. Davidson JM. *Localization by X Rays and Stereoscopy*. London, U.K.: H. K. Lewis; 1916.
7. Munz Y, Moorthy K, Dosis A, Hernandez JD, Bann S, Bello F et al. The benefits of stereoscopic vision in robotic-assisted performance on bench models. *Surg Endosc* 2004;18(4):611–616.
8. Korean Standards Association. *3D Standard and Patent Investigation Report*. Seoul, South Korea: Korean Standards Association; 2012.
9. Hounsfield GN. Computerized transverse axial scanning (tomography): Part I. Description of system. *Br J Radiol* 1973;46:1016–1022.
10. Carr H. Field gradients in early MRI. *Phys Today* 2004;2:83.
11. Lauterbur PC. Autobiography. Nobel Prize official website. 2003. Retrieved October 11, 2012.
12. Hidalgo DA. Fibula free flap: A new method of mandible reconstruction. *Plast Reconstr Surg* 1989;84(1):71–79.
13. Antony AK, Chen WF, Kolokythas A, Weimer KA, Cohen MN. Use of virtual surgery and stereolithography-guided osteotomy for mandibular reconstruction with the free fibula. *Plast Reconstr Surg* 2011;128(5):1080–1084.
14. Sink J, Hamlar D, Kademani D, Khariwala SS. Computer-aided stereolithography for presurgical planning in fibula free tissue reconstruction of the mandible. *J Reconstr Microsurg* 2012;28(6):395–403.
15. Roser SM, Ramachandra S, Blair H, Grist W, Carlson GW, Christensen AM et al. The accuracy of virtual surgical planning in free fibula mandibular reconstruction: Comparison of planned and final results. *J Oral Maxillofac Surg* 2010;68(11):2824–2832.
16. Rozen WM, Ashton MW, Stella DL, Phillips TJ, Grinsell D, Taylor GI. The accuracy of computed tomographic angiography for mapping the perforators of the deep inferior epigastric artery: A blinded, prospective cohort study. *Plast Reconstr Surg* 2008;122(4):1003–1009.
17. Phillips TJ, Stella DL, Rozen WM, Ashton M, Taylor GI. Abdominal wall CT angiography: A detailed account of a newly established preoperative imaging technique. *Radiology* 2008;249(1):32–44.
18. Rozen WM, Phillips TJ, Ashton MW, Stella DL, Gibson RN, Taylor GI. Preoperative imaging for DIEA perforator flaps: A comparative study of computed tomographic angiography and Doppler ultrasound. *Plast Reconstr Surg* 2008;121:9.
19. Rozen WM, Ashton MW, Stella DL, Phillips TJ, Taylor GI. Stereotactic image-guided navigation in the preoperative imaging of perforators for DIEP flap breast reconstruction. *Microsurgery* 2008;28:417.
20. Lui KW, Hu S, Ahmad N, Tang M. Three-dimensional angiography of the superior gluteal artery and lumbar artery perforator flap. *Plast Reconstr Surg* 2009;123(1):79–86.
21. Gacto P, Barrera F, Sicilia-Castro D, Miralles F, Collell M, Leal S et al. A three-dimensional virtual reality model for limb reconstruction in burned patients. *Burns* 2009;35(7):1042–1046.
22. Suarez C, Acha B, Serrano C, Parra C, Gomez T. VirSSPA – A virtual reality tool for surgical planning workflow. *Int J Comp Assist Radiol Surg* 2009;4(2):133–139.
23. Marsh JL, Vannier MW, Stevens WG. Surface reconstructions from computerized tomographic scans for evaluation of malignant skull destruction. *Am J Surg* 1984;148:530.
24. Cutting C, Oliker A, Haring J, Dayan J, Smith D. Use of three-dimensional computer graphic animation to illustrate cleft lip and palate surgery. *Comput Aided Surg* 2002;7:326.
25. Nkenke E, Benz M, Maier T, Wiltfang J, Holbach LM, Kramer M et al. Relative en- and exophthalmometry in zygomatic fractures comparing optical non-contact, non-ionizing 3D imaging to the Hertel instrument and computed tomography. *J Craniomaxillofac Surg* 2003;31:362.

26. Ferrario VF, Dellavia C, Serrao G, Sforza C. Soft-tissue facial areas and volumes in individuals with ectodermal dysplasia: A three-dimensional noninvasive assessment. *Am J Med Genet* 2004;126A:253.
27. Ji Y, Zhang F, Schwartz J, Stile F, Lineaweaver WC. Assessment of facial tissue expansion with three-dimensional digitizer scanning. *J Craniofac Surg* 2002;13:687.
28. Pallanch J. 3D and the next dimension for facial plastic surgery. *Facial Plast Surg Clin North Am* 2011;19(4):xix–xxi.
29. Markiewicz MR, Bell RB. The use of 3D imaging tools in facial plastic surgery. *Facial Plast Surg Clin North Am* 2011;19:655–682.

10 Digital Thermographic Photography for Preoperative Perforator Mapping

Vachara Niumsawatt, Warren M. Rozen, and Iain S. Whitaker

CONTENTS

10.1 OVERVIEW

In planning flap reconstruction, it is crucial to be able to identify a suitable perforator. It has been well recognised that preoperative localisation of the involved perforating arteries in the planning of musculocutaneous or fasciocutaneous flaps can lead to a higher survival rate of the whole skin island. With the introduction of freestyle reconstruction flaps comes a need for a safe and reliable method of perforator mapping. Wei et al. described *freestyle* flaps when a flap is raised after a perforator was identified in an unfamiliar region; flap harvest can still be done, by surgically exploring the region for vessels of suitable size.[1] This had led to an increase in the number of flaps available. The need for an accurate and simple imaging modality has become increasingly important. Several imaging technologies have been developed and utilised by reconstructive surgeons in helping to identify this crucial information prior to flap design. Doppler ultrasound yields a low sensitivity and is operator dependent for both identifying and interpretation of results. Cutaneous perforators can be mapped by magnetic resonance imaging (MRI), computed tomographic angiography (CTA), and digital subtraction angiography (DSA), each of which is not without morbidity and can be associated with radiation exposure, risk of contrast reactions and extravasation, and/or nephrotoxicity. These modalities, while providing accurate and precise information on the details of vascular anatomy, can be time-consuming and expensive. The need for non-invasive, inexpensive, sensitive, accurate bedside devices with minimal or no adverse effects has pushed radiologists and reconstructive surgeons into seeking alternative imaging technologies. Several papers in the literature have analysed the use of digital infrared (IR) thermography in preoperative flap reconstruction planning.

10.2 HISTORY OF THERMOGRAPHY

10.2.1 Early Thermography Development

IR radiation was discovered in 1800 by Sir Frederick William Herschel, a German-born British astronomer, while he was measuring the temperature of the various components of visible light spectrum created by a white light passing through a prism. He measured the temperature of each visible light band and holding a thermometer just beyond the red end of the visible spectrum. This thermometer was meant to be a control to measure the ambient air temperature in the room. To his amazement, he noticed that when the thermometer was placed beyond the red band of the visible spectrum, there was a further increase in temperature.[2] Herschel called this invisible light *infrared*.[3] His only son, Sir John Herschel, carried on some of his experiment. He was a keen photographer and successfully created the first thermographic image using solar radiation. He created an evaporograph image of the heating rays of IR using carbon suspension in alcohol and named it *thermogram*, hence laying the foundations of thermal imaging based on IR rays.[4]

A major development in IR technology is in early 1929 by a Hungarian physicist Kalman Tihanyi. He was credited for inventing the first IR-sensitive camera for British anti-aircraft defence after the Great War.[4] This is based on the idea that all objects emit a heat signal in the form of IR radiation. The higher the object's temperature, the more IR radiation emitted. An IR thermographic camera can detect this radiation in a similar way to an ordinary camera that can detect visible light. IR thermography in human physiology was first used in 1934, with an earlier work by the American physiologist James Hardy who showed that regardless of skin colour or ethnicity, the human body is a highly efficient radiator with an emissivity, at 0.98, close to that of a perfect black body.[5]

10.2.2 History of IR Imaging in Medicine

The major development of IR technology remained dominant in military use, not until the 1950s when the first electronic sensor for IR radiation could be used to produce thermal imaging. Physicians around the world started to recognise the potential benefit of IR technology in medicine and physiology. The first practice of diagnostic thermography was carried out in 1957 by R. Lawson when he detected that the skin overlying breast tumour has an increase in temperature compared to normal tissue.[6,7] The use of IR thermography in medicine was adopted from the principle that increase in body temperature causes a higher amount of radiation emitted. Hence, an increase in vascularity, which is a hallmark of many pathological changes such as inflammation or neoplasms with increased metabolic activity, leads to an increase in temperature, which can be detected by an IR thermographic camera.

The first medical thermal image was very crude with the images displayed in black and white. Before the arrival of the computer and analytical software, much discussion was needed between physicians and physicists for the interpretation of results using a subjective thermogram score.[5,6] By the mid-1970s, the first image processing computer for medical thermography was installed in Bath, UK. The use of a coloured screen was provided to display the digitalised image.[6] Further improvement in software and photographic technology has expanded around the international scientific community. Improving technology has allowed for an improve, detection temperature sensitivity of <0.1°. Modern imaging systems offer real-time digital image capture in combination with advanced computer software to assist in image analysis.[8] It allowed for application for colour coding with different temperatures represented. The digital images can be viewed as both static (single image) and dynamic (real time) to monitor the changes in temperature depending on the time and pathophysiological response.

10.3 PHYSIOLOGY OF HEAT TRANSPORT IN THE SKIN

It has long been established that body temperature is an indicator of health condition. Since Hippocrates around 480 BC, wet mud was used to cover patients' bodies and observation of the drying mud was made as the moisture evaporated. This allowed the ancient physicians to detect increase in temperature changes as a useful indicator of a bodily dysfunction. The human body is *homoeothermic*, meaning that they are capable of regulating the core temperature in a constantly changing environment. The main mechanisms in which the human body maintains the thermal balance are by way of inhibition and stimulation of the sympathetic centre, containing within the posterior hypothalamus.[9] During heat exposure or intense exercise, skin blood flow can be increased to provide greater heat dissipation across skin surface. This mechanism is achieved by inhibition of the sympathetic response resulting in vasodilation of the peripheral blood vessel. Under hyperthermic conditions, whether be environmental or physiological, the skin combines with vital anatomical structure and functions to protect and defend the body from a dangerous level of thermal stress by regulating heat transfers between the core, skin, and environment. When exposed to a cool environment, the temperature control system institutes exactly opposite procedures. The sympathetic response is stimulated resulting in peripheral vasoconstriction to preserve heat and metabolic energy for internal vital organs. The skin surface is nearly eliminated of blood flow and becomes an excellent insulator. This emitting or omission of heat dissipation as a response to change in vascularity can be detected by IR thermography.

The vascular anatomy of an individual has also played a crucial role in thermography and its basis. The vessels that supply blood to the flap are isolated perforators. These perforators may pass either through or in between the deep tissues (i.e. muscle or septum).[10] The anatomy of skin circulation is described as the separation of horizontal and vertical components. The horizontal component consists of several vascular plexuses that lie in parallel to the skin surface (subpapillary, subdermal, and prefascial plexus). The vertical components are perforators that arise from deeper arteries and veins. These vessels then anastomose with the prefascial, subdermal, and subpapillary plexuses.[11] Thermography is used to detect these vertical perforators as perfusion of blood courses through the vasculature.

From these bases, the application of IR thermography has expanded into oncology (including establishment of the early breast cancer detection and demonstration projects),[12,13] neuropathy,[14,15] arthritis, rheumatism, Raynaud's phenomenon,[16,17] monitoring and diagnosing vascular disorders (diabetes, deep venous thrombosis), assessment of burn injury,[18,19] dermatological disorder, monitoring efficacy of therapeutic drugs, skeletal muscle kinetic and recovery in sports medicine, and assessment of blood perfusion in flap reconstruction planning, assessment, and monitoring.

10.4 USE OF DIRT IN ASSESSING AND MAPPING PERFORATORS IN PREOPERATIVE FLAP RECONSTRUCTION

Preoperative imaging to assess the vasculature has been an area of interest to reconstructive surgeons since the early days of microsurgery. In the past, the imaging modality most frequently used was the handheld Doppler probe which has been proved to yield a low sensitivity.[20,21] With the current technique of perforator-based flap reconstruction evolved a demand for more accuracy in identifying smaller and finer vessels. CTA and MRI have been the workhorse in preoperative flap reconstruction planning for resolution and objectivity in imaging. However, a quest to find a simpler, convenient, inexpensive, and widely available mode of imaging has resulted in the development and improvement of IR thermography.

In flap surgery, the perfusion and reperfusion of the flap are crucial for successful surgery. It is these that make IR thermography an ideal tool in detecting these changes. Several key papers in the literature have proposed the use of IR thermography in predicting and identifying vessels for the pre-planning of flap reconstruction. Theuvenet et al. used the digital thermograph camera (Philip) with a photovoltaic liquid nitrogen-cooled InSb detector to evaluate the marking of perforators in various areas that could be harvested as musculocutaneous or fasciocutaneous flaps.[22] First, he performed a dynamic IR thermography (DIRT) using cadaveric lower limb to investigate the perforator for tensor fascia lata (TFL) flap design. The cadaver skin underwent a cold challenge with a metal drum filled with water of 5°C. A warm NaCl 0.9% at 60°C was then injected into the femoral artery. DIRT was then used to video record the reperfusion of the cutaneous skin. Areas of hotspots were then marked with insoluble ink and dissection was performed to identify correlating perforators. From four TFL specimens, a total of 31 out of 36 perforators that were detected by DIRT were located. The five perforators which were not visualised with DIRT as hotspots seem to have been obstructed in their distal portion of the vessels. A further 16 living volunteers had their perforators analysed after cold challenge, with or without the use of exsanguination and tourniquet. After rewarming or release of the tourniquet, hotspots can be detected with DIRT. The areas investigated include trunk for visualising latissimus dorsi area and extremities for TFL flap design. Interestingly, one patient with known severe atherosclerosis of the lower limb has shown minimal hotspots which reflect the underlying peripheral vascular disease.[22]

Many international centres have since demonstrated benefit from the use of IR thermographic camera to detect perforators of the abdomen for pre-planning of transverse rectus abdominis musculocutaneous (TRAM) flap and deep inferior epigastric pedicle (DIEP) free flap. Salmi performed a series of thermographic study on the abdomen for eight free TRAM flap reconstructions. DIRT (Inframetrics Model 600) was used to measure the temperature changes from different phases of flap reconstruction including preoperative, induction, dissection/ligation of pedicle, and post-operative recovery period. Without using the cold challenge, a video recording of the perfusion stages was taken at four different points. In the preoperative stage, the hotspot was located close to the periumbilical region with a higher temperature of 1.4°C ± 0.52°C than the rest of the abdomen, which corresponds to the pedicle identified during dissection. During the induction, there is a flush reaction and the flap has increased in temperature by 0.9°C ± 0.57°C; this is likely due to the vasodilation effect from general anaesthetic. After the pedicle has been cut, the hotspots vanished and the whole flap temperature decreased by 3.4°C ± 1.05°C. After a re-established flow, the hotspot can be detected with a mean of 17 min has lapse.[23] This study demonstrated the potential for DIRT to detect physiological change during interruption and re-establishment of perfusion in flap reconstruction.

A unique feature of DIRT compared to other investigative modalities is the ability to provide information regarding the flow characteristics of the perforator. It has the added value of the rate and pattern of rewarming of the hotspots that represents the quality of the perforators. This information cannot be achieved with a conventional multi-detector computer tomography (MDCT) or MRI but rather a 4D CT imaging.[24,25] De Weerd used not only static thermographic images but also a dynamic image while the skin reperfused. This additional information of perforator characteristics included its calibre and length. It seems logical that DIRT has the ability to highlight the perforator with the largest calibre, shortest course with highest flow rate and represent it as the brightest hotspot on the skin that appears rapidly after a cold challenge. In this study, a total of 23 patients underwent a delay breast reconstruction after mastectomies were recruited. Deep inferior epigastric artery (DIEA) perforators were located using a handheld Doppler probe, and these perforators were then marked for comparison with DIRT images. They were then given a cold challenge with a desktop fan blown over the abdomen for 2 min. DIRT camera (Nikon Laird S270) was used to detect reperfusion of abdominal skin. From the study, they were able to observe the differences in the rate of rewarming and brightness of different hotspots. These rapid reperfusion hotspots seem to correlate with the most audible sound detected by Doppler probe. All of the DIEA free flaps were based on the perforators which appeared first upon reperfusion seen by DIRT. They were all deemed suitable for free flap reconstruction. A total of eight patients underwent MDCT to compare the result of IR thermography with respect to localisation and quality of the selected arterial perforator. All perforators detected by DIRT were clearly visible on the MDCT scan. All of the flaps survived where three suffered a partial flap loss. Furthermore, the DIEA perforators detected as most suitable by DIRT are all based on lateral row.[24] The finding is consistent with reports by Itoh and Arai which found that in 88.2%, the most dominant branch of the DIEA is the lateral branches (although not related to the specific zone of supply).[26]

10.5 COLD CHALLENGE

Thermography uses IR rays reflected by an object to produce an image based on temperature differences. Conventional thermography without the use of cold challenges provides vague and unclear images as the blood perfused across the capillary of the skin surface. This dermal capillary network produces a uniform heat across the entire skin surface which will be detected by the IR thermography. This makes the identification of specific perforators difficult with no useful information obtained.[27] In order to identify a flow of perfusion through the perforators, the flow of blood through the area of interest needs to be eliminated or cooled. Various techniques have been used to establish a baseline background image before a reperfusion to identify *hotspots*.

Theuvenet used exsanguination and pneumatic tourniquet to interrupt the flow of blood into the distal extremities. After applying the tourniquet, the entire skin was then cooled with cold water at 5°C for 7 min. Baseline IR thermographic images were then taken. Blood was then allowed to flow back into the extremity as the tourniquet was released. Hotspots of reperfusing perforators can then be detected with IR thermography. Using this technique, they were able to accurately locate perforators, with patients however reporting some discomfort from the use of the tourniquet. There was no long-term complication observed. For the trunk and proximal extremities where the tourniquet cannot be used, a metal barrel filled with cold water at 5°C was rolled on the skin in an up and fro manner for a total of 7 min. This allows for the skin surface to cool, and through it, the weight partly interrupted the arterial blood flow. Again, the technique can accurately identify perforators. However, patients reported pain and one patient sustained superficial skin necrosis from extreme cold.[22] Itoh, Chijiwa, and Whitaker all have employed the use of vinyl bag filled with ice to cool the skin surface to obtain baseline images. Itoh placed the ice-filled bag onto patient skin for 5–10 s, Chijiwa for 25 s, and Whitaker for 10 min.[27–29] None of the studies report any complication or complaint from their subjects group. De Weerd used a very simple method of cold challenge. He placed a desktop fan over the abdominal area for 2 min before capturing the baseline thermographic image.[24,25] From these studies, there is not any uniform cold challenge method or cooling period to obtain baseline IR thermography image.

It is necessary to establish an optimal temperature to create a baseline cooling temperature rendered the hotspots. Zetterman et al. attempted to find the ideal cooling period of cold challenges. Their study focussed on the cooling period used, to provide the ideal length of time where the perforators were visible for flap planning. Half of their patients (N = 8 in each group) were subjected to cooling of 30 s while the other half to 300 s (or 5 min). After 30 s of cold challenge, hotspots are visible and continue to be observed for 4 min thereafter. However, a longer (300 s) cooling period gives a 3.4 times larger temperature difference between the hotspots and the baseline than a shorter cooling period did (30 s). The perforators were more clearly identified for a longer period, of up to 10 min, giving plenty of time for the operating surgeon to design the flap.[30] Appearance of a hotspot was more rapid in the 300 s than 30 s groups, 150 s versus 180 s, respectively, after removal of the cold cushions from the skin. Furthermore, after 300 s, the whole abdominal skin became isothermic, making this a more ideal time for baseline. None of the recruited volunteers felt uncomfortable even with a cooling period of 300 s. Zetterman's study demonstrated that a cold challenge of at least 30 s is sufficient to identify the perforators. However, a longer cooling time of up to 300 s (or 5 min) can provide more information regarding the rate of perfusion and give more time in which to plan the flap.[30]

10.6 COMPARISON OF DIRT TO OTHER MODALITIES IN PREOPERATIVE PERFORATOR MAPPING FOR FLAP PLANNING

10.6.1 DIRT versus Doppler Probe

When comparison is made between DIRT and conventional handheld Doppler probe, it has been found that the number of hotspots found by thermography was higher than those found by Doppler probe. Sixty-seven to eighty percent of perforators found by DIRT are matched with their corresponding flow Doppler signal. The distance between the cutaneous mark of the vessels found by flow Doppler and the closest hotspot found by thermography was an average of 0 mm to 12 mm ± 4.3 mm.[24] The distance in discrepancy of the location of perforator is believed to have been the result of perforator vessels with oblique trajectories in the subcutaneous tissue.[24,31] Studies by both Tenorio and De Weerd demonstrate that Doppler can better locate vessels in the deeper layer where they exited the muscular fascia and thermography detected their location underneath the skin.[25,31] DIRT takes less time to perform than Doppler probe with the average of examination time of 20 min compared to 45 min.[24] Another feature of DIRT is the intensity and rate of recovery that is directly proportional to the diameter of perforators. This is possible because of the dynamic feature in which handheld Doppler probe cannot attain.[24,31]

10.6.2 DIRT versus CTA

Although CTA has revolutionised preoperative imaging by accurately identifying and assessing the diameter and course of perforators, it still has a number of drawbacks which IR thermography can address. The attributes of CTA and DIRT are shown in Table 10.1.[29] The use of DIRT in comparison to CTA was demonstrated initially by De Weerd in 2009. It was found that the selected DIEA perforators from DIRT can be clearly visualised on axial MDCT images. Upon dissection of the flap, the size and precious location of these perforators again can be seen and was select for flap pedicle.[24,25] Whitaker et al. further developed this technique with comparison made with the use of 3D CTA imaging prior to flap reconstruction (see Figure 10.1). The image of DIRT was used

TABLE 10.1
Comparison of the Attributes of DIRT versus CTA

CTA	DIRT
Detects 100% of perforators	Detects clinically significant perforators >1 mm diameter
Locates to <1 mm	Locates to <1 cm
Associated with radiation exposure	Radiation-free
Uses intravenous contrast anaphylactic risk	Non-invasive, repeatable
Separate hospital visit	Single visit performed in clinic
30 min CT appointment with technician	10 min procedure
3D recon and report by specialist	Image reported by surgeon
Delay between scan and report	Immediate report in clinic
Static images	Temporal information regarding perfusion
Cost of scanner >£1 million	Cost of camera >£20,000

Source: Whitaker, I.S. et al., *J. Plast. Reconstr. Aesthet. Surg.*, 65, 130, 2012.

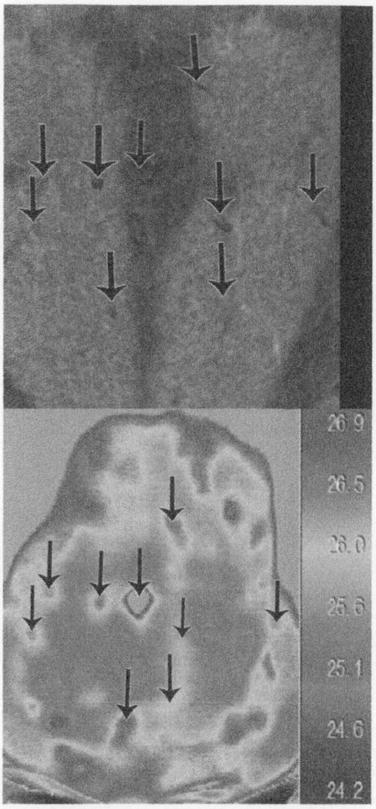

(a)

(b)

FIGURE 10.1 (a) CTA of the abdominal wall vasculature, highlighting the location of DIEA perforators. (b) Digital thermographic photograph of the abdominal wall of the same patient, demonstrating concordance in localising perforators. The thermographic image has been taken 1 min after removal of a cold challenge. Arterial perforators have preferentially rewarmed the skin in a pattern that highlights their distribution. The scale on the right demonstrates increasing thermal activity from blue to red. (Reproduced from Chubb, D. et al., *Ann. Plast. Surg.*, 66, 324, 2011. With permission.)

to demonstrate hotspots of the perforator within the designed DIEA flap (Figure 10.2a and b). The superimposed images of DIRT and 3D CTA show a direct and accurate correlation of major and minor abdominal perforators (Figure 10.2c). The intensity of the temperature reflected the size of the perforator as the largest perforator has the highest intensity in thermal imaging.[29] Both of these studies were also able to identify even smaller perforators that might not be suitable to be used as anastomosing vessels for flap reconstruction.[24,29] These smaller perforators have shown a slower reperfusion with less degree of temperature differences compared to the surrounding skin surface. Although the 3D CTA provides information on the perforator's diameter, its location, and the course it takes, thermography records temperature changes which are a direct result of rates of blood flow that can somewhat be an interpretation of individual vessel characteristic. This allows for the change in blood flow especially in the changes of vascular tone.[29,32] Furthermore, DIRT is portable and can be repeated on the same patient without causing an adverse outcome. The accuracy of these findings has been compared not only to CTA but also to operative findings, confirming in vivo flow dynamics to be associated with thermography (see Figure 10.2d). De Weerd had demonstrated the benefit of intra-operative and post-operative flap monitoring of the device. This tool can provide an immediate feedback for the operative surgeon and allow appropriate action to be taken at the most effective time.[25] These studies suggest that DIRT can be used in conjunction with CTA to improve free flap surgery planning.

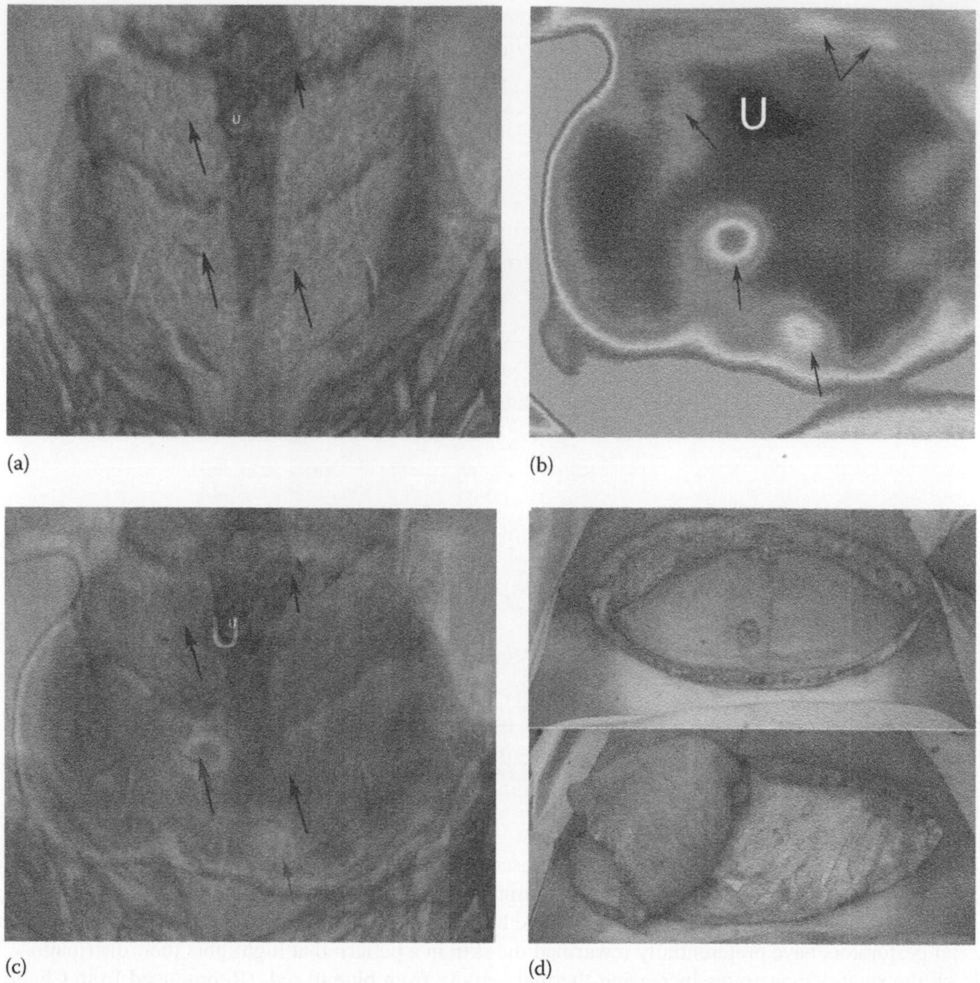

FIGURE 10.2 (a) Preoperative CTA showing one suitable single medial row perforator supplying the right hemi-abdomen, with a diameter of 2 mm. The other perforators were felt to be insufficient to supply a flap. This image shows one small perforator to the right of the umbilicus and two small perforators just to the left of the midline. (b) Thermal image after 10 min of cold challenge using a water pack at 5°C showing the presence of one *hotspot* confirming the presence of the dominant perforator on the right and the lack of visible hotspots on the left. (c) Preoperative thermal image overlying the preoperative CTA, showing the correlation between the findings of the two modalities (black arrows). (d) Intra-operative photographs showing the raised DIEP flap, with the marked perforator of choice on the right hemi-abdomen. The left hemi-abdomen had no perforators of note. (Reproduced from Whitaker, I.S. et al., *J. Plast. Reconstr. Aesthet. Surg.*, 65, 130, 2012. With permission.)

In our unpublished series, we undertook a prospective clinical analysis of consecutive cases of patients undergoing microvascular free flap breast reconstruction and utilised a combination of preoperative CTA, preoperative thermography, and intra-operative perforator detection. We sought to assess outcomes including a quantitative analysis of the accuracy of DIRT, a cost-saving analysis, and a subjective assessment of the ease of imaging interpretation and implementation into operative planning. To these ends, we found in our early cases that DIRT was highly sensitive for perforators over 1.2 mm (100%); there was poor sensitivity for periumbilical perfs, with umbilical branches lighting up, and a poor sensitivity for perforators <1 mm. We have largely decided to abandon the use of DIRT as a means of achieving our aims in the course of such investigations and use it as an adjunct to other imaging modalities (particularly CTA). We have felt that DIRT has not yet reached the efficacy of the current gold standard, CTA, despite its ease of use and lack of morbidity. The ongoing work of our units and those that continue to publish in the field suggests that with improvements in technique and resolution, its role in preoperative imaging may yet evolve.

10.7 IR THERMOGRAPHY: PROCEDURE AND PROTOCOL

10.7.1 Pre-Examination Preparation

- Detailed history is taken, in particular assessing for known pathology which can increase or decrease blood flow in the examination area such as inflammation, infection, trauma, burn, neoplasm, peripheral vascular disease, and deep vein thrombosis.
- Explanation about the procedure is given to patients; this includes the understanding that
  - Thermography technology does not see into the body and does not image any structure deeper than the skin
  - The study does not necessarily indicate that there is no abnormality and an abnormal
  - There is no risk of exposure to radiation from thermographic camera
- All questions and concerns about any aspect of the examination should be addressed.
- Informed consent obtained.
- No strenuous exercise for at least 3 h before the examination.
- No lotions, creams, powders, or makeup on the area of examination on the day of the exam.
- Avoid shaving the area on the day of the examination.
- Avoid extended sun or heat exposure the day before and the day of the exam.
- No bathing or exposure to cold closer than 1 h before the examination.

10.7.2 Procedure

- Preset the thermographic camera as per institute protocol including the diagnostic software.
- Environmental controls
  - Examination should be performed in a room where ambient temperature is controlled.
  - Avoid draughts and exposure to significant external or internal heat sources (e.g. sunlight, incandescent lighting).
  - Ventilation systems should be designed to avoid airflow onto the patient.
- The thermal imaging room should ideally be kept between 20°C and 23°C to avoid altering the patient's physiology, that is, shivering or perspiring.
- Patient is asked not to touch the examined body part to prevent heat transfer.
- Patient is placed in a comfortable position so that the maximum surface area is exposed to the thermographic camera.
- Cold challenge
  - There are several cold challenge techniques:
  - Desktop fan[24,25]
- A desktop fan is used to blow cold air on the area to be examined for 2 min.
  - Plastic bag filled with ice or water pack at 5°C[27,29]
- A plastic bag or water pack kept in a refrigerator at cold temperature (5°C) is placed on the area to be examined for 2–5 min.
- IR imaging
  - After the cold challenges, static or dynamic IR thermographic images can be taken over 10 min.

10.7.3 Reporting

- Interpreting thermologists need to assure that all pre-imaging preparation and office protocols are followed.
- Any deviation from the protocol should be charted by the technician.
- A full patient history needs to be available to the interpreting thermologists.
- Information regarding to the quality and quantity of hotspots is documented including the following:
  - Presence of hotspot
  - Time of reperfusion
  - Degree of heat intensity
  - Area of reperfusion

10.8 SUMMARY

DIRT technology allows assessment of perfusion and reperfusion in real time. It is inexpensive, repeatable, without adverse effect, simple to implement, and interpreted as an investigative tool. It can be used as an alternative or in collaboration with other diagnostic interventions to map and characterise perforators in designing cutaneous and musculocutaneous flaps, by the presence of hotspots. It has a similar sensitivity and specificity in detecting cutaneous perforators as CTA and better sensitivity than Doppler probe.[23,24] However, while the CTA provides information on all the perforators in the area, giving a precise location of less than 1 mm vessel calibre and additionally giving the exact course of the vessel, helping surgeons choose the perforator that requires the least intramuscular dissection, DIRT can provide the information regarding the quality and in vivo flow dynamics of the perforators.[24,25,29] De Weerd et al. described the characteristics of the hotspots seen in IR thermography as significant in choosing the perforators as the pattern and rate of hotspots rewarming are important in qualitative assessment.[25] Furthermore, the availability as a portable device allows DIRT to be operated intra-operatively and as a bedside post-operative assessment. This allows the reconstructive surgeon to take an immediate appropriate action if issues arise with perfusion. Although some DIRT devices do not require the use of a cold challenge, due to its high sensitivity in detecting temperature differences (<0.1°C),[33] it is still recommended with all current

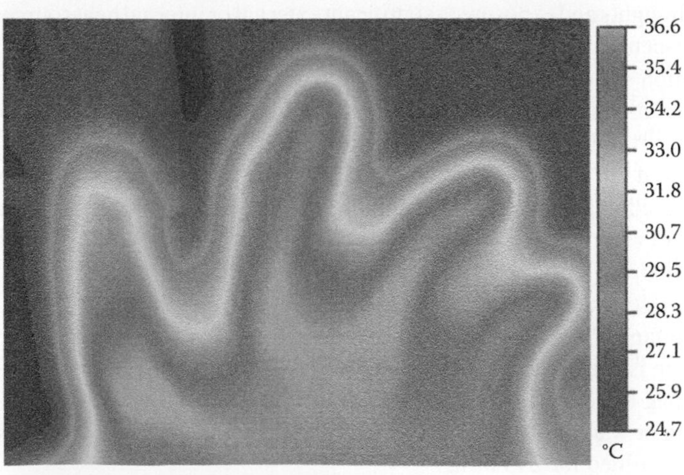

FIGURE 10.3 Post-operative digital thermograph of a replanted index finger. Thermography was used as an adjunct to post-operative monitoring and demonstrates the presence of active blood flow, albeit at altered thermographic levels to the rest of the fingers and hand.

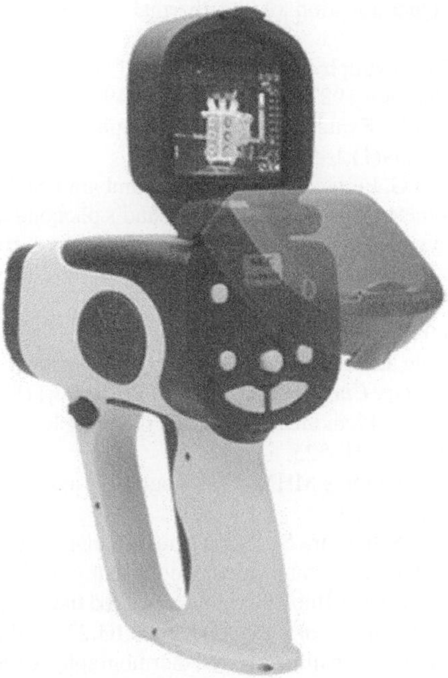

FIGURE 10.4 The digital thermographic camera (Thermo Tracer TH 7800, NEC Avio Infrared Technologies, Tokyo). (Image retrieved from http://www.namicon.com/products.xpg?catid=121&prodid=575 on December 27, 2012.)

models based on the current literature. This cold challenge has been shown to improve accuracy and allow for detection of rate of perfusion. With this technology applicable in a range of scenarios in reconstructive surgery, including flap planning, flap monitoring, replantation monitoring (see Figure 10.3), and intra-operative guidance, there is sure to be an explosion in its utility in plastic and reconstructive surgery. Advances in the hardware and software alike (see Figure 10.4) continue to contribute to the evolution of DIRT.

REFERENCES

1. Wei FC, Mardini S. *Flaps and Reconstructive Surgery*. Elsevier; 2009.
2. Ring EFJ. The discovery of infrared radiation in 1800. *Imaging Sci J* 2000;48:1–8.
3. Herchel W. Observations of the powers of prismatic colours to heat and illuminated objects. *Philos Trans B* 1800;90:255–283.
4. Ring EFJ. The historical development of thermometry and thermal imaging in medicine. *J Med Eng Tech* 2006;30(4):192–198.
5. Hardy JD. Radiation of heat from the human body. The human skin as a black body radiator. *J Clin Invest* 1934;13:593–620.
6. Jaing LJ, Ng EYK, Yeo ACB, Wu S, Pan F, Yau WY, Chen JH, Yang Y. A perspective on medical infrared imaging. *J Med Eng Tech* 2005;20(6):257–267.
7. Ring EFJ, Ammer K. Infrared thermal imaging in medicine. *Physiol Meas* 2012;33:R33–R46.
8. De Weerd L, Mercer JB, Weum S. Dynamic infrared thermography. *Clin Plast Surg* 2011;38(2):277–292.
9. Guyton AC, Hall JE. *Textbook of Medical Physiology*. Elsevier; 2006.
10. Blondeel P. The "Gent" consensus on perforator flap terminology: Preliminary definitions. *Plast Reconstr Surg* 2003;112:1378–1383.
11. Cormack G. *The Arterial Anatomy of Skin Flaps*. Second edition. Churchill Livingstone; 1994.
12. Saxena A, Willital G. Infrared thermography: Experience from a decade of pediatric imaging. *Eur J Pediatr* 2008;167:757–764.

13. Centigul MP, Herman C. Quantification of the thermal signature of a melanoma. *Int J Therm Sci* 2011;50:421–431.
14. Herrick RT, Herrick SK. Thermography in the detection of carpal tunnel syndrome and other compressive neuropathies. *J Hand Surg Am* 1987;12(5 Pt 2):943–949.
15. So YT, Olney RK, Aminoff MJ. Evaluation of thermography in the diagnosis of selected entrapment neuropathies. *Neurology* 1989;39(1):1–5.
16. Caramaschi P, Codella O, Poli G, Perbellini L, Biasi D, Bambara LM, Corrocher R, De Sandre G. Use of computerized digital thermometer for diagnosis of Raynaud's phenomenon. *Angiology* 1989;40:863–871.
17. Ammer K. Diagnosis of Raynaud's phenomenon by thermography. *Skin Res Technol* 1996;2:182–185.
18. Anselmo V, Zawacki B. Infrared photography as a diagnostic tool for the burn ward. *Proc Soc Photo-Optical Instr Eng* 1973;8:181.
19. Liddington M, Shakespeare P. Timing of the thermographic assessment of burns. *Burns* 1996;22:26–28.
20. Yu P, Youssef A. Efficacy of the handheld Doppler in preoperative identification of the cutaneous perforators in the anterolateral thigh flap. *Changgeng Yi Xue Za Zhi* 2006;118:928–933, discussion 934–935.
21. Khan UD, Miller JG. Reliability of handheld Doppler in planning local perforator-based flaps for extremities. *Aesthet Plast Surg* 2007;31:521–525.
22. Theuvenet WJ, Koeyers GF, Borghouts MHM. Thermographic assessment of perforating arteries. *Scand J Plast Reconstr Surg* 1986;20:25–29.
23. Salmi AM, Tukiainen E, Asko-Seljavaara S. Thermographic mapping of perforators and skin blood flow in the free transverse rectus abdominis musculocutaneous flap. *Ann Plast Surg* 1995;35:159–164.
24. De Weerd L, Weum S, Mercer J. The value of dynamic infrared thermography (DIRT) in perforator selection and planning of free DIEP flaps. *Ann Plast Surg* 2009;63:274–279.
25. De Weerd L, Mercer JB, Weum S. Dynamic infrared thermography. *Clin Plast Surg* 2011;38(2):277–292.
26. Itoh Y, Arai K. The deep inferior epigastric artery free skin flap: Anatomic study and clinical application. *Plast Reconstr Surg* 1993;91:853–863.
27. Itoh Y, Arai K. Use of recovery-enhanced thermography to localize cutaneous perforators. *Ann Plast Surg* 1995;34(5):507–511.
28. Chijiwa T, Arai K, Miyazaki N, Igota S, Yamamoto N. Making of a facial perforator map by thermography. *Ann Plast Surg* 2000;44:596–600.
29. Whitaker IS, Lie KH, Rozen WM, Chubb D, Ashton MW. Dynamic infrared thermography for the preoperative planning of microsurgical breast reconstruction: A comparison with CTA. *J Plast Reconstr Aesthet Surg* 2012;65(1):130–132.
30. Zetterman E, Salmi AM, Suominen S, Karonen A, Asko-Seljavaara S. Effect of cooling and warming on thermographic imaging of the perforating vessels of the abdomen. *Eur J Plast Surg* 1999;22:58–61.
31. Tenorio X, Mahajan A, Wettstein R. Early detection of flap failure using a new thermographic device. *J Surg Res* 2009;151:15–21.
32. Chubb D, Rozen WM, Whitaker IS, Asthon MW. Images in plastic surgery: Digital thermographic photography ("Thermal imaging") for preoperative perforator mapping. *Ann Plast Surg* 2011;66(4):324–325.
33. Alderson JKA, Ring EFJ. "Sprite" high resolution thermal imaging system. *Thermol* 1995;1:110–114.

11 Stereotactic Image-Guided Surgery

Vachara Niumsawatt, Warren M. Rozen, Mark W. Ashton, Alberto Alonso-Burgos, and Iain S. Whitaker

CONTENTS

11.1 OVERVIEW

Interest in the development of stereotactic surgery in humans had been documented in the literature as early as the nineteenth century.[1–4] The idea is to accurately localise anatomical structure within the human body. It was recognised that this can be achieved by recreating a 3D construct using three planes designated X (horizontal), Y (coronal), and Z (sagittal).[2] A coordinate can then be used to localise structures with precious positioning. However, a rigid fixation is needed, as slight movement could result in displacement of coordination. A rigid frame was then developed which is fixed to a known external landmark to create stability which provided the most accurate positioning. This novel technique is termed *stereotaxy* or *stereotactic guidance*. These terms are derived from the Greek words stereos meaning *three dimension* and *taxis* meaning *orderly arrangement*.[2,5] The word *tactic* originated from a Latin word meaning *to touch*.[5,6] Several prototypes of stereotactic frames have been developed around the world, but their benefit remained within the neurosurgery and head/neck surgery community. The modern era of stereotactic technology was marked by the development of radio-imaging technology such as computer technology (CT) and magnetic resonance imaging (MRI), computer software, and digital signalling. These technologies have allowed stereotactic techniques to become frameless. This was able to allow the instrument to be used anywhere on the human body without the need to fixate patients into a rigid frame. The ability to see fine soft tissue anatomical detail with the use of CT and MRI coupled with navigation tools allow localisation and detail descriptions of vessel perforators. Rozen et al. have taken the idea and expanded the potential use of stereotactic image guidance in preoperative flap reconstruction planning. CT-guided stereotaxy has improved the accuracy and provided real-time navigation systems for reconstructive surgeons in performing flap reconstructions.[7–9]

11.2 HISTORY OF STEREOTACTIC IMAGE-GUIDED NAVIGATION

11.2.1 Early Stereotaxy Development

The use of navigation techniques to accurately map anatomical structures has been pioneered since the late 1800s. It is heavily utilised in the field of neurosurgery. It began with Dittmar who in 1873 used a guiding device in mice to create bulbar vasomotor centres in rats.[1] In 1889, Zernove, a Russian anatomist, developed an encephalometer that allows mapping of surface topography for the localisation of the cranial sutures and cerebral sulci.[3] The advancement in stereotaxy arrived in 1908, by Sir Victor Horsley, a British neurophysiologist and neurosurgeon, and his associate Robert Clarke, a mathematician.[2] Their work was originally to answer the question whether or not the cerebellar cortex is directly connected to the peduncles and spinal cord. In order to identify the pathway of connection, they needed to cause a destruction of the cerebellar nuclei. If the pathway existed, then the nerve fibre of the peduncles and spinal cord should not undergo degenerative changes. One major obstacle remained: How can a discrete and accurate destruction be made to the cerebellar nuclei without damaging the surrounding structure? The answer is through a navigation instrument. Horsley and Clarke developed the Horsley–Clarke frame, which allowed an accurate placement of an insulated needle which delivered electrode electrocoagulation into the nuclei resulting in cerebral tissue necrosis.[4] The device utilises three planes: a line connecting the lower margin of the orbit and the external auditory meatus is the horizontal reference, the frontal (coronal) line passes through the two auditory canals, and the sagittal line bisects the head between these two planes. The frame is screwed onto the skull with the orientation along the horizontal plane. The frontal and sagittal planes can be created by adjusting the perpendicular and bisecting lines, respectively. Their experiments on the animal heads allowed an extraordinary precious mapping of the relationship between the intra-cranial and extra-cranial structures in a 3D form.[2,4]

Despite the success of their work and patency by Clarke, the development of a human model stereotactic apparatus had never been constructed. It was not until 1918 when Aubrey Mussen, a Canadian neuroanatomist and neurophysiologist, modified the original Horsley–Clarke apparatus to be useable in humans.[4,10–12] He designed a rectangular brass frame attached to the patient's head by ear bars, which were able to be inserted into the external auditory canals, and a clamp fixed to the infraorbital ridge. Mussen also developed the first human stereotactic atlas based on cranial landmarks that was similar to Clarke's animal stereotactic atlas. However, Mussen's stereotactic instrument was used only in laboratory experiment and never used in the clinical setting.[4,6] His work remained unnoticed for many years and had not been mentioned in the scientific community at the time. The work was not resurrected until 30 years later, in 1947 with Spiegel, an American neurologist who began developing his own stereotactic device for humans in the clinical setting. The device was much similar to that of Horsley and Clarke apparatus which fixed onto the patient's skull. However, an intraoperative radiography was incorporated into the procedure to help in localising intra-cranial structures.[4] In 1952, Spiegel and Wycic developed the first stereotactic atlas of the human brain which allowed them to perform a targeting localisation with précised sectioning of the brain, a procedure which they termed *stereoencephalotomy*.[1,4] The procedure avoids the need for an open neurosurgical operation which carried a high mortality rate due to it precise identification of affected lesion which prevents unnecessary destruction of the cerebral tissue. Since then, several designs of stereotactic frames have been developed in various international centres. These innovations have paved the way for a modern era of stereotactic technology.

11.2.2 Modern Stereotactic and Its Expansion in Medicine

The leap in modern development of stereotactic guidance was incorporated with radio-imaging technologies (CT and MRI) and digital signalling technologies (positioning sensor probes). The improvement of computer software has allowed the use of CT in conjunction with stereotactic apparatus. This has dramatically improved target localisation with additional information regarding the structure of surrounding tissue. These radiographic modalities provided the ability to see and interpret human anatomy in a 3D format. The first use of CT in collaboration with stereotactic techniques was first described by Bergstrom and Greitz in 1976. A modification of the Leksell stereotactic frame is placed on the patient's head and attached to the CT scanner. The images were then used to map out cerebral lesions with given coordinates for preoperative planning of radiosurgical and conventional neurosurgery procedures.[13,14]

With continued advances in computer software and the development of digital signalling technology, the idea of a frameless navigation system was developed. Frameless stereotactic uses a position sensor maker rather than a fixed rigid stereotaxic frame to determine real-time coordinates. In 1986, the first frameless stereotactic technology was performed by David Roberts, an American neurosurgeon, using fiducial markers (FMs) on the scalp.[15,16] These radiopaque markers were placed on the patients' scalp prior to undergoing CT imaging. The outlined contours and FM position were then stored and reformatted to match the optical image seen from a modified operating microscope. During the operation, the CT images were superimposed through the optical microscope which outlined the interested boundaries. This technique had allowed a precious accuracy ranging from 0.8 to 6 mm and a mean of less than 2 mm.[15] A newer model of frameless stereotactic navigation utilised articulated arms (localiser) which provided intraoperative reference points. The articulated arms consist of sterile surgical probes connected to multi-jointed and articulated arms with free movement. The information regarding the arm position is transmitted to the navigator system where the analogue data are converted into digital formats and correlated with the preoperative image data. The information can be transmitted via a connected cable or by ultrasonic emitters attached to the articulated arms which can be detected by digitiser (an overhead-fixation system).[17,18] The latter technology allowed more freedom for the operating surgeon. Frameless stereotaxy has proven to be minimally invasive, more flexible, faster, and safer with improved accuracy than the previous frame technology.[15,19–21]

The ability to use FMs and articulated arms has overcome the need for a fixed frame, thus allowing the stereotactic technique to be used on other parts of the body (see Figure 11.1). The benefit and

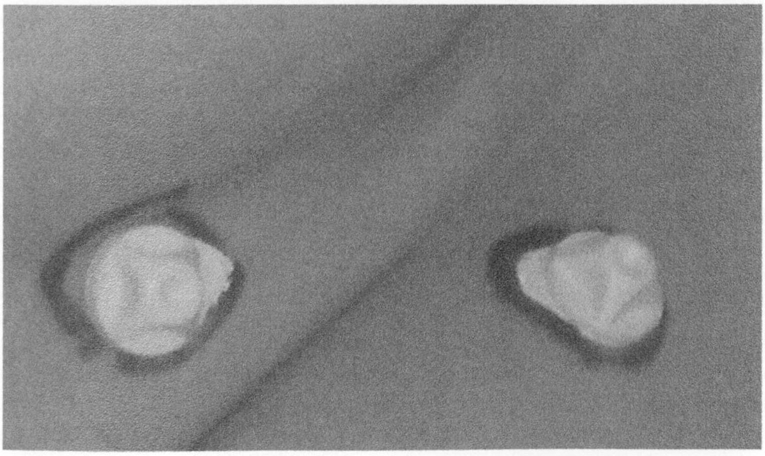

FIGURE 11.1 FM placed on the skin surface.

potential of this technology have been recognised by other surgical specialities with use in otolaryngology, head and neck surgery, skull base surgery, and mid-face reconstruction.[22–24] In cardiology, the technology has been used to navigate wire placement in percutaneous coronary intervention.[25] In total joint arthroplasty where precise placement of prosthesis is crucial, the stereotactic technology has shown to improve success and has been adopted by several orthopaedic surgeons.[26,27] Stereotactic guidance in conjunction with preoperative radiological imaging has been utilised for accurate breast biopsy and providing radiotherapy.[28–32] The use of stereotaxy in soft tissue and identification of perforators in flap reconstruction has been explored in the work of Rozen et al.[7–9] These studies have shown that stereotactic image-guided studies can increase operative accuracy and allow for preoperative planning which decreases operative mortality and morbidity.

11.3 STEREOTACTIC IMAGING NAVIGATION IN PREOPERATIVE FLAP RECONSTRUCTION

The use of stereotactic guidance is based on the marking of known bony landmarks, which has largely limited its use. In more than other surgical specialties, this restriction has limited the expansion of the stereotactic technique in soft tissue localisation. Stereotactic techniques in soft tissue without bony landmark localisation were first used in the diagnosis and biopsy of breast tissue. This technique has been explored since the early 1990s (Parker). It has been shown to have a sensitivity of 1.2%–4.0% in the literature.[33] Diaz and Mitnick have found the technique to be an alternative investigative tool when conventional ultrasound (US)-guided core biopsy could not identify the lesion. Both studies have shown that the use of stereotactic biopsy is an accurate and reliable method in localising breast lesions, particularly for otherwise difficult to identify breast lesions such as nonpalpable lesions, small breasts, or breasts with prosthetic implants.[28,34–39] However, it must be noted that stereotaxy with radiographic imaging in the form of x-ray was employed in these cases with several limitations. X-ray imaging provides little information with regard to soft tissue detail and is therefore unreliable in detecting small lesions.

The new technology which incorporated the use of computed tomography angiography (CTA) and MRI with surface-marking stereotaxy can overcome this issue. Kuhl et al. have evaluated the usefulness of preoperative MRI-guided stereotactic localisation and core biopsy of suspicious breast lesions that are not visible on US. He has found that MRI can provide detail in soft tissue anatomy, thereby avoiding damage to vital structures during the procedure. A lesion of up to 4 mm in size can be accurately detected with a 98% success rate of localisation.[40] The potential of CT and MRI to be used in conjunction with stereotaxy provides an alternate and accurate means of obtaining 3D mapping of soft tissue. This potential has expanded into the field of plastic and reconstructive surgery with the work of Rozen et al. in 2008. It is a general consensus that preoperative awareness of perforator location and course can permit improved flap design, operative safety, and planning of dissection. Rozen et al. utilised the capability of CTA to identify arterial anatomy in relation to surrounding soft tissue for pre-planning of deep inferior epigastric perforator (DIEP) and anterior lateral thigh (ALT) flap reconstruction. Three types of stereotactic methods of CT-guided stereotaxy were used in the identification of perforators: fiducial marking technique, *soft-touch* registration, and *Z-touch* surface-matching registration.[9]

11.3.1 Fiducial Marking Technique

Fiducial marking has provided an alternative means to create reference points which are crucial in the navigation system for stereotaxy (see Figure 11.1). These markers create reference points for the computer software which can then be displayed as digital images. The technique requires CTA or MRI, radiological imaging software, FMs, a reference star (RS) (articulated arms), navigation software, digitiser (an overhead sensor), and navigator station (see Figures 11.1 through 11.6).

Patients first undergo CTA or MRI. In the Rozen et al. study, prior to CTA, FMs were placed within the operated field within the scanning range on superficial bony landmark with least mobile skin to provide a reliable fixation point. They have recommended at least six FMs for DIEP and nine for ALT flap reconstruction.[7–9] CTA was then performed with images reformatted into maximum intensity projection (MIP) and 3D volume-rendered technique (VRT) images using commercially available software. The image files were then transferred to navigation software. Patients were then placed in a supine position mimicking both the position during CTA scanning and intraoperative positioning.

An *RS* (articulated arms) was attached to the patient's thigh to aid in registration. This acts to communicate the spatial positioning of the patient to the navigator computer system. It was placed on the patient's thigh as the device is needed to be outside the area of perforator identification but close enough for the information to relay to the navigator computer. The navigation software then registers the position of the FMs and the RS. This process involves the operator pointing a stereotactic pointer (ward) at the centre of each FM. The location of each individual marker can then be incorporated on the 3D CTA-reconstructed images. The operator can then use the stereotactic pointer to mark out the perforator on the patient's skin as identified by the navigator reconstructed images.

From Rozen et al. study, they were able to identify over 63 perforators in 10 patients using this technique. All 63 perforators were located with a 100% correlation between conventional CTA preoperative marking and CT-guided stereotaxy. When compared to operative finding, all perforators located by CT-guided stereotaxy were again located (100% sensitivity). There was, however, a single false positive from an ALT perforator which resulted in a positive predictive value of 98.4%. There was a mean of 2 mm discrepancy in the location of the actual perforators. It seems that the use of CT-guided stereotaxy with FMs is a reliable and an accurate method for preoperative flap reconstruction planning.[9]

11.3.2 Surface Landmark: *soft-touch* Registration and *Z-touch* Surface-Matching Registration

Two further techniques were used and analysed by Rozen et al. in CT-guided stereotaxy preoperative flap planning. These techniques relied on anatomical landmarks as reference points such as the anterior superior iliac spine (ASIS), greater trochanter (GT), or pubic symphysis. A wireless handheld device was then used to collect data points on the patient's skin. In the *soft-touch* technique, the registration was made by using a *soft-touch pointer* equipped with two navigation points attached to the device. The two navigation points signal its position which is picked up by an overhead digitiser. After calibration with known landmarks, the collection of data is done by gently placing the tip of the instrument on the patient's skin. The digitiser, which is mounted to the navigation station, detected the movement of the two navigation points and displayed the information on the monitor. Z-touch provides a touchless registration through automatic recognition of laser reflections by the infrared cameras. This device is swept over the skin of the patient with a visible laser detecting surface contours, and the information is transmitted directly to the navigation system via infrared signal. These make patient registration quick and easy by simply touching the patient's skin with either a pointer or a laser. Lorenz et al. found that they took a mean of 5.8 min to set up the navigator station, 4.1 min to use z-touch, and 8.2 min to use soft touch in registering patients for an endoscopic paranasal sinus surgery.[41] Because both devices register CT and MR images without frames or markers, scans taken only for registration purposes can be avoided, helping to reduce costs. Although the use of surface landmarks with the handheld device has shown to produce precise and accurate results in neurosurgery and ENT surgery with average discrepancy of 1.5–2.3 mm, a less successful result has been observed in soft tissue navigation.[41] Rozen et al. have found the system to be difficult to use. Most of the surface-matching registration failed the registration process despite using multiple points, including the same landmarks used with success during FM registration.[9]

11.4 CLINICAL USE IN PREOPERATIVE FLAP RECONSTRUCTION IMAGING

11.4.1 Use of Stereotactic Image-Guided Preoperative Imaging for DIEP Flaps

DIEP flaps have become a workhorse flap for autologous breast reconstruction, as they have proven over the years that they are a versatile flap with low donor site morbidity. However, one perceived limitation of the flap is its reliance on deep inferior epigastric artery perforators which can be variable in their anatomy. CTA has gained increasing acceptance by plastic and reconstructive surgeons to be a routine preoperative imaging modality of choice to identify the anatomy to assist in raising the flap. The issue still remains the need for transposition of images and data from the virtual world to reality. Currently, surgeons need to estimate the location of the perforators from a known landmark such as an umbilicus or the linea alba. This method is subjective, with interpretation depending on the experience and knowledge of the surgeon and/or interpretation of imaging. Rozen et al. have adapted the use of CT-guided stereotactic imaging into navigation for DIEP flap reconstruction. They have found that all major perforators (>1 mm in diameters) were identified by the stereotactic image-guided navigation technique with a distance discrepancy of only 2 mm (see Figures 11.2 through 11.7). When compared to conventional CTA, CT-guided stereotaxy demonstrated better correlation with perforator location (2 mm vs. 5 mm).[8] Their technique and protocol is described as follows.

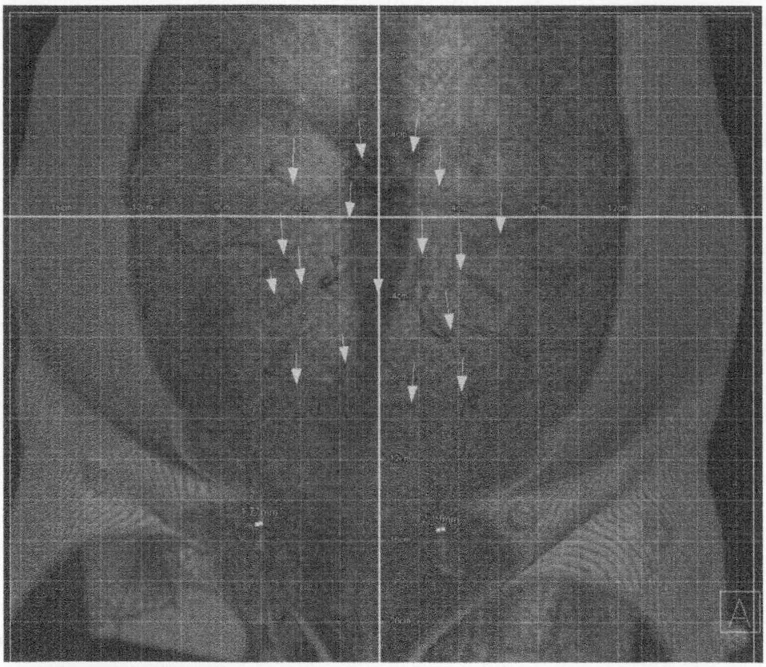

FIGURE 11.2 CTA with VRT image of the abdominal wall vasculature, demonstrating multiple perforators (location of emergence from the anterior rectus sheath is at the tip of the arrowhead). Blue arrows represent perforators of greater than 1 mm diameter. Yellow perforators, those less than 1 mm, were not included in the current study. The scaled grid is centred on the umbilicus as a reference point. (Reproduced from Rozen, W.M. et al., *Microsurgery*, 28(6), 417, 2008. With permission.)

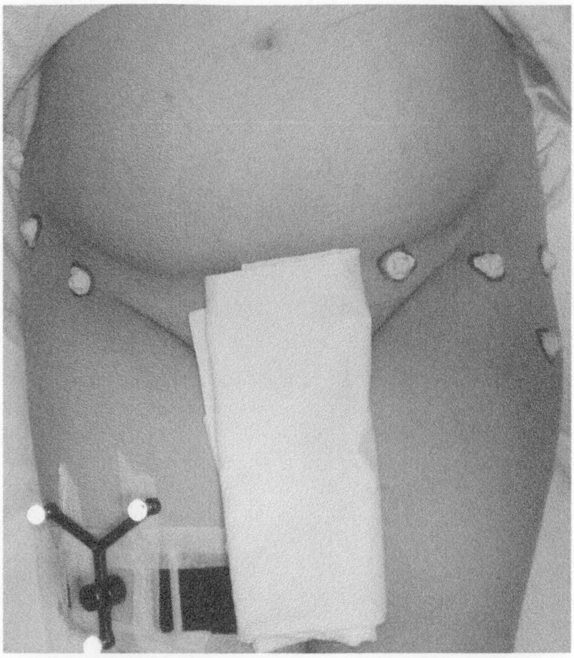

FIGURE 11.3 FM and *RS* placement, for fiducial-point patient registration. (Reproduced from Rozen, W.M. et al., *Microsurgery*, 28(6), 417, 2008. With permission.)

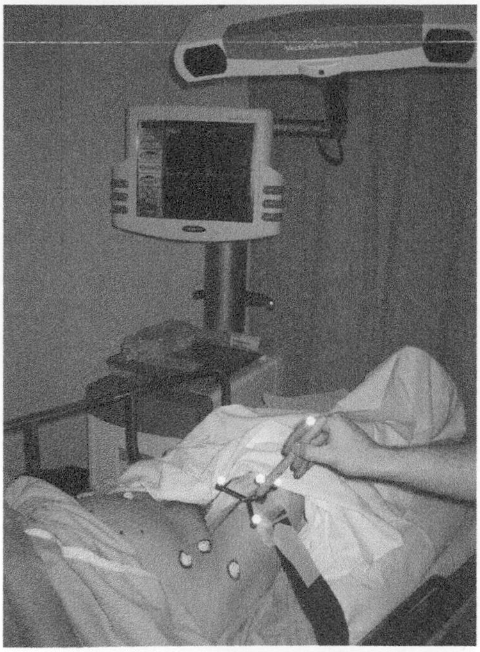

FIGURE 11.4 Navigation station for registration and localisation of patient data, by means of fiducial-point registration, utilising a *pointer*, *RS*, and FMs. (Reproduced from Rozen, W.M. et al., *Microsurgery*, 28(6), 417, 2008. With permission.)

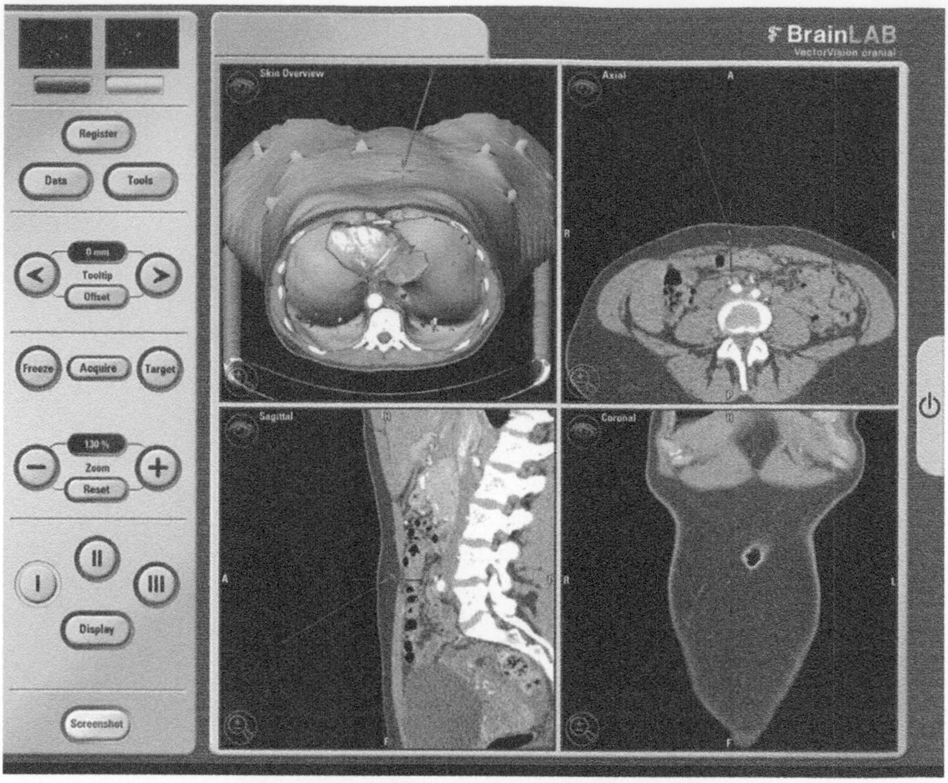

FIGURE 11.5 3D reconstructed images as seen on BrainLAB VectorVision Cranial software, demonstrating coronal, sagittal, and axial planes of a CTA of the abdominal wall vasculature. (Reproduced from Rozen, W.M. et al., *Microsurgery*, 28(6), 417, 2008. With permission.)

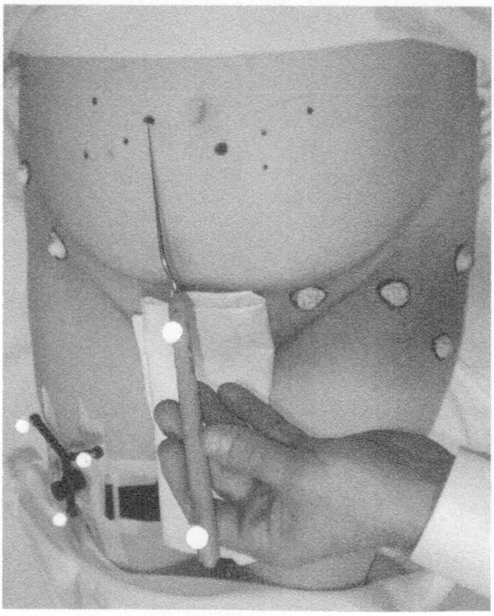

FIGURE 11.6 Localisation of perforators on the abdominal wall skin with the *pointer*, documenting with a blue mark, the location on the skin of the exact point of emergence of each perforator from the anterior rectus sheath. (Reproduced from Rozen, W.M. et al., *Microsurgery*, 28(6), 417, 2008. With permission.)

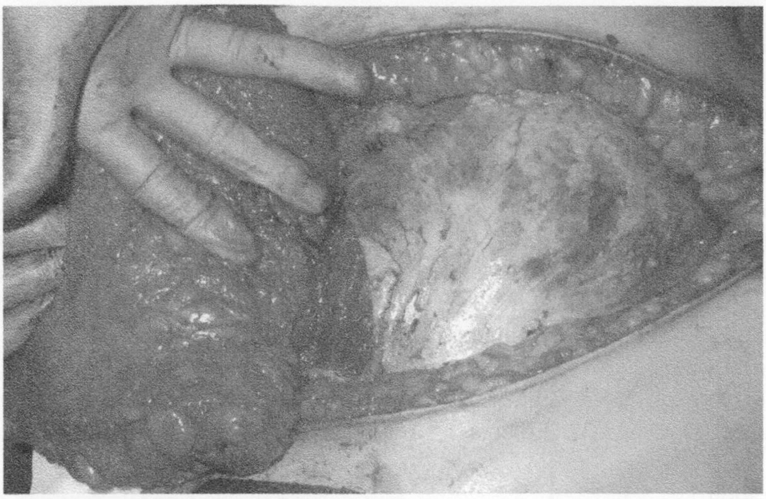

FIGURE 11.7 Intraoperative photograph highlighting a large perforator, seen preoperatively with both conventional CTA techniques and CT-guided stereotactic imaging. (Reproduced from Rozen, W.M. et al., *Microsurgery*, 28(6), 417, 2008. With permission.)

11.4.2 Procedure

- Preoperative imaging is performed within 24 h of the operation to reduce the change in patient's physique/habitus. This change can cause discrepancy in FM position and thus displace the navigation coordinates. Fluid balance, diet, and/or medications can all have a potential influence.
- The patient is placed on the CT scanner in the supine position similar to that of an intra-operative position.
- FMs are placed on the patient's bony landmarks of the hip and abdominal wall (or relevant body part). A minimum of six locations are recommended:
  - ASIS × 2
  - Anterior inferior iliac spine × 1–2
  - Pubic symphysis
  - GTs × 2
- The patient then undergoes CTA scanning of the anterior abdominal wall (or relevant body part):
  - Scanning protocol
- CTA settings as per Table 11.1.

TABLE 11.1
CT Scan Settings

Scan Type	Dynamically Timed Helical Multidetector Row CTA
Slice thickness	64 detector row × 0.6 mm collimator width
Helical detector pitch	0.9
Gantry rotation speed	0.37 s
Tube potential	120 kV
Tube current	180 mA

Sources: Rozen, W.M. et al., *Microsurgery*, 28, 227, 2008; Rozen, W.M. et al., *Microsurgery*, 28, 417, 2008; Rozen, W.M. et al., *Surg. Radiol. Anat.*, 31, 401, 2009.

- The study range is from 4 cm above the umbilicus to the pubic symphysis in a caudo-cranial direction.
- An intravenous contrast (Omnipaque 350 100 ml IVI) is given at the rate of 4 mL/s with bolus trigger point from the common femoral artery (100 HU, minimum delay).
- The image is reconstructed with 1 mm/0.7 mm overlapping axial images:
  - CTA reporting
- CTA images are reformatted into MIP and 3D VRT images using commercially available computer software.
- The perforators are marked on a 2D representation with an overlying scaled grid.
- The umbilicus is used as a reference point with measurement of the size of perforators and the distance between the perforators and umbilicus taken.
- Thin axial images are exported as *digital imaging and communications in medicine* (DICOM) file format and are loaded onto the stereotactic navigation software. The images are 3D reconstructed, demonstrating the anatomy in coronal, sagittal, and axial planes (see Figure 11.5).
- At operation
  - The patient is placed in supine position to replicate the patient position in the CT scanner.
  - An *RS* is attached firmly to the patient's upper thigh using a Velcro strap (see Figures 11.3 and 11.6).
  - A digitiser mounted on the navigation station is placed focusing over the patient's lower abdomen including all of the FMs and the RS (see Figure 11.4).
  - Patient registration (calibration) is done by placing the stereotactic pointer (ward) to the centre of each FM (see Figure 11.4).
  - Localisation of perforators is done by slow manoeuvring of the pointer to each perforator as displayed on the navigation station (see Figure 11.6).
  - Each perforator is then marked on the abdominal wall skin.

11.4.3 Use of Stereotactic Image-Guided Preoperative Imaging for ALT Flaps

Similar to the DIEP flap in autologous breast reconstruction, the ALT flap is an increasingly popular reconstructive option in extremity, head, and neck reconstruction despite the uncertainty in its perforator anatomy. Rozen et al. have proposed the use of CT-guided stereotactic imaging in improving the accuracy of identifying perforators and assisting in preoperative ALT flap design. They have found a similar result to that of their DIEP flap study, with CT-guided stereotactic imaging demonstrating all perforators >1 mm in diameter with precise localisation (see Figures 11.8 through 11.13). Further benefit of CT-guided stereotaxy is the ability to identify perforators' courses. Musculocutaneous and septocutaneous perforators can be seen prior to the operation which prevented unnecessary dissection and better planning. This allowed for minimisation of donor site morbidity and avoidance of failed flap harvest. CT-guided stereotaxy is a more accurate and reliable method of perforator mapping when compared to Doppler US or CTA alone.[7] Their technique and protocol is described in the following.

11.4.4 Procedure

- The procedure is done similar to that of the DIEP flap protocol described in the 'Use of Stereotactic Image-Guided Preoperative Imaging for DIEP' section.
- Preoperative imaging is performed within 24 h of the operation.
- The patient is placed on the CT scanner in supine position similar to that of an intraoperative position.

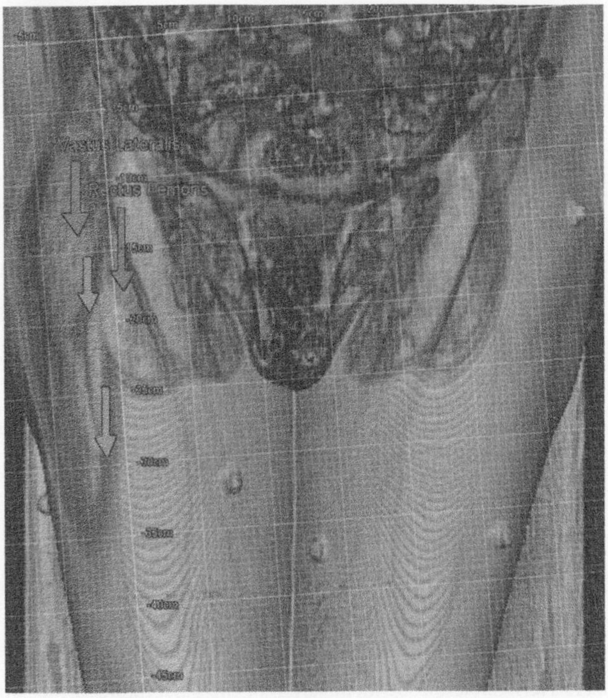

FIGURE 11.8 CTA with VRT image of the perforators supplying the anterolateral thigh of the right leg of a patient, prior to stereotactic navigation. Two large perforators are identified, each greater than 1 mm luminal diameter, with the blue arrowheads at the location of fascial penetration. (Reproduced from Rozen, W.M. et al., *Microsurgery*, 28(4), 227, 2008. With permission.)

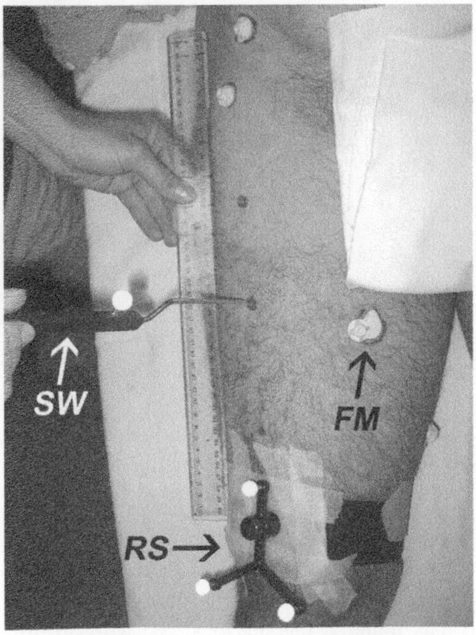

FIGURE 11.9 Localisation of perforators on the skin of the right thigh with a stereotactic wand (SW), documenting with a blue mark the location on the skin of the exact point of emergence of each perforator from the fascia lata of the same patient. FMs and *RS* marker, used for fiducial-point patient registration, are in place. (Reproduced from Rozen, W.M. et al., *Microsurgery*, 28(4), 227, 2008. With permission.)

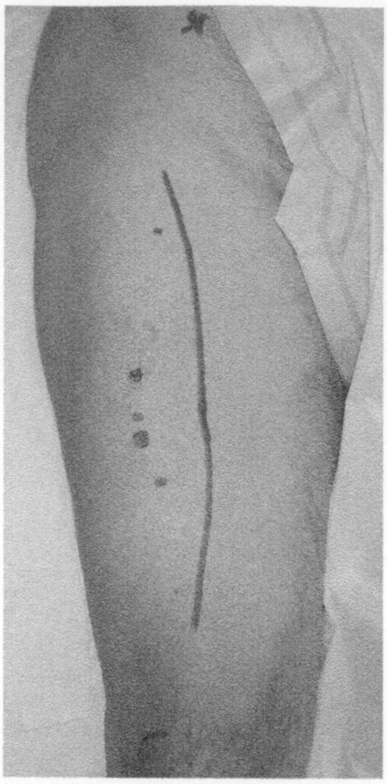

FIGURE 11.10 Intraoperative Doppler probe localisation of the perforators of the same patient. Black markings highlight the ASIS, the supero-lateral border of patella, and the middle thirds of the line between these bony landmarks. The medial border of the flap is also highlighted in black. Perforators localised on Doppler are marked with blue dots. (Reproduced from Rozen, W.M. et al., *Microsurgery*, 28(4), 227, 2008. With permission.)

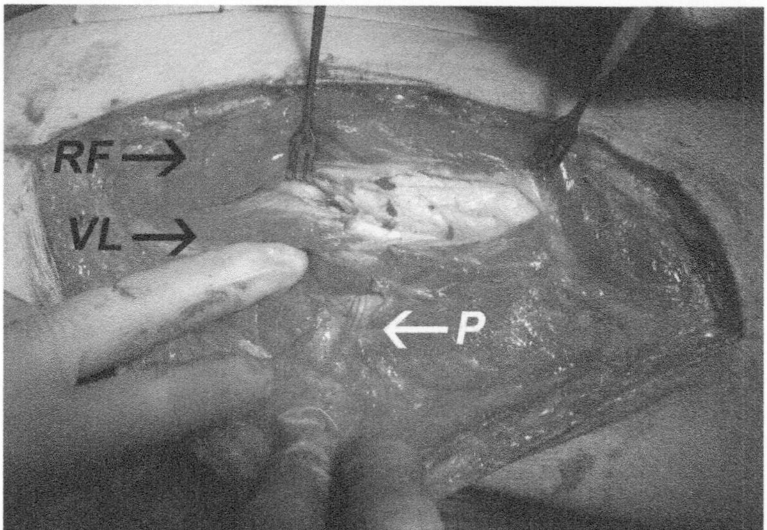

FIGURE 11.11 Intraoperative photograph demonstrating a large musculocutaneous perforator supplying the planned anterolateral thigh flap, found at the site localised with all three imaging modalities utilised. P = perforator; RF = rectus femoris; VL = vastus lateralis. (Reproduced from Rozen, W.M. et al., *Microsurgery*, 28(4), 227, 2008. With permission.)

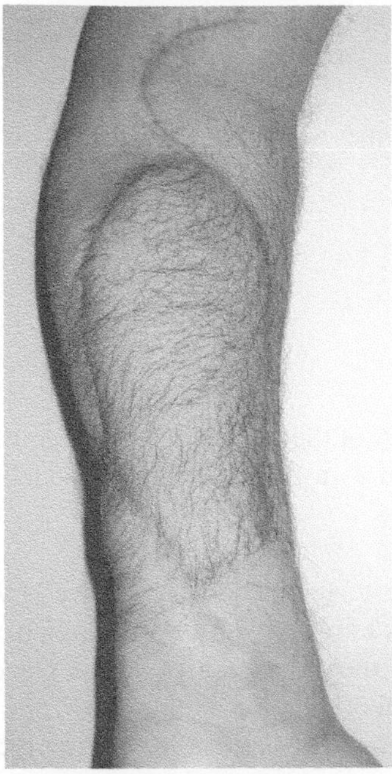

FIGURE 11.12 Post-operative photograph of the recipient site (left forearm) of the anterolateral thigh flap of the same patient, at 10 weeks post-operatively. (Reproduced from Rozen, W.M. et al., *Microsurgery*, 28(4), 227, 2008. With permission.)

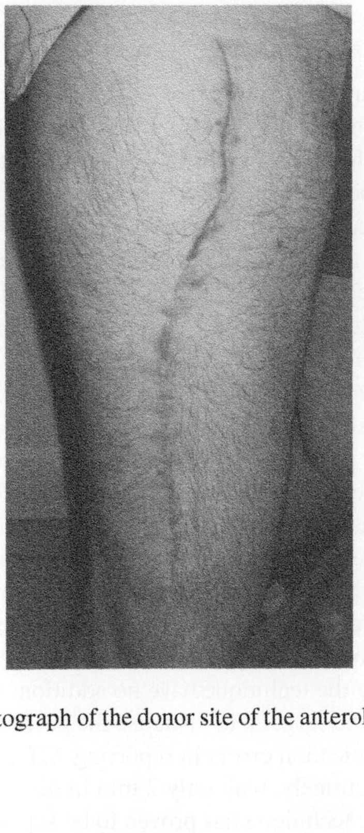

FIGURE 11.13 Post-operative photograph of the donor site of the anterolateral thigh flap of the same patient, at 10 weeks post-operatively.

1. FMs are placed on the patient's bony landmark of the hip and thigh. A minimum of nine locations are recommended:
   - ASIS
   - Anterior inferior iliac spine
   - Pubic symphysis
   - Pubic tubercle
   - GTs
   - Medial epicondyle
   - Lateral epicondyle
   - Medial malleolus
   - Lateral malleolus
2. Patients then underwent CTA of the leg with the same setting as DIEP.
3. Thin, axial images exported as a DICOM file are loaded onto a stereotactic navigation software.
4. At operation
   - The patient is placed in supine position (see Figure 11.9).
   - An *RS* is attached firmly to the patient's lower thigh (see Figure 11.9).
   - A digitiser mounted on the navigation station is placed overhead focusing over the patient's leg including all of the FMs and the RS.
   - Patient registration (calibration) is done by placing the stereotactic pointer (ward) to the centre of each FM.
   - Localisation of perforators is done with a slow manoeuvring of the pointer to each perforator as displayed on the navigation station.
   - Each perforator is then marked on the skin of the thigh (Figure 11.11 shows intraoperative perforator identified with CT-guided stereotaxy).

11.5 SUMMARY

The use of the stereotactic technique has evolved over the past century, with much of the work focused in the field of neurosurgery. It has much benefit in being able to locate the precise position of anatomical structures within the human body, in a 3D construct. The technology and its potential were adapted in many areas of medicine, laying the groundwork for its introduction into reconstructive surgery. CTA-guided stereotaxy was used in plastic surgery in identifying perforators for preoperative flap planning by Rozen et al. in 2008. It has proven to be a reliable, reproducible, and accurate method, helping to identify the location, size, and course of each individual perforator, which assists in flap design. It allows for an identification of potential pitfalls prior to the operation, which helps avoid causing donor site morbidity to patient[7]. Being able to use stereotaxy during the operation, surgeons can have real-time visual guides when dissecting out perforators and are able to navigate through the surrounding tissue safely. The technique can directly facilitate a minimal amount of dissection during tracing individual perforators through the soft tissue, intramuscular septa, or muscle. This can further reduce operative time, decrease donor site morbidity, and avoid failed flap harvest over routine imaging alone. The use of CT-guided stereotaxy is a non-invasive procedure which adds no morbidity over routine imaging alone, and there is minimal extra time for setting up or undertaking the procedure. Evolution of the techniques used within stereotaxy (see Figure 11.14) has led to improved protocols, and the more recent published techniques in multi-planar mapping and patient registration (see Figure 11.15) have led to optimisation of the technique. While there is a hardware cost, individual episodes of using the technique have no additional financial cost over routine imaging alone. The procedure allows the surgeon to visualise the perforators independent of a radiologist, making it quick and less communication errors in reporting. CT-guided stereotaxy can identify perforators of greater than 1 mm accurately, with only 2 mm in discrepancy in distance from operative findings (see Figure 11.16).[8,9] The technique has proven to be superior to CTA and Doppler US.[7]

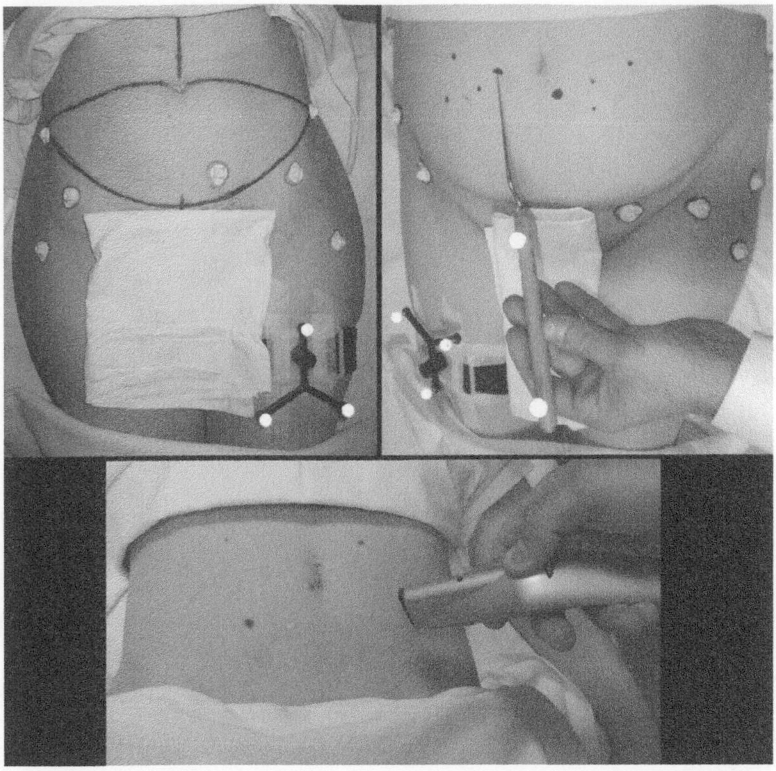

FIGURE 11.14 The three techniques used for *registration* during image-guided stereotactic navigation: *fiducial-point* registration (top left); *soft-touch, surface-matching* pointer registration (top right); and *z-touch surface-matching* laser registration (bottom). (Reproduced from Rozen, W.M. et al., *Surg. Radiol. Anat.*, July; 31(6), 401, 2009. With permission.)

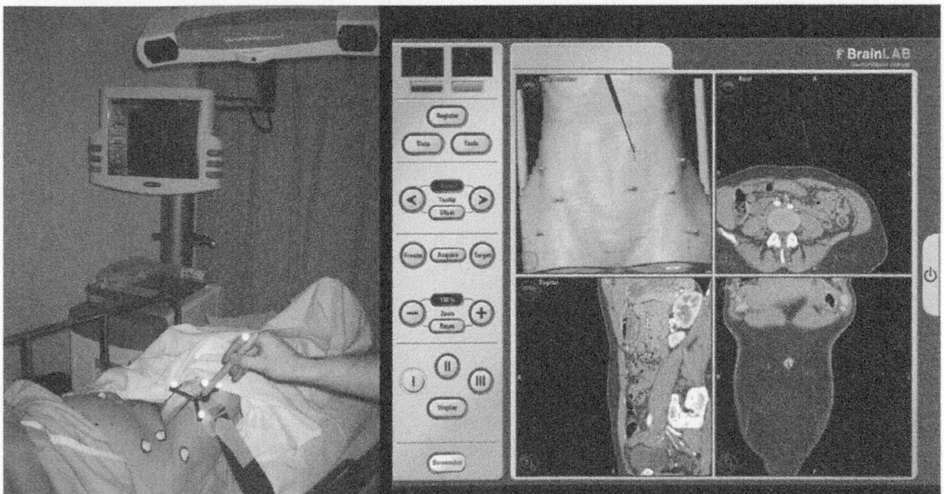

FIGURE 11.15 Left: Navigation station for registration and localisation of patient data, by means of fiducial-point registration, utilising a *stereotactic pointer, RS*, and FM for the abdominal wall donor site. Right: 3D multi-planar reconstruction images, as seen on BrainLAB *VectorVision Cranial* software, demonstrating coronal, sagittal, and axial planes during stereotactic navigation of a CTA of the abdominal wall vasculature. (Reproduced from Rozen, W.M. et al., *Surg. Radiol. Anat.*, July; 31(6), 401, 2009. With permission.)

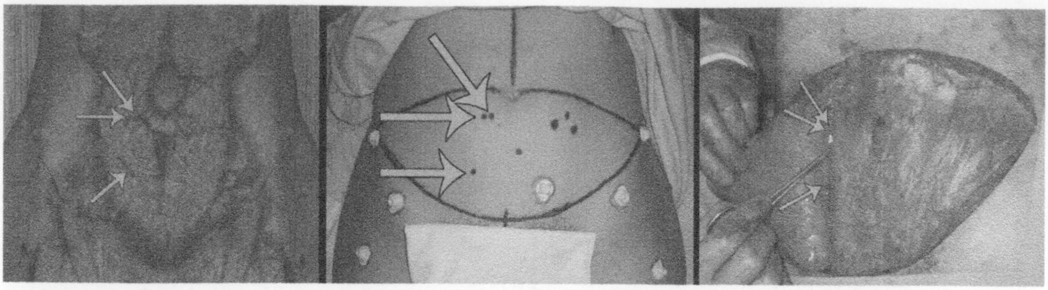

FIGURE 11.16 Correlation of CTA (left), CTA-guided stereotaxy (middle), and operative findings (right), demonstrating concordance for the three largest perforators selected preoperatively (blue arrows). (Reproduced from Rozen, W.M. et al., *Surg. Radiol. Anat.*, July; 31(6), 401, 2009. With permission.)

REFERENCES

1. Spiegel EA. *History of Human Stereotaxy (Stereoencephalotomy): Stereotaxy of the Human Brain*, 2nd edn. Stuttgart/New York: Georg Thieme Verlag, 1982, pp. 3–10.
2. Horsely V, Clark RH. The structure and functions of the cerebellum examined by a new method. *Brain* 1908;31:45–124.
3. Picard C, Olivier A, Bertrand G. The first human stereotaxic apparaturs: The contribution of Audrey Mussen to the field of stereotaxis. *J Neurosurg* 1983;59:673–676.
4. Lasak JM, Gorecki JP. The history of stereotactic radiosurgery and radiotherapy. *Otolaryngol Clin N Am* 2009;42:593–599.
5. Rahman M, Murad GJA, Mocco J. Early history of the stereotactic apparatus in neurosurgery. *Neurosurg Focus* 2009;27:1–5.
6. Gildenberg PL. *Stereotactic Surgery: Present and Past" Stereotactic Neurosurgery,* M. Peter Heilbrun (ed.). Baltimore, MD: Williams & Wilkins, 1988.
7. Rozen WM, Ashton MW, Ferris S, White D, Stella DL, Phillips, TJ, Taylor GI. Developments in perforator imaging for the anterolateral thigh flap: CT angiography and CT-guided stereotaxy. *Microsurgery* 2008;28:227–232.
8. Rozen WM, Ashton MW, Stella DL, Phillips TJ, Taylor GI. Stereotactic image-guided navigation in the preoperative imaging of perforators for DIEP flap breast reconstruction. *Microsurgery* 2008;28:417–423.
9. Rozen WM, Buckland A, Ashto MW, Stella DL, Phillips TJ, Taylor GI. Image-guided, stereotactic perforator flap surgery: A prospective comparison of current techniques and review of the literature. *Surg Radiol Anat* 2009;31:401–408.
10. Bullard DE, Nashold BSJ. Evolution of principles of stereotactic neurosurgery. *Neurosurg Clin N Am* 1995;6:27–41.
11. Jensen RL, Stone JL, Hayne R. Use of the Horsley-Clarke stereotactic frame in humans. *Stereotact Funct Neurosurg* 1995;65:194–197.
12. Jensen RL, Stone JL, Hayne RA. Introduction of the human Horsley-Clarke stereotactic frame. *Neurosurg* 1996;38:563–567.
13. Bergstrom M, Greitz T. Stereotaxis and tomography. A technical note. *Am J Roentagenoli* 1976;127:167–170.
14. Gildenberg P. The history of stereotactic neurosurgery. *Neurosurg Clin N Am* 1990;1:765–780.
15. Roberts DW, Strohbehn JW, Hatch JF, Murray W, Hettenberger H. A frameless stereotaxic integration of computerized tomographic imaging and the operating microscope. *J Neurosurg* 1986;65:545–549.
16. Wolfsberger S, Rossler K, Regatschnig R, Ungersbock K. Anatomical landmarks for image registration in frameless stereotactic neuronavigation. *Neurosurg Rev* 2002;25:68–72.
17. Barnett GH, Kormos DW, Steiner CP et al. Intraoperative localization using an armless, frameless stereotactic wand: Technical note. *J Neurosurg* 1993;78:510–514.
18. Barnett GH, Kormos DW, Steiner CP et al. Use of a frameless, armless stereotactic wand for brain tumor localization with two-dimensional and three-dimensional neuroimaging. *Neurosurgery* 1993;33:674–678.
19. Quiñones-Hinojosa A, Ware ML, Sanai N, McDermott MW. Assessment of image guided accuracy in a skull model: Comparison of frameless stereotaxy techniques vs. frame-based localization. *J Neurooncol* 2006;76:65–70.

20. Tessman C. Exploring frameless stereotactic image guided surgery. *AORN J* 1999;69:498–512.
21. White E, Boswell W, Whang G, Mandelin P, Astrahan M, Duddalwar V. CT-guided fiducial marker placement for stereotactic radiosurgery. *Appl Rad* 2011;5:23–31.
22. Hohlweg-Majert B, Schon R, Schelzeisen R, Gellrich NC, Schramm A. Navigational maxillofacial surgery using virtual models. *World J Surg* 2005;29:1530–1538.
23. Nyachhyon P, Kim PC. Intraoperative stereotactic navigation for reconstruction in zygomatic-orbital trauma. *J Nepal Med Assoc* 2011;51:37–40.
24. Hanasono MM, Jacob RF, Bidaut L, Robb GL, Skoracki RJ. Midfacial reconstruction using virtual planning, rapid prototype modelling, and stereotactic navigation. *Plast Reconstr Surg* 2010;126:2002–2006.
25. Krause K, Adamu U, Weber M, Hertting K, Hamm C, Kuck KH, Hoffmann R, Kelm M, Blindt R. German stereotaxis-guided percutaneous coronary intervention study group: First multicentre real world experience. *Clin Res Cardiol* 2009;98:541–547.
26. Kim KI, Ramteke AA, Bae DK. Navigation–assisted minimal invasive total knee arthroplasty in patients with extra-articular femoral deformity. *J Arthroplasty* 2010;25:658e17–658e22.
27. Dunbar NJ, Roche MW, Park BH, Branch SH, Conditt MA, Banks SA. Accuracy of dynamic tactile-guided unicompartmental knee arthroplasty. *J Arthroplasty* 2012;27:803–808.
28. Diaz ML, Noguera JJ, Alonso-Burgos A, Dominguez P, Pina LJ, Zornoza G, Martínez-Regueira F. Stereotactic-guided excisional biopsy: A new technique for very thin breasts. *Breast J* 2006;12:566–568.
29. Purdie TG, Bissonnette JP, Franks K et al. Cone-beam computed tomography for on-line image guidance of lung stereotactic radiotherapy: Localization, verification, and intrafraction tumor position. *Int J Radiat Oncol Biol Phys* 2007;68:243–252.
30. Van der Voort van Zyp N, Prqvost JB, Hoogeman MS et al. Stereotactic radiotherapy with real-time tumor tracking for non-small cell lung cancer: Clinical outcome. *Radiother Oncol* 2009;91:296–300.
31. Nguyen NP, Garland L, Welsh J et al. Can stereotactic fractionated radiation therapy become the standard of care for early stage non-small cell lung carcinoma. *Cancer Treat Rev* 2008;34:719–727.
32. Helbich TH, Matzek W, Fuchsjager MH. Stereotactic and ultrasound-guided breast biopsy. *Eur Radiol* 2004;14:383–393.
33. Jackman RJ, Noweis KW, Soto JR, Marzomi FA, Finkelstein SI, Shepard MJ. Stereotactic, automated, large-core needle biopsy of nonpalpable breast lesions: False-negative and histologic underestimation rates after long term follow-up. *Radiology* 1999;210:799–805.
34. Mitnick JS, Vazquez MF, Roses DF, Harris MN, Colen SR, Colen HS. Stereotactic localisation for fine needle aspiration biopsy in patients with augmentation prostheses. *Ann Plast Surg* 1992;29:31–35.
35. Parker SH, Lovin JD, Jobe WE et al. Stereotactic breast biopsy with a biopsy gun. *Radiology* 1990;176:741–747.
36. Parker SH, Lovin JD, Jobe WE, Burke BJ, Hopper KD, Yakes WR. Nonpalpable breast lesions: Stereotactic automated large-core biopsies. *Radiology* 1991;180:403–407.
37. Elvecrog EL, Lechner MC, Nelson MT. Non palpable breast lesions: Correlation of stereotaxic large-core needle biopsy and surgical biopsy results. *Radiology* 1993;188:453–455.
38. Gisvold JJ, Goelln er JR, Gran t CS et al. Breast biopsy: A comparative study of stereotaxically guided core and excisional techniques. *Am J Radio* 1994;162:815–820.
39. Brenner RJ, Fajardo L, Fisher PR et al. Percutaneous core biopsy of the breast: Effect of operator experience and number of samples on diagnostic accuracy. *Am J Radio* 1996;166:341–346.
40. Kuhl CK, Elevelt A, Leutner CC, Gieseke J, Pakos E, Schild HH. Interventional breast MR imaging: Clinical use of a stereotactic localization and biopsy device. *Radiology* 1997;204:667–675.
41. Lorenz KJ, Frühwald S, Maier H. The use of the BrainLAB Kolibri navigation system in endoscopic paranasal sinus surgery under local anaesthesia. An analysis of 35 cases. *HNO* 2006;54:851–860.

12 Lymphatics
Anatomy, Mapping, and Evolving Imaging Technologies

Ramin Shayan, Iain S. Whitaker, Cara Michelle Le Roux, and Tara Karnezis

CONTENTS

12.1 INTRODUCTION

The lymphatic system is an intricate, hierarchically arranged network of vessels that is vital for interstitial fluid balance (Shayan et al., 2006). The lymphatics also form part of the first element of the body's defences to interact with pathogens or malignant cells attempting to infiltrate the peripheral tissues of the body (Kinmonth, 1972). Lymphatics are vital to cellular movement within the immune system (Johnson et al., 2006), but these lymphatic channels may be hijacked as potential routes of cancer spread and dissemination (Haagensen et al., 1972). They may also become compromised by acquired physical insults such as surgery or parasitic infection or be congenitally deficient or defective at birth – all resulting in lymphoedema (Kinmonth, 1972). With improving technologies, researchers have been able to hone in on the intricacies of the microanatomy of the lymphatic vessel subtypes and differentiate these distinct vessel entities even further (Shayan et al., 2007, 2012). With this refinement, the study of *macro* lymphatic vessel patterning and layout has become one of mapping drainage of vessels for that individual and in the particular area of the body in question (e.g. draining a tumour in a certain anatomical location), rather than a quest to describe a specific pattern of lymphatic vessels that may be generalised to a larger population. As discussed in Chapter 7, numerous techniques for injection and intra-operative mapping of lymphatic vessels have been described; these are not discussed in this chapter, which focuses exclusively on techniques for deriving an image of the lymphatic vessels.

12.2 LYMPHATIC DEVELOPMENT

In understanding lymphatic vessel anatomy and macroscopic patterning, it is important to be aware of the origins and development of the lymphatic system. There is evidence that the lymphatic vasculature originates from the blood vascular system (Oliver and Harvey, 2002; Francois et al., 2008). Blood vessels develop and remodel in a series of early developmental processes, known as vasculogenesis and angiogenesis, which give rise to the blueprint of the blood vascular system (Oliver and Harvey, 2002). Lymphatic vessels originate from this template in a process known as lymphangiogenesis (Shayan et al., 2006), in which venous endothelial cells in the anterior cardinal vein begin to express lymphatic markers and become polarised to migrate laterally to form primitive lymph nodes and lymphatics (Francois et al., 2008).

Several critical advances in research into the lymphatic system were made in the 1990s. The first was the characterisation of the lymphangiogenic subfamily of the VEGF family of protein growth factors, VEGF-C (Joukov et al., 1996) and VEGF-D (Achen et al., 1998). The cloning of these genes and development of antibodies against them have enabled researchers to create animal models for lymphangiogenesis and cancer metastasis and to study these growth factors in human disease (Stacker et al., 2001). The second advance was the discovery of molecular markers with specificity for lymphatic endothelium, which enabled researchers to identify and visualise lymphatic vessels (hitherto indistinguishable from blood vessels using histopathology alone) immunohistochemically (Banerji et al., 1999). The advent of these key tools in the study of lymphatics led to the realisation that lymphatic vessels are fundamental to cancer metastasis (Matsumoto et al., 2013) and also to many other pathological processes (Alitalo, 2011). The lymphatic vasculature has become the subject of intense clinical and scientific interest as a potentially valuable therapeutic target in these conditions (Shayan et al., 2006). They have also enabled us to refine our understanding of the lymphatic vascular anatomy and improve techniques for visualising and predicting the *macro-anatomy* and drainage patterns of lymphatics in patients.

12.3 LYMPHATIC ANATOMY

Since the 1990s, our conceptualisation of lymphatic vessel subtypes has evolved. In addition to the obvious locational, morphological, and anatomical differences in the subtypes of the lymphatic vasculature, key functional and molecular profile distinctions are also emerging (Shayan et al., 2007; Wang et al., 2010; Karnezis 2012a,b; Shayan, 2013). The intricate network of thin-walled vessels which constitutes the lymphatic vasculature commences within the superficial dermis of the skin as highly permeable, blind-ending sacs, known as *initial lymphatics* or *lymphatic capillaries* (Figure 12.1) (Casley-Smith and Florey, 1961; Leak and Burke, 1966; Leak, 1976; Oliver and Detmar, 2002; Oliver and Harvey, 2002) – approximately 60 μm in diameter in humans (Skobe and Detmar, 2000; Scavelli et al., 2004; Witte et al., 2006) and ranging from 6 μm cell thickness in the region of the nucleus to 50–100 nm away from the nucleus (Skobe and Detmar, 2000). These superficial, thin-walled vessels are devoid of pericytes (Jain, 2003) or basement membrane (Leak, 1976; Leak and Jones, 1993) and act as the entry point or *on-ramp* to the lymphatic system, performing a role as the chief absorptive lymphatic vessel subtype (Leak, 1976). These lymphatics consist of a lymphatic endothelial cell (LEC) monolayer (Leak, 1976), anchored to the extracellular matrix (ECM) with which they are structurally continuous (Gerli et al., 1991), by hollow actin and glycoprotein microfibril filaments that are approximately 100 Å in width (Casley-Smith and Florey, 1961; Leak and Burke, 1966; Leak and Burke, 1968b; Solito et al., 1997).

These filaments translate interstitial fluid volume expansion into radial tension on the vessel and lateral endothelial cell displacement, to create temporary inter-cellular fenestrations or *clefts* (Leak, 1976; Solito et al., 1997; Gerli, 2000). Glycoproteins that form the fibrillin anchoring filaments

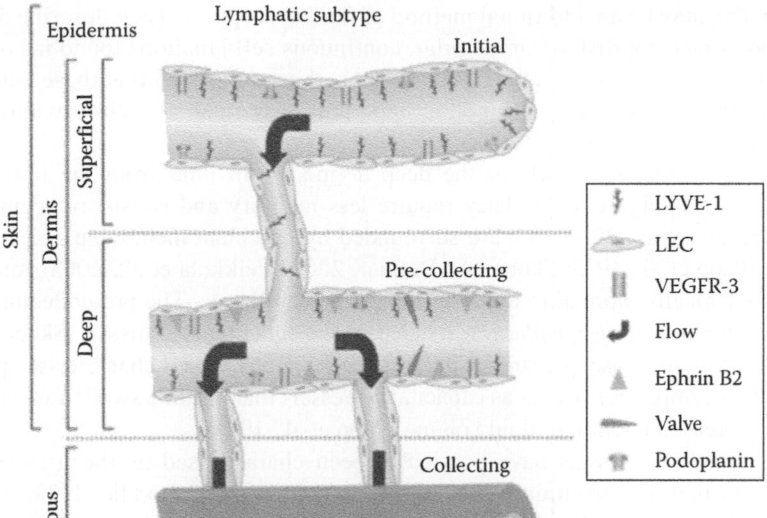

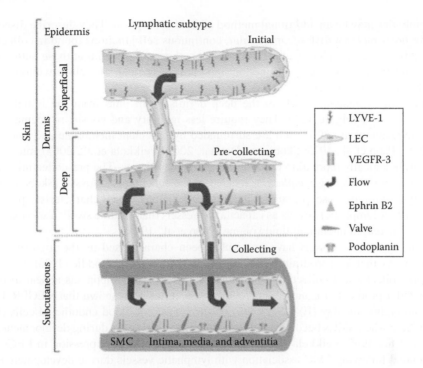

FIGURE 12.1 Schematic representation of lymphatic vessel subtypes in the skin. Lymphatic vessels commence in the superficial area of case the skin as initial lymphatics that absorb interstitial fluid and cells to drain into the more deeply located pre-collector lymphatics. These in turn drain into the collecting lymphatic vessels, which are located in the subcutaneous tissues and propel lymphatic fluid to the lymph nodes by the muscular contraction of their pacemaker cells. Whilst initial lymphatics consist only of a monolayer of LECs that are connected to the ECM by actin filaments, the more deeply located vessel subtypes become progressively complex in their mural structure, culminating in the collecting lymphatics that have an intima, media, and adventitia and consist of a collagen basement membrane, pericytes, and SMCs. Whilst there is not currently a specific histological marker for the individual lymphatic vessel subtypes, the subtypes are further delineated by their differential expression of a range of molecular markers that are known to be expressed on LECs. Common examples include LYVE-1 and podoplanin. Whilst initial lymphatics express both of these markers, collecting lymphatics stain strongly for podoplanin but only weekly express LYVE-1. Therefore, the combination of morphological features, anatomical location, and molecular profiles makes it increasingly possible to differentiate the lymphatic vessel subtypes in tissues. (Adapted from Shayan, R. et al., *Carcinogenesis*, 27(9), 1729, 2005. With permission.)

include Arg-Gly-Asp (RGD) residues, which are capable of binding integrin family transmembrane glycoproteins, which in turn induce intracellular signalling to alter the cytoskeletal structure and enhance lymphatic permeability (Solito et al., 1997; Scavelli et al., 2004).

The lack of a continuous basement membrane (Leak and Burke, 1966) around the initial lymphatics also encourages entry of interstitial fluid plasma proteins and cells into these vessels and so restoration of normal interstitial volume (Casley-Smith and Florey, 1961; Leak and Burke, 1968a; Leak, 1976). Once fluid volumes in surrounding ECM are normalised, anchoring filaments slacken, returning LECs to their overlapping resting position.

In addition to this mechanical method, several other methods of fluid absorption also aid interstitial fluid absorption. They include pinocytosis (trafficking *through* the LEC itself) (Leak, 1976) and cytoskeletal structural alterations that further aid fluid influx, mediated by ECM signalling (Weber et al., 2002). It has also been shown that cytoskeletal responses to the lymphangiogenic growth factors may vary according to which receptor is stimulated (Veikkola et al., 2003). Most recently, Baluk and colleagues postulated that novel junctions between LECs of initial lymphatics may be an additional method of fluid absorption. They describe discontinuous *button-like junctions* that differ from regular, continuous cell junctions found in collecting lymphatics and blood vessels (Baluk et al., 2007). The authors suggested that these button junctions facilitate fluid uptake and that the junction apparatus may open and close without disturbing junctional integrity (Baluk et al., 2007).

Pre-collecting lymphatic vessels in the deep dermis drain fluid from the initial lymphatics (Sacchi et al., 1997) (Figure 12.1). They require less mobility and consist of segments containing valves (Scavelli et al., 2004) and are surrounded by basement membrane and smooth muscle cells (SMCs) (Papp et al., 1975; Skobe and Detmar, 2000; Veikkola et al., 2003), alternating with regions morphologically more akin to initial lymphatic capillaries. The pre-collecting lymphatics, in turn, drain into *collecting lymphatics*, located in the subcutaneous tissue (Skobe and Detmar, 2000). Early electron microscopic studies in lymphoedematous tissues characterised pre-collecting (or *post-capillary* lymphatic) vessels as capacitance vessels that became swollen *sac-like sinuses* in the setting of increased interstitial fluid volume (Papp et al., 1975).

Collecting lymphatic vessels have previously been characterised as the high-velocity, high-volume *freeways* that lead to draining lymph nodes (McHale and Roddie, 1983). In the case of both the pre-collector and collecting lymphatics, the structural components appear also to relate to the molecular profile. For example, in blood vessels, it has been shown that VEGFR-3, which is present from embryonic day (E) 8.5 (mouse) on the surface of blood endothelial cells (BECs), is down-regulated when SMCs become associated with the vessel walls during development at E10-16 (Kaipainen et al., 1995; Veikkola et al., 2003). Similarly, LYVE-1 expression in LECs becomes down-regulated following SMC association with lymphatic vessels during development (Makinen et al., 2005, 2007). Thus, more SMCs associated with collecting lymphatics compared with pre-collecting vessels, given the inverse relationship between SMCs and LYVE-1 expression, could explain the relative levels of LYVE-1 expression that differentiates these vessels (Pepper and Skobe, 2003; Makinen et al., 2005).

Those collecting lymphatics that are over 200 μm in diameter also have arterial-type mural intima, media, and adventitia (Pullinger and Florey, 1935; Papp et al., 1975; Scavelli et al., 2004) and pericytes (Petrova et al., 2004; Tammela et al., 2007). They propel lymph at an average rate of 10 μm/s, mostly by intrinsic wall motion (generated by specialised pacemaker – SMCs) and to a lesser degree by extrinsic compression by adjacent arterial pulsation and skeletal muscle contraction (McGeown et al., 1987b, 1988a,b), eventually returning lymph to the central veins. The SMCs consist of thin actin-type and thick myosin-type myofilaments (Papp et al., 1975).

Larger collecting lymphatics coalesce into lymphatic trunks, then intra-thoracic ducts. Whilst animals such as toads possess *lymphatic hearts* (Jones et al., 1997), larger mammals rely on collecting lymphatic vessels to generate surges up to 100 μm/s, several times per minute, to drain lymph to a lymph node within 20 min (Thornbury et al., 1989, 1990; McHale, 2005). Flow alterations may occur due to changes in the levels of nitric oxide (Shirasawa et al., 2000; Padera, 2005) within the LECs that in turn produce SMC dilatation. They may also be under autonomic control, as shown by splanchnic stimulation effecting thoracic duct flow (Bulekbaeva and Akhmetbaeva, 1982) and sympathetic stimulation (McGeown et al., 1987a; Thornbury et al., 1990), especially mediated via the alpha-adrenoceptors (Thornbury et al., 1989, 1993) and in response to adrenaline or noradrenaline (McHale and Roddie, 1983). It has also been suggested that acetylcholine may enhance luminal dilatation via nitric oxide release (Koller et al., 1999). Further to these mechanisms, there are independent *endothelium-mediated* vasomotor adaptations that compensate for increased lymph volumes that may be regulated by prostaglandins (PGs) (Koller et al., 1999; Karnezis, 2012a,b). It is via PGs that collecting lymphatics may also dilate in response to tumour-derived VEGF-D, potentially increasing the lymph flow and capacity to transport tumour cells to lymph nodes (Karnezis, 2012a,b).

12.4 LYMPHATIC MAPPING

Lymphatic mapping relates to understanding the drainage patterns and gross layout of the lymphatic vessels. Since Kinmoth's radiographic injection studies, lymphatic mapping has largely been performed using some variation of radiological or nuclear medicine imaging. For the purposes of discussion, description of radiological techniques will largely be reserved in the Evolving Imaging Technologies section.

Lymph fluid passes through a series of lymph nodes or other secondary lymphoid organs (gastro-respiratory submucosal lymphoid aggregations such as Peyer's patches and tonsils) (Cupedo et al., 2002). Afferent lymph node ducts divide before passing beneath the capsule of the node into cortical sinuses and then pass through a reticuloendothelial cell filter (Cupedo et al., 2002). Lymphatics transport antigen-presenting cells (APCs), such as dendritic cells, from their primary location (throughout the interstitial tissues where they interact with foreign pathogens) to the lymph nodes, where they present epitope fragments to the lymphocytes. This antigen presentation triggers the lymphocytes, the main effector cells of the immune system, to clonally expand and form antigen-specific helper and cytotoxic T cell populations and antigen-specific antibody-secreting B cell populations, respectively (Cupedo and Mebius, 2005). Thus, it is tailored as an individualised *antigen-specific* immune response to a pathogen and an element of *memory* is developed.

The memory of antigens consists of maintaining residual lymphocytes with the ability to recognise the original epitope, in order to generate an efficient and rapid immune response, should the particular pathogen be re-encountered (Cupedo and Mebius, 2005). Whilst lymph continues to flow through the medullary sinus to the hilar region of the lymph node and into efferent ducts, tumour cells may become trapped and proliferate or spread further to distal organs (McHale, 2005).

For many years, clinical understanding of the lymphatic drainage patterns was largely based on Sappey's 1874 atlas, which included highly detailed anatomical drawings of the lymphatic vessels in many regions of the body. Sappey performed these studies using mercury injections, which have never been repeated due to the hazards of mercury toxicity. The atlas compiled from these studies contained a combination of observed patterning and ideas extrapolated from visualised vessels; one example of the latter was the female breast, in which lymphatic vessels were drawn radiating out centrifugally from the nipple (Sappey, 1874). Despite these shortcomings, and in the absence of superior alternatives, these concepts remained the mainstay of our understanding until recently (Last, 1998).

In terms of the skin, Sappey's atlas suggested that lymphatic drainage was distributed in quadrants, in the body, joining at a watershed area that could drain in either direction; however, lymph from one side of the body would never drain from a region of skin completely across the midline of the body or through a horizontal line drawn around the waist through the umbilicus. These concepts were in contradiction to clinical observations of the behaviour of melanoma in some patients, in whom metastases would appear in areas unexpected according to Sappey's outlines – leading to the adage that *melanoma can do anything*.

It was not until the advent of the techniques of lymphoscintigraphy (LS) (Figure 12.2) that incorporated a functional component that inconsistencies between the time-honoured lymphatic maps and the clinical reality began to emerge (Sherman and Ter-Pogossian, 1953). Using this technique, clinicians began to develop a working understanding of the lymphatics in cancer. In so doing, clinicians were also able to use the radioisotope LS injection maps to simultaneously elucidate a more clear understanding of the regional lymph node groups that drained different regions of the body. Early imaging studies by Turner-Warwick and Kinmonth were the first modern studies that enabled meaningful comparison with Sappey's work; however, they neither specifically confirmed nor challenged the traditional view of lymphatic drainage patterns. They used radioactive gold LS and non-radioisotopic radiopaque dye to image the lymphatic vasculature of living humans (Turner-Warwick, 1955; Kinmonth, 1972). Kinmonth demonstrated the collecting lymphatic vessel pathways in normal and diseased individuals, particularly in the upper and lower limbs.

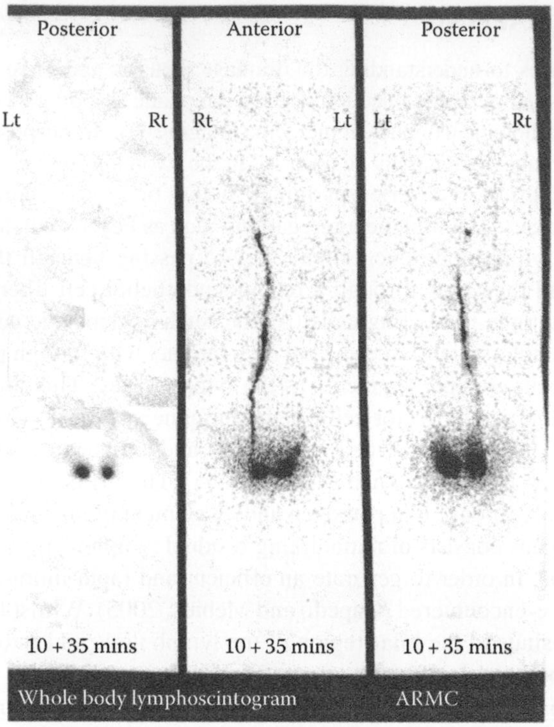

FIGURE 12.2 LS of bilateral lower limbs. Reproduced image from gamma camera views of bilateral lower limb, derived from whole-body LS study. Images were taken at 0 min (left), 30 min (centre), and 90 min (right) following injection of technetium-99 radiolabelled colloid into the first webspace of the foot bilaterally. Lower focal collection of the tracer represents a higher concentration of the tracer at the injection sites, and linear structures extending proximally indicate the pathways of the major collecting lymphatic vessels. No draining lymph nodes are visualised.

From this point onwards, imaging would become integral to the study of the lymphatic system. These methodologies would come to form the basis for modern LS and sentinel lymph node (SLN) biopsy. For a full discussion on SLN biopsy (SLNB), see Chapter 7.

This concept of SLNB was first described by Cabanas for use in squamous cell carcinoma of the penis in the 1970s (Cabanas, 1977). The method was later modified by Morton and Cochrane for use in melanoma patients and later for breast and other epithelial tumours from the 1990s. Some proponents of the SLN tracing technique believed that the injection of dyes such as India ink or Patent Blue V (which is a particle size that is selectively taken up and retained by initial lymphatics) is the optimum technique of identifying blue lymph nodes either by visualising a blue SLN through the skin or by performing an open operative approach to the lymph nodes thought empirically to be the most likely nodal basin to drain the area of skin in which the tumour was detected. Others advocated a nuclear medicine approach, in which a technetium-labelled colloid would be injected around the primary tumour in question and a series of images taken: one at the time of injection and then images at incremental time points for a set time thereafter (Figure 12.2). The injection of radiolabelled colloid would usually take place in the morning prior to an afternoon operating list or in the night before a morning operating list. In addition to these LS images obtained using nuclear imaging, a handheld intra-operative gamma probe emitting gamma irradiation readings and audible tone as it nears the areas of higher radiolabelled colloid was also added to the standard technique of SLNB, and large population comparisons demonstrated that this improved detection rates of the true SLN for a particular injection site, from 70%–80% to 95% (Carlson et al., 2002; Leong, 2004).

Amongst the foremost proponents of the SLNB techniques, the Sydney Melanoma Unit led by Thompson and Uren was amongst the most well respected and prolific. Their early work on melanoma LS studies demonstrated that although most cases exhibited typical ipsilateral drainage patterns, certain cases exhibited more unexpected contralateral drainage that contradicted Sappey's drawings (Uren et al., 1998a). As experience with SLNB improved, so too did the confidence with which observed patterns of lymphatic drainage were seen to contradict predictions of where lymphatics from different anatomical locations should drain, according to the original Sappey model. A notable example of this phenomenon is melanoma metastasis from a primary tumour located on the lower posterior trunk region, through deep para-aortic lymph nodes located deep within the retroperitoneal (Uren et al., 1998a) or thoracic cavities (Uren et al., 1999). This drainage pattern bypasses the inguinal lymph nodes to which this area of skin is expected to drain and suggests that there may be previously unknown direct communications between the lower back and intra-thoracic/abdominal lymph nodes. Other examples of aberrant were of forearm lesions draining to the supraclavicular lymph nodes (Uren et al., 1996), central inter-scapular primary lesions, or lesions on one or other side of the midline draining across the traditional watershed areas to the contralateral or bilateral axillary lymph node basins (Uren et al., 2003).

In performing LS, there are a number of variable factors to consider, which may be responsible for any observed variations. These include the tracer radioisotope and dosage used, the location(s) chosen to inject the tracer, and the imaging protocol(s) implemented. The technique espoused by most major melanoma units utilises filtered sulphur colloid tagged with technetium-99m radionuclide. SLNB facilitates the mapping of lymphatic pathways that drain a particular area of tissue, and it identifies the lymph nodes into which they drain (Leong, 2004); it has resulted in the detection and location of potentially metastatic draining lymph nodes in unexpected sites (Uren et al., 1995, 1998b; Thompson and Uren, 2001a); this occurs at a rate of up to 30% (Uren et al., 2006). Regardless of whether the draining nodal basin is expected or in an unusual location, any clinical benefits to the patient lie in the accurate detection and sampling of the true draining SLN (Uren et al., 2006).

As a result of the improved understanding of the peculiarities of the lymphatic drainage in certain areas of the body, as demonstrated by Thompson and Uren – and thus the limitations of the traditional anatomical description – Taylor and colleagues set about to address some of the clinical questions raised by unexpected observations made in clinical SLNB studies. To this end, they adapted previous methods of cadaveric vascular injection studies, to develop a reliable method of cadaveric lymphatic mapping. Initially, two techniques were used by Taylor and colleagues to elucidate the lymphatic anatomy and variations therein. Firstly, with the use of hydrogen peroxide mixed with India ink injected both intradermally and subcutaneously, the tissues could be examined macroscopically and photographed. The second technique was adapted from cadaveric radiographic anatomical injection studies previously used by the Taylor group, which itself is adapted from Salmon's technique of vascular delineation from the 1930s (Rees and Taylor, 1986). Hydrogen peroxide (6%) was injected directly into the tissues to inflate the lymphatic vessels located within the subcutaneous tissues. The collecting lymphatic vessels were cannulated and subsequently injected with a radiopaque lead oxide mixture and radiographic images obtained (Suami et al., 2005).

In 2007, refinements of the cadaveric injection technique led to improvements in the investigation of lymphatics in cadaveric anatomical studies in which an extruded glass tube instead of a 30-gauge needle was used to cannulate smaller collecting lymphatic vessels. The injection mixture was also modified, using milk powder to suspend the lead oxide (Suami et al., 2007).

Advances in imaging technologies provided another opportunity to enhance the outcomes of lymphatic anatomical studies, and as such, both computed tomography and magnetic resonance imaging (MRI) were incorporated into cadaveric studies of lymphatics (Pan et al., 2008). The use of clinical contrast media in cadaveric radiographic studies for lymphangiography was also attempted (Pan et al., 2009); however, the effectiveness of this method was limited due to the lack of a living circulation.

In combination, these minor refinements facilitated several detailed cadaveric studies not previously performed. The Taylor group studied the lymphatic territories of the upper limb including documenting changes in an individual cadaver's lymphatic anatomy following ipsilateral axillary dissection in that specimen (Suami et al., 2007). These studies demonstrated numerous parallel and irregularly interconnecting collecting lymphatic pathways that drained in an unpredictable manner into a variable array of lymph nodes in the axilla. Parallel multiple studies of the collecting lymphatics emanating from the breast were performed (Suami et al., 2008; Pan et al., 2009). The findings of these studies challenged the conception, illustrated in drawings based on earlier mercury injection studies, that the collecting lymphatics draining the breast radiated from the nipple. They also challenged the conception held by many proponents of breast surgeon SLNB that the injections of Patent Blue V dye and radiolabelled colloid should be performed in a peri-areolar location. Certainly, these injections will drain an SLN – the primary node draining the area of the areola into which the injections were performed. However, this may not necessarily drain the area of tissue in which the clinician is interested – the drainage of the area surrounding the tumour itself. Therefore, to obtain a true and accurate understanding of the drainage of a tumour in the breast – and therefore enabling sampling and histological analysis of the node to which the tumour is most likely to drain – the Taylor group advocated a *peri-tumoural* rather than a *peri-areolar* injection of Patent Blue V dye or radiocolloid tracer. This represented a significant advance both in our anatomical understanding of the collecting lymphatic drainage patterns and in the clinical application of this understanding in SLNB. Studies of the upper torso were also performed, demonstrating a more variable anatomy than previously thought (Suami et al., 2008). Similar variations in the drainage routes of the lower limb were also demonstrated with alternative drainage routes noted from the heel to the inguinal lymph nodes (Pan et al., 2011).

The lymphatic drainage of the superficial tissues of the head and neck was also investigated to try and explain emerging reports of unexpected clinical and LS findings (Pan et al., 2008). The lymphatic drainage of the nasal fossae and nasopharynx in a series of fresh cadaveric dissections was described in 2009 (Pan et al., 2009) followed by studies of the external ear (Pan et al., 2011), all clinically important for understanding patterns of tumour spread from common sites of cutaneous and mucosal tumour occurrence. From the database of cadaveric studies amassed, the variability of the drainage patterns in lymphatic vessels of the human head and neck (Pan et al., 2010) – even between two sides of the same cadaver (Pan et al., 2011) – illustrated an important principle also highlighted in previous lymphatic injection studies. This principle was that there is a significant difference between the ideal of outlining a definite and predictable drainage pattern that is reproducible between individual patients and a study performed in a particular patient that identifies their unique pattern of drainage (whether influenced by individual developmental nuances or acquired alterations due to tumour blockage, trauma, or surgery). There may be so much inherent variability between individuals, if not between the equivalent contralateral areas – and, indeed, in the *same* area assessed under different physiological or pathological conditions – that it may be impossible to accurately predict an empirical drainage pattern for a particular tumour in a particular patient. Instead, if clinicians are to elucidate the drainage pattern that is useful for identification of tumour metastasis and therefore patient prognostication and potentially improved patient outcomes (local disease control and survival), then it is critical that preconceived ideas of potential drainage sites be suspended in favour of documented and objective mapping of the pattern of collecting lymphatic vessels and SLN sampling.

12.5 EMERGING TECHNIQUES OF LYMPHATIC MAPPING

Recently, Reynolds and co-workers (Reynolds et al., 2007, 2009) developed computational models to provide improved visualisation and analysis of the functional lymphatic anatomy of the skin and to assess historical assumptions about lymphatic anatomy. In their studies, accumulated 2D melanoma LS data were used from over 5000 patients with cutaneous melanoma treated at the Sydney Melanoma Unit, Australia. The 2D LS data were mapped onto an anatomically based 3D computer model of the skin and lymph nodes. Spatial analysis was then carried out to visualise the relationship between primary melanoma sites and the locations of draining SLNs, which collectively showed patterns of skin lymphatic drainage.

Heat maps were produced to visualise the patterns of drainage from the skin to each node field, which highlighted the inter-patient variability in skin lymphatic drainage and showed the skin regions in which highly variable drainage would occur (Reynolds et al., 2007, 2010). Results indicated that the most variable drainage patterns included skin on the torso close to Sappey's lines (Sappey, 1874) and skin on the head and neck and that, overall, the commonly used Sappey's lines were not effective in predicting lymphatic drainage. Results also showed that although lymphatic drainage of the head and neck is highly complex and clinically unpredictable, there were still clear patterns of drainage shown in the data. Some node fields drained relatively circumscribed areas of skin, particularly the preauricular and occipital node fields, which drained large regions of the head and neck. Overall, the 3D models developed by Reynolds et al. quantitatively updated the knowledge of lymphatic drainage of the skin, demonstrating how they differed from traditional anatomical descriptions and are available to view online at www.bioeng.auckland.ac.nz/melanoma and www.bioeng.auckland.ac.nz/head.

Furthermore, Reynolds and colleagues conducted a thorough statistical analysis to move beyond anatomically based definitions of lymphatic drainage of the skin based largely on variants of Sappey's lines towards a purely data-driven approach (Reynolds et al., 2009). Results indicated that most skin regions showed symmetric lymphatic drainage about the coronal midline of the body. Subsequent cluster analysis showed a clear anatomic division of the skin into nine separate clusters, primarily grouping regions of skin according to the dominant draining node fields: the axilla, groin, cervical level II, and preauricular node fields. Interestingly, the clusters draining primarily to axillary and groin node fields divided the trunk into regions comparable to Sappey's lines (Reynolds et al., 2010). Even though there was variability of lymphatic drainage on the torso between individuals, Sappey's lines appeared to conform to the most likely drainage behaviour of these data.

LS imaging has also been used to determine SLN locations in patients with breast cancer, demonstrating lymphatic drainage patterns of the breast. In 2011, Blumgart et al. conducted studies into lymphatic drainage of the breast using aggregated LS data from 2304 patients from the Royal Prince Alfred Hospital, Sydney, Australia (Reynolds et al., 2010). Their study aimed to test commonly held assumptions of breast lymphatic anatomy, where results confirmed the left and right breasts are likely to have symmetric drainage patterns and that there is likely no statistically significant difference between the draining breast lymphatics of males and females. Furthermore, results showed that direct lymphatic drainage of the breasts is likely to be independent between node fields.

These breast LS data were also modelled and mapped onto a 3D computational model of the breast and sentinel node field locations (Blumgart et al., 2011a,b). The likelihood of drainage to each node field from the whole breast and from each breast region was calculated using Bayesian inferential techniques. Patterns were observed in the drainage where regions anatomically close to each node field showed an increased drainage to that node field. In addition, as expected, the breast almost always drained to the axillary node field (98.2%) and frequently to the internal mammary node field (35.3%). Additional draining node fields included the infraclavicular, supraclavicular, and interpectoral node fields with 1.7%, 3.1%, and 0.7% patients, respectively. These results are available to visualise online at www.abi.auckland.ac.nz/breast-cancer.

In parallel with these important clinical developments, molecular biologists have also made significant advances in the areas of lymphatic imaging. Utilising the recent capacity to stain lymphatic vessels in tissues using antibodies against specific markers located on the surface of lymphatic endothelium, secondary fluorescent-tagged antibodies could then be used to detect these primary markers, and fluorescent microscopy was used to visualise the highlighted vessels (Shayan et al., 2007). Specific quantification protocols were then developed to allow accurate delineation between normal and diseased lymphatics (Shayan et al., 2007; Lokmic and Mitchell, 2011). So far, such techniques are yet to be adapted to human application.

12.6 LYMPHATIC IMAGING

When considering the interaction of the clinician with the lymphatic system and certainly in the case of lymphatic imaging, it is critical to bear in mind that this takes place almost exclusively at the level of the collecting lymphatic vessels. Hitherto, and with the exception of the initial or capillary lymphatic vessels visualised in immunohistochemically labelled lymphatics in tumour or other tissue paraffin sections, and the vessels observed in the molecular labelling techniques (see above) – which currently remain in experimental models – the collecting lymphatics are the vessels that clinicians image using available imaging technologies.

12.7 EVOLVING TECHNOLOGIES

The computational models developed by Reynolds et al. and Blumgart et al. provide novel 3D frameworks for visualising lymphatic drainage patterns of the skin and breast (Reynolds et al., 2010; Blumgart et al., 2011a). The heat maps and the interactive software could be a new resource for clinicians to use in preoperative discussions with patients with cancers that can metastasise to the lymph nodes and could be used in the identification of SLN fields during follow-up of such patients. This visualisation framework may be extended in the future to enable the addition of LS data from multiple centres in real time, as well as include data from other imaging modalities such as single-photon emission computed tomography (SPECT). This modality is a nuclear medicine tomographic imaging technique using gamma rays in a similar manner to conventional nuclear medicine planar imaging with a gamma camera. In addition, however, it can provide true 3D information presented as cross-sectional slices that may be reformatted or manipulated as required. Whilst gamma cameras have been used traditionally during LS imaging, recent software advances have been made, utilising them in combination with SPECT/CT imaging to accurately locate SLNs to which higher concentrations of tracer drain. This hybrid imaging technology allows the nuclear medicine physician to determine the exact anatomical position of the SLN during preoperative LS in patients.

Due to the precise anatomical detail available in SPECT/CT, knowledge of the lymphatic anatomy can be further refined. For example, in a study by Uren et al., the anatomy of the axillary node field draining the breast was reassessed using such images.[7] Historically, it was suggested that the lymphatic drainage of the breast was to lymph nodes lying in the antero-pectoral group of nodes in the axilla just lateral to the pectoral muscles. Uren and colleagues used SPECT/CT LS to show that the breast does not always drain to the anterior group of level I lymph nodes in the axilla but may instead drain to the mid-axilla and/or posterior group in about 50% of patients with breast cancer, regardless of the location of the cancer within the breast.

12.8 MAGNETIC RESONANCE AND OTHER RECENT METHODS OF LYMPHANGIOGRAPHY

Whilst MRI has been in clinical use for many years, it has only recently been applied to the imaging of lymphatic vessels (Liu et al., 2009). Notohamiprodjo and colleagues compare lymphangiography with traditional LS for the imaging of lymphatic vessels. Thirty patients with unilateral or bilateral lymphoedema and lymph vessel transplants of lower limbs were examined using 3.0 T fat-saturated 3D gradient-echo MR following gadopentetate dimeglumine injections (Notohamiprodjo et al., 2012). The results of both techniques were reviewed separately by a nuclear physician and a radiologist who rated delay and drainage pattern, enhancing levels, and quality of images of depiction of lymph nodes and lymph vessels. They found that lymphatic vessels were clearly visualised with MR lymphangiography, whilst they were not detectable with LS (Notohamiprodjo et al., 2012). MR lymphangiography and LS show a clear concordance.

Visualisation of the inguinal lymph nodes was superior with LS. In contrast, MR lymphangiography provided superior lymphatic vessel depiction including a higher level of accuracy in identifying morphologic features of lymphatic vessel abnormalities. MR lymphangiography showed a higher sensitivity for lymphatic vessel abnormalities and lower specificity for lymph node abnormalities. Two similar studies comparing the same modalities for use in the investigation of extremity lymphoedema were conducted by the same authors, 5 years apart (Liu et al., 2005, 2010). In the earlier study, 39 patients with lymphoedema of the lower limb, abdominal wall, or external genitalia underwent LS and MR lymphangiography. Assessment of the imaging studies included the degree and quality of visualisation of the malformations of the collecting lymphatics, lymphatic trunks, lymph nodes, and tissue oedema. MR clearly detected dilated superficial collecting lymphatics and deeper lymphatic trunks, as well as the accumulation of chyle and node enlargements. In patients with lymphatic hypoplasia or aplasia, LS displayed a pattern of dermal backflow in the form of radiotracer filling dermal lymphatics or isotope stagnation at the injection point. MR images demonstrated the extent of tissue fluid accumulation and distinguished oedema fluid from subcutaneous fat. In patients with peripheral and central lymphatic malformations, LSG provided images representative of the function of the lymphatic vessels but failed to give detailed information regarding anatomy, whereas 3D MRI provided extensive information on the anatomy of the lymph stagnated vasculature as well as on the effects of lymphatic dysfunction on local structures and tissue composition. In the later study by the same group, a sample of 16 patients primary extremity lymphoedema (Liu et al., 2010). Their LS technique incorporated the use of the tracer (99)Tc-labelled dextran, whereas the MR protocol used gadobenate dimeglumine as the contrast agent. Both the state of morphological abnormalities and the functional state of the lymphatic systems of affected limbs were compared. The authors found that MR detected inguinal nodes in 16 of 17 patients, whereas LS revealed inguinal nodes in 9. Further, MR revealed more precise information about structural and functional abnormalities of lymph vessels and nodes than LS by real-time measurement of lymph flow in vessels and nodes, making the former a more sensitive and accurate investigation than LS for detecting anatomical and functional abnormalities in the lymphatic system in patients with extremity lymphoedema.

In a Japanese study, four diagnostic imaging modalities of the lymphatic system were compared: MRI, CT, LS, and indocyanine green (ICG) lymphography. ICG is a fluorescent cyanine dye originally developed for use in hepatic and cardiac functional assessment that was later adapted for use in angiography in the optic fundus. It was also found that due to its high rate of binding to plasma proteins, ICG could remain within the blood vessels and lymphatics due to low extravasation rates, thus making it ideal for visualising superficial lymphatic vessels in subcutaneous tissues when stimulated with fluorescent and laser light. This application has led to the field of so-called fluorescence image-guided surgery (FIGS). The application of light of the desired wavelength allows the clinician to visualise the vessels in real time, intra-operatively (Hirche et al., 2010).

In their study of 21 female patients (42 arms) with unilateral mild upper limb lymphoedema, the investigators found MR and ICG lymphography were superior to LS or CT for diagnosis of lymphoedema. Whilst LS could demonstrate some abnormal lymphatic vessels, some significantly deranged lymphatic vessels (determined clinically) were not identified on LS, presumably due to their inability to traffic the tracer in sufficient concentration to be detectable using the gamma camera technology. In these cases, whilst ICG lymphography was similarly unable to identify the collecting lymphatic vessels, it did demonstrate dermal backflow pattern. The authors suggest therefore that dual investigations for examination of the lymphatic system using ICG lymphography and evaluation of oedema in subcutaneous fat tissue using MRI be undertaken as the optimal diagnostic combination. Finally, a study undertaken in China to assess the role of gadolinium contrast-enhanced MR lymphangiography in the clinical setting of 32 patients with breast carcinoma found that this technique enabled clinicians to visualise the lymphatic system, identify SLNs, and differentiate between metastatic and non-metastatic lymph nodes (Lu et al., 2013).

12.9 FUTURE QUANTITATIVE IMAGING TECHNIQUES

Animal models have been generated to explore the role of lymphatics and lymphangiogenic growth factors in immunity and interstitial fluid homeostasis, as well as diseases such as lymphoedema and metastatic cancer, and to study lymphatic development. Hitherto, lymphatic vessel analysis has primarily been restricted to counting lymphatics in 2D tissue slices, due to a lack of more sophisticated methodologies, or to simple descriptive studies. In order to accurately examine lymphatic dysfunction in these models and analyse the effects of lymphangiogenic growth factors on the lymphatic vasculature, it was essential to quantify the morphology and patterning of the distinct lymphatic vessel types in 3D tissues. Shayan and colleagues developed a method for performing such analyses, integrating user-operated image-analysis software (a plug-in for image-J [Shayan et al., 2007]) with an approach that considers important morphological, anatomical, and patterning features of the distinct lymphatic vessel subtypes, depicted in whole-mounted immunofluorescent staining of full-thickness mouse skin. This efficient, reproducible technique was validated by analysing healthy and pathological tissues from mice and awaits application in humans (Shayan et al., 2007).

REFERENCES

Achen, M.G., Jeltsch, M., Kukk, E., Makinen, T., Vitali, A., Wilks, A.F., Alitalo, K., and Stacker, S.A. (1998). Vascular endothelial growth factor D (VEGF-D) is a ligand for the tyrosine kinases VEGF receptor 2 (Flk1) and VEGF receptor 3 (Flt4). *Proc Natl Acad Sci USA 95*, 548–553.

Alitalo, K. (2011). The lymphatic vasculature in disease. *Nat Med* November 7; *17* (11), 1371–1380.

Baluk, P., Fuxe, J., Hashizume, H., Romano, T., Lashnits, E., Butz, S., Vestweber, D. et al. (2007). Functionally specialized junctions between endothelial cells of lymphatic vessels. *J Exp Med 204*, 2349–2362.

Banerji, S., Ni, J., Wang, S.-X., Clasper, S., Su, J., Tammi, R., Jones, M., and Jackson, D.G. (1999). LYVE-1, a new homologue of the CD44 glycoprotein, is a lymph-specific receptor for hyaluronan. *J Cell Biol 144*, 789–801.

Blumgart, E.I., Uren, R.F., Nielsen, P.M.F., Nash, M.P., and Reynolds, H.M. (2011a). Lymphatic drainage and tumour prevalence in the breast: A statistical analysis of symmetry, gender and node field independence. *J Anat 218*, 652–659.

Blumgart, E.I., Uren, R.F., Nielsen, P.M.F., Nash, M.P., and Reynolds, H.M. (2011b). Predicting lymphatic drainage patterns and primary tumour location in patients with breast cancer. *Breast Cancer Res Treat 130*, 699–705.

Bulekbaeva, L.E. and Akhmetbaeva, N.A. (1982). Development of sympathetic influences on lymph flow in the postnatal ontogeny of dogs. *Zh Evol Biokhim Fiziol 18*, 140–143.

Cabanas, R.M. (1977). An approach for the treatment of penile carcinoma. *Cancer Cell 39*, 456–466.

Carlson, G.W., Murray, D.R., Thourani, V., Hestley, A., and Cohen, C. (2002). The definition of the sentinel lymph node in melanoma based on radioactive counts. *Ann Surg Oncol 9*, 929–933.

Casley-Smith, J.R. and Florey, H.W. (1961). The structure of normal small lymphatics. *Quart J Exp Physiol and Cognate Med Sci 46*, 101–106.

Cupedo, T., Kraal, G., and Mebius, R.E. (2002). The role of CD45+CD4+CD3- cells in lymphoid organ development. *Immunol Rev 189*, 41–50.

Cupedo, T. and Mebius, R.E. (2005). Cellular interactions in lymph node development. *J Immunol 174*, 21–25.

François, M., Caprini, A., Hosking, B., Orsenigo, F., Wilhelm, D., Browne, C., Paavonen, K., Karnezis, T., Shayan, R., Downes, M., Davidson, T., Tutt, D., Cheah, K.S., Stacker, S.A., Muscat, G.E., Achen, M.G., Dejana, E., and Koopman, P. (2008). Sox18 induces development of the lymphatic vasculature in mice. *Nature*. Dec 4; *456* (7222), 643–647.

Gerli, R., Ibba, L., and Fruschelli, C. (1991). Ultrastructural cytochemistry of anchoring filaments of human lymphatic capillaries and their relation to elastic fibers. *Lymphology 24*, 105–112.

Haagensen, C.D., Feind, C.R., Herter, F.P., Slanetz, C.A., and Weinberg, J.A. (1972). *The Lymphatics in Cancer*, 1st edn. Philadelphia, PA: W.B. Saunders.

Hirche, C., Dresel, S., Krempien, R., and Hünerbein, M. (2010). Sentinel node biopsy by indocyanine green retention fluorescence detection for inguinal lymph node staging of anal cancer: Preliminary experience. *Ann Surg Oncol 17* (9), 2357–2362.

Jain, R.K. (2003). Molecular regulation of vessel maturation. *Nat Med.* June; *9* (6), 685–693.

Johnson, L.A., Clasper, S., Holt, A.P., Lalor, P.F., Baban, D., and Jackson, D.G. (2006). An inflammation-induced mechanism for leukocyte transmigration across lymphatic vessel endothelium. *J Exp Med 203*, 2763–2777.

Jones, J.M., Gamperl, A.K., Farrell, A.P., and Toews, D.P. (1997). Direct measurement of flow from the posterior lymph hearts of hydrated and dehydrated toads (Bufo marinus). *J Exp Biol 200*, 1695–1702.

Joukov, V., Pajusola, K., Kaipainen, A., Chilov, D., Lahtinen, I., Kukk, E., Saksela, O., Kalkkinen, N., and Alitalo, K. (1996). A novel vascular endothelial growth factor, VEGF-C, is a ligand for the Flt-4 (VEGFR-3) and KDR (VEGFR-2) receptor tyrosine kinases. *EMBO J 15*, 290–298.

Kaipainen, A., Korhonen, J., Mustonen, T., van Hinsbergh, V.W., Fang, G.H., Dumont, D., Breitman, M., and Alitalo, K. (1995). Expression of the fms-like tyrosine kinase 4 gene becomes restricted to lymphatic endothelium during development. *Proc Natl Acad Sci USA 92*, 3566–3570.

Karnezis, T., Shayan, R., Caesar, C., Roufail, S., Ardipradja, K., Harris, N.C., Farnsworth, R.H. et al. (2012b). VEGF-D promotes tumour metastasis by regulating prostaglandins produced by the collecting lymphatic endothelium. *Cancer Cell 21*, 181–195.

Karnezis, T., Shayan, R., Fox, S., Achen, M.G., and Stacker, S.A. (2012a). The connection between lymphangiogenic signaling and prostaglandin biology: A missing link in the metastatic pathway. *Oncotarget* August; *3* (8), 890–903. Epub August 19.

Kinmonth, J.B. (1972). *The Lymphatics: Diseases, Lymphography, and Surgery*, 1st edn. London, U.K.: Edward Arnold.

Koller, A., Mizuno, R., and Kaley, G. (1999). Flow reduces the amplitude and increases the frequency of lymphatic vasomotion: Role of endothelial prostanoids. *Am J Physiol Regul Integr Comp Physiol 277*, 1683–1689.

Last, R.J. (1998). *Last's Anatomy: Regional and Applied*, 9th edn. Edinburgh, U.K.: Churchill Livingstone.

Leak, L.V. (1976). The structure of lymphatic capillaries in lymph formation. *Fed Proc 35*, 1863–1871.

Leak, L.V. and Burke, J.F. (1966). Fine structure of the lymphatic capillary and the adjoining connective tissue area. *Am J Anat 118*, 785–809.

Leak, L.V. and Burke, J.F. (1968a). Electron microscopic study of lymphatic capillaries in the removal of connective tissue fluids and particulate substances. *Lymphology 1*, 39–52.

Leak, L.V. and Burke, J.F. (1968b). Ultrastructural studies on the lymphatic anchoring filaments. *J Cell Biol 36*, 129–149.

Leak, L.V. and Jones, M. (1993). Lymphatic endothelium isolation, characterization and long-term culture. *Anat Rec 236*, 641–652.

Leong, S.P. (2004). Sentinel lymph node mapping and selective lymphadenectomy: The standard of care for melanoma. *Curr Treat Options Oncol 5*, 185–194.

Liu, N.F., Lu, Q., Jiang, Z.H., Wang, C.G., and Zhou, J.G. (2009). Anatomic and functional evaluation of the lymphatics and lymph nodes in diagnosis of lymphatic circulation disorders with contrast magnetic resonance lymphangiography. *J Vasc Surg* April; *49* (4), 980–987.

Liu, N.F., Lu, Q., Liu, P.A., Wu, X.F., and Wang, B.S. (2010). Comparison of radionuclide lymphoscintigraphy and dynamic magnetic resonance lymphangiography for investigating extremity lymphoedema. *Br J Surg 97*, 359–365.

Liu, N.F., Wang, C., and Sun, M. (2005). Noncontrast three-dimensional magnetic resonance imaging vs lymphoscintigraphy in the evaluation of lymph circulation disorders: A comparative study. *J Vasc Surg 41* (1), 69–75.

Lokmic, Z. and Mitchell, G.M. (2011). Visualisation and stereological assessment of blood and lymphatic vessels. *Histol Histopathol* June; *26* (6), 781–796.

Lu, Q., Hua, J., Kassir, M.M., Delproposto, Z., Dai, Y., Sun, J., Haacke, M., and Hu, J. (2013). Imaging lymphatic system in breast cancer patients with magnetic resonance lymphangiography. *PLoS ONE* July 5; *8* (7), e69701.

Makinen, T., Adams, R.H., Bailey, J., Lu, Q., Ziemiecki, A., Alitalo, K., Klein, R., and Wilkinson, G.A. (2005). PDZ interaction site in ephrinB2 is required for the remodeling of lymphatic vasculature. *Genes Dev 19*, 397–410.

Makinen, T., Norrmen, C., and Petrova, T.V. (2007). Molecular mechanisms of lymphatic vascular development. *Cell Mol Life Sci 64*, 1915–1929.

Matsumoto, M., Roufail, S., Inder, R., Caesar, C., Karnezis, T., Shayan, R., Farnsworth, R.H., Sato, T., Achen, M.G., Mann, G.B., and Stacker, S.A. (2013). Signaling for lymphangiogenesis via VEGFR-3 is required for the early events of metastasis. *Clin Exp Metastasis* Aug; *30* (6), 819–832.

McGeown, J.G., McHale, N.G., and Thornbury, K.D. (1987a). The effect of electrical stimulation of the sympathetic chain on peripheral lymph flow in the anaesthetized sheep. *J Physiol 393*, 123–133.

McGeown, J.G., McHale, N.G., and Thornbury, K.D. (1987b). The role of external compression and movement in lymph propulsion in the sheep hind limb. *J Physiol 387*, 83–93.

McGeown, J.G., McHale, N.G., and Thornbury, K.D. (1988a). Arterial pulsation and lymph formation in an isolated sheep hindlimb preparation. *J Physiol 405*, 595–604.

McGeown, J.G., McHale, N.G., and Thornbury, K.D. (1988b). Effects of varying patterns of external compression on lymph flow in the hindlimb of the anaesthetized sheep. *J Physiol 397*, 449–457.

McHale, N.G. (2005). Lymph circulation and lymph propulsion. *Proceedings 1st International Symposium on Cancer Metastasis and the Lymphovascular System: Basis for Rational Therapy*, 4.

McHale, N.G. and Roddie, I.C. (1983). The effect of intravenous adrenaline and noradrenaline infusion of peripheral lymph flow in the sheep. *J Physiol 341*, 517–526.

Notohamiprodjo, M., Weiss, M., Baumeister, R.G., Sommer, W.H., Helck, A., Crispin, A., Reiser, M.F., and Herrmann, K.A. (2012). MR lymphangiography at 3.0 T: Correlation with lymphoscintigraphy. *Radiology* July; *264* (1):78–87.

Oliver, G. and Detmar, M. (2002). The rediscovery of the lymphatic system: Old and new insights into the development and biological function of the lymphatic vasculature. *Genes Dev 16*, 773–783.

Oliver, G. and Harvey, N. (2002). A stepwise model of the development of lymphatic vasculature. *Ann N Y Acad Sci 979*, 159–165; Discussion 188–196.

Padera, T. (2005). Lymphatic pathophysiology and metastasis. *Proceedings 1st International Symposium on Cancer Metastasis and the Lymphovascular System: Basis for Rational Therapy.*

Pan, W.R., le Roux, C.M., Levy, S.M., and Briggs, C.A. (2010). The morphology of the human lymphatic vessels in the head and neck. *Clin Anat* September; *23* (6), 654–661.

Pan, W.R., le Roux, C.M., Levy, S.M., and Briggs, C.A. (2011). Lymphatic drainage of the external ear. *Head Neck* January; *33* (1), 60–64.

Pan, W.R., Le Roux, C.M., and Rozen, W.M. (2009). The use of clinical contrast media for lymphangiography in cadaveric studies. *Lymphat Res Biol 7* (3), 169–172.

Pan, W.R., Suami, H., and Taylor, G.I. (2008). Lymphatic drainage of the superficial tissues of the head and neck: Anatomical study and clinical implications. *Plast Reconstr Surg* May; *121* (5), 1614–1624.

Papp, M., Viragh, S., and Ungvary, G. (1975). Structure of cutaneous lymphatics propelling lymph. *Acta Med Acad Sci Hung 32*, 311–320.

Pepper, M.S. and Skobe, M. (2003). Lymphatic endothelium: Morphological, molecular and functional properties. *J Cell Biol 163*, 209–213.

Petrova, T.V., Karpanen, T., Norrmen, C., Mellor, R., Tamakoshi, T., Finegold, D., Ferrell, R. et al. (2004). Defective valves and abnormal mural cell recruitment underlie lymphatic vascular failure in lymphedema distichiasis. *Nat Med 10*, 974–981.

Pullinger, B.D. and Florey, H.W. (1935). Some observations on the structure and functions of lymphatics: Their behavior in local edema. *16*, 49–61.

Rees, M.J. and Taylor, G.I. (1986). A simplified lead oxide cadaver injection technique. *Plast Reconstr Surg* January; *77* (1), 141–145.

Reynolds, H.M., Dunbar, P.R., Uren, R.F., Thompson, J.F., and Smith, N.P. (2007). Three-dimensional visualisation of lymphatic drainage patterns in patients with cutaneous melanoma. *Lancet Oncol 8*, 806–812.

Reynolds, H.M., Smith, N.P., Uren, R.F., Thompson, J.F., and Dunbar, P.R. (2009). Three-dimensional visualization of skin lymphatic drainage patterns of the head and neck. *Head and Neck 31*, 1316–1325.

Reynolds, H.M., Walker, C.G., Dunbar, P.R., O'Sullivan, M.J., Uren, R.F., Thompson, J.F., and Smith, N.P. (2010). Functional anatomy of the lymphatics draining the skin: A detailed statistical analysis. *J Anat 216*, 344–355.

Sacchi, G., Weber, E., Agliano, M., Raffaelli, N., and Comparini, L. (1997). The structure of superficial lymphatics in the human thigh: Precollectors. *Anat Rec A Discov Mol Cell Evol Biol 247*, 53–62.

Sappey, P.C. (1874). *Anatomy, Physiology and Pathology of Lymphatic Vessels in Man and Vertebrates.* Paris, France: DeLahaye, A.

Scavelli, C., Weber, E., Agliano, M., Cirulli, T., Nico, B., Vacca, A., and Ribatti, D. (2004). Lymphatics at the crossroads of angiogenesis and lymphangiogenesis. *J Anat 204*, 433–449.

Shayan, R., Achen, M.G., and Stacker, S.A. (2006). Lymphatic vessels in cancer metastasis: Bridging the gaps. *Carcinogenesis 27*, 1729–1738.

Shayan, R., Inder, R., Karnezis, T., Caesar, C., Paavonen, K., Ashton, M.W., Mann, G.B., Taylor, G.I., Achen, M.G., and Stacker, S.A. (2013). Tumor location and nature of lymphatic vessels are key determinants of cancer metastasis. *Clin Exp Metastasis*. Mar; *30* (3), 345–356.

Shayan, R., Karnezis, T., Murali, R., Wilmott, J., Ashton, M.W., Taylor, G.I., Thompson, J.F., Hersey, P., Achen, M.G., Scolyer, R.A., and Stacker, S.A. (2012). Lymphatic vessel density in primary melanomas predicts sentinel lymph node status and risk of metastasis. *Histopathology,* May 17; *61* (4), 702–710. doi: 10.1111/j.1365-2559.2012.04310.x.

Shayan, R., Karnezis, T., Tsantikos, E., Williams, S.P., Runting, A., Ashton, M.W., Achen, M.G., Hibbs, M.L., and Stacker, S.A. (2007). A system for quantifying the patterning of the lymphatic vasculature. *Growth Factors 25*, 417–425.

Sherman, A.I. and Ter-Pogossian, M. (1953). Lymph-node concentration of radioactive colloidal gold following interstitial injection. *Cancer 6*, 1238–1240.

Shirasawa, Y., Ikomi, F., and Ohhashi, T. (2000). Physiological roles of endogenous nitric oxide in lymphatic pump activity of rat mesentery in vivo. *Am J Physiol Gastrointest Liver Physiol 278*, G551–G556.

Skobe, M. and Detmar, M. (2000). Structure, function, and molecular control of the skin lymphatic system. *J Invest Dermatol Symp Proc 5*, 14–19.

Solito, R., Alessandrini, C., Fruschelli, C., Pucci, A.M., and Gerli, R. (1997). An immunological correlation between the anchoring filaments of initial lymph vessels and the neighboring elastic fibres: A unified morphological concept. *Lymphology 30*, 194–202.

Stacker, S.A., Caesar, C., Baldwin, M.E., Thornton, G.E., Williams, R.A., Prevo, R., Jackson, D.G., Nishikawa, S., Kubo, H., and Achen, M.G. (2001). VEGF-D promotes the metastatic spread of tumor cells via the lymphatics. *Nat Med 7*, 186–191.

Suami, H., Pan, W.R., Mann, G.B., and Taylor, G.I. (2008). The lymphatic anatomy of the breast and its implications for sentinel lymph node biopsy: A human cadaver study. *Ann Surg Oncol* March; *15* (3), 863–871. Epub 2007 Nov 28.

Suami, H., Taylor, G.I., O'Neill, J., and Pan, W.R. (2007). Refinements of the radiographic cadaver injection technique for investigating minute lymphatic vessels. *Plast Reconstr Surg* July; *120* (1), 61–67.

Suami, H., Taylor, G.I., and Pan, W.R. (2005). A new radiographic cadaver injection technique for investigating the lymphatic system. *Plast Reconstr Surg* June; *115* (7), 2007–2013.

Tammela, T., Saaristo, A., Holopainen, T., Lyytikka, J., Kotronen, A., Pitkonen, M., Abo-Ramadan, U., Yla-Herttuala, S., Petrova, T.V., and Alitalo, K. (2007). Therapeutic differentiation and maturation of lymphatic vessels after lymph node dissection and transplantation. *Nat Med 13*, 1458–1466.

Thompson, J.F. and Uren, R.F. (2001a). Anomalous lymphatic drainage patterns in patients with cutaneous melanoma. *Tumori 87*, S54–S56.

Thornbury, K.D., Harty, H.R., McGeown, J.G., and McHale, N.G. (1993). Mesenteric lymph flow responses to splanchnic nerve stimulation in sheep. *Am J Physiol 264*, H604–H610.

Thornbury, K.D., McHale, N.G., and McGeown, J.G. (1989). Alpha-and beta-components of the popliteal efferent lymph flow response to intra-arterial catecholamine infusions in the sheep. *Blood Vessels 26*, 107–118.

Thornbury, K.D., McHale, N.G., and McGeown, J.G. (1990). Contribution of lymph formation in the popliteal node to efferent lymph flow following stimulation of the sympathetic chain in the sheep. *Exp Physiol 75*, 75–80.

Turner-Warwick, R.Y. (1955). The demonstration of lymphatic vessels. *Lancet 2*, 1371.

Uren, R.F., Howman-Giles, R., and Thompson, J.F. (1998a). Lymphatic drainage from the skin of the back to retroperitoneal and paravertebral lymph nodes in melanoma patients. *Ann Surg Oncol 5*, 384–387.

Uren, R.F., Howman-Giles, R., and Thompson, J.F. (1999). Direct lymphatic drainage from a melanoma on the back to paravertebral lymph nodes in the thorax. *Clin Nucl Med 24*, 388–389.

Uren, R.F., Howman-Giles, R., and Thompson, J.F. (2003). Patterns of lymphatic drainage from the skin in patients with melanoma. *J Nucl Med 44*, 570–582.

Uren, R.F., Howman-Giles, R., Thompson, J.F., and Quinn, M.J. (1996). Direct lymphatic drainage from the skin of the forearm to a supraclavicular node. *Clin Nucl Med 21*, 387–389.

Uren, R.F., Howman-Giles, R.B., Thompson, J.F., Roberts, J., and Bernard, E. (1998b). Variability of cutaneous lymphatic flow rates in melanoma patients. *Melanoma Res 8*, 279–282.

Uren, R.F., Howman-Giles, R.B., Thompson, J.F., Shaw, H.M., and McCarthy, W.H. (1995). Lymphatic drainage from peri-umbilical skin to internal mammary nodes. *Clin Nucl Med 20*, 254–255.

Uren, R.F., Thompson, J.F., Howman-Giles, R., and Chung, D.K. (2006). The role of lymphoscintigraphy in the detection of lymph node drainage in melanoma. *Surg Oncol Clin N Am* April; *15* (2), 285–300.

Veikkola, T., Lohela, M., Ikenberg, K., Makinen, T., Korff, T., Saaristo, A., Petrova, T., Jeltsch, M., Augustin, H.G., and Alitalo, K. (2003). Intrinsic versus microenvironmental regulation of lymphatic endothelial cell phenotype and function. *FASEB J 17*, 2006–2013.

Wang, Y., Nakayama, M., Pitulescu, M.E., Schmidt, T.S., Bochenek, M.L., Sakakibara, A., Adams, S. et al. (2010). Ephrin-B2 controls VEGF-induced angiogenesis and lymphangiogenesis. *Nature 465*, 483–486 doi:10.1038.

Weber, E., Rossi, A., Solito, R., Sacchi, G., Agliano, M., and Gerli, R. (2002). Focal adhesion molecules expression and fibrillin deposition by lymphatic and blood vessel endothelial cells in culture. *Microvasc Res 64*, 47–55.

Witte, M.H., Jones, K., Wilting, J., Dictor, M., Selg, M., McHale, N., Gershenwald, J.E., and Jackson, D.G. (2006). Structure function relationships in the lymphatic system and implications for cancer biology. *Cancer Metastasis Rev 25*, 159–184.

13 Vascular Anomalies in Children
Tumours and Vascular Malformations

Luigino Santecchia, Piergiorgio Falappa, and Mario Zama

CONTENTS

Peripheral vascular anomalies are very common (Greene et al. 2011). One in three infants has cutaneous birthmarks at birth or immediately after, but only 1% of these require subsequent monitoring and therapeutic management (Fevurly and Fishman 2012). Notwithstanding the high incidence of vascular anomalies, our understanding of this pathology is still incomplete and the large number and complexity of classification systems proposed has not helped improve our understanding (Behr and Johnson 2013a,b; Britney 2007). The major barrier to elucidating the clinical and pathophysiological mechanisms underlying the development and regression of vascular anomalies has been the lack of a definitive classification system with a universally accepted nomenclature that is recognised by all specialists involved in its management (El-Merhi et al. 2013; Enjolras et al. 2007; Garzon and Frieden 2007). This lack of an accepted nomenclature is evidenced by the terms frequently used incorrectly to describe vascular anomalies from cavernous, strawberry, and tuberous angioma to red fleck and port-wine stain birthmarks (Redondo 2004).

In 1982, Mulliken and Glowacki (Finn et al. 1983; L. S. M. D et al. 2013) proposed a classification system based on two main groups – haemangiomas and vascular malformations – which for the first time took into account biological, histopathological, and clinical characteristics of the condition (Table 13.1). Importantly with this classification, vascular tumours and vascular malformations have a number of clinical, immunohistochemical, and biological differences (Table 13.2). The increasing body of evidence from studies on tumour angiogenesis and major advances in imaging techniques prompted the International Society for the Study of Vascular Anomalies (ISSVA) to produce an updated classification (Table 13.3) (Enjolras et al. 2007). Included in this classification are certain vascular tumours not present in older classifications including congenital vascular tumours that are present at birth (A.G. MD and MD 2011; Finn et al. 1983; Ramundo 2005) to be distinguished from infantile haemangiomas (IHs) that are not evident at birth and rarely seen before the second to third week of life but that grow quickly thereafter (Drolet et al. 2008; I et al. 2002; Perman et al. 2012). Congenital haemangiomas of which there are two types – rapidly involuting congenital haemangiomas (RICHs) (Dina 2006; Mueller and P 2007; North et al. 2006; Richter and Friedman 2012) and noninvoluting congenital haemangiomas (NICHs) (D.M.A. MD 2011; North et al. 2001, 2006; Wassef et al. 2006) – as well as kaposiform haemangioendotheliomas (KHs) (A.G. MD and MD 2011; D.M.A. MD 2011; L.L. L et al. 2004) and tufted haemangiomas (THs) (A.G. MD and MD 2011; Alex and Aryeh 2002; Enjolras et al. 2001; Requena and Omar 2007) through a process called platelet trapping related to their peculiar histological structure can lead to severe conditions

TABLE 13.1
First *Biological* Classification of Vascular Anomalies

Vascular Tumours	*Vascular Malformations*
Infantile haemangioma	Slow-flow vascular malformations
	Capillary malformation (CM)
	Venous malformation (VM)
	Lymphatic malformation (LM)
	Fast-flow vascular malformations
	Arterial malformation (AM)
	Arteriovenous fistula (AVF)
	Arteriovenous malformation (AVM)

Source: Reproduced from Enjolras, O. et al., *Color Atlas of Vascular Tumors and Vascular Malformations*, Cambridge University Press, Paris, 2007. With permission.

TABLE 13.2
Main Differences between the Very Common Vascular Tumour, Infantile Haemangioma, and Vascular Malformations

	Infantile Haemangioma	*Vascular Malformations*
Age of occurrence and course	Infancy and childhood	Everlasting if not treated
Course	Three stages: proliferating, involuting, involuted	Commensurate growth or slow progression
Sex prevalence	3–9 girls/1 boy	1 girl/1 boy
Cellular	Increased endothelial cellular turnover. Increased mastocytes. Thick basement membrane	Normal cellular turnover. Normal number of mastocytes. Normal thin basement membrane
Immunohistochemical expression	Proliferating haemangioma: PCNA +++, VEGF +++, bFGF +++, collagenase IV +++, urokinase ++, TIMP-1 –, mast cells –, LYVE-1/CD31 +++, PROX1 – Involuting haemangioma: PCNA –, VEGF +, bFGF ++, collagenase IV –, urokinase ++, TIMP-1+++, mast cells +++, LYVE-1/CD31 –, PROX1 –	Barely detectable: PCNA, VEGF, bFGF, urokinase; not detectable: collagenase IV, variable staining for TIMP 1
Factors causing flare	None (or unknown)	Trauma, hormonal changes
Pathology	Distinctive aspects of the three phases of the tumour. GLUT1 +	CM, VM, LM, AVM, depending on the type. GLUT1 –
Radiological aspects on MRI	Well-delineated tumour with flow voids	Hypersignal on T2 sequences with VM or LM. Flow voids without parenchymal staining with AVM
Treatment	Spontaneous involution, or pharmacological treatment, or surgery, or lasers	Lasers, or surgery and/or embolisation/sclerotherapy depending on the type

Source: Reproduced from Enjolras, O. et al., *Color Atlas of Vascular Tumors and Vascular Malformations*, Cambridge University Press, 2007. With permission.

Notes: VEGF, vascular endothelial growth factor; bFGF, basic fibroblast growth factor; TIMP, tissue inhibitor matrix proteinase; GLUT1, glucose transporter 1; CM, capillary malformation; VM, venous malformation; LM, lymphatic malformation; AVM, arteriovenous malformation; MRI, magnetic resonance imaging.

such as Kasabach–Merritt syndrome (Bing et al. 2006; Le Nouail et al. 2007; Masashi et al. 2006; Wakabayashi et al. 2011).

Although the diagnosis of vascular anomalies is mainly clinical (Ballah et al. 2011; Fevurly and Fishman 2012; Greene et al. 2011; Marler et al. 2002; Redondo et al. 2011; Theiler et al. 2013; Weibel 2011), diagnostic imaging also plays an important role in monitoring progression and in therapeutic management (Table 13.4) (Degrugillier-Chopinet et al. 2011; Flors et al. 2011). The use of different imaging techniques is essential to determine the haemodynamic features of the anomalies to confirm that classification is appropriate, to establish size, and to assess effects on non-vascular components, such as muscle and bone tissue. It is necessary to adhere to a precise diagnostic protocol that allows a therapeutic decision to be made, for example, to proceed with a surgical intervention or regular and watchful observation over time (Chalouhi et al. 2011; Conway and Hosking 2012; Restrepo 2013; Thawait et al. 2013).

TABLE 13.3
Updated Classification of Vascular Anomalies by the International Society for the Study of Vascular Anomalies (ISSVA)

Vascular Tumours	***Vascular Malformations***
Infantile haemangiomas	*Slow-flow vascular malformations*
Congenital haemangiomas (RICH and NICH)	
Tufted angioma (with or without Kasabach–Merritt syndrome)	Capillary malformation (CM): Port-wine stain, telangiectasia, angiokeratoma
Kaposiform haemangioendothelioma (with or without Kasabach–Merritt syndrome)	
Spindle cell haemangioendothelioma	Venous malformation (VM): Common sporadic VM, Bean syndrome, familial cutaneous and mucosal venous malformation (VMCM), glomuvenous malformation (GVM) (glomangioma), Maffucci syndrome
Other, rare haemangioendotheliomas (epithelioid, composite, retiform, polymorphous, Dabska tumour, lymphangioendotheliomatosis, etc.)	
Dermatologically acquired vascular tumours (pyogenic granuloma, targetoid haemangioma, glomeruloid haemangioma, microvenular haemangioma, etc.)	
	Lymphatic malformation (LM)
	Fast-flow vascular malformations
	Arterial malformation (AM)
	Arteriovenous fistula (AVF)
	Arteriovenous malformation (AVM)
	Complex-combined vascular malformations
	CVM, CLM, LVM, CLVM, AVM-LM, CM-AVM

Source: Reproduced from Enjolras, O. et al., *Color Atlas of Vascular Tumors and Vascular Malformations*, Cambridge University Press, 2007. With permission.

Notes: C, capillary; V, venous; L, lymphatic; AV, arteriovenous; M, malformation; RICH, rapidly involuting congenital haemangioma; NICH, noninvoluting congenital haemangioma.

TABLE 13.4
Diagnostic Imaging Devices and the Various Vascular Anomalies

	Infantile Haemangioma	***CM***	***VM***	***LM***	***AVM***
Ultrasonography/doppler	+++	++	++	++	+++
Plain radiographs	–	–	++ (phleboliths, bone)	± (bone)	+ (bone)
MRI, MRA, MRV	++	–	+++	+++	++
CT	+	–	+	+	+
Angio-CT scans	–	–	+	–	++
Lymphoscintigraphy	–	–	–	+	–
Biopsy	+	+	+	+	+
Angiography	–	–	+	–	+++

Source: Reproduced from Enjolras, O. et al., *Color Atlas of Vascular Tumors and Vascular Malformations*, Cambridge University Press, 2007. With permission.

Notes: MRI, magnetic resonance imaging; MRA, magnetic resonance angiography; MRV, magnetic resonance venography; CT, computed tomography; CM, capillary malformation; VM, venous malformation; LM, lymphatic malformation; AVM, arteriovenous malformation.

13.1 VASCULAR TUMOURS

13.1.1 Infantile Haemangioma

IHs are the most common vascular tumours in infants with 10%–12% occurring in the first year of life; they develop the following proliferation of angiogenic tissue during the perinatal phase (Bruckner and Frieden 2006; Richter and Friedman 2012). Haemangiomas can be superficial or deep or a combination of the two. Superficial haemangiomas involve the superficial papillary derma and appear as red, nodular, well-demarcated lesions with a coarse-grained surface that are hot to touch and have an elastic texture. The size and consistency of these lesions increases with exertion or crying and they do not disappear with finger pressure (Bauland et al. 2006; Régnier et al. 2007). Deep haemangiomas located under the skin in the deep dermal and hypodermal layers present as a protrusion with an overlying bluish tint or telangiectasia that are hot and elastic to touch. In general, these types of lesions regress more slowly than superficial haemangiomas (Elluru 2013; Reinisch 2011). Compound haemangiomas with both superficial and deep part are usually larger and present with an overlying bluish tint (Vikkula et al. 1998) (Figure 13.1). Haemangiomas have three distinct developmental phases (A.G. MD and MD 2011; Mueller and P 2007):

- *Proliferative*: Normally, the lesion appears during the first month of life and grows rapidly until the sixth to eighth month. During this period, there is a rapid increase in tumour size with hyperplasia of endothelial cells forming syncytial masses and thickened, multilaminated basement membranes.
- *Quiescence*: This is a slower growth phase in parallel with the child's growth that lasts up to 16–18 months.
- *Involution*: This starts with a slow and spontaneous regression (apoptosis) of endothelial cells, with fibro-fatty substitution and thin monolayer basement membrane (Figure 13.2).

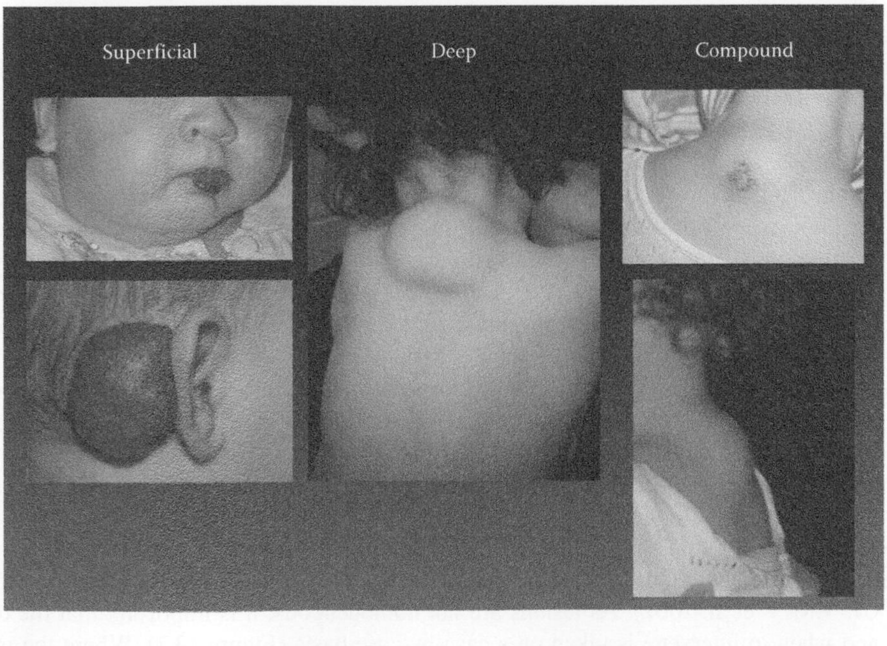

FIGURE 13.1 In the left side, two infantile haemangiomas (IHs) to surface manifestation are shown. Top left is an IH of the lower lip to exophytic development. Bottom left is an IH behind the ear, pushing forward the pavilion. In the center, totally subcutaneous IH is shown. The right side is a mixed form with a subcutaneous prevalence.

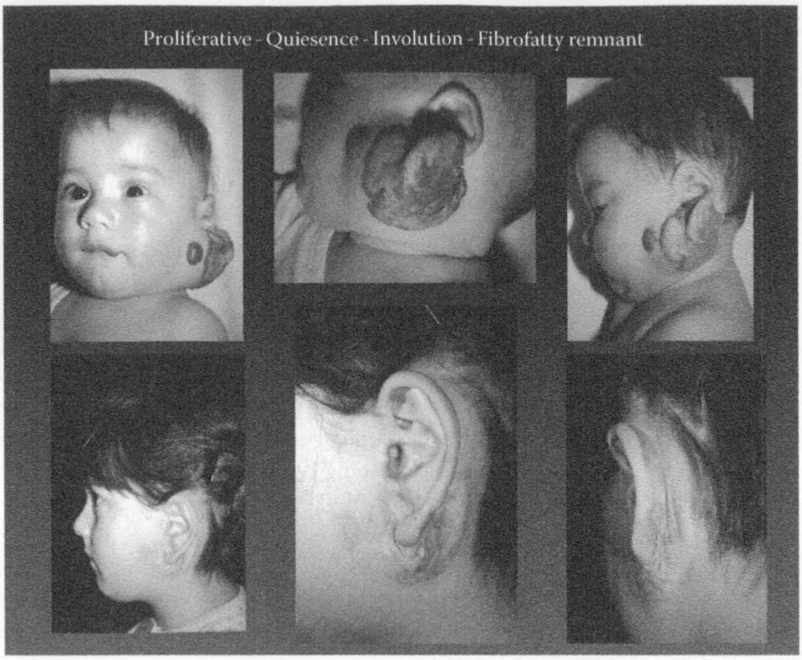

FIGURE 13.2 Evolutionary phases of a typical infantile IH over 6 years. The lesion goes through various stages of growth before, with endothelial proliferation and rapid flourishing and visible increase in volume, in the upper left. Stability phase is in the top center. Initial regression is in the upper right. Slow resorption over 5–6 years with residual fibrofatty and redundancy skin, below.

13.2 VASCULAR TUMOURS: INDICATIONS AND TIMING FOR MANAGEMENT

The decision on when and how best to intervene depends on the patient's overall clinical picture including his or her age, the location and size of the tumour, the presence of co-morbidities, and timings of vaccinations (Eivazi and Werner 2013; MMSc 2011; Richter and Friedman 2012; W.I.E. F et al. 2000). Historically, haemangiomas were managed by close observation during their natural life cycle until the end of the involution phase. Surgical intervention to remove the sequelae – fibro-fatty remnants of involuted haemangiomas and excess dyschromic/dystrophic tissue – was carried out only when necessary (Maguiness and Frieden 2010). More recently, an increasing number of surgeons recommend early surgical intervention, in particular when the haemangioma is in an easily accessible position (Santecchia et al. 2013; Spector et al. 2008). However, the majority of physicians still only recommend surgery when other medical interventions have failed or the child has a life or function-threatening haemangioma (Akcay et al. 2012; Geh et al. 2007; H.E.H. M et al. 2010). In general, a decision on surgical excision of haemangiomas and/or fibro-fatty remnants is taken before the child starts primary school rather than waiting until the end of the involution phase unless there are complications that necessitate an earlier intervention (Eivazi and Werner 2013; Hassan et al. 2013; Kivelev et al. 2012a,b; Maguiness and Frieden 2010) (Figures 13.3 through 13.5).

Some lesions such as ulcerated haemangiomas of the lip (Figure 13.6a and b) do not follow these general rules and early surgical intervention during the proliferative phase is required (Salins et al. 2007; V.M. P et al. 2002). As lesions are not homogeneous, it is important that the decision on how and when to intervene is taken on a case-by-case basis (Figure 13.7). Where the management approach is unclear, for example, when the haemangioma is without complications or when complications have yet to be observed, prevention is vital using a *watchful waiting* approach (Beck and Gosain 2009; MMSc 2011).

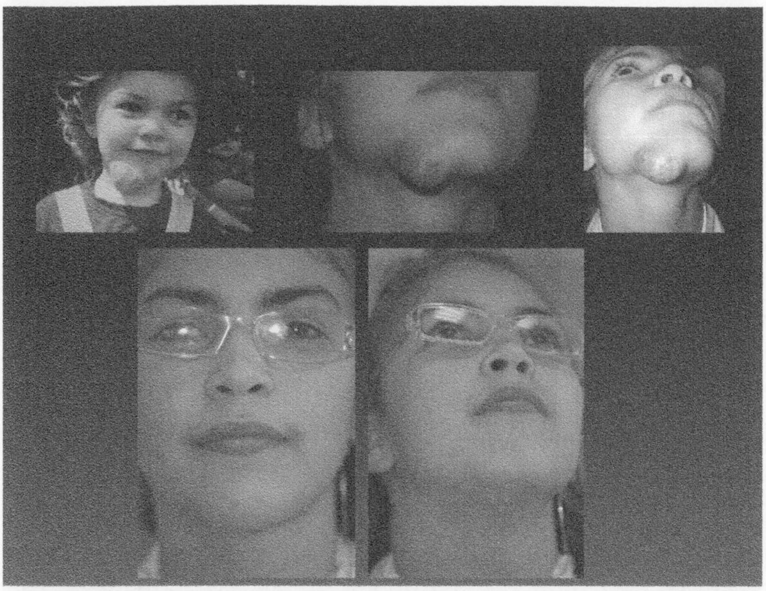

FIGURE 13.3 Mixed IH of the right chin area in the stable phase. Fibrofatty remnant well represented. At the bottom of the long-term result after late surgical removal.

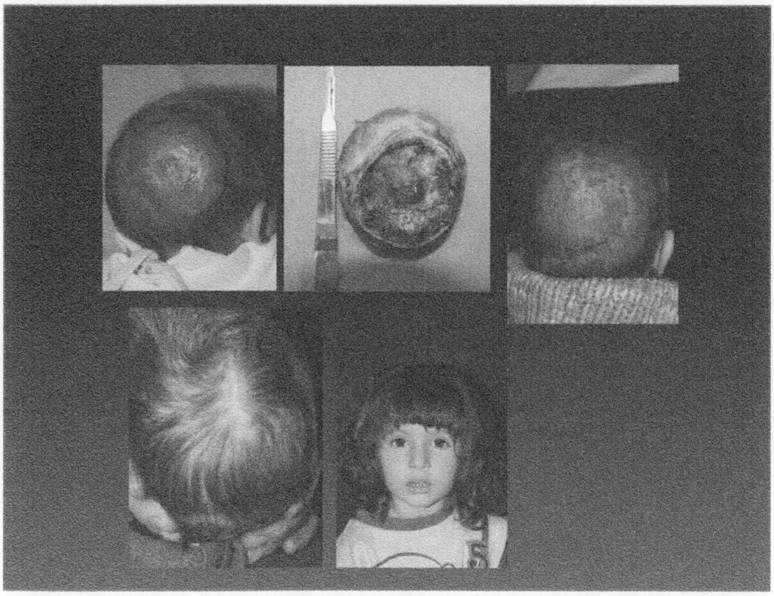

FIGURE 13.4 Top left is a giant infantile IH of the scalp in the growing-up phase. In the top center, the lesion is completely removed. In the upper right, the surgical result after double flap rotation. At the bottom, long-term result shows no significant residual areas of alopecia.

Three main therapeutic objectives are agreed by most specialists with some modifications based on individual patient needs (Enjolras 2004; Maguiness and Frieden 2010):

1. Prevent, reduce, or eliminate pain and eliminate functional impairment.
2. Prevent or reduce scars and/or physiognomic and dysmorphodynamic damage.
3. Prevent, reduce, or eliminate complications in life- and function-threatening haemangiomas.

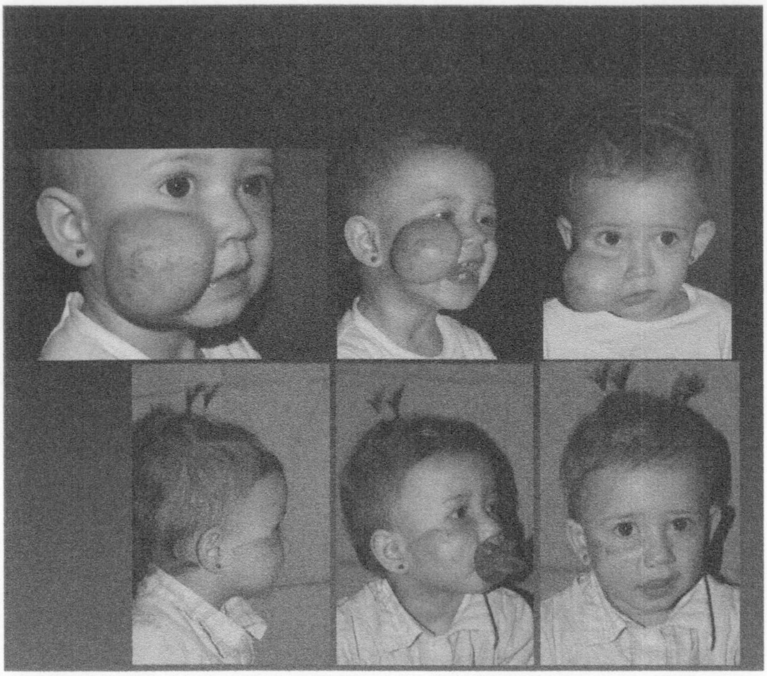

FIGURE 13.5 Massive IH of the right cheek after 6 months of medical therapy with propranolol. At the top right, you will notice the aesthetic and functional deformity with the pushdown of the right buccal rhyme. At the bottom, the functional and aesthetic result after the complete surgical removal of residual deficit and cover with medially advancement Mustardè flap.

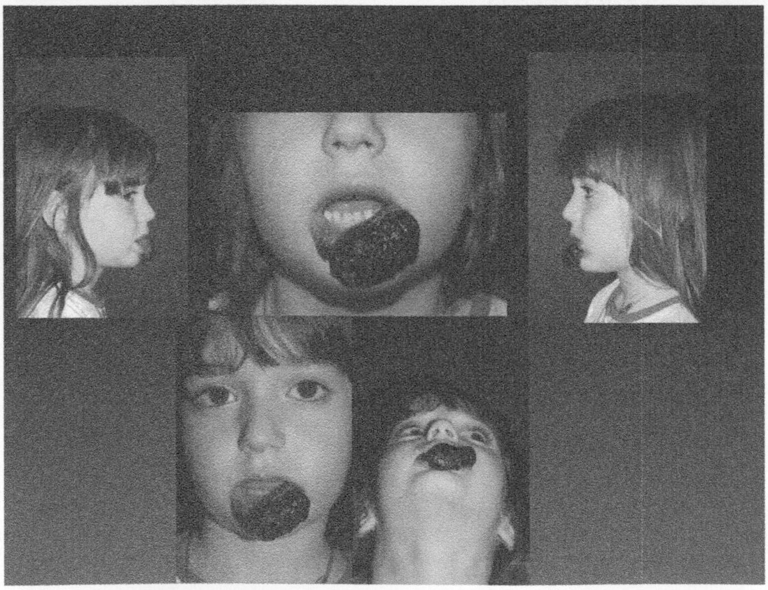

(a)

FIGURE 13.6 (a) Infantile IH of the lower lip ulcerated and infected with crusted surface and bleeding from dripping. The lesion appeared smelly and prevented the normal diet of the patient orally. *(Continued)*

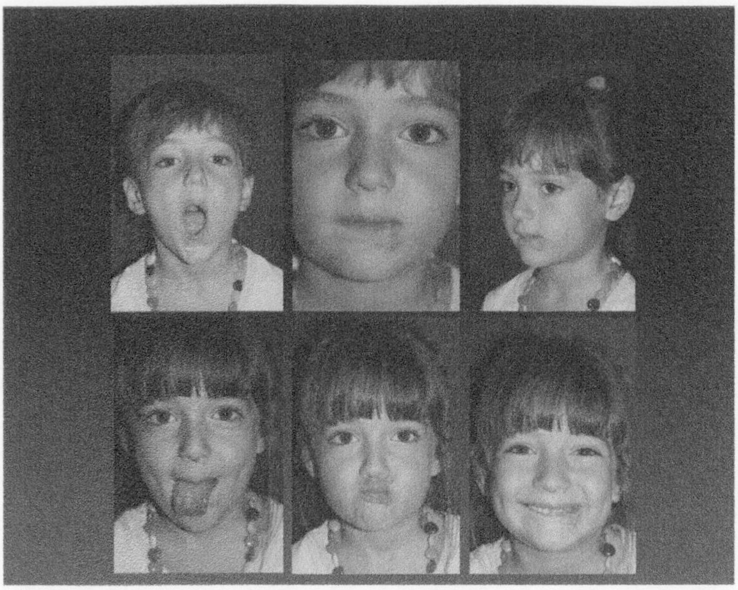

(b)

FIGURE 13.6 (*Continued*) (b) Result after surgical removal in two stages lower lip reconstruction using full thickness cross-lip flap taken from the upper lip. Note the complete return of the aesthetic and functional vermilion and the ring of orbicularis oris muscle preservation with no signs of incontinence.

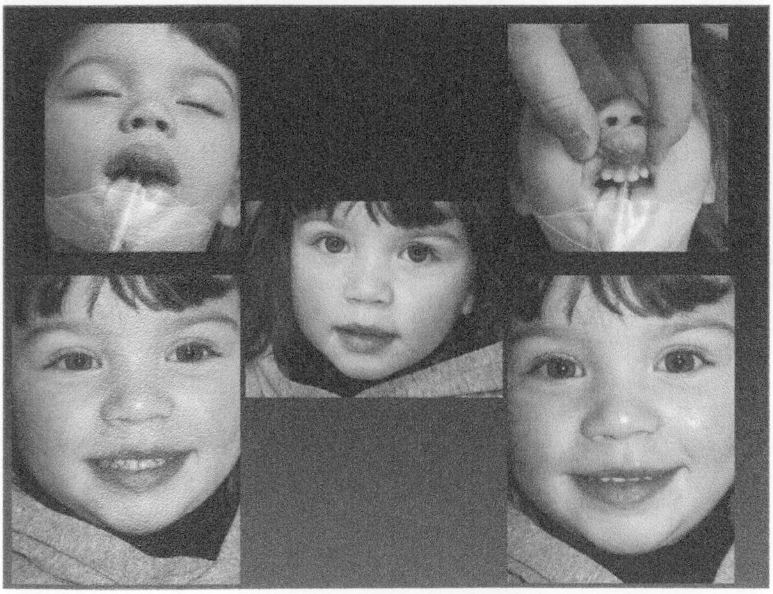

FIGURE 13.7 Infantile IH of the central portion of the upper lip without ulceration of the mucosa. Brief follow-up at the bottom after surgical removal through an intraoral mucosal access in the upper vestibule.

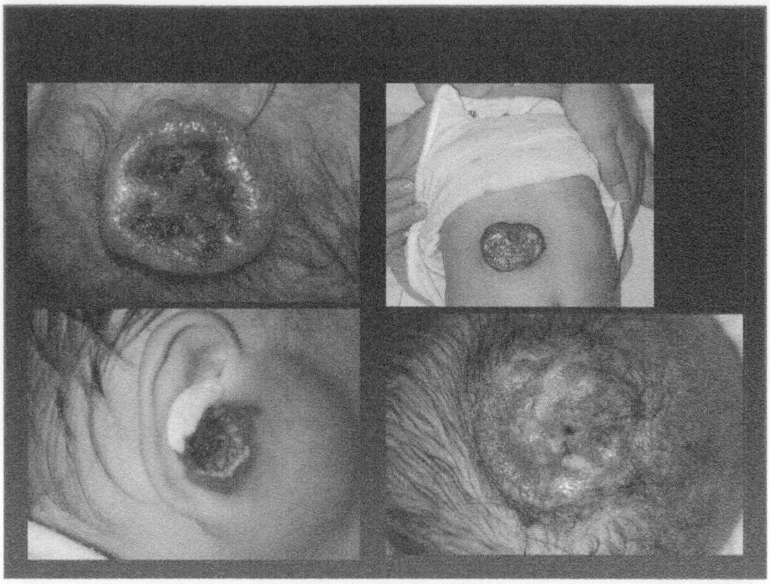

FIGURE 13.8 Ulcerated IHs of the scalp seen at the top left; at the top right is ulcerated IH of the abdomen; another IH in the pre-auricular region at the bottom left, and finally a wide infected and bleeding lesion of the vertex of the scalp.

In the *first group*, the most common complication is *ulceration* (Brandie et al. 2004) but with the use of up-to-date wound care techniques (guided scarring and use of advanced wound-healing dressings) (Metry 2004) with or without pharmacological therapies, laser treatment (dye laser 598 nm) (A. F et al. 2009; Brandie et al. 2004), surgical excision (stepwise or preferably complete excision), functional improvements, and pain relief can be achieved (Theologie-Lygidakis et al. 2012) (Figure 13.8).

The *second group* includes haemangiomas mainly on the upper body and face where surgery is vital to avoid the development of a dysmorphic disorder which can occur in patients with large and growing facial haemangiomas or to improve the aesthetic outcome for patients (A. F et al. 2009). The site, size, growing/involution rate, and degree of deformity of facial features determine the timing and nature of surgery, taking into account the psychological distress over time for the patient and his or her family (Madana et al. 2012; RUGGERI 2004) (Figure 13.9).

The *third group* includes rare and serious forms that can cause loss of function and/or death without immediate intervention. Among these are peri- and intra-orbital haemangiomas with involvement of the eyelids that can result in vision impairment (Haggstrom 2006) (Figure 13.10); airway haemangiomas involving the posterior glottis and the subglottis that can cause airway obstruction (A. F et al. 2009; I.N.J. MD and MD 2011; R.M.B. MD et al. 2011) (Figure 13.11); hepatic haemangioma associated with heart failure (Boon et al. 2007); diffuse miliary angiomatosis with secondary hypothyroidism (Christine 2008) (Figure 13.12); haemangiomas with thrombocytopenia or Kasabach–Merritt's syndrome (Bing et al. 2006) (Figure 13.13); and some high-flow giant haemangiomas of the head and neck often associated with congestive heart failure (Agrawal et al. 2012; Jhawar et al. 2012).

13.3 SURGICAL REMOVAL OF HAEMANGIOMAS

Vascular anomalies can be successfully treated, but an in-depth knowledge of the pathology is necessary as well as an up-to-date awareness of the medical and surgical options available which can be either used alone, sequentially, or in combination as part of an integrated approach over

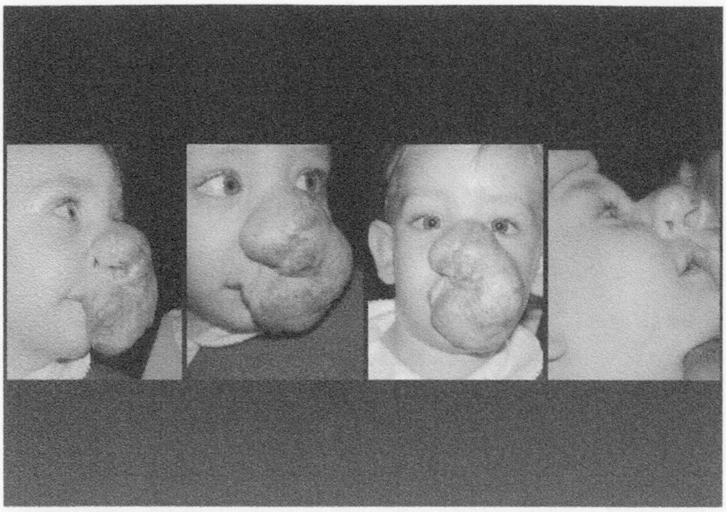

FIGURE 13.9 Haemangiomatous very extensive lesions of the face can cause severe dysmorphic changes when multiple drives simultaneously affect aesthetic. The dysmorphodinamic damage is the distortion in the overgrowth and worsening of the normal structures, otherwise not affected by the primary vascular lesion.

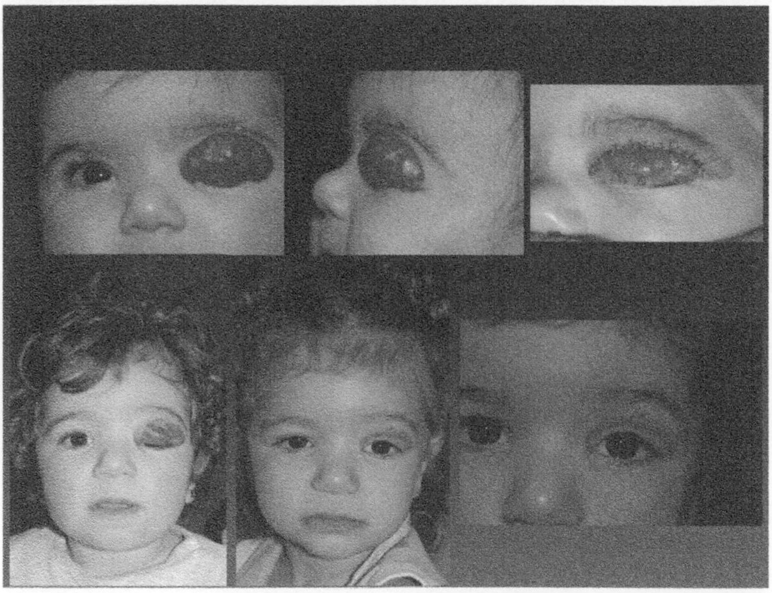

FIGURE 13.10 Periorbital IHs can involve the eyelid alone but often tend to extend into the orbital cavity through the septum and the periorbital fat, up to the extrinsic muscle and intraconal fat tissues. Surgical mass reduction represents a function-threatening procedure to be performed in emergency if other medical therapies are slow in achieving the desired effect. In these cases, medical and surgical therapies have to be integrated if the vascular abnormality of the orbital cone portions are interested as both intra- and extraconal. The later treatment or abstention from therapy involves the onset of serious secondary problems related to the axis of view (reduction or asymmetry of the visual field), the extrinsic motility of the eyeball (residual strabismus), refractive errors (astigmatism), and the extreme degree of the amblyopia by extrinsic compression of the optic nerve.

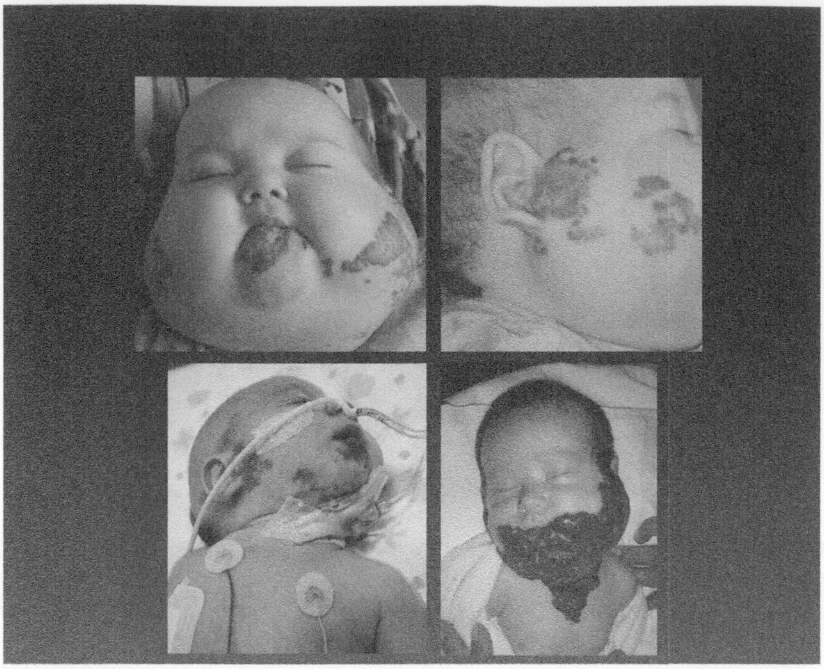

FIGURE 13.11 Haemangiomas located on the midline, although apparently minor, indicate the possible involvement of the respiratory tract and the glottis, even in the absence of respiratory symptoms at the time of the visit. At the top is a voluminous IH of the face without reported respiratory symptoms. At the bottom left is a vascular lesion apparently contained that it causes severe airway obstruction with respiratory failure. At the bottom right is a distribution in the so-called beard area, which is often associated with acute respiratory syndromes.

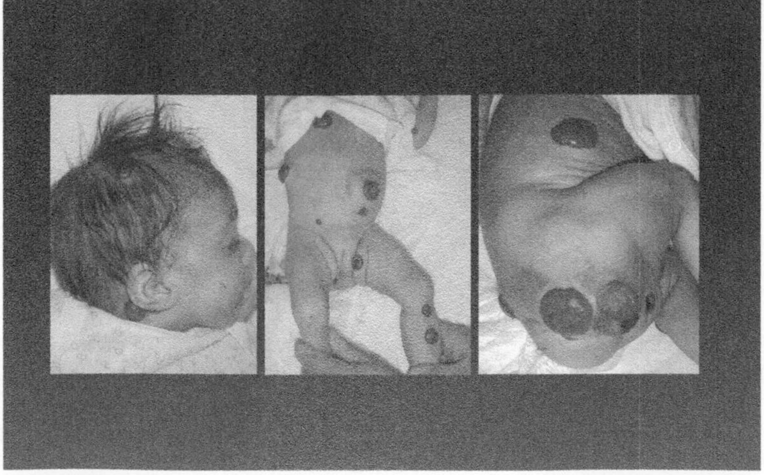

FIGURE 13.12 The diffuse haemangiomatosis or miliaris IHs occurs when five or more vascular lesions spread over several dermatomes. Often, internal organs are also involved, including the liver. A deficiency of thyroid hormones can be associated with clinical hypothyroidism.

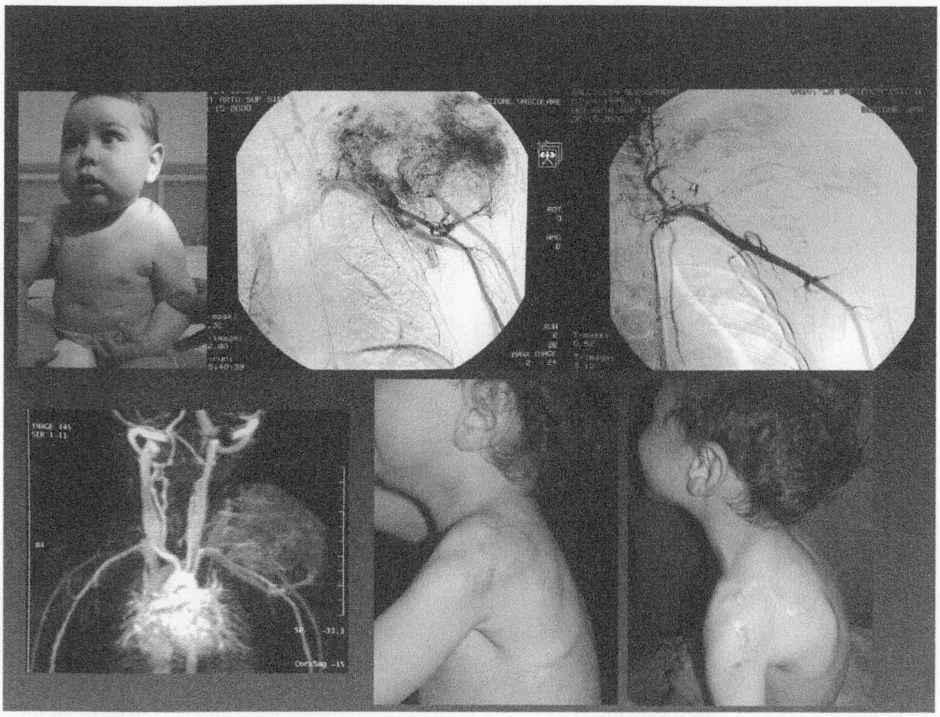

FIGURE 13.13 Kasabach-Merritt syndrome, in most cases supported by particular histologically vascular tumors, is referred to as tufted IHs or kaposiform haemangiotelioma. For their particular structure, they act as networks that remain trapped in the erythrocytes, especially the thrombocytes, with framework clinical anemia and bleeding risk. At the top left is the patient presented with the swelling of the shoulder girdle hardwood left and thrombocytopenia associated with the deterioration of coagulation. In the upper center and right is represented the embolization procedure that preceded a 48 h surgery. Platelets have increased from 5000/mm^3 to 265.000/mm^3 after 24 h from treatment. At the bottom left, supplementary magnetic resonance imaging (MRI) of the same lesion shows a diffuse and homogeneous enhancement after contrast medium. At the bottom center and right are post-operative images after complete removal of the lesion, performed after transthoracic insertion of a tourniquet in the left subclavian artery, surgically placed for intraoperative haemostatic purposes.

time (Geh et al. 2007; Jablecki et al. 2013; Waner and O 2013). Successful management requires extensive and specific experience in specific complex area in order to establish the diagnosis and accurately define the overall syndrome in order to reduce the possibility of diagnostic error and improve the efficacy of managing any complications that may arise (Spector et al. 2008). There is no universally accepted gold standard on the optimal management of haemangiomas, and therefore treatment choices on how, when, and why surgical options should be considered instead of observation alone are based on individual and shared knowledge/experience (Eivazi and Werner 2013). For example, based on currently available data, physicians are in agreement that haemangiomas in the orbital area and airway and glottis haemangiomas are potentially life-threatening and require urgent management to 'respect life and health' (*quoad vitam et valetudinem*) (ENJOLRAS 2008; Nolan et al. 2012). Hepatic haemangiomas with hepatic failure and diffuse angiomatosis are examples of haemangiomas with potentially serious consequences (Zhu and Ma 2013).

In addition, although early surgical intervention is not mandatory in patients with haemangiomas that cause severe cosmetic disfigurement, it should be considered in patients with facial haemangiomas involving the nose, lip, cheek, ear, or scalp (Adouani et al. 2008) (Figure 13.14). Surgical intervention is frequently recommended in patients with slow-healing ulcers or to stop bleeding; the latter is the most common complication in patients with booming haemangiomas (Gallarreta et al. 2013).

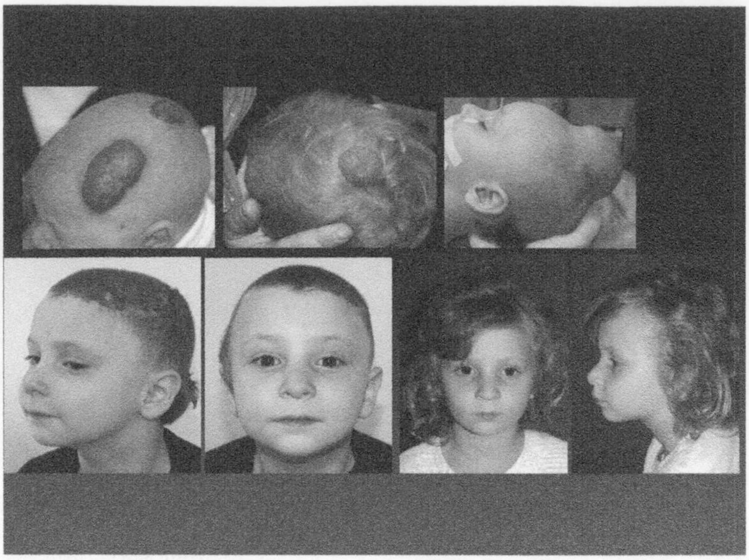

FIGURE 13.14 Multiple IHs of the scalp. Multiple or extended vascular lesions of the scalp require frequently considerable amount of skin, sufficient to cover the loss of substance after surgical removal. In this case, a skin expander positioned in a first surgical time on the subgaleal vertex of the scalp was used. After 2 months, the skin obtained allowed the complete removal of the IHtous lesions and the simultaneous coverage with expanded pedicle flap right side. The final scar is an inch inside the edge of the scalp and virtually invisible.

In most cases, bleeding can be stopped by applying gentle pressure for a few minutes to the blood vessels that make up haemangioma. In rare cases, emergency surgical intervention is required, when an ulcer causes major bleeding from a large vessel (S.J.F. MD et al. 2004). Nevertheless, in general, ulcerated haemangiomas are painful, in particular those in the genito-urinary area, where they are repeatedly soiled with urine and faeces (Choi et al. 2011) (Figure 13.18).

Other haemangiomas that normally require surgery are those occurring in the salivary glands, in particular parotid haemangiomas; as with giant forms, there is the possibility of a narrowing/obstruction of the auditory canal and secondary otitis media due to cerumen impaction and subsequent transient conductive hearing loss (Weibel 2011) (Figure 13.11). Facial haemangiomas can have a major psychosocial impact, and it is entirely understandable that parents may put pressure on clinicians to conduct early surgery which they hope will be effective and they can start afresh (W.I.E. F et al. 2000). However, it should be remembered that up to the 60% of haemangiomas at certain sites resolve spontaneously over time and that scars caused by surgery are permanent, although generally acceptable from an aesthetic point of view. If an aggressive approach to management is adopted, many children will undergo surgery and may have permanent scarring for haemangiomas that, otherwise, may have resolved spontaneously. Before any surgical intervention, a careful risk assessment needs to be carried out as, although it might be the only treatment that can produce guaranteed psychological benefits both for the patient and his or her parents, it is not without risks even if minimal (Maguiness and Frieden 2010). Clearly, in these cases, surgery is only employed when there is a low risk of bleeding and complications and, therefore, can be carried out if the perceived need is great enough. In contrast, there are cases in which the scar resulting from early surgery may be preferably to that which will result if the condition is allowed to take its natural course. In these situations, surgical intervention should not be delayed and physicians should recommend that parents make a quick decision in order to obtain the best possible outcome (Santecchia et al. 2013; Shaul et al. 2005) (Figure 13.14).

The timing of surgery has implications according to the four developmental stages of haemangioma (J. P et al. 2002; MMSc 2011):

1. *Proliferative phase* – during rapid growth, increased blood flow in the area of the lesion makes control of haemostasis problematic, with possible sudden and considerable intraoperative bleeding (the patient's age and body weight need to be included in the risk assessment). Patients undergoing surgery on very large lesions or on haemangiomas in high blood flow areas, such as the head and neck, may require a blood transfusion(s).
2. *Early involutional phase* – in this phase, the haemangioma that has reached its maximum size shows the first signs of cutaneous regression but it still has significant blood flow. If pressure is applied to the edges, it empties of blood, but once the pressure is released, the lesions rapidly fill up again. From a surgical point of view, the risk is lower than that for Stage 1 but it very much depends on the site and level of vascularisation.
3. *Mid-involutional phase* – in this phase, the haemangioma has lost most of its initial turgor and redness, with typical multifocal merging hypochromic greyish spots. It has a soft/spongy consistency and, after manual compression, it still fills up with blood although less rapidly than in Stage 2.
4. *Late involutional phase* – in this phase, the haemangioma has very little or no residual blood flow. The hypochromic cutaneous residue resembles a translucent, inelastic empty sack that does not refill after compression.

Patients seeking surgical treatment in the late involutional stage (Phase 4) are excellent candidates for debulking surgery or scar revision as further improvement is not to be expected. In these patients, surgery is relatively bloodless since the haemangioma is composed mostly of fatty scar tissue. However, most of these children are already attending school, as the average is 5–7 years of age, facing embarrassment and psychological issues, in particular for facial haemangiomas (Waner and O 2013). Surgery can be performed during the proliferative phase in patients with ulcerated, bleeding haemangiomas, because they will almost certainly result in redundant skin or scars that will eventually benefit from surgical intervention. Furthermore, these haemangiomas cause pain, insomnia, and continuous bleeding (often leading to iron-deficiency anaemia), causing a worsening of the patient's conditions (Wakabayashi et al. 2011; Rhea et al. 2002). Although quite often parents push for treatment in the early- to mid-involutional phase, early surgery may be inappropriate in certain cases. One such case is large haemangiomas, which cannot be completely removed and may present a significant risk during both the growing and late stage (Salins et al. 2007). Further contraindications for early surgery are as follows: the risk of excessive bleeding, facial nerve injury, and a significant surgical scar or residual asymmetry which may become more evident as the child grows (Arita et al. 2012; Cheng et al. 2006; Norman et al. 2010).

With reference to the three aforementioned therapeutic objectives, the approach should be as follows.

13.3.1 Prevent, Reduce, or Eliminate Pain; Remove Functional Impairment

Ulceration is the most common complication occurring in approximately 15%–25% of haemangiomas in patients with an average age of 4 months (Hassan et al. 2013; Sadykov et al. 2013). Risk factors include an increased cell turnover, large, segmental lesions with a superficial component, as well as those on mucosal sites (such as the lips and anogenital areas) or intertriginous sites (such as the neck, perineum, and areas in close contact with the diaper) (Brandie et al. 2004). Although strategies for prevention of ulceration have not yet been established, irritation, friction, and the use of tight fitting clothes should be avoided. Use of emollients to improve skin elasticity at sites of risk is recommended (I et al. 2002). In haemangiomas with superficial ulceration, pain as a result of the natural healing process is the major cause of morbidity (Jablecki et al. 2013). In addition, there is also the risk of wound infections which can lead to them increasing in size and a delay in the healing process (Alex and Aryeh 2002). Ulceration at periorificial sites (perioral, anogenital, and perinasal areas) is most concerning because of the obvious functional and aesthetic consequences due to the higher risk of infection and stenosis (Brandie et al. 2004).

Bleeding is a surprisingly uncommon complication, with severe bleeding occurring in only about 1% of cases (Nolan et al. 2012); severe bleeding is life-threatening in the first year of life, but only large haemangiomas in areas where trauma is more likely to occur such as the scalp, face, and limbs (S.J.F. MD et al. 2004). Blood dripping or spotting, although relatively common, is frequently not diagnosed as it develops most often in areas not routinely monitored by parents (nose, pharynx, upper gastrointestinal [GI] tract, and airways) (Yoo 2011). Left untreated, chronic anaemia with fatigue, depletion of reserves, and poor growth can result (Pavlov et al. 2013).

13.3.1.1 Function-Threatening Haemangiomas of the Eyelids and Orbit

Total and partial obstruction of the visual axis with a haemangioma can lead to complications, for example, strabismus and astigmatism, and in extreme cases to amblyopia and visual impairment (Rosca et al. 2006) (Figure 13.15). Even when the haemangioma does not completely occlude the eyelid and the visual axis, it can increase intra-orbital pressure, and the presence of a *mass* on the eye can cause astigmatism, diplopia and proptosis, and, in severe cases, loss of vision due to compression of the optic nerve (Christine et al. 2008). Segmental haemangiomas of the eyelids, those at the edge of the eyelashes and those on the upper eyelids, have the greatest risk of complications (MMSc 2011). We believe that all eyelid haemangiomas >1 cm in diameter with visible changes in the normal make-up should be removed by the first year of age in order to prevent deformity, as the lesions gets progressively bigger permanently altering the tarsal conjunctiva coating the internal surface of the eyelids. In these cases, delaying treatment means that excessive tissue growth during the proliferative phase may reduce function even if vision is not compromised (Soldatskii et al. 2012) (Figure 13.16). Patients with haemangiomas of the eyelids and orbit should have regular eye tests conducted by an experienced ophthalmologist from the age of 3 to 4 months, and if visual impairment is suspected/detected, systemic therapy with propranolol or prednisone should be started before surgical debulking (Conway and Hosking 2012; Geh et al. 2007; Sadykov et al. 2013) (Figure 13.17).

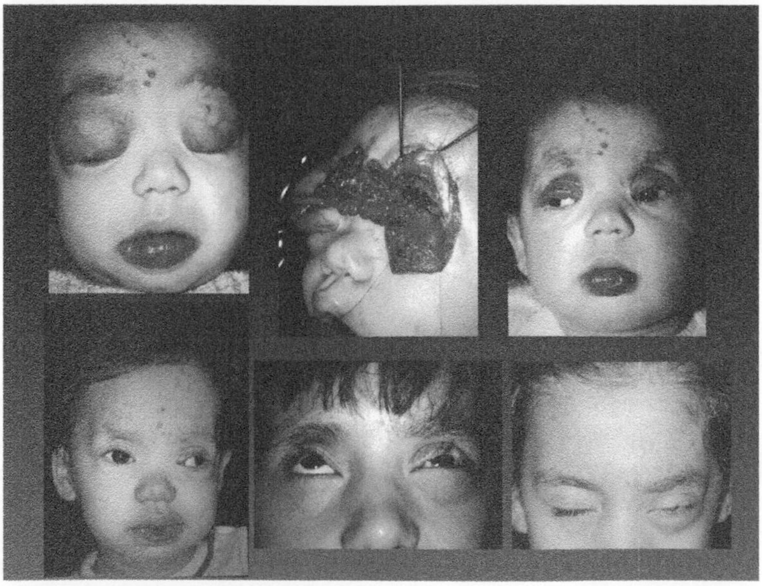

FIGURE 13.15 Bilateral periorbital IHs removed through eyelid surgical approach. We note residual strabismus due to intraconal involvement of the extrinsic muscles weakened by vascular injury.

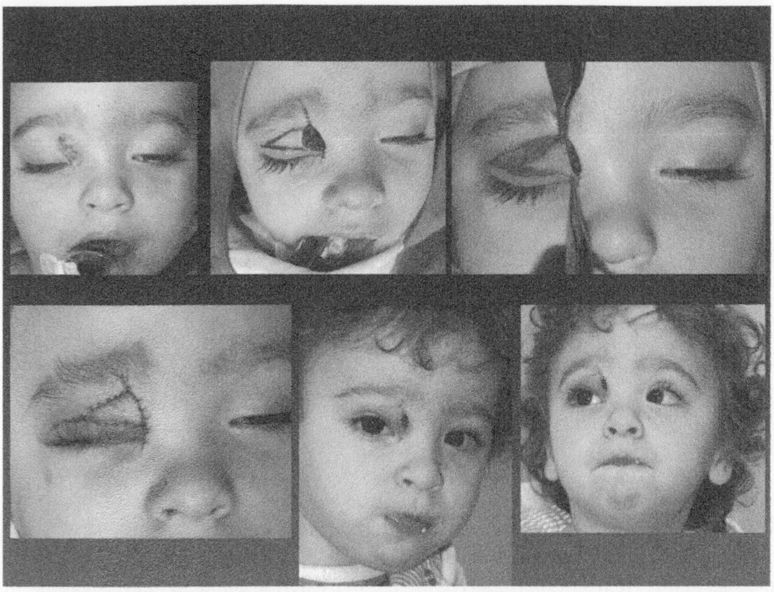

FIGURE 13.16 Haemangioma of the internal right eyelid. The surgical removal, while simple to perform, has required in this case the preparation of a sliding composite flap, medialized on a subcutaneous pedicle to fill the loss of substance. At the right bottom is the short follow-up with mild eyelid lymphoedema after surgery.

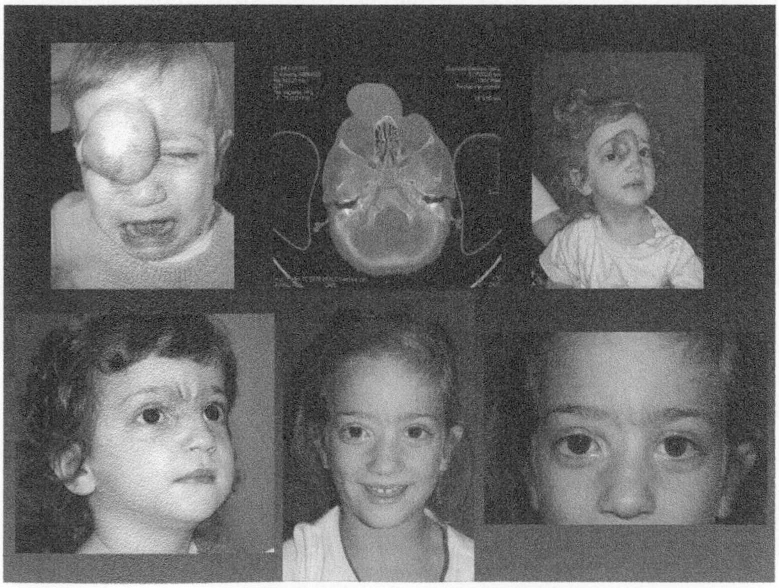

FIGURE 13.17 Massive haemangioma of the fronto-glabellar region. Top middle, computed tomography (CT) imaging showing the bone surface is not communicating with the vascular lesion. At the bottom left, follow-up at 1 month and down the center and right at 6 months after surgery.

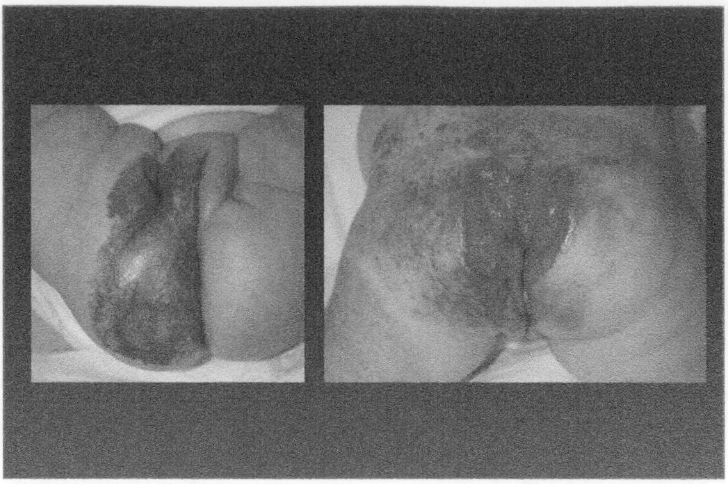

FIGURE 13.18 In the left side, Large perineal haemangiomas may constitute a distinctive group of associated anorectal, neurologic, renal, or urinary tract and genital defects. The acronym PELVIS syndrome emphasizes the characteristic findings of this syndrome: perineal haemangioma, external genitalia malformations, lipomyelomeningocele, vesicorenal abnormalities, imperforate anus, and skin tag. In the right side, SACRAL syndrome: spinal dysraphism, anogenital, cutaneous, renal, and urologic anomalies, associated with an IH of lumbosacral localization.

13.3.1.2 Lumbosacral Haemangiomas, Possible Spinal Dysraphism, or Structural Anomalies

Spinal dysraphism (including cauda equina, spina bifida, lipomyelomeningocele) has been reported in association with segmental haemangiomas of the lumbosacral area and structural anomalies of the genito-urinary system (Bruckner and Frieden 2006). The constellation of structural anomalies in this region is known by a number of acronyms such as *SACRAL* (*s*pinal dysraphism, *a*nogenital, *c*utaneous, *r*enal and urological, *a*ngioma of *l*umbosacral localization) (Britney 2007) and *PELVIS* (*p*erineal haemangioma, *e*xternal genitalia malformations, *l*ipomyelomeningocele, *v*escicolo-renal abnormalities, *i*mperforate anus, *s*kin tags) (D.M.A. MD 2011) (Figure 13.18) and is considered by some to be the lower-body equivalent of the upper body *PHACES* (*p*osterior fossae abnormalities, *h*aemangioma, *a*rterial/*a*ortic anomalies, *c*ardiac anomalies, *e*ye abnormalities, *s*ternal/*s*upraumbilical raphe) syndrome (Drolet: 2006f; Heyer 2006; MariaCGarzon 2007; Soto, Sandoval 2012).

13.3.1.3 Segmental Extremity Haemangiomas

Segmental or regional haemangiomas on an extremity can be a cause for concern because they tend to cover a large surface area and as such are prone to ulceration (Lanoel et al. 2012). Where possible, intervention is indicated to prevent ulceration that causes pain and distress for the patient and his or her family. Some patients with extensive leg and perineal haemangiomas also have vascular structural abnormalities with dermatomeric or median involvement of the genito-urinary tract, pelvis, and abdomen (Haggstrom 2006).

13.3.2 Prevent or Reduce Scars and/or Physiognomic and Dysmorphodynamic Damage

IHs can cause permanent dystrophic scars with facial disfigurement. During the involution phase, changes in the vascular tissue can result in inelastic, fibro-fatty skin. Certain areas of the face and neck (such as the nose, nasal pyramid, cheeks, and ears) are prone to dystrophic scarring, while surgery to remove very large scalp haemangiomas can result in large areas of alopecia (Meijer-Jorna et al. 2012; Mueller and P 2007) (Figure 13.19).

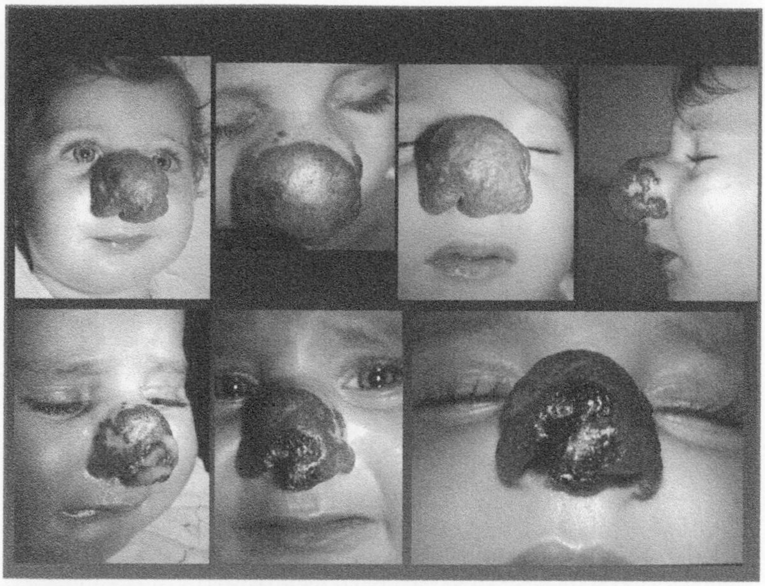

FIGURE 13.19 Ulceration of the nostrils with continuous irritation, rhinitis, and excess drainage of mucus and/or bleeding. Surgery is required in these patients possibly after the first year of age as there is a high risk of infection and alar cartilage reabsorption.

13.3.2.1 Exophytic Haemangiomas and Skin Structural Alterations

Exophytic, sessile, or pedunculated angiomatous lesions with a thick dermal component can cause significant permanent skin changes, particularly if they occur on the head and neck (Eivazi and Werner 2013). Following involution, as the skin is stretched over time, destruction of the elastic tissue modifies dermal structural components which can cause permanent damage. Early surgical intervention is recommended in these cases for cosmetic and physiognomic reasons (Brauer and Geronemus 2013; Singh 2006) (see Figure 13.9).

13.3.2.2 Nasal Tip Haemangioma and 'Cyrano de Bergerac' Nose Deformity

Nasal tip haemangiomas have unusual characteristics – the nasal cartilage is deformed and displaced and the tip of the nose has a round bulbous appearance (Arneja et al. 2010; McCarthy et al. 2001) (Figure 13.19). In some patients, ulceration of the nostrils can cause continuous irritation and rhinitis may develop with excess drainage of mucus and/or bleeding. Surgery is required in these patients after the first year of age as there is a high risk of infection and reabsorption of the alar cartilage (Burget 2009) (Figure 13.20). Deformities due to complications of this condition are disfiguring, with a poor cosmetic and psychological outcome, and therefore it is imperative to carry out debulking surgery when the patient is >1 year old following systemic or intralesional steroid therapy as the condition does not resolve naturally (McCarthy et al. 2001). Surgical excision should be completed before school age to prevent permanent damage to self-esteem and body image. Cosmetic surgery using techniques, such as lipofilling, may be delayed to late adolescence (S.I. MD et al. 2011).

13.3.2.3 Segmental Facial Haemangioma and PHACE Syndrome and/or Skin Textural Changes

Patients with large segmental facial haemangiomas not only risk poor aesthetic outcomes but also associated structural anomalies, such as the PHACE syndrome (Heyer et al. 2006). The diagnostic workup for this syndrome includes magnetic resonance imaging (MRI) and magnetic resonance angiography (MRA) of the head and neck, MRI of the mediastinum and aortic arch, echocardiogram, eye tests, and thyroid investigations (Carinci et al. 2012; Metry et al. 2013) (Figure 13.21).

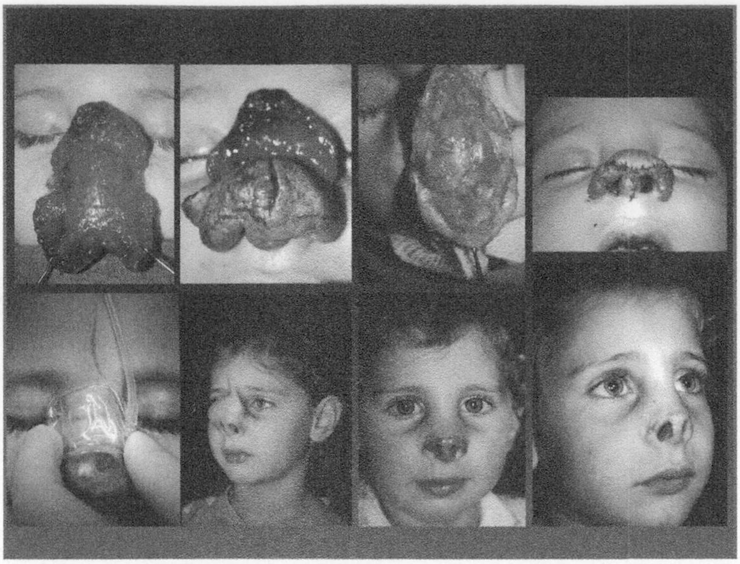

FIGURE 13.20 The patient above was submitted to first surgical reduction of the angiomatous ulcerated skin of the nasal pyramid, as seen in the series at the top. The series below shows instead the two surgical times after that, first involving the use of a skin expander placed on the nasal dorsum and then slip the skin expanded as obtained by classical technique.

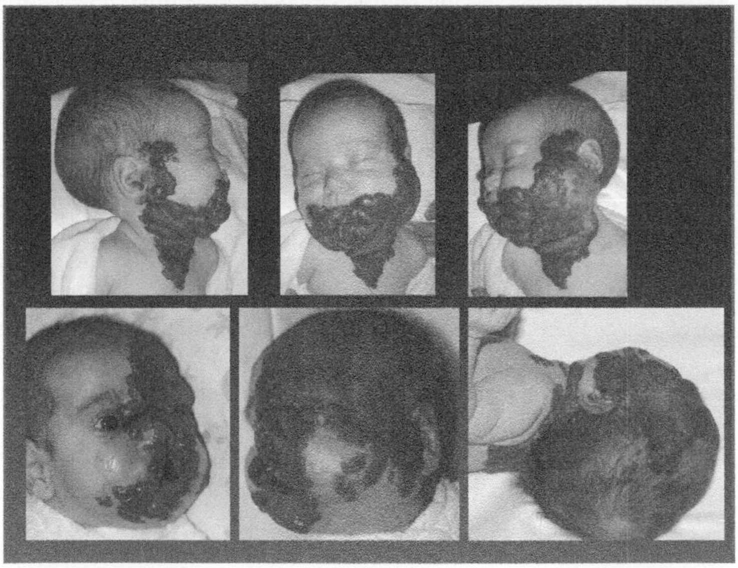

FIGURE 13.21 PHACE syndrome. It is the uncommon association between large infantile haemangiomas, usually of the face, and birth defects of the brain, heart, eyes, skin, and/ or arteries. It is an acronym that stands for the medical names of the parts of the body. It often impacts the following: P—posterior fossa abnormalities and other structural brain abnormalities; H—haemangioma(s) of the cervical facial region; A—arterial cerebrovascular anomalies; C—cardiac defects, aortic coarctation, and other aortic abnormalities; and E—eye anomalies.

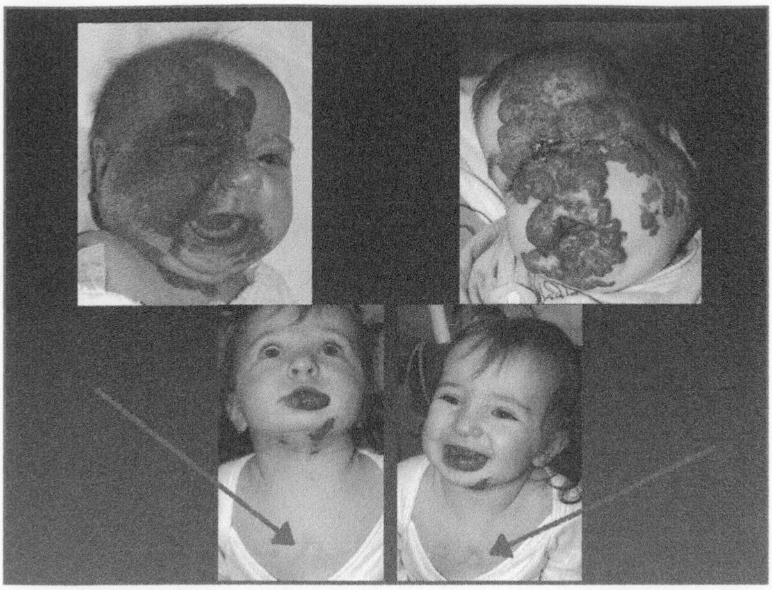

FIGURE 13.22 Sometimes, an S is added, making it PHACES, with S standing for Sternal defects and/or Supraumbilical raphe. The association of anomalies was first coined by Dr. Ilona Frieden in 1996, making it a relatively new syndrome, which had been unheard of before. A diagnosis is generally made from a physical examination, along with the imaging of the head and chest, and an eye examination. PHACES is most common among female infants. Long-term quality of life varies. Sometimes, it is fatal; other times, children have a rough for a first few years and then lead more normal lives. In addition to the obvious visual characteristic (IH), PHACE children often suffer from strokes and seizures (which are generally at their worst when haemangioma is in its growth phase).

Patients with the PHACE syndrome have an increased risk of stroke in the first 4 years of life compared to those with isolated IH (Andrea and Paolo 2006; Bronzetti et al. 2004; Drolet 2006; Hernandez-Martin et al. 2012; Metry et al. 2013) (Figure 13.22).

13.3.3 Prevent, Reduce, or Eliminate Function and Life-Threatening Complications

13.3.3.1 Airway and Glottis Haemangioma

Patients with segmental/dermatomeric haemangiomas in the mandibular area and in the median line even small have a high risk of associated airway and glottis involvement (Haugen et al. 2012). Babies 4–12 weeks old typically present with noisy breathing, high-pitched wheezing, and a hoarse cry that is often mistakenly diagnosed as laryngitis, bronchospasm, or epiglottitis (Figure 13.23). Airway haemangioma is one of the most serious, potentially *life-threatening* complications of IHs, and the input of a multidisciplinary team in conjunction with paediatric otolaryngology by fibrolaryngoscopy is vital (Akcay et al. 2012; ENJOLRAS 2008). First-line treatment is usually high-dose oral propranolol or steroids or followed by steroid infiltration during fibroscopy with CO_2 ablative or Nd:Yag laser as adjunct therapy (A. F et al. 2009; Poetke and Berlien 2005). The use of interferon is decreasing due to tolerability issues, and currently, vincristine (Alex and Aryeh 2002; Masashi et al. 2006) or bleomycin (Pienaar et al. 2006) is the preferred option. In patients with giant haemangioma that do not respond to this therapy, tracheotomy may be used as a temporary measure in patients at high risk during the first year of life (I.N.J. MD and MD 2011; Yue et al. 2013; Zur et al. 2005).

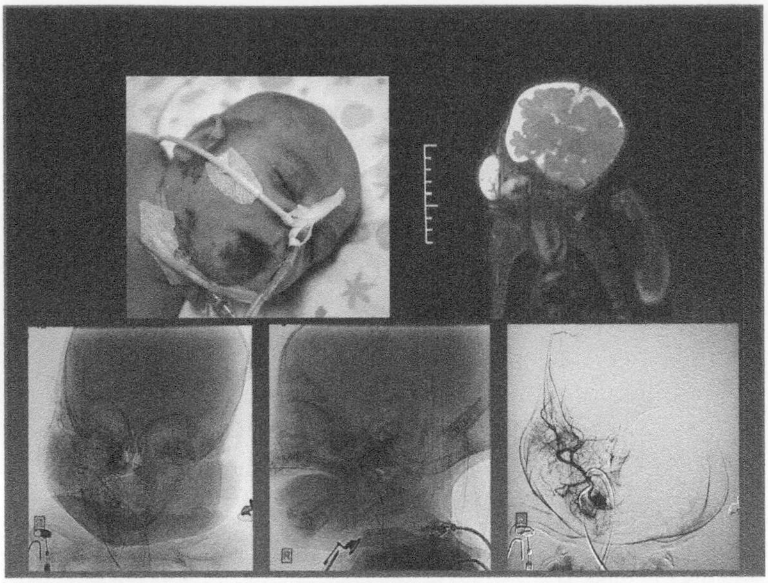

FIGURE 13.23 Subglottic haemangiomas may form a large mass in the subglottic airway, causing varying degrees of airway obstruction. However, not every subglottic haemangioma will shrink completely. Many require active intervention because of their life-threatening nature in the airway. Haemangiomas of the larynx or trachea are often seen in children who have multiple haemangiomas appearing in a particular dermatomal region (one of the four regions of the body associated with a particular spinal nerve). They may be associated with haemangiomas in other non-airway sites such as the skin of the scalp or back. Symptoms include croup-like cough, noisy breathing when inhaling and exhaling, and difficulty breathing. To diagnose a subglottic haemangioma, the child will first have a plain neck X-ray. The X-ray alone may show a mass in his airway. Flexible laryngoscopy may also be enough to reveal that a haemangioma is causing the respiratory symptoms. There are many potential treatments for subglottic haemangiomas depending on the severity of the child's case. Propranolol shows promise in the rapid reduction of airway symptoms. Other treatment options include tracheostomy, intralesional laser, steroid injections, microdebrider excision, and open surgical excision, the choice of which is based on the severity of the clinical case.

13.3.3.2 Symptomatic Liver Haemangiomas

The liver is the most common extracutaneous site of multilocational angiomatous lesions (1%) (Dubois et al. 2007). Hepatic haemangiomas are often asymptomatic but a small proportion can cause co-morbidities and in rare cases are life-threatening. The most common multifocal liver haemangiomas can cause hepatic failure and congestive heart failure, while diffuse liver haemangiomas – which can occupy the entire liver and cause abdominal compartment syndrome – and a severe form of hypothyroidism attributable to tumour-related deiodination of thyroxine are rarer (Boon et al. 2007). A third type of hepatic haemangioma, the solitary liver haemangioma, often presents at birth with arteriovenous shunting and in most cases is not a true haemangioma but a form of RICH (A.G. MD and MD 2011; Choi et al. 2011; Perman et al. 2012).

13.4 DIAGNOSTIC RADIOLOGY FOR HAEMANGIOMAS

X-rays rarely show evidence of dystrophic or hypertrophic bone alterations, except in the case of cranial haemangiomas which can depress the cranial plates and cause upper maxillary asymmetry and orbital dystopia (R.A. MD and ChB 2011) (Figure 13.25). Doppler or colour Doppler ultrasonography show haemangiomas as well-defined masses with non-homogeneous echo-structure, multiple diastolic fast-flow vascular formations, and fast venous flow (Degrugillier-Chopinet et al. 2011) (Figure 13.24). Ultrasound examination in the transition from the proliferation to the involution

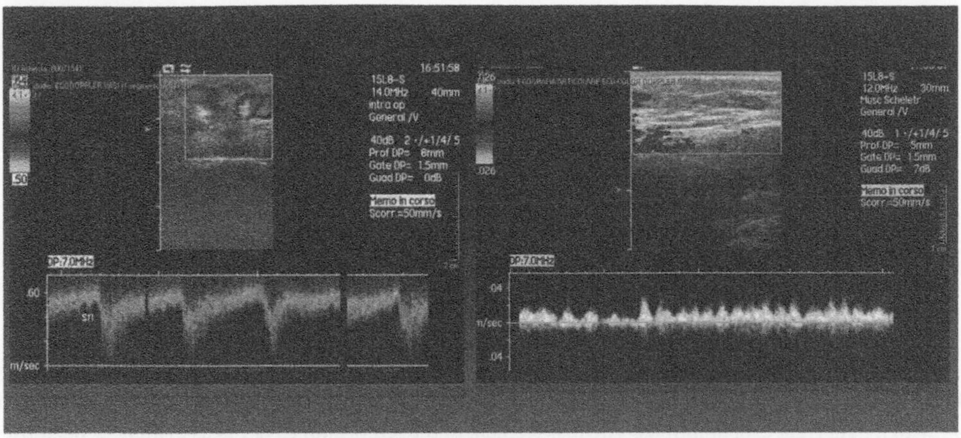

FIGURE 13.24 Typical AVM that demonstrates feeding arteries, draining veins, and dilated vessels depicts low resistance arterial flow above the baseline and pulsatile venous flow below the baseline, consistent with AV shunting.

phase shows an increase in the fatty component and a progressive reduction of the vascular component, with specific changes in the ultrasound signal (Berzigotti and Piscaglia 2011; Marler et al. 2002; R.A. MD and ChB 2011).

Computed tomography scan during the proliferation phase shows a well-defined mass with extensive homogeneous impregnation following administration of a contrast medium. In the involution phase, the intensity of the contrast medium becomes patchy and heterogeneous. CT is useful to determine the extent of compression caused by the haemangioma on critical anatomic regions (such as the trachea and mediastinum region) which may have structural and/or functional malformations (Wassef et al. 2006) (Figure 13.25).

The ability of MRI to provide multidimensional images, to differentiate between muscle and fat, and to visualise vessels makes it particularly useful in evaluating haemangiomas. MRI is the diagnostic method of choice, in particular in very young patients, as ionising radiation is not used (Restrepo 2013; Yilmaz et al. 2011). Haemangiomas have a parenchymal intensity at T1, a modest signal enhancement at T2, and a strong signal enhancement after injection of paramagnetic contrast medium (Anon. 2001) (Figure 13.26).

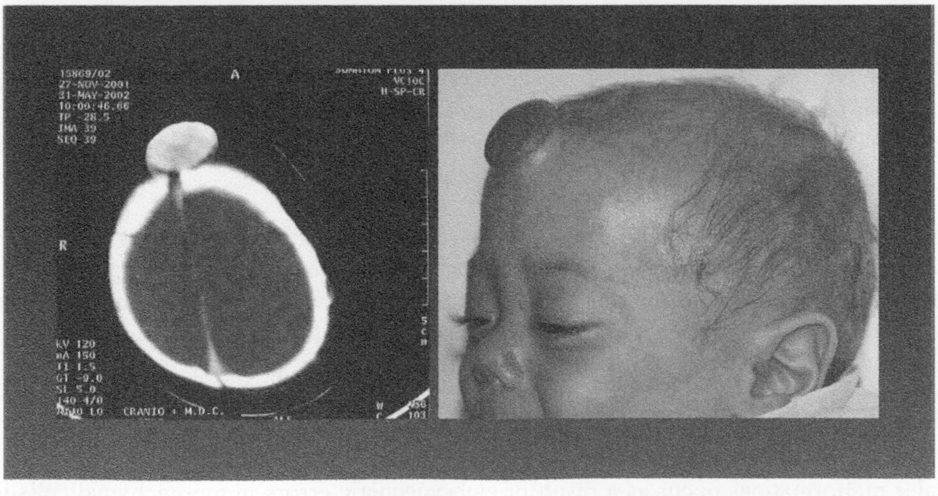

FIGURE 13.25 CT scan and related clinical case. Haemangioma of the frontal midline with a full thickness defect of the ossification of the skull on the fronto-parietal suture line.

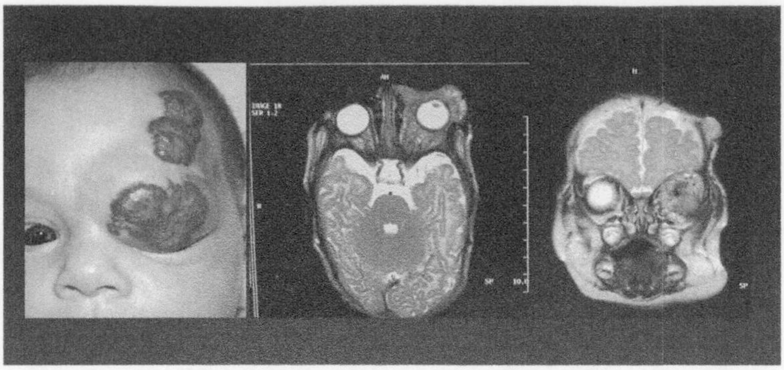

FIGURE 13.26 Case report and its MRI in axial and frontal view of the infantile IH of the fronto-periorbital region with a light right exophthalmos. The involvement of the left orbital cavity is as evident as the intra- and extraconal tissues.

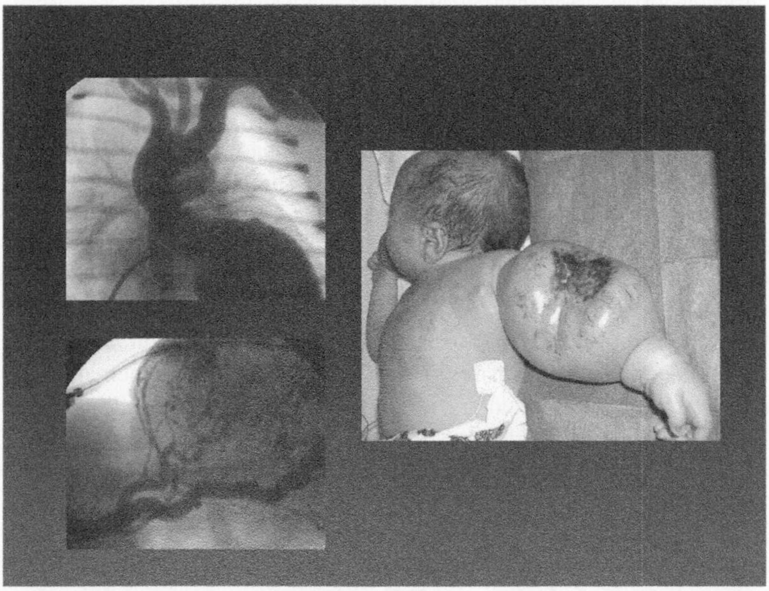

FIGURE 13.27 Ulcerated giant RICH (rapidly involuting congenital haemangioma) of the left arm. Arteriography overview shows a marked hypertrophy of the subclavian artery with well-represented ipsilateral hypertrophic arterial circle.

Angiography is considered to be useful only in certain rare haemangioma cases. This technique allows the visualisation of a mass with an early fast flow, a parenchymographic opacisation phase which persists also during the observation of the draining veins with opacisation. In general, a number of afferent arterial vessels are dilated and/or contorted and there is an increase in the diameter of veins (Ballah et al. 2011; C et al. 2004) (Figure 13.27).

13.5 VASCULAR MALFORMATIONS

Vascular malformations occur as a result of embryogenetic errors in mesenchymal cells forming vessels and, although present at birth, may not be picked up during neonatal development or in the first days of life (Gloviczki et al. 2009; Hochman et al. 2011; J.U. MD et al. 1999).

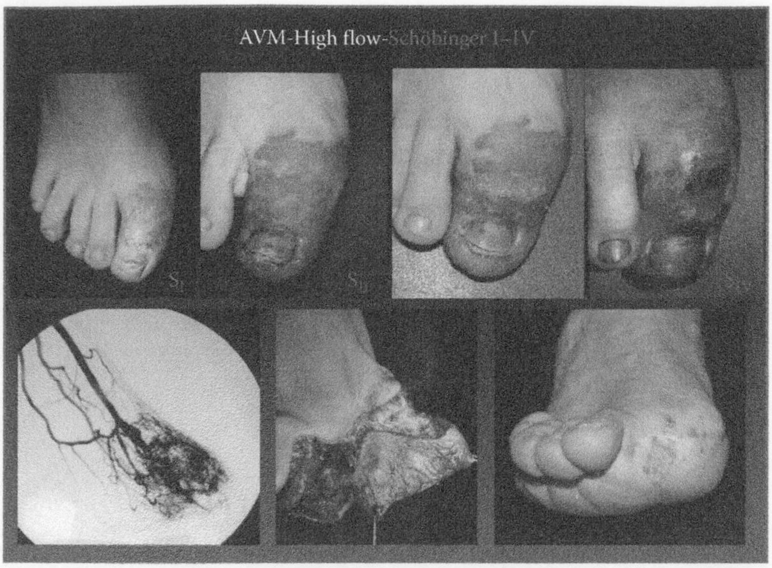

FIGURE 13.28 AVMs are categorized according to Schöbinger clinical staging: stage I (quiescence), stage II (expansion), stage III (destruction). Stage IV malformation leads to heart failure, if not treated (decompensation). Stage I lesions remain stable for long periods. Expansion (stage II) is usually followed by pain, bleeding, and ulceration (stage III). Once present, these symptoms and signs indicate that the lesion inevitably progresses until the malformation is surgically resected.

Interestingly, some malformation may only become evident during adolescence or even in adult age as they may go through a *quiescent* phase which can last many years (Garzon et al. 2007). However, most malformations are identified early in life and they grow with the child but do not have the characteristic proliferation and involution phases of haemangiomas and of vascular tumours in general. Most often, growth is gradual and progressive, but in rare cases, their growth is rapid. Very often vascular malformations may appear suddenly or increase in size after trauma, infection, and fever and during periods of hormonal changes (puberty, pregnancy, and menopause) but frequently appear without a specific trigger (Garzon and Frieden 2007; Meijer-Jorna et al. 2012; Richter and Friedman 2012) (Figure 13.28). On histological examination, they do not show endothelial cell proliferation but are composed of large vascular lacunae covered with flat endothelium on a thin basal membrane. Compared with vascular tumours, they have a regular number of mastocytes (A.G. MD and MD 2011; T et al. 2004).

Vascular malformations are never composed of a single vessel but by a patchy cluster of vessels, with or without fistulae, and a possible arterial, venous, or lymphatic predominance. The majority of these malformations do not spontaneously regress and continue to grow if not treated appropriately (El-Merhi et al. 2013; Fevurly and Fishman 2012) (Figure 13.29).

Vascular malformations can be distinguished according to their clinical and *haemodynamic characteristics*:

- Predominantly capillary malformations (CMs)
- Predominantly venous malformations (VMs)
- Predominantly lymphatic malformations (LMs)
- Complex-combined vascular malformations (CVMs or CLVs)
- Arteriovenous malformations (AVMs)

In addition, based on their haemodynamic features, they can be classified as *slow-flow* and *fast-flow* malformations. Slow-flow malformations include CMs, VMs, LMs, CVMs, and CLVs, while

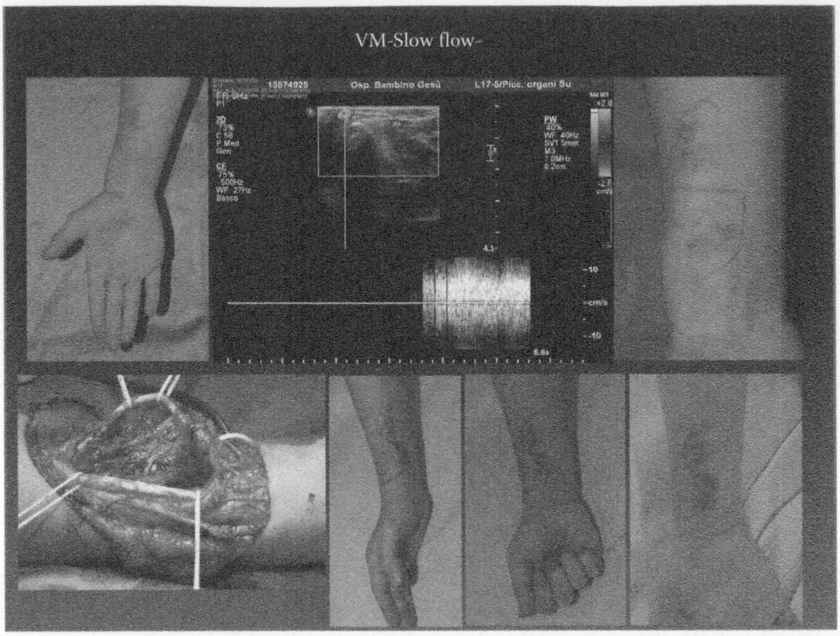

FIGURE 13.29 Venous malformations (VMs) are made of dysplastic vessels with no cellular proliferation. Low-flow or slow-flow malformations (lf/sfVM) consist predominantly of venous and/or lymphatic vessels. VMs are the most common vascular malformations. Doppler ultrasonography should be the initial imaging modality and demonstrates the absence of flow or low-velocity venous flow.

fast-flow malformations include arterial aneurysms, ectasias, stenosis, fistulas, and AVMs with shunts (Arneja and Gosain 2008; Wollina et al. 2012). In the latter group, it is necessary to evaluate carefully the risk of haemodynamic overload and cardiac failure (A.S. Liu et al. 2010; MMSc and PhD 2011) (Figure 13.30). Finally, there are complex both slow- and fast-flow forms that are typically associated with the growth of bone and soft tissues, such as the Parkes Weber syndrome (A.M.K. MD and MD 2011; Schook et al. 2011) and Klippel–Trenaunay syndrome (Goksu et al. 2012; Lefebvre et al. 2004; Notarnicola et al. 2012) (Figure 13.31).

13.6 DIAGNOSIS

After obtaining a detailed medical history, the first-level diagnostic test is either a Doppler or colour Doppler ultrasonography, which provides useful information on fast or slow flow (El-Merhi et al. 2013; Legiehn and Heran 2006; Redondo et al. 2011; Restrepo 2013). Plain x-rays easily underline the presence of the phleboliths in the soft tissues, that is, a typical expression of the VMs (Casanova et al. 2006) (Figure 13.32). Comparative x-rays are necessary to underline the dysmetria of the limbs (Figures 13.33 and 13.34). Second-level tests include MRI and MRA and CT with contrast medium.

Angiography (arteriography, phlebography, varicography) is a third-level test to be used after less invasive techniques. However, it constitutes the preliminary examination foreseeing a treatment of interventional radiology (Ballah et al. 2011; Hasiloglu et al. 2013; Jarrett et al. 2013) (Figure 13.46).

In very young paediatric patients, CT, MRI, MRA, and angiography should be carried out on sedation or under general anaesthesia. In most cases, intravascular contrast medium is necessary to evaluate in detail AVMs, CMs, and VMs (Kakimoto et al. 2005).

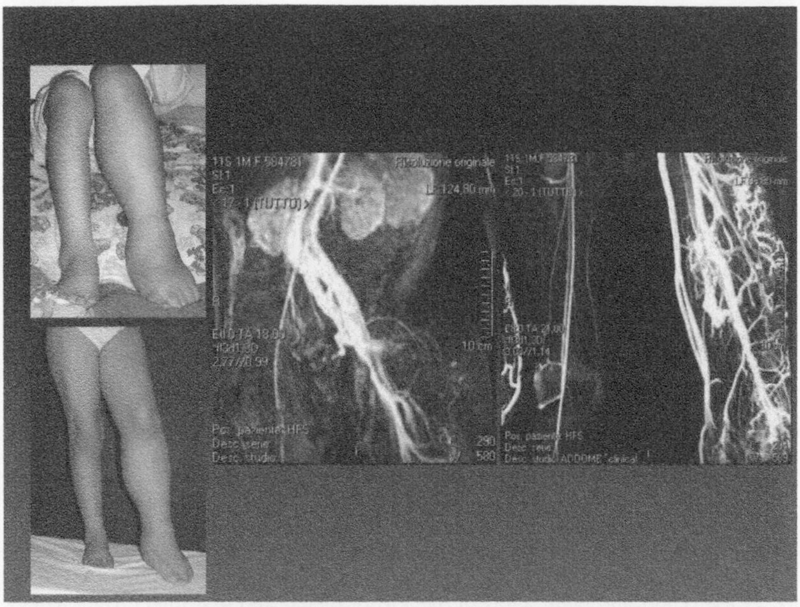

FIGURE 13.30 Parkes Weber syndrome (PWS). This syndrome is characterized by Klippel-Trénaunay (KT) abnormalities combined vascular anomalies (hemi-hypertrophy, port wine stain, and varicose veins) along with arteriovenous Fistulae, resulting in dyspnea and congestive heart failure.

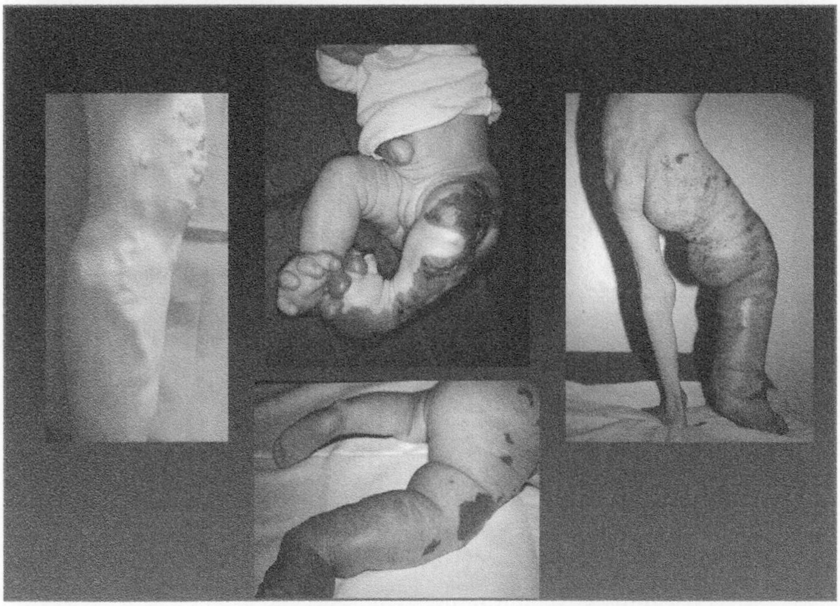

FIGURE 13.31 Klippel-Trénaunay syndrome (KTS) is a rare congenital anomaly classically defined as the triad of vascular stain, soft tissue and/or bony hypertrophy, and venous varicosities (sometimes residual marginal vein). KT syndrome has a complex constellation of anomalies that includes cutaneous capillary malformation (usually on an affected limb), abnormal development of deep and superficial veins, and limb asymmetry, usually bone and soft tissues enlargement. Mixed vascular malformations may be present and include capillary, venous, and lymphatic systems.

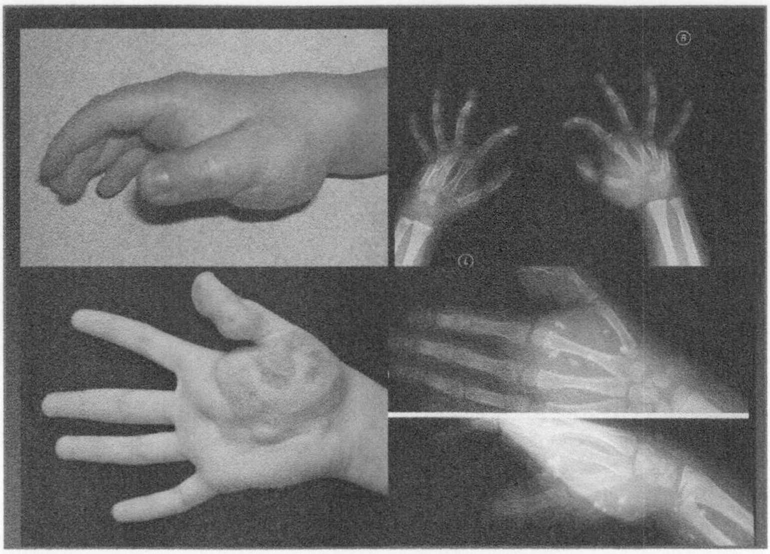

FIGURE 13.32 Case report and plain X-ray of the VM of thenar and first finger, right hand and ipsilateral distal third of the forearm. You can see the characteristic and pathognomonic phleboliths, round shaped in various sizes that were not present on standard X-ray in early childhood (top right).

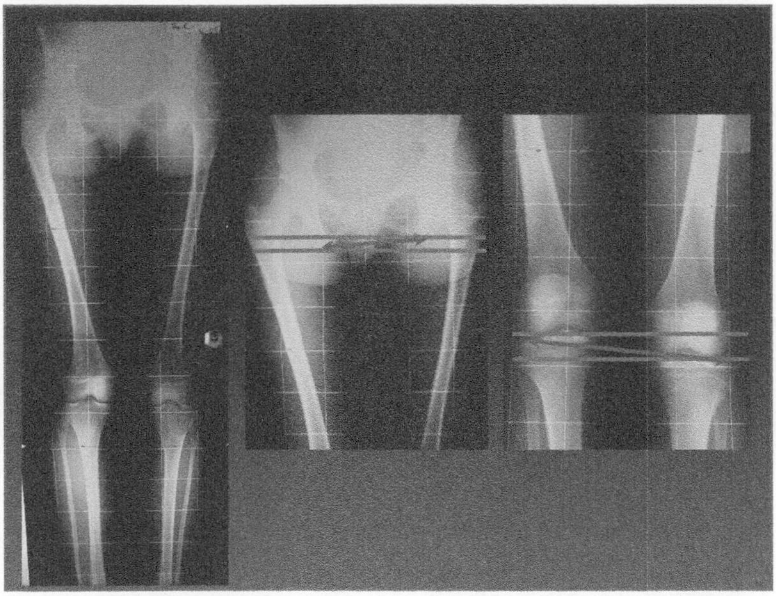

FIGURE 13.33 Standard X-rays with the meter of the lower limbs. It is clear a longitudinal asymmetry of the lower right, mainly due to the elongation of the femur. Note the compensatory rotation of the basin.

13.7 MANAGEMENT

To establish the optimal treatment for lesions that do not regress spontaneously and continue to grow over time, it is useful to determine the predominant vascular type, location, size, depth, and the involvement of underlying organs and structures before beginning therapy (Meijer-Jorna et al. 2012; Wassef 2011a). Slow-flow forms on lower limbs may benefit from graduated compression stockings that, if correctly prescribed and regularly worn, can prevent malformations getting worse

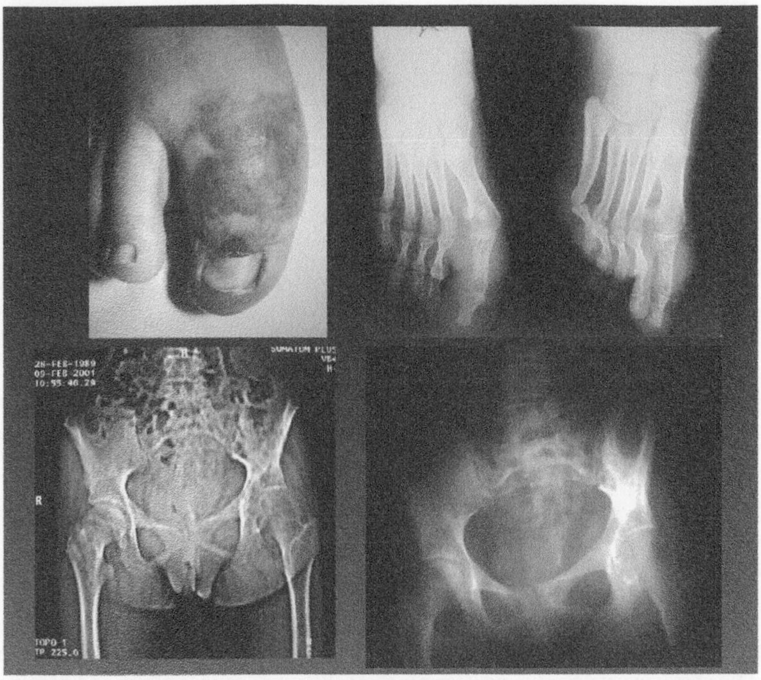

FIGURE 13.34 Two clinical cases with structural bone rarefaction of the first phalanx of the big toe (top) in an AVM and of the left hemipelvis in an LM (bottom).

(MMSc and MSc 2011). The response to flash pulse dye laser is generally favourable for superficial CMs of the upper body and less beneficial for malformations in the lower limbs. The most complex and deep forms can be removed surgically only when first treated with angioradiological sclerotisation or embolisation (Stefan et al. 2003). This combined radiological and surgical approach allows for easier excision, with reduced intraoperative bleeding and risk of complications (Tyagi et al. 2006). Slow-flow malformations cause primitive venous stasis, and diffuse malformations can trigger intravascular loco-regional coagulopathy (Hermans et al. 2006) with mild thrombocytopenia that is otherwise proper to certain syndromes, such as Kasabach–Merritt's syndrome (Le Nouail et al. 2007; Lei et al. 2011). Vascular malformations may also induce skeletal abnormalities, for example, deformations, hypertrophy, and hypoplasia in the slow-flow forms and, in the fast-flow forms, erosions, deformations, and hyperplasia (H et al. 2001). Some rare intraosseous locations of high-flow malformations are resembling a worm-holed aspect of the bony spongiosa (Linfante et al. 2012; R et al. 2001; Zhao-Hui et al. 2008) (Figure 13.34).

13.8 DIAGNOSTIC RADIOLOGY FOR VASCULAR MALFORMATIONS

13.8.1 Capillary Malformations

CMs are sporadic lesions consisting of slow-flow CMs commonly called *port-wine stains* or *naevus flammeus* (Ercan et al. 2013; Poetke and Berlien 2005; S.M.M. MD and MD 2011; Savas et al. 2013) (Figure 13.35). They are often associated with LMs and may be part of a group of neurocutaneous syndromes called *phakomatoses* (Kim et al. 2012; R.A. M et al. 2004). Doppler or colour Doppler ultrasonography is used to exclude a venous/arteriovenous component; for the differential diagnosis of Klippel–Trenaunay, Parkes Weber, or Sturge–Weber syndromes, MRI, CT, and, in some cases, digital subtraction angiography are performed (Phi et al. 2012).

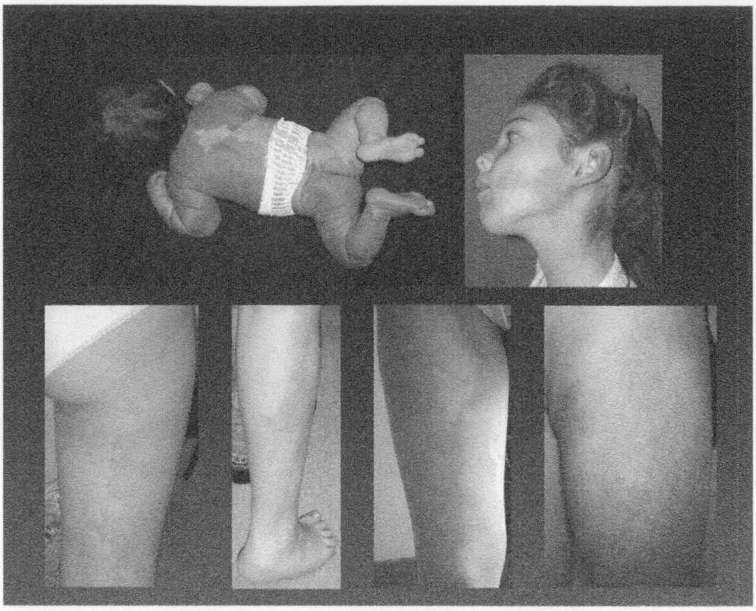

FIGURE 13.35 The designation capillary malformation (CM) is widely used for what was formerly called a nevus flammeus or port wine stain. This new terminology, however, is inaccurate and ambiguous. There are at least nine different skin disorders fulfilling the criteria of a CM. Examples include nevus anemicus, cutis marmorata telangiectatica congenita, angiokeratoma circumscriptum, and several vascular lesions that do not represent nevi, such as the nuchal or glabellar salmon patch and the cutaneous changes of Rendu–Osler disease. We should use CM as an umbrella term and not as a name for a specific cutaneous entity. (From Rudolf Happle, "What is a capillary malformation?" *Journal of the American Academy of Dermatology* vol.59:6 Dec 2008, pp. 1077–1079.)

13.8.2 Lymphatic Malformations

LMs include localised forms (superficial or deep) (Figure 13.36), diffuse forms (Figure 13.37), and cystic lymphangioma (Azizkhan et al. 2006) (Figure 13.38). They present as localised tumefactions or oedematous areas (elephantiasis in the extremities in late lymphoedema). LMs are compressible in their early stages when subcutaneous fibrosis is not present but become progressively incompressible due to fibrosis secondary to chronic oedema caused by leakage of protein into the interstitial space (E et al. 2006; Güvenç et al. 2005), while cystic lymphangioma initially presents as a compressible tumefaction on the face and neck with cervico-facial localisation (cystic hygroma) (Figure 13.39). CT scans of LMs show multilobular cystic formations that, with contrast, are limited to intralocular septa. Bone hypertrophy, frequent in LMs, may also be visible on CT scans.

Among the imaging methods, MRI provides the most detailed outcome and allows the possibility of distinguishing between the lymphatic component (isointense signal at T1 that increases moderately and consistently at T2) and the cystic component (distinguishable at T2 due to the homogenous and hyperintense signal) (Kadota et al. 2011; Theiler et al. 2013) (Figure 13.40). Differential diagnosis of cystic lymphangiomas and LMs with MRI is performed using paramagnetic contrast medium that enhances only the walls of the cystic cavities and not the complete mass as in VMs (Navarro 2011). When the cystic cavity is perforated, lymph comes out, but if intracystic haemorrhage has occurred, the fluid is coffee coloured. In cases where the cavities are small, as in microcystic lymphangioma fluid, aspiration and sclerotherapy are not possible.

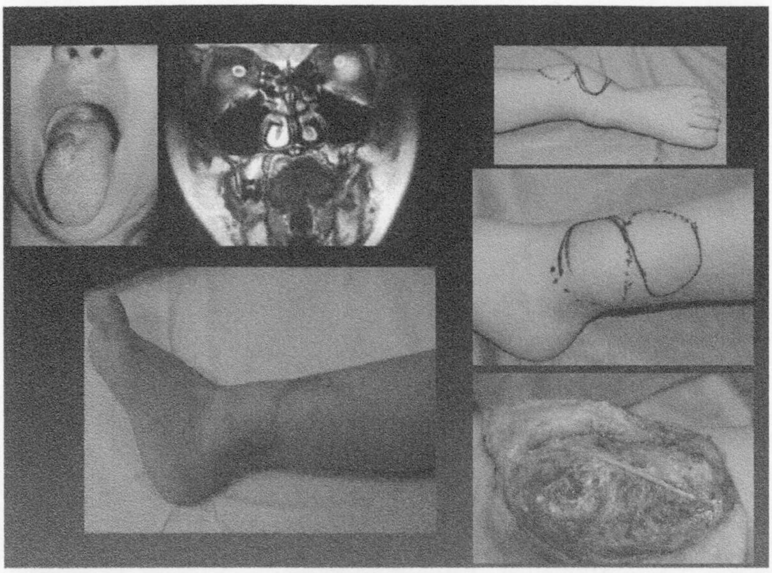

FIGURE 13.36 Two cases of localized LM: top left, a lesion involving the right portion of the body of the tongue with its representation in T2-MRI. On the right and bottom LM of the distal third of the leg since the external framework with intraoperative and short distance post-operative.

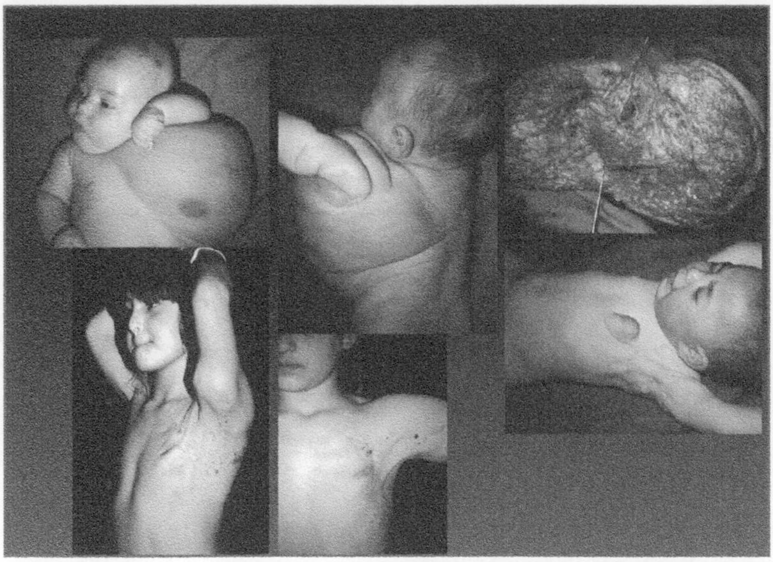

FIGURE 13.37 Giant LM of the axilla and right hemithorax. Intraoperative picture and result in short- and long-distance follow-up (8 years) after extensive surgical excision.

13.8.3 Venous Malformations

VMs take many forms including abnormalities of the number, course, aplasia, hypoplasia, or ectasia of a series of veins (H.K. D et al. 2002). They can also occur as a result of valvular and venous anomalies from single/multiple venous spaces dilated post-capillary and characterised by stagnant flow (Stefan et al. 2003) (Figure 13.41).

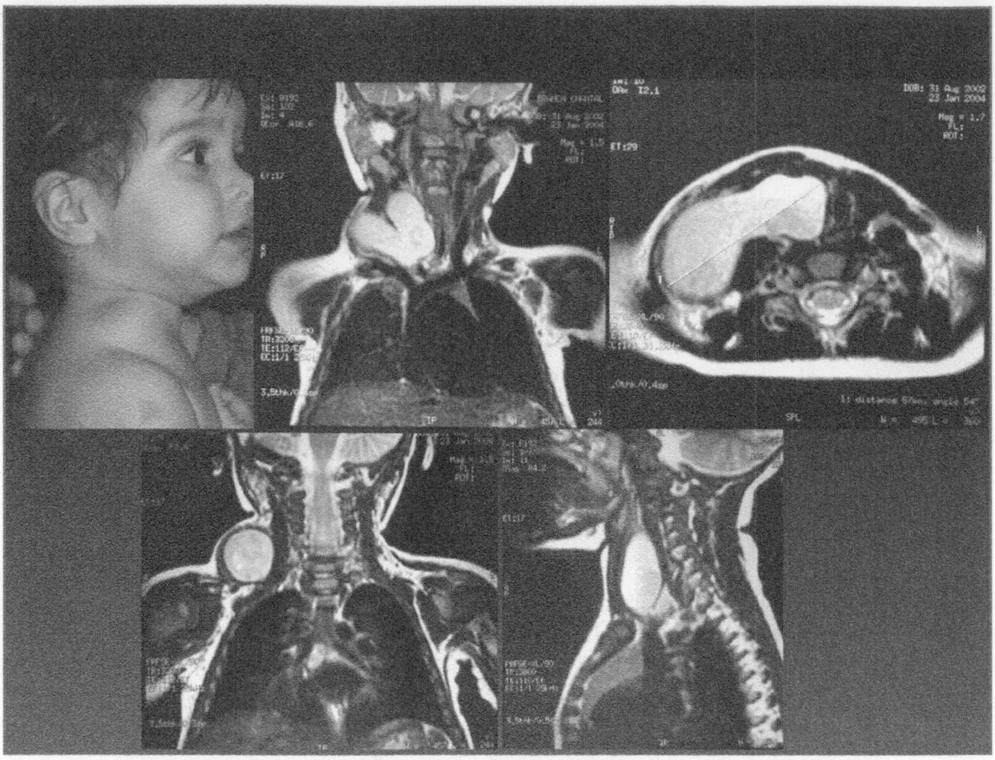

FIGURE 13.38 Clinical presentation and MRI of right localized supraclavicular LM to the lower third of the neck. At the top are coronal and axial T2-MRI images. At the bottom is the coronal and sagittal T2-weighted image of the same lesion.

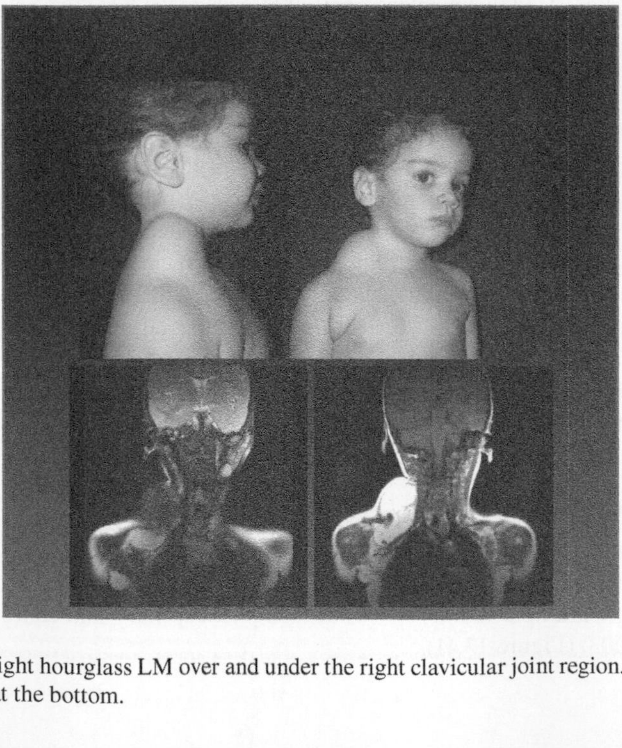

FIGURE 13.39 Upright hourglass LM over and under the right clavicular joint region. Coronal T1-MRI and T2-weighted images at the bottom.

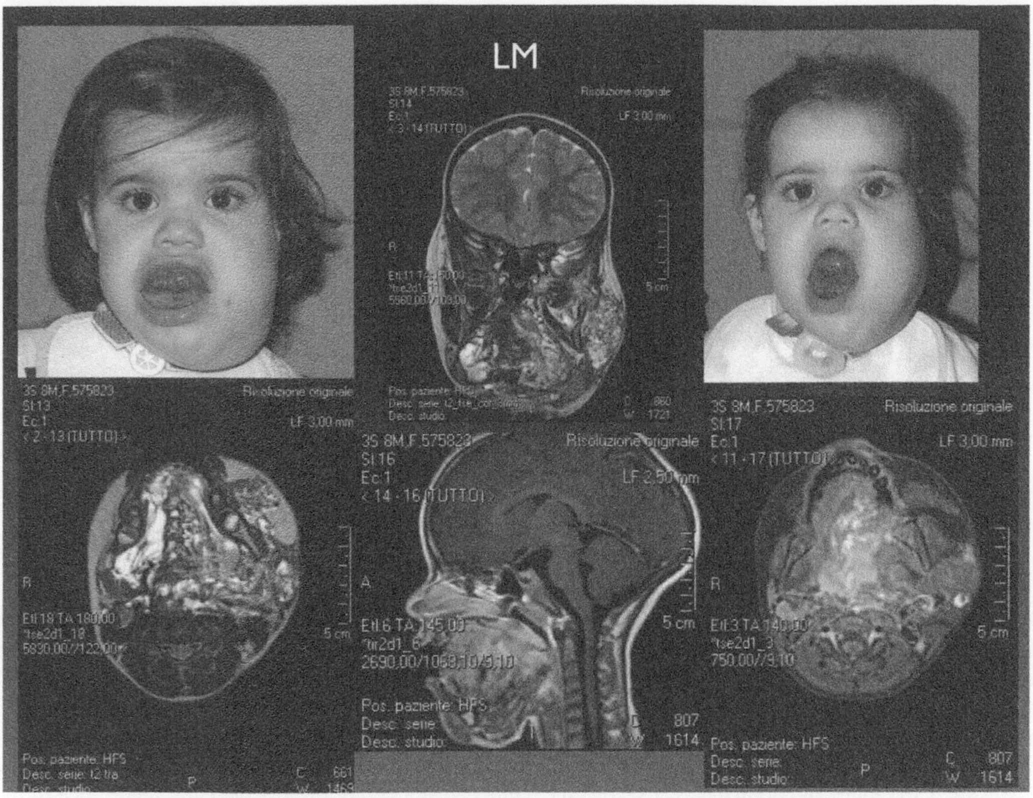

FIGURE 13.40 Microcystic LM. Coronal view on MRI in the top center and axial and sagittal projections (bottom). The patient has undergone tracheostomy due to the narrowing of the upper airways, as clearly visible on MRI in sagittal projection at the bottom center.

Clinical features of localised VMs are as follows:

- Overlying skin has dark-blue or purple colouration.
- Malformation increases in size when the affected region is lowered or when the Valsalva manoeuvre is performed.

Swelling of the soft tissues and presence of phleboliths are evident on standard x-ray (Figures 13.32 through 13.41). When VMs occur in the limbs, bone involvement is frequent while skeletal hypertrophy is more common in venous capillary conditions as in the Klippel–Trenaunay syndrome (see Figure 13.31).

In order to make timely decisions on treatment, patients with longitudinal dysmetria of the limbs, are carefully measured for bone length and width, comparing with the controlateral limb (Lefebvre et al. 2004) (Figure 13.33). Isolated venous lesions present as osteolytic lacunae not clearly differentiated from other benign tumours (Zhao-Hui et al. 2008). Often multiple bone malformations are associated with skin alterations and a disease entity characterised by rapidly growing multiple osteolytic areas, with spontaneous fractures, phleboliths, and shortening of the limb otherwise known as the Gorham–Stout syndrome (Nakatsuka et al. 2012).

Doppler ultrasonography shows different pictures according to the type of dysplasia. On one hand, localised ectasia and rare venous aneurism are easily documented, while on the other hand, hypoplasia, aplasia, and the persistent anomaly of a marginal vein external to the lower limb are

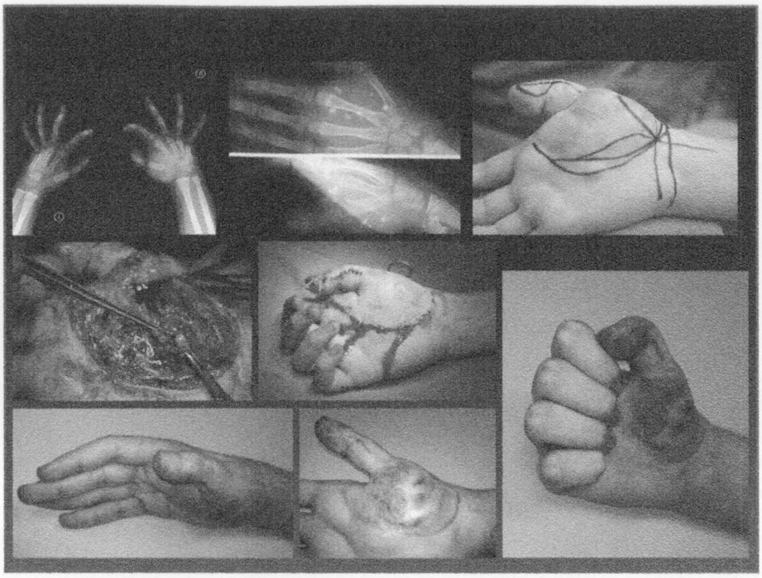

FIGURE 13.41 Low-flow venous malformation (lfVM) of the thenar space with lots of phleboliths highlighted to standard X-rays. The images show the intraoperative release of vascular phleboliths from the inside of the caves, once logged surgery. In this case, a careful surgical removal is done by preserving structures, tendon, muscle, and nerves, scrupulously avoiding the motor branch of the median nerve to the thenar eminence. Bottom result after 2 months, with optimal functional recovery. The patient is advised to wear a customized lightweight elastic glove (grade I corresponding to about 15 mmHg), for the next 6–8 months at least 12 h per day. This is to reduce the occurrence of secondary lymphoedema and/or of possible early recurrence of the malformation.

difficult to interpret (Casanova et al. 2006) (see Figure 13.31). The key role of Doppler/colour Doppler ultrasonography is the differential diagnosis with arteriovenous fistulas. Typically, vascular lacunae present as multiple, partially confluent non-echogenic areas, often without signal during Doppler sonography at rest, but with signal with respiratory or compressive manoeuvres.

13.8.4 Venous Malformations with Continuous Flow

CT allows a quick and easy diagnosis of *phleboliths*, a pathognomonic sign of VM (R.A. MD and ChB 2011). In syndromes localised in bone, CT allows a more accurate evaluation of malformations than MRI (Wu et al. 2012). While MRI in contrast shows better results for the evaluation of soft tissues, muscles and areas of malformation present with homogeneous intensity making a problematic evaluation of the extent and depth of the VM in relation with surrounding tissues (Kakimoto et al. 2005) (Figure 13.42).

MRI allows a better differentiation of soft tissues than CT and, as a result, may produce more accurate data on the extent of the malformation and its relationship with the surrounding structures. The use of paramagnetic medium is particularly useful in the differential diagnosis of LM when the uptake of medium involves the complete malformation and not just the walls of the cystic cavity (Anon. 2001). Venous lacunae are hyperintense areas at T2-weighted sequences and thus are easily distinguishable from muscles and subcutaneous fat (Figure 13.43). In addition, vessels for venous drainage that characteristically have slow blood flow are typically hyperintense areas which can be easily observed. Unlike AVMs, VMs are homogeneously hyperintense at T2, without areas where signal is absent (Anon. 2001; T. F et al. 2001). In partial or total thrombosis, the signal is extremely variable depending on the time from thrombus formation (Figure 13.44). Occasionally, it is possible to observe small marginal areas with highly hypointense signal at T1- and T2-weighted MRI, due to the presence of

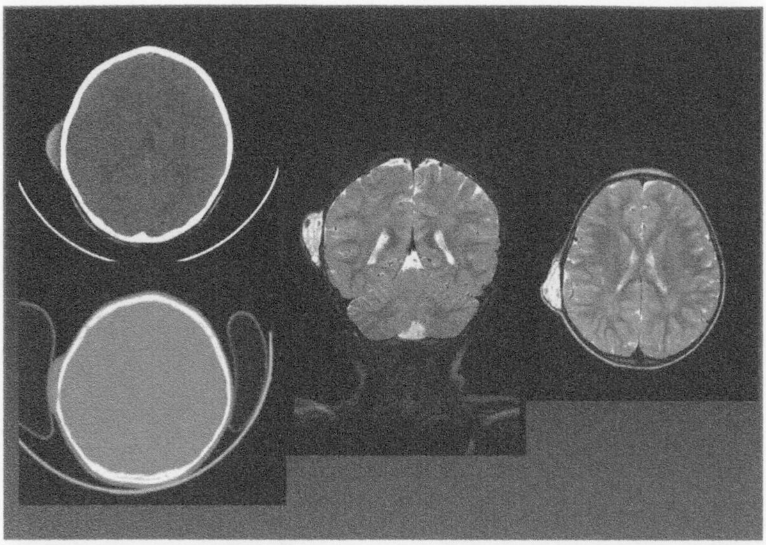

FIGURE 13.42 VM of the right temporal region. CT shows a full thickness lack of ossification of the skull, corresponding to an intracranial vascular communication (left). Representation in the coronal and axial T2-weighted MRI on the right. Note the better definition of soft tissue in MRI on the right than CT. In any case, CT shows more precisely the skeletal defect.

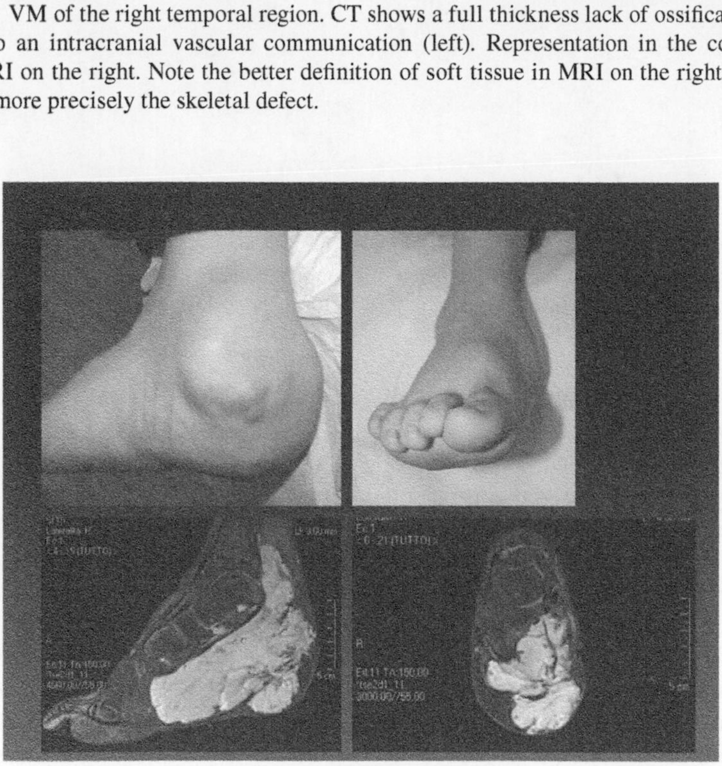

FIGURE 13.43 CT and MRI are used primarily for the pretreatment evaluation of lesion extension. These lesions are usually isointense on T1-weighted MR images and markedly hyperintense on T2-weighted images with variable gadolinium enhancement. Direct phlebography helps confirm the diagnosis. Three distinct phlebographic patterns (cavitary, spongy, and dysmorphic) have been identified. In most cases, conservative treatment is recommended. Sclerotherapy with or without surgery is useful in cases of functional impairment or significant aesthetic prejudice, even if recurrences are frequent. Direct phlebography is performed when a more detailed assessment of the vascular pattern is needed or as part of sclerotherapy. The use of the appropriate imaging technique is critical in establishing the diagnosis, evaluating extension, and planning appropriate treatment.

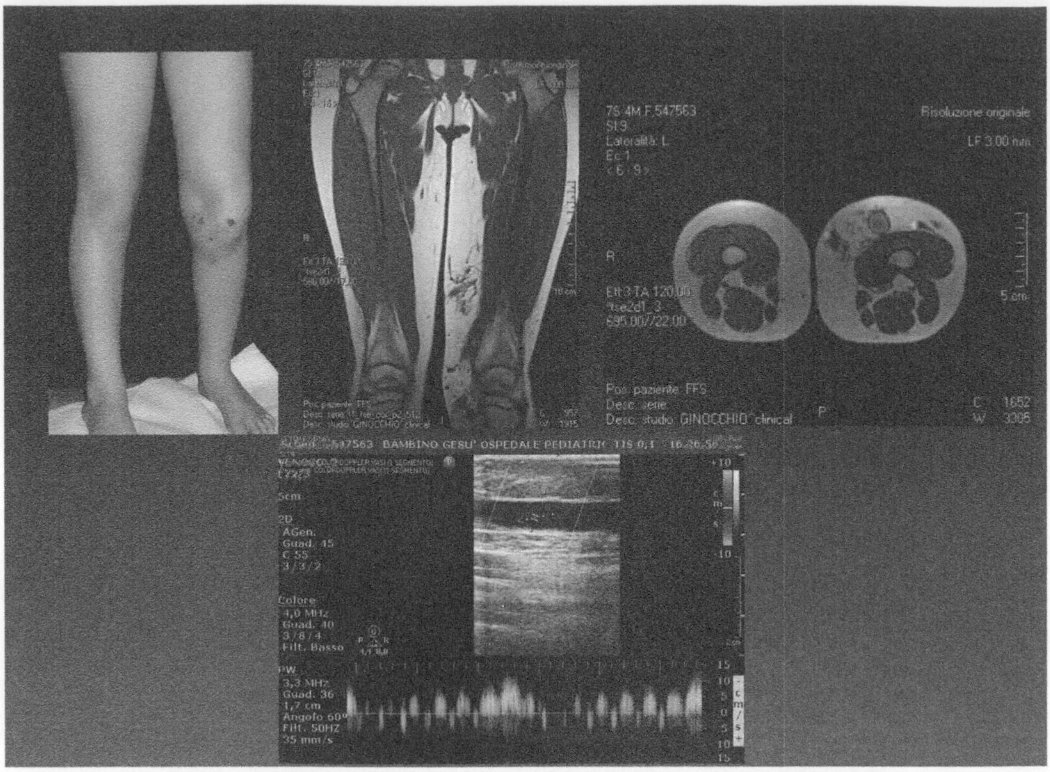

FIGURE 13.44 Case report and its coronal and axial T1-MRI on the top right of dysmorphic appearance VM, with subcutaneous cavity of the distal-medial thigh region and the knee. In ultrasonography, you notice a thrombosis of a venous collector of large caliber, which shows no intraluminal flow and does not appear deprimibile to compression.

haemosiderin. Anomalous superficial venous vessels or venous ectasias can be easily identified by MRI for the high-intensity signal at T2 due to slow blood flow (Finley et al. 2005) (Figure 13.45).

Angiography of VMs is based mainly on the study of venous vessels in the area. Frequently, the late phase of arteriography is non-significant, showing incorrect evidence of normality or in some cases of a poor and partial uptake (Murakami et al. 2012). Ascending and descending phlebography is necessary to show the functioning of deep veins (mainly for CVMs) and possible anomalies of the superficial venous circle (C.P. D 2007; Hegde et al. 2012; R et al. 2001).

Superficial localised venous dysplasia cannot be evaluated since the flow through dilated veins is slower than that in normal veins and, as such, can only be observed using the direct puncture technique (Figure 13.46). Occasionally, to evaluate the VM as a whole, multiple direct punctures under ultrasound or fluoroscopic guidance are required to avoid injecting contrast medium into the interstitial space between the irregular cavities. The malformation can be characterised either by an apparent absence of drainage and connections with the regional venous system or by the presence of different size connections and the escape of contrast medium to the superficial and deep system.

13.8.5 Arteriovenous Malformations

AVMs present as localised, warm, and pulsating tumefactions. The main finding on standard x-ray examination is swelling of soft tissues with vascular ectasia in the region of the arteriovenous fistula

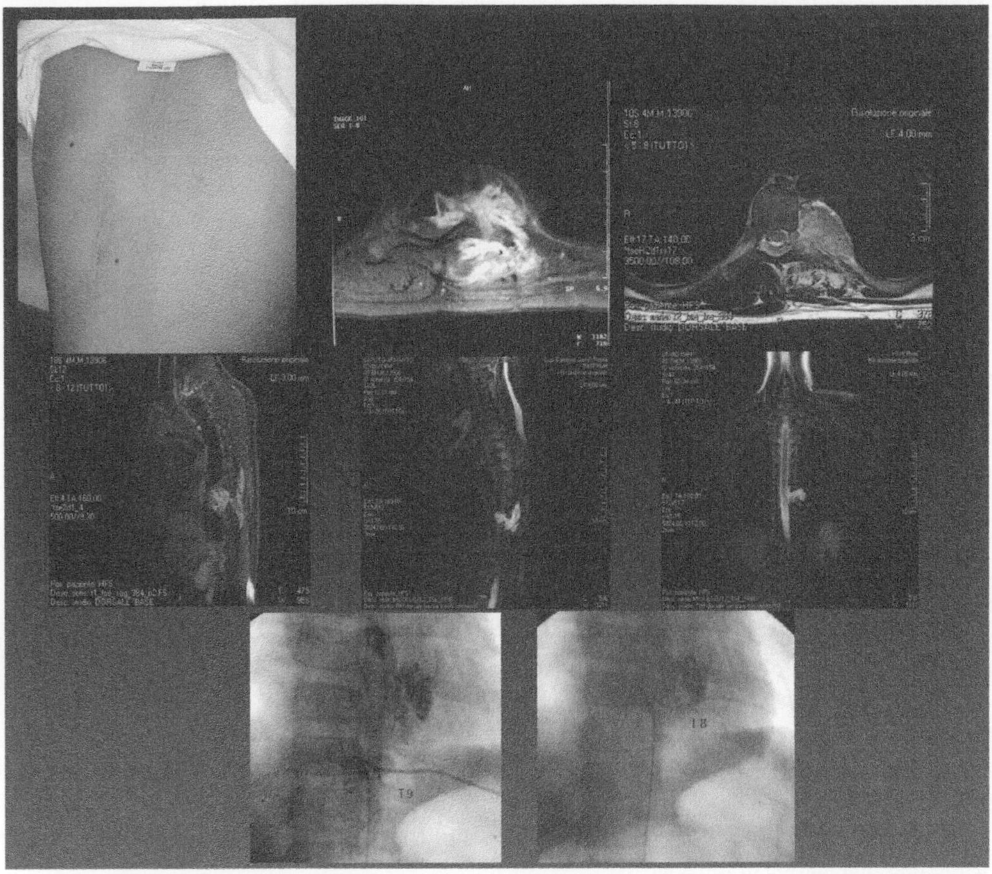

FIGURE 13.45 Surgical scar in the paravertebral back seat in previous suspicion of lipomatous lesion detected elsewhere to examination ultrasonography. Intervention in other structure interrupted by copious intraoperative bleeding. The subsequent study in greater detail Sat Fat suppressed T2-axial MRI (top) and in the sagittal and coronal (bottom left) and intercostal selective arteriography at an early stage and advanced, MV showed a deep intramuscular and intra-thoracic spine with intracanal footprint on the bone. Clinically, the patient presented intense pain and paresthesias in the dorsal region in various episodes repeated.

as a result of large vein flow (Jablecki et al. 2013; Pompa et al. 2011; Wassef 2011b). Occasionally, regional bones may also show increased volume.

Colour Doppler ultrasonography is the elective diagnostic test for AVMs (Figure 13.47). It shows a typical colourimetric signal due to the presence of fast arterial flows with a variable course and turbulence. Pulsed Doppler shows a high pick rate and diastolic rate related to the low resistance in the fistula. Flow metre findings of afferent arterial vessels may provide information on the haemodynamic relevance of the fistula and are particularly useful for follow-up therapy. Colour Doppler ultrasonography gives also useful information on muscular involvement (Orhan et al. 2012; Pompa et al. 2012; Somasundaram et al. 2013) (Figure 13.48).

CT scan may be particularly useful to identify concomitant cerebral, abdominal, or deep pelvic vascular malformations as well as to determine the size of larger and deeper malformations (Kakimoto et al. 2005; R.A. MD and ChB 2011). AVMs appear as a tangled web of serpiginous tubular structures on MRI with the absence of signal in both arterial and venous fast-flow vessels. The signal intensity in T2-weighted sequences may indicate the flow rate in the centre of the malformation (JF et al. 2002) (Figure 13.49). Slow-flow areas appear as small hyperintense dots within the lesion, while although the AVM centre is at fast flow, the absence of signal does not allow a clear

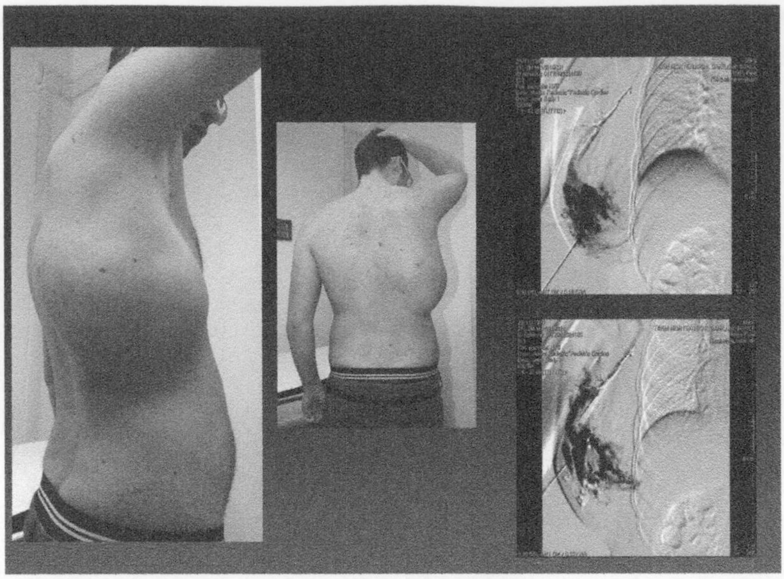

FIGURE 13.46 Clinical presentation and direct puncture venography of the chest wall extended right VM has already undergone previous arterial embolization to no avail. Spongy appearance of dysmorphic and malformation.

differentiation between the centre and the other parts of the malformation. The clear differentiation between muscle and fat by MRI allows to accurately determine the extension of the AVM into the surrounding anatomical areas (Restrepo 2013). It is limited by not being able to distinguish between invasion and dislocation of muscle.

Rapid sequence angiography of AVMs allows the observation of branch arteries and draining veins and localisation of fistulas. Arterious branches appear hypertrophic, contorted with rapid flow and with evident fistulas, and should be evaluated selectively (occasionally via coaxial catheters). There is no evidence of parenchymal opacisation that is typical of haemangiomas. Draining venous vessels are also contorted and dilated (A.M.K. MD and MD 2011; Pompa et al. 2012) (Figure 13.50).

13.9 INTERVENTIONAL RADIOLOGY IN VASCULAR ANOMALIES

Interventional radiology is a newer treatment option for vascular anomalies that is minimally invasive and, where possible, avoids post-surgical scars (Pompa et al. 2011, 2012). Angioradiological intervention is a type of endovascular surgery which in the main includes

- Embolisation
- Sclerotherapy
- Scleroembolisation

to manage pathologies where it is necessary to occlude/reduce cavities or pathological communications. Angioplasty and stenting can be used, albeit infrequently, for the treatment of venous congenital stenoses (Anon. 2009). Loco-regional thrombolytic therapy may be used in certain exceptions when it is necessary to reduce thrombus size and also during the acute phase of treatment (Richard and Julie 2010).

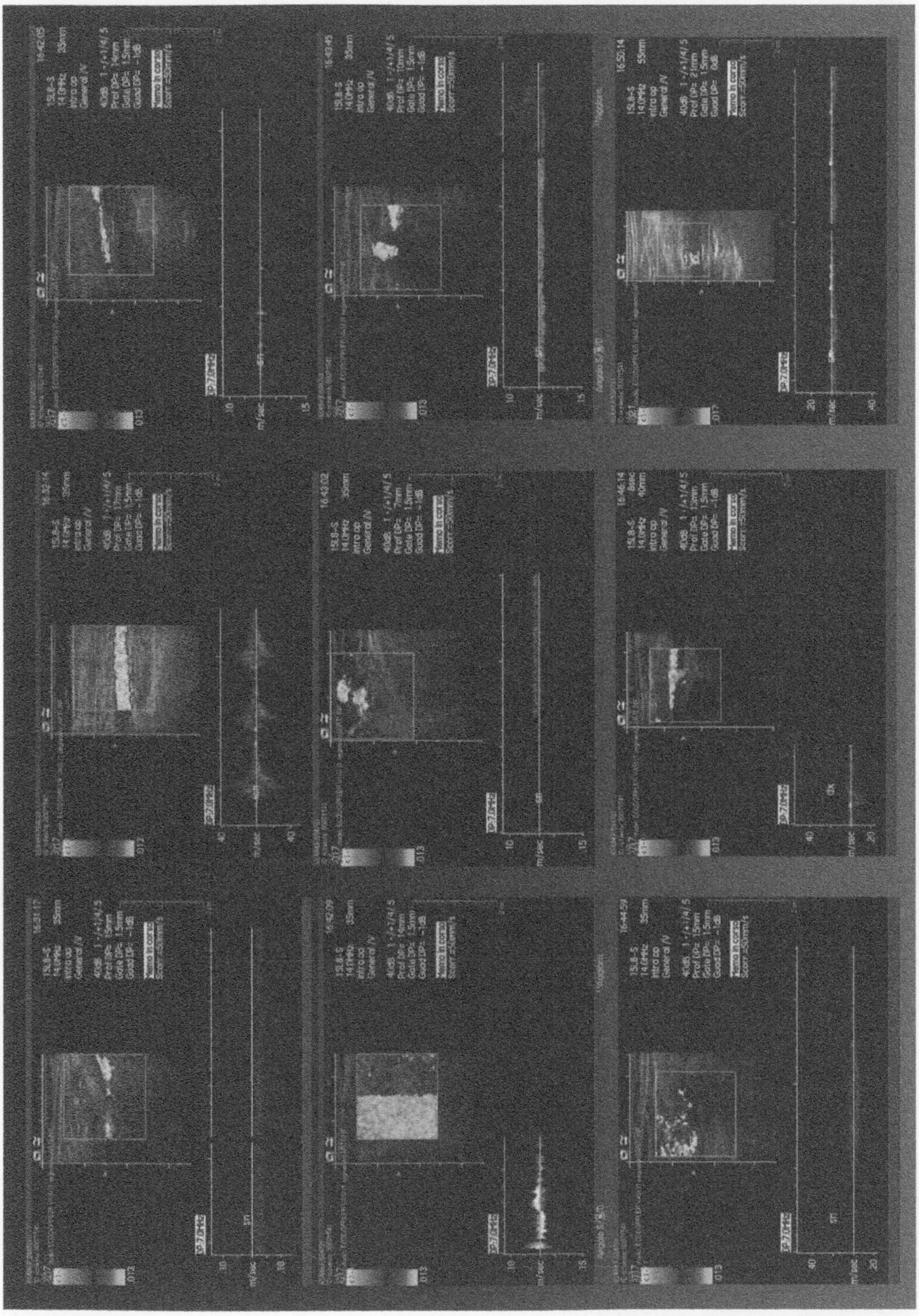

FIGURE 13.47 Ultrasonography of AVM in several sequential samplings.

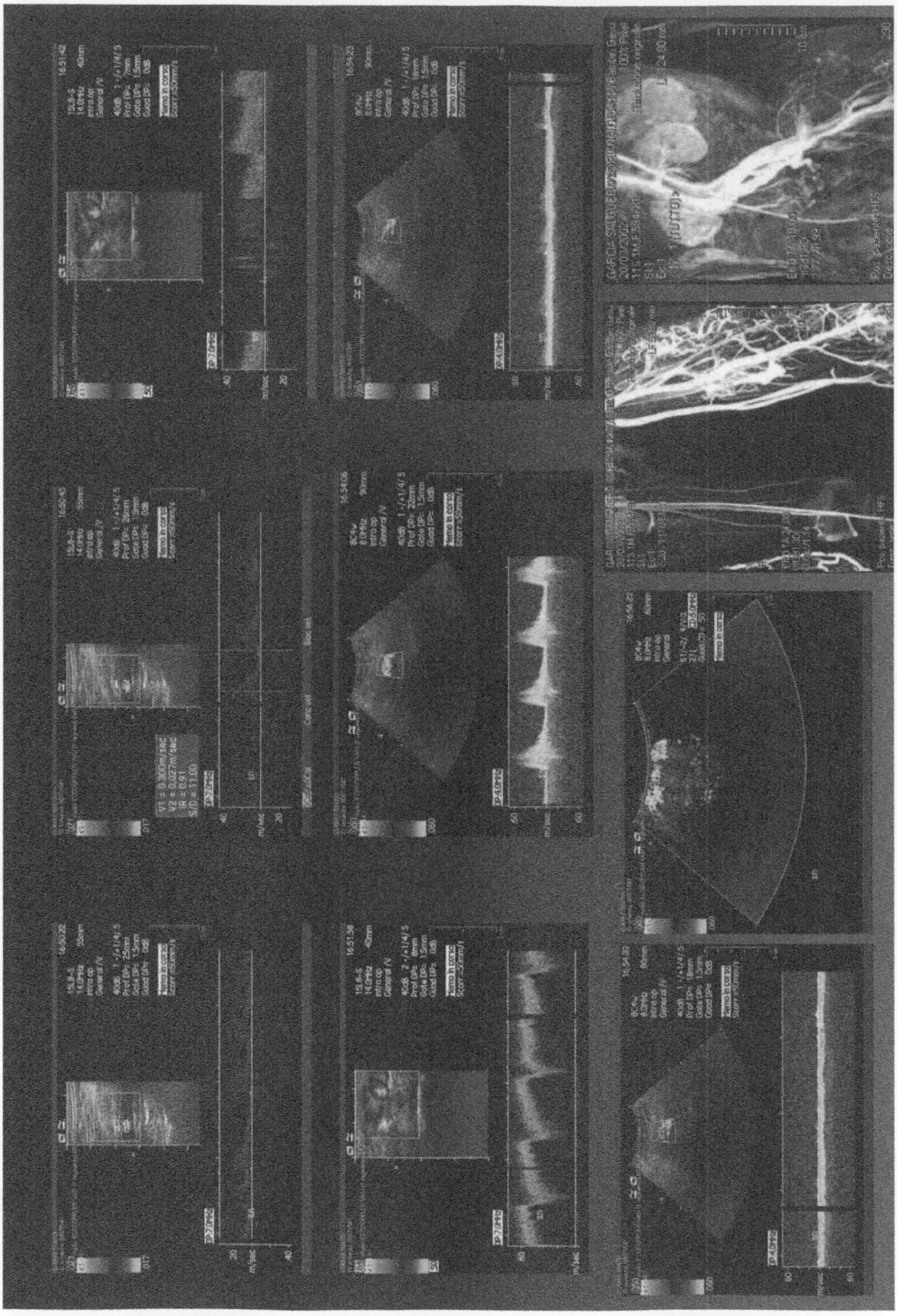

FIGURE 13.48 Same case as previous figure, with integration in the lower right of MRA.

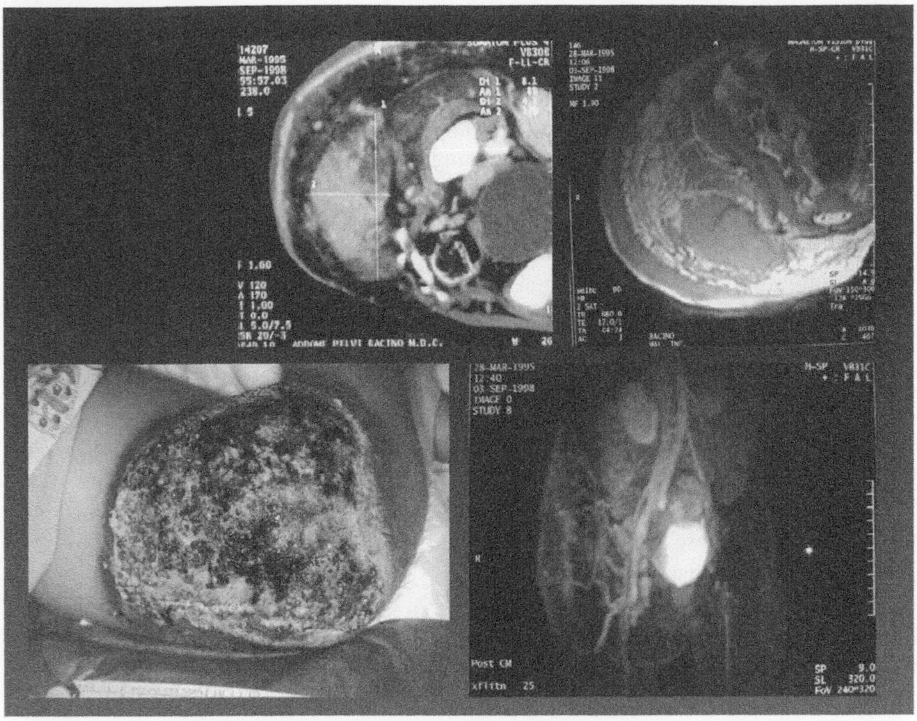

FIGURE 13.49 Ulcerated and infected AVM of the right gluteal region at the bottom left. Deterioration of the general condition of the child. Axial MRI (top) and MRA (lower right).

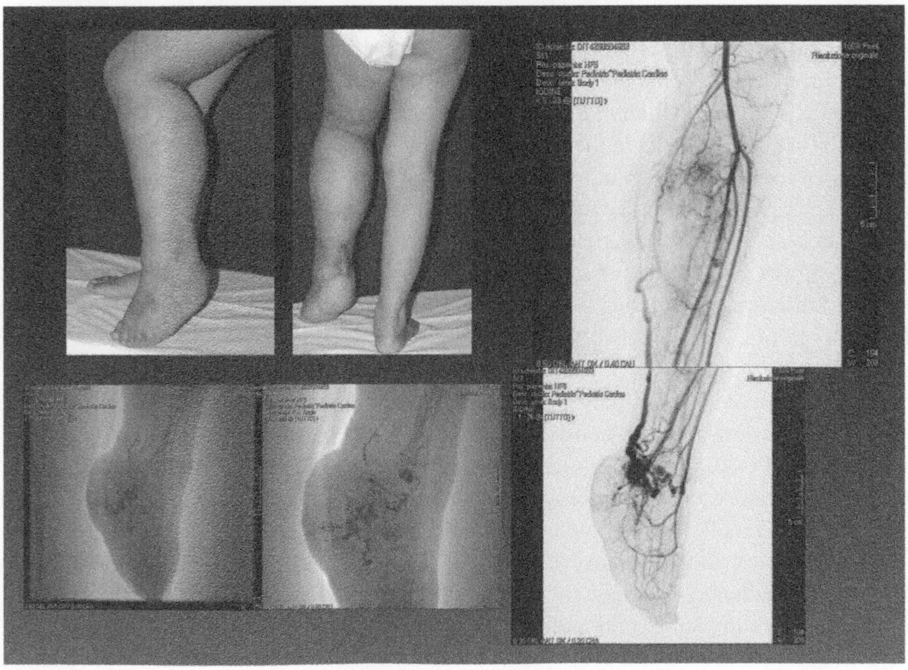

FIGURE 13.50 Lower limb AVM from the leg to the foot. At the bottom left, you can see the Onyx emboli in calcaneal region. On the right image is the subtraction angiography (digital subtraction angiography) after an initial embolization of the most distal portion involving the calcaneal region.

13.9.1 Embolisation (or Embolotherapy)

All the occlusive procedures may be used alone, preoperatively as an adjuvant to surgery, or postoperatively (Stefan et al. 2003). Haemangioma embolisation does not usually produce good long-term outcomes for the haemodynamic characteristics of this pathology. Embolisation may act as a palliative therapy to control symptoms in haemangiomas that are resistant to medical therapy or when congestive heart failure due to increased flow develops (Bhavsar et al. 2012; Lazic et al. 2012; MMSc and PhD 2011; Pompa et al. 2012). In these cases, particularly in liver multiple localisations, the goal is to reduce shunt until the beginning of the involution phase.

Interventional radiology for vascular malformations has two approaches:

1. Arterial by superselective catheterisation and embolisation
2. Venous by percutaneous puncture or venous catheterisation

In exclusively or predominantly venous malformations, the venous approach is preferred. While in the management of AVMs, one or both approaches may be employed when necessary. The arterial route requires distal catheterisation to reach the centre, and therefore the use of specific catheters (occasionally coaxial), tailored for each case and of suitable embolisation materials, is mandatory (Pompa et al. 2011).

Materials used in embolisation include

- Liquids
- Particles
- Coils and plugs
- Detachable balloons

Liquids – the tissue adhesives *N*-butyl-2-cyanoacrylate (NBCA), a patented ethylene vinyl alcohol (EVOH) often referred to as *glues*, are frequently used (C.P. D 2007; Eivazi and Werner 2013). Glues are rapidly hardening liquids that polymerise on contact with blood. They are not radiopaque per se but may be mixed with other opaque substances such as LIPIODOL® (ethyl esters of iodised fatty acids of poppyseed oil) and tantalum (E et al. 2006). One of the advantages of these substances in addition to their fluidity which makes injection even into microcatheters easier is that they provide the possibility of regularising the time of polymerisation with the addition of substances such as LIPIODOL or iophendylate (Pantopaque). Thus, it is possible to calculate the time taken to reach the centre following injection of a contrast medium and to modulate the time of polymerisation.

Onyx is a non-adhesive liquid embolic agent used for embolisation of arteriovenous malformations (bAVM). Onyx is composed of an EVOH copolymer dissolved in dimethyl sulfoxide (DMSO) and suspended micronised tantalum powder to provide contrast for visualisation under fluoroscopy. Onyx is available in two product formulations, Onyx 18 (6% EVOH) and Onyx 34 (8% EVOH) (Figure 13.50).

Particles are biocompatible, accurately calibrated particles that can either be resorbable or nonresorbable according to their composition. Resorbable microspheres are composed of fibrin sponge particles (SPONGOSTAN) used in preoperative embolisations, and their occlusive effect is limited to 48 h. Nonresorbable microspheres are composed of solid polymers such as polyvinyl alcohol (DuPont, Elvanol), hydroxylated polyvinyl acetal (PVAc) sponge (IVALON), Contour PVA Embolization Particles, and PVA particles (Embospheres) and have a range of particle sizes to meet the differing requirements to occlude the fistula under examination (Figure 13.51).

To render them radiopaque, they are mixed with contrast medium during embolisation under fluoroscopic control to ensure that the correct amount is used and to stop the procedure when occlusion has occurred. To obtain a longer-lasting effect, it is possible to use a mixture of resorbable and nonresorbable particles together with small quantities of ethanol and iodine contrast medium to attain a result similar to that obtained with glues but with a much reduced inflammatory reaction.

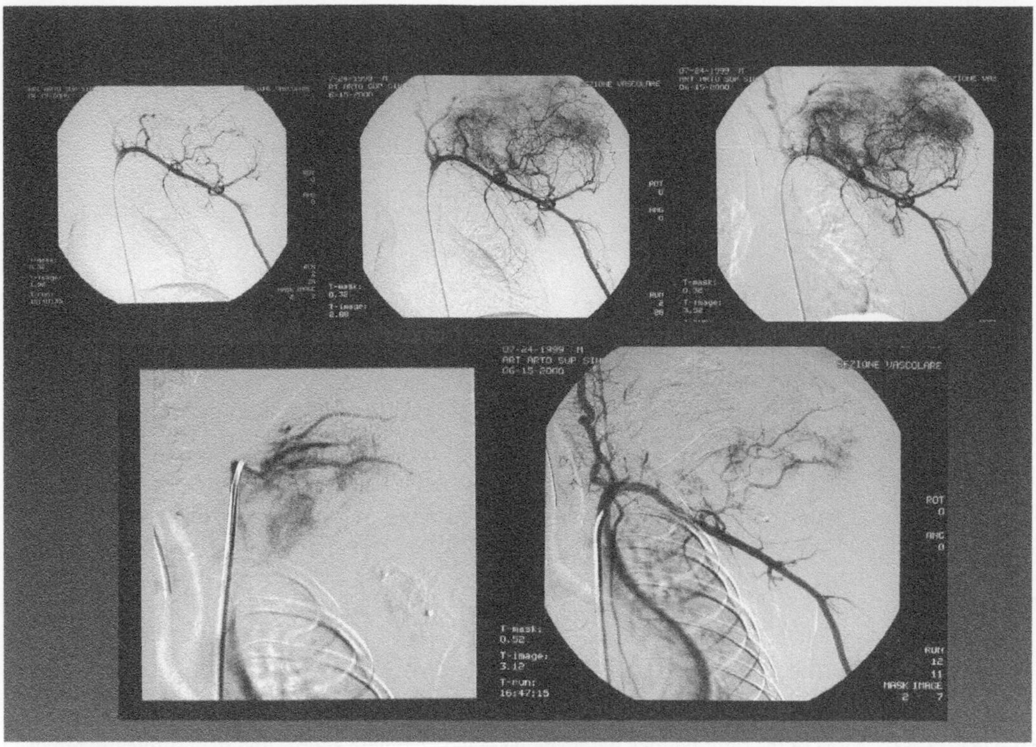

FIGURE 13.51 Kasabach–Merritt syndrome caused by tufted IH of the left shoulder girdle. Digital subtraction angiography at the top and result at the bottom after embolization, performed with PVA particles.

Metal coils are devices generally made of metals such as platinum that when introduced into the human body are compatible with subsequent MRI examinations (Alex and Aryeh 2002). Coils are introduced as strings inside catheters that coil around to form a plug after reaching their position in the target vessel. Occlusion with single or multiple coils is equivalent to a surgical ligature of the same vessel. Coils are available in many types with different sizes and forms, and certain types have fibre tails to produce a greater occluding effect and allow fibrin deposition on their surface. They may be introduced through a catheter already in situ and together with liquid polymerising glues to obtain immediate occlusion (Anon. 2010; M.E. L et al. 2001; MMSc and PhD 2011) (Figure 13.52).

Detachable balloons are catheter-delivered devices that can be inflated under radioscopic control and detached in the selected place to result in immediate vessel occlusion. Balloons are available in a wide range of sizes and may be used also for occlusion of large fistulas with a single feeding artery (Buttarelli et al. 2011). Currently, the plugs are in increasing development, which are devices of nitinol nester of various diameters, introduced in the target desired through catheters, and freed only when it holds to have reached the centre of the lesion and the desirable effect (Herbreteau 2007; R et al. 2001) (Figures 13.53 and 13.54).

Materials used in embolisation are in continuous evolution as is the development of new techniques and new approaches. Therefore, a new perspective for the management of these pathologies is opening, as interstitial laser therapy (Brauer and Geronemus 2013; Poetke and Berlien 2005; SPENDEL et al. 2001) and radio-frequency ablation (A.M.K. MD and MD 2011; MMSc et al. 2011), to be performed always under ultrasonographic, fluoroscopic guidance. In AVMs, the approach to the venous vessels, with or without arterial embolisation, seems to be more effective in both the medium and long term (J.U. MD et al. 1999).

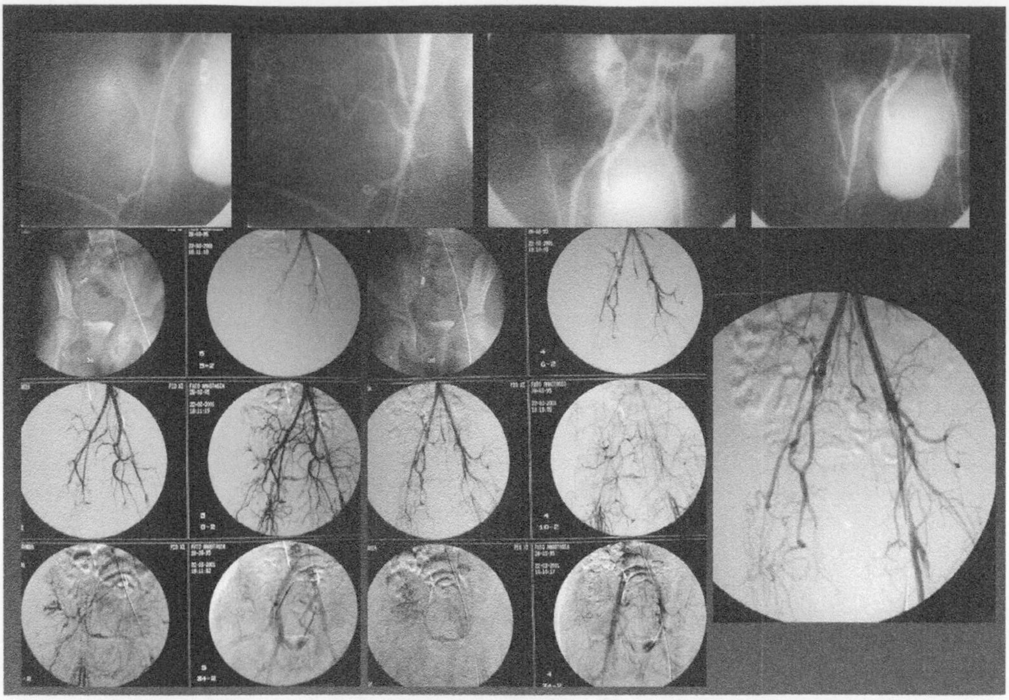

FIGURE 13.52 AVM of the right buttock before being embolized with spirals and then surgically removed.

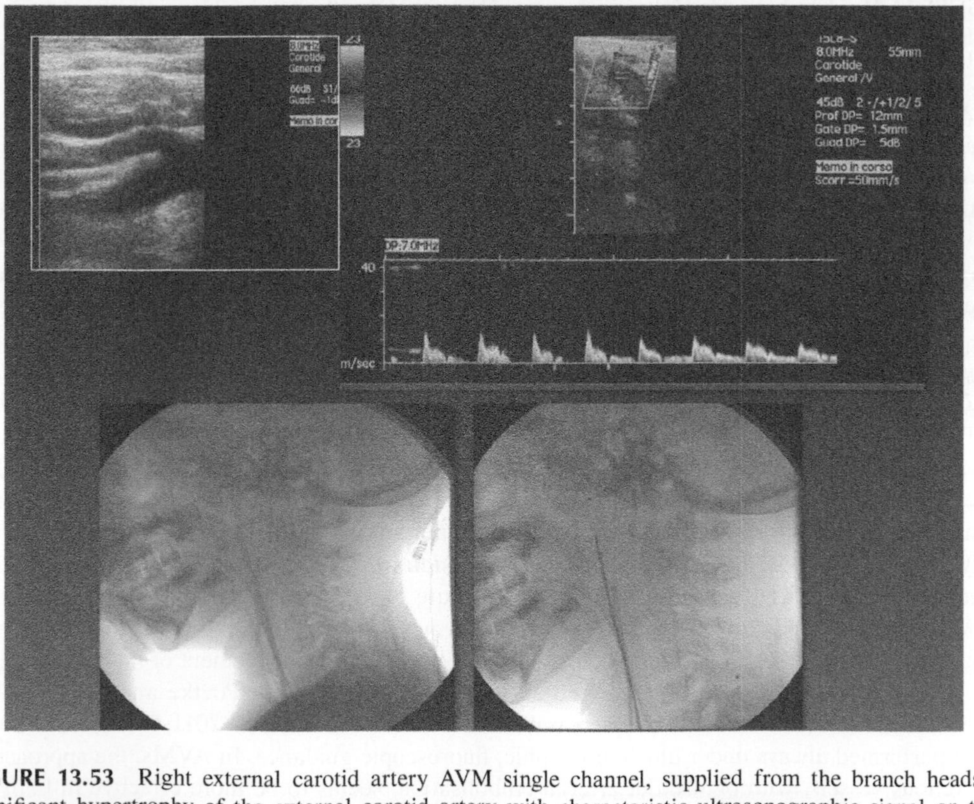

FIGURE 13.53 Right external carotid artery AVM single channel, supplied from the branch headset. Significant hypertrophy of the external carotid artery with characteristic ultrasonographic signal on top. Angiographic images during the procedure with the Amplatzer™ embolization (bottom).

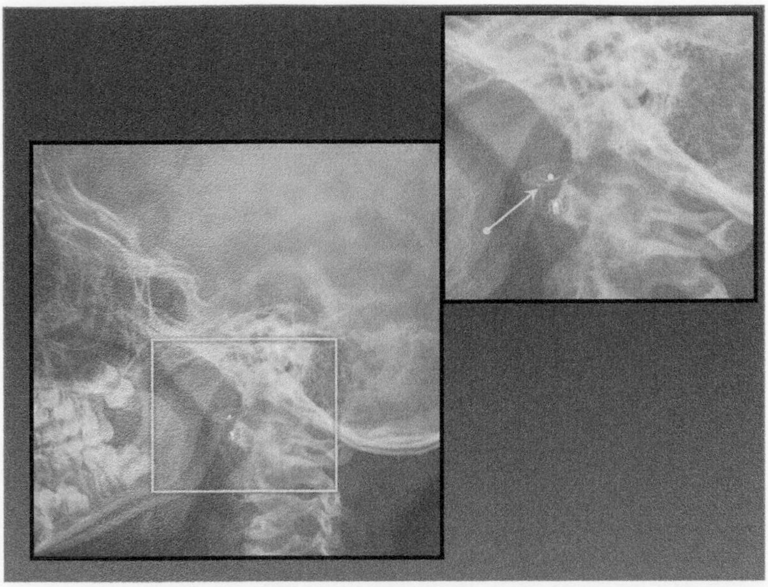

FIGURE 13.54 Same case as the previous image. Check the Amplatzer™ Plug after 8 months. The latter remained in the released position with the definitive closure of the fistula.

Occlusion of venous vessels eliminates low-pressure varices that are not treated by arterial embolisation and as a result may improve treatment of small arterial pedicles that may have left after each embolisation. The venous approach produces excellent results as demonstrated by post-embolisation arteriography and in addition may also be safer – mainly for limb malformations – as vascular spasms and the possible embolisation of digital branches are avoided.

13.10 SCLEROTHERAPY

Sclerotherapy is the direct or retrograde injection of an irritant agent into venous and lymphatic lesion (Batista Rodrigues Johann et al. 2005; Mariano et al. 2011). Compounds used in sclerotherapy include sodium tetradecyl sulphate (STS) (Fibro-Vein™) and polidocanol (Asclera® and Aethoxysklerol®), available in different concentrations. The STS is approved in several countries as foam to increase the volume and enhance effects on vascular walls. Opacisation requires combination with iodine contrast medium, which allows observation during injection (Figure 13.55). These irritant agents are particularly useful in VMs and superficial/submucosal LMs to reduce the risk of chemical necrosis and the subsequent development of cutaneous or mucosal ulcers. The same agents at lower concentrations are also used as sclerotherapy of lower extremity varices (Figure 13.56).

13.11 SCLEROEMBOLISATION

Scleroembolisation is a therapeutic procedure using mainly Ethibloc® and absolute ethanol. Ethibloc (Ethnor Laboratories/Ethicon, Norderstedt, Germany) is a semi-liquid, radiopaque mixture of four agents that have occludent and sclerosant activity (zein, alcohol, oleum papaveris, propylene glycol, and a contrast medium) (Stefan et al. 2003; Tyagi et al. 2006). Ethibloc emulsion precipitates after contact with blood and has a sustained effect after approximately 30–60 days on the vascular wall before reabsorption. It should be injected subcutaneously under fluoroscopic control into dysplastic cavities (R et al. 2001). Multiple needles distributed on the whole lesion can also be employed (Figures 13.57 and 13.58). Following treatment antibiotic and anti-inflammatory

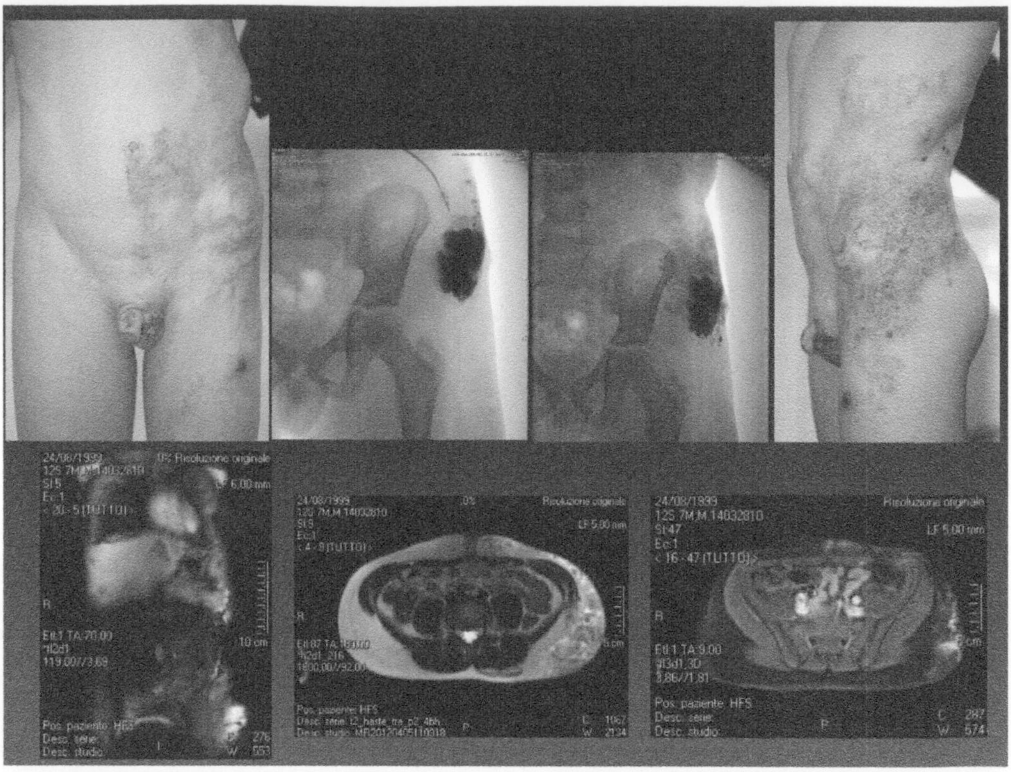

FIGURE 13.55 Wide VM of the left thoraco-abdominal wall. Direct puncture venography and sclerotherapy with STS 3% on center top. Coronal and axial MRI showing the extensive subcutaneous location of the malformation at the bottom.

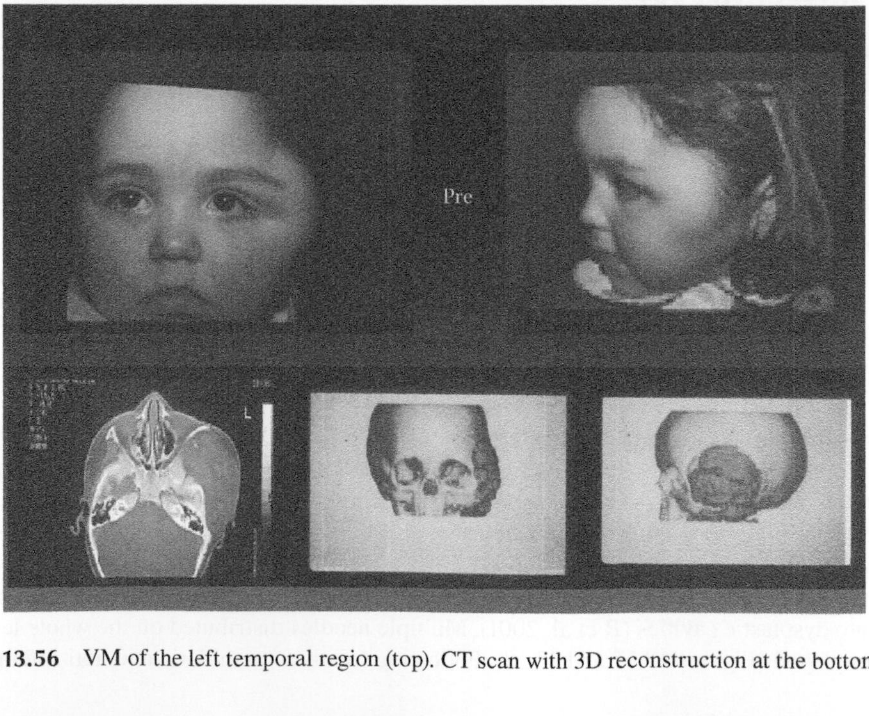

FIGURE 13.56 VM of the left temporal region (top). CT scan with 3D reconstruction at the bottom right.

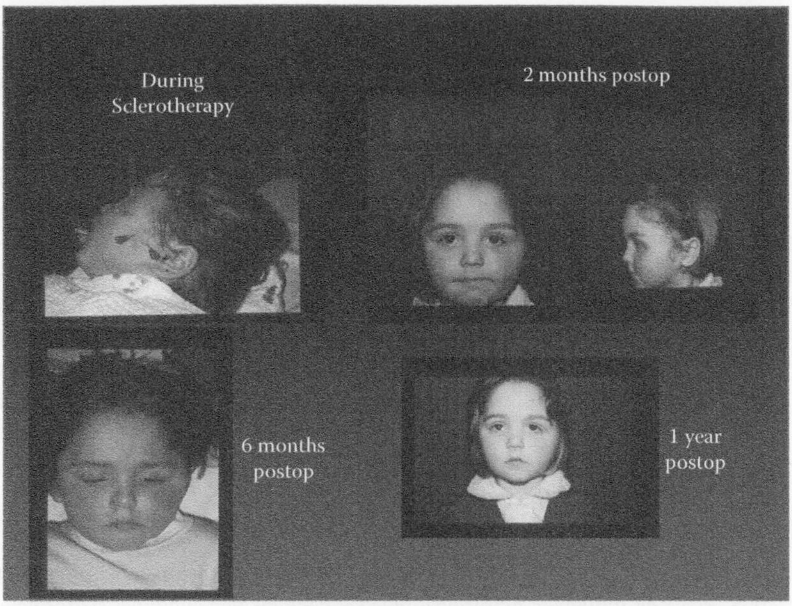

FIGURE 13.57 Same case during scleroembolization with ethibloc, through multiple stings (top left). Top right is two months follow-up after treatment. Bottom left is 6 months and bottom right after 1 year follow-up.

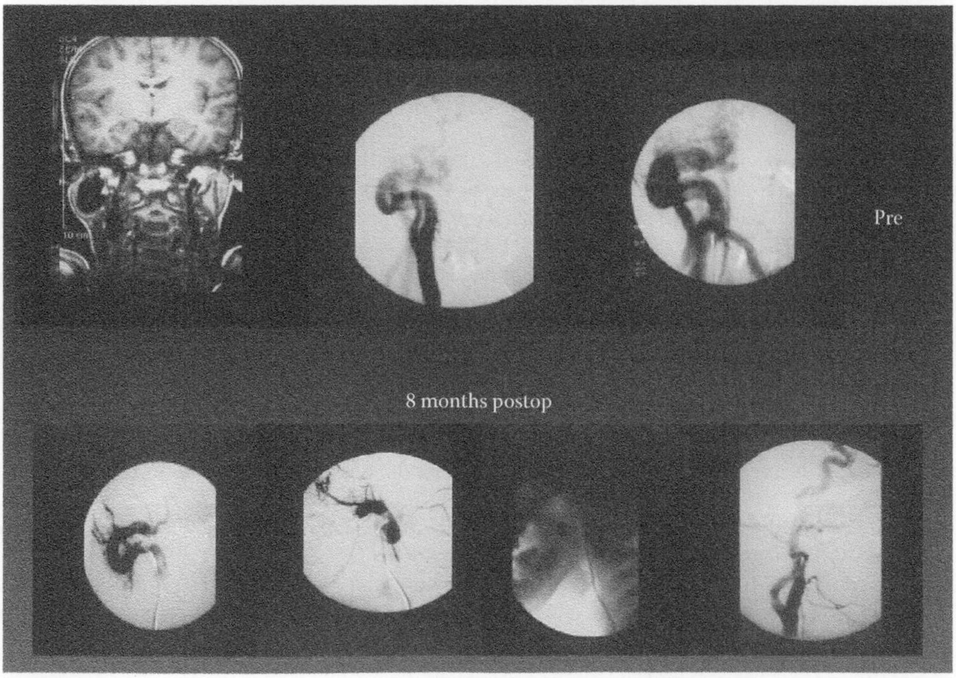

FIGURE 13.58 Right ear region AVM single channel. T1-MRI, top left. Right carotid angiography and selective external carotid artery in the upper right, prior to treatment. Bottom left are phases of intraoperative embolization performed with spirals. In the lower right, 8 months follow-up of the right carotid artery, which shows the complete disappearance of the fistula with a reduction of the caliber of the external carotid artery.

agents are recommended, the former due to the risk of infection and formation of abscesses and the latter because of the risk of irritation/inflammation of the vascular walls. Recently, Ethibloc was used also as percutaneous therapy of aneurysmal bone cysts that can be considered intraosseous VM. Currently, Ethibloc® is not in commerce anymore.

Absolute ethanol (95% or 96%), a highly aggressive agent used in the treatment of VMs, causes instant coagulation of the cavity into which it is injected (Eivazi and Werner 2013; Guéro 2007). When combined with a small quantity of iodine contrast medium, the extent of the malformation can be visualised. The advantages of this procedure include the lack of allergic reactions and uncomplicated metabolisation, but care should be taken to avoid it entering the venous circle as it is toxic to the myocardium and the recommended dosage of <0.5 mL/kg of body weight given in divided dosages should be closely adhered to. Due to the risk of nerve damage, its use near main nervous branches, mainly of the lower limbs, should be avoided as ethanol has effects on the vasa nervorum – small arteries that provide blood supply to peripheral nerves (Laurian et al. 2004; Mariano et al. 2011).

REFERENCES

Adams, M.D. January 1, 2011. Special considerations in vasculara: Hematologic management. *Clinics in Plastic Surgery* 38(1): 153–160.

Adouani, A., J. Bouguila, M.A. Abdelali, M. Ben Aicha, A. Landolsi, M. Hellali, K. Zitouni, I. Mahri, and I. Zairi. 2008. Place du traitement chirurgical précoce dans les hémangiomes périorificiels de la face. *Annales De Chirurgie Plastique Esthétique* 53(5): 435–440.

Agrawal, A., P. Banode, and S. Shukla. 2012. Giant cavernous hemangiomas of the brain. *Asian Journal of Neurosurgery* 7(4): 220–222.

Akcay, A., Z. Karakas, E.T. Saribeyoglu, A. Unuvar, C. Baykal, M. Garipardic, S. Anak, L. Agaoglu, G. Ozturk, and O. Devecioglu. 2012. Infantile hemangiomas, complications and follow-up. *Indian Pediatrics* 49(10): 805–809.

Alex, Z. and M. Aryeh. 2002. Hemangiomas and vascular malformations: Unapproved treatments. *Clinics in Dermatology* 20: 660–667.

Andrea, R. and T.-D. Paolo. 2006. Agenesis carotid in FHACE. *American Journal of Neuroradiology* 9: 1062.

Angiero, F., S. Benedicenti, A. Benedicenti, K. Arcieri, and E. Bernè. August 24, 2009. Head and neck hemangiomas in pediatric patients treated with endolesional 980-nm diode laser. Ed. Mary Ann Liebert, Inc. *Photomedicine and Laser Surgery* 00: 1–7.

Anon. 2001. Magnetic resonance imaging findings of vascular malformations of the lower extremity. 1–7.

Anon. 2009. Antithrombotics: Indications and management. 1–74.

Anon. 2010. Trattamento chirurgico delle malformazioni vascolari superficiali e degli emangiomi della faccia. 1–18.

Arita, H., H. Kishima, K. Hosomi, K. Iwaisako, N. Hashimoto, Y. Saitoh, and T. Yoshimine. 2012. Hemifacial spasm caused by intra-axial brainstem cavernous angioma with venous angiomas. *British Journal of Neurosurgery* 26(2): 281–283.

Arneja, J.S., H. Chim, B.A. Drolet, and A.K. Gosain. 2010. The cyrano nose: Refinements in surgical technique and treatment approach to hemangiomas of the nasal tip. *Plastic and Reconstructive Surgery* 126(4): 1291–1299.

Arneja, J.S. and A.K. Gosain. 2008. Vascular malformations. *Plastic and Reconstructive Surgery* 121(4): 195e–206e.

Arnold, R. and G. Chaudry. 2011. Diagnostic imaging of vascular anomalies. *Clinics in Plastic Surgery* 38(1): 21–29.

Azizkhan, R.G., M.J. Rutter, R.T. Cotton, L.H.Y. Lim, A.P. Cohen, and J.L. Mason. 2006. Lymphatic malformations of the tongue base. *Journal of Pediatric Surgery* 41(7): 1279–1284.

Ballah, D., A.M. Cahill, L. Fontalvo, A. Yan, J. Treat, D. Low, and M. Epelman. 2011. Vascular anomalies: What they are, how to diagnose them, and how to treat them. *Current Problems in Diagnostic Radiology* 40(6): 233–247.

Batista Rodrigues Johann, A.C., M.C.F. Aguiar, M.A. Vieira do Carmo, R.S. Gomez, W.H. Castro, and R.A. Mesquita. 2005. Sclerotherapy of benign oral vascular lesion with ethanolamine oleate: An open clinical trial with 30 lesions. *Oral Surgery, Oral Medicine, Oral Pathology, Oral Radiology, and Endodontology* 100(5): 579–584.

Bauland, C.G., M.A.M. van Steensel, P.M. Steijlen, P.N.M.A. Rieu, and P.H.M. Spauwen. 2006. The pathogenesis of hemangiomas: A review. *Plastic and Reconstructive Surgery* 117(2): 29e–35e.

Beck, D.O. and A.K. Gosain. 2009. The presentation and management of hemangiomas. *Plastic and Reconstructive Surgery* 123(6): 181e–191e.
Behr, G.G. and C. Johnson. 2013a. Vascular anomalies: Hemangiomas and beyond – Part 1, Fast-flow lesions. *American Journal of Roentgenology* 200(2): 414–422.
Behr, G.G. and C.M. Johnson. 2013b. Vascular anomalies: Hemangiomas and beyond – Part 2, Slow-flow lesions. *American Journal of Roentgenology* 200(2): 423–436.
Berzigotti, A. and F. Piscaglia. 2011. Ultrasound in portal hypertension – Part 1. *Ultraschall in Der Medizin (Stuttgart, Germany: 1980)* 32(6): 548–568 – quiz 569–571.
Bhavsar, T., J. Wurzel, and N. Duker. 2012. Myometrial cavernous hemangioma with pulmonary thromboembolism in a post-partum woman: A case report and review of the literature. *Journal of Medical Case Reports* 6(1): 397.
Bing, H., L. Ralph, P. Jeffrey, P. Shi-Kaung, and S. Lance. 2006. Kasabach–Merritt syndrome-associated kaposiform hemangioendothelioma successfully treated with cyclophosphamide, vincristine, and actinomycin D. *Journal of Pediatric Hematology/Oncology Endocrinology and Metabolism* 20(12): 567–569.
Boon, L.M., P.E. Burrows, H.J. Paltiel, D.P. Lund, R.A. Ezekowitz, J. Folkman, and J.B. Mulliken. 2007. Hepatic vascular anomalies in infancy: A twenty-seven-year experience. *The Journal of Pediatrics* 129: 346–354.
Brandie, M., R. Melissa, L.M. Levy, and D.W. Metry. 2004. Response of ulcerated perineal hemangiomas of infancy to becaplermin gel, a recombinant human platelet-derived growth factor. *Archives of Dermatological Research* 140(2): 1–4. http://www.archdermatol.com.
Brauer, J.A. and R.G. Geronemus. 2013. Laser treatment in the management of infantile hemangiomas and capillary vascular malformations. *Techniques in Vascular and Interventional Radiology* 16(1): 51–54.
Breugem, C.C., M. Maas, J.A. Reekers, and C.M.A.M. van der Horst. September 15, 2001. Use of magnetic resonance imaging for the evaluation of vascular malformations of the lower extremity. *Plastic and Reconstructive Surgery* 108(4): 870–877.
Britney. 2007. Vascular anomalies: Classification and update, Personal oral communication in California University of San Francisco, 1–60.
Bronzetti, G., A. Giardini, A. Patrizi, D. Prandstraller, A. Donti, R. Formigari, M. Bonvicini, and F.M. Picchio. 2004. Ipsilateral hemangioma and aortic arch anomalies in posterior fossa malformations, hemangiomas, arterial anomalies, coarctation of the aorta, and cardiac defects and eye abnormalities (PHACE) anomaly: Report and review. *Pediatrics* 113(2): 412–415.
Bruckner, A.L. and I.J. Frieden. 2006. Infantile hemangiomas. *Journal of the American Academy of Dermatology* 55(4): 671–682.
Burget, G.C. 2009. Preliminary review of pediatric nasal reconstruction with detailed report of one case. *Plastic and Reconstructive Surgery* 124(3): 907–918.
Burke, R.M., R.J. Morin, C.A. Perlyn, B. Laure, and S.A. Wolfe. January 1, 2011. Special considerations in vascular anomalies: Operative management of craniofacial osseous lesions. *Clinics in Plastic Surgery* 38(1): 133–142.
Buttarelli, L., E. Capocasale, C. Marcato, M.P. Mazzoni, M. Iaria, and C. Rossi. 2011. Embolization of pancreatic allograft arteriovenous fistula with the amplatzer vascular plug 4: Case report and literature analysis. *Transplantation Proceedings* 43(10): 4044–4047.
C, V.J., B. Joaquim, and V. Miguel. 2004. MR and MR angiography characterization of soft tissue vascular malformations. *Current Problems in Diagnostic Radiology* 8: 1–10.
Carinci, S., S. Tumini, N.P. Consilvio, P. Cipriano, A. Di Stefano, N. Vercellino, P. Dalmonte, and F. Chiarelli. 2012. A case of congenital hypothyroidism in PHACE syndrome. *Journal of Pediatric Endocrinology and Metabolism* 25(5–6): 603–605.
Casanova, D., L.M. Boon, and M. Vikkula. 2006. Les malformations veineuses: Aspects cliniques et diagnostic différentiel. *Annales De Chirurgie Plastique Esthétique* 51(4–5): 373–387.
Chalouhi, N., A.S. Dumont, C. Randazzo, S. Tjoumakaris, L.F. Gonzalez, R. Rosenwasser, and P. Jabbour. 2011. Management of incidentally discovered intracranial vascular abnormalities. *Neurosurgical Focus* 31(6): E1.
Cheng, N.-C., D.-M. Lai, M.-H. Hsie, S.-L. Liao, and Y.-B.T. Chen. 2006. Intraosseous hemangiomas of the facial bone. *Plastic and Reconstructive Surgery* 117(7): 2366–2372.
Choi, Y.J., S.R. Jee, K.S. Park, C.H. Ryu, H.R. Seo, S.I. Ha, S.H. Lee, and K.S. Ok. 2011. Involvement of splenic hemangioma and rectal varices in a patient with klippel: Trenaunay syndrome. *The Korean Journal of Gastroenterology Taehan Sohwagi Hakhoe Chi* 58(3): 157–161.
Christine, L.L., De la Roque Eric Dumas, and H. Thomas. 2008. Propranolol for severe hemangiomas of infancy. *New England Journal of Medicine* 6(12): 2649–2651. http://www.nejm.org.
Christine, L.L. 2008. Quels angiomes faut-il surveiller et traiter? *Journal de Pediatrie et de Puericulture* 11: 395–399.

Conway, M. and S.L. Hosking. 2012. Investigation of ocular hemodynamics in Sturge–Weber syndrome. *Optometry and Vision Science: Official Publication of the American Academy of Optometry* 89(6): 922–928.

Corr, P.D. September 27, 2007. Cirsoid aneurysm of the scalp. *Singapore Medical Journal* 48(10): 268–269.

D, C.P. 2007. Cirsoid aneurysm of the scalp. *Singapore Medical Journal* 48(10): 268–269.

D, H.K., J. P, H.P. Kozakewich, J.U. MD, and P.E. Burrows. 2002. Venous malformations of skeletal muscle. *Plastic and Reconstructive Surgery* 110: 1–11.

Degrugillier-Chopinet, C., A. Bisdorff-Bresson, C. Laurian, G.-M. Breviere, D. Staumont, P. Fayoux, D. Lenica, and C. Gautier. 2011. Role of duplex doppler for superficial "angiomas". *Journal Des Maladies Vasculaires* 36(6): 348–354.

Drolet, B.A., E.A. Swanson, and I.J. Frieden. 2008. Infantile hemangiomas: An emerging health issue linked to an increased rate of low birth weight infants. *The Journal of Pediatrics* 153(5): 712.e1–715.e1.

Drolet, B.A. 2006. Early stroke and cerebral vasculopathy in children with facial hemangiomas and PHACE association. *Pediatrics* 117(3): 959–964.

Dubois, J., G. Laurent, G. Andrée, P.T.F.R.C.S.A.D.J.D.F.D.S.R.C.S.F.R.C. S, T.J. David, L.C. Laberge, F. Denis, and J. Powell. 2007. Imaging of hemangiomas and vascular malformations in children. *Academic Radiology* 5(5): 390–400.

Eivazi, B. and J.A. Werner. 2013. Management of vascular malformations and hemangiomas of the head and neck - An update. *Current Opinion in Otolaryngology and Head and Neck Surgery* 21(2): 157–163.

El-Merhi, F., D. Garg, M. Cura, and O. Ghaith. 2013. Peripheral vascular tumors and vascular malformations: Imaging (magnetic resonance imaging and conventional angiography), pathologic correlation and treatment options. *The International Journal of Cardiovascular Imaging* 29(2): 379–393.

Elluru, R.G. 2013. Cutaneous vascular lesions. *Facial Plastic Surgery Clinics of NA* 21(1): 111–126.

Enjolras, O. 2004. Anomalies vasculaires superficielles («angiomes»). *EMC – Pédiatrie* 1(2): 129–151.

Enjolras, O. 2004. Dermatologue, responsable des consultations des angiomes Anomalies vasculaires superficielles («angiomes») Superficial vascular anomalies («angiomas»). *Pédiatrie* 1: 129–151.

Enjolras, O. 2008. The Main Misdiagnosis in a Vascular Anomalies Personal communication Hôpital Lariboisière & Hôpital d'enfants Armand Trousseau, Paris, France.

Enjolras, O., A. Picard, and V. Soupre. August 2006. Hémangiomes Congénitaux Et Autre Tumeurs Vasculaires Infantiles Rares. *Annales De Chirurgie Plastique Esthétique* 51(4): 339–346.

Enjolras, O., J.P. L.M.B.M. PhD, M. Wassef, H.P. Kozakewich, and P.E. Burrows. 2001. Noninvoluting congenital hemangioma: A rare cutaneous vascular anomaly. *Plastic and Reconstructive Surgery* 107: 1647–1654.

Ercan, T.E., F. Oztunc, T. Celkan, M. Bor, O. Kizilkilic, M. Vural, Y. Perk, C. Islak, and B. Tuysuz. 2013. Macrocephaly-capillary malformation syndrome in a newborn with tetralogy of fallot and sagittal sinus thrombosis. *Journal of Child Neurology* 28(1): 115–119.

F, A., B. S, B. A, A. K, and B. E. 2009. Head and neck hemangiomas in pediatric patients treated with endolesional 980-Nm diode laser. *Photomedicine and Laser Surgery* 00: 1–7.

F, T., M. S, A. S, H. N, and H. A. 2001. Les malformations artérioveineuses médullaires chez l'enfant. *Archives De Pédiatrie* 8: 508–511.

F, W.I.E., S. P, D. M, M. K, M.C. Mihm Jr, and S. L. 2000. Hemangiomas in infants and children. *Archives of Facial Plastic Surgery* 2(Apr–June): 103–111. http://www.archfacial.com.

Fevurly, R.D. and S.J. Fishman. June 2012. Vascular anomalies in pediatrics. *The Surgical Clinics of North America* 92(3): 769–800, x.

Finley, A.C., J.R. Hosey, T.C. Noone, D.M. Shackelford, and S. Varadarajulu. 2005. Multiple focal nodular hyperplasia syndrome: Diagnosis with dynamic, gadolinium-enhanced MRI. *Magnetic Resonance Imaging* 23(3): 511–513.

Finn, M.C., J. Glowacki, and J.B. Mulliken. 1983. Congenital vascular lesions: Clinical application of a new classification. *Journal of Pediatric Surgery* 18(6): 894–900.

Fishman S.J., P.E. Burrows, A.M. Leichtner, and P. John. May 28, 2004. Gastrointestinal manifestations of vascular anomalies in childhood: Varied etiologies require multiple therapeutic modalities. Ed. W.B. Saunders. *Journal of Pediatric Surgery* 33(7): 1–5.

Flors, L., C. Leiva-Salinas, I.M. Maged et al. 2011. MR Imaging of soft-tissue vascular malformations: Diagnosis, classification, and therapy follow-up. *Radiographics* 31(5): 1321–1340; discussion 1340–1341.

Gallarreta, F.W. de M., K.A.M. Grecca Pieroni, C.P.T. Mantovani, F.W.G. de Paula Silva, P. Nelson-Filho, and A.M. de Queiroz. 2013. Oral changes stemming from hemangioma of the tongue. *Pediatric Dentistry* 35(2): 75–78.

Garzon, M.C., M.O. Enjolras, and I.J. Frieden. December 14, 2007. Vascular tumors and vascular malformations: Evidence for an association: 1–5.

Garzon, M.C., J.T. Huang, O. Enjolras, and I.J. Frieden. 2007. Vascular malformations Part II: Associated syndromes. *Journal of the American Academy of Dermatology* 56(4): 541-564.

Geh, J.L.C., V.S.Y. Geh, B. Jemec, A. Liasis, J. Harper, K.K. Nischal, and D. Dunaway. 2007. Surgical treatment of periocular hemangiomas: A single-center experience. *Plastic and Reconstructive Surgery* 119(5): 1553–1562.

Gloviczki, P., A. Duncan, M. Kalra, G. Oderich, J. Ricotta, T. Bower, M. McKusick, H. Bjarnason, and D. Driscoll. 2009. Vascular malformations: An update. *Perspectives in Vascular Surgery and Endovascular Therapy* 21(2): 133–148.

Goksu, E., E. Alpsoy, T. Ucar, and R. Tuncer. 2012. Multiple spinal cavernous malformations in Klippel–Trenaunay–Weber syndrome. *Neurologia I Neurochirurgia Polska* 46(5): 496–500.

Greene, A.K. January 1, 2011. Management of hemangiomas and other vascular tumors. *Clinics in Plastic Surgery* 38(1): 45–63.

Greene, A.K. and A.I. Alomari. January 1, 2011. Management of venous malformations. *Clinics in Plastic Surgery* 38(1): 83–93.

Greene, A.K. and D.B. Orbach. January 1, 2011. Management of arteriovenous malformations. *Clinics in Plastic Surgery* 38(1): 95–106.

Greene, A.K., A.S. Liu, J. Mulliken, K. Chalache, and S.J. Fishman. 2011. Vascular anomalies in 5,621 patients: Guidelines for referral. *Journal of Pediatric Surgery* 46(9): 1784–1789.

Greene, A.K., Chad A. Perlyn, and Ahmad I. Alomari. January 1, 2011. Management of lymphatic malformations. *Clinics in Plastic Surgery* 38(1): 75–82.

Grisey, A., P. Roth, A. Martin, A. Czorny, C. Riehl-Duvinage, R. Maillet, and J.-P. Schaal. 2006. Diagnostic prénatal et prise en charge d'un cas d'hémangiome congénital du cuir chevelu. Revue de la littérature. *Journal de Gynecologie, Obstetrique et Biologie de la Reproduction* 35: 405–410.

Guéro, S. 2007. Tumeurs et malformations vasculaires des membres. *Chirurgie De La Main* 26(6): 278–287.

Gupta, A. and H. Kozakewich. January 1, 2011. Histopathology of vascular anomalies. *Clinics in Plastic Surgery* 38(1): 31–44.

Güvenç, B.H., G. Ekingen, A. Tuzlacı, and U. Şenel. 2005. Diffuse neonatal abdominal lymphangiomatosis: Management by limited surgical excision and sclerotherapy. *Pediatric Surgery International* 21(7): 595–598.

H, D., F. J, M. P, F.-B. D, and G. F. 2001. Cavernous hemangioma of the sphenoid sinus: Case report and review of the literature. *Surgical Neurology* 55: 1–5.

Haggstrom, A.N. 2006. Patterns of infantile hemangiomas: New clues to hemangioma pathogenesis and embryonic facial development. *Pediatrics* 117(3): 698–703.

Hasiloglu, Z.I., M. Asik, O. Kizilkilic, S. Albayram, and C. Islak. February 2013. Cavernous hemangioma of the cavernous sinus misdiagnosed as a meningioma: A case report and MR imaging findings. *Clinical Imaging* 37(4): 744–746.

Hassan, Y., A.K. Osman, and A. Altyeb. 2013. Noninvasive management of hemangioma and vascular malformation using intralesional bleomycin injection. *Annals of Plastic Surgery* 70(1): 70–73.

Haugen, T.W., W.E. Wood, and C. Helwig. 2012. Postcricoid vascular abnormalities: Hemangiomas, venous malformations, or anatomic variant. *International Journal of Pediatric Otorhinolaryngology* 76(6): 805–808.

Hegde, A.N., S. Mohan, and C.C.T. Lim. 2012. CNS cavernous haemangioma: "Popcorn" in the brain and spinal cord. *Clinical Radiology* 67(4): 380–388.

Herbreteau, D. 2007. Indications et limites des techniques d'embolisation dans les malformations vasculaires pédiatriques. *Archives De Pédiatrie* 14(6): 712–714.

Hermans, C., B. Dessomme, C. Lambert, and V. Deneys. 2006. Malformations veineuses et coagulopathie. *Annales De Chirurgie Plastique Esthétique* 51(4–5): 388–393.

Hernandez-Martin, S., J.C. Lopez-Gutierrez, S. Lopez-Fernandez, M. Ramirez, M. Miguel, J. Coya, D. Marin, and J.A. Tovar. 2012. Brain perfusion SPECT in patients with PHACES syndrome under propranolol treatment. *European Journal of Pediatric Surgery* 22(1): 54–59.

Heyer, G.L., W.S. Millar, S. Ghatan, and M.C. Garzon. 2006. The neuro-logic aspects of PHACE: Case report and review of the literature. *Pediatric Neurology* 35: 419–424.

Hochman, M., D.M. Adams, and T.D. Reeves. 2011. Current knowledge and management of vascular anomalies, II: malformations. *Archives of Facial Plastic Surgery* 13(6): 425–433.

I, M.M., S.-C. Ignacio, P.E. North, and M.C. Mihm Jr. 2002. Infantile hemangioma. *Archives of Dermatology* 138: 881–884.

Immerman, S., W.M. White, and M. Constantinides. February 1, 2011. Cartilage grafting in nasal reconstruction. *Facial Plastic Surgery Clinics of NA* 19(1): 175–182.
Jablecki, J., Elsevier, J. Kaczmarzyk, and L. Kaczmarzyk. 2013. Surgical treatment of hemangiomas and arteriovenous malformations in upper extremity. *Polski Przeglad Chirurgiczny* 85(3): 107–113.
Jacobs, I.N. and A.M. Cahill. January 1, 2011. Special considerations in vascular anomalies: Airway management. *Clinics in Plastic Surgery* 38(1): 121–131.
Jarrett, D.Y., M. Ali, and G. Chaudry. 2013. Imaging of vascular anomalies. *Dermatologic Clinics* 31(2): 251–266.
JF, M., N. F, D. D, G. M, T. D, N. S, M. L, G.-H. S, and F. D. 2002. Radioanatomie des malformations arterioveineuses cerebrales. *Cancer/Radiothérapie* 2: 173–179.
Jhawar, S., T. Nadkarni, and A. Goel. 2012. Giant cerebral cavernous hemangiomas: A report of two cases and review of the literature. *Turkish Neurosurgery* 22(2): 226–232.
John, P., G.F. Rogers, and J.J. Marler. March 19. Circular excision of hemangioma and purse-string closure: The smallest possible scar. *Plastic and Reconstructive Surgery* 15: 1544–1554.
Kadota, Y., T. Utsumi, T. Kawamura, M. Inoue, N. Sawabata, M. Minami, and M. Okumura. August 2011. Lymphatic and venous malformation or "Lymphangiohemangioma" of the anterior mediastinum: Case report and literature review. *General Thoracic and Cardiovascular Surgery* 59(8): 575–578.
Kakimoto, N., K. Tanimoto, H. Nishiyama, S. Murakami, S. Furukawa, and S. Kreiborg. 2005. CT and MR imaging features of oral and maxillofacial hemangioma and vascular malformation. *European Journal of Radiology* 55(1): 108–112.
Kaneko, T.I., M. Ueda, M. Negoro, J. Yoshida, and Y. Yamada. September 11, 2001. Curative treatment of central hemangioma in the mandible by direct puncture and embolisation with n-butyl-cyanoacrylate (NBCA). Edited by Elsevier Inc. *Oral Oncology* 37: 605–608. http://www.elsevier.com/locate/oraloncology.
Kim, K.H., S.-B. Chung, D.-S. Kong, H.-J. Seol, and H.J. Shin. February 2012. Neurocutaneous melanosis associated with dandy-walker complex and an intracranial cavernous angioma. *Child's Nervous System* 28(2): 309–314.
Kivelev, J., E. Koskela, K. Setala, M. Niemela, and J. Hernesniemi. August 2012. Long-term visual outcome after microsurgical removal of occipital lobe cavernomas. *Journal of Neurosurgery* 117(2): 295–301.
Kivelev, J., M. Niemela, and J. Hernesniemi. April 2012. Treatment strategies in cavernomas of the brain and spine. *Journal of Clinical Neuroscience: Official Journal of the Neurosurgical Society of Australasia* 19(4): 491–497.
Kulungowski, A.M. and S.J. Fishman. January 1, 2011. Management of combined vascular malformations. *Clinics in Plastic Surgery* 38(1): 107–120.
L, L.L., P.E. North, M.-M.L. Fernand, S.M. H, F.A. L, and W.S. W. 2004. Kaposiform hemangioendothelioma. *American Journal of…* 28(5): 559–568.
L, M.E., G.I. Taylor, H.N. D, M.J. Peter, B. Alan, and R. Diego. 2001. The angiosome concept applied to arteriovenous malformations of the head and neck. *Plastic and Reconstructive Surgery* 107: 633–646.
Lanoel, A., V. Tosi, M. Bocian, F. Lubieniecki, S.B. Poblete, H.O. Garcia, and A.M. Pierini. 2012. Perianal ulcers on a segmental hemangioma with minimal or arrested growth. *Actas Dermo-Sifiliograficas* 103(9): 820–823.
Laurian, C., F. C, D. Herbreteau, and O. Enjolras. 2004. Surgical treatment of vascular malformations of lower limbs. *EMC-Chirurgie 1* 1: 100–124. http://www.elsevier.com/locate/emcchi.
Lazic, M., J. Hadzi-Djokic, D. Basic, and M. Acimovic. 2012. Congenital arteriovenous fistula of the horseshoe kidney with multiple hemangiomas. *Srpski Arhiv Za Celokupno Lekarstvo* 140(7–8): 508–510.
Le Nouail, P., V. Viseux, and O. Enjolras. 2007. Phénomène de kasabach-merritt . *Annales de Dermatologie et de Vénéréologie* 134: 1–8.
Lee, S., S.-B. Lee, H.Y. Chung, J.M. Lee, and S. Huh. August 2011. Current drug therapies for infantile hemangioma: Focused on beta blocker. *Journal of the Korean Medical Association* 54(8): 876–883. DOI:10.5124/jkma.2011.54.8.876.
Lefebvre, D., A. Elias, P. Léger, F. Marson, V. Chabert, H. Rousseau, and H. Boccalon. 2004. Anomalies veineuses congénitales des membres inférieurs. *EMC – Radiologie* 1(3): 317–341.
Legiehn, G.M. and M.K.S. Heran. 2006. Classification, diagnosis, and interventional radiologic management of vascular malformations. *Orthopedic Clinics of North America* 37(3): 435–474.
Lei, H.-Z., B. Sun, D.-K. Liu, X.-N. Guo, Y.-C. Ma, J.-B. Qiao, and C.-X. Dong. 2011. Combined and sequential therapy for Kasabach–Merritt syndrome. *Zhonghua Yi Xue Za Zhi* 91(36): 2538–2541.
Linfante, I., F. Tari Capone, G. Dabus, S. Gonzalez-Arias, P.E. Lau, and E.A. Samaniego. 2012. Spinal arteriovenous malformation associated with spinal metameric syndrome: A treatable cause of long-term paraplegia? *Journal of Neurosurgery. Spine* 16(4): 408–413.
Liu, A.S., J. Mulliken, D. Zurakowski, S.J. Fishman, and A.K. Greene. 2010. Extracranial arteriovenous malformations: Natural progression and recurrence after treatment. *Plastic and Reconstructive Surgery* 125(4): 1185–1194.

M, H.E.H., P.H.M. Spauwen, and P.N.M.A. Rieu. 2010. Surgical treatment of hemangiomas and vascular malformations in functional areas. *Pediatric Surgery International* 11: 308–311.

M, R.A., E. A, and S. L. 2004. Vascular malformations as syndromic markers. *Anales del sistema sanitario de Navarra* 27: 45–46.

Madana, J., D. Yolmo, S. Gopalakrishnan, and S.K. Saxena. 2012. Development of hemangioma in a tongue harboring long-standing angiokeratoma circumscriptum. *Ear, Nose, and Throat Journal* 91(11): E7–E10.

Maguiness, S.M. and I.J. Frieden. 2010. Current management of infantile hemangiomas. *Ysder* 29(2): 106–114.

Maguiness, S.M. and M.G. Liang. January 1, 2011. Management of capillary malformations. *Clinics in Plastic Surgery* 38(1): 65–73.

Mariano, F.V., P.A. Vargas, R. Della Coletta, and M.A. Lopes. 2011. Sclerotherapy followed by surgery for the treatment of oral hemangioma: A report of two cases. *General Dentistry* 59(3): e121–e125.

Marler, J.J., S.J. Fishman, J. Upton, P.E. Burrows, H.J. Paltiel, R.W. Jennings, and J. Mulliken. 2002. Prenatal diagnosis of vascular anomalies. *Journal of Pediatric Surgery* 37(3): 318–326.

Martinez, M., S.-C. Ignacio, P.E. North, and M.C. Mihm. June 14, 2002. Infantile hemangioma. *Archives of Dermatology* 138: 881–884.

Masashi, T., O. Chiai, Y. Atsuki, K. Miwako, K. Noriaski, Y. Takashi, H. Takeshi, A. Miho, H. Yasuo, and M. Junichi. 2006. Successful treatment with vincristine of an infant with intractable Kasabach–Merritt syndrome. *Pediatrics International* 48: 82–84.

McCarthy, J.G., L.J. Borud, and S. J. 2001. Hemangiomas of the nasal tip. *Plastic and Reconstructive Surgery* 31: 31–39.

MD, A.G. and H.K. MD. 2011. Histopathology of vascular anomalies. *Clinics in Plastic Surgery* 38(1): 31–44.

MD, A.M.K. and S.J.F. MD. 2011. Management of combined vascular malformations. *Clinics in Plastic Surgery* 38(1): 107–120.

MD, D.M.A. 2011. Special considerations in vascular anomalies: Hematologic management. *Clinics in Plastic Surgery* 38(1): 153–160.

MD, I.N.J. and A.M.C. MD. 2011. Special considerations in vascular anomalies: Airway management. *Clinics in Plastic Surgery* 38(1): 121–131.

MD, J.U., C.J. Christopher, J. P, P.E. Burrows, and P.S.M. D. 1999. Vascular malformations of the upper limb: A review of 270 patients. *The Journal of Hand Surgery* 24(5): 1019–1035.

MD, R.A. and G.C.M. ChB. 2011. Diagnostic imaging of   Vascular anomalies. *Clinics in Plastic Surgery* 38(1): 21–29.

MD, R.M.B., R.J.M. MD, C.A.P.M. PhD, B.L. MD, and S.A.W. MD. 2011. Special considerations in vascular anomalies: Operative management of craniofacial osseous lesions. *Clinics in Plastic Surgery* 38(1): 133–142.

MD, S.I., W.M.W. MD, and M.C. MD. 2011. Cartilage grafting in nasal reconstruction. *Facial Plastic Surgery Clinics of NA* 19(1): 175–182.

MD, S.J.F., P.E. Burrows, L.A. M, and J. P. 2004. Gastrointestinal manifestations of vascular anomalies in childhood: Varied etiologies require multiple therapeutic modalities. *Journal of Pediatric Surgery* 33(7): 1–5.

MD, S.M.M. and M.G.L. MD. 2011. Management of capillary malformations. *Clinics in Plastic Surgery* 38(1): 65–73.

Meder, J.F., F. Nataf, D. Delvat, M. Ghossoub, D. Trystram, S. Nagi, L. Merienne, S. Godon-Hardy, and D. Fredy. March 11, 2002. Radioanatomie des malformations arterioveineuses cerebrales. Ed. Paris Elsevier. *Cancer/ Radiotherapie* 2: 173–179.

Meijer-Jorna, L.B., E. Aronica, C.M. van der Loos, D. Troost, and A.C. van der Wal. 2012. Congenital vascular malformations–cerebral lesions differ from extracranial lesions by their immune expression of the glucose transporter protein GLUT1. *Clinical Neuropathology* 31(3): 135–141.

Meijer-Jorna, L.B., C.M. van der Loos, P. Teeling, O.J. de Boer, S. Florquin, C.M.A.M. van der Horst, and A.C. van der Wal. June 2012. Proliferation and maturation of microvessels in arteriovenous malformations—Expression patterns of angiogenic and cell cycle-dependent factors. *Journal of Cutaneous Pathology* 39(6): 610–620.

Metry, D. 2004. Update on hemangiomas of infancy. *Current Opinion in Pediatrics* 16: 373–377.

Metry, D., I.J. Frieden, C. Hess et al. 2013. Propranolol use in PHACE syndrome with cervical and intracranial arterial anomalies: Collective experience in 32 infants. *Pediatric Dermatology* 30(1): 71–89.

MMSc, A.K.G.M. 2011. Management of hemangiomas and other vascular tumors. *Clinics in Plastic Surgery* 38(1): 45–63.

MMSc, A.K.G.M., and A.I.A.M. MSc. 2011. Management of venous malformations. *Clinics in Plastic Surgery* 38(1): 83–93.

MMSc, A.K.G.M., and D.B.O.M. PhD. 2011. Management of arteriovenous malformations. *Clinics in Plastic Surgery* 38(1): 95–106.

MMSc, A.K.G.M., C.A.P.M. PhD, and A.I.A.M. MSc. 2011. Management of lymphatic malformations. *Clinics in Plastic Surgery* 38(1): 75–82.

Mueller, B.U. and P. John. December 14, 2007. The infant with a vascular tumor. Edited by W B Saunders Company. *Seminars in Perinatology* 23(4): 332–340.

Murakami, K., T. Endo, and T. Tominaga. 2012. An analysis of flow dynamics in cerebral cavernous malformation and orbital cavernous angioma using indocyanine green videoangiography. *Acta Neurochirurgica* 154(7): 1169–1175.

Nakatsuka, S.-I., N. Shigeta, Y. Ojima, H. Kimura, T. Nagano, and K. Ito. 2012. A large retroperitoneal cystic venous malformation mimicking bilateral ovarian cystic tumors. *Archives of Gynecology and Obstetrics* 286(4): 1011–1014.

Navarro, O.M. 2011. Soft tissue masses in children. *Radiologic Clinics of North America* 49(6): 1235–1259; vi–vii.

Nolan, M., C.W.J. Hartin, J. Pierre, and D.E. Ozgediz. 2012. Life-threatening hemorrhage from a congenital hemangioma caused by birth trauma. *Journal of Pediatric Surgery* 47(5): 1016–1018.

Norman, W., C. Gloria, J.W. Polley, C. Fady, S. Harish, and D. Gerard. 2010. Arteriovenous malformation of the forehead, anterior scalp, and nasal dorsum. *Plastic and Reconstructive Surgery* 105(7): 2433–2439.

North, P.E., M. Waner, C.A. James, M. A, I.J. Frieden, and M.C. Mihm Jr. 2001. Congenital nonprogressive hemangioma. *Archives of Dermatological Research* 137: 1607–1620.

North, P.E., M. Waner, L. Buckmiller, C.A. James, and M.C. Mihm Jr. 2006. Vascular tumors of infancy and childhood: Beyond capillary hemangioma. *Cardiovascular Pathology* 15(6): 303–317.

Notarnicola, A., V. Pesce, G. Maccagnano, G. Vicenti, and B. Moretti. 2012. Klippel–Trenaunay syndrome: A rare cause of disabling pain after a femoral fracture. *Archives of Orthopaedic and Trauma Surgery* 132(7): 993–996.

Odile Enjolras. Life-Threatening «Angiomas» Personal Communication Hôpital Lariboisière, Paris & Hôpital d'enfants Armand Trousseau, Paris, France.

Odile Enjolras. The Main Misdiagnosis in a Vascular Anomalies Clinic Personal communication Hôpital Lariboisière & Hôpital d'enfants Armand Trousseau, Paris, France.

Orhan, K., M. Icen, S. Aksoy, H. Avsever, and G. Akcicek. 2012. Large arteriovenous malformation of the oromaxillofacial region with multiple phleboliths. *Oral Surgery, Oral Medicine, Oral Pathology and Oral Radiology* 114(4): e147–e158.

P, J., R.G. F, and J.J. Marler. 2002. Circular excision of hemangioma and purse-string closure: The smallest possible scar. *Plastic and Reconstructive Surgery* 15: 1544–1554.

P, V.M., D.P. A, P. A, V. Soupre, and O. Enjolras. 2002. Les lèvres angiomateuses angiomatous lips. *Annales De Chirurgie Plastique Esthétique* 47: 561–579.

Pavlov, N., B.M. Strebel, A.K. Brill, J. Schmidtko, P. Cottagnoud, and A.N. Stucki. 2013. 28-year-old patient with iron deficiency anemia. *Praxis* 102(4): 233–236.

Perman, M.J., L. Castelo-Soccio, and M. Jen. 2012. Differential diagnosis of infantile hemangiomas. *Pediatric Annals* 41(8): 1–7.

Phi, J.H., S.-K. Kim, A. Cho, D.G. Kim, S.H. Paek, S.-H. Park, and K.-C. Wang. 2012. Intracranial capillary hemangioma: Extra-axial tumorous lesions closely mimicking meningioma. *Journal of Neuro-Oncology* 109(1): 177–185.

Pienaar, C., R. Graham, S. Geldenhuys, and D.A. Hudson. 2006. Intralesional bleomycin for the treatment of hemangiomas. *Plastic and Reconstructive Surgery* 117(1): 221–226.

Poetke, M. and H.P. Berlien. 2005. Laser treatment in hemangiomas and vascular malformations. *Medical Laser Application* 20(2): 95–102.

Pompa, V., E. Brauner, L. Bresadola, S. Di Carlo, V. Valentini, and G. Pompa. 2012. Treatment of facial vascular malformations with embolisation and surgical resection. *European Review for Medical and Pharmacological Sciences* 16(3): 407–413.

Pompa, V., V. Valentini, G. Pompa, S. Di Carlo, and L. Bresadola. 2011. Treatment of high-flow arteriovenous malformations (AVMs) of the head and neck with embolization and surgical resection. *Annali Italiani Di Chirurgia* 82(4): 253–259.

R, K., T. I, U. M, N. M, Y. J, and Y. Y. 2001. Curative treatment of central hemangioma in the mandible by direct puncture and embolisation with N-butyl-cyanoacrylate (NBCA). *Oral Oncology* 37: 605–608. http://www.elsevier.com/locate/oraloncology.

Ramundo, S. 2005. (11262)Yan (November 15): 1–20.

Redondo, P. 2004. Clasificación de las lesiones vasculares congénitas. *An. Sist. Sanit. Navar.* 1–17.

Redondo, P., L. Aguado, and A. Martinez-Cuesta. 2011. Diagnosis and management of extensive vascular malformations of the lower limb: Part I. Clinical diagnosis. *Journal of the American Academy of Dermatology* 65(5): 893–906.

Redondo, P. and M. Fernàndez. April 22, 2004. Protocol for the treatment of haemangiomas and/or vascular malformations. *Anales del Sistema Sanitario de Navarra Navarre* 27: 45–46.

Régnier, S., N. Dupin, C. Le Danff, M. Wassef, O. Enjolras, and S. Aractingi. 2007. Endothelial cells in infantile haemangiomas originate from the child and not from the mother (a fluorescence in situ hybridization-based study). *British Journal of Dermatology* 157(1): 158–160.

Reinisch, J.F. April 2011. Discussion: Untreated hemangiomas: Growth pattern and residual lesions. *Plastic and Reconstructive Surgery* 127(4): 1649.

Requena, L. and P.S. Omar. 2007. Cutaneous vascular anomalies. Part I hamartomas, malformations, and dilatation of preexisting vessels. *Journal of the American Academy of Dermatology* 37: 523–549.

Restrepo, R. March 2013. Multimodality imaging of vascular anomalies. *Pediatric Radiology* 43(Suppl 1): S141–S154.

Rhea, Y., L. Osmann, O. Selahattin, A. Omur, C. Seyhan, A. Kenan, and C. Cemalettin. 2002. Unilateral cleft lip complicated by a hemangioma. *Plastic and Reconstructive Surgery* 110(4): 1084–1087.

Richard, L. and B. Julie. 2010. Clinical guidelines for stroke management 2010, pp. 1–172. http://www.strokefoundation.com.

Richter, G.T. and A.B. Friedman. 2012. Hemangiomas and vascular malformations: Current theory and management. *International Journal of Pediatrics* 2012: 645678.

Rosca, T.I., M.I. Pop, M. Curca, T.G. Vladescu, C.S. Tihoan, A.T.T. Serban, E.A. Bontas, and G. Gherghescu. (February 2006). Vascular tumors in the orbit—Capillary and cavernous hemangiomas. *Annals of Diagnostic Pathology* 10(1): 13–19.

Ruggeri, C. August 2004. Hemangiomas and vascular malformations of head and neck. *Otolaryngology—Head and Neck Surgery* 131(2): P256.

Ruggeri, C.S., A. Nicassio, and F.A. Urquiola. August 2004. Hemangiomas and vascular malformations of head and neck otolaryngology. *Head and Neck Surgery* 131(2): P256.

Sadykov, R.R., F. Podmelle, R.A. Sadykov, K.R. Kasimova, and H.R. Metellmann. April 2013. Use of propranolol for the treatment infantile hemangiomas in the maxillofacial region. *International Journal of Oral and Maxillofacial Surgery* 42(7): 863–867.

Salins, P.C., S. Kumar, and C.B. Rao. 2007. Management of large vascular lesions of the lip: Case reports. *Int. J. Oral Maxillofac. Surg*. 26: 45–48.

Santecchia, L., M.F. Bianciardi Valassina, G. Ciprandi, R. Fruhwirth, and M. Zama. March 2013. The use of interstitial echo-guided diode laser 980-nm for deep vascular anomalies in pediatric patients: A preliminary study. *Surgical Techniques and Development* 3(1): 5–8.

Santecchia, L., M.F. Bianciardi Valassina, F. Maggiulli, G. Spuntarelli, R. De Vito, and M. Zama. March 2013. Early surgical excision of giant congenital hemangiomas of the scalp in newborns: Clinical indications and reconstructive aspects. *Journal of Cutaneous Medicine and Surgery* 17(2): 106–113.

Savas, J.A., J.A. Ledon, K. Franca, A. Chacon, and K. Nouri. 2013. Pulsed dye laser-resistant port-wine stains: Mechanisms of resistance and implications for treatment. *British Journal of Dermatology* 168(5): 941–953.

Schook, C.C., J. Mulliken, S.J. Fishman, A.I. Alomari, F.D. Grant, and A.K. Greene. 2011. Differential diagnosis of lower extremity enlargement in pediatric patients referred with a diagnosis of lymphedema. *Plastic and Reconstructive Surgery* 127(4): 1571–1581. http://eutils.ncbi.nlm.nih.gov/entrez/eutils/elink.fcgi?dbfrom=pubmed&id=21187804&retmode=ref&cmd=prlinks.

Shaul, D.B., H.L. Monforte, M.A. Levitt, A.R. Hong, and A. Peña. 2005. Surgical management of perineal masses in patients with anorectal malformations. *Journal of Pediatric Surgery* 40(1): 188–191.

Sheilagh, M. 2007. Vascular anomalies: Classification and update. Personal Oral Communication in California University of San Francisco, San Francisco, CA.

Singh, D.J. 2006. Hemangiomas. *Children's Craniofacial Association* 1: 9.

Smolinski, K.N. and A.C. Yan. 2005. Hemangiomas of infancy: Clinical and biological characteristics. *Clinical Pediatrics* 44: 747–766.

Soldatskii, I.L., V.V. Roginskii, A.G. Nadtochii, and O.P. Blisniukov. 2012. On the classification of vascular structures in children. *Vestnik Otorinolaringologii* 2: 36–39.

Somasundaram, S.K., G. Akritidis, S. Alagaratnam, T.V. Luong, and O.A. Ogunbiyi. 2013. Extraluminal colonic arteriovenous haemangioma: An unusual cause of chronic lower gastrointestinal bleeding. *Annals of the Royal College of Surgeons of England* 95(2): e44–e46.

Soto-Sandoval, J.F. and J. Cortés-Gómez. May–June 2012. Patient with PHACE syndrome. Clinical case and literature review. *Acta Ortopédica Mexicana* 26(3): 202–206.

Spector, J.A., F. Blei, and B.M. Zide. 2008. Early surgical intervention for proliferating hemangiomas of the scalp: Indications and outcomes. *Plastic and Reconstructive Surgery* 122(2): 457–462.

Spendel, S., E.-C. Prandl, M. Uggowitzer et al. 2001. Ultrasound-navigated interstitial Nd:YAG laser coagulation of congenital vascular disorders. *Medical Laser Application* 16: 121–127. http://www.urbanfischer.de/journals/lasermed.

Stefan, P., H. Aref, C. Valerie, B. Beatrice, and B. Francis. 2003. Classification of venous malformations in children and implications for sclerotherapy. *Pediatric Radiology* 33: 99–103.

T, T.S., R.A. Wallis, Y. He, and P.F. Davis. 2004. Mast cells and hemangioma. *Plastic and Reconstructive Surgery* 113(3): 999–1011.

Thabet, F., S. Mrad, S. Abroug, N. Hattab, and A. Harbi. May 15, 2001. Les Malformations Artérioveineuses Médullaires Chez L'enfant. *Archives De Pédiatrie* 8: 508–511.

Thawait, S.K., K. Puttgen, J.A. Carrino, L.M. Fayad, S.E. Mitchell, T.A.G.M. Huisman, and A. Tekes. 2013. MR imaging characteristics of soft tissue vascular anomalies in children. *European Journal of Pediatrics* 172(5): 591–600.

Theiler, M., R. Walchli, and L. Weibel. 2013. Vascular anomalies – A practical approach. *Journal Der Deutschen Dermatologischen Gesellschaft* 11(5): 397–405.

Theologie-Lygidakis, N., O.K. Schoinohoriti, F. Tzerbos, and I. Iatrou. 2012. Surgical management of head and neck vascular anomalies in children: A retrospective analysis of 42 patients. *Oral Surgery, Oral Medicine, Oral Pathology and Oral Radiology.*

Tyagi, I., R. Syal, and A. Goyal. 2006. Management of low-flow vascular malformations of upper aero digestive system – Role of N-butyl cyanoacrylate in peroperative devascularization. *British Journal of Oral and Maxillofacial Surgery* 44(2): 152–156.

Upton, J., C.J. Coombs, P. John, P.E. Burrows, and P. Stephen. October 12, 1999. Vascular malformations of the upper limb: A review of 270 patients. *The Journal of Hand Surgery* 24(5): 1019–1035.

Vazquez, P.M., P.A. Diner, A. Picard, V. Soupre, and O. Enjolras. October 8, 2002. Les Lèvres Angiomateuses Angiomatous Lips. *Annales De Chirurgie Plastique Esthétique* 47: 561–579.

Vikkula, M., L.M. Boon, J.B. Mulliken, and B.R. Olsen. 1998. Molecular basis of vascular anomalies. *Trends in Cardiovascular Medicine* 8(7): 281–292.

Wakabayashi, S., K. Yamaguchi, T. Kugimiya, and E. Inada. 2011. Successful anesthetic management for resection of a giant hepatic hemangioma with Kasabach–Merritt syndrome using FloTrac system. *Masui* 60(11): 1326–1330.

Waner, M. and T.M.-J. O. 2013. The role of surgery in the management of congenital vascular anomalies. *Techniques in Vascular and Interventional Radiology* 16(1): 45–50.

Wassef, M., R. Vanwijck, P. Clapuyt, L. Boon, and G. Magalon. 2006. Tumeurs et malformations vasculaires, classification anatomopathologique et imagerie. *Annales De Chirurgie Plastique Esthétique* 51(4–5): 263–281.

Wassef, M. 2011a. Vascular tumors and pseudo-tumors. Common venous malformation. *Annales De Pathologie* 31(4): 281–286.

Wassef, M. 2011b. Vascular tumors and pseudo-tumors. Arteriovenous malformation. *Annales De Pathologie* 31(4): 292–296.

Weibel, L. 2011. Vascular anomalies in children. *VASA. Zeitschrift Fur Gefasskrankheiten* 40(6): 439–447.

Wierzbicka, E., D. Herbreteau, R.M. Bersin, and G. Lorette. 2006. Malformations lymphatiques kystiques. *Arch Dermatol Venereol* 133: 597–601.

Williams III, E.F., P. Stanislaw, M. Dupree, K. Mourtzikos, M.C. Mihm, and L. Shannon. May 2, 2000. Hemangiomas in infants and children. *Archives of Facial Plastic Surgery: Official Publication for the American Academy of Facial Plastic and Reconstructive Surgery, Inc. and the International Federation of Facial Plastic Surgery Societies* 2(April–June): 103–111. http://www.archfacial.com.

Wollina, U., L. Unger, G. Haroske, and B. Heinig. 2012. Classification of vascular disorders in the skin and selected data on new evaluation and treatment. *Dermatologic Therapy* 25(4): 287–296.

Wu, B., W. Liu, and Y. Zhao. 2012. Coexistence of extra-axial cavernous malformation and cerebellar developmental venous anomaly in the cerebellopontine angle. *World Neurosurgery* 78(3–4): 375.e5–375.e9.

Yilmaz, K.B., H.I. Canter, I. Vargel, T. Ormeci, U. Can, A. Turk, and O. Saygili. 2011. Use of three-dimensional MRI-angiography in preoperative evaluation and postoperative management of hemangiomas of head and neck region. *The Journal of Craniofacial Surgery* 22(5): 1814–1818.

Yoo, S. 2011. GI-associated hemangiomas and vascular malformations. *Clinics in Colon and Rectal Surgery* 24(3): 193–200.

Yue, H., J. Qian, V.M. Elner, J. Guo, Y.-F. Yuan, R. Zhang, and Q. Ge. 2013. Treatment of orbital vascular malformations with intralesional injection of pingyangmycin. *The British Journal of Ophthalmology* (April).

Zhao-Hui, D., X. Chun-Di, and C. Shun-Nian, eds. 2008. Diagnosis and treatment of blue rubber bleb nevus syndrome in children. *World Journal of Pediatrics* 4: 70–73.

Zhu, D.-M. and G.-F. Ma. 2013. Hepatic hemangiomas and vascular malformations. *Clinical Nuclear Medicine*.

Zur, K.B., R.E. Wood, and R.G. Elluru. 2005. Pediatric postcricoid vascular malformation: A diagnostic and treatment challenge. *International Journal of Pediatric Otorhinolaryngology* 69(12): 1697–1701.

14 Imaging and Surgical Principles for Maxillary Reconstruction

Riccardo Cipriani, Rossella Sgarzani, Luca Negosanti, Achille Tarsitano, Claudio Marchetti, and Emilia Pascali

CONTENTS

14.1 RADIOLOGICAL ANATOMY OF MAXILLA

The radiological anatomy of maxilla is described on multislice spiral computer tomography images.

14.1.1 3D Reconstruction of Computer Tomography Scan

Maxilla (long and thin arrow) is a voluminous, paired bone that is fused anteriorly, under the piriform aperture (1) and consists of a body (2) and four processes: frontal (3), zygomatic (4), palatal (5) and alveolar (6). The palatal process (5) is shown clearly in the three-dimensional (3D) reconstruction of the axial plane (Figure 14.1).

The body of the maxilla (2) has a superior surface (orbital, 7) that is part of the orbital floor together with the zygomatic bone (8); a medial surface (9) that forms most part of the lateral wall of the nasal cavity (1); an anterior surface with the infraorbital foramen (10), which forms the outlet of the eponymous canal which transmits the infraorbital nerve, a branch of the maxillary nerve (V2). On the anterior surface of maxilla under piriform aperture (1) is present the anterior nasal spine (arrow 11), which is formed by the union of the same process of contralateral maxillary bone; the anterior nasal spine represents the inferior border of the piriform aperture and, together with the contralateral bone, forms the anterior border of the nasal cavities.

The frontal process (3) is located superiorly and articulates at the top with the frontal bone (12), anteriorly with the nasal bone (13), and posteriorly with the lacrimal bone (14). The zygomatic process (4) is the apex of the body (2) and articulates with the zygomatic bone (8). The palatal process (5) and the alveolar process (6) are below, and the palatal process is in relationship with the horizontal plate of the palatine bone (19) (Figure 14.2).

The posterior surface of the body of the maxilla (arrow 15) presents an eminence at the bottom, the maxillary tuberosity (16), which is part of the pterygopalatine fossa (17). On this plane we can also see the anterior nasal spine (11), the frontal process (3), the alveolar process (6), the infraorbital foramen (10), the zygomatic bone (8), the nasal bone (13), the frontal bone (12), and the mandible (18).

The palatal process of the maxilla (5) is articulated posteriorly with the horizontal plate of the palatine bone (19). The posterior nasal spine (20) is formed by the union of the posterior edges of the horizontal plates of the palatines bones; the incisive foramen (arrow 21) is located in the median front end of the palatal process (5) (Figure 14.3).

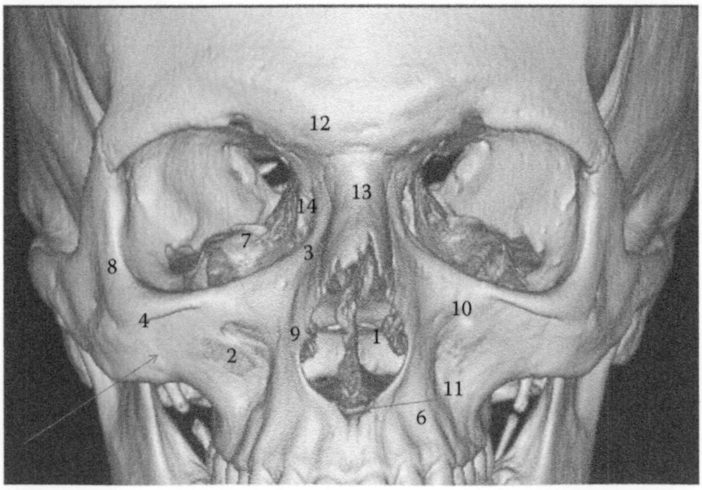

FIGURE 14.1 3D reconstruction on coronal plane.

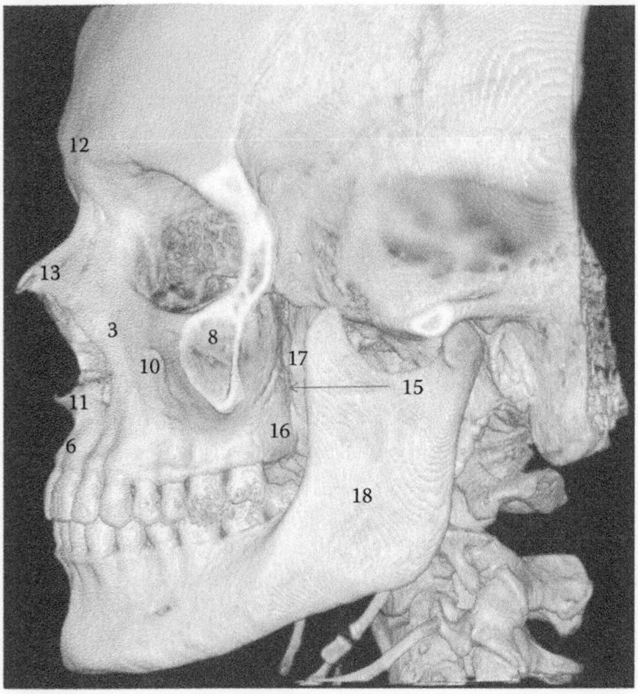

FIGURE 14.2 3D reconstruction on sagittal plane.

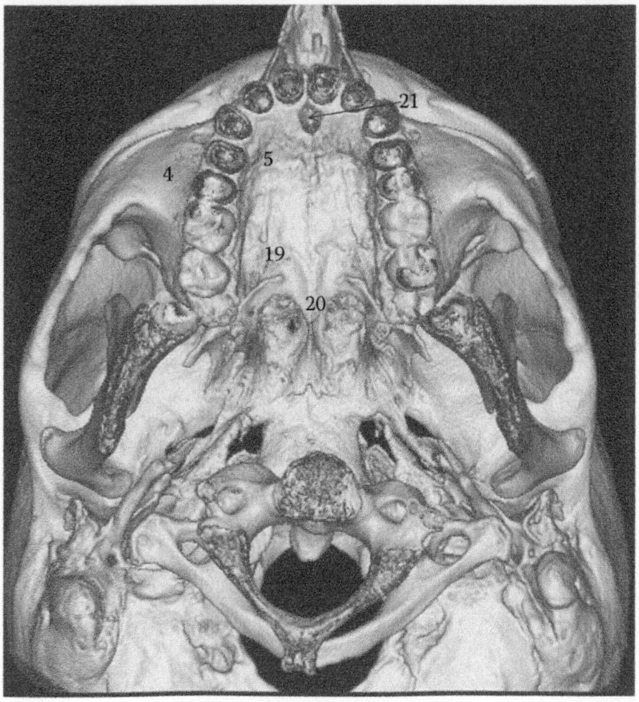

FIGURE 14.3 3D reconstruction on axial plane, from the bottom view.

14.1.2 Non-Contrast CT Scan Reconstructed with a Bone Filter on Axial Plane, Presented in Cranio–Caudal Direction

The maxillary sinus (antrum of Highmore – 22) is contained inside the body of the maxilla and is laterally bordered by the lamina papyracea of the ethmoid bone (arrow 23). Together with the greater wing of the sphenoid bone (24), it posteriorly delimits the inferior orbital fissure (arrow 25), a channel in the floor of the orbit bone through which pass the infraorbital nerve and the zygomatic nerve (V2) and the infraorbital artery (Figure 14.4).

This slot allows communication between the orbit (26) and the pterygopalatine fossa (17), which communicates anteriorly and posteriorly, and continues medially with a dell that turns into the infraorbital canal.

The foramen rotundum (27) is below and posterior to the inferior orbital fissure (arrow 25), located in the greater wing of the sphenoid (24) and crossed by the maxillary division of the trigeminal nerve, which after being detached from the Gasser ganglion exits from the Meckel cave engaging in the side wall of the cavernous sinus and reaches the foramen rotundum, through which it leaves the cranial cavity. It then penetrates into the pterygopalatine fossa (17) where, in the upper part of the pit, is contained the sphenopalatine ganglion to which it gets attached; it passes through the inferior orbital fissure and runs into the infraorbital canal, where it takes the name of infraorbital nerve (terminal branch) and emerges from the infraorbital foramen, where it divides into several cutaneous branches.

The foramen rotundum connects the cranial cavity with the pterygopalatine fossa.

The nasal bone (13) and the lacrimal bone (14) form the lacrimal sac fossa (28), the beginning of the corresponding nasolacrimal duct. The nasal bony septum is formed by the perpendicular plate of the ethmoid (29), which forms its posterosuperior part, and the vomer (30), which forms its posteroinferior part. The ethmoidal cells (31), the sphenoid sinus (32), the zygomatico-sphenoid sutures (arrow 33), and the horizontal segment of the petrous internal carotid canal (34) are seen.

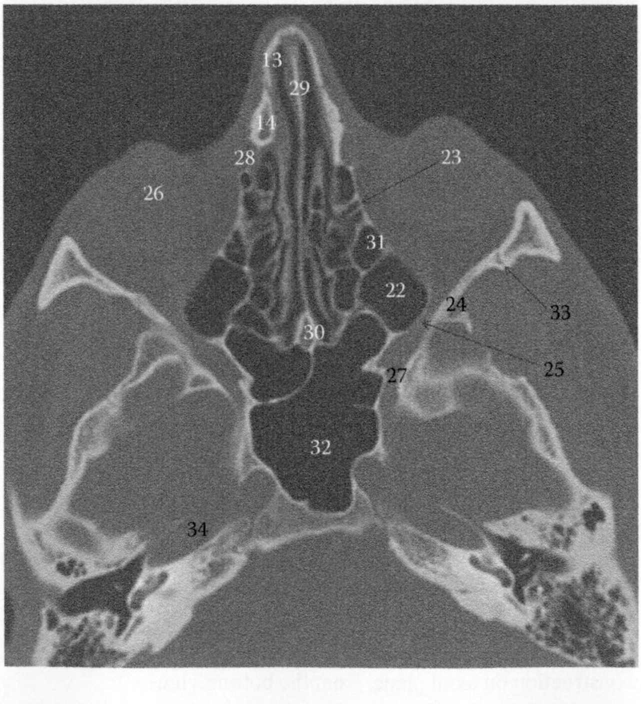

FIGURE 14.4 Non-contrast CT scan reconstructed with a bone filter on axial plane.

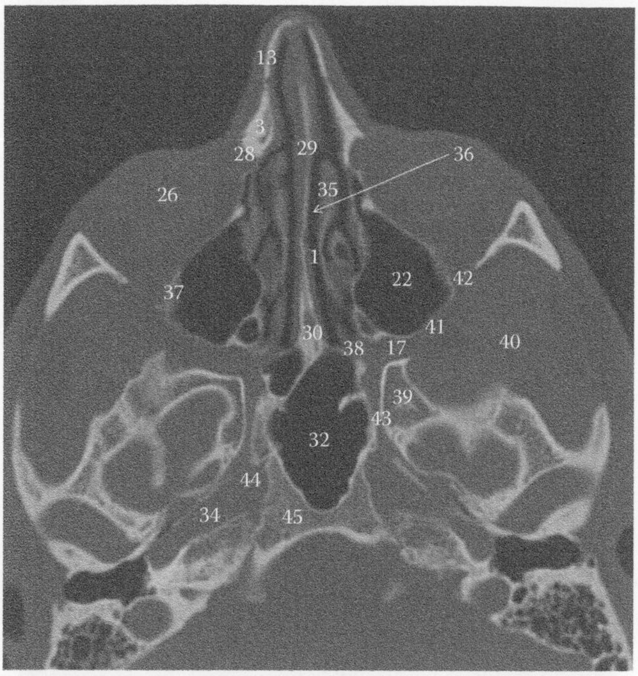

FIGURE 14.5 Non-contrast CT scan reconstructed with a bone filter on axial plane.

The image put in evidence the maxillary sinus (22), the medial wall of which forms the side wall of the nasal cavity (1), which is a triangle divided at midline by the nasal septum (29,30), within which is located the middle turbinate (35), which delimits the middle meatus (arrow 36) (Figure 14.5).

The upper wall of the maxillary sinus constitutes part of the floor of the orbit (26) and on it runs the infraorbital canal (37); the rear wall of the maxillary sinus is the anterior limit of the pterygopalatine fossa (17). The pterygopalatine fossa is a small, deep cavity located behind the maxilla, which contains the pterygopalatine or sphenopalatine Meckel ganglion, and branches of the maxillary nerve; it is bounded medially by the perpendicular plate of palatine bone that articulates with the upper body of sphenoid bone forming the sphenopalatine foramen (38), crossed by sphenopalatine nerves and vessels. The sphenopalatine foramen (38) is located on the medial wall of the pterygopalatine fossa (17) and allows communication with the nasal cavity (1).

The posterior limit of the pterygopalatine fossa (17) is formed by the pterygoid process (39) of the sphenoid bone. The lateral border is formed by the communication with the infratemporal fossa (40) through the pterygomaxillary fissure (41), which transmits the internal maxillary artery and branches of the mandibular nerve. The superior aspect of the pterygopalatine fossa (17) is in direct continuity with the sphenomaxillary fissure (42), which is continuous with the inferior orbital fissure (arrow 25). Posteriorly it continues with the vidian (pterygoid) canal (43) between the palatine bone, maxillary bone, and the pterygoid process, which contains the vidian nerve, which arises from a branch of the facial nerve (large superficial petrosal nerve) and pertains to the sphenopalatine (pterygopalatine) ganglion.

The vidian canal (43) connects with the pterygopalatine fossa (17), anteriorly, and to carotid canal floor (foramen lacerum), posteriorly. The foramen lacerum (44) represents the cartilaginous anteromedial floor of the horizontal segment of the internal carotid canal (34).

The pterygopalatine fossa opens inferiorly to the posterolateral corner of the hard palate, in correspondence with the greater palatine foramen, through which pass the palatine nerves and the descending palatine artery. The greater palatine foramen connects the pterygopalatine fossa with the oral cavity (Figures 14.6, 14.25, and 14.26).

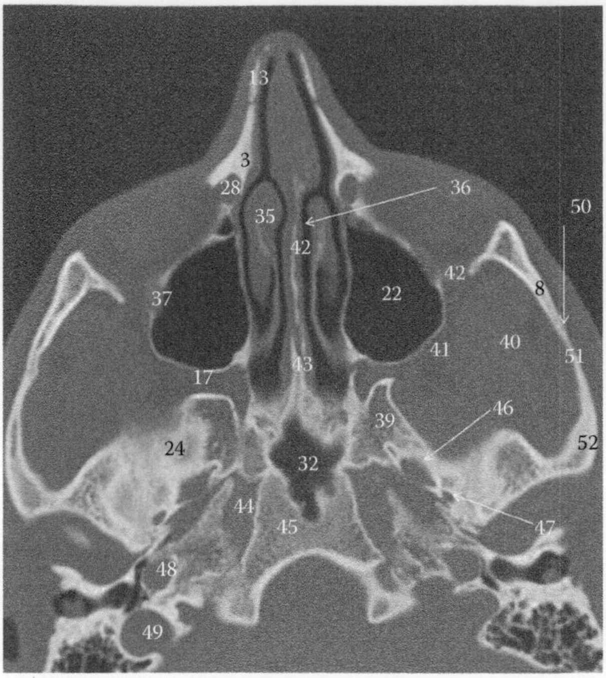

FIGURE 14.6 Non-contrast CT scan reconstructed with a bone filter on axial plane.

The pterygopalatine fossa is therefore an important crossroads of the deep face of maxilla, because it serves as a potential pathway for disease spread between the orbit, the intracranial cavity, the sinonasal cavity, the masticator space, and the oral cavity.

In the figure are also indicated the nasal bone (13), the frontal process of the maxilla (3), which delimits the nasolacrimal duct (28), the sphenoid sinus (32), and the clivus (45).

In the figure are also shown the maxillary sinus (22), the pterygopalatine fossa (17), the pterygomaxillary fissures (41), the infratemporal fossa (40), the sphenomaxillary fissures (42), the foramen ovale (arrow 46), the foramen spinosum (arrow 47), the pterygoid process (39), the clivus (45), the foramen lacerum (44), the vertical petrous internal carotid artery canal (48), the jugular bulb (49), the zygomatico-temporal suture (arrow 50), the zygomatic arch (51) formed by the zygomatic bone (8) and the zygomatic process of temporal bone (52), the nasal bone (13), the frontal process of the maxilla (3), the nasolacrimal duct (28), the middle turbinate (35), which delimits the middle meatus (arrow 36), and the sphenoid sinus (32). The infraorbital canal (37) runs on the upper wall of the maxillary sinus. The foramen ovale (arrow 46) gives passage to the mandibular nerve (V3). The foramen spinosum (arrow 47) gives passage to the middle meningeal artery. Foramen ovale and foramen spinosum are both contained in the greater wing of the sphenoid bone (24).

The figure shows the maxillary sinus (22), the zygomatico-temporal foramen (arrow 53) which runs in the zygomatic bone (8) and gives passage to the zygomatic nerve (V2), the zygomatic process of the temporal bone (52), the zygomatico-temporal sutures (arrow 50), the mandibular condyle (54), the pterygoid process (39) which constitutes the posterior limit of the pterygopalatine fossa (17), the pterygomaxillary fissures (41), the infratemporal fossa (40), the infraorbital canal (37), the nasal septum (29,30), the perpendicular plate of the palatine bone (55) which delimits the medial wall of pterygopalatine fossa (17), the middle turbinate (35), the middle meatus (arrow 36), the nasal bone (13), the frontal process of the maxilla (3), the nasolacrimal duct (28), the vertical petrous internal carotid artery canal (48), the jugular bulb (49), and the clivus (45) (Figure 14.7).

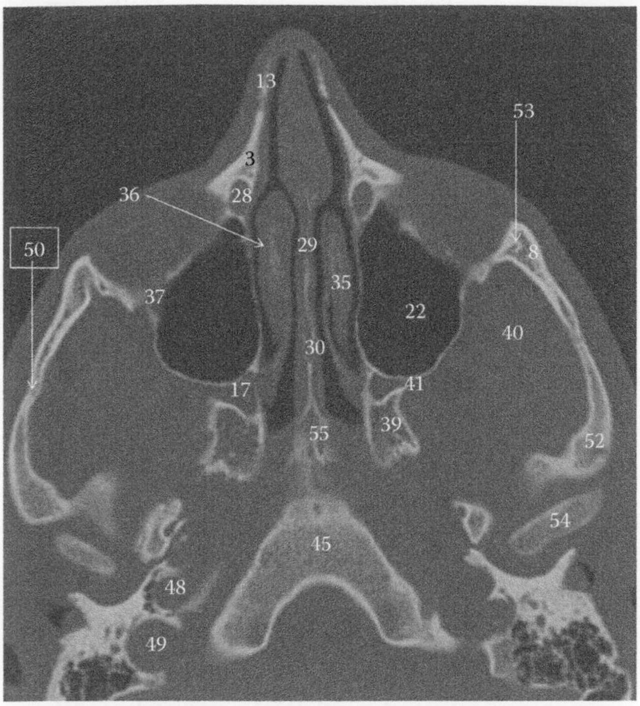

FIGURE 14.7 Non-contrast CT scan reconstructed with a bone filter on axial plane.

On the anterior surface of the maxillary sinus (22) is the infraorbital foramen, the outlet of its eponymous channel (arrow 10), from which emerges the infraorbital nerve; the frontal process of maxilla (3); and the medial (56) and lateral (57) pterygoid plates. The greater palatine nerve emerges from the pterygopalatine fossa (Figure 14.6 coronal, sagittal, 4 and 5) and is a branch of the pterygopalatine ganglion; it descends through the greater palatine channel (arrow 58) and emerges upon the hard palate through the greater palatine foramen, which opens close to the lateral border of the palate, immediately behind the palate maxillary sutures. It continues in a groove of the hard palate toward the incisor teeth.

In the figure are also shown the zigomaticomaxillary sutures (59), the articulation between the apex of the zygomatic process of the maxilla and the zygomatic bone; the body of the zygomatic bone (8), the mandibular ramus (60), the infratemporal fossa (40), the retromaxillary fat pad (61), the masticator space (62), the outlet of the nasolacrimal duct (28) below the inferior turbinate (63) in the inferior meatus (64), the choanae (65), the mucosal nasopharyngeal space (66), the vomer (30), and C1 (67) which articulates with the condyle of the occipital bone (68) (Figure 14.8).

The greater (arrow 69) and the lesser (arrow 70) palatine foramina transmit the greater and lesser palatine nerves from the pterygopalatine fossa, inferiorly, to the palate, together with the eponymous vessels. The lesser palatine foramina are usually two on each side and are situated behind the greater palatine foramen; these are best seen on axial CT scan. The channel of the anterior superior alveolar nerve (arrow 71), a branch of the maxillary nerve, originates from the anterior part of the infraorbital canal and runs in the thickness of the bone until it reaches the dental alveoli over the upper canine and incisor teeth. The anterior alveolar vessels and nerves (branches of maxillary nerve) also run in this channel. In the figure are also shown the zigomaticomaxillary sutures (59), the body of the zygomatic bone (8), the inferior turbinate (63), the inferior meatus (64), the frontal process of the maxilla (3), the vomer (30), the medial (56) and lateral (57) pterygoid plates, the choanae (65), the mucosal nasopharyngeal space (66), the retromaxillary fat pad (61), the masticator space (62), the mandibular ramus (60), C1 (67) which articulates with the occipital condyle (68), and the odontoid process (C2) (72) (Figure 14.9).

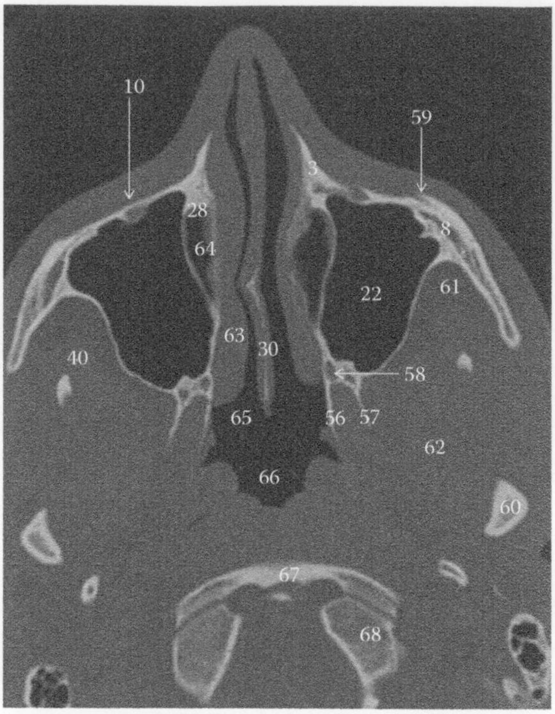

FIGURE 14.8 Non-contrast CT scan reconstructed with a bone filter on axial plane.

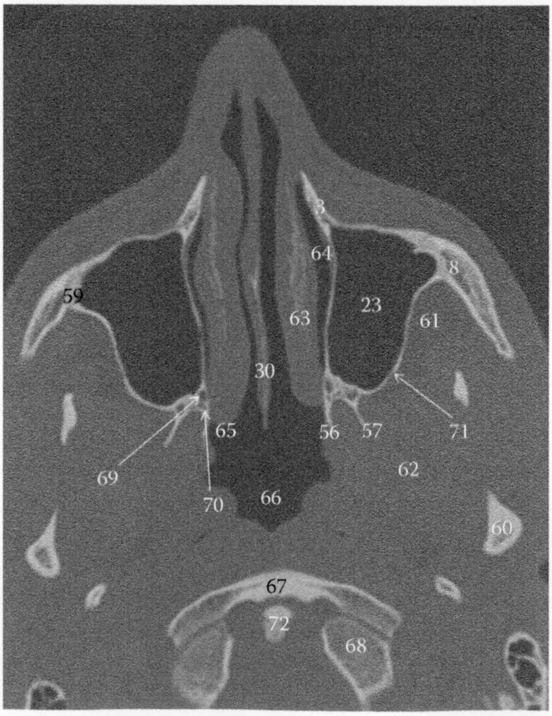

FIGURE 14.9 Non-contrast CT scan reconstructed with a bone filter on axial plane.

The image shows the palatal process of the maxilla (5) which, together with the contralateral process, forms the hard palate; the upper face constitutes the floor of the nasal cavity and the lower face forms a large part of the roof of the oral cavity and continues into the alveolar process. The palatal process of the maxilla (5) is separated from the horizontal plate of the palatine bone (19) by the transverse suture (arrow 73) and the right and the left halves of the palatine bones are separated by the median palatine suture (arrow 74). At the level of the hard palate the groove for the greater palatine nerve (58) and the second lesser palatine foramen (arrow 70) are seen. We also see separately the openings of the left and right nasal palatine channel (arrow 75); the most caudal part of the maxillary sinus (22), just over the alveolar process (arrow 6); the medial (56) and lateral (57) pterygoid plate, the anterior nasal spine (11), the posterior nasal spine (20), the mandibular ramus (60), the masticatory space (62), the nasopharyngeal mucosal space (66), C1 (67), C2 (72), and the occipital condyle (68) (Figure 14.10).

The palatal process of the maxilla (5) presents the openings of the nasopalatine (incisive) canals, separately right and left (arrow 75), which are crossed by the nasopalatine and the sphenopalatine nerves (ramus of the maxillary nerve) and open into nasal cavities. The figure shows the alveolar process (arrow 6), the mandibular ramus (60), the mandibular foramen (arrow 76) in which runs the inferior alveolar nerve, the mucosal nasopharyngeal space (66), the oral cavity (77), C1 (67), and C2 (72) (Figure 14.11).

The palatal process of the maxilla (5) presents the median incisive foramen (arrow 78) in the centre, located at the front end of the median palatine suture. The incisive foramen is the common opening of the right and left nasopalatine (incisive) channels in the oral cavity. The nasopalatine channel puts into communication the oral and the nasal cavities.

The image also shows the alveolar process of the maxilla (arrow 6), which contains the alveoli and, together with the contralateral process, forms the upper alveolar arch; the mandibular ramus (60) with the mandibular foramen (arrow 76); the oral cavity (77); the oropharyngeal mucosal space (79); and C2 (72) (Figure 14.12).

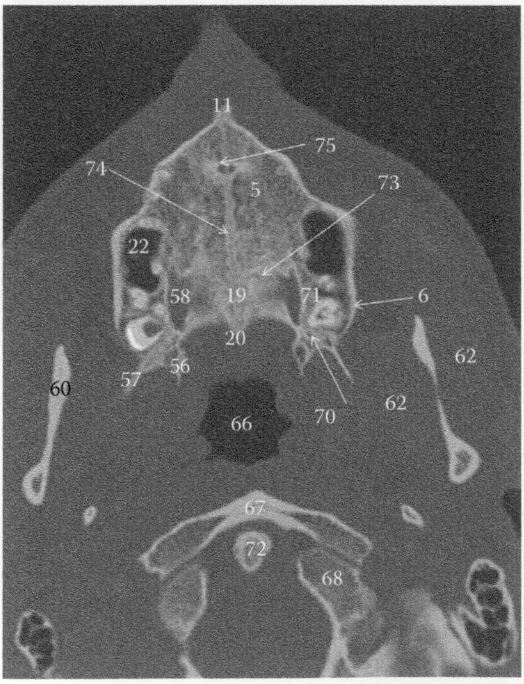

FIGURE 14.10 Non-contrast CT scan reconstructed with a bone filter on axial plane.

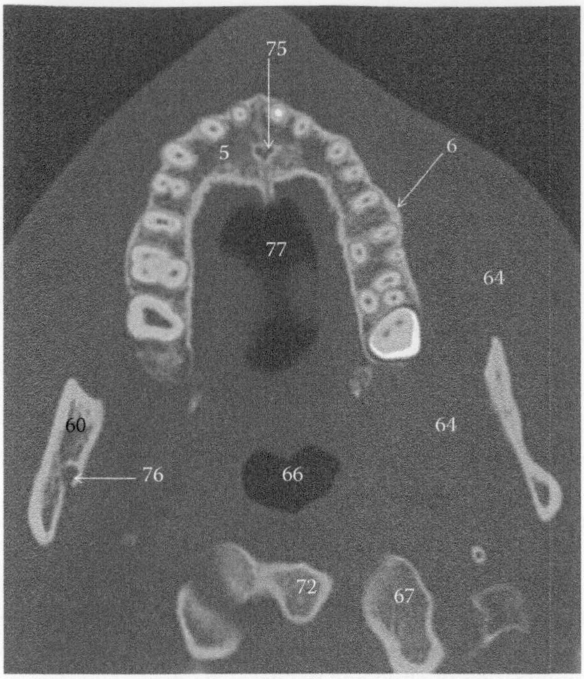

FIGURE 14.11 Non-contrast CT scan reconstructed with a bone filter on axial plane.

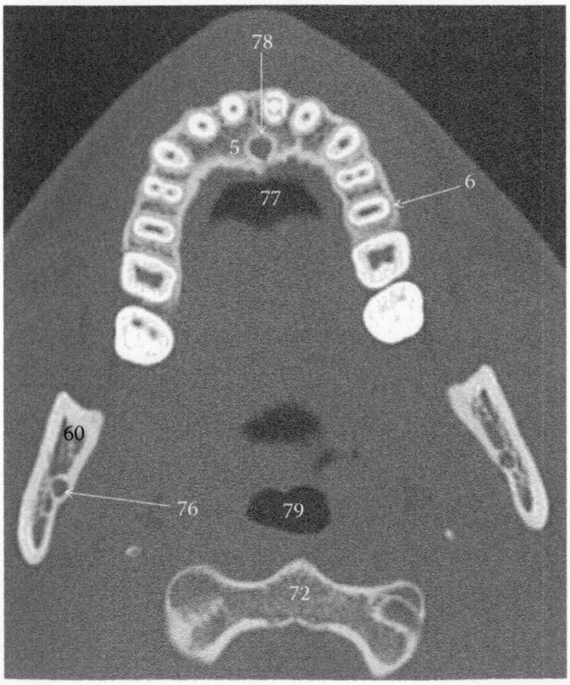

FIGURE 14.12 Non-contrast CT scan reconstructed with a bone filter on axial plane.

14.1.3 Non-Contrast CT Scan Reconstructed with a Bone Filter on Coronal Plane, Presented in Front–Rear Direction

The image shows the frontal process of the maxilla (3) that articulates with the frontal bone (12), the frontal sinus (80), the anterior portion of the inferior turbinate (63), the middle (36) and inferior (64) meatus, the perpendicular plate of the ethmoid (nasal septum) (29) with normal bifid appearance about the septal cartilage (81), the septal process of the maxilla (82) corresponding to the articulation between the palatal process and vomer, the palatal process (5) and the maxillary alveolus (6), and the orbit (26) (Figure 14.13).

The image shows the maxillary sinus (22), the nasolacrimal duct (28), the orbit (26), the lamina papyracea (arrow 23) of the ethmoid bone, the frontal bone (12), the frontal sinus (80), the anterior ethmoid cell (83), the middle (35) and inferior (63) turbinates, the middle (36) and inferior (64) meatus, the crista galli (84), the perpendicular plate of the ethmoid bone (nasal septum) (29), the septal cartilage (81), the vomer (30) (nasal septum), the incisive canal (75) and the incisive foramen (arrow 78), the palatal process (5), the maxillary alveolus (6), the oral cavity (77), the zygomatic process of the body of the maxilla (4), the zygomatico-maxillary suture (59), and the infraorbital foramen (arrow 10) (Figure 14.14).

The outlet of the nasolacrimal duct (28) is in the inferior meatus (64); the middle (35) and inferior (63) turbinates, the middle (36) meatus, the orbit (26), the lamina papyracea (arrow23) of the ethmoid bone, the crista galli (84) and the cribriform plate (arrow 85) of the ethmoid that forms the medial side of anterior cranial fossa, the frontal bone (12), the frontal sinus (80), the anterior ethmoidal cell (83), the perpendicular plate of the ethmoid bone (nasal septum) (29), the vomer (30) (nasal septum), the maxillary sinus (22), the descending portion of the infraorbital canal (arrow 37), the zygomatic process of the body of the maxilla (4), the zygomatico-maxillary sutures (arrow 59), the palatal process (5), and the oral cavity (77) are seen (Figure 14.15).

The figure shows the osteomeatal complex, which is an anatomic area superolateral to the middle meatus (36) that receives drainage of the frontal, anterior ethmoid, and maxillary sinuses. The osteomeatal complex includes the superomedial maxillary sinus (22), the maxillary infundibulum (arrow 86), the ethmoid bulla, the dominant ethmoid air cell of the anterior ethmoid complex (83), the hooked process (87), just inferior to the ethmoid bulla, which defines the medial wall of the

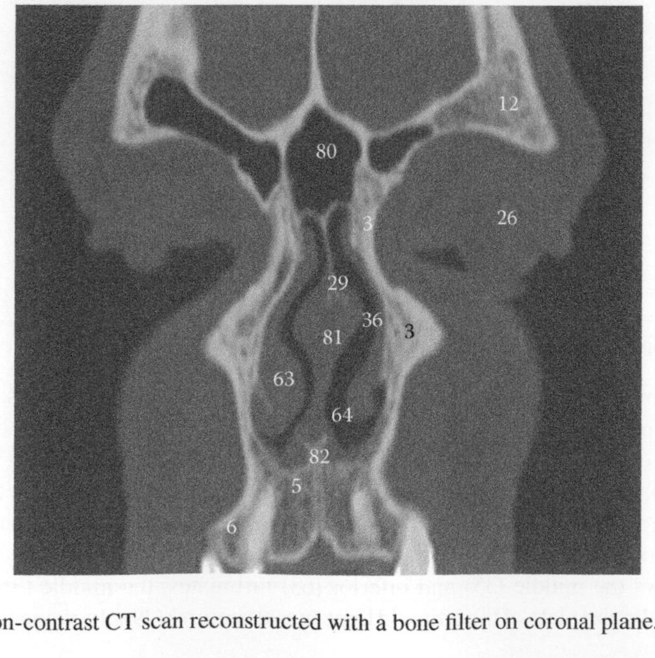

FIGURE 14.13 Non-contrast CT scan reconstructed with a bone filter on coronal plane.

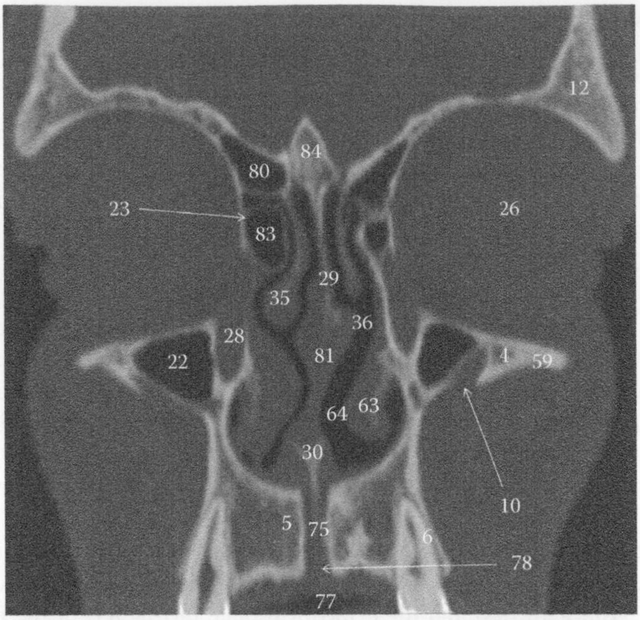

FIGURE 14.14 Non-contrast CT scan reconstructed with a bone filter on coronal plane.

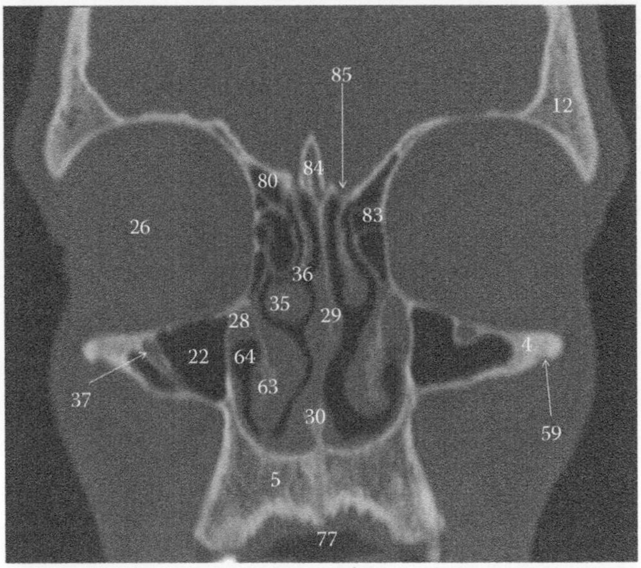

FIGURE 14.15 Non-contrast CT scan reconstructed with a bone filter on coronal plane.

maxillary infundibulum, and the hiatus semilunaris (arrow 88), which appears as a groove in the lateral wall of the middle meatus. The middle (35) and inferior (63) turbinates, the inferior meatus (64), the perpendicular plate of the ethmoid bone (nasal septum) (29), the vomer (30) (nasal septum), the crista galli (84), the cribriform plate (arrow 85) of the ethmoid, the orbit (26), the lamina papyracea (arrow 23), the frontal bone (12), the zygomatic bone (8), the infraorbital canal (37), the palatal process (5) and maxillary alveolus (6), and the oral cavity (77) are also indicated (Figure 14.16).

The figure shows the middle (35) and inferior (63) turbinates, the middle (36) and inferior (64) meatus, the perpendicular plate of the ethmoid bone (nasal septum) (29), the vomer (30) (nasal septum),

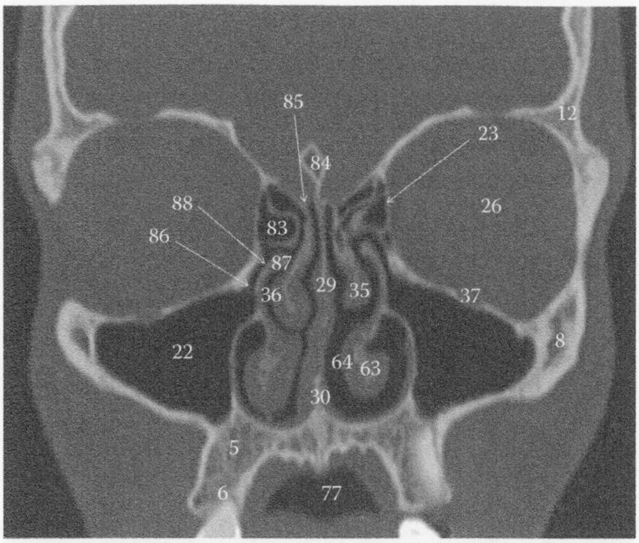

FIGURE 14.16 Non-contrast CT scan reconstructed with a bone filter on coronal plane.

the middle ethmoid cell (89), the cribriform plate (arrow 85), the orbit (26), the lamina papyracea (arrow 23), the greater wing of the sphenoid bone (24), the zygomatic bone (8), the infraorbital canal (37), the anterior superior alveolar nerve canal (arrow 71), the palatal process (5) and the maxillary alveolus (6), and the oral cavity (77) (Figure 14.17).

The figure shows the communication between the pterygopalatine fossa (17) and the inferior orbital fissure (25), the infratemporal fossa (40), the pterygopalatine fissures (41), the sphenopalatine foramen (38), and the greater palatine canal (58). The superior orbital fissure (90), which serves as a communication between the middle cranial fossa and the orbital cavity is also seen. The opthalmic division of the trigeminal nerve (V1), the oculomotor nerve, the trochlear nerve, the abducens nerve, and the opthalmic veins pass through the superior orbital fissure (90). The optic canal (91) is contained in the lesser wing (arrow 92) of the sphenoid bone and gives passage to the optic nerve.

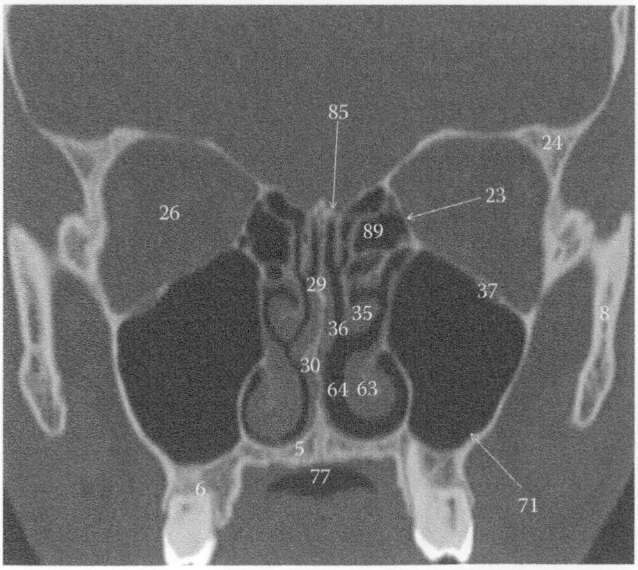

FIGURE 14.17 Non-contrast CT scan reconstructed with a bone filter on coronal plane.

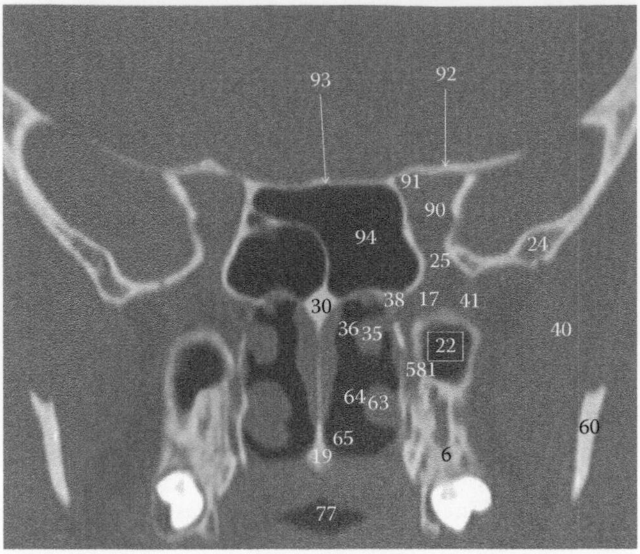

FIGURE 14.18 Non-contrast CT scan reconstructed with a bone filter on coronal plane.

In Figure 14.6 are also present the greater (24) wing of sphenoid bone, the sphenoidal planum (arrow 93), the maxillary sinus (22), the sphenoidal sinus (94), the vomer (30), the horizontal plate of the palatine bone (19), the rear end of the middle (35) and inferior (63) turbinate, the inferior meatus (64), the choanae (65), the maxillary alveolus (6), the oral cavity (77), and the mandibular ramus (60) (Figure 14.18).

The figure shows, in the coronal view, the anterior clinoid process (95), that is the medial aspect of the lesser wing of sphenoid bone, the optic canal (91), the foramen rotundum (arrow 27), the vidial canal (arrow 43), the medial (56) and lateral (57) pterygoid plates of the pterygoid process (39) of the sphenoid bone, the greater wing (24) of sphenoid that articulates with the temporal bone (96), the infratemporal fossa (40), the masticator space (62), the perpendicular plate of the palatine bone (55), the sphenoidal sinus (94), the choanae (65), the mandibular ramus (60), and the oral cavity (77) (Figure 14.19).

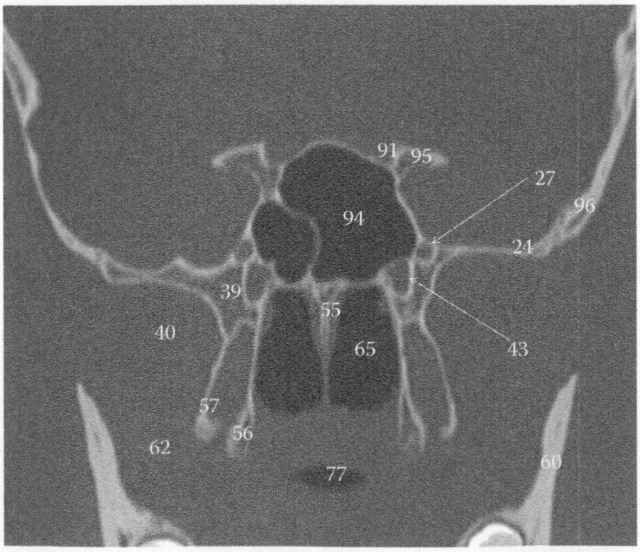

FIGURE 14.19 Non-contrast CT scan reconstructed with a bone filter on coronal plane.

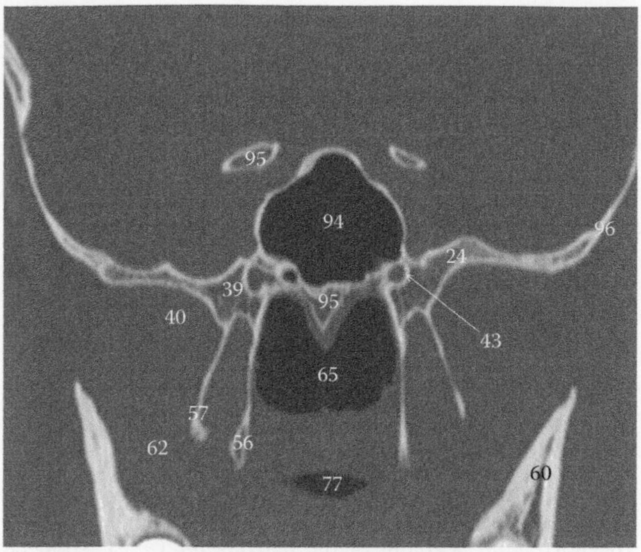

FIGURE 14.20 Non-contrast CT scan reconstructed with a bone filter on coronal plane.

The figure shows the anterior clinoid process (95), the vidial canal (arrow 43), the medial (56) and lateral (57) pterygoid plate of pterygoid process (39) of sphenoid bone, the greater wing (24) of the sphenoid that articulates with the temporal bone (96), the perpendicular plate of the palatine bone (55), the sphenoidal sinus (94), the choanae (65), the mandibular ramus (60), the infratemporal fossa (40), the masticator space (62), and the oral cavity (77) (Figure 14.20).

The figure shows the sphenoidal sinus (94), the posterior clinoid process (97) of the body of the sphenoid bone, the foramen lacerum (44), the foramen ovale (46), the greater wing (24) of the sphenoid, which is connected with the temporal bone (96), the nasopharyngeal mucosal space (66), the oropharyngeal mucosal space (79), the mandibular ramus (60), and the masticator space (62) (Figure 14.21).

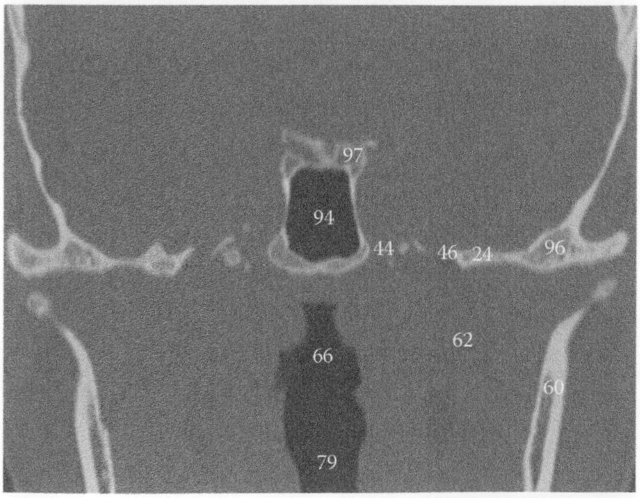

FIGURE 14.21 Non-contrast CT scan reconstructed with a bone filter on coronal plane.

14.1.4 Non-Contrast CT Scan Reconstructed with a Bone Filter on Sagittal Plane, Presented in Medial to Lateral Direction

The figure shows the body of the maxilla with internal maxillary sinus (22), the inferior orbital fissure (arrow 25), the groove for the superior alveolar nerve (arrow 71), the foramen spinosum (arrow 47), the bony eustachian tube (arrow 98), the horizontal segment of the petrous internal carotid canal (arrow 34), the infraorbital canal (arrow 37) that runs on the superior surface of the body of the maxilla, the orbit (26), the greater wing of sphenoid bone (24) and the frontal bone (12) (Figure 14.22).

The figure shows the maxillary sinus (22), the pterygomaxillary fissure (41), the foramen ovale (arrow 46), the horizontal segment of the petrous internal carotid canal (arrow 34), the maxillary tuberosity (16), bulging lower extremity of the root behind the last molar tooth, the infraorbital canal (arrow 37), the orbit (26), the frontal bone (12), the greater wing of sphenoid (24), and the lateral plate of the pterygoid process (57) (Figure 14.23).

The figure shows the infraorbital foramen (arrow 10), the maxillary sinus (22), the maxillary tuberosity (arrow 16), the alveolar process of maxilla (arrow 6), the lateral plate of the pterygoid process (arrow 57), the pterygoid process (39), the pterygomaxillary fissure (41), the superior orbital fissure (arrow 90), the horizontal segment of the petrous internal carotid canal (arrow 34), the orbit (26), and the frontal bone (12) (Figure 14.24).

The figure has been acquired according to an oblique sagittal plane to show the communication between the pterygopalatine fossa (17) and the inferior orbital fissure (25), with the foramen rotundum (arrow 27) and with the greater palatine channel (arrow 58), which flows across the palate in the greater palatine foramen (arrow 69). There are also shown the medial plate of pterygoid process (arrow 56), the superior orbital fissure, the apex of the orbit (26), the pterygoid process (39), the lesser wing of the sphenoid bone (92), the anterior clinoid process (95), the frontal bone (12), the frontal sinus (80), the maxillary sinus (22), the sphenoidal sinus (94), the posterior ethmoidal cell (99), the frontal process (3), the palatine process (5), the maxillary alveolus (6), the inferior turbinate (63), and the inferior meatus (64) (Figure 14.25).

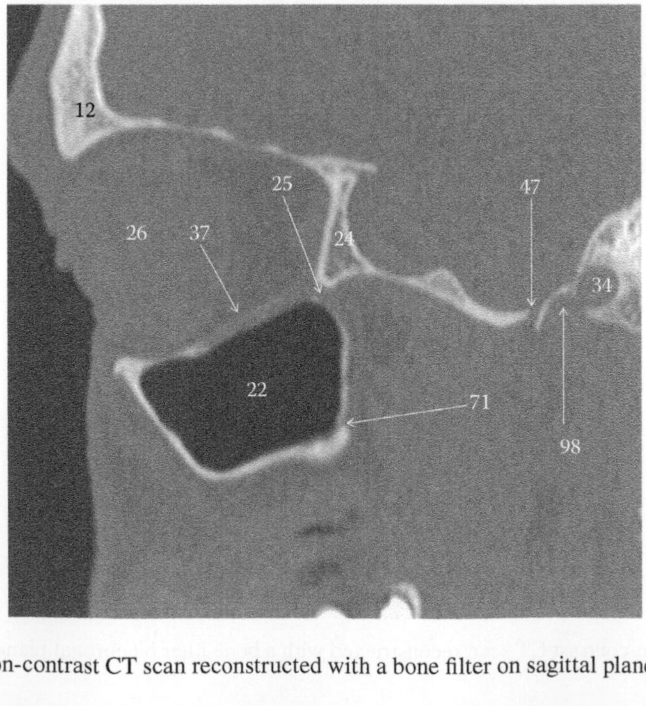

FIGURE 14.22 Non-contrast CT scan reconstructed with a bone filter on sagittal plane.

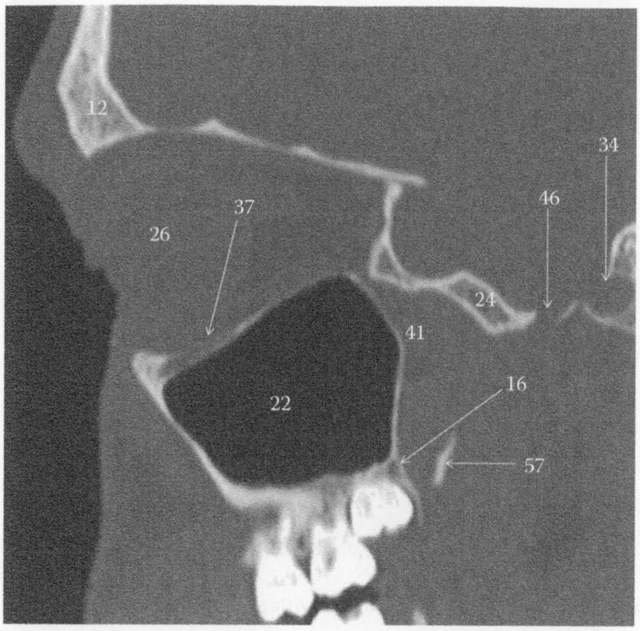

FIGURE 14.23 Non-contrast CT scan reconstructed with a bone filter on sagittal plane.

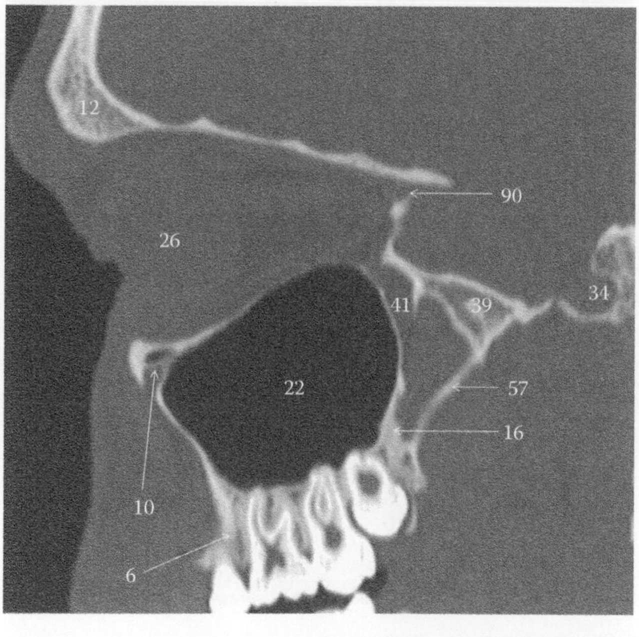

FIGURE 14.24 Non-contrast CT scan reconstructed with a bone filter on sagittal plane.

The figure shows the communication between the pterygopalatine fossa (17) and the vidian canal (arrow 43), the greater palatine channel (arrow 58), the greater palatine foramen (arrow 69), the maxillary sinus (22), the sphenoidal sinus (94), the middle (89) and posterior (99) ethmoidal cells, the inferior meatus (64), the medial plate (56) of the pterygoid process (39), the anterior clinoid process (95), the frontal bone (12), the frontal sinus (80), the frontal process (3), and the maxillary alveolus (arrow 6) (Figure 14.26).

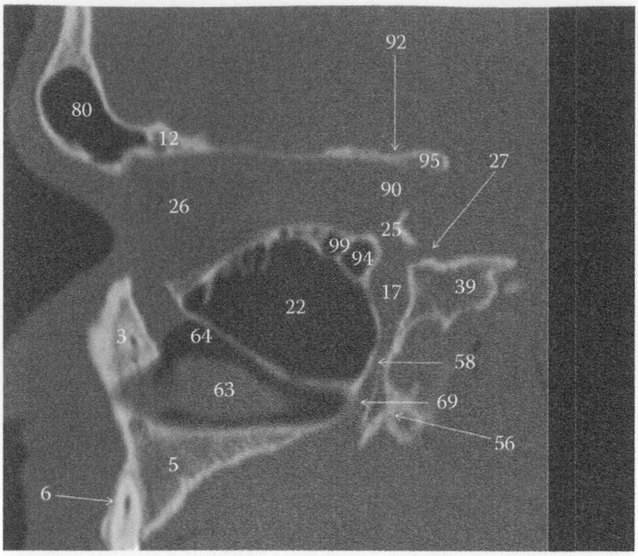

FIGURE 14.25 Non-contrast CT scan reconstructed with a bone filter on sagittal plane.

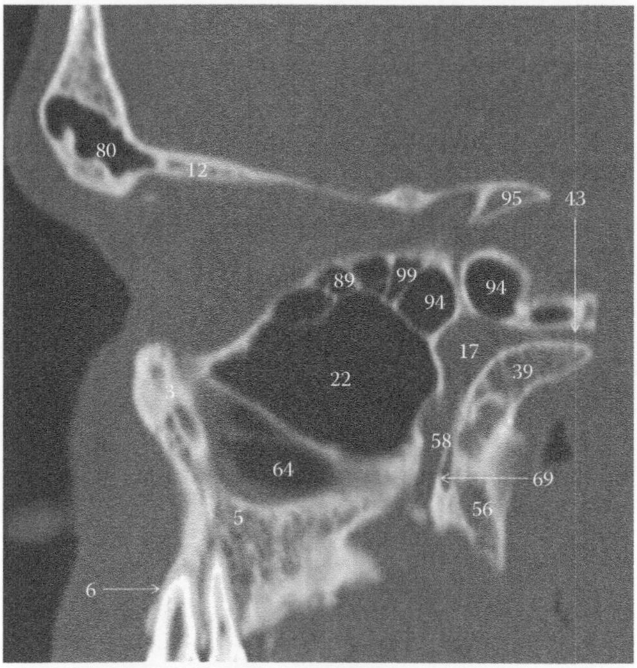

FIGURE 14.26 Non-contrast CT scan reconstructed with a bone filter on sagittal plane.

The figure has been acquired according to an oblique sagittal plane to show the frontal process (3) of the maxilla in its entirety and its articulation with the nasal bone (13) and the alveolar process of the maxilla (6). There are also shown the maxillary sinus (22), the inferior meatus (64), the anterior (83), middle (89), and posterior (99) ethmoidal cells, the sphenoidal sinus (94), the frontal bone (12), the frontal sinus (80), the anterior clinoid process (95), and the pterygopalatine fossa (17) (Figure 14.27).

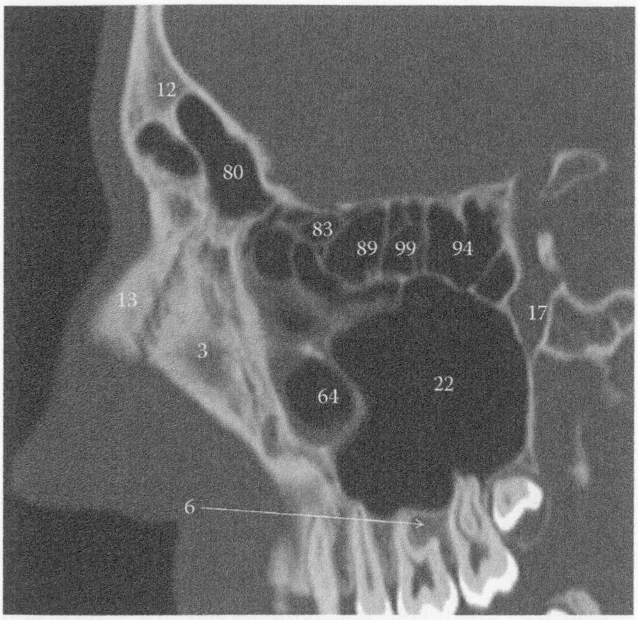

FIGURE 14.27 Non-contrast CT scan reconstructed with a bone filter on sagittal plane.

The figure shows the middle (35) and inferior (63) turbinates (36) together with the middle and inferior (64) meatus, the choanae (65), the nasal bone (13), the frontal process (3) of the maxilla, the frontal bone (12), the frontal sinus (80), the anterior clinoid process (95), the anterior (83), middle (89), and posterior (99) ethmoidal cells, the sphenoidal sinus (94), the palatine process (5), the maxillary alveolus (6), and the oral cavity (77) (Figure 14.28).

The figure shows the palatine process (5), which articulates with the horizontal plate of palatine bone (19), the perpendicular plate of palatine bone (95), the vomer (30), the perpendicular plate of the ethmoid (29), the planum sphenoidal (arrow 93), the cribriform plate (arrow 85), the nasal

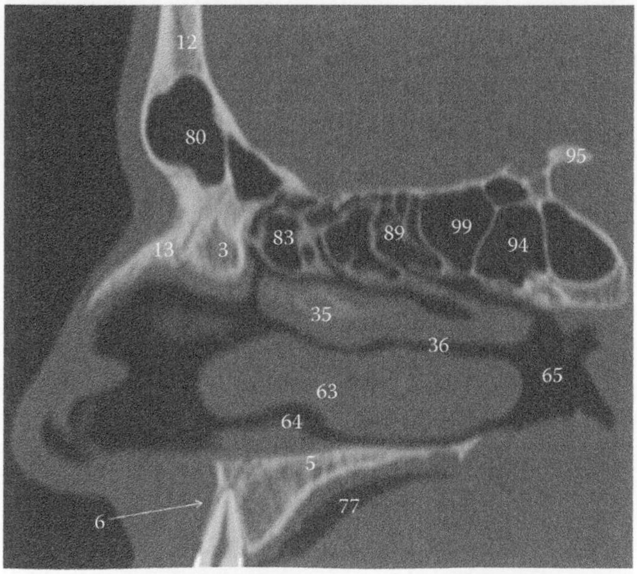

FIGURE 14.28 Non-contrast CT scan reconstructed with a bone filter on sagittal plane.

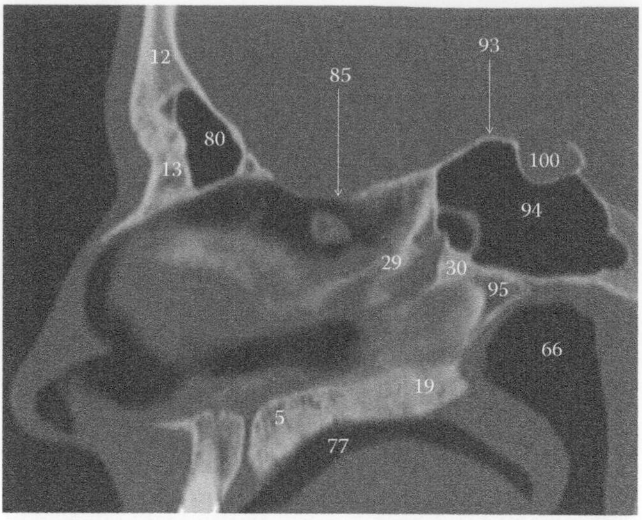

FIGURE 14.29 Non-contrast CT scan reconstructed with a bone filter on sagittal plane.

bone (13), the frontal bone (12), the frontal sinus (80), the sphenoidal sinus (94), the pituitary fossa (100), the oral cavity (77), and the nasopharyngeal mucosal space (66) (Figure 14.29).

14.1.5 T1-Enhanced MR Image

The axial T1-enhanced MR image shows the cephalad aspect of pterygopalatine fossa (arrow 17) with the entrance of the maxillary nerve inside the foramen rotundum (arrow 27), the maxillary sinus (22), the sphenoidal sinus (94), the Meckel cave (101), the cavernous internal carotid artery (102), the temporalis muscle in the infratemporal fossa (40), the middle turbinate (35) and the middle meatus (36), the sphenoidal sinus (94), and the maxillary sinus (22) (Figure 14.30).

The axial T1-enhanced MR image shows the maxillary sinus (22), the pterygopalatine fossa (17), inside which is the internal maxillary artery (arrow 103), the mandibular nerve in the foramen ovale (46), the horizontal petrous internal carotid artery (arrow no 34), the vidian nerve

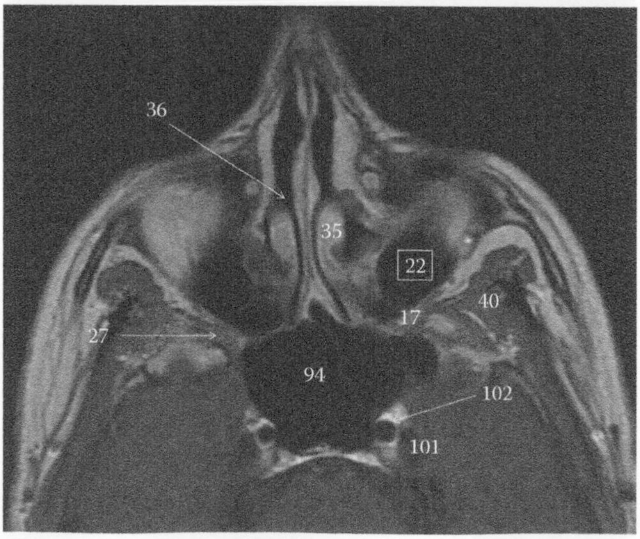

FIGURE 14.30 Axial T1 enhanced MR image.

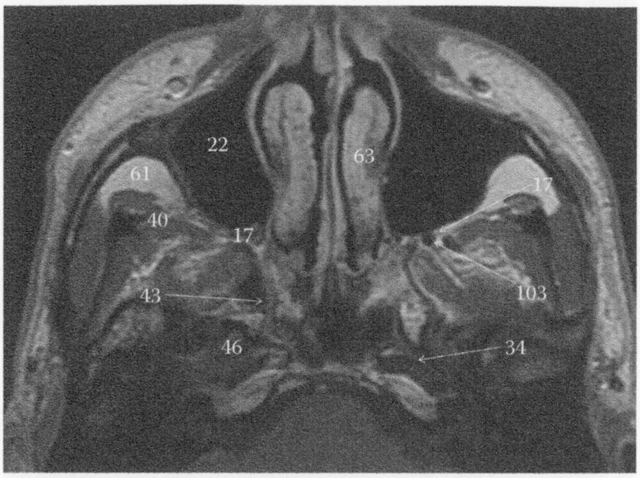

FIGURE 14.31 Axial T1 enhanced MR image.

in the eponymous canal (arrow 43), the inferior turbinate (63), the temporalis muscle in the infratemporal fossa (40), and the retromaxillary fat pad (61) (Figure 14.31).

In the coronal-enhanced MR image are shown the maxillary nerve in the foramen rotundum (arrow 27), the vidian nerve in the eponymous channel (arrow 43), the inferior orbital fissure (arrow 25), the masticator space (62) with the medial (104) and lateral (105) pterygoid muscles, the sphenoidal sinus (94), the nasopharyngeal mucosal space (66), the oropharyngeal mucosal space (79), the mandibular ramus (60), and the parapharyngeal space (106) (Figure 14.32).

The coronal-enhanced MR image shows the mandibular nerve in the foramen ovale (arrow 46), the Meckel hollow (101), the cavernous internal carotid artery (102), the temporalis muscle in the infratemporal fossa (40), the pituitary gland (106), the medial (104) and lateral pterygoid muscles (105), the mandibular ramus (60), the nasopharyngeal mucosal space (66), and the parapharyngeal space (106) (Figure 14.33).

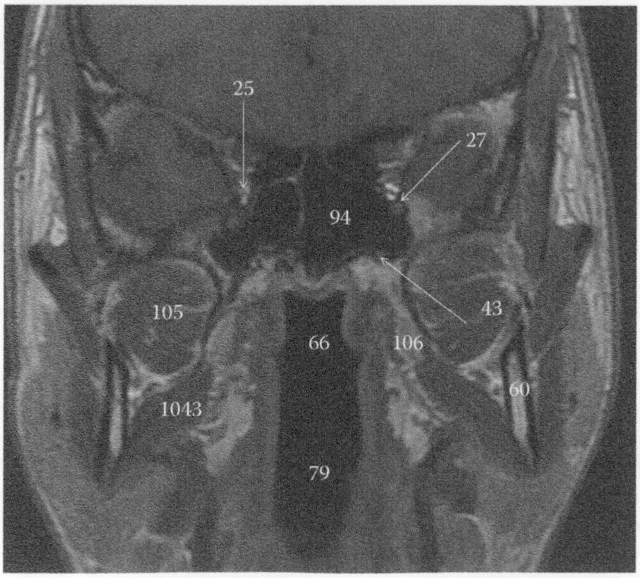

FIGURE 14.32 Coronal enhanced MR image.

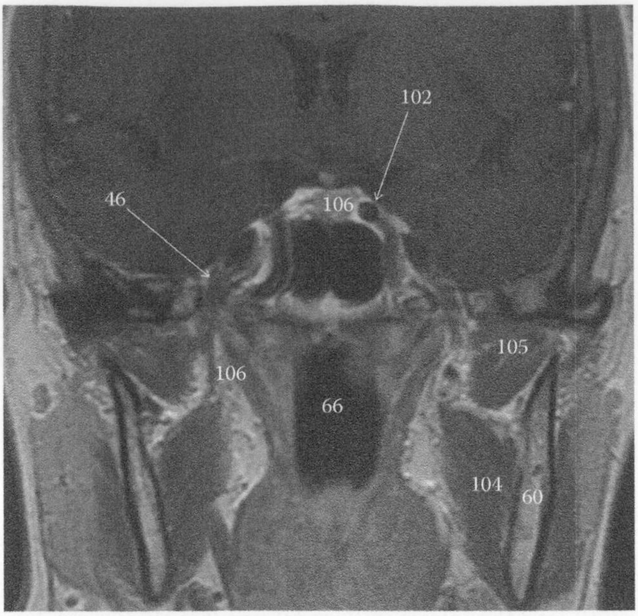

FIGURE 14.33 Coronal enhanced MR image.

14.2 ROLE OF MAXILLA

Maxilla is a fusion of two bones along the palatal fissure that forms the upper jaw. It represents the functional and aesthetic cornerstone of the midface [1,2].

Maxilla is the structural support between the skull base and the occlusal plane and plays several important functional roles. It has a fundamental role in mastication because the alveolar process (maxillary arch) holds the upper teeth and because several masticatory muscles insert on it. Furthermore maxilla has a central role in swallowing and speech, allowing the hard palate–tongue contact and forming a barrier between the nasal and oral cavity. It has also a central role in nasal respiration, forming the floor and the lateral walls of the nasal antrum.

Maxilla is interposed between the central nervous system and nasal, oral, and sinus cavities, and its integrity prevents central nervous system infection.

The roof of the maxilla forms the orbital floor and supports the ocular globe preventing entropion; its symmetry allows a binocular vision without diplopia.

Furthermore, maxilla plays a major role in facial aesthetics, determining first of all midface projection and giving support to midface structures as superior lip, nasal tip, and columella.

The anterior surface of the maxilla gives attachment to mimetic muscles, which serve as a key point of mimetic movements and dynamic aesthetics.

14.3 MAXILLARY DEFECTS

14.3.1 Aetiology

Defects of the head and neck can be caused by the resection of tumours, congenital anomalies, and traumatic reasons. Among them, oncology is the most frequent indication for reconstruction.

Maxillary tumours [3] are a heterogeneous group of diseases. Head and neck cancers rarely lead to metastatic diffusion, and morbidity and mortality are usually linked to local extension and invasion. Surgery and radiotherapy can control the disease locally and therefore they are the base of a successful treatment. Local control in this region is difficult for the anatomic complexity and proximity of vital structures. Increased surgical margins have many consequences and can lead to a decreased function, an increased disfigurement, and a lower quality of life.

Despite improvement in neoadjuvant therapies, the primary treatment approach is often surgery. In localised disease (T1, T2), radiotherapy and surgery demonstrate similar good results. In patients with more advanced cancer or with regional lymph nodes metastasis, a more aggressive treatment is required, including both surgery and radiotherapy. The association of these treatments lead to better disease control but have dramatic consequences, because the effects induced by the resection are amplified by the negative effects of radiations, such as sclerosis or microvascular occlusion. Reconstructive surgery allows to increase surgical margins and therefore the possibility to restore anatomy and function of the resected area.

Congenital anomalies that involve the maxilla and require a reconstructive procedure are mainly represented by facial clefts, which will not be discussed in this chapter, and facial asymmetries, such as Romberg disease, hemifacial microsomia, and Goldenhar syndrome [4]. In asymmetries, the loss of soft tissues and muscles and bone hypotrophy are the main indication for surgical correction. Similar defects can be found in acquired anomalies due to previous radiotherapy or surgical treatments.

Maxillary traumas are nowadays often treated with conservative techniques (osteosynthesis) and complex defects with loss of bone and soft tissues are less and less frequent, and produce defects similar to those that can be found in acquired anomalies due to previous radiotherapy or surgical treatments [5].

14.3.2 Type of Defect

Maxillary region defects can involve only bone, or bone and soft tissues in case of composite defects.

Bone defects alone are sometimes post-traumatic, as in comminute fractures with loss of bony segments, and more rarely post-oncologic.

Usually oncologic resections include at least bone and mucosa and can be therefore classified as composite defects. Also congenital defects are usually composite defects, and express themselves as tissue hypotrophy rather than the lack of bone segments or soft tissue.

Maxillary defects can be otherwise classified as defects causing aesthetic impairment only and defects causing both functional and aesthetic impairment.

Congenital mild maxillary defects, for example, often cause aesthetical impairment only. Surgical correction can be indicated as midface volume and maxillary projection have a major aesthetic value. Maxillary bone hypoplasia or malposition can be corrected by upper maxillary advancement or combined osteotomies, or bone distraction. Composite tissue atrophy are nowadays frequently treated with lipofilling. Lipofilling is a useful and low-risk technique that allows a satisfactory camouflage of composite tissue atrophy with a staged volume restoration.

Oncologic resection causes both aesthetic and functional impairment. Depending on the resected part of the maxilla, functional impairment can affect vision with bulbar displacement and diplopia, mastication, swallowing, phonation, and respiration. Aesthetic impairment can express itself as ectropion, asymmetry, and lack of projection. The goal of reconstruction is to restore both aesthetics and function, and in most of the cases only a free tissue transfer allows to achieve both these goals. The entity and the site of the defect determine what is the most appropriate flap, as it will be discussed later.

14.3.3 Classifications

Many classification systems [6–9] have been proposed for maxillary defects but none of them is accepted universally.

The main schemes have been published between 2000 and 2001, and all of them report interesting aspects. The most accepted ones are those proposed by Brown and Cordeiro in 2000.

Brown et al. [6] develop a scheme of defects caused by maxillectomy by independent vertical and horizontal components. Classes I–IV describe the increasing extent of the maxillary defect in the vertical dimension, while classes V and VI represent orbitomaxillary and nasomaxillary defects,

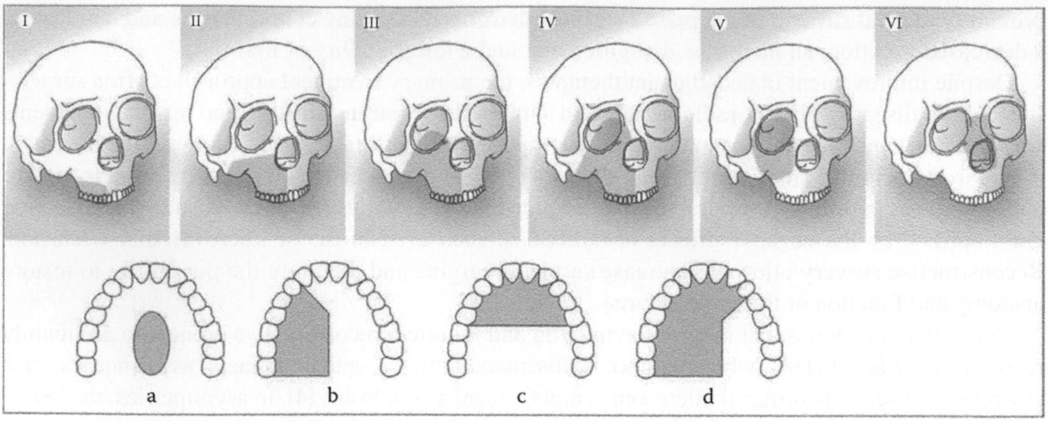

FIGURE 14.34 Brown's classification. Vertical classes: I, maxillectomy not causing an oronasal fistula; II, not involving the orbit; III, involving the orbital adnexae with orbital retention; IV, with orbital enucleation or exenteration; V, orbitomaxillary defect; VI, nasomaxillary defect. Horizontal classes: (a) palatal defect only, not involving the dental alveolus; (b) less than or equal to 1/2 unilateral; (c) less than or equal to 1/2 bilateral or transverse anterior; (d) greater than 1/2 maxillectomy. (From Brown, J.S. et al., *Head Neck*, 22, 17, 2000.)

respectively. The addition of letter a–c to vertical classes II–IV qualifies the horizontal aspect of the defect, including the amount of palate and alveolar ridge sacrifice (Figure 14.34).

The vertical component tends to be related to the aesthetical outcome, while the horizontal one has much greater functional consequences.

Deficit of the inferior section has greater impact on dentition, mastication, and speech articulation. The superior region has a greater aesthetical impact due to the loss of midface projection and disruption of nasal region, and a functional impact related to loss of sinonasal and orbital support.

Brown reported a reconstructive algorithm linked to the classification system (Table 14.1).

TABLE 14.1
Recommended Method of Reconstruction According to Brown's Classification System

	I	II	III	IV	V	VI
Obturation	+	+	–	–	–	–
Local pedicled flaps						
Temporalis, temporoparietal	+	+(b)	–	–	–	–
Soft tissue free flaps						
RF, ALT	+	+(a,b)	–	–	+	–
RA, LD	–	–	–	+	–	–
Hard tissue or composite flaps						
Radial	+	+(b,c)	–	–	+	+
Fibula	–	+	–	–	–	–
DCIA	–	+	+	+	–	–
Scapula	–	+	+	+	–	–
TDAA	–	+	+	+	+	+

Source: Brown, J.S. et al., *Head Neck*, 22, 17, 2000.

Note: +, recommended; –, not recommended; RF, radial forearm flap; ALT, anterolateral thigh flap; RA, rectus abdominis flap; LD, latissimus dorsi flap; DCIA, deep circumflex iliac artery, supplies the iliac crest; TDAA, thoracodorsal angular artery, supplies the scapula tip.

In class I defects, either obturation and reconstruction with local flaps from temporal region or free radial forearm flap are indicated. In class II, obturation can be used for IIa–b defects, while reconstruction can be achieved with local flaps (IIb) or free radial forearm or anterolateral thigh flaps (IIa–b), considering the need of soft tissues. Bone reconstruction is not imperative, because zygomatic implants or the use of ipsilateral incisors/canine, often retained, allowed to restore dental aesthetics, even in larger dental defects (IId). For class IIC we have to consider the loss of height of the perinasal maxilla. In case of large bone defects, composite bone free flaps might be used to restore oronasal support.

In class III defects we have a loss of orbital and cheek support and dental arch. The reconstruction might provide support to the orbit and facial skin and sufficient bone to obtain union between the alveolar remnant and the zygomatic buttress. A soft tissue only free flap provides good closure of oronasal defects but requires bone grafts. A composite flap is well indicated. Class IV defects often involve patients with stage IV disease. The poor prognosis should be taken into account in the choice of the reconstructive method. Composite flaps are well indicated in these cases, if possible considering patient's general conditions.

Class V defect involve the exenteration of the orbit, while the palate remains intact and bone is not generally required. The aim of reconstruction is to create a sufficient depth to provide an orbital prosthesis. For unilateral defects, local flaps may be an option, while, for larger skin loss, the anterolateral thigh or the radial forearm flaps are the best choices. Nasomaxillary defects are at great risk of cerebrospinal fluid leak. In these cases, the radial forearm osteocutaneous flap provides a bone segment to support the flap and reconstruct the nasal region.

Cordeiro and Santamaria [7] described a classification that consider, the maxilla as a hexahedrium in which the roof is the floor of the orbit, the floor is the hard palate, the other walls are the vertical buttresses, and the antrum is contained within the six walls.

This classification provides a good accuracy to determine the surface-area-to-volume requirement and the need for palatal closure and orbital reconstruction. The main disadvantage is the lack of attention to functional dental reconstruction.

Type I defect is consequent to limited maxillectomy and involves one or two walls, excluding the palate. Type II is the consequence of subtotal maxillectomy and involves the loss of inferior five walls with preservation of the orbital floor. Type III defect results after total maxillectomy and includes resection of all six walls of the maxilla and is subdivided in IIIa and IIIb depending on preservation or not of the orbital content (Figure 14.35).

The reconstructive approach described by Cordeiro considers the amount of loss of surface area and volume of the defect.

Type I presents large surface area/low volume defects. The radial forearm fasciocutaneous flap provides in these cases multiple skin islands to resurface anterior cheek and medial nasal lining. Type II defects have a large surface area/medium volume loss. In these cases, the radial forearm osteocutaneous flap provides a large skin island that is folded on itself to include the bone that reconstructs the anterior maxillary arch. Type IIIa presents a defect with medium surface area/medium volume. Bone is required to reconstruct the orbital floor. Cranial or rib bone graft can be used in combination with the rectus abdominis myocutaneous flap. The skin island of the flap recreates the palate while soft tissues fill the defect and cover the bone graft. An alternative can be the temporalis muscle flap. Type IIIb presents a large surface area/large volume defect. The rectus abdominis myocutaneous flap provides soft tissue to fill the defect and multiple skin islands to resurface external skin, palatal defect, and lateral wall of nose. Also in orbitomaxillectomy there is a large surface/large volume defect. The rectus abdominis myocutaneous flap with a single skin island allows filling the defect and recreating the external surface.

Less used classifications are those published by Triana in 2000 and Okay in 2001 [8,9].

Triana et al. [8] classify defects subsequent to inferior partial maxillectomy or total maxillectomy (Figures 14.36 and 14.37). Inferior maxillary defects are subdivided based on the extent of palate loss, while total maxillary defects are subdivided based on the loss of orbit, malar bone, and zygomatic arch. Considering this classification, the need of bone transfer depends on the amount of palate and alveolar arch lost and on the integrity of the remaining dentition.

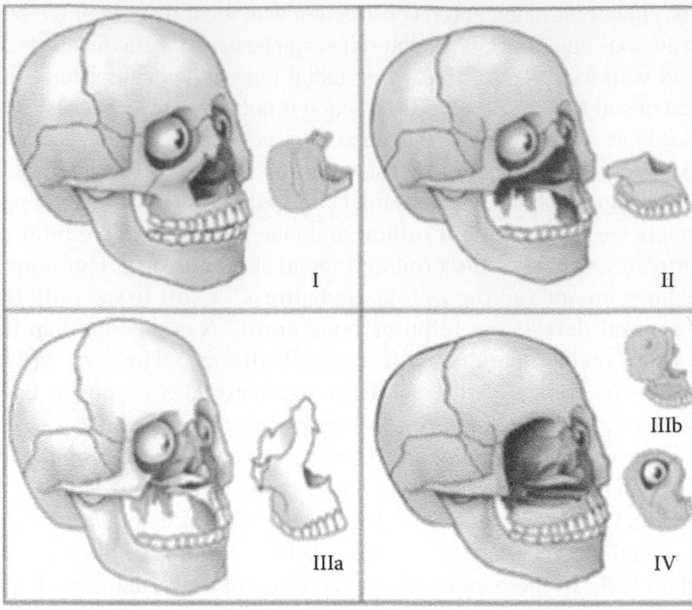

FIGURE 14.35 Cordeiro's classification. (From Cordeiro, P.G. and Santamaria, E., *Plast. Reconstr. Surg.*, 105, 2331, 2000.)

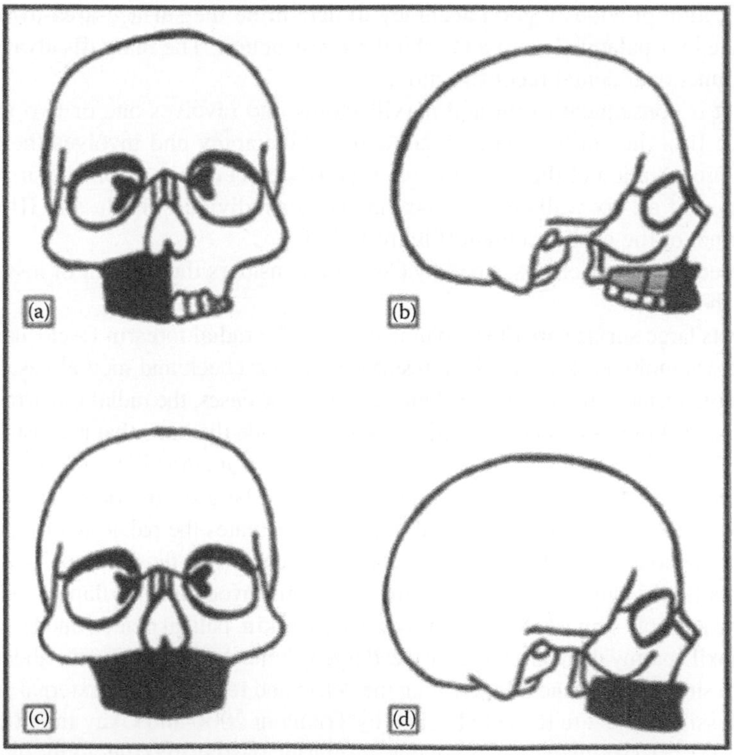

FIGURE 14.36 Partial maxillectomy defect according to Triana. (a and b) Anteroposterior and lateral view of an inferior partial maxillectomy. Hatched lines indicate additional palate resection. (c and d) Anteroposterior and lateral view of an inferior partial maxillectomy with total palate resection. (From Triana, R.J. et al., *Arch. Facial Plast. Surg.*, 2, 91, 2000.)

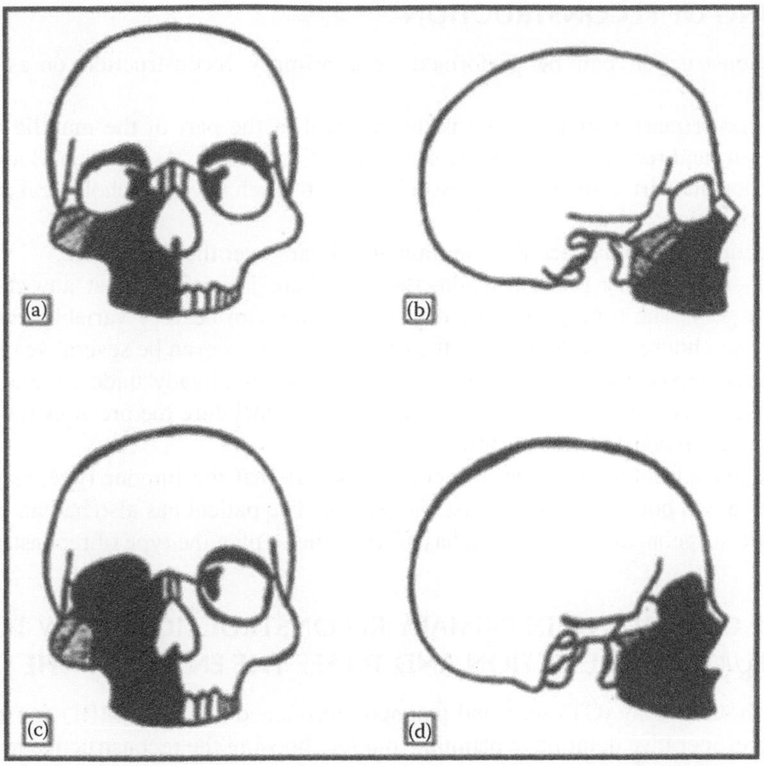

FIGURE 14.37 Total maxillectomy according to Triana. (a and b) Anteroposterior and lateral view of total maxillectomy. (c and d) Anteroposterior and lateral view of total maxillectomy with orbital exenteration. Hatched lines indicate additional malar bone and zygomatic arch resection. (From Triana, R.J. et al., *Arch. Facial Plast. Surg.*, 2, 91, 2000.)

Okay et al. [9] proposed a classification based on the amount of the defect in both horizontal and vertical plane. This system considers the biomechanical properties for obturator stability and retention. In class Ia are included defects that involve the hard palate with preservation of the tooth-bearing alveolus. Class Ib includes defects involving any portion of the maxillary alveolus and dentition posterior to the canines or the premaxilla. Class II defects involves any portion of the tooth-bearing maxillary alveolus but only one canine. Class III includes defects that involved any portion of the tooth-bearing maxillary alveolus and included canines, total palatectomy defects, and anterior transverse palatectomy that involves more than half of the palatal surface. Okay considers two subclasses: subclass f for defects that involve the inferior orbital rime and subclass z for defects that involve the body of the zygoma.

For each class, different methods of reconstruction are proposed considering the possibility to achieve a good closure with an obturator, if a sufficient amount of bone to stabilise it is present, or with local or free flaps in all other cases. The algorithm proposed by Okay is summarised in Table 14.2.

TABLE 14.2
Reconstructive Algorithm Proposed by Okay et al.

	Prosthetic Obturation	Soft Tissue Reconstruction	Vascularized Bone-Containing Free Flap
Class I	X	X	
Class II	X		X
Class III			X

Source: Okay, D.J. et al., *J. Prosthet. Dent.*, 86, 352, 2001.

14.4 TIMING OF RECONSTRUCTION

Maxillary reconstruction can be performed as a primary reconstruction or as a secondary reconstruction.

Immediate or primary reconstruction is the removal of the part of the maxilla involved by a tumour, with surgical reconstruction at the same operative session. As a patient does not wake up without an important part of his face, it is associated with much lower psychological morbidity than delayed reconstruction.

Primary reconstruction has become the standard of care over the last decade.

In delayed or secondary reconstruction, the procedure is performed at any stage following the ablative surgery. The timing of delayed reconstruction can be very variable. From that point onwards, one can choose when to perform the procedure. It may even be several years later.

Often delayed reconstruction is requested if a patient has already undergone a breast reconstruction with unsatisfactory results. During this surgical procedure the previous reconstruction is removed and a new reconstruction performed.

One important advantage of delayed reconstruction is that the tumour type, staging, and the prognosis are known both to the oncologist and patient. The patient has also had an opportunity to choose a plastic surgeon, and the surgeon has all the time to plan the type of reconstruction.

14.5 ROLE OF IMAGING IN PRIMARY RECONSTRUCTION: HOW TO EVALUATE THE RESECTION AND TO SEE THE ENTITY OF THE DEFECT

Computerised tomography (CT) scan and magnetic resonance imaging (MRI) are today the gold standard for pre-operative demolitive planning and for choosing the reconstructive method.

The planning of complex osteotomies in craniomaxillofacial surgery requires a high degree of experience and expertise to achieve the best result. Many reports about 3D CT imaging and 3D visualisation of an individual model of the skeleton have opened up new opportunities, especially in craniofacial surgery after the first concept of 3D planning in craniofacial surgery was described by Cutting et al. [10].

The use of 3D CT and biomodels has made the planning and execution of complex craniomaxillofacial cases more precise [11]. Many reports during the past decade about 3D CT imaging dealt with craniomaxillofacial surgery and its planning [12], but making an osteotomy biomodel as lifelike as possible and to transfer the plan to the operation itself is a challenging work and a valuable aid in composite total maxillectomy reconstruction.

Typically the examination will be done in the axial plane. For examination including the oral cavity or the oropharynx, it is advisable to orient the plane of the occlusal surface to the plane of the gantry; particularly in patients with dental fillings, this helps to reduce the number of sections degraded by metal artefacts. Any gaps in the imaging series resulting from such artefacts can be compensated for by acquiring a few sections as appropriate at a slightly different angle. Axial slices allow good evaluation of the extension of the maxillary tumour in the axial plane, but the extension in the cranio–caudal direction can only be estimated. Problems can arise from partial volume effects and artefacts, especially caused by bone and metal. Further problems arise from the anatomical situation itself. Many structures which are clearly evident in coronal or sagittal sections may be missed in axial sections, where they may be cut tangentially and not in cross section. Areas where such difficulties are apt to occur include the skull base, the palate, the orbital floor, and the paranasal sinuses. Imaging in the coronal or semicoronal plane has become standard in CT for evaluation of diseases of the maxilla, paranasal sinuses, or orbital floor [13] (Figure 14.38).

Axial view is useful to assess the anterior/posterior and transversal dimension. Coronal and sagittal images are useful for cranio–caudal evaluation of tumour spread and for skull base invasion.

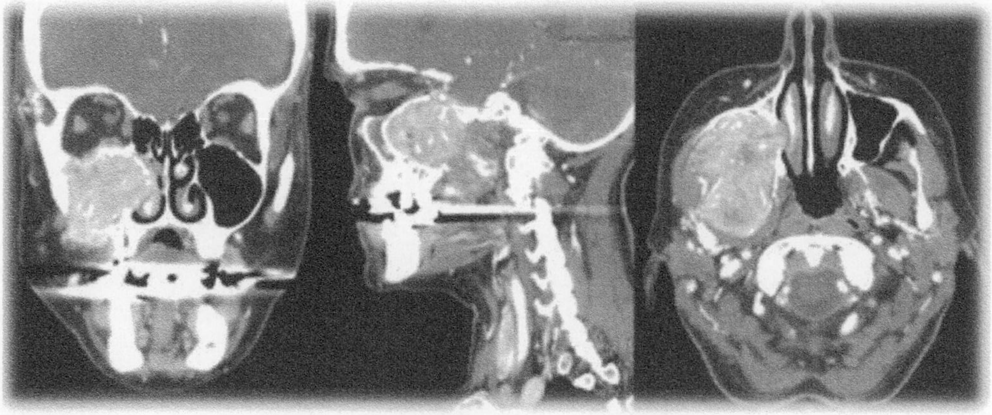

FIGURE 14.38 Coronal, sagittal, and axial CT scan views of a malignant tumour of midface.

According to Brown classification [14] (Figure 14.34), the vertical defect should be assessed using the coronal view of CT scan; the involvement of maxillary sinus, orbital floor, skull base, and oro-nasal fistula are fundamental parameters for demolitive surgical planning.

In Figure 14.39, we present a typical case of maxillary resection type Ib according to Brown classification.

In Figure 14.40, we show a surgical resection of alveolar bone, zygoma, and maxillary sinus in a patient affected by an oral squamous cell carcinoma (OSCC). In this case, the orbital floor was not involved by the tumour (type IIb).

When the CT scan or MRI shows a tumour involvement of the orbital floor, a type III or type IV resection should be performed (Figure 14.41).

Figure 14.42 shows maxillary resections type V and VI.

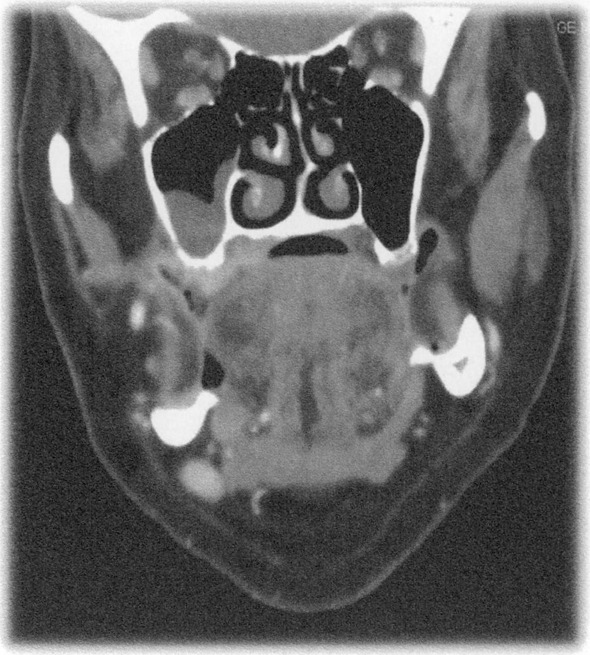

FIGURE 14.39 Oral squamous cell carcinoma of maxillary alveolar gingiva. The surgical resection in this case can be classified as a type Ib according to Brown classification.

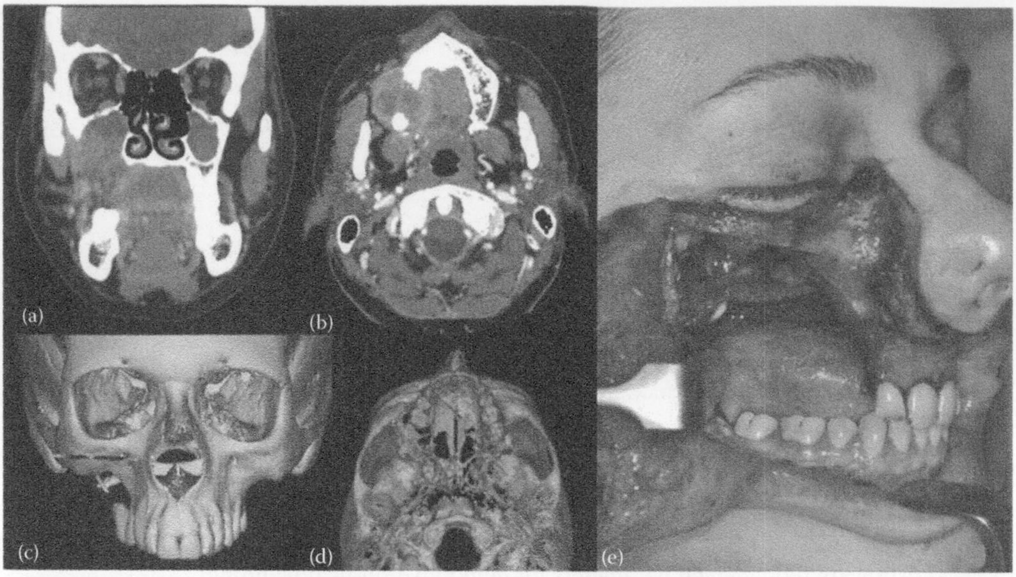

FIGURE 14.40 Axial (a) and coronal (b) view of an OSCC involving the alveolar bone, zygoma, and maxillary sinus (type IIb). The 3D surgical planning of resection is performed using 3D CT DICOM data in coronal (c) and palatal (d) view. Image (e) shows the surgical resection via Weber–Ferguson access.

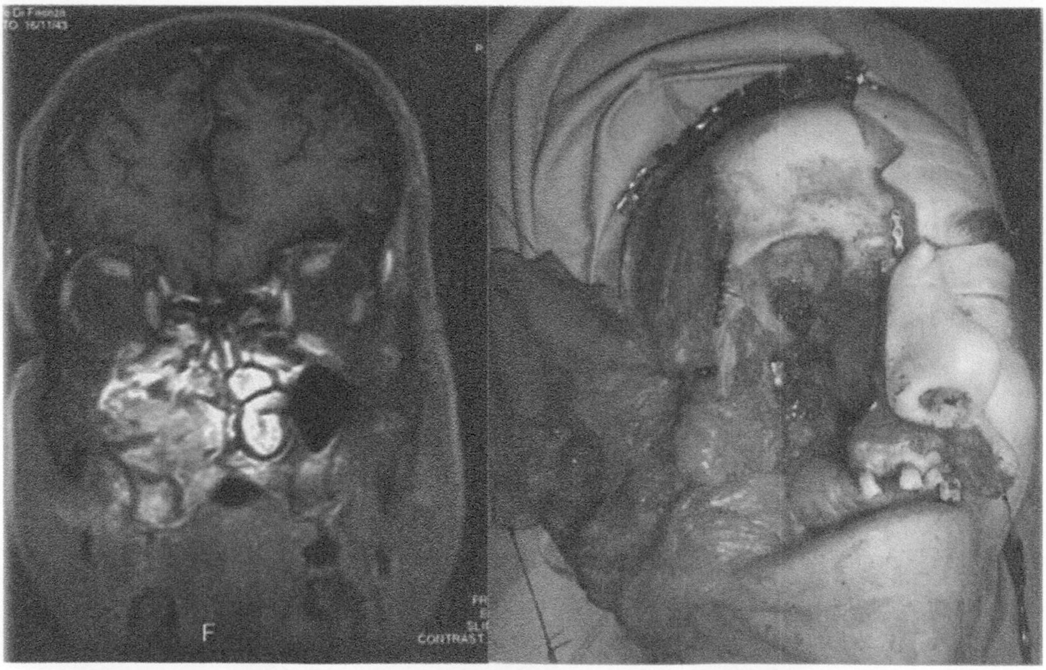

FIGURE 14.41 Radiological (MRI) and clinical images of a maxillary resection associated with an exenteratio orbitae (type IVb) for an adenoid cystic carcinoma originating from minor salivary glands of the palate.

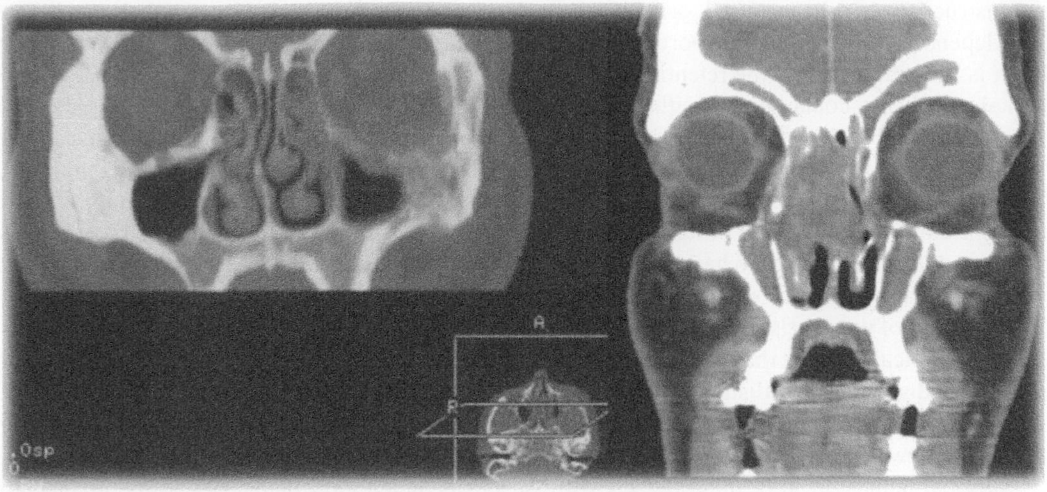

FIGURE 14.42 On the left side is a CT scan shown an adenoid cystic carcinoma involving the orbit and zygoma (resection type V). On the right side the CT scan shows a naso-ethmoidal adenocarcinoma (resection type VI).

14.5.1 Neural Spread Assessment

Perineural spread of head and neck tumours is a form of metastatic disease in which the tumour disseminates to noncontiguous regions along the endoneurium or perineurium. Both CT and MR imaging can help detect perineural spread, although MR imaging is the modality of choice because of its multiplanar capability, its superior soft tissue contrast, and the decreased amount of artefact from dental hardware. Perineural spread most commonly occurs in adenoid cystic carcinoma [15] and squamous cell carcinoma through trigeminal nerve branches. Nerve enlargement may lead to foraminal enlargement and, ultimately, to foraminal destruction, findings that are best seen on CT. Extension through the foramen ovale and involvement of the Meckel cave is best seen on coronal T1-weighted MR images, and nerve enhancement is best seen on fat-suppressed T1-weighted MR images. Other radiologic findings include obliteration of fat planes at foraminal openings, neuropathic atrophy, cavernous sinus enlargement, and replacement of the trigeminal subarachnoid cistern with soft tissue. The pathway of perineural tumour spread is predictable with knowledge of the pertinent cranial nerve anatomy; however, patients with radiologically or pathologically proved perineural spread may have normal nerve function at clinical examination. Therefore, it is imperative that the radiologist be familiar with both normal cranial nerve anatomy and the radiologic appearance and assessment of perineural tumour extension.

14.6 FLAPS FOR MAXILLARY RECONSTRUCTION

14.6.1 History of Maxillary Reconstruction

The main goals to achieve in maxillary reconstruction are to obtain a healed wound; separate nasal and oral cavities; restore maxillary buttresses; maintain a patent nasal airway; restore functional dentition, deglutition, and mastication; and reestablish globe position or address an exenterated cavity cosmetically. From a more aesthetical point of view, the reconstruction has to suspend a dynamic facial soft tissue and restore midfacial contour, in particular midface projection.

Maxillary defects have been traditionally obturated by placement of a maxillary prosthesis, obtaining the oronasal separation, which is fundamental for speaking and swallowing [16,17]. This approach has a low surgical complexity and the length of the procedure is less than with tissue reconstruction. Maxillary, nasal, orbital, and ocular defects can be restored by prosthesis and their use depends on substantial support from native tissues, and the status of the canine and molar teeth is very important to the retention of the prosthesis. Depending on the defect, orbitofacial and dental prostheses could be used either alone or in addition to surgical flaps [18,19]. Nevertheless, prosthetic rehabilitation has substantial shortcomings and patients might become dissatisfied for several reasons. First of all prosthesis need to be removed and cleaned regularly. Denture bulkiness, poor residual dentition, and poor retentive surfaces lead to poor retention, leakage, and oronasal regurgitation [20,21]. In case of loss of the zygomatic prominence, the stability of the prosthesis is decreased. Radiotherapy also has a negative effect on the comfort and retention of the obturator and the underlying tissues that supports it.

Initial use of prosthesis does not preclude future tissue reconstruction, but immediate reconstruction is technically easier than is a secondary procedure and reduces substantial psychological and emotional distress due to disfigurement [22]. The advantage in detection of recurrent tumour with prostheses compared with flap coverage remains unproven, and the accuracy of modern imaging methods allows accurate assessment of the resection bed without direct inspection [23].

Surgical management of these defects with various pedicled flaps dates back to the nineteenth century. Von Langenbeck described in 1862 [24] the use of local palatal flaps for small defects; it was later revisited by Gullane in 1977 [23]. In the twentieth century, local flaps from nasal septum, tongue, cheek, upper lip, pharynx, turbinate, forehead, and neck were described [25–32]. In the 1960s and 1970s, these techniques were largely replaced by pedicled myocutaneous flaps [24,33] that accommodated large defects by providing a sufficiently large volume of well-vascularised tissue. However, this type of reconstruction was not ideal because myocutaneous flaps tended to be bulky and poorly pliable.

The great improvement in head and neck reconstruction was in the 1980s thanks to the development of microvascular anastomotic techniques. Microsurgery allowed composite free tissues transfer, one stage procedures, and no limitations of reach and orientation of regional myocutaneous pedicled flaps. The introduction of microsurgery [34,35] allowed to reconstruct wide defects, even in the presence of damages induced by complementary treatment, restoring function and an acceptable aesthetic in most cases.

The principal advantages of free flaps are the high number of possible donor sites, the possibility to shape the flap obtaining a 3D reconstruction, and the contemporary work by two equipes reducing surgery time. The advent of perforator flaps also introduced another advantage, the low donor site morbidity.

Various donor sites for free tissue transfer have been described for defects after maxillectomy, including radial forearm [36–40], rectus abdominis [41–43], fibula [44–49], scapular system [50–55], and iliac crest [56,57].

14.6.2 Flaps Indicated in Maxillary Reconstruction

Several free flaps were described in maxillary reconstruction. In our experience, we think that three principal flaps are indicated for soft tissue reconstruction: radial forearm, rectus abdominis, and anterolateral thigh (ALT). In case of composite defects that require bone restoring, we found the fibula free flap the ideal method of reconstruction, due to the possibility to plan the insetting preoperatively by CAD-CAM techniques. Iliac crest is an option in case of need of a large volume of bone.

14.6.2.1 Radial Forearm

The radial forearm flap was first described in China by Goufan and Yuzhi in 1981 for hand reconstruction [58] and was so called 'Chinese' flap. It was immediately used in head and neck reconstruction; in particular Shaw used it for the nose [59] and Soutar in intraoral reconstruction [60,61]. It can be harvested as a fasciocutaneous or an osseofasciocutaneous flap.

Midface restoration is one of the better indications for this flap, but it has many applications, including reconstruction of the tongue, lip, oral floor, pharynx, larynx, and cervical oesophagus.

The radial artery is the dominant vascular supply and provides a long pedicle up to 20 cm [62,63]. The thin and pliable fasciocutaneous paddle makes it ideal for lining the oral mucosa and the flap can be folded to recreate the gingivobuccal sulcus or tubed for hypopharyngeal reconstruction.

Allen test [64] must be performed before flap harvesting to ensure adequate blood flow to the distal upper extremity via the ulnar artery.

In osseocutaneous flap, no more than one third of the radius (10 cm) should be harvested.

Donor-site morbidity is historically the major disadvantage of the radial forearm flap, because the defect is often large and requires a skin graft. Donor-site graft loss occurs at rates as low as 2% [65]. Some technical tricks were described to reduce donor site morbidity; in particular closure with an advanced flap based on ulnar artery perforator branches seems to be a better solution [66].

In case of osseocutaneous flap, the radius weakness is another reported consequence and a plate must be prophylactically placed.

14.6.2.2 Rectus Abdominis and DIEAP Flap

The rectus abdominis free flap is a muscle or musculocutaneous flap useful for defects that include the orbits, tongue, cheeks, posterior mandible, and the cranial base [67]. It was described after the anatomical study upon its pedicle made by Taylor and Daniel in 1974 [68].

The flap is based on the deep inferior epigastric vessels that supply the entire central abdominal wall. Several skin islands can be harvested based on that pedicles [69]. The muscle itself measures approximately 25 cm × 6 cm and gives a large amount of soft tissue to fill dead spaces.

Better advantages of rectus abdominis flap are its easy access, manipulability, and size. It can be performed simultaneously and quickly while the head and neck resection is being performed. The donor-site morbidity is related to the risk of hernia and the loss of abdominal wall strength [70,71].

To avoid this risk, deep inferior epigastric perforator flap (DIEAP) flap can be harvested based on the same pedicle.

Caution must be used in patients who have undergone abdominal surgery as the blood supply may be compromised.

Nowadays we think that the DIEAP flap and the anterolateralthigh flap (ALT) flap can be a better alternative with a lower donor site morbidity, useful in most of the indications of rectus abdominis flap.

14.6.2.3 ALT and Tensor Fascia Lata Flap

Anterolateral thigh is fasciocutaneous perforator flap introduced by Song in 1984 [72] commonly used in head and neck reconstruction. Nowadays it is often preferred to radial forearm and rectus abdominis because of the lower donor site morbidity.

The vascular base [72–74] is the descending branch of the lateral circumflex femoral artery. The pedicle can be found along the medial edge of the vastus lateralis and multiple septocutaneous or musculocutaneous perforators can be founded in the lateral thigh septum or on the vastus lateralis itself.

The flap is thin and pliable, and can be easily shaped to restore tridimensional defects. The main disadvantage is the origin from a hair-bearing area. The subcutaneous tissue can be bulky but it is possible to thin it obtaining a very thin flap [75].

Skin grafts are required for donor sites greater than 9 cm in width [76,77]. The donor site morbidity is very low [78].

ALT flap can be easily converted to tensor fascia lata flap if perforators are considered not reliable. The tensor fascia lata is based along the ascending branch of the lateral circumflex femoral artery and can be harvested with iliac bone. The pedicle of the tensor fascia lata is shorter than that of the anterolateral thigh flap, and the donor site is more difficult to close, often requiring a skin graft [79].

14.6.2.4 Fibula

The fibula free flap can be harvested as an osseous, osteomuscular, osteocutaneous, or osteomyocutaneous flap. It was firstly described in leg reconstruction by Ueba and Fujikawa in the 1970s [80]. Hidalgo introduced it in mandibular reconstruction [81]. Its vascular pedicle is represented by the peroneal artery.

It provides up to 40 cm of bone with excellent quality that can tolerate multiple osteotomies because of its segmental blood supply.

The presence of septocutaneous and musculocutaneous perforating vessels derived from the peroneal artery allows harvesting a skin paddle from the lateral leg independently from the bone.

A small cuff of the soleus and flexor hallucis longus must be preserved around the fibula to preserve the vascularisation and the cutaneous perforators that may pass through these muscles.

Although a skin island up to 14 cm wide may be used, defects greater than 5 or 6 cm will require a skin graft for closure.

Flap shaping must be done prior to pedicle section to reduce ischemia time. Particular attention must be taken to protect the vascular pedicle during bone drilling.

Post-operative morbidity of the fibula free flap is relatively low [82]. A preoperative angiogram is not always necessary but it must be considered in patients with peripheral vascular disease or previous lower leg trauma.

14.6.2.5 Iliac Crest

The iliac crest free flap was first introduced by Dr. G. Taylor in 1979 [56] and introduced for use in midface reconstruction by Brown [57].

The pedicle is based on the deep circumflex iliac artery and is usually generous in length and in diameter.

The dissection begins along the inguinal crease from the femoral pulse laterally to the anterior superior iliac spine. The dissection is performed through the external oblique and tensor fascia lata muscles, and the medial retraction of the inguinal ligament provides access to the iliac crest. A composite flap can be harvested using part of the internal oblique muscle. A meticulous layered closure can prevent the occurrence of an abdominal hernia. A careful dissection and preservation of the lateral cutaneous nerve of the thigh, which runs medial to the anterior superior iliac spine, can prevent neuroma formation and sensory loss to the lateral thigh.

Some authors have discouraged the use of this flap in the maxilla owing to its large bulk, limited skin paddle mobility, shorter pedicle length, and slightly higher donor-site morbidity. However, it remains a viable second-line option for structural reconstruction of the mandible and midface.

14.7 CAD-CAM TO PLAN MAXILLARY RECONSTRUCTION WITH FREE FLAP

The use of virtual planning to restore tissue that was lost due to tumour surgery is becoming more popular in reconstructive surgery. Particularly in complex anatomical situations involving different sorts of tissue, the use of CAD-CAM applications facilitates planning and execution.

This method is widespread in craniomaxillofacial surgery, but also other specialties are using this technique in their clinical routine [83].

The rapid prototyping approach allows the creation of any desired 3D design, which is created virtually using computer software. Models and templates built through rapid prototyping allow the surgeon to bring the planning to the operating theatre and close the gap between set-up and execution. Here, we report a case of reconstruction with a special technique for virtual planning, rapid prototyping, and reconstructive CAD-CAM plate sintering in order to support the microvascular reconstruction. We also want to demonstrate the ability to plan and execute the restoration of an anatomically complex area with functional demands.

14.7.1 Primary Reconstruction: A Case Example

We report a case of a 17-year-old male affected by a tumour involving his left maxilla (Figure 14.43).

In Figure 14.44 we show the 3D CT surgical osteotomies planned.

A computer tomography scan of the patient's leg was performed, and the necessary bony shape was virtually inserted in the 3D surgical planning using Surgicase® software (Leuven, Belgium, EU). A CAD-CAM titanium mesh was created using a laser-sintering system (Figure 14.45).

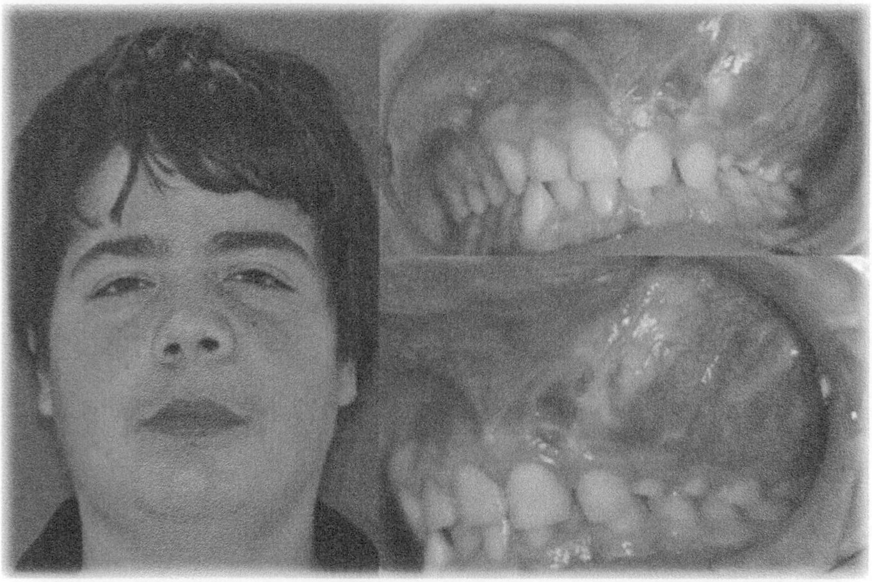

FIGURE 14.43 Extraoral and oral view of a young patient affected by a large left maxillary tumour.

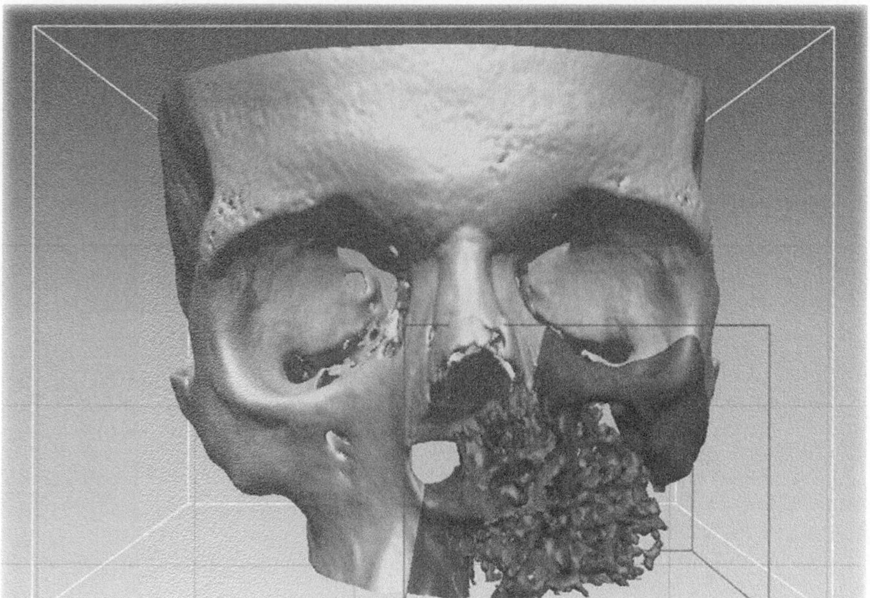

FIGURE 14.44 3D CT surgical osteotomies planned: the orbital floor is also removed.

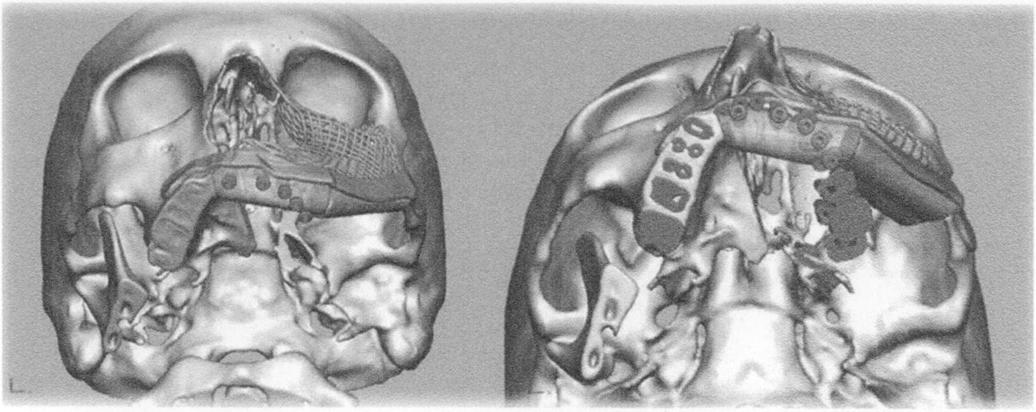

FIGURE 14.45 3D CT showing the virtual reconstructive planning using the microvascular fibula flap supported by a custom-made titanium mesh to reconstruct the anterior maxillary sinus wall and the left orbital floor. In the right image, it is possible to see the simulation of the dental implant inserted in the fibula bone in order to obtain a prosthetic rehabilitation.

A cutting bone guide was created in order to obtain precise osteotomy lines both for the maxilla and the fibula (Figure 14.46).

The patient had a left maxillectomy involving the alveolar bone, maxillary sinus, the orbital floor, and the zygomatic arch, via Weber–Ferguson access (Figure 14.46a). The microvascular fibula flap was cut using the cutting guide and supported by the CAD-CAM titanium mesh (Figure 14.46b).

The post-operative clinical view (Figure 14.47a) and the 3D CT scan show a good aesthetical and functional short-term result (Figure 14.48).

14.7.1.1 Conclusions

The reported case demonstrates that the CAD-CAM technique can be of great value in planning and executing the reconstruction of resected or damaged tissue. The bone and the titanium mesh

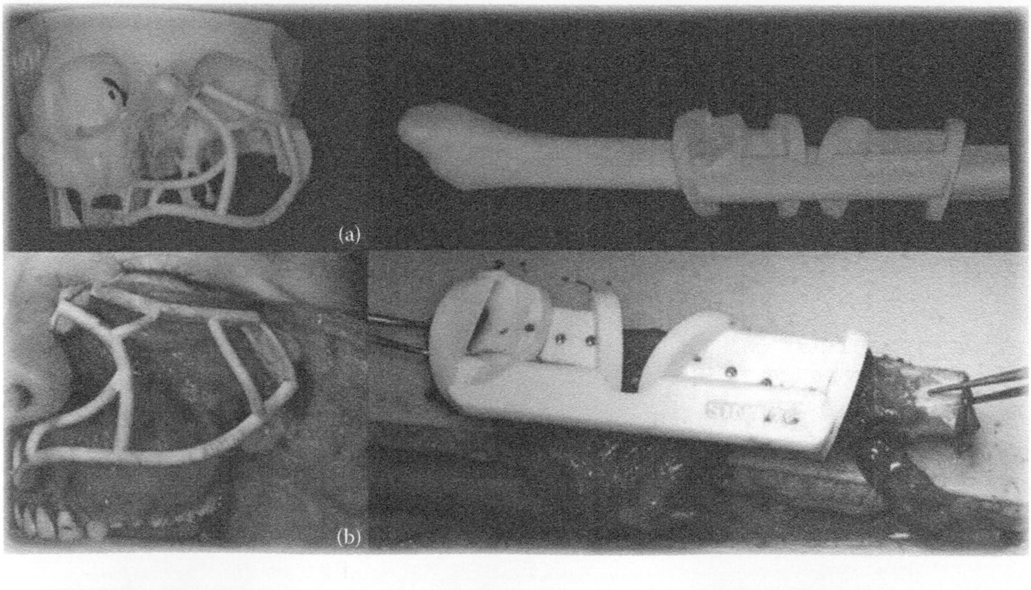

FIGURE 14.46 Stereolithographic models (a) and clinical view (b) of cutting bone guides for maxilla and fibula.

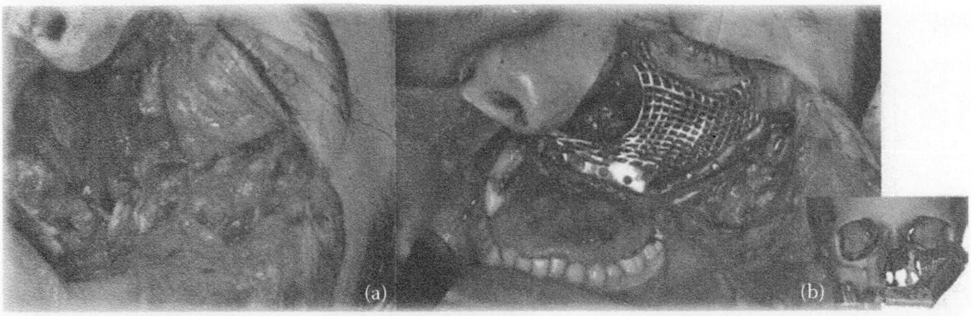

FIGURE 14.47 Intraoperative images showing the tumour resection (a) and the fibula flap insetting (b) supported by a CAD-CAM titanium mesh, in order to obtain a 3D reconstruction of the anterior wall of the maxillary sinus, the zygomatic arch, and the orbital floor.

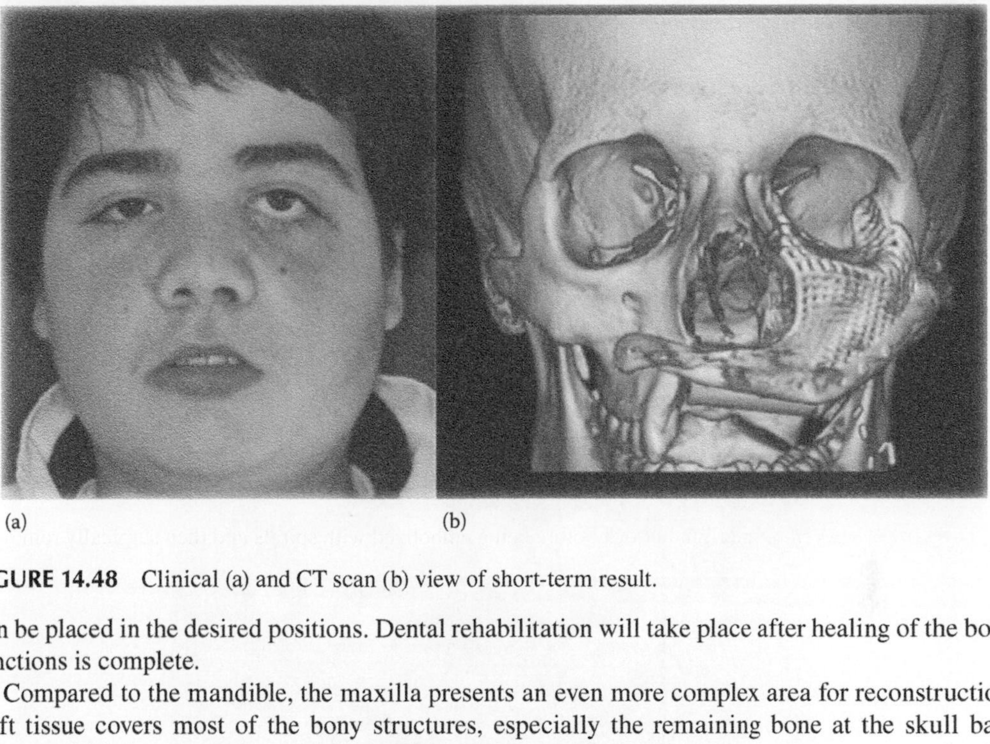

(a) (b)

FIGURE 14.48 Clinical (a) and CT scan (b) view of short-term result.

can be placed in the desired positions. Dental rehabilitation will take place after healing of the bony junctions is complete.

Compared to the mandible, the maxilla presents an even more complex area for reconstruction. Soft tissue covers most of the bony structures, especially the remaining bone at the skull base region, which is necessary for bone fixation. The anatomical proximity to vital structures further complicates the process of reconstruction.

We regard 3D models as a reasonable amendment in craniofacial reconstruction that offers multiple advantages. They facilitate surgical planning by demonstrating the anatomical characteristics of the tissue to be operated upon. By adding a haptic sensation, this approach optimises preoperative planning. The surgeon achieves a better impression of the anatomical situation, the actual amount of bone, and the demands on the reconstruction, which will result in a safer operation, shorter operation time, and a more predictable result.

14.7.2 Delayed Reconstruction: A Case Example

We report the case of a 73-year-old male with an important maxillary defect. At the age of 70, an OSCC was diagnosed, and the patient underwent a total maxillectomy. The surgical defect was covered using a pedicled temporalis muscle flap (Figure 14.49).

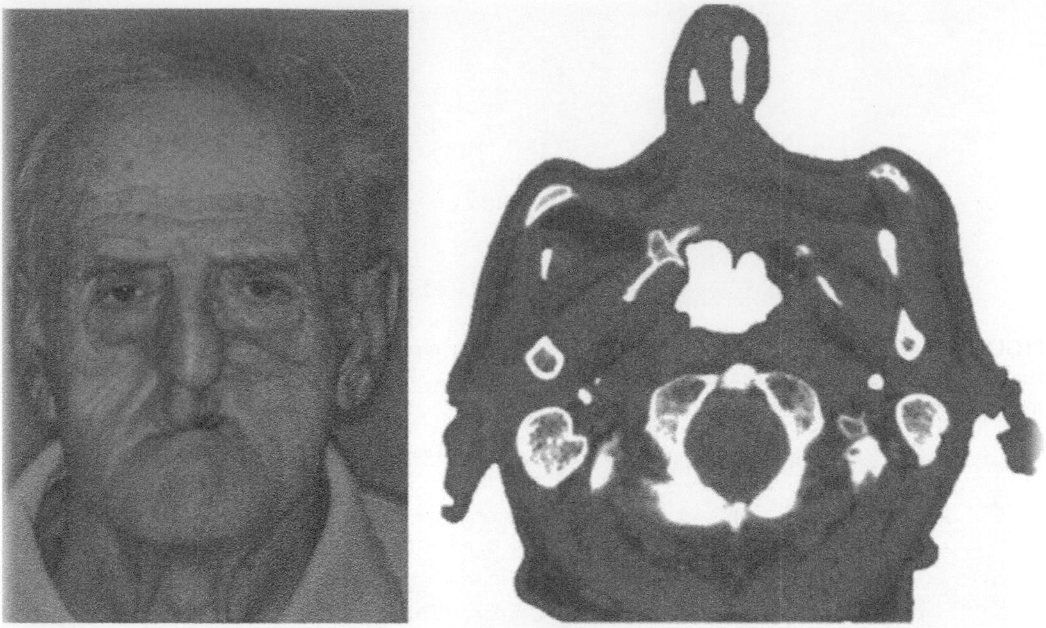

FIGURE 14.49 Clinical and radiological images after total maxillary resection for OSCC.

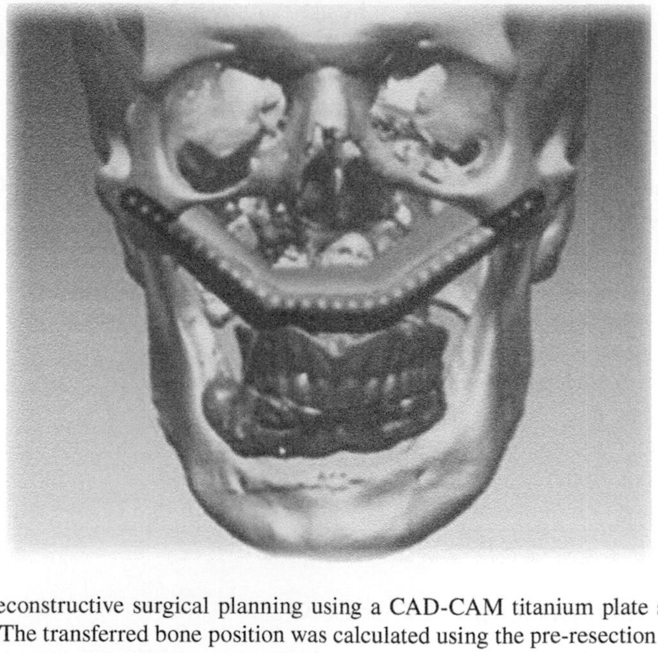

FIGURE 14.50 Reconstructive surgical planning using a CAD-CAM titanium plate supporting a microvascular fibula flap. The transferred bone position was calculated using the pre-resection prosthesis imported into the planning.

To reduce the defect and to reconstruct the processus alveolaris, a microvascular fibula flap was selected for transfer. An individually pre-molded titanium mesh was used to support the fibula flap.

'Backward' planning was used to find the best position of the bony part. The position of the jaws was defined using the prosthesis which the patient used before the surgical resection (Figure 14.50).

A CT scan of the left leg was performed, and the necessary bony shape was virtually matched with the patient's fibula. To achieve the desired lengths and angles at the fibula's resection and split sites, a rapid prototype template was fabricated (Figure 14.51).

The titanium plate was obtained from CT scan DICOM data using a laser-sintering method.

Figure 14.52 shows the fibula flap with skin paddle supported by the titanium plate.

Post-operative 3D CT scan shows a satisfactory aesthetical result. Four zygomatic implants were inserted in order to support the prosthetical rehabilitation (Figure 14.53).

This case demonstrates that CAD-CAM techniques can be of great value in planning and executing the reconstruction of resected or damaged tissue. The bone and the titanium mesh can be placed in the desired positions. Dental rehabilitation will take place after healing of the bony junctions is complete.

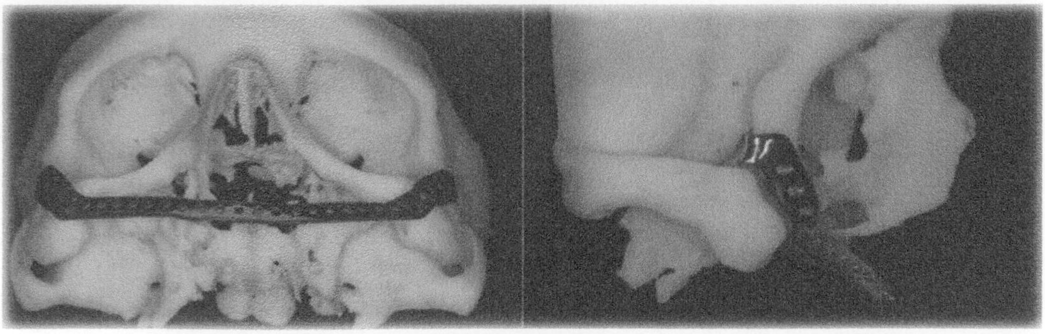

FIGURE 14.51 Frontal and lateral view of the stereolithographic model with the CAD-CAM titanium plate.

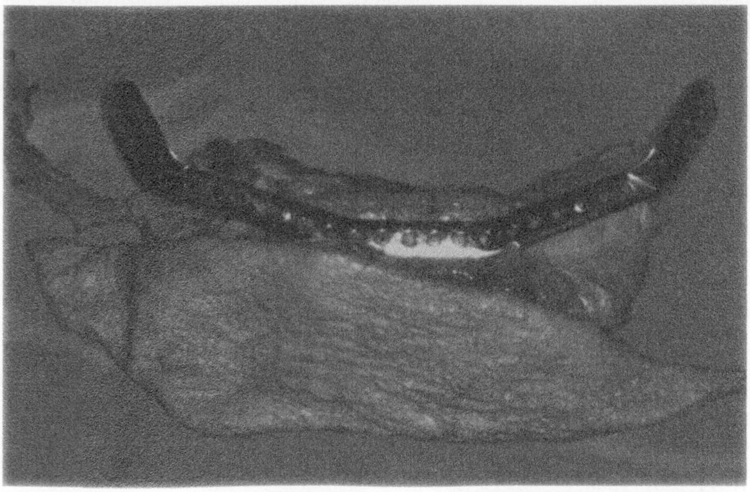

FIGURE 14.52 Fibula free flap supported by CAD-CAM titanium plate.

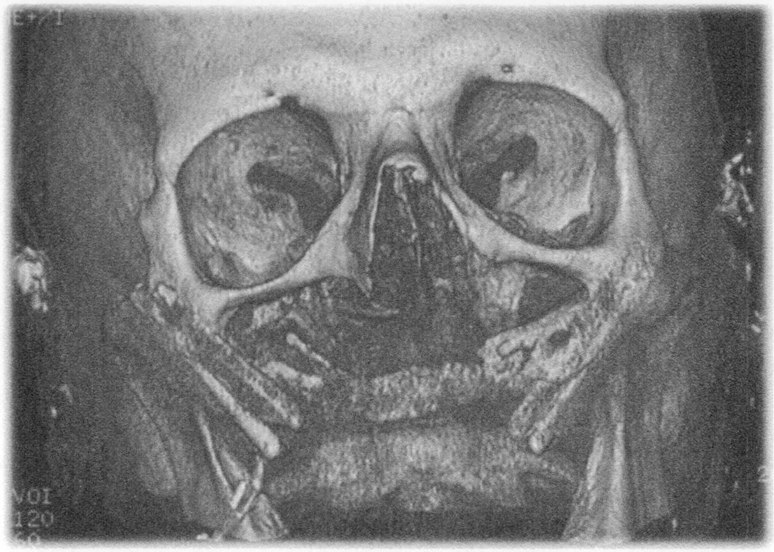

FIGURE 14.53 3D CT scan showing a good restoration of maxillary contour. Four zygomatic implants were inserted after the titanium plate removal.

REFERENCES

1. Hurvitz KA, Kobayashi M, Evans GR. Current options in head and neck reconstruction. *Plast Reconstr Surg* 2006;118(5):122e–133e. Review.
2. Gurtner GC, Evans GR. Advances in head and neck reconstruction. *Plast Reconstr Surg* 2000;106(3):672–682; quiz 683.
3. Mathes SJ, Ed. *Plastic Surgery*. Philadelphia, PA: Saunders, 2006. Vol. V, pp. 91–254.
4. Longaker MT, Siebert JW. Microvascular free-flap correction of severe hemifacial atrophy. *Plast Reconstr Surg* 1995;96(4):800–809.
5. Lee JC, St-Hilaire H, Christy MR, Wise MW, Rodriguez ED. Anterolateral thigh flap for trauma reconstruction. *Ann Plast Surg* 2010;64(2):164–168.
6. Brown JS, Rogers SN, McNally DN, Boyle M. A modified classification for the maxillectomy defect. *Head Neck* 2000;22:17–26.
7. Cordeiro PG, Santamaria E. A classification system and algorithm for reconstruction of maxillary and midfacial defects. *Plast Reconstr Surg* 2000;105:2331–2346.
8. Triana RJ, Uglesic V, Virag M et al. Microvascular free flap reconstructive options in patients with partial and total maxillectomy defects. *Arch Facial Plast Surg* 2000;2:91–101.
9. Okay DJ, Genden E, Buchbinder D, Urken M. Prosthodontic guidelines for surgical reconstruction of the maxilla: A classification system of defects. *J Prosthet Dent* 2001;86:352–363.
10. Cutting C, Bookstein FL, Grayson B, Fellingham L, McCarthy JG. Three-dimensional computer-assisted design of craniofacial surgical procedures: Optimization and interaction with cephalometric and CT-based models. *J Plast Reconstr Surg* 1986;77:877–887.
11. Rose EH, Norris MS, Rosen JM. Application of high-tech three dimensional imaging and computer-generated models in complex facial reconstructions with vascularised bone grafts. *Plast Reconstr Surg* 1993;91:252–264.
12. Marchetti C, Bianchi A, Bassi M, Gori R, Lamberti C, Sarti A. Mathematical modeling and numerical simulation in maxillofacial virtual surgery (VISU). *J Craniofac Surg* 2006;17:661–667.
13. Baum U, Greess H, Lell M, Nömayr A, Lenz M. *Eur J Radiol* 2000;33:153–160.
14. Brown J, Shaw R. Reconstruction of the maxilla and midface: Introducing a new classification. *Lancet Oncol* 2010;11:1001–1008.
15. Tarsitano A, Pizzigallo A, Gessaroli M, Sturiale C, Marchetti C. Intraoperative biopsy of the major cranial nerves in the surgical strategy for adenoid cystic carcinoma close to the skull base. *Oral Surg Oral Med Oral Pathol Oral Radiol* 2011;113(2):214–221.

16. Robb GL, Marunick MT, Martin JW, Zlotolow IM. Midface reconstruction: Surgical reconstruction versus prosthesis. *Head Neck* 2001;23:48–58.
17. Ali A, Fardy MJ, Patton DW. Maxillectomy: To reconstruct or obturate? Results of a UK survey of oral and maxillofacial surgeons. *Br J Oral Maxillofac Surg* 1995;33:207–211.
18. Funk GF, Arcuri MR, Frodel JL Jr. Functional dental rehabilitation of massive palatomaxillary defects: Cases requiring free tissue transfer and osseointegrated implants. *Head Neck* 1998;20:38–48.
19. Gliklich RE, Rounds MF, Cheney ML, Varvares MA. Combining free flap reconstruction and craniofacial prosthetic techniques for orbit, scalp, and temporal defects. *Laryngoscope* 1998:108:482–487.
20. Gillespie CA, Kennan PD, Ferguson BJ. Hard palate reconstruction in maxillectomy. *Laryngoscope* 1986;96:443–444.
21. Futran ND, Haller JR. Considerations for free-flap reconstruction of the hard palate. *Arch Otolaryngol Head Neck Surg* 2005;125:665–669.
22. Olsen KD, Meland NB, Ebersold MJ et al. Extensive defects of the sino-orbital region: Results with microvascular reconstruction. *Arch Otolaryngol Head Neck Surg* 1992;118:828–833.
23. Gullane PJ, Arena S. Palatal island flap for reconstruction of oral defects. *Arch Otolaryngol* 1977;103:598–599.
24. Ariyan S. The pectoralis major myocutaneous flap: A versatile flap for reconstruction in the head and neck. *Plast Reconstr Surg* 1979;63:73–81.
25. Edgerton MT, DeVito RV. Closure of palatal defects by means of a hinged nasal septum flap. *Plast Reconstr Surg* 1963;31–33:537–540.
26. Wallace AF. Esser's skin flap for closing large palatal fistulae. *Br J Plast Surg* 1966;19:322–326.
27. Chambers RG, Jaques DA, Mahoney WD. Tongue flaps for intraoral reconstruction. *Am J Surg* 1969;118:783–786.
28. Muzaffar AR, Adams WP, Hartog JM et al. Maxillary reconstruction: Functional and aesthetic considerations. *Plast Reconstr Surg* 1999;104:2172–2183.
29. Elliott RA Jr. Use of nasolabial skin flap to cover intraoral defects. *Plast Reconstr Surg* 1976;58:201–205.
30. Guerrerosantos J, Altamirano JT. The use of lingual flaps in repair of fistulas of the hard palate. *Plast Reconstr Surg* 1966;38:123–126.
31. Miller TA. The Tagliacozzi flap as a method of nasal and palatal reconstruction. *Plast Reconstr Surg* 1985;76:870–875.
32. Komisar A, Lawson W. A compendium of intraoral flaps. *Head Neck Surg* 1985;8:91–97.
33. Baker SR. Closure of large orbito-maxillary defects with free latissimus dorsi myocutaneous flaps. *Head Neck Surg* 1984;6:828–832.
34. Lyons AJ. Perforators flaps in head and neck surgery. *Int J Oral Maxillofac Surg* 2006;35:199–207.
35. Taylor GI, Palmer JH. The vascular territories (angiosomes) of the body: Experimental study and clinical applications. *Br J Plast Surg* 1987;40(2):113–141.
36. Cordeiro PG, Bacilious N, Schantz S, Spiro R. The radial forearm osteocutaneous "sandwich" free flap for reconstruction of the bilateral subtotal maxillectomy defect. *Ann Plast Surg* 1998;40:397–402.
37. McLoughlin PM, Gilhooly M, Phillips JG. Reconstruction of the infraorbital margin with a composite microvascular free flap. *Br J Oral Maxillofac Surg* 1993;31:227–229.
38. Chepeha DB, Moyer JS, Bradford CR et al. Osseocutaneous radial forearm free tissue transfer for repair of complex midfacial defects. *Arch Otolaryngol Head Neck Surg* 2005;131:513–517.
39. Genden EM, Wallace DI, Okay D, Urken ML. Reconstruction of the hard palate using the radial forearm free flap: Indications and outcomes. *Head Neck* 2004;26:808–814.
40. Marshall DM, Amjad I, Wolfe SA. Use of the radial forearm flap for deep, central, midfacial defects. *Plast Reconstr Surg* 2003;111:56–64.
41. Pribaz JJ, Morris DJ, Mulliken JB. Three-dimensional folded freeflap reconstruction of complex facial defects using intraoperative modeling. *Plast Reconstr Surg* 1994;93:285–293.
42. Yamamoto Y, Nohira K, Minakawa H et al. "Boomerang" rectus abdominis musculocutaneous free flap in head and neck reconstruction. *Ann Plast Surg* 1995;34:48–55.
43. Brown JD, Burke AJC. Benefits of routine or maxillectomy and orbital reconstruction with the rectus abdominis free flap. *Otolaryngol Head Neck Surg* 1999;121:203–209.
44. Nakayama B, Matsuura H, Ishihara O et al. Functional reconstruction of a bilateral maxillectomy defect using a fibula osteocutaneous flap with osseointegrated implants. *Plast Reconstr Surg* 1995;96:1201–1204.
45. Yim KK, Wei FC. Fibula osteoseptocutaneous free flap in maxillary reconstruction. *Microsurgery* 1994;15:353–357.

46. Nakayama B, Matsuura H, Hasegawa Y et al. New reconstruction for total maxillectomy defect with a fibula osteocutaneous free flap. *Br J Plast Surg* 1994;47:247–249.
47. Anthony JP, Foster RD, Sharma AB et al. Reconstruction of a complex midfacial defect with the folded fibular free flap and osseointegrated implants. *Ann Plast Surg* 1996;37:204–210.
48. Kazaoka Y, Shinohara A, Yokou K, Hasegawa T. Functional reconstruction after a total maxillectomy using a fibula osteocutaneous flap with osseointegrated implants. *Plast Reconstr Surg* 1999;103:1244–1246.
49. Futran ND, Wadsworth JT, Villaret D, Farwell DG. Midface reconstruction with the fibula free flap. *Arch Otolaryngol Head Neck Surg* 2002;128:161–166.
50. Swartz WM, Banis JC, Newton ED et al. The osteocutaneous scapular flap for mandibular and maxillary reconstruction. *Plast Reconstr Surg* 1986;77:530–545.
51. Granick MS, Ramasastry SS, Newton ED et al. Reconstruction of complex maxillectomy defects with the scapular-free flap. *Head Neck* 1990;12:377–385.
52. Schusterman MA, Reece GP, Miller MJ. Osseous free flaps for orbit and midface reconstruction. *Am J Surg* 1993;6:341–345.
53. Coleman JJ III. Osseous reconstruction of the midface and orbits. *Clin Plast Surg* 1994;1:113–124.
54. Holle J, Vinzenz K, Wuringer E et al. The prefabricated combined scapula flap for bony and soft-tissue reconstruction in maxillofacial defects: A new method. *Plast Reconstr Surg* 1996;98:542–552.
55. Uglesic V, Virag M, Varga S et al. Reconstruction following radical maxillectomy with flaps supplied by the subscapular artery. *J Craniomaxillofac Surg* 2000;28:153–160.
56. Taylor G, Townsend P, Corlett R. Superiority of the deep circumflex iliac vessels as the supply for free groin flaps. Clinical work. *Plast Surg Reconstr* 1979;64:745.
57. Brown JS. Deep circumflex iliac artery free flap with internal oblique muscle as a new method of immediate reconstruction of maxillectomy defects. *Head Neck* 1996;18:412–421.
58. Yang GF, Chen PJ, Gao YZ, Liu XY, Li J, Jiang SX. Forearm free skin flap transplantation: A report of 56 cases. 1981. *Br J Plast Surg* 1997;50(3):162–165.
59. Shaw WL. Microvascular reconstruction of the nose. *Clin Plast Surg* 1981;8:471.
60. Soutar DS, Scheker LR, Tanner NSB, McGregor IA. The radial forearm flap in intra-oral reconstruction: A versatile method for intra-oral reconstruction. *Brit J Plast Surg* 1983;36:1.
61. Soutar DS, McGregor IA. The radial forearm flap in intra-oral reconstruction: The experience of 60 consecutive cases. *Plast Reconstr Surg* 1986;78:1.
62. Mathes SJ, Nahai F. *Reconstructive Surgery: Principles, Anatomy and Techniques*. New York: Churchill Livingstone, 1997.
63. Timmons MJ. The vascular basis of the radial forearm flap. *Plast Reconstr Surg* 1986;77:80.
64. Allen EV. Thromboangiitis obliterans: Methods of diagnosis of chronic obstructive occlusive arterial lesions distal to the wrist with illustrative cases. *Am J Med Sci* 1929;178:237.
65. Emerick KS, Deschler DG. Incidence of donor site skin graft loss requiring surgical intervention with the radial forearm free flap. *Head Neck* 2007;29:573.
66. Bardsley AF, Soutar DS, Elliot D, Batchelor AG. Reducing morbidity in the radial forearm flap donor site. *Plast Reconstr Surg* 1990;86(2):287–292; discussion 293–294.
67. Moyer J, Chepeha D, Teknos T. Contemporary skull base reconstruction. *Curr Opin Otolaryngol Head Neck Surg* 2004;12:294.
68. Taylor GI, Daniel RK. The anatomy of several free flap donor sites. *Plast Reconstr Surg* 1975;56:243.
69. Pennington DG. The rectus abdominis myocutanoeous free flap. *Brit J Plast Surg* 1980;33:277.
70. Kroll S, Baldwin B. Head and neck reconstruction with the rectus abdominis free flap. *Clin Plast Surg* 1994;21:97.
71. Cordeiro P, Disa J. Challenges in midface reconstruction. *Semin Surg Oncol* 2000;19:218.
72. Song YG, Chen GZ, Song YL. The free thigh flap: A new free flap concept based on the septocutaneous artery. *Br J Plast Surg* 1984;37:149–159.
73. Ali RS, Bluebond-Langner R, Rodriguez ED, Cheng MH. The versatility of the anterolateral thigh flap. *Plast Reconstr Surg* 2009;124(6 Suppl):e395–e407. Review.
74. Lueg E. The anterolateral thigh flap: Radial forearm's "big brother" for extensive soft tissue and head and neck defects. *Arch Otolaryngol Head Neck Surg* 2004;130:813.
75. Yu P. Characteristics of the anterolateral thigh flap in a Western population and its application in head and neck reconstruction. *Head Neck* 2004;26:759.
76. Kimata Y, Uchiyama K, Ebihara S, Nakatsuka T, Harii K. Anatomic variations and technical problems of the anterolateral thigh flap: A report of 74 cases. *Plast Reconstr Surg* 1998;102:1517.
77. Kawai K, Imanishi N, Nakajima H, Aiso S, Kakibuchi M, Hosokawa K. Vascular anatomy of the anterolateral thigh flap. *Plast Reconstr Surg* 2004;144:1108–1117.

78. Kimata Y, Uchiyama K, Ebihara S et al. Anterolateral thigh flap donor-site complications and morbidity. *Plast Reconstr Surg* 2000;106:584–589.
79. Coskunfirat O, Ozkan O. Free tensor fascia lata perforator flap as a backup procedure for head and neck reconstruction. *Ann Plast Surg* 2006;57:159.
80. Liu J, Kumar VP. The first description of the free vascularized bone transplant. *Plast Recosntr Surg* 1997;99(1):270–272.
81. Hidalgo DA. Fibula free flap: A new method of mandible reconstruction. *Plast Reconstr Surg* 1989;84(1):71–79.
82. Hidalgo D, Rekow A. A review of 60 consecutive fibula free flap mandible reconstructions. *Plast Surg Reconstr* 1995;96:585.
83. Metzger MC, Hohlweg-Majert B, Schon R, Teschner M, Gellrich NC, Schmelzeisen R, Gutwald R. Verification of clinical precision after computer-aided reconstruction in craniomaxillofacial surgery. *Oral Surg Oral Med Oral Pathol Oral Radiol Endod* 2007;104:e1–e10.

15 Imaging for Jaw Reconstruction

Wei F. Chen, Steven Lo, Anuja K. Antony, and Fu Chan Wei

CONTENTS

15.1 INTRODUCTION

Mandibular reconstruction for oncologic and non-oncologic defects was revolutionised with the inception and popularisation of the fibula osteoseptocutaneous flap, allowing stable vascularised bone graft especially for restoration of mandibular integrity and occlusion.

Imaging has played an important part in the evolution in the approach to both tumour resection and jaw reconstruction. In terms of determination of bone invasion, previous reliance on physical examination and conventional radiography has been superseded with advances in single-photon emission computed tomography (SPECT) bone scintigraphy, MRI, and more recently PET/CT. This has allowed a more accurate preoperative planning of mandibular resection and a reduction in unnecessary segmental mandibulectomies. Furthermore, although we continue to perform the majority of our mandibular reconstructions at Chang Gung Memorial Hospital freehand and design the neomandibular construct in situ, advances in 3D CT planning may in the future allow the use of *virtual surgery*. This may allow a more accurate reconstruction of the mandible and minimise inter-operator variation in results, particularly in low-volume oncology centres.

Finally, in adjunct to jaw reconstruction such as osseointegrated teeth or concomitant functional muscle reconstruction, imaging plays a vital part in preoperative planning. A number of cases are presented herein that demonstrate the utility of 3D CT reconstruction and MRI.

15.2 ONCOLOGIC JAW RECONSTRUCTION

With standard mandibular reconstruction, no planning is normally made with 3D CT or models unless osseointegrated teeth are planned. Soft tissue and bone resection margins are determined by a combination of preoperative imaging and intraoperative examination and after frozen section is complete.

Imaging in the context of oncological mandibular reconstruction has three main diagnostic purposes: the determination of bone invasion, the assessment of degree of local tumour spread (e.g. tumour stage IVa vs. IVb) and resectability, and the assessment of regional and distant spread. This section focuses on the determination of bone invasion by imaging, as an aid to surgical resection and reconstructive planning, and will not cover aspects related to regional or distant spread.

15.2.1 Determination of Bone Invasion

15.2.1.1 Physical Examination and Conventional Radiography

Accurate determination of bone invasion is a prerequisite for planning of the surgical resection and reconstruction, allowing preparation for a vascularised bone transfer in mandibulectomy cases. It is no longer acceptable in most major oncology centres to base the surgical plan on physical examination and conventional radiographs alone, when newer imaging modalities provide greater diagnostic information that may aid both surgical planning and patient counselling.

Van Cann et al. studied the sensitivity and specificity of physical examination compared to various imaging techniques in 67 oral squamous cell cancer patients (Van Cann et al. 2008). The sensitivity and specificity of both physical examination and conventional radiographic examination (Panorex) was poor and would in the present age be insufficient grounds on which to confidently base definitive surgical planning (clinical examination sensitivity 59%, specificity 74%, conventional radiography sensitivity 61%, specificity 61%). The low sensitivity of these tests may result to inadequate bone resection (high false negative), whilst the low specificity may conversely result in increased morbidity due to unnecessary mandibular resection (high false positive). Physical examination and conventional radiography were subsequently compared in Van Cann et al.'s study with bone scintigraphy, CT, PET/CT, and MRI, as discussed in the following.

15.2.1.2 Bone Scintigraphy, CT, PET/CT, and MRI

Bone scintigraphy with SPECT allows 3D reconstruction of the mandible and has previously been shown to have a very low false-negative rate (high sensitivity) and may reduce unnecessary mandibulectomies. Van Cann et al. confirmed these previous findings by demonstrating that SPECT has a sensitivity of 100% (no false negatives) but a specificity of only 57% (high false positives). CT scanning has traditionally been viewed in conventional surgical teaching as being one of the best modalities for bone imaging, but in head and neck cancer, this is not necessarily true. CT cannot be used in isolation due to artefacts from dental fillings and has been shown to have a relatively poor sensitivity and specificity for bone invasion in oral squamous cell carcinoma. MRI likewise has a number of drawbacks in bone imaging, with motion artefacts and local inflammation or oedema producing false positives. Van Cann et al. found a sensitivity and specificity for CT of 58% and 96% and MRI of 63% and 100%, respectively. This study concludes by presenting a number of imaging algorithms in their study, but these are not the ones that we follow in our institution.

More recently, PET in conjunction with CT has been utilised to provide more data than standard PET alone (which provides uptake data but poor morphological and anatomical localisation) or CT alone (which provides morphological data only). In brief, PET utilises the principle of increased uptake of glucose in malignant cells, due to an oncogene-related increase in membrane transporter proteins for glucose. A study from our own institution compared PET/CT with MRI in 114 patients with oral squamous cell carcinoma (Abd El Hafez et al. 2011). Diagnostic imaging accuracy was compared with the reference standard of histopathological examination. In this study, PET/CT was shown to be more specific than MRI (specificity 83% vs. 61%, $p = 0.0015$). However, sensitivity with PET/CT was lower than MRI (sensitivity 78% vs. 97%, $p = 0.04$).

Given the very high sensitivity of MRI at 97%, it is recommended that an MRI scan is performed first to exclude bone invasion. A negative MRI can therefore confidently exclude the presence of bone marrow invasion and therefore aid the surgical resection and reconstructive planning. PET/CT at present plays a complementary role to MRI, as the specificity is much higher and may confirm that signs of bone marrow invasion on MRI are indeed due to tumour invasion. It should be noted that both sensitivity and specificity are poorer in edentulous patients and caution must be taken in interpreting the results in this sub-cohort. Thus, our present algorithm specifies that in the presence of positive MRI for possible bone marrow invasion, a true positive may be confirmed by a subsequent PET/CT. Higher rates of false positives with MRI in the Taiwanese population have been attributed to betel nut chewing that may result in trismus, submucous fibrosis, and local inflammation, which, as we have alluded to previously, result in difficulties in interpretation of true bone invasion.

15.2.2 Imaging of the Donor Site

Is CT angiography of the donor fibula necessary? At this time, routine preoperative vascular imaging of the lower extremity in preparation for free fibula transfer remains controversial (Karanas et al. 2004). Theoretical advantages of preoperative CT angiography of the donor fibula include delineation of the vascular anatomy of the skin paddle and detection of vascular anomalies such as arteria peronea magna. In the setting of virtual surgical planning of mandible reconstruction using free fibula flap, preoperative CT scan provides the added advantage of allowing virtual planning using patient-specific virtual fibula. Counter-intuitively, the use of patient-specific virtual fibula does not lead to further increase in accuracy compared to the use of generic virtual fibula, as demonstrated by Roser et al. (2010). Whilst different opinions exist in the literature with regard to the consistency of the peroneal artery perforator anatomy (Ribuffo et al. 2009), many authors feel that the anatomy of a fibula osteocutaneous flap is sufficiently consistent that routine CT angiography for the purpose of evaluating perforator anatomy is not warranted (Wei et al. 1994, Yu et al. 2011). Finally, since vascular anomalies such as arteria peronea magna when pedal exam is normal are unlikely, the palpation of the pedal pulses can be safely used as a preliminary test to indicate further vascular imaging (Lutz et al. 1999). Surgeon preference determines the need for CT angiography, and it can be used routinely for simultaneous evaluation of lower extremity vasculature and 3D virtual surgery imaging or more selectively in cases of (1) patients with abnormal pedal pulses and (2) patients with significant lower extremity trauma.

15.3 3D IMAGING AND VIRTUAL SURGERY IN JAW RECONSTRUCTION

The fibula microvascular free flap is uniquely suited for reconstruction of the mandible. Its dual periosteal and endosteal blood supply allows for multiple fibular osteotomies in order to recreate the intricate 3D geometry of a mandible. The soft tissue components of the osteocutaneous and osteomyocutaneous modifications of the flap allow for resurfacing of associated intraoral mucosa, external face and neck defects, and obliteration of dead space. Furthermore, its favourable osseous characteristics allow primary or secondary insertion of dental implants for optimal prosthodontic rehabilitation. Since its introduction by Hidalgo in 1989, it has rapidly become the flap of choice for mandibular reconstruction (Hidalgo 1989). Its utility was further broadened with Wei's demonstration in 1994 that fibula flap's septocutaneous skin paddle is anatomically consistent and reliable (Wei et al. 1994).

The steep learning curve associated with mandible reconstruction using the free fibula flap stems not only from the technical expertise required for microsurgery but also from the skill required to obtain the precise geometrical contour of the neomandible in order to achieve favourable functional and aesthetic outcomes. Interestingly, despite its pivotal importance, the contouring is classically performed with a freehand approach, which is relatively imprecise and time consuming and has low reproducibility. Successful reconstruction then depends largely on surgeon experience, intraoperative judgement, and having a keen perception of three dimensionality.

New technologies have allowed reconstructive surgeons to decrease the abstract nature of fibular contouring (Casap et al. 2008, Cohen et al. 2009, Hirsch et al. 2009, Yamanaka et al. 2010,

Antony et al. 2011, Zheng et al. 2012). An exhaustive discussion of each of these technologies is beyond the scope of this chapter. Instead, we will focus on virtual surgical planning in combination with stereolithographic model-guided surgery that may increase operative precision and efficiency.

15.3.1 Virtual Surgical Simulation with Stereolithographic Model-Guided Surgery

High-definition CT scans of the maxillofacial skeleton and lower extremities are obtained and forwarded to Medical Modeling, Inc. (Golden, Colorado), for 3D rendering (Figure 15.1) using the Materialise software (Leuven, Belgium). A web-based teleconference is held between a biomedical engineer and the extirpative and reconstructive surgical teams. Surgical simulation begins with the ablative surgeon directing a virtual mandibulectomy. The virtual resection can be repeated as many times as needed to facilitate appropriate margins.

Upon achieving satisfactory mandible resection, the reconstructive surgeon begins the virtual reconstruction. This is performed by superimposing the patient's own 3D reconstructed fibula on the mandibular defect. Alternatively, a generic virtual fibula can be used without incurring significant inaccuracy (Roser et al. 2010). Virtual osteotomies determine the angle of the cutting planes, number and length of the fibula segments, and overall contour of the neomandible (Figure 15.2). This is a trial-and-error process and, as in the case of virtual resection, can be repeated until a satisfactory result is achieved. The restoration of native mandibular contour is confirmed by superimposing the ipsilateral mandible on the reconstructed segments (Figure 15.3). If the ipsilateral mandible is pathologically deformed, a mirror image of the contralateral mandible can be used for this purpose.

With data obtained from the virtual simulation, stereolithographic models of the neomandible, mandibular, and fibular cutting guides (Figures 15.4 and 15.5) and a plate-bending template (Figure 15.6) are manufactured. A reconstruction plate is contoured preoperatively against the neomandible model using the plate-bending template as a guide or a prebent plate can be manufactured preoperatively. The mandibular and fibular cutting guides and the reconstruction plate are sterilised for later intraoperative use.

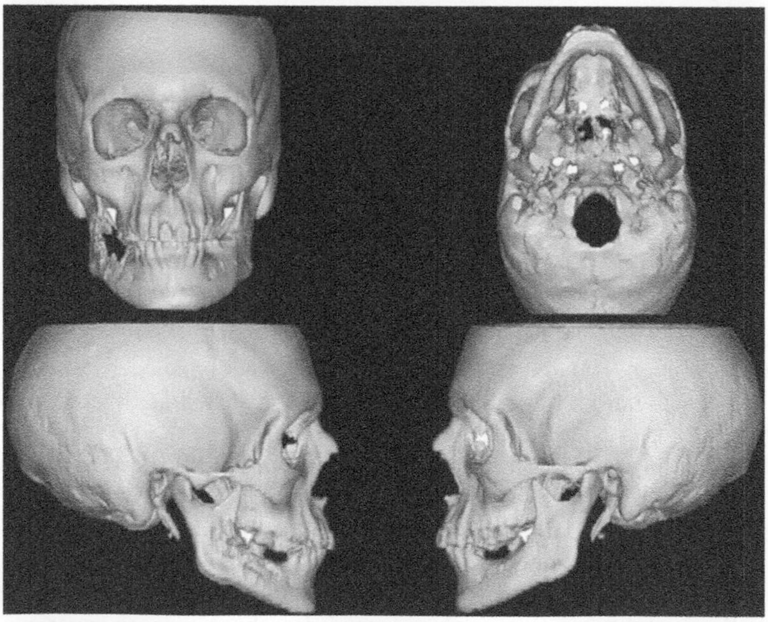

FIGURE 15.1 High-definition CT scans of the maxillofacial skeleton with 1 mm slice thickness are obtained and sent to Medical Modeling, Inc. (Goden, Colorado), in uncompressed DICOM format. Three-dimensional rendering is performed with the Materialise software (Leuven, Belgium).

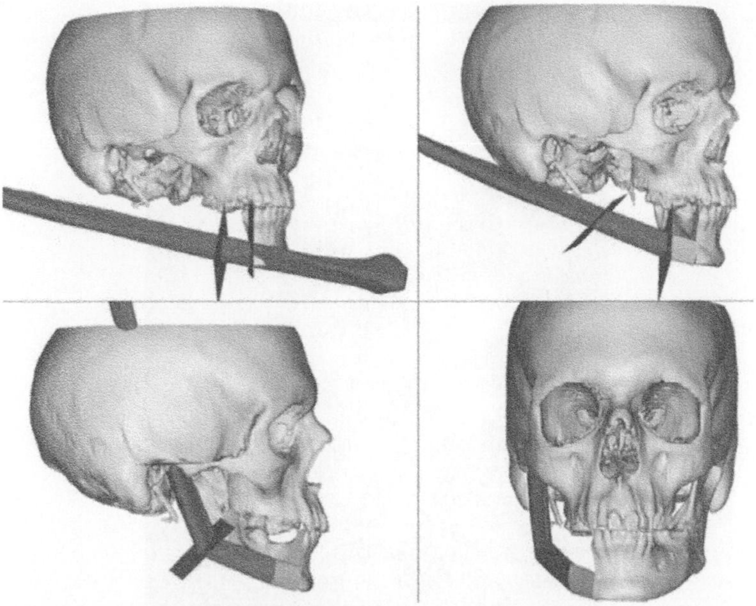

FIGURE 15.2 Virtual reconstruction begins with superimposition of a virtual fibula over the mandibular defect. Either the patient's own or a generic virtual fibula can be used. Osteotomy is performed sequentially in a medial-to-distal fashion. The process can be repeated until the optimal number of fibular segment, cutting planes, and neomandibular contour is achieved.

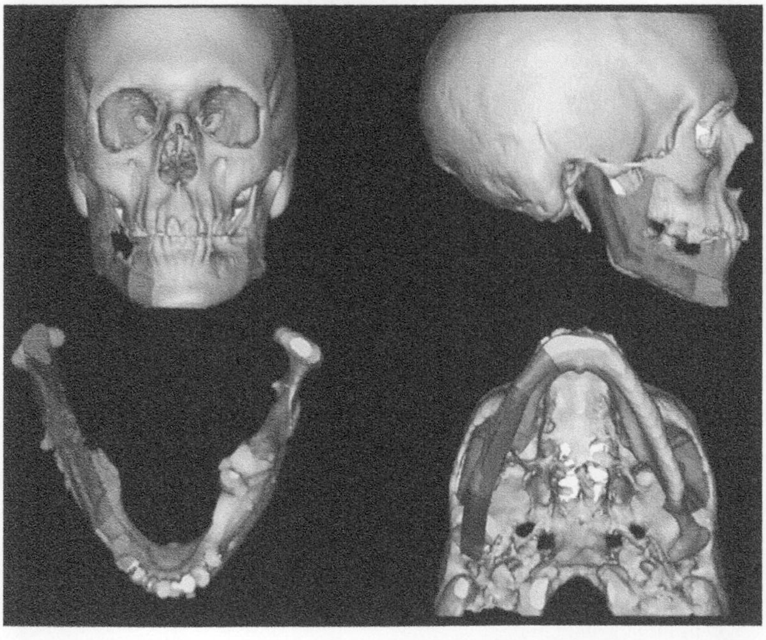

FIGURE 15.3 Superimposition of the reconstructed neomandible over the ipsilateral native mandible allows confirmation of adequate restoration of preoperative contour. If the ipsilateral mandible is too pathologically deformed for comparison, a mirror image of the contralateral mandible can be used for this purpose.

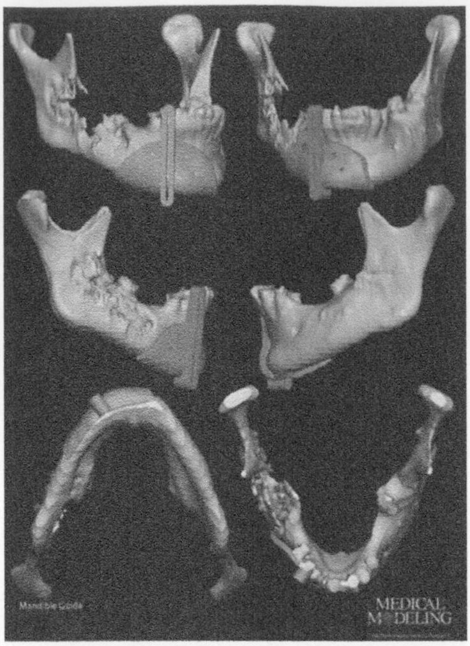

FIGURE 15.4 Mandibular cutting guide allows the virtual resection to be replicated on the patient's mandible, producing a mandibular defect that is identical to what was planned virtually.

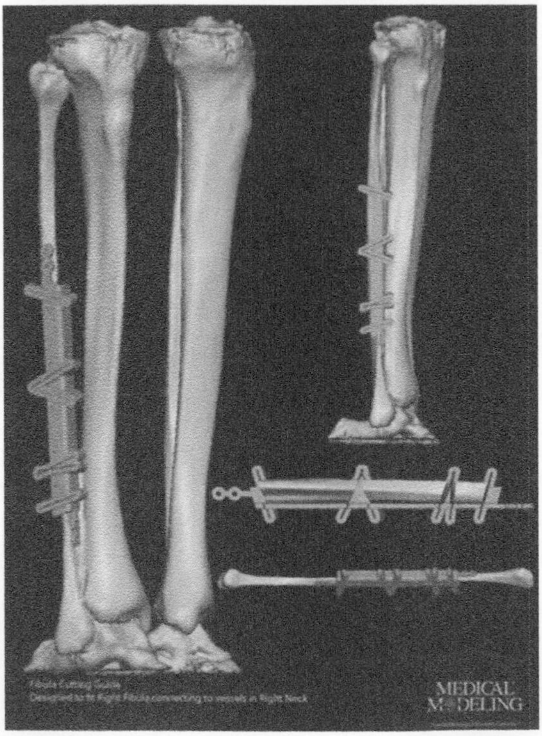

FIGURE 15.5 Fibular cutting guide allows straightforward osteotomy. One simply osteotomises along the cutting slots on the guide. This greatly accelerates the processes of fibular osteotomy and the assembly of fibular segments into a neomandible.

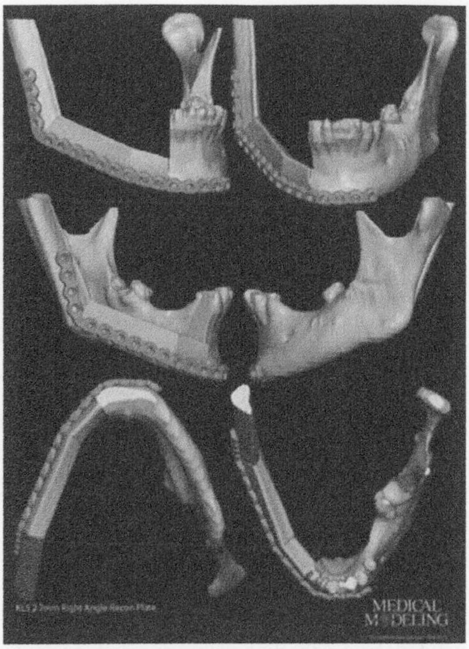

FIGURE 15.6 A plate-bending template is designed virtually and stereolithographically modelled. Plate bending is performed preoperatively against the neomandible model using the plate-bending template as a guide.

15.3.2 Surgical Technique

Mandible resection and fibula flap harvest proceed simultaneously with a two-team approach. After sufficient mandibular exposure is obtained and with the patient in maxillomandibular fixation, pilot holes are drilled on the mandible using the pre-contoured reconstruction plate as a template. The plate is then removed and sterilised. The mandibular cutting guide is fixed to the mandible with unicortical screws. Osteotomies performed with the cutting guide effectively replicate the virtual mandibular resection pattern, generating a defect precisely as planned.

The fibula flap is harvested with a standard lateral approach (Hidalgo 1989, Wei et al. 1994). The fibular cutting guide is fixed to the fibula. The cutting guide placement can be adjusted cephalad or caudad to avoid injury to septocutaneous vessels. With the peroneal pedicle protected with a small malleable retractor, cutting guide–directed osteotomies are performed. The resulting fibular segments are assembled and fixed to the reconstruction plate in situ to minimise ischaemia time (Figure 15.7). The neomandible/reconstruction plate construct is transferred as a unit and secured to the mandibular remnant at its predetermined optimal position (Figure 15.8). The microvascular anastomoses, soft tissue inset, and donor wound closure are completed in standard fashion.

15.3.3 Advantages Virtual Surgery Techniques

Reconstructive surgeons have long sought a technique that would make mandible reconstruction using free fibula flap more methodical. Templates made from paper, acrylic plastic, and metal have been designed to facilitate the process of fibular/neomandible contouring (Hidalgo 1991, Rohner et al. 2003, Strackee et al. 2004, Wang et al. 2009). Virtual surgical simulation with stereolithographic model-guided surgery represents a progression from these predecessor techniques, offering enhanced planning accuracy and technical sophistication.

Reconstruction plate contouring against a stereolithographically manufactured model or a prebent plate offers the ability for meticulous plate shaping without the need for wide intraoperative

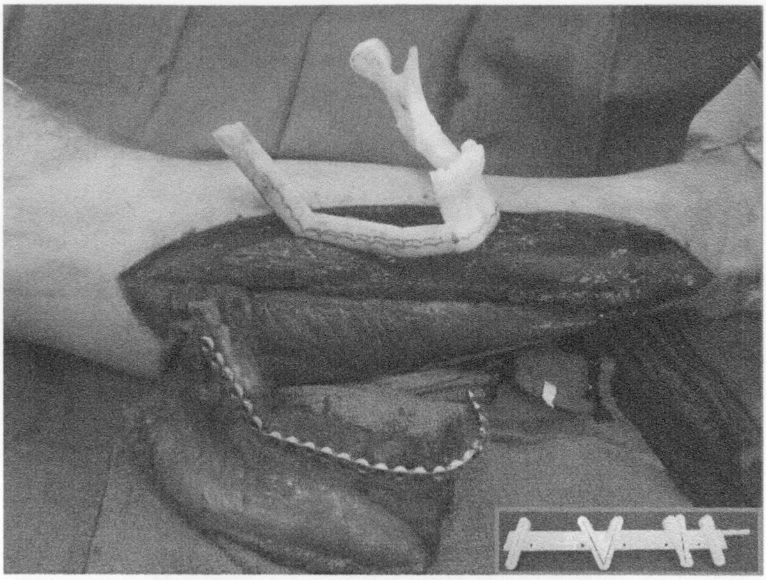

FIGURE 15.7 The fibular segments are assembled and fixed to the prebent reconstruction plate in situ to minimise ischaemia time. The neomandible/reconstruction plate construct is then transferred as a unit to the mandibular defect. Alternatively, the process can be performed safely at a side table, because both the osteotomy and assembly of the fibular segments proceed relatively quickly in comparison to the standard freehand technique.

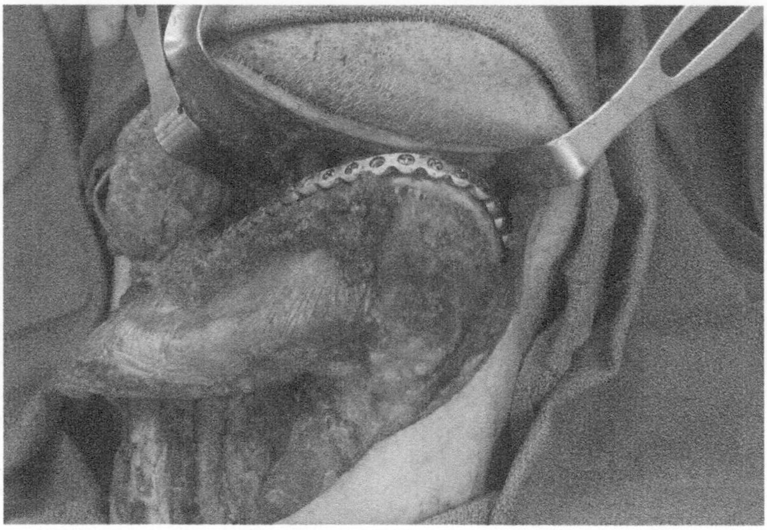

FIGURE 15.8 The neomandible/reconstruction plate construct is transferred and insetted to the mandibular defect. The need for adjustment osteotomy to achieve an adequate fit is minimal to none.

bony exposure and the interference from adjacent soft tissue or a deforming lesion. The cutting guide–directed osteotomy yields excellent bone-to-bone contacts and minimises the need for further adjustment osteotomy or burring. These factors translate into a reduction in operative time, turning experience gained virtually into efficiency in the operating room (Figure 15.9). How accurate are the virtual surgery and cutting guide–directed osteotomy? Roser et al. studied 19 mandibular and 44 fibular osteotomies and found discrepancies of 1–2 mm between the planned and

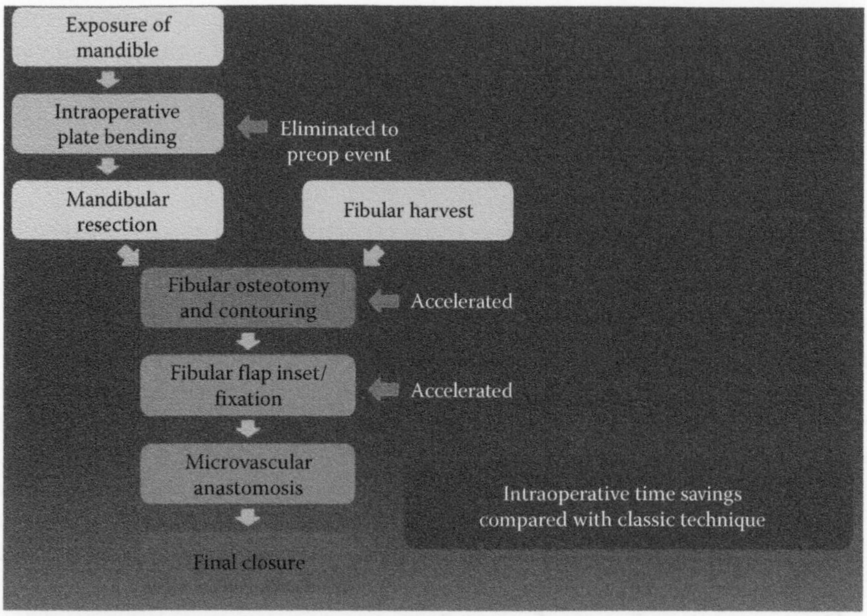

FIGURE 15.9 This diagram demonstrates three key steps from which intraoperative time is saved. Plate bending is turned into a preoperative event and therefore completely eliminated. Fibular osteotomy is accelerated because it is directed by a cutting guide and no intraoperative measurements are necessary. Fibular osseous flap inset is accelerated as well because the fibular segments are already precisely osteotomised and the need of further adjustment to inset is minimal.

actual mandibular and fibular osteotomies (Roser et al. 2010). Interestingly, the largest discrepancy (58.7% overlap) was seen between the virtually shaped reconstruction plate and the manually bent reconstruction plate, reflecting the imprecise nature of manual plate bending.

15.3.4 Limitations of Virtual Surgery

There are a number of limitations to the use of virtual surgery. Caution must be taken as although the bone can be shaped virtually, this does not account for the restricting factor of skin paddle tethering, position of the skin paddle vessels, rotation of the skin flap, and pedicle length. These must be checked prior to final contouring of the neomandible in situ. Furthermore, the final inset of the flap skin paddle must be assessed against the resection defect, as virtual surgery is limited in planning the inset of soft tissue components and may not account for tethering to the bone component. The correct side on which to place the reconstruction plate, although determined preoperatively with virtual surgery, should be reassessed once the flap and resection defect are complete. Highly restrictive soft tissue tethering to the skin paddle may limit or require alterations to the surgical plan.

Although virtual surgery results in greater accuracy in execution of osteotomies, it remains to be seen whether minor inaccuracies in occlusion and inset actually translate into significant functional differences for the patient. Studies that use validated scoring systems such as the European Organisation for Research and Treatment of Cancer (EORTC) head and neck module are warranted to assess comparative outcomes. Inaccuracies in reconstruction plate contour with freehand techniques may be addressed with virtual surgery, although newer preformed reconstruction plates may offer a simpler solution, as we discuss later.

Although virtual surgery may be a worthy alternative to the standard freehand approach, with potential for increased operative efficiency, the main drawbacks of the technique include the additional cost incurred, effort spent on the virtual planning, and the limited utility in addressing the soft tissue component of the reconstruction. Furthermore, functional superiority of virtual planning versus freehand planning has yet to be demonstrated using validated scoring systems.

15.3.5 Preformed Reconstruction Plates: An Alternative to Virtual Surgery

Commercially available preformed reconstruction plates can be used in the reconstruction of the neomandible, offering an alternative and lower-cost approach than virtual surgery. Moreover, reducing the metal fatigue associated with repeated bending may minimise the risk of plate fracture, a problem common to load-bearing mandible reconstruction. The concept of preformed plates has been successful for many years in distal radius fractures, where tolerances in the articular congruity of less than 2 mm are necessary. Mandibular data have been collected on a sample of 925 Caucasians and 960 Chinese patients, and although there are statistical differences between ethnic populations, clustering of the ramus length into three sizes allows preformed reconstruction plates to fit the majority of patients (Metzger et al. 2011). A recent study involving 71 patients with a 2-year follow-up suggests acceptable fitting accuracies, reduced operative time, and minimised risk of fatigue fractures (Probst et al. 2012). It therefore holds promise as an alternative technique to freehand reconstruction plate contouring with the significant twofold advantages of reduced operative time and lower rates of implant failure.

15.3.6 Osseointegrated Teeth in Fibular Reconstruction

At Chang Gung Memorial Hospital, 3D imaging in jaw reconstruction is mainly reserved for cases involving primary osseointegrated teeth, where accuracy of placement of implants is of paramount importance. Primary osseointegrated teeth have been used predominantly in non-oncologic cases of ameloblastoma segmental mandibulectomies (Chang et al. 2011). A 3D modelling in this context may allow a more accurate placement of dental implants versus freehand techniques. We have previously described this technique in 10 cases (7 benign tumours, 3 cases osteoradionecrosis).

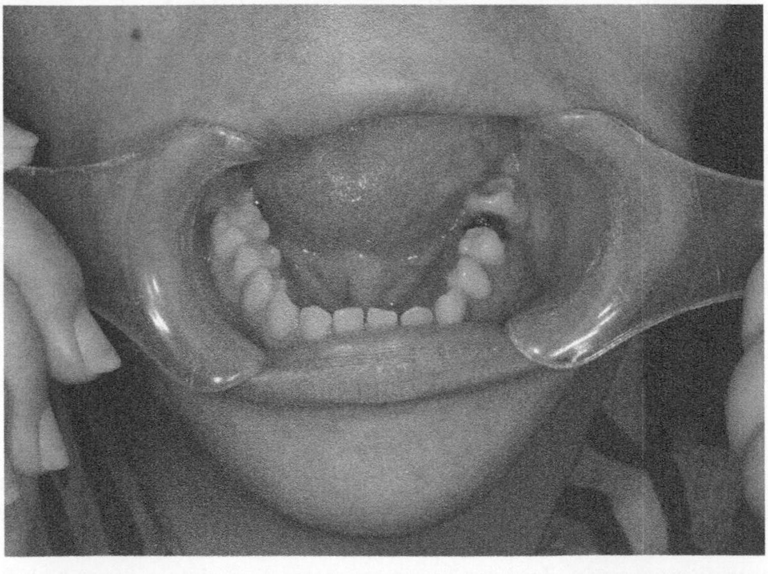

FIGURE 15.10 Preoperative view of a 24-year-old female with primary left ameloblastoma confirmed on biopsy. CT showed a lesion 2.1 × 3.2 × 2.2 in the left mandibular body with cortical thinning (Figure 15.13). Reconstruction was performed with a left free fibula osteoseptocutaneous flap, double-barrelled strut, and primary osseointegrated teeth (Figures 15.14 and 15.15). Figure 15.16 and the final figure shows the fibula skin paddle in situ, with the dental implants remaining subcutaneous at this stage, until stages 2 and 3 as discussed earlier (Figure 15.18).

Briefly, the technique involves three stages. In the first stage, 3D CT is used to create a wax model, on which a reconstruction plate can be preformed to accurately restore occlusion. After tumour ablation and temporary intermaxillary fixation, the preformed reconstruction plate is inserted. The fibula osteoseptocutaneous flap is osteotomised to produce a double-barrelled segment, with the lower barrel fixed to the reconstruction plate and the upper segment adjusted with the dental implants in situ. Testing screws 10 mm in size are temporarily fixed into the dental implants to allow accurate positioning and inclination of the upper barrel. The test screws mimic the final length of the dental prostheses which are fitted at a later stage. The testing screws are then removed and implant cover screws placed. At the second stage at 12 months, the cover screws are removed and replaced with healing abutments. To facilitate mucosal integration, a strip of fibula skin is removed around the abutments and a palatal mucosal graft performed. The third stage involves the fabrication and placement of the dental implants. In our series, the flap success was 100% and all patients completed successful implant rehabilitation of all 25 implants in 10 patients. A case example is illustrated in Figures 15.10 through 15.18.

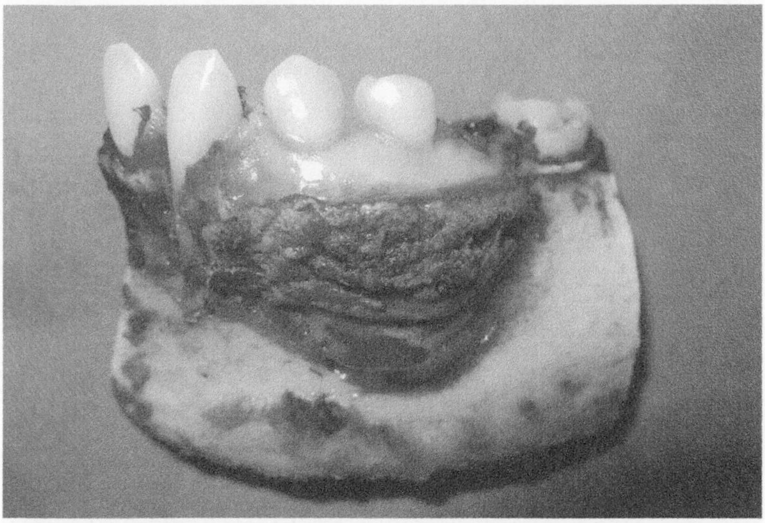

FIGURE 15.11 Resection involved a left segmental mandibulectomy with sacrifice of the inferior alveolar nerve.

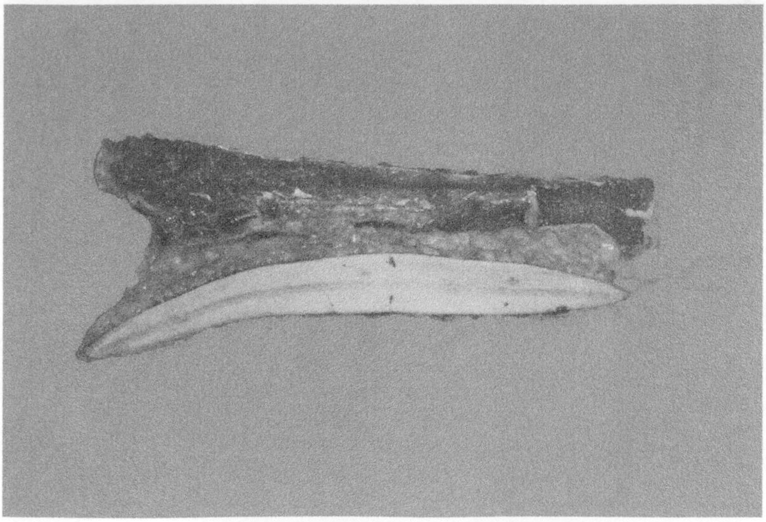

FIGURE 15.12 Fibula osteoseptocutaneous flap prior to osteotomies.

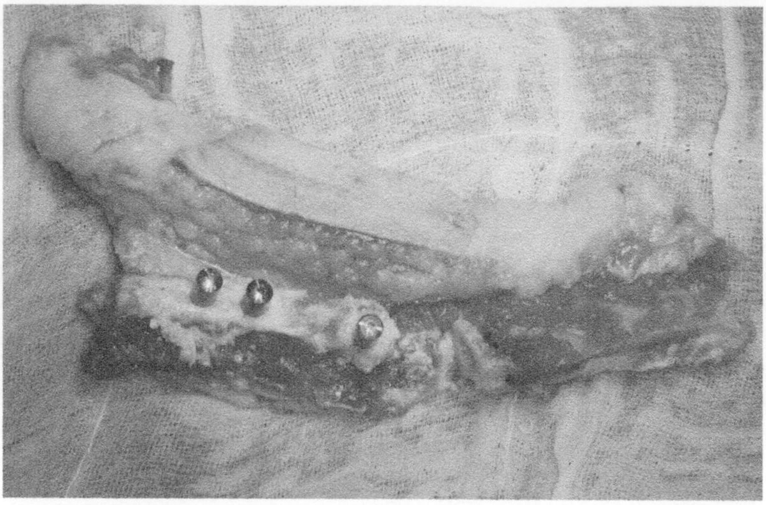

FIGURE 15.13 Post-osteotomy with dental implants and temporary test screws in the upper barrel.

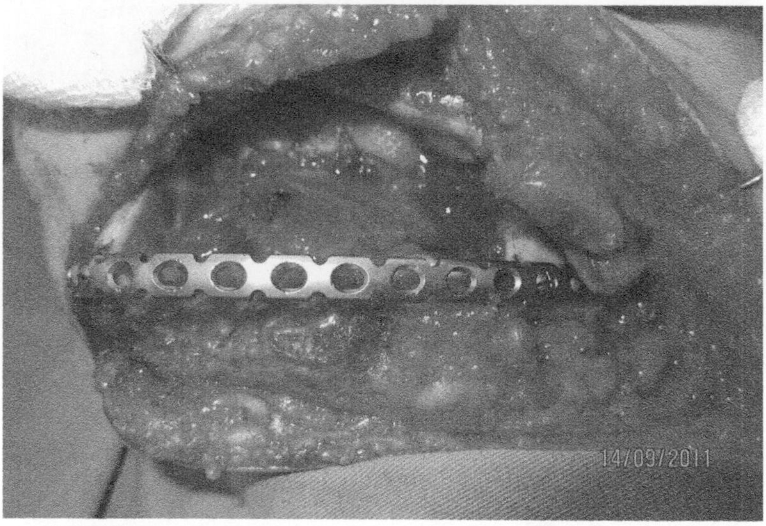

FIGURE 15.14 Preformed reconstruction plate.

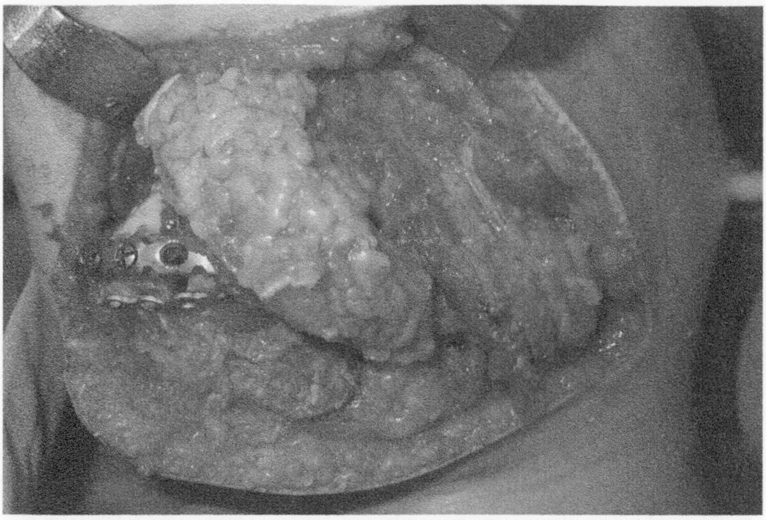

FIGURE 15.15 The lower barrel is fixed to the preformed reconstruction plate. Miniplate fixation is used for the upper barrel to allow finer adjustments. The upper barrel is precisely aligned using the test screws, which are subsequently removed.

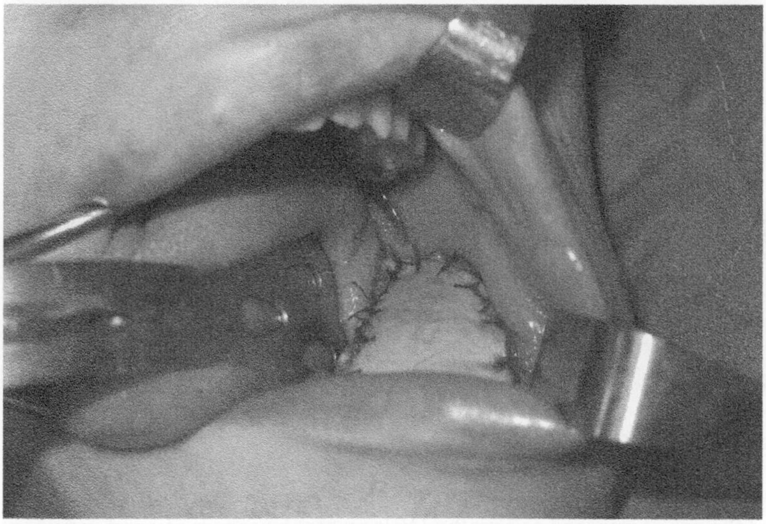

FIGURE 15.16 Skin paddle with dental implants subcutaneously buried, ready for the second and third stages.

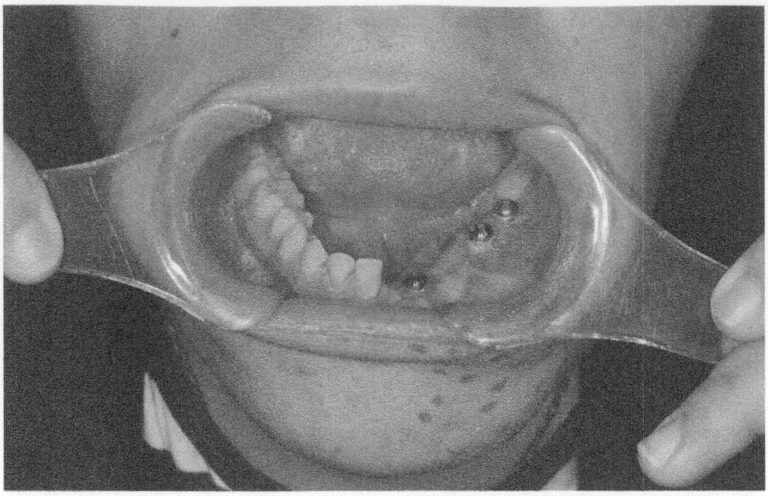

FIGURE 15.17 Dental implants exposed and healing abutments in situ. The red shading indicates the sensory area of the inferior alveolar nerve. The nerve was reconstructed at the time of surgery and sensation is gradually returning.

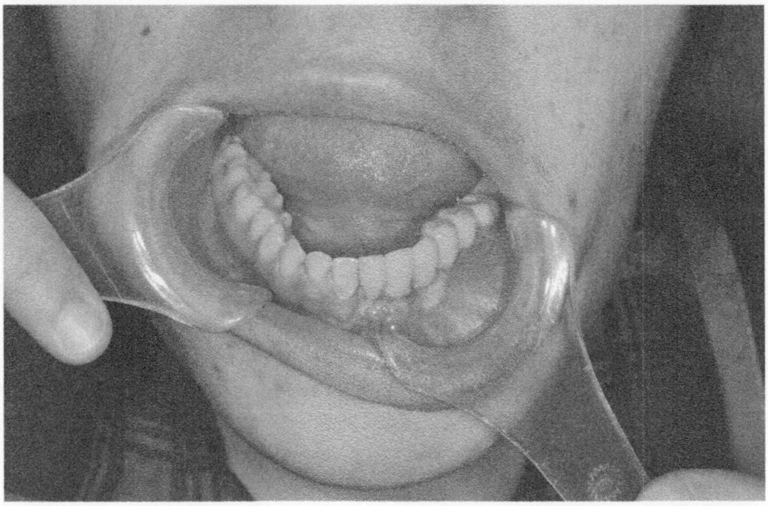

FIGURE 15.18 With the dental bridge in place. Note the similarity with the preoperative view in Figure 15.10.

15.4 CONCLUSIONS

As imaging evolves, so do our capabilities to *pre-plan* the reconstructive surgery. In this chapter, we have discussed the use of imaging as a method to increase the sensitivity and specificity of mandibular bone invasion and hence allow not only a reduction in false negatives but also in false positives, resulting in a reduced morbidity for the patient. Reliance on simple physical examination and conventional radiographs has been superseded. The importance in being able to exclude bone invasion with a highly sensitive MRI scan is supported by a more specific CT/PET that allows confirmation of positive MRI scan results. The future of mandibular reconstruction is exciting and in a stage of transition. *Virtual surgery* is a technique that is immediately visual and may in the future become the norm in certain oncological centres and allows a great degree of accuracy in the preoperative planning. Its application may include both oncologic and non-oncologic applications and may find further use in adjunctive procedures such as primary osseointegrated teeth.

15.5 SUMMARY POINTS

- Bone invasion cannot be accurately determined with physical examination and conventional radiography alone.
- MRI can be used to rule out bone invasion, given its high sensitivity of 97%.
- A positive MRI should be followed by PET/CT imaging to exclude false positives due to its higher specificity.
- Virtual surgery may offer an alternative and more efficient method of fibula contouring of the neomandible.
- Caution must be exercised in performing contouring with virtual surgery due to the restrictive nature of the skin paddle inset and vascular pedicle.
- The functional superiority of virtual surgery over freehand osteotomies has not been demonstrated using validated scoring systems.
- Commercially available preformed reconstruction plates may provide an alternative to virtual surgery as a means to increasing contouring efficiency and reducing implant fracture.

REFERENCES

Abd El-Hafez YG, Chen CC, Ng SH et al. Comparison of PET/CT and MRI for the detection of bone marrow invasion in patients with squamous cell carcinoma of the oral cavity. *Oral Oncol* 2011;47(4):288–295.

Antony AK, Chen W, Kolokythas A et al. Use of virtual surgery and stereolithography-guided osteotomy for mandibular reconstruction with the free fibula. *Plast Reconstr Surg* 2011;128(5):1080–1084.

Casap N, Wexler A, Eliashar R. Computerized navigation for surgery of the lower jaw: Comparison of 2 navigation systems. *J Oral Maxillofac Surg* 2008;66(7):1467–1475.

Chang YM, Wallace CG, Tsai CY et al. Dental implant outcome after primary implantation into double-barreled fibula osteoseptocutaneous free flap-reconstructed mandible. *Plast Reconstr Surg* 2011;128(6):1220–1228.

Cohen A, Laviv A, Berman P et al. Mandibular reconstruction using stereolithographic 3-dimensional printing modeling technology. *YMOE* 2009;108(5):661–666.

Hidalgo DA. Fibula free flap: A new method of mandible reconstruction. *Plastic Reconstr Surg* 1989;84(1):71.

Hidalgo DA. Aesthetic improvements in free-flap mandible reconstruction. *Plastic Reconstr Surg* 1991;88(4):574–585; discussion 586–587.

Hirsch DL, Garfein ES, Christensen AM et al. Use of computer-aided design and computer-aided manufacturing to produce orthognathically ideal surgical outcomes: A paradigm shift in head and neck reconstruction. *YJOMS* 2009;67(10):2115–2122.

Karanas YL, Antony A, Rubin G et al. Preoperative CT angiography for free fibula transfer. *Microsurgery* 2004;24(2):125–127.

Lutz BS, Wei FC, Ng SH et al. Routine donor leg angiography before vascularized free fibula transplantation is not necessary: A prospective study in 120 clinical cases. *Plastic Reconstr Surg* 1999;103(1):121–127.

Metzger MC, Vogel M, Hohlweg-Majert B et al. Anatomical shape analysis of the mandible in Caucasian and Chinese for the production of preformed mandible reconstruction plates. *J Craniomaxillofac Surg* 2011;39(6):393–400.

Probst FA, Mast G, Ermer M et al. MatrixMANDIBLE preformed reconstruction plates—A two-year two-institution experience in 71 patients. *J Oral Maxillofac Surg* 2012;70(11):e657–e666.

Ribuffo D, Atzeni M, Saba L et al. Clinical study of peroneal artery perforators with computed tomographic angiography: Implications for fibular flap harvest. *Surg Radiol Anat* 2010;32(4):329–334.

Rohner D, Jaquiry C, Kunz C et al. Maxillofacial reconstruction with prefabricated osseous free flaps: A 3-year experience with 24 patients. *Plast Reconstr Surg* 2003;112(3):748–757.

Roser SM, Ramachandra S, Blair H et al. The accuracy of virtual surgical planning in free fibula mandibular reconstruction: Comparison of planned and final results. *J Oral Maxillofac Surg* 2010;68(11):2824–2832.

Strackee SD, Kroon FHM, Spierings PTJ et al. Development of a modeling and osteotomy jig system for reconstruction of the mandible with a free vascularized fibula flap. *Plast Reconstr Surg* 2004;114(7):1851–1858.

Van Cann EM, Koole R, Oyen WJ et al. Assessment of mandibular invasion of squamous cell carcinoma by various modes of imaging: Constructing a diagnostic algorithm. *Int J Oral Maxillofac Surg* 2008;37(6):535–541.

Wang TH, Tseng CS, Hsieh CY et al. Using computer-aided design paper model for mandibular reconstruction: A preliminary report. *YJOMS* 2009;67(11):2534–2540.

Wei FC, Seah CS, Tsai YC et al. Fibula osteoseptocutaneous flap for reconstruction of composite mandibular defects. *Plast Reconstr Surg* 1994;93(2):294–304.

Yamanaka Y, Yajima H, Kirita T et al. Mandibular reconstruction with vascularised fibular osteocutaneous flaps using prefabricated stereolithographic mandibular model. *Br J Plast Surg* 2010;63(10):1751–1753.

Yu P, Chang EI, Hanasono MM. Design of a reliable skin paddle for the fibula osteocutaneous flap: Perforator anatomy revisited. *Plast Reconstr Surg* 2011;128(2):440–446.

Zheng G, Su Y, Liao G et al. Mandible reconstruction assisted by preoperative virtual surgical simulation. *Oral Surg Oral Med Oral Pathol Oral Radiol* 2012;113(5):604–611.

16 Imaging in Surgical Strategies for Facial Reconstruction

Francesco Stagno d'Alcontres, Gabriele Delia, Flavia Lupo, Marcello Longo, Francesca Granata, and Philippe Pelissier

CONTENTS

Facial reconstruction has always been a *challenge* for plastic surgeons and has represented one of the major boosts for the development of the speciality.

Many difficulties are linked to anatomical facial features, such as the small amount of local tissue available for reconstruction, the concept of aesthetic unity, and the essential balance between aesthetics and functionality.

The anatomical knowledge of tissues and their vascularisation is of primary importance for the reconstructive planning.

The French anatomist and surgeon Michel Salmon was the first to take an interest in cutaneous vascularisation.

In his book *Les artères de la peau* (1936), he focused on the extremely rich vascularisation of head skin (Figure 16.1).

Today, *imaging procedures* allow us to study preoperatively the patients' vascular anatomy, giving a tridimensional mapping of the surgical site (Figures 16.2 and 16.3).

16.1 HISTORICAL BACKGROUND

Until the 1970s, the reconstruction of facial defects was achieved by the easiest closure, often neglecting aesthetic and functional purposes, and the results obtained were often poor.

However, the twentieth century represented a turning point for theoretical and technical innovations, with plastic surgery developing as well.

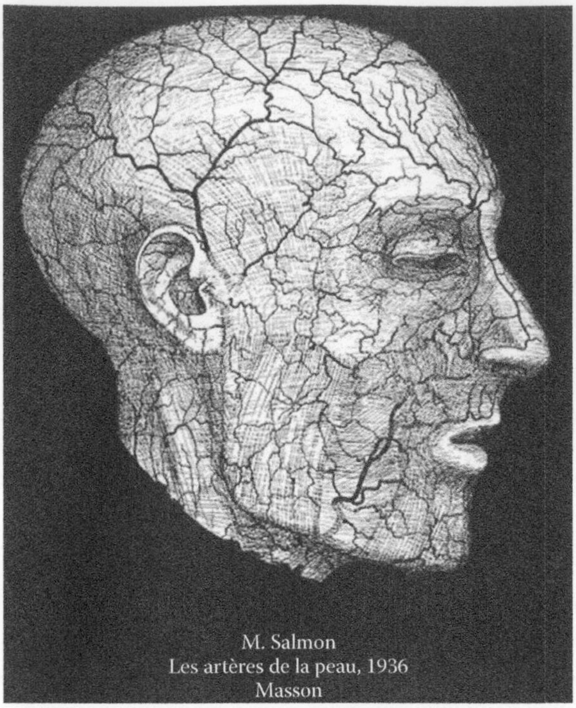

FIGURE 16.1 The blood supply to the skin of the head. (From Salmon M., *Les Artères de la peau*, Masson, Paris, France, 1936.)

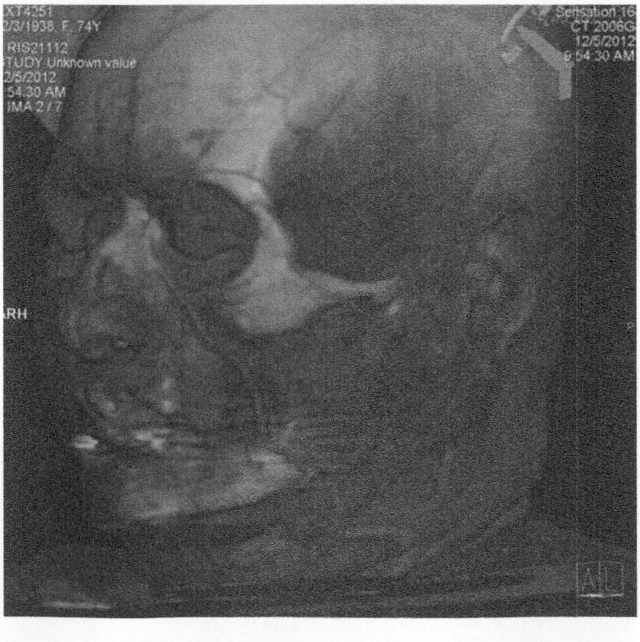

FIGURE 16.2 Computed tomography angiography of a 68-year-old patient. Post-processed volume rendered image shows the arterial and venous supply of the face.

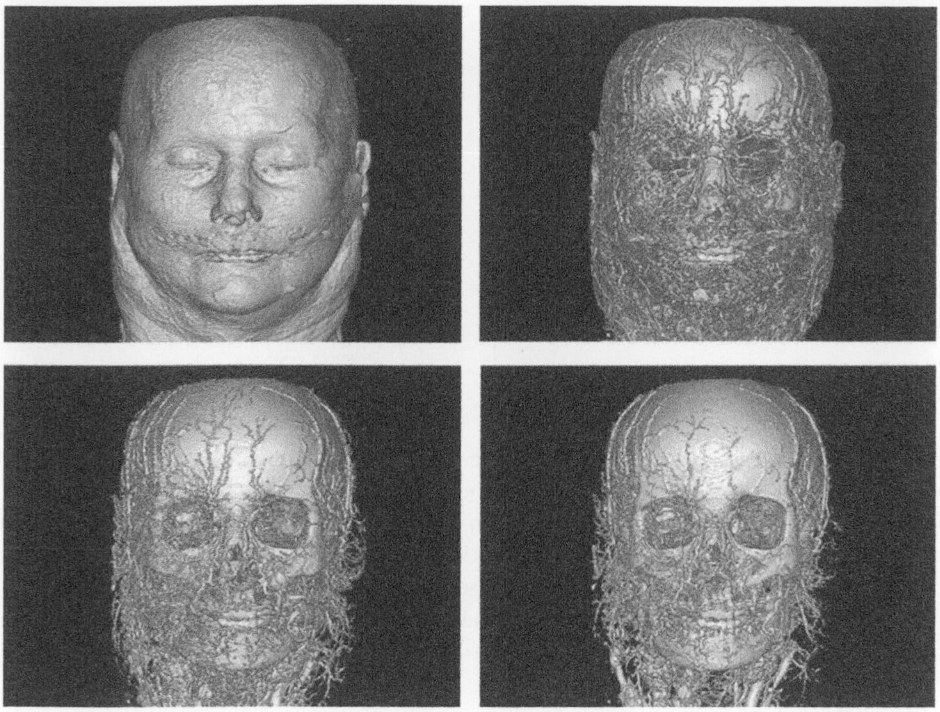

FIGURE 16.3 Modern imaging of the blood supply to the head and neck skin.

In 1944, Aufrict introduced some of the most important concepts in facial reconstruction – the aesthetic units. In 1954, Gonzalez and Ulloa clearly defined the edge of each aesthetic unit:

1. Chin area
2. The frontal region
3. Upper lip
4. Lower lip
5. Lobule of the nose
6. Dorsum of the nose
7. Cheeks
8. Neck
9. Eyelids

In 1998, Menick clearly defined the guidelines for a successful facial reconstruction:

- Restoration of facial contour and skin texture
- Restoration of entire unit, not only small defects, to avoid the *lost and replaced effect*
- Hiding the incision line at the edge of the aesthetic unit

16.2 CLASSICAL VASCULARISATION PRINCIPLES: RANDOM FLAP

The majority of flaps involved in facial reconstruction are random-pattern vascularised flaps.

In the various regions of human body, the relationship between the base and the length of a cutaneous flap must not exceed the ratio of 1:1/1.5 (Figure 16.4).

Thanks to its extraordinary vascular abundance, the skin of the head allows random flaps with a ratio of 1/3 and even more.

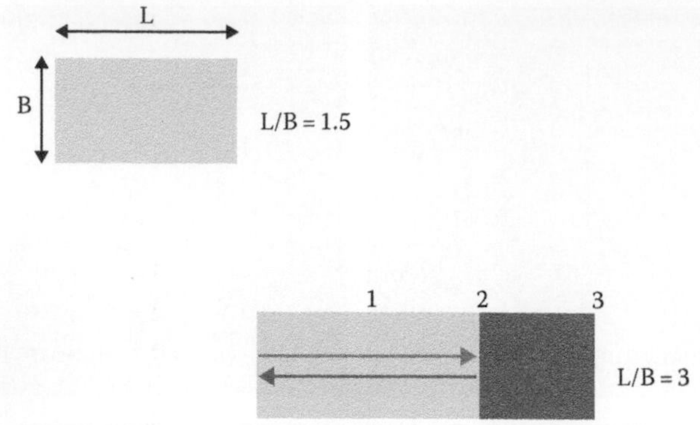

FIGURE 16.4 The length to width ratio for planning skin flaps.

This concept can be used and extended with more confidence knowing the precise vascular anatomy of the territories in which we design a local flap.

In this sense, advanced radiologic methods can be very useful in such applications. In addition, a perfect knowledge of the vascularisation of the skin used in the reconstructions offers better results while minimising the risks of necrosis due to hypoperfusion.

While planning a reconstruction in the facial region, we also have to consider additional parameters according to the aesthetic outcome:

- Direction of skin incisions
- Limit of aesthetic units of the face
- Localisation of main arteries
- Direction of blood drainage (low venous pressure regions)
- Texture and thickness of tissues (similar with similar)

Sometimes, a little loss of substance requires a huge reconstruction to gain the best aesthetic and functional results (Figure 16.5).

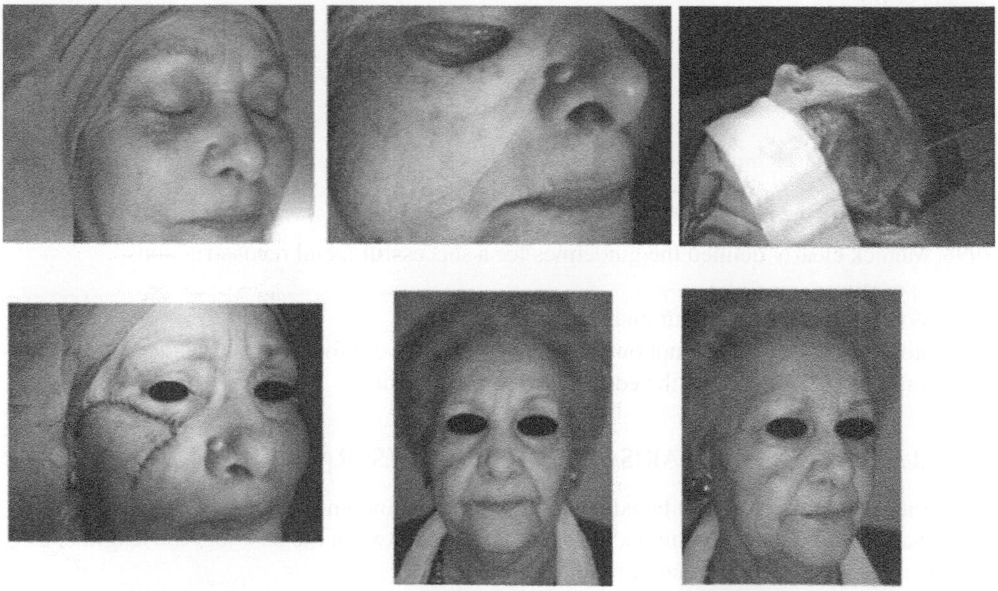

FIGURE 16.5 Reconstruction of a lower eyelid defect with a rotation advancement skin flap.

In this chapter, will focus on the importance of modern imaging techniques in the planning of the most common local flap in clinical practice for facial reconstruction.

The different aesthetic and sub-aesthetic units will be considered separately in order to make the transmission of information easier and more schematic.

16.2.1 Reconstruction of the Nose

The skin of the nose is vascularised by the branches of the facial and internal maxillary artery. These branches anastomose each other forming a rich vascular network with a *honeycomb* pattern. The alar region and the base of the nose are vascularised by the septal branch and by the lateral nasal branch and the side walls and the dorsum by the angular artery (facial artery branch), by the supratrochlear branch of the ophthalmic artery, and by the infraorbital branch of the internal maxillary artery (Figure 16.6).

16.2.2 Nasolabial Flap

This is one of the most used flaps for nasal reconstruction, the gold standard for the alar and lateral wall of the nasal pyramid. It has a reliable anatomy, as its vasculature is based on the angular artery, a branch of the facial artery that anastomoses with the ophthalmic artery distally (Figure 16.7).

The flap is harvested from the nasolabial region homolateral to the side of reconstruction. Usually, if well designed, aesthetic sequelae are minimal, scaring problems of the donor site are rare, and the scar is hidden in the neo-nasolabial fold. The amount of tissue that can be taken, above all in elderly patients, is considerable (Figures 16.8 through 16.10).

The rotation and the transposition flaps based on random vascularisation from the angular artery are very useful in the reconstruction of the nose sidewall (Figures 16.11 and 16.12).

In double transposition flap – *bilobed flap* – the first flap closes the loss of substance, while the second closes the harvesting site of first flap. The harvesting region is closed directly (Figures 16.13 and 16.14).

16.2.3 Rieger–Marchac Flap

Very common for the reconstruction of nasal tip and nasal dorsum defects, this flap is both a rotational and VY advancement flap, which takes advantage of skin laxity in the glabellar region.

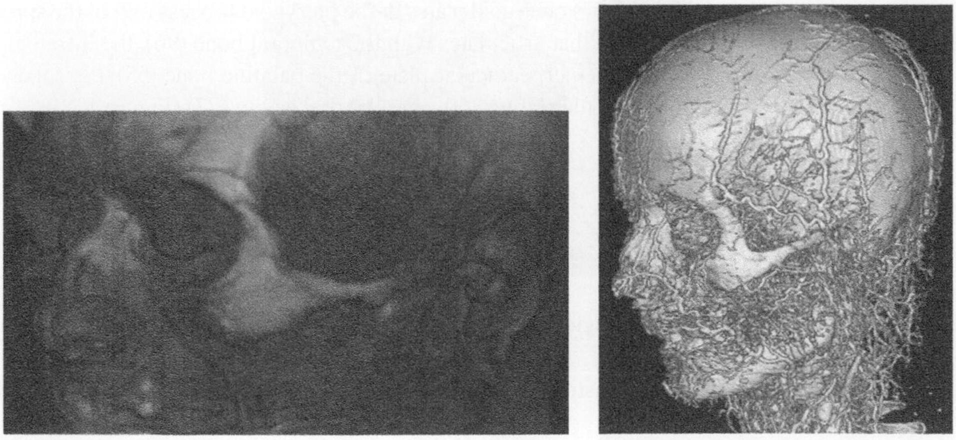

(a) (b)

FIGURE 16.6 Details of the blood supply to the nose.

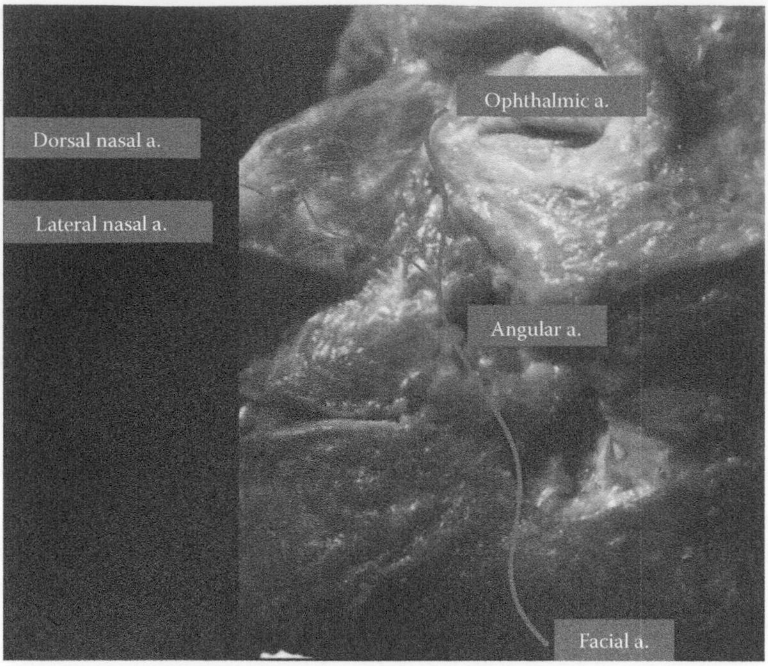

FIGURE 16.7 Anatomical view of the vessels on which the nasolabial flap is based.

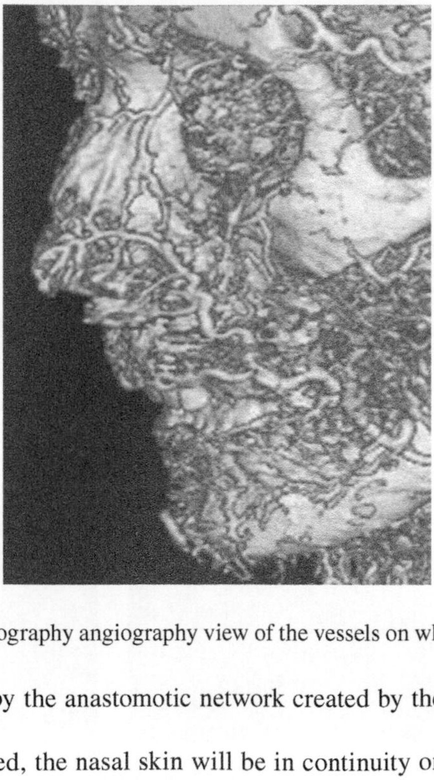

FIGURE 16.8 Computed tomography angiography view of the vessels on which the nasolabial flap is based.

The flap is vascularised by the anastomotic network created by the dorsal nasal artery and the lateral nasal artery.

All the skin is undermined, the nasal skin will be in continuity only from one lateral margin. The skin flap is repositioned and the glabellar region is closed like the VY flap (Figures 16.15 and 16.16).

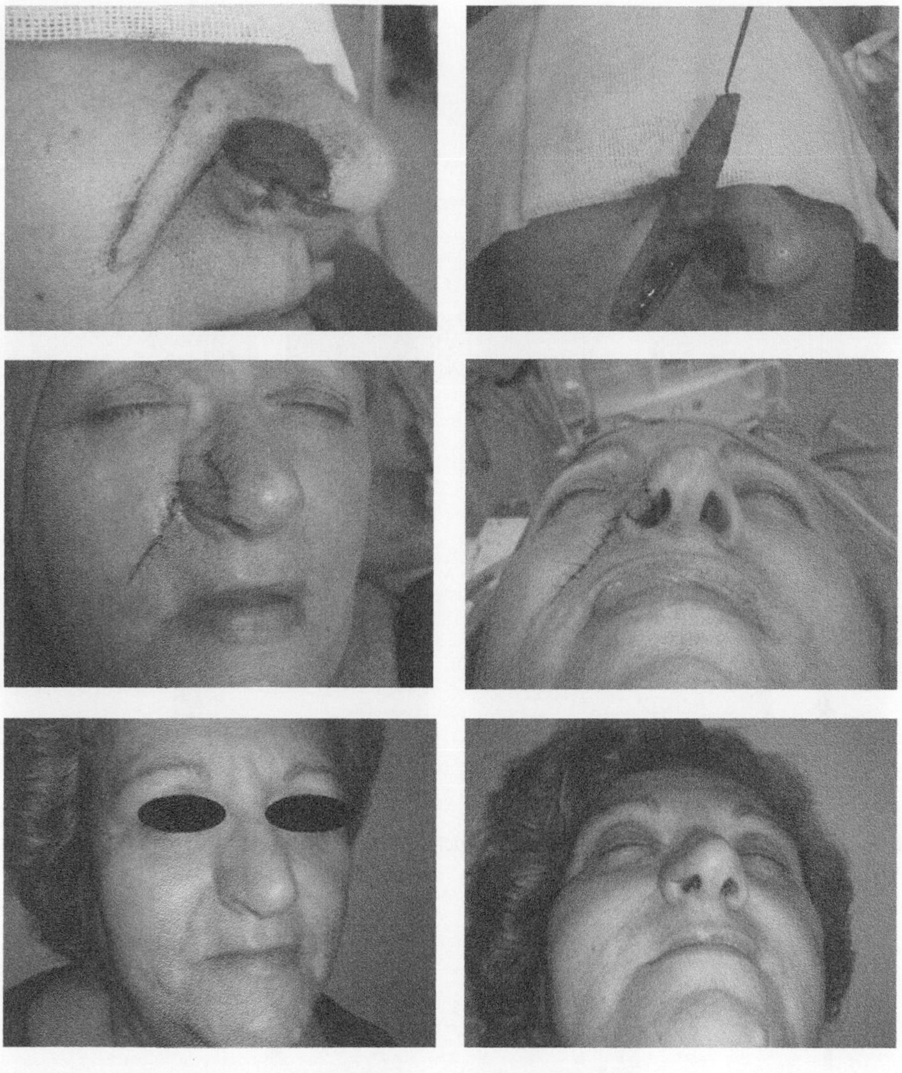

FIGURE 16.9 Use of the nasolabial flap to reconstruct a defect of the lateral wall of the nose in a 68-year-old female patient.

16.2.4 Frontal Flap

The frontal flap is the key flap in plastic surgery, first described about 2800 years ago.

It is still the gold standard in rhinopoiesis and in all complex reconstructions of the nasal pyramid.

The flap is designed along the course of one of the supratrochlear arteries. It is always used as a local flap; 3 weeks is necessary for the autonomisation, and then the pedicle is cut and reshaped. Exact artery localisation provided by imaging techniques allows us to design our edge in a precise manner, minimising the tissue around the artery without reducing the vascular safety (Figures 16.17 and 16.18).

16.2.5 Lip Reconstruction

Lips are vascularised by the labial artery and branches of the facial artery.

The superior labial artery originates from the facial artery at 12 mm more or less from the oral commissure. The mean diameter is 1.8 mm. It runs along the inferior border of the lip, between the mucosa and orbicularis oris muscle. At the midline, the artery anastomoses with the contralateral artery.

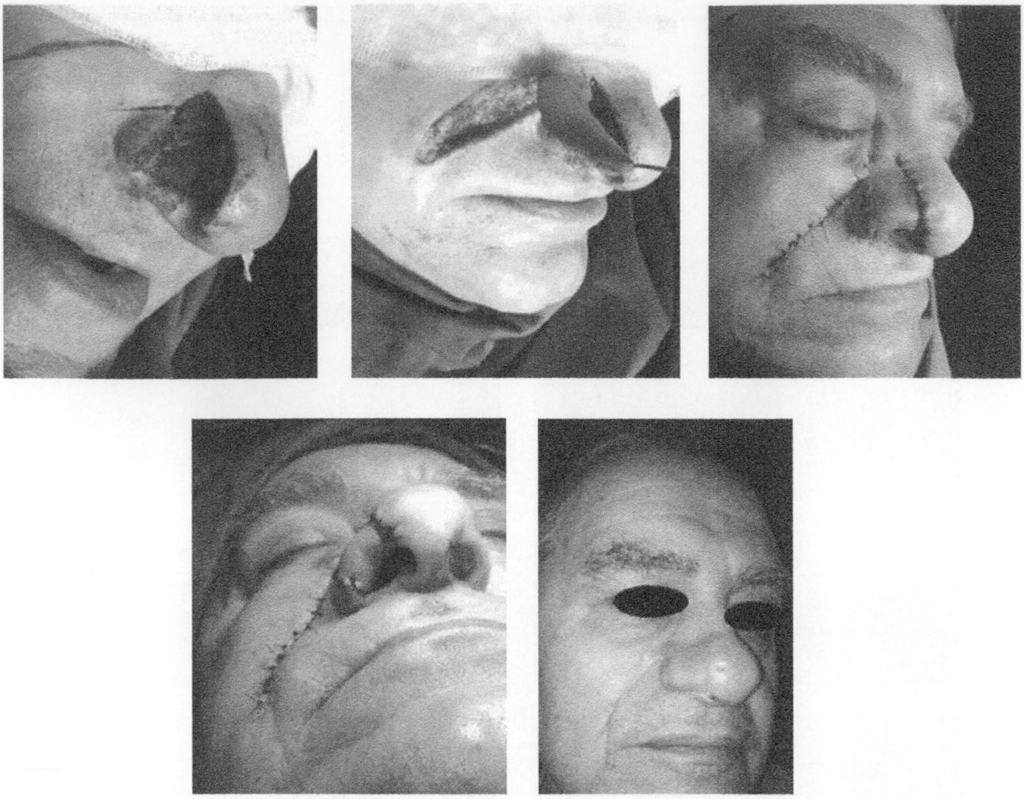

FIGURE 16.10 Use of the nasolabial flap to reconstruct a defect of the lateral wall of the nose in a 61-year-old male patient.

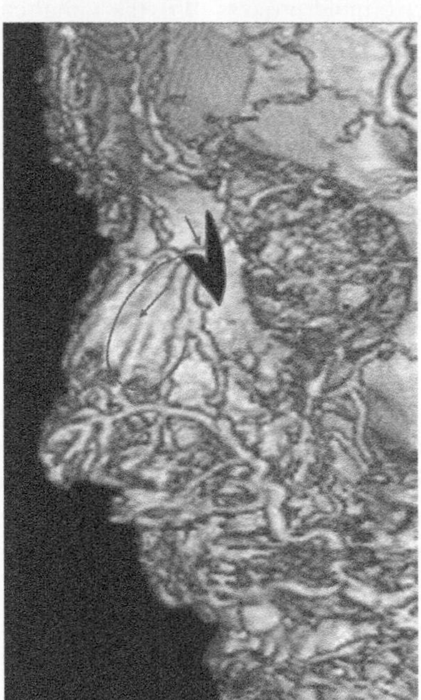

FIGURE 16.11 CTA imaging performed before the rotation flap to the nose.

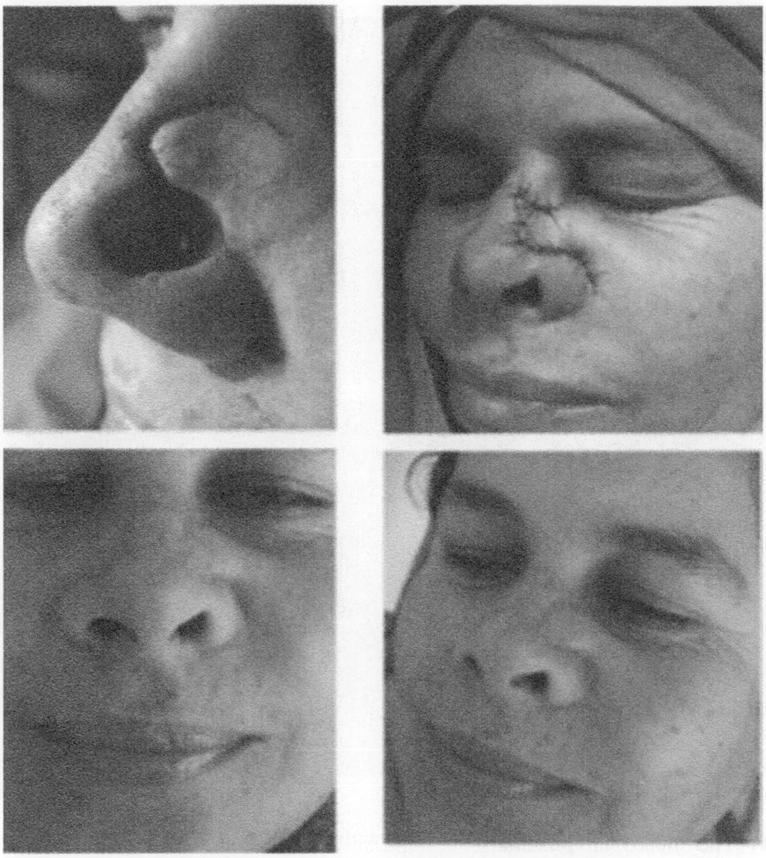

FIGURE 16.12 Rotation flap to the nose.

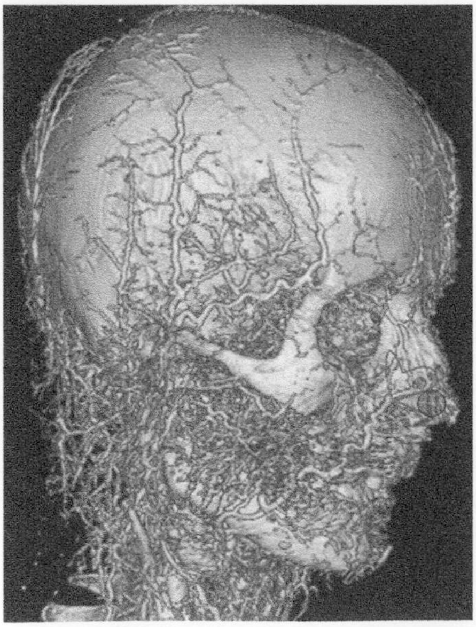

FIGURE 16.13 CTA imaging performed before the bilobed flap procedure.

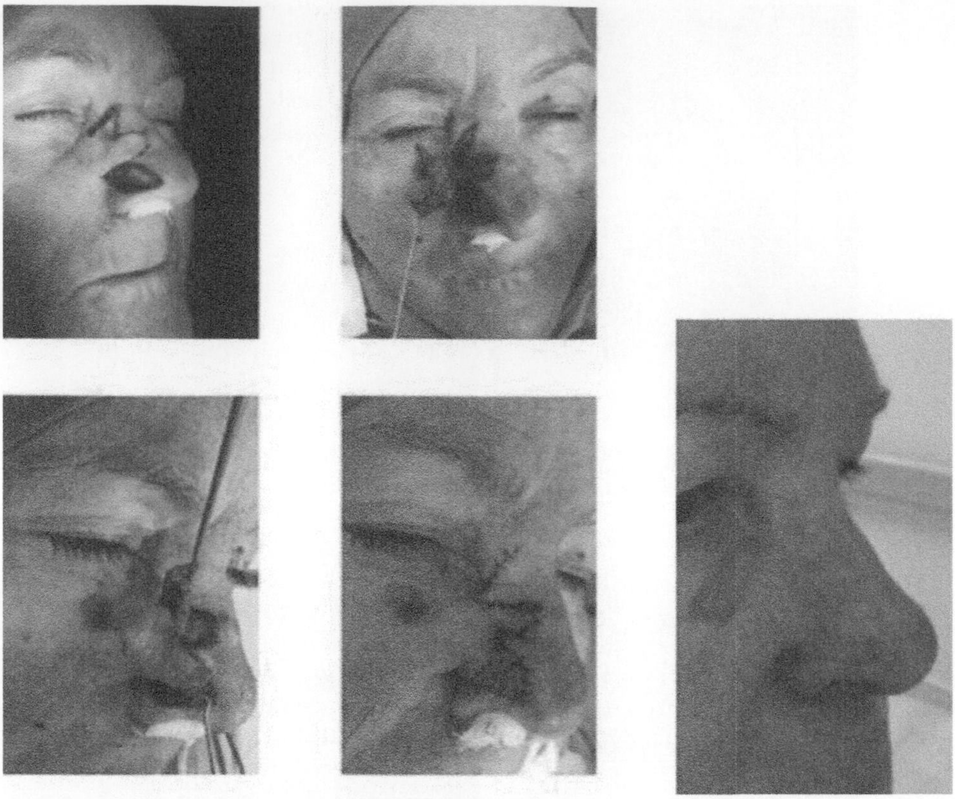

FIGURE 16.14 The bilobed flap procedure.

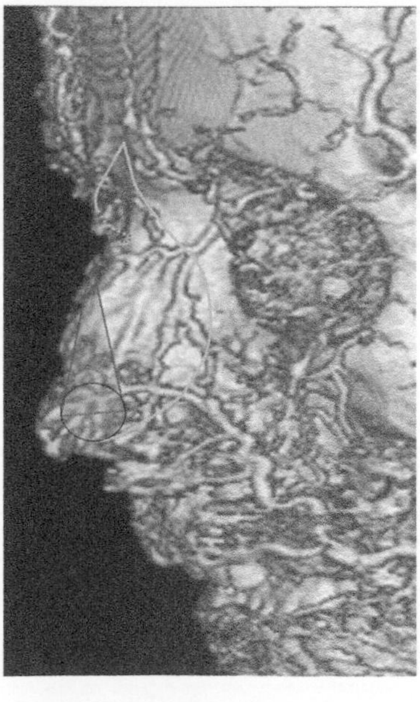

FIGURE 16.15 CTA imaging performed before the Marchac flap procedure.

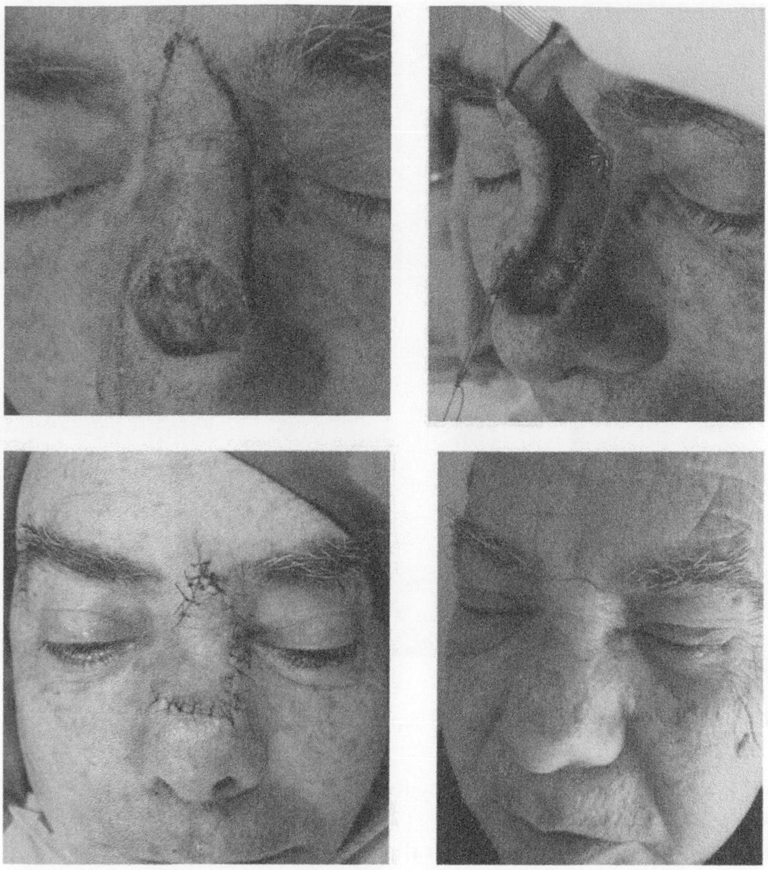

FIGURE 16.16 The Marchac flap procedure.

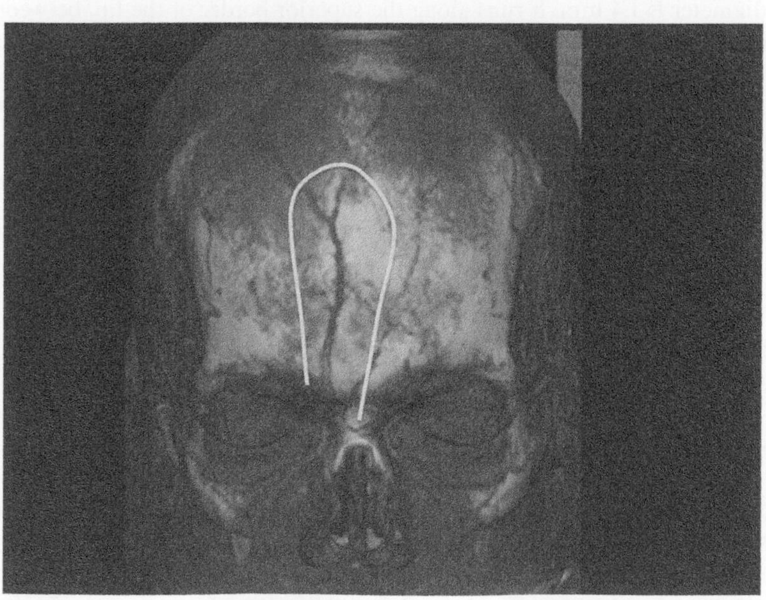

FIGURE 16.17 Imaging of the blood supply of the frontal flap.

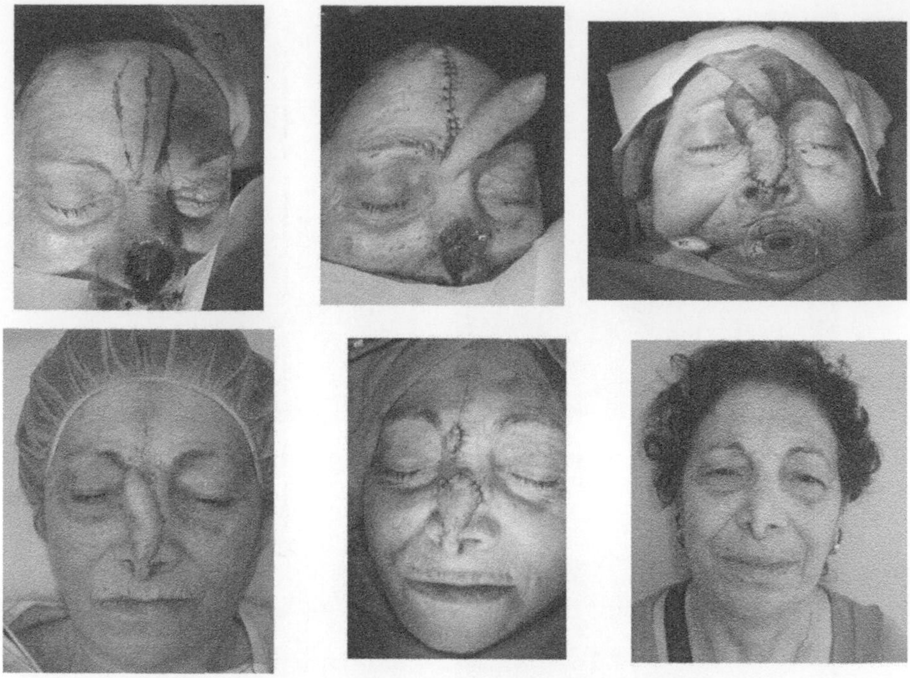

FIGURE 16.18 Clinical application of the blood supply of the frontal flap.

The superior labial artery is the main artery for superior lip vascularisation, also irrorated by the sub-alar and subseptal branches.

The superior labial artery also vascularises the alar cartilages (alar branches), the inferior region of the septum membranosum (septal branches), and the columella.

The inferior labial artery originates from the facial artery at 24 mm approximately from the oral commissure.

The main diameter is 1.4 mm. It runs along the superior border of the lip, between the mucosa and orbicularis oris muscle. The main field of irroration is the inferior lip, which is also irrorated by the labiomental artery branches of the facial artery.

The horizontal branch of the labiomental artery runs between the musculus depressor labii inferioris and orbicularis oris muscle.

The vertical branch of the labiomental artery arises from the submental artery.

16.2.6 Facial Artery Anatomical Variations

The facial artery anatomy and distribution pattern can be summarised in five different types:

Type A (48%): The facial artery bifurcates in the superior labial artery and the lateral nasal artery (which produces the superior and inferior alar branches) that anastomoses with the angular artery.

Type B (38%): It is similar to Type A but the nasal artery ends with superior alar branches, and the angular artery is not present.

Type C (8%): The facial artery ends with the superior labial artery.

Type D (4%): The facial artery ends with the superior alar artery; the angular artery arises directly from the principal artery trunk.

Type E (2%): The facial artery is only rudimental; no ramifications arise from the artery (Figures 16.19 and 16.20).

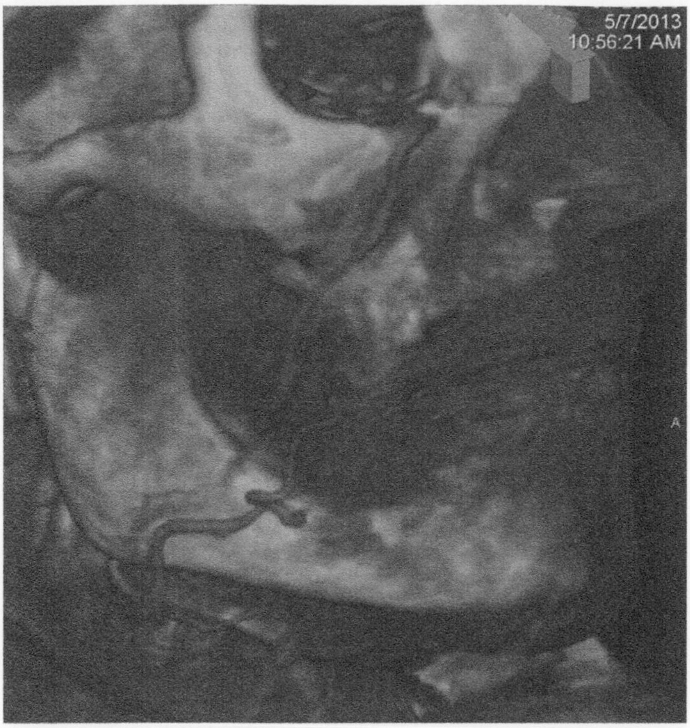

FIGURE 16.19 Imaging of the facial artery.

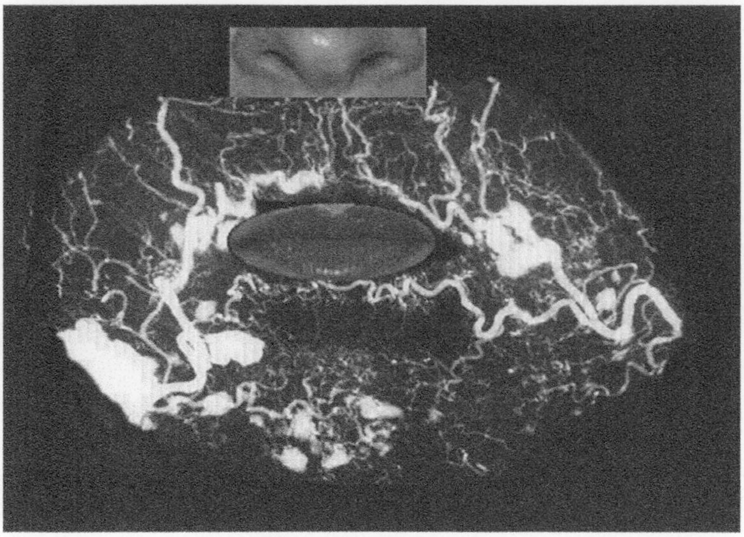

FIGURE 16.20 Imaging of the facial artery.

16.2.7 Burow's Flap

It is mainly used for central reconstruction of the upper lip. It is basically a double advancement flap of residual lip. The advancement is facilitated by the removal of two triangles from the nasolabial region. The two flaps are sutured on the midline (Figures 16.21 and 16.22).

The same technique is applicable to the inferior lip (Figures 16.23 and 16.24).

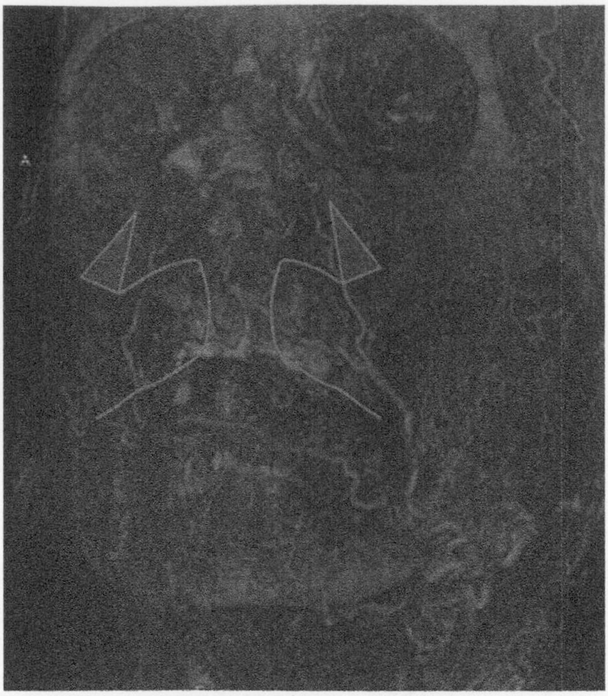

FIGURE 16.21 CTA imaging of blood supply derived from superior labial artery, branch of facial artery.

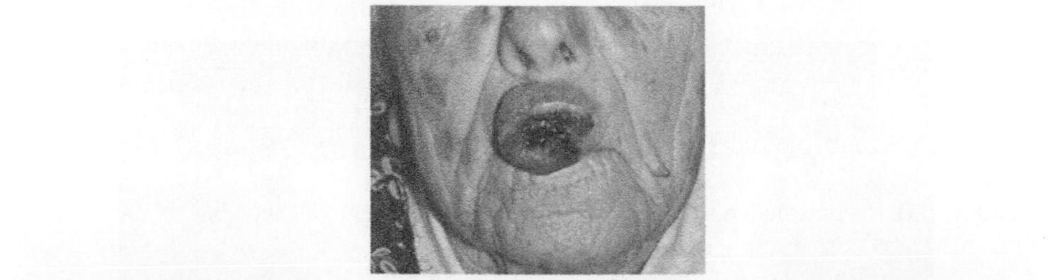

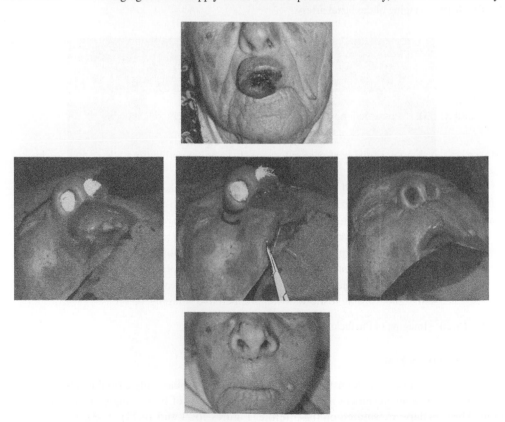

FIGURE 16.22 Burow's flap.

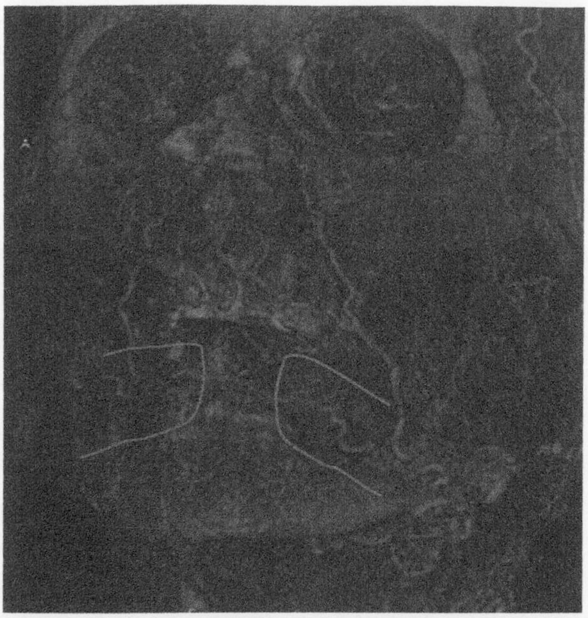

FIGURE 16.23 CTA imaging of the blood supply derived from inferior labial artery, branch of facial artery.

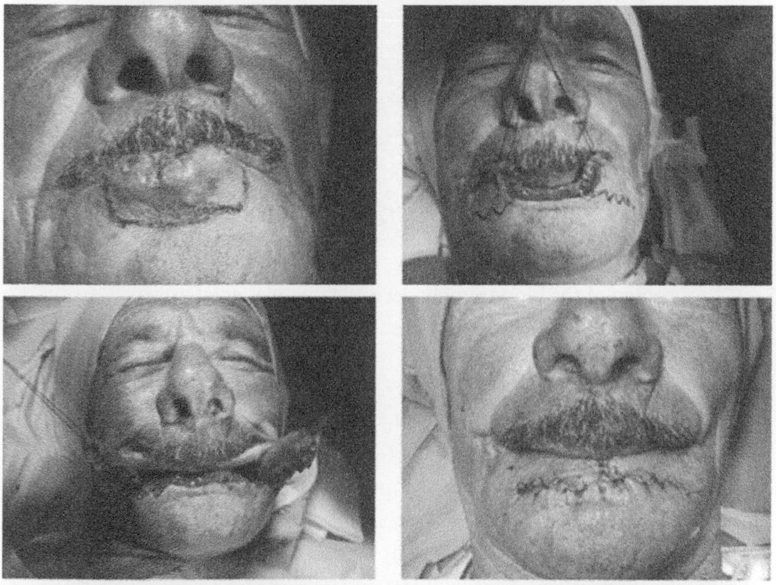

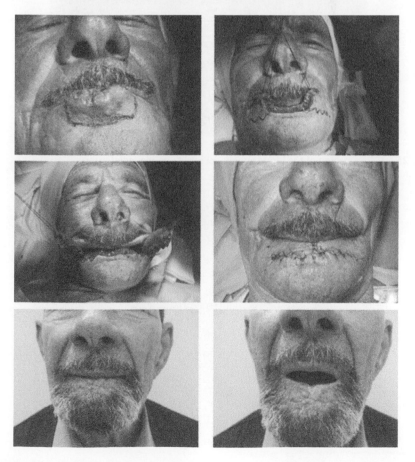

FIGURE 16.24 Burow's flap.

For bigger losses of substance, a good alternative is the Gillies flap, which is a local rotation-advancement flap based on the labial artery (Figures 16.25 through 16.27).

Other rotation-advancement flaps are based on the same principles, and they are commonly used in lip reconstruction, for example, the Karapandzic flap (Figures 16.28 and 16.29).

The von Bruns flap is a good alternative for huge lateral defects. It is a pedicled transposition flap based on the facial artery (Figures 16.30 and 16.31).

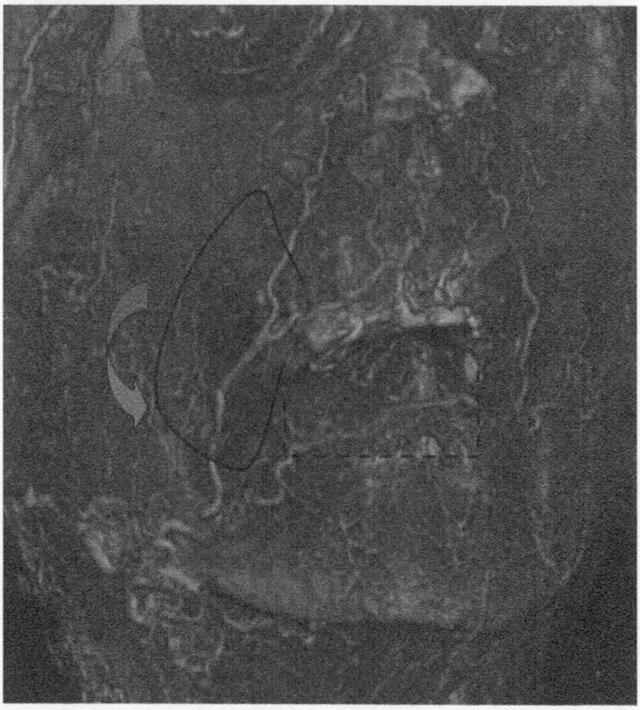

FIGURE 16.25 CTA imaging of the blood supply derived from the facial artery.

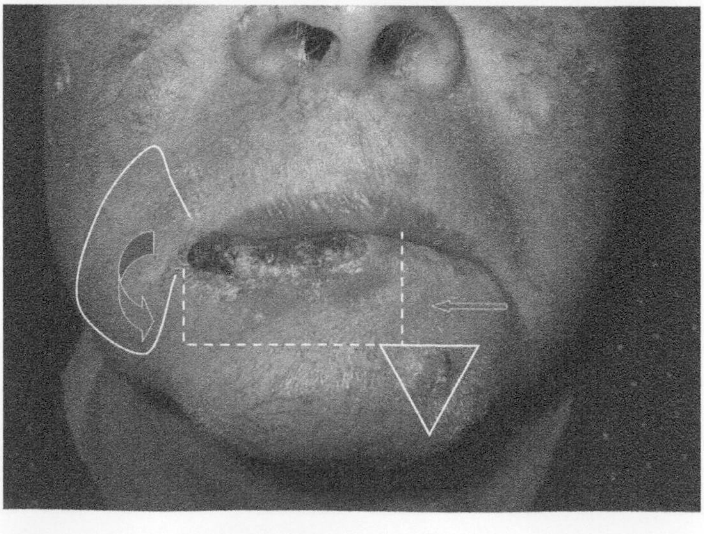

FIGURE 16.26 Lesion of the lower lip in a 66-year-old male patient.

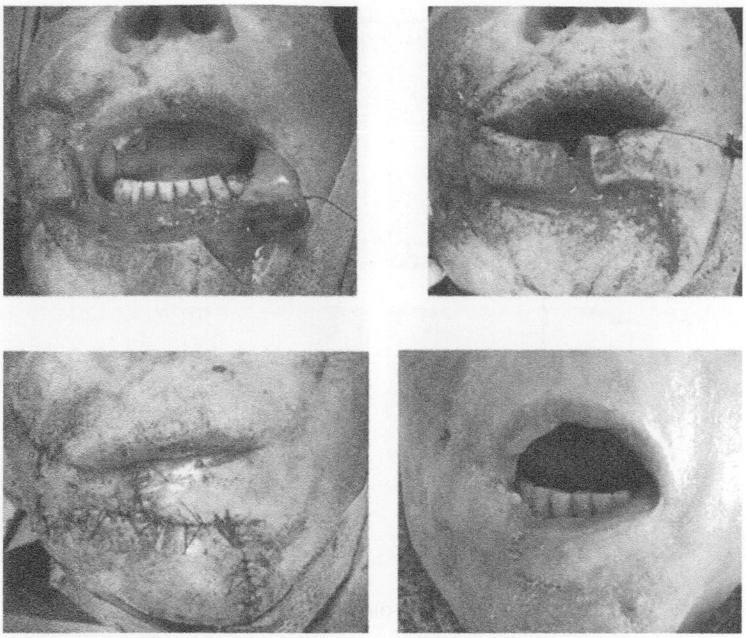

FIGURE 16.27 Gillies' flap.

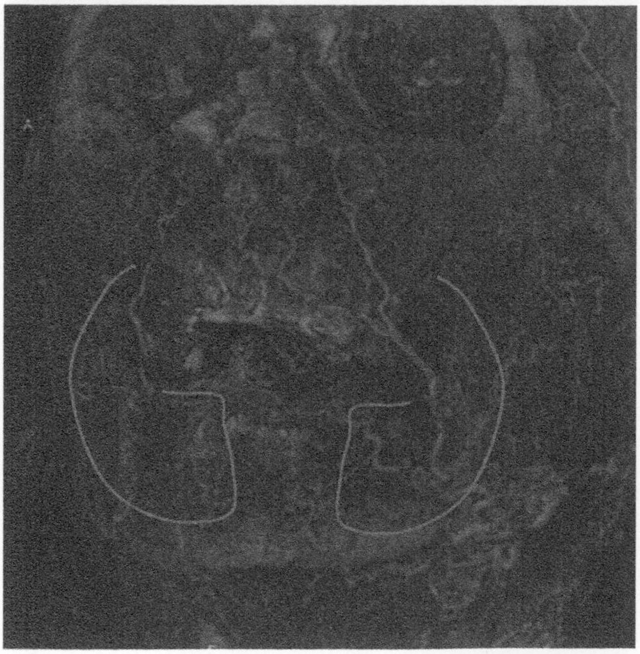

FIGURE 16.28 CTA imaging of the blood supply from the facial artery in a 76-year-old male patient.

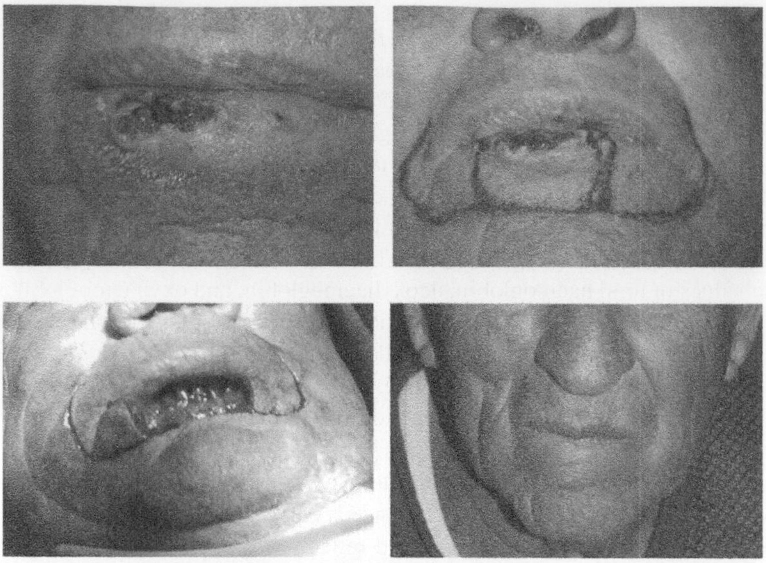

FIGURE 16.29 The Karapandzic flap in a 76-year-old male patient.

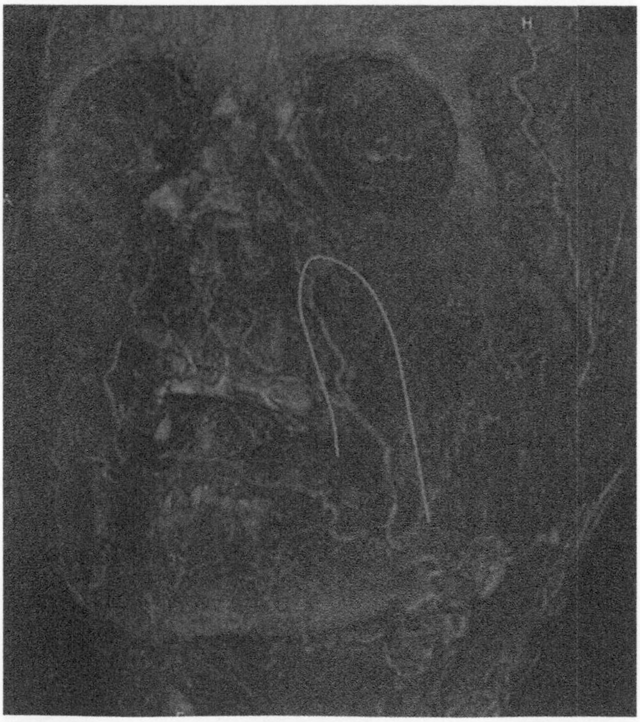

FIGURE 16.30 CTA imaging of the blood supply from the facial artery.

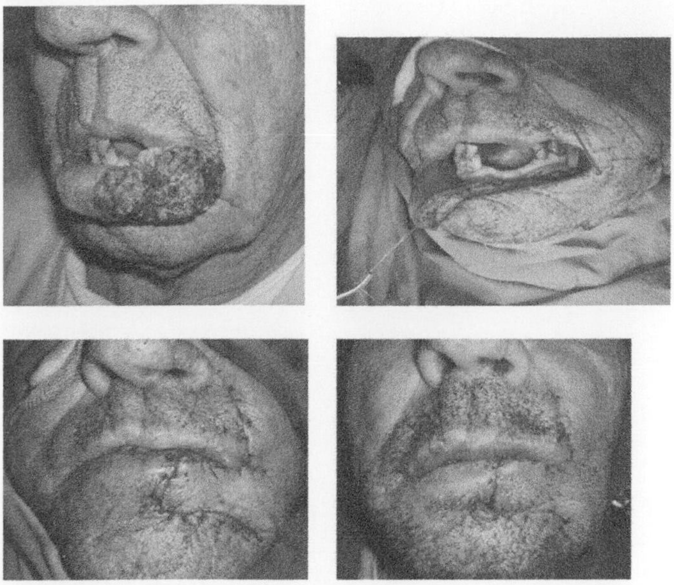

FIGURE 16.31 Von Brun's flap in a 71-year-old male patient.

BIBLIOGRAPHY

Aufricht G., Evaluation of pedicle flap versus skin graft, reconstruction of surface defects and scar contractures of the chin, cheeks and neck. *Surgery* 1944;15:1.

Gonzales-Ulloa M., Castillo A., Stevens E., Alvarez Fuertes G., Leonelli F., and Ubaldo F., Preliminary study of total restoration of the facial skin. *Plastic and Reconstructive Surgery* 1954;13:151–161.

Lupo F. and OrtizMonasterio F., Le schisi facciali rare: Revisione di una casistica di 490 pazienti. *Rimango a disposizione pe rulteriori chiarimenti* (Minerva) 2006;19:201–206.

Menick F.J., Artistry in aesthetic surgery. Aesthetic perception and the subunit principle. *Clinics in Plastic Surgery* 1987;14(4):723–735.

Menick F.J., Facial reconstruction with local and distant tissue: The interface of aesthetic and reconstructive surgery. *Plastic and Reconstructive Surgery* 1998;102(5):1424–1433.

Ortiz-Monasterio F., Analysis estetica de la cara. In F. Ortiz Monasterio and F. Molina (eds.), *Cirugı´a Estetica del esqueletofacial.* Buenos Aires, Argentina: Panamericana, 2005.

Ortiz Monasterio F., The concept of aesthetic units for the correction of facial cleft. In D. David (ed.), *Craniofacial Surgery 11.* Bologna, Italy: Medimond, 2005.

Ortiz Monasterio F. and Taylor J., Major craniofacial clefts: Case series and treatment philosophy. *Plastic and Reconstructive Surgery* 2008;122(2):434–443.

Salmon M., *Les Artères de la peau.* Paris, France: Masson, 1936.

17 Imaging and Surgical Strategies for Cutaneous Neoplasm of the Scalp

Luca Andrea Dessy, Matteo Atzeni, Andrea Conversi, Luca Saba, Manfredi Greco, and Diego Ribuffo

CONTENTS

17.1 INTRODUCTION

Scalp reconstruction has always been a challenging task, in particular after oncological demolition. Diverse and complex set of scalp defects can be distinguished mainly in two types. In case of small to moderately sized defects in patients with good general health, full closure is achieved easily.[1] Aesthetic aspects, including the preservation of eyebrow symmetry and hairline as well as avoidance of alopecia, are the challenge in those cases.[2] Besides, large defects in patients with poor general performance status require full closure, which is the ultimate and challenging goal.[3]

Tumours attributed to actinic damage show a constant rise in incidence, and the exposed location of the scalp leaves it as one of the primary regions for skin cancer.[4] Rarer malignancies are soft-tissue sarcomas, primary adnexal cancers, and secondary malignancies.[5] Because of the apparent location of the tumour, patients usually are seen at an early stage of the disease, when simple resection with primary closure is possible, leading to an excellent prognosis.

The oncological radicality should be pursued especially in large infiltrating tumours, although the extent of the residual defect after excision may result in technical difficulties for the reconstruction.

Although the reconstructive challenges increase exponentially with local tumour advancement, the modern methods of reconstructive surgery allow for radical resection and reconstruction of virtually any extent of scalp tumour. The limitation to this rule more strongly depends on invasion into deeper structures than on the extent of infiltration of scalp tissue by the tumour.[6]

Scalp reconstruction after malignancies may be suboptimal when insufficient oncologic radicality is used,[7] when inadequate reconstructive procedures are selected leading to prolonged recovery and/or unstable scars, and when patients delay consultation until the tumour has reached extensive dimensions.

Surgical excision with adequate margins is the standard treatment for scalp malignancies. For instance, it has been evidenced that for node-negative primary scalp melanoma, subperiosteal resection can significantly decrease in-transit/satellite recurrence when compared with subgaleal resection.[8] Adjunctive treatments such as irradiation, chemotherapy, and immunotherapy have to be considered as adjuvant therapies or second options if surgery is impossible or not desired.[9,10]

Surgical treatment of scalp neoplasm requires a precise diagnostic evaluation. Clinical assessment is often sufficient to assess small lesions involving scalp superficial layers and leaving deep layers intact; this is clearly proven by the possibility to mobilise the lesion on the cranium. Larger lesions that show to be adherent to deep planes require a diagnostic imaging to define local and distant involvement. Once the diagnostic evaluation is completed, the more appropriate treatment modality can be selected, taking into account patient's age, condition, and will.

The loss of skin envelope has been one of the oldest yet most frequent and costly problems in our health-care system. To restore functional and aesthetic integrity in patients for oncological reasons, an armamentarium of reconstructive surgical procedures including autogenous, allogenous, and xenogenous tissue transfer as well as implantation of alloplastic materials has been favoured. The best replacement for scalp tissue is scalp tissue. There is no other donor site in the body that will approximate the same hair-bearing qualities of scalp tissue.

The proper choice of a reconstructive technique is affected by several factors: the size and location of the defect, the presence or absence of periosteum, the quality of surrounding scalp tissue, the presence or absence of hair, the location of the hairline, and patient co-morbidities. Successful reconstruction of these defects requires a detailed knowledge of scalp anatomy, hair physiology, skin biomechanics, and the variety of possible local tissue rearrangements. In nearly total defects, local tissues may be inadequate and tissue expansion or free tissue transfer may be the only alternatives.

However, especially in the case of elderly patients with poor performance status and large wounds, new options for wound bed preconditioning, like artificial dermis or topical negative-pressure therapy, have to be taken into consideration.[11] Tissue engineering combines advances in cell culture technology to medical and surgical advances in science to allow for new solutions though synthetic substitutes increasingly effective and efficient.

This chapter gives an overview of the diagnostic imaging for tumours of the scalp and the state of the art in scalp reconstruction strategies.

17.1.1 Anatomy of the Scalp

The scalp is defined as the anatomic area overlying the skull between the superior orbital rims anteriorly and the superior nuchal line posteriorly. Soft and hard tissues within this region are commonly divided into six layers: skin, subcutaneous tissue, galea, loose areolar tissue, calvarial periosteum (pericranium), and calvarial bone. The skin of the scalp is the thickest in the body, ranging from 8 mm thick in the occipital area and decreasing in thickness as one moves anteriorly and temporally (3 mm). It is attached by firm, fibrous septa that run through the subcutaneous to the underlying galea. The subcutaneous layer of dense connective tissue and fat binds the skin to the underlying galea. The subcutaneous layer contains the principal arteries and veins of the scalp, as well as the sensory nerves and lymphatics. Because of the fibrous septa, this layer is inelastic and firm. The blood vessels embedded in this layer bleed freely when transected presumably because they are less able to retract.

The galea aponeurotica is the tough fibrous layer of the scalp. It is extensive in its attachments and is a part of the subcutaneous musculoaponeurotic system (SMAS) of the face. It connects the occipitalis muscle posteriorly with the frontalis muscle anteriorly and the temporoparietal fascia (superficial temporal fascia) in one temporal region with the same layer on the contralateral side. The loose areolar plane beneath the galea is composed of thin, avascular connective tissue and has been termed in various ways (innominate fascia, subaponeurotic layer, subgaleal fascia[12,13]). This plane is easily dissected. The laxity of this layer contributes for the mobility of the scalp.

The innermost layer of the scalp, the pericranium, is densely adherent to the outer table of the skull. The pericranium contains a rich vascular network that allows it to serve as a recipient bed for skin grafts or as a flap.

The scalp has a rich blood supply arising from four principal arteries and lesser contributing vessels. The occipital and superficial temporal arteries on each side are the main vascular afferents. Lesser contributions to the scalp are made by the posterior auricular artery, small branches of the external carotid artery, and the supraorbital and supratrochlear vessels. These vessels travel in the subcutaneous layer and form abundant anastomoses, such that the entire scalp can survive one major vessel.[14]

The scalp has multiple sensory nerves. The anterior portion of the scalp is supplied by the supraorbital and supratrochlear nerves. A branch of the second or third cervical nerve, the lesser occipital nerve, supplies the posterior scalp. The great auricular nerve provides sensation to the posterior auricular region, earlobe, and angle of the jaw. The temporal region receives sensory input from the auriculotemporal nerve, a branch of the mandibular division of the trigeminal nerve. This nerve can be found accompanying the superficial temporal artery just above the zygomatic arch.

17.1.2 Radiological Imaging

Imaging techniques represent an optimal tool to study the cancer affecting the skull. Nowadays, it is possible to use three different radiological procedures: ultrasound (US) assessment, computed tomography (CT), and magnetic resonance (MR). The information obtained from each one of these procedures is different and should be understood.

US imaging is based on the difference in acoustic impedance of the tissues; the physics of US is beyond the purposes of this chapter, but one fundamental rule is that the US cannot offer detailed information about the bones, because of the big acoustic impedance of this structure. Therefore, it is possible to identify the neoplasm and to assess its dimension, but no correct information about the bone involvement can be obtained.[15,16] A further limit of US is the low inter-observer reproducibility that is demonstrated in previous studies. To study skin neoplasm, it is important to use 10 MHz frequency probes that allow to have a high spatial resolution of the tissues closer to the probe. Other authors suggested to use a high-frequency probe (20 MHz) that may help in assessing positive skin tumours, in differentiating them, and in precising, before histological examination, the exact location of the lesion within the different skin layers and its origin.[15]

CT imaging nowadays represents the first-line tool in the staging of the skin neoplasms of the skull because of its potentiality to assess the bone involvement. CT imaging is based on the x-ray attenuation of the tissues and the bones determines a significant x-ray attenuation: this allows CT to be extremely sensitive in the bone involvement. The spatial resolution of the newer scanner is about 0.4 mm with isotropic voxels that allow to post-process the data in multiple spatial planes and with volumetric software.[17] CT exams should be performed before and after the administration of contrast material in order to assess the vascular pattern of the neoplasm.[18] In fact, it is also possible to identify the arterial and venous routes of the tumour in case of a voluminous tumour. In particular, it is mandatory to perform a CT angiography with a delay time of about 25 s followed by a second acquisition after 70 s to map the venous vessels to identify the arterial phase. CT is an extremely reproducible technique with very high inter- and intra-observer agreement. One limit of CT relies in the impossibility to exactly quantify the meningeal involvement that can be observed when a destructive neoplasm completely involves the skull bone.[19]

Magnetic resonance imaging (*MRI*) represents the gold standard procedure because it allows to detect the neoplasm and to quantify its extension from the skin plane to the meningeal level. The MR exam should be performed before and after administration of the contrast material for two reasons: The first one is that usually these neoplasms show a significant and heterogeneous contrast enhancement in the T1-weighted images acquired after administration of the contrast material. Secondly, when there is a cancer involvement of the meninges, usually these become thickened and show an intense and homogeneous contrast enhancement.[20] The vascular analysis of the neoplasm is not excellent using the MRI, compared to the CT, because of its minor spatial resolution that is about 1 mm.

In some cases also, the use of nuclear medicine can be helpful in identifying the neoplasm and its spread, particularly the perineural spread. A recent publication showed in a 66-year-old man that underwent 2-F-18 fluoro-2-deoxy-D-glucose (FDG) positron emission tomography (PET) after the excision of a skin neoplasm the perineural spread of the neoplasm that was visible only using the FDG-PET.[21] Obviously, this approach cannot be considered routinely because of the economic and biologic cost of the FDG-PET.

In conclusion, the imaging techniques allow to correctly identify the skin neoplasms of the skull and to obtain all the information necessary to plan the correct surgical approach, particularly vascular analysis and bone and meningeal involvement.

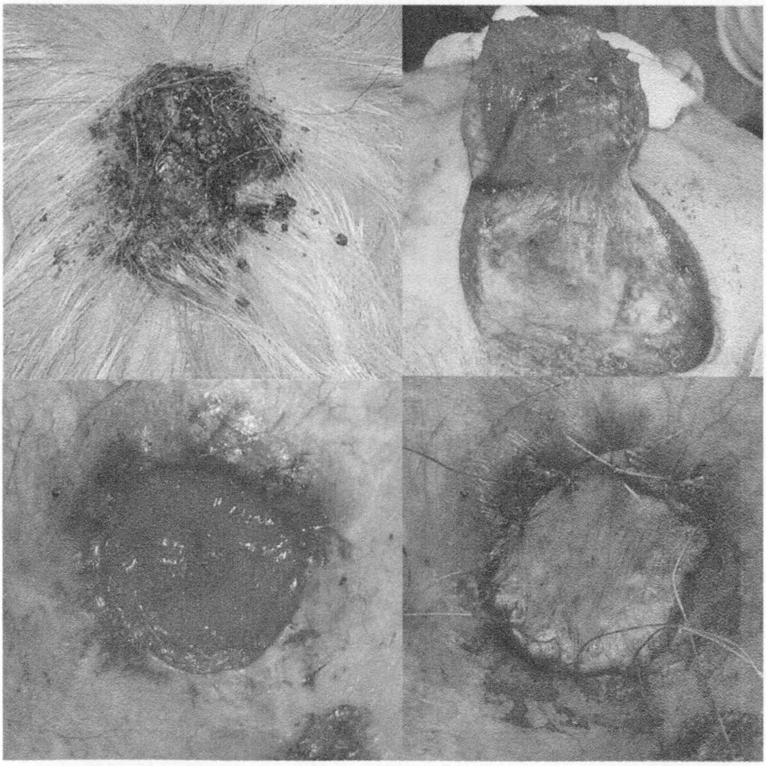

FIGURE 17.1 Top left, preoperative view of a 70-year-old male, affected by a basal cell carcinoma of the scalp; top right, intraoperative view showing subgaleal cancer excision; bottom left, intraoperative view showing scalp defect after cancer excision and round block suture to reduce defect dimension; bottom right, intraoperative view showing skin grafting of the scalp defect.

17.1.3 Surgical Strategies in Scalp Reconstruction

When the lesion does not extend beyond the galea, the surgical excision is performed in the subgaleal plan (Figure 17.1). In cases of deeper tumour extension and suspicious external cortical bone involvement, the external calvarium requires to be removed en block together with the lesion (Figures 17.2 and 17.3). More advanced tumours infiltrating the diploic bone require a full-thickness calvarium demolition (Figure 17.4). Therefore, reconstruction of the scalp depends on the structures missing.

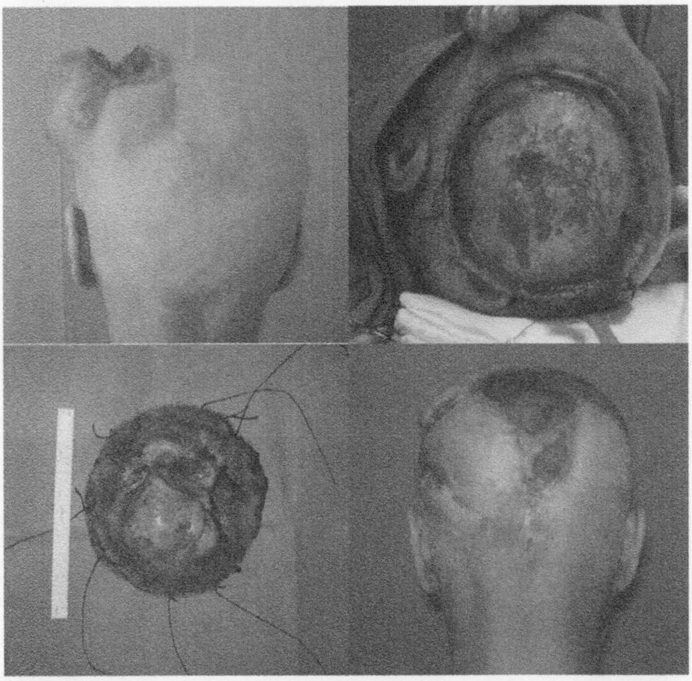

(a)

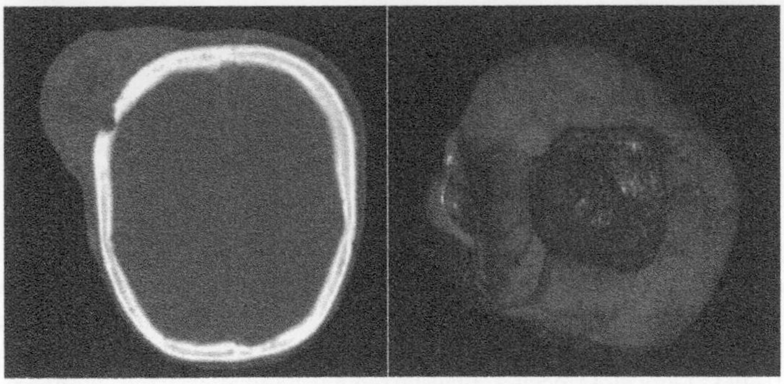

(b)

FIGURE 17.2 (a) Top left, preoperative view of a 51-year-old female, affected by a relapsing squamous cell carcinoma of the scalp; top right, intraoperative view after cancer excision and bone milling; bottom left, scalp cancer after excision; bottom right, early postoperative view after reconstruction by cutaneous pedicled flap and skin graft. (b) Same patient as in (a): left, CT imaging showing bone involvement by skin cancer; right, 3D CT reconstruction showing the cancer and its vascularisation.

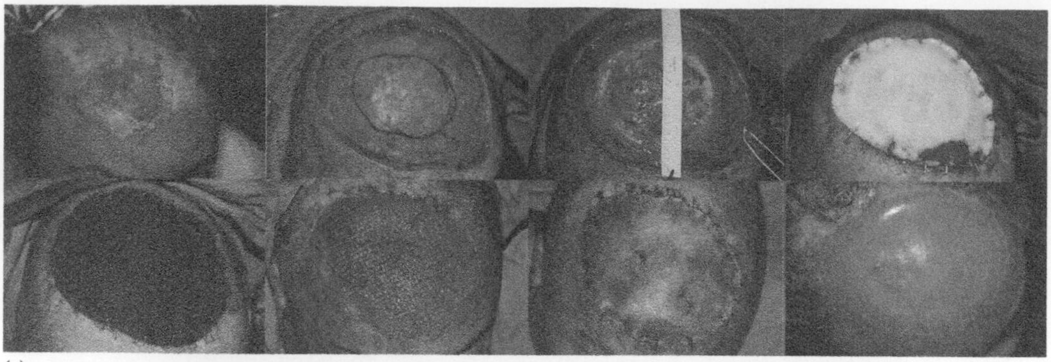

(a)

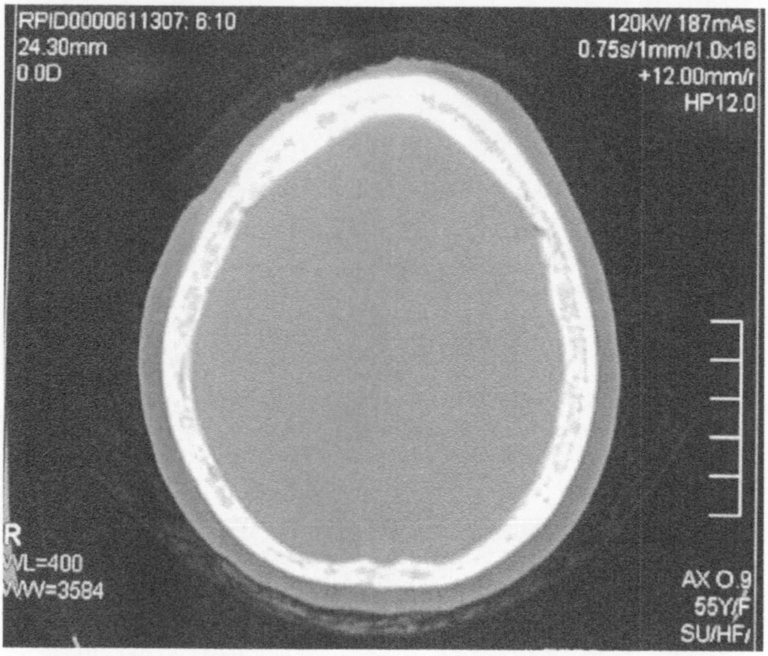

(b)

FIGURE 17.3 (a) Top extreme left, preoperative view of a 71-year-old female, affected by a relapsing infiltrating basal cell carcinoma of the scalp with suspicious external cortical bone involvement; top centre left, intraoperative view showing wide tumour excision with 15 mm of surgical skin margins; top centre right, intraoperative view showing the defect after resection of the external cortical bone and round block suture with Gore-Tex CV-0 (W.L. Gore & Associates, Flagstaff, AZ, United States); top extreme right, defect covered with a 10 × 10 cm Hyalomatrix® template; bottom extreme left, defect covered with a polyurethane sponge applied on the Hyalomatrix template; bottom centre left, postoperative complete wound coverage with granulation tissue 2 weeks after the application of Hyalomatrix on the diploic bone after tumour resection; bottom centre right, intraoperative view after partial-thickness skin grafting 3 weeks after tumour resection; bottom extreme right, postoperative aspect 1.5 years after skin grafting. (b) Same patient as in (a): preoperative CT image of the scalp showing initial external cortical bone tumour infiltration.

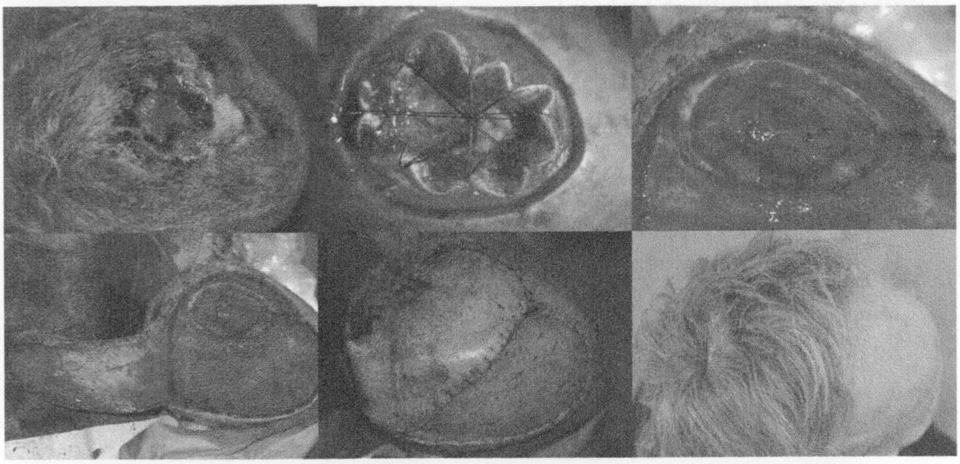

(a)

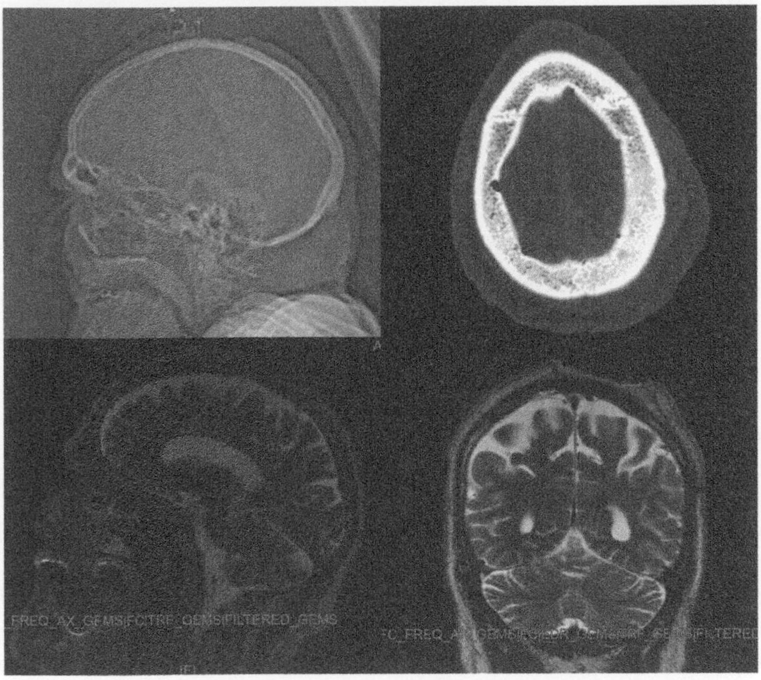

(b)

FIGURE 17.4 (a) Top left, preoperative view of a 75-year-old male, affected by a relapsing infiltrating squamous cell carcinoma of the scalp with suspicious diploic bone infiltration; top centre, intraoperative view showing wide tumour excision with 15 mm of surgical skin margins; top right, intraoperative view showing the defect after cancer resection with an area of external cortical bone excision and a central area with a full-thickness bone excision and dura mater exposure; bottom left, intraoperative view showing the elevation of an axial scalp flap base on the right occipital artery; bottom centre, intraoperative view showing the scalp defect covered with the described flap and the flap donor area with a partial-thickness skin graft; bottom right, postoperative aspect 1 year after reconstruction. (b) Same patient as in (a): top left, preoperative lateral view radiogram of the skull not clearly evidencing bone infiltration; top right, preoperative transversal view of CT imaging showing initial external cortical bone tumour infiltration; bottom left, preoperative sagittal view of MRI showing initial external cortical bone tumour infiltration and dura mater preservation; bottom right, coronal view of MRI showing initial diploic bone infiltration and dura mater preservation.

17.2 PARTIAL-THICKNESS DEFECTS

Coverage with a skin graft is usually only an option superficial to the temporalis muscle or if oncologic radicality allows for the periosteum to remain intact (Figure 17.1). Furthermore, skin transplants frequently result in unstable, depressed, and unsightly scars, which have to be rated as poor from both functional and aesthetic standpoints. The lesions are relatively small (from 2 to 5 cm in diameter). Hair transplantation may be required for secondary scalp reconstruction.

17.3 FULL-THICKNESS DEFECTS

Full-thickness defects are subject to necrosis and sequestration of dried exposed bone. Skin grafting is not a practicable option without an intact pericranium. Thus, a more aggressive approach is required.

In case of a full-thickness skull bone defect, reconstruction is not always necessary or recommended. It is sometimes convenient to defer the wound coverage after final histology is obtained with confirmation of margin clearance, reconstructing in conditions of oncological safety.[6–9] In addition, reconstruction must be a process of restoring form and function.

Size and location of the bone defect and expected intracranial pressure are important determinants for considering bone reconstruction in the acute stage. Larger bone defects can result in a spectrum of complaints ranging from headaches and motion intolerance to seizures and aesthetic concerns. There are no firm rules on defect diameters and bone replacement requirements. Defects with a diameter of 5–7 cm are considered as medium. Morcelised bone can be used for small skull defects and calvarial bone or rib grafts are suitable for medium-sized defects. The harvest of calvarial bone grafts is not favoured in these generally older oncology patients for oncologic reasons.[22] Patients with a recent history of infection and necrosis and patients who are likely to receive postoperative irradiation are excluded for nonvascularised bone grafts or prosthetic material, such as polymethylmethacrylate, hydroxyapatite cement, or titanium (Figure 17.6), as reconstructive options at the time of ablative surgery. Vascularised ribs for structural support in combination with the latissimus dorsi muscle can be used to cover large defects.[23] In the case of dural defects, fibrin glue is only used to close small dural defects. Artificial patches (e.g. Gore-Tex [W. L. Gore & Associates, Flagstaff, Arizona], Neuro-Patch [B. Braun Melsungen AG, Melsungen, Germany]) and nonvascularised fascia grafts are mainly, but not exclusively, used in nonirradiated areas to reduce the risk of infection. Vascularised fascia lata (in a musculocutaneous anterolateral thigh flap) is an option for reconstructing dural defects that have been previously irradiated.[22]

With the advent of new dermal substitutes, the choice of more demanding reconstructive procedures (i.e. pedicle or free flaps) becomes less compelling and the possibility to cover the exposed bone with a dermal matrix makes the reconstructive procedure easier and less cumbersome for the patient, reducing the costs of care and hospitalisation. These biomaterials are opening up to easier and less stressful possibilities of reconstruction for the patient (less lengthy interventions, lack of morbidity of the donor areas, and faster postoperative rehabilitation).

Currently, many authors have contributed their expertise on the possibility of using dermal matrix on loss of substance with bone exposure.[10–15]

Some authors have integrated the use of negative-pressure therapy with the use of the dermal matrix to increase the local blood supply.[13,15–17]

Generally, the wounds that do not contain a sufficient blood flow to the survival of a graft, with exposed bone or tendon, require the use of flaps. Especially at the calvarium, the amount of dermis influences the durability and functional and aesthetic properties of the skin graft. If the wound does not result in a well-vascularised granulation bed, then local, distant, or free-flap coverage may be necessary, because the skin graft has a certain degree of failure of skin take, depending entirely on the re- and neovascularisation coming from the wound bed.[18,19] Even today, for most patients, flaps remain the ideal treatment, but some of them are not candidates for more demanding reconstructive surgery; moreover, often these procedures are associated with long hospitalisations, risk of infection, thrombosis, and loss of flaps.[20]

Surgical strategies vary with the cause and size of the defect and the quality of the surrounding local tissue, taking into consideration the patient's health condition, age, and will.

The following are the basic methods used to cover exposed bone.

17.3.1 Outer-Table Removal with Direct or Delayed Grafting

Immediate skin grafting after removal of the outer table results in a bumpy coverage that is prone to ulceration. Delayed grafting after granulation of the wound created by removal of the outer table is reported to yield a stable graft with minimal chance of skin graft breakdown.[24]

17.3.2 Local Scalp Flap(s) with Galeal Scoring

17.3.2.1 Small Defects (<6 cm)

The use of local flaps is generally the best method to close these wounds. The flaps are raised above the pericranium and are based on the major nutrient blood supply. The nonstretchable scalp can be made to cover a larger area by scoring the galea perpendicular to the direction of the tension. Great care must be taken to avoid injuring the vessels in the supragaleal plane.[25] If the flap must be widened, the galea can be cross-hatched to relieve tension. Almost all flaps require galeal scoring to provide successful closure. If the scalp loss is in a conspicuous area (i.e. hairline), it is wise to transpose a hair-bearing flap from a location that can be more easily camouflaged. In small defects, the donor area can be closed primarily or, if necessary, covered with a split-thickness skin graft. These flaps should be designed to take advantage of neck skin laxity. Mobilisation of the scalp adjacent to the donor defect, with galeal scoring, may aid in donor site reduction.

17.3.2.2 Medium-Sized Defects

When dealing with these larger defects, the principles of closure remain the same. The best choice is usually a large scalp flap with skin grafting of the donor pericranium.

In some cases, the use of multiple axial flaps is helpful. This concept was initially described as a four-flap technique, utilising the entire remaining scalp to close the defect.[25] This technique was then modified to a three-flap technique in which two smaller flaps adjacent to the defect are used to provide primary wound closure and a third larger flap, consisting of the entire remaining scalp, is used to close the donor defect following rotation of the two smaller flaps. These flaps are based on known vascular territories and can be used to cover defects up to one-third of the scalp surface area.

The width of the two smaller flaps should be at least one-half the width of the primary defect so that, when mobilised and juxtaposed, they automatically cover the raw surface. The larger flap includes the rest of the scalp. If the defect is lateral to the midline, the base of the pedicle of the large scalp flap should be based on the contralateral side of the defect. These flaps are elevated in the loose areolar plane and will require extensive undermining of the remaining scalp, forehead, and nape of the neck. Care must be taken when performing lateral dissection so as to avoid injury to the vascular pedicles as they enter the scalp.

17.3.2.3 Large Defects (8–10 cm)

When the defect is large, anterior, and off to one side, a subtotal scalp flap can be raised (Figures 17.2a and 17.4a). Based on the superficial temporal and posterior auricular arteries, the remaining scalp can be transposed with a large donor deficit that must be grafted. The back cut in the occipital region may require special attention (e.g. padding), as it may break down if the patient lies on it. Better results are obtained with a free flap.

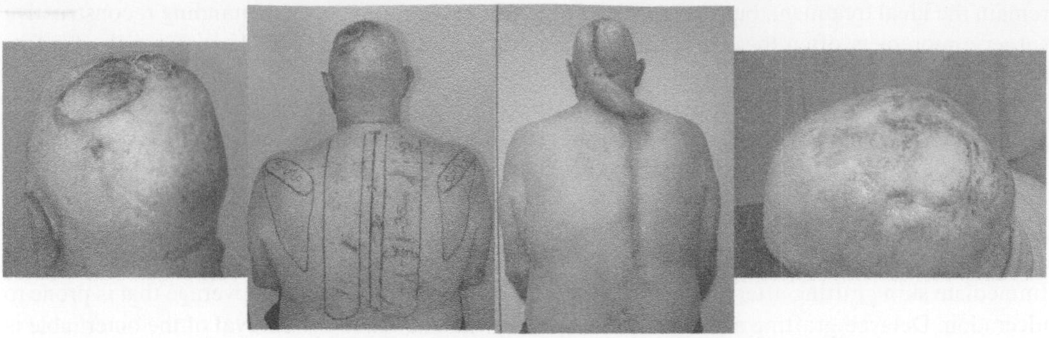

FIGURE 17.5 Extreme left, preoperative view of a 78-year-old male, affected by radiodermatitis with bone exposure after radiotherapy for cerebral neoplasm; centre left, preoperative markings for extended trapezium flap reconstruction before surgical delay; centre right, postoperative view of pedicled trapezium flap after 4 weeks; extreme right, postoperative view of final reconstruction after section of pedicle.

17.3.2.4 Pericranial Flaps and Overlying Skin Grafts or Local Flaps

Pericranial flaps are endowed with a rich vascular network that allows them to be used as pedicled flaps (Figure 17.5) to cover denuded bone and act as a bed for skin grafting.

Pericranial flaps should be designed larger than the recipient site because of their elastic properties. In addition, the random anastomoses that vascularise these flaps are weakest between major vascular territories. Thus, they must be based on major vascular territories that do not cross the midline. The advantages of the pericranial flaps are their minimal donor site morbidity and dependability as a bed for skin grafting. However, these flaps should be laid down in a manner that reduces pressure (i.e. bolster dressings). The maximum defect size that can be covered by this flap is 7 cm × 12 cm.[26]

17.3.2.5 Tissue Expansion Followed by Local Flap Closure

This technique is an acceptable method of closure without visible change in hair thickness.

Temporary coverage of exposed bone must be obtained before expansion.

Approximately 50% of the scalp can be reconstructed with expanded scalp tissue.[27] It does require staged operations with a lengthy interval period and is potentially associated with expander complications.[28] Stable scalp coverage must be obtained during the expansion process to prevent calvarial desiccation and subsequent osteomyelitis. If the periosteum is intact, it can be primarily skin grafted.

When using tissue expansion, the largest expander possible should be placed in a subgaleal position. The shape of tissue expander bases affects the amount of tissue gain. The appropriately sized and shaped expander should be selected on the basis of the individual patient's defect (Figure 17.6).[29] A single large expander is preferred over multiple smaller expanders, as this will give the greatest gain in tissue per volume of expansion and minimise the infectious risk by limiting the number of operative sites. However, in scalp reconstruction, multiple expanders are frequently used in a single setting to gain the greatest amount of expansion per operative procedure. The incision should be small and placed at a distance from the defect, the pocket, and the future flap. Intraoperative filling of the expander reduces the need for drains by preventing hematoma and seroma formation. A good estimation of flap length is twice the height of the expander above the skin surface. Overexpansion by 30%–50% makes the procedure more reliable.

External tissue expanders may be an alternative to internal expansion in selected cases. They provide constant tension across a wound to accomplish wound closure through less invasive methods. There are many available external tissue expanders utilising hooks, sutures, metal footplates, or elastomer-based adhesive strips for adherence to the skin.[30–32]

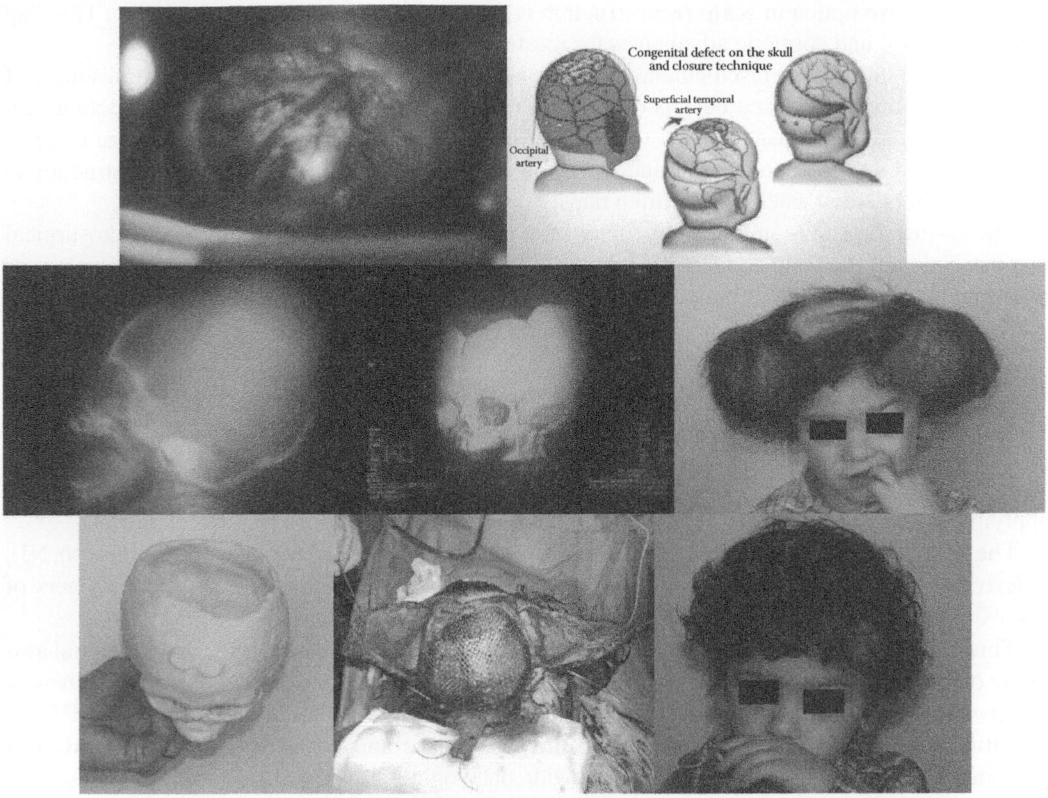

FIGURE 17.6 Top left, aplasia cutis congenita with calvarial bone involvement; top right, drawings of immediate reconstruction with extended occipital flap to cover the skin defect; centre left and centre, x-ray and CT scan of the bone defect before final reconstruction; centre right, postoperative view after bilateral skin expansion; bottom left, 3D custom model of bone defect; bottom centre, intraoperative view of final reconstruction by titanium mesh and pre-expanded skin flap; bottom right, postoperative view after 5 months.

17.3.2.6 Microvascular Flap Coverage

When local flaps are not an option, management of large scalp frequently requires free-flap coverage. Free tissue transfer is the only available option for full-thickness defects of the entire scalp. Several free-flap options are available for scalp and forehead reconstruction. These choices depend on different factors such as patient characteristics, defect variables, and surgeon preference.[33–37]

Free tissue transfer allows for successful reconstruction in high-risk patients in whom local reconstructive techniques would likely fail. Although many of these patients will eventually die as a result of their disease, reconstruction can provide a good quality of life.[38]

McClean and Bunke[39] described the free vascularised omental transfer for scalp coverage. The omentum was moulded to the scalp defect and then covered with a split-thickness skin graft. The necessity of laparotomy and the availability of less morbid flaps have limited the usefulness of this transfer. The latissimus dorsi muscle, which can be transferred as a myocutaneous unit or as a free muscle only and covered with a split-thickness skin graft, was first used in 1978 to cover a scalp defect.[40] The muscle is large enough to cover the entire scalp and is reliable in its anatomy. In addition, the thoracodorsal artery and vein provide a long pedicle that aids in the utility of this flap.

The parascapular flap is more bulky than the latissimus dorsi flap but does not sacrifice a functional muscle. It cannot cover the entire scalp. These flaps are unsatisfactory from an aesthetic standpoint and do not restore hair-bearing tissue to the scalp.

An alternative option in scalp reconstruction is the use of the anterolateral thigh flap. This flap offers structural and cosmetic advantages for most scalp defects.[41]

The fascial layer of the fasciocutaneous anterolateral thigh flap can easily be used as a source of vascularised fascia to replace defects of the dura mater.[42] The well-vascularised fascia component will be useful in the management of wound healing of the dura and will prevent leakage of cerebrospinal fluid and infection of the underlying cerebral tissues. Also, total scalp reconstruction is possible with bilateral anterolateral thigh flaps.[43]

The aesthetic result is an important factor affecting the quality-of-life outcome of microsurgical reconstruction of the scalp and forehead. Disadvantages in aesthetic outcome such as skin colour or texture mismatch and excess bulk of the flap are readily noticeable.

17.3.2.7 Bioresorbable Dermal Substitute

Patients affected by infiltrating large tumours of the scalp and American Society of Anesthesiologists (ASA) class III may not be candidates for any of the previously described aggressive surgical procedures.

In this category of patients, during the same surgical procedure, the defect can be covered by applying dermal substitutes on the pericranium, the diploic bone or dura (Figure 17.3).[44–49]

The dermal regeneration template for excellence is Integra® (Integra LifeSciences, Plainsboro, NJ), a derivative of organic synthesis; it consists of bovine collagen polymerised with copolymers of glycosaminoglycan (GAG). It is the most widely used dermal substitute.

This dermal regeneration template allows obtaining an appropriate coverage and an optimal aesthetic outcome. In the absence of autologous dermis, staged reconstruction with a dermal equivalent or dermal regeneration template may offer a good reconstructive option in selected cases.[45–48,50]

Advantages in using these templates are the ease of use and the ability to induct neodermis formation to obtain optimal graft take after wide oncological demolitions. First, this conduct can assure surgical radicality reducing the possibility of relapse, even in the most aggressive and infiltrating tumours. Second, reconstruction can restore form and function. Good bone coverage with recovery of a sufficient soft-tissue thickness and a good morphology can be achieved. Moreover, patients requiring oncologic surgery of the scalp are often elderly, with co-morbid illness, so that a complex reconstruction is not always recommended, and sometimes surgery has to be abandoned in favour of radiotherapy.[51]

The use of these dermal templates is a valid technical option that gives a good result, is accepted by patients, and is easy to be applied. Dermal substitutes have enormous potential to allow an increase in therapeutic options available to the surgeon and the patient's benefit.

REFERENCES

1. Dalay C, Kesiktas E, Yavuz M et al. Coverage of scalp defects following contact electrical burns to the head: A clinical series. *Burns* 2006;32:201–207.
2. Blackwell KE, Rawnsley JD. Aesthetic considerations in scalp reconstruction. *Facial Plast Surg* 2008;24:11–21.
3. Angelos PC, Downs BW. Options for the management of forehead and scalp defects. *Facial Plast Surg Clin North Am* 2009;17:379–393.
4. Wells MD. Scalp reconstruction. In: Mathes SJ, Vincent RH, eds., *Plastic Surgery*. Philadelphia, PA: Saunders; 2005, pp. 607–632.
5. Horch RE, Stark GB, Beier JP. Unusual explosive growth of a squamous cell carcinoma of the scalp after electrical burn injury and subsequent coverage by sequential free flap vascular connection: A case report. *BMC Cancer* 2005;5:150.
6. Soma PF, Chibbaro S, Makiese O. Aggressive scalp carcinoma with intracranial extension: A multidisciplinary experience of 25 patients with long-term follow-up. *J Clin Neurosci* 2008;15:988–992.
7. Hussussian CJ, Reece GP. Microsurgical scalp reconstruction in the patient with cancer. *Plast Reconstr Surg* 2002;109:1828–1834.

8. Pannucci CJ, Collar RM, Johnson TM, Bradford CR, Rees RS. The role of full-thickness scalp resection for management of primary scalp melanoma. *Ann Plast Surg* 2012;69:165–168.
9. Nedea EA, DeLaney TF. Sarcoma and skin radiation oncology. *Hematol Oncol Clin North Am* 2006;20:401–429.
10. Urosevic M, Dummer R. Role of imiquimod in skin cancer treatment. *Am J Clin Dermatol* 2004;5:453–458.
11. Chang KP, Lai CH, Chang CH et al. Free flap options for reconstruction of complicated scalp and calvarial defects: Report of a series of cases and literature review. *Microsurgery* 2010;30:13–18.
12. Casanova R, Cavalcante D, Grotting JC et al. Anatomic basis for vascularized outer-table calvarial bone grafts. *Plast Reconstr Surg* 1986;78:300.
13. Tolhurst DE, Carstens MH, Greco RJ, Hurwitz DJ. The surgical anatomy of the scalp. *Plast Reconstr Surg* 1991;87:603.
14. Leedy JE, Janis JE, Rohrich RJ. Reconstruction of acquired scalp defects: An algorithmic approach. *Plast Reconstr Surg* 2005;116:54e.
15. Clément A, Hoeffel C, Fayet P, Benkanoun S, Sahut D'izarn J, Oudjit A, Legmann P, Gorin I, Escande J, Bonnin A. Value of high frequency (20 MHz) and Doppler ultrasound in the diagnosis of pigmented cutaneous tumors. *J Radiol* 2001;82(5):563–571.
16. Schmid-Wendtner MH, Burgdorf W. Ultrasound scanning in dermatology. *Arch Dermatol* 2005;141(2):217–224.
17. Marin D, Nelson RC, Rubin GD, Schindera ST. Body CT: Technical advances for improving safety. *AJR Am J Roentgenol* 2011;197(1):33–41.
18. Bae KT. Intravenous contrast medium administration and scan timing at CT: Considerations and approaches. *Radiology* 2010;256(1):32–61.
19. Xie CM, Liu XW, Li H, Zhang R, Mo YX, Li JP, Geng ZJ, Zheng L, Lv YC, Wu PH. Computed tomographic findings of skull base bony changes after radiotherapy for nasopharyngeal carcinoma: Implications for local recurrence. *J Otolaryngol Head Neck Surg* 2011;40(4):300–310.
20. Maroldi R, Ambrosi C, Farina D. Metastatic disease of the brain: Extra-axial metastases (skull, dura, leptomeningeal) and tumour spread. *Eur Radiol* 2005;15(3):617–626.
21. Conrad GR, Sinha P, Holzhauer M. Perineural spread of skin carcinoma to the base of the skull: detection with FDG PET and CT fusion. *Clin Nucl Med* 2004;29(11):717–719.
22. van Driel AA, Mureau MA, Goldstein DP, Gilbert RW, Irish JC, Gullane PJ, Neligan PC, Hofer SO. Aesthetic and oncologic outcome after microsurgical reconstruction of complex scalp and forehead defects after malignant tumor resection: An algorithm for treatment. *Plast Reconstr Surg* 2010;126(2):460–470.
23. Seitz IA, Gottlieb LJ. Reconstruction of scalp and forehead defects. *Clin Plast Surg* 2009;36:355–377.
24. Stuzin JM, Zide BM. *Grabb and Smith's Plastic Surgery*, 4th edn. Boston, MA: Little, Brown; 1991, p. 401.
25. Orticochea, M. New three-flap scalp reconstruction techniques. *Br J Plast Surg* 1971;24:184.
26. Terranova, W. The use of periosteal flaps in scalp and forehead reconstruction. *Ann Plast Surg* 1990;24:450.
27. Manders ER, Schenden MJ, Furrey JA et al. Skin expansion to eliminate large scalp defects. *Plast Reconstr Surg* 1984;74:493.
28. Azzolini A, Riberti C, Caalca D. Skin expansion in head and neck reconstructive surgery. *Plast Reconstr Surg* 1992;90:799.
29. Marcks KM, Trevaskis A, Nauss TJ. Scalp defects and their repair. *Plast Reconstr Surg* 1951;7:237.
30. Dal Cin A, Seal SKF. Scalp expansion with the Canica wound closure system: First case report. *Can J Plast Surg* 2006;14(4):233–235.
31. Concannon MJ, Puckett CL. Wound coverage using modified tissue expansion. *Plast Reconstr Surg* 1998;102(2):377–384.
32. Laurence VG, Martin JB, Wirth GA. External tissue expanders as adjunct therapy in closing difficult wounds. *J Plast Reconstr Aesthet Surg* 2012;65:e297–e299.
33. Lutz BS, Wei FC, Chen HC, Lin CH, Wei CY. Reconstruction of scalp defects with free flaps in 30 cases. *Br J Plast Surg* 1998;51:186–190.
34. Pennington DG, Stern HS, Lee KK. Free-flap reconstruction of large defects of the scalp and calvarium. *Plast Reconstr Surg* 1989;83:655–661.
35. Earley MJ, Green MF, Milling MA. A critical appraisal of the use of free flaps in primary reconstruction of combined scalp and calvarial cancer defects. *Br J Plast Surg* 1990;43:283–289.
36. McCombe D, Donato R, Hofer SO, Morisson W. Free flaps in the treatment of locally advanced malignancy of the scalp and forehead. *Ann Plast Surg* 2002;48:600–606.
37. Losken A, Carlson GW, Culbertson JH et al. Omental free flap reconstruction in complex head and neck deformities. *Head Neck* 2002;24:326–331.

38. Wang HT, Erdmann D, Olbrich KC, Friedman AH, Levin LS, Zenn MR. Free flap reconstruction of the scalp and calvaria of major neurosurgical resections in cancer patients: Lessons learned closing large, difficult wounds of the dura and skull. *Plast Reconstr Surg* 2007;119:865.
39. McClean D, Bunke H. Autotransplant of omentum to a large scalp defect with microsurgical revascularization. *Plast Reconstr Surg* 1972;49:268.
40. Maxwell P, Steuber K, Hoopes J. A free latissimus dorsi myocutaneous flap. *Plast Reconstr Surg* 1978;62:462.
41. Ozkan O, Coskunfirat OK, Ozgentas HE, Derin A. Rationale for reconstruction of large scalp defects using the anterolateral thigh flap: Structural and aesthetic outcomes. *J Reconstr Microsurg* 2005;21(8):539–545.
42. Koshima I, Fukuda H, Yamamoto H et al. Free anterolateral thigh flaps for reconstruction of head and neck defects. *Plast Reconstr Surg* 1993;92:421–428.
43. Kwee MM, Rozen WM, Ting JW, Mirkazemi M, Leong J, Baillieu C. Total scalp reconstruction with bilateral anterolateral thigh flaps. *Microsurgery* 2012;32:393–396.
44. Spector JA, Glat PM. Hair-bearing scalp reconstruction using a dermal regeneration template and micrograft hair transplantation. *Ann Plast Surg* 2007;59(1):63–66.
45. Koenen W, Goerdt S, Faulhaber J. Removal of the outer table of the skull for reconstruction of full-thickness scalp defects with a dermal regeneration template. *Dermatol Surg* 2008;34(3):357–363.
46. Corradino B, Di Lorenzo S, Leto Barone AA, Maresi E, Moschella F. Reconstruction of full thickness scalp defects after tumour excision in elderly patients: Our experience with Integra dermal regeneration template. *J Plast Reconstr Aesthet Surg* 2010;63(3):e245–e247.
47. Abbas Khan MA, Chipp E, Hardwicke J, Srinivasan K, Shaw S, Rayatt S. The use of Dermal Regeneration Template (Integra®) for reconstruction of a large full-thickness scalp and calvarial defect with exposed dura. *J Plast Reconstr Aesthet Surg* 2010;63(12):2168–2171.
48. Khan MA, Ali SN, Farid M, Pancholi M, Rayatt S, Yap LH. Use of dermal regeneration template (Integra) for reconstruction of full-thickness complex oncologic scalp defects. *J Craniofac Surg* 2010;21(3):905–909.
49. Mueller CK, Bader RD, Ewald C, Kalff R, Schultze-Mosgau S. Scalp defect repair: A comparative analysis of different surgical techniques. *Ann Plast Surg* 2012;68(6):594–598.
50. Dessy LA, Mazzocchi M, Rizzo MI, Onesti MG, Scuderi G. Scalp reconstruction using Dermal Induction Template: State of the art and personal experience. *In Vivo* 2013;27(1):153–158.
51. Finco G, Atzeni M, Musu M et al. Greater occipital nerve block for surgical resection of major infiltrating lesions of the posterior scalp. *Plast Reconstr Surg* 2010;125:52e–53e.

18 Surgical Strategies and Imaging for Regional Flaps in the Head and Neck

Gary Xia Vern Tan, Warren M. Rozen, Vachara Niumsawatt, Alberto Alonso-Burgos, and Edmund W. Ek

CONTENTS

18.1 OVERVIEW

Surgical reconstruction of the head and neck is predominantly required after tumour resections but also in cases of trauma, infection, and congenital abnormalities.[41] In today's ageing population, a large proportion of head and neck reconstruction is performed to correct complex defects created by surgical resection of advanced head and neck cancers. Free-flap reconstruction of such defects may not be ideal in such patients given their advanced age and co-morbidities. Local and regional flaps provide reconstructive options with comparatively less morbidity and operative risk.[5] Furthermore, local and regional flaps provide like-for-like tissue, which is well matched in terms of texture and colour to the recipient site.[33] This is particularly advantageous in the head and neck where cosmesis is especially important given the visibility of this area and the associated psychosocial implications.

18.2 HISTORY OF HEAD AND NECK RECONSTRUCTION

Head and neck reconstruction dates as far back as the sixth century BC during which the ancient Indians used local flaps for nasal reconstruction.[47] Until the mid-twentieth century, the lack of understanding of the vascular supply of flaps resulted in head and neck reconstruction methods being restricted to direct closure and random flaps (local flaps and delayed flaps performed over multiple surgeries), all of which had limited use in the reconstruction of larger defects.[50] This was revolutionised by Milton who revealed that flap viability was dependent on the pattern of blood supply rather than arbitrary length-to-width ratios.[30] This formed the basis of regional pedicled flaps, first described in 1955 by Owens who reconstructed a mandibular defect using a latissimus dorsi flap.[34] However, the use of regional flaps for head and neck reconstruction only achieved widespread use after 1979, when Ariyan described the pedicled pectoralis major myocutaneous flap.[3] In the late 1980s, free-flap reconstruction began to gain popularity as they were not limited by pedicle length and provided a wider range of donor-site options, enabling surgeons to tailor flaps to better match the form and function required at the defect site.[50] This was further augmented through the development of perforator flaps, which enabled tissue to be harvested from anywhere in the body with an adequate blood vessel (perforator) to supply the flap whilst minimising donor-site morbidity.[14] Although free-flap reconstruction has become one of the primary techniques used in major head and neck reconstruction, advancements in imaging technology, anatomical knowledge, and surgical methods have enabled the refinement of local and regional flap techniques, which may be more useful in certain head and neck reconstructions.

18.3 LOCAL FLAP RECONSTRUCTION IN THE HEAD AND NECK

Local flaps utilise tissue directly adjacent to the defect for reconstruction. Small local flaps are commonly based on a random pattern of blood supply. Larger local flaps, particularly those including deeper layers, would rely on perforators for their blood supply (Figure 18.1). Knowledge of available perforators in the head and neck allows for safer and better planning of flap design for optimal

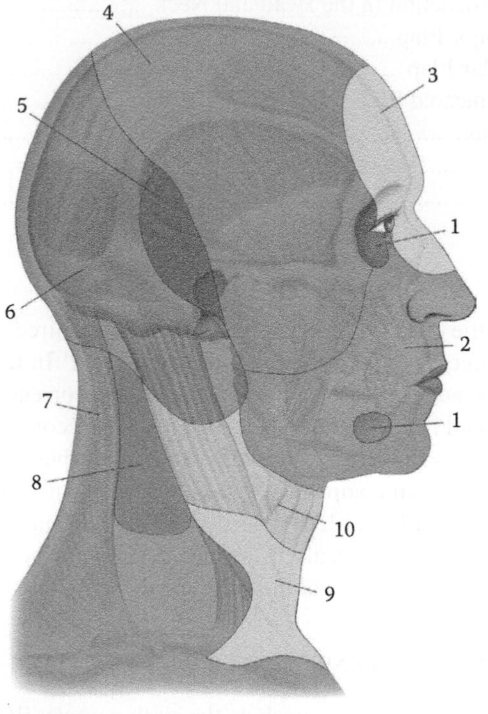

FIGURE 18.1 The angiosomes of the head and neck, highlighting the angiosomes of the inferior thyroid artery (zone 9) and superior thyroid artery (zone 10). (Reproduced from Houseman, N.D. et al., *Plast. Reconstr. Surg.*, 105, 2287, 2000. With permission.)

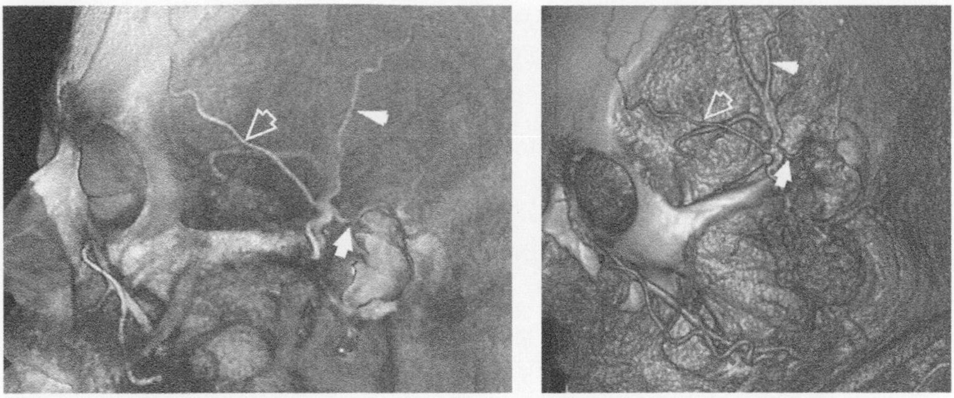

(a) (b)

FIGURE 18.2 (a, b) Head and neck carotid CTA with maximum intensity projection (MIP) reconstruction (a) and volume-rendered (VR) reconstruction (b) reformats from external views where branches of the superficial temporal artery can be seen: anterior auricular artery (arrow), frontal branch (open arrow), and parietal branch (arrowhead).

functional and cosmetic reconstruction with minimal donor-site morbidity.[14] Doppler ultrasonography has been used to localise these perforators in preoperative planning, particularly for freestyle perforator flaps.[45] More recently, computed tomographic angiography (CTA) has enabled a more detailed preoperative analysis of available perforators for head and neck reconstruction.[48]

The head and neck region is broadly supplied by two major arteries, namely, the common carotid (branching into the external and internal carotids) and the subclavian (Figure 18.2). A number of branches of these arteries give off perforators which supply the skin of the head and neck, which can be used as source vessels for local flaps.

18.3.1 Superior Thyroid Artery

The superior thyroid artery is the first branch arising from the anterior aspect of the external carotid artery. It gives off sternocleidomastoid (SCM) and superior laryngeal branches and then travels as a single vessel to enter the upper pole of the thyroid gland. In a large dissection study by Hurwitz et al., the superior thyroid artery was shown to supply the anterior neck skin via a direct cutaneous branch in 80% of their dissections.[17] Similarly, Wilson et al. described the superior thyroid artery perforator (STAP) fasciocutaneous flap based on a perforator consistently found within 2 cm of the midpoint at the anterior border of SCM, along with its venae comitantes (Figure 18.3).[48] The STAP flap procedure provided a well-matched tissue for facial reconstructions and also tightening of the neck skin, which was ideal for use in elderly patients[48]. Intraoperatively, the STAP flap was raised from distal to proximal in the deep subcutaneous plane until the midline and subsequently in the subplatysmal plane.[48] The flap was islanded and then transposed to reconstruct the periauricular defect.[48] Preoperative characterisation of a dominant perforator (greater than 0.8 mm) and flap planning via CTA and Doppler ultrasonography allowed surgeons to identify its course, allowing a more targeted dissection.[48] It also enabled the design of the STAP flap with a long skin paddle extending across the neck midline, which could provide good reach (Figure 18.4).[48] Furthermore, Wilson et al. highlighted the importance of CTA for surgical planning through their experience of accidental intraoperative damage to a perforator when preoperative planning CTA was not performed (Figure 18.5).[48]

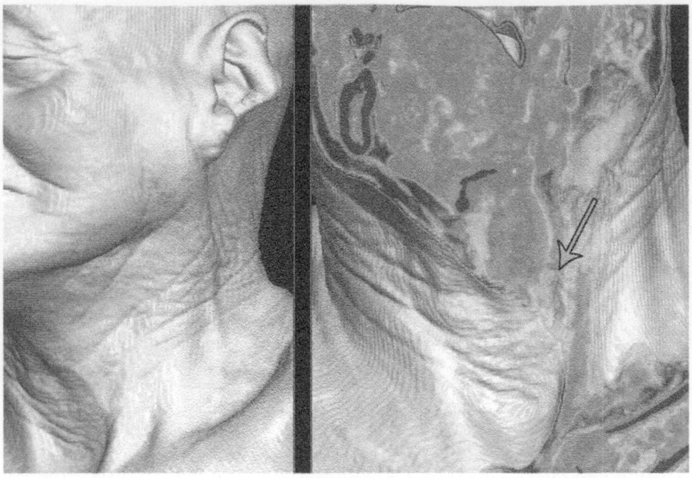

FIGURE 18.3 Preoperative CTA of a patient undergoing periauricular reconstruction with a STAP flap. Skin surface-rendered view on the left and cropped view demonstrating the STAP (arrow) on the right, with the perforator seen to emerge between the layers of the investing layer of fascia forming the epimysium of SCM and traverse a short subplatysmal course, before perforating the platysma within the ipsilateral neck and traversing an axial (transverse) subcutaneous course up to the midline, adjoining the axial course of the STAP of the contralateral side of the neck. (Reproduced from Wilson J.L. et al., *Plast. Reconstr. Surg.*, 129, 641, 2012. With permission.)

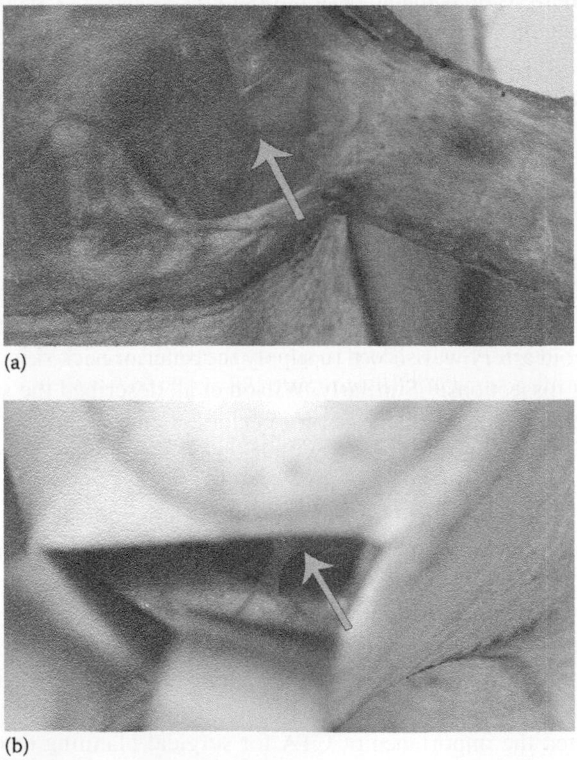

FIGURE 18.4 (a) Intraoperative identification of the same STAP as shown in Figure 18.2, confirming the position, course, and use of the axial course of this perforator as the vascular basis of the STAP flap. (b) Another patient, undergoing a neck lift, with endoscopic identification of a STAP. (Reproduced from Wilson J.L. et al., *Plast. Reconstr. Surg.*, 129, 641, 2012. With permission.)

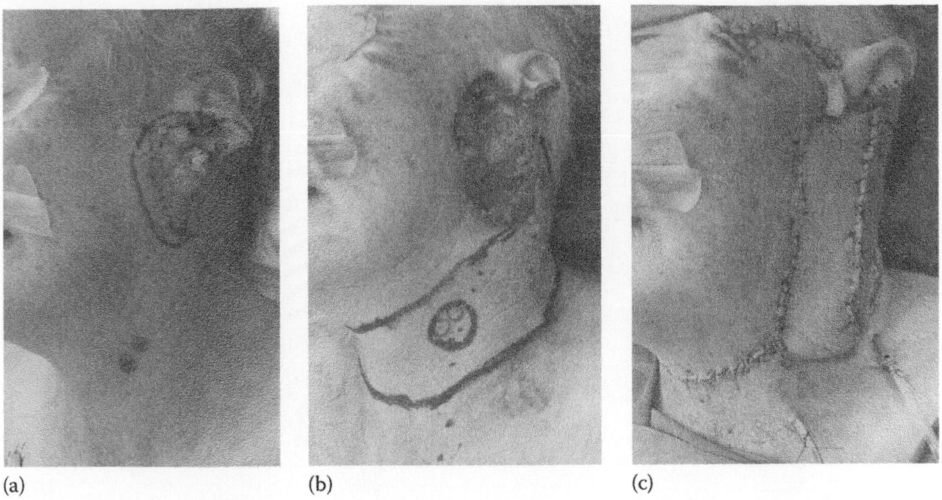

FIGURE 18.5 Operative series of the same patient in Figures 18.2 and 18.3. (a) The lesion for excision is marked and perforators marked. (b) The defect is created and the STAP flap marked. (c) The flap is transposed and inset. *Note*: a rotation flap is also performed above the external auditory meatus (EAM) to maintain patency of the EAM. (Reproduced from Wilson J.L. et al., *Plast. Reconstr. Surg.*, 129, 641, 2012. With permission.)

18.3.2 Facial Artery

The facial artery emerges from the external carotid artery and exits the neck by hooking around the inferior border of the mandible, anterior to the masseter muscle. Just prior to crossing the inferior border of the mandible, it gives off the submental artery, which supplies the skin over the submandibular and submental triangles (Figure 18.6).[43] It then passes superiorly towards the nasolabial region, giving off terminal branches including the inferior and superior labial, lateral nasal, and angular arteries. The high degree of vascularity within the facial artery angiosome makes it an ideal source for perforators in the facial region.[20]

The submental artery flap, first described by Martin et al.[27] in 1993, has been well recognised for its versatility in terms of tissue constituents (myocutaneous,[19] osteomuscular,[6] osteomyocutaneous[12], adipoplatysmal)[44] and reconstructive applications to a wide variety of head and neck defects,[32]

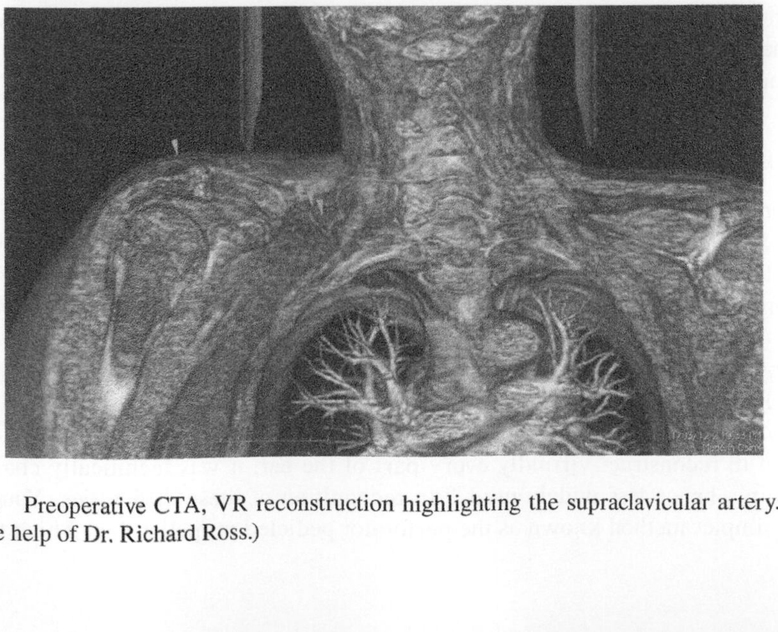

FIGURE 18.6 Preoperative CTA, VR reconstruction highlighting the supraclavicular artery. (Image produced with the help of Dr. Richard Ross.)

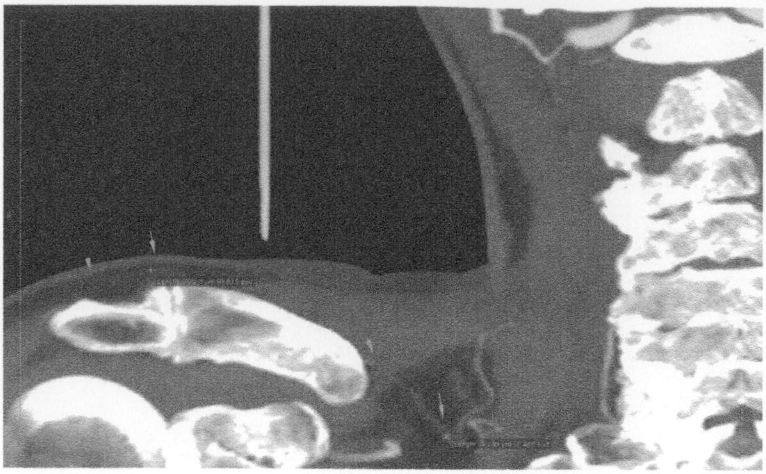

FIGURE 18.7 Preoperative CTA, MIP reconstruction highlighting the supraclavicular artery. (Image produced with the help of Dr. Richard Ross.)

including intra-oral,[39] laryngeal,[40] and periorbital.[21] The submental flap provides well-matched skin for facial reconstructions in terms of texture and colour.[33] Furthermore, the skin laxity at the donor site allows for direct closure with a well-hidden scar in the submental area.[33] Behan et al. described a variation named the cervico-submental (CSM) keystone island flap, which is based on perforators from multiple vascular territories supplying the anterior neck skin, thus creating a versatile flap with robust blood supply.[5] Although preoperative imaging was not routine in planning the CSM keystone island flap, Behan et al. suggested identification of perforators via CTA for flap planning in cases where previous neck dissections had been performed.[5]

In 2005, Hofer et al. introduced the idea of the facial artery perforator flap as a more refined local flap for perioral reconstructions.[15] In a subsequent case series, Kannan and Mathur further classified facial artery perforator flaps based on its terminal branches and three progressively cranial anatomical levels in the face (Level I, submental artery; Level II, inferior and superior labial arteries; Level III, lateral nasal and angular arteries), highlighting the gradual decrease in perforator size in more cranial branches.[20] Handheld Doppler was used for preoperative identification of perforators at Levels I and II, but this was not applicable to perforators at Level III given their small size and correspondingly weak Doppler signals.[20] The development of multidetector CTA (MDCTA) has enabled higher-resolution imaging,[8] which could be used to identify such small perforators for more detailed preoperative flap planning (Figure 18.7).

18.3.3 Posterior Auricular Artery

The posterior auricular artery originates from the external carotid artery and travels in the sulcus between the auricular cartilage and the mastoid process of the temporal bone. In 1972, Masson introduced the retroauricular island flap (RIF) for reconstruction of conchal defects.[28] More recently, Cordova et al. classified the RIF into three subtypes based on their pedicle: superior pedicle RIF (SP-RIF), perforator RIF (P-RIF), and inferior pedicle RIF (IP-RIF).[10] The SP-RIF is supplied by the superior auricular artery which branches off the superficial temporal artery, whereas the P-RIF and IP-RIF are supplied by the posterior auricular artery.[10] From their experience, Cordova et al. found that although the posterior auricular artery-based IP-RIF could potentially be used to reconstruct virtually every part of the ear, it was technically challenging and time consuming, hence less widely used.[10] In recognition of these difficulties, Youn et al. have developed a simpler method known as the perforator pedicled propeller flap, which they used for reconstruction of a helical rim defect.[51] This method involved the preoperative identification of perforators using a handheld Doppler and elevation of the flap only enough to allow tension-free mobilisation without having to dissect the posterior auricular artery.[51] Youn et al. have also suggested that this technique could be applied to any helical rim reconstructions in a freestyle perforator flap fashion through the identification of any perforators via handheld Doppler mapping, regardless of the source artery.[51]

18.3.4 Superficial Temporal Artery

The superficial temporal artery is a terminal branch of the external carotid artery, which originates superior to the digastric muscle and then passes through the parotid gland. It then runs behind the ascending ramus of the mandible and divides into the anterior and posterior branches approximately 3 cm above the zygomatic arc. This artery forms the basis of the widely recognised workhorse flap, the temporoparietal fascia flap (TPFF), with applications including ear reconstruction, hair-bearing flaps for eyebrow or moustache reconstruction, skull base reconstruction, and orbital reconstruction post-exenteration.[9] The temporoparietal fascia is a continuation of the galea aponeurotica superiorly and the superficial musculoaponeurotic system (SMAS) inferiorly.[31] The thin, pliable, and vascular nature of the TPFF enables it to be easily moulded onto a variety of irregular defects as well as to serve as a reliable bed for skin grafting.[9]

Traditionally, the TPFF is raised via a pre-auricular facelift incision extending to the hairline, with subsequent lifting of anterior and posterior scalp flaps to reveal the underlying temporoparietal fascia.[9] Preoperative handheld Doppler mapping can be used to mark the course of the superficial temporal artery.[15] The posterior branch of the superficial temporal artery is preferentially used as the vascular pedicle for the TPFF as dissection of the anterior branch endangers the frontal branch of the facial nerve.[50] Venous drainage of the TPFF occurs via the superficial temporal vein which commonly lies close to the superficial temporal artery but has been shown to lie as far as 3 cm away.[31] This pedicle can be dissected down to the root of the helix, providing a large arc of rotation for the TPFF, allowing extension to the midface, mandible, and oral cavity.[9] Endoscopic harvest of the TPFF has also been described with the benefits of less scarring, alopecia, and operative time.[9] Preoperative Doppler mapping of the superficial temporal artery may be more important in these endoscopic approaches given the limited intraoperative field of view.

18.4 REGIONAL FLAP RECONSTRUCTION IN THE HEAD AND NECK

Regional flaps are designed from tissue distant from the defect site whilst maintaining its original blood supply via a pedicle. As described earlier, regional pedicled flaps were the preferred method of reconstruction in the 1980s as they enabled reconstruction at distant sites and provided a wider range of tissue options, which could not be achieved with local flaps. With advancements in microsurgical techniques, free tissue transfer has now become the preferred method for head and neck reconstruction with benefits including better functional recovery, less donor-site morbidity, and improved cosmesis.[26] However, regional pedicled flaps may be still warranted in certain clinical situations. For example, a regional flap may be chosen over free-flap reconstruction in an elderly patient with multiple medical co-morbidities to minimise the operative risk or in a salvage procedure for a failed free flap.[26]

18.4.1 Pectoralis Major Flap

After it was described by Ariyan in the 1970s, the pectoralis major flap became a workhorse flap for post oncological head and neck reconstruction, given its reliable vascular supply and easy harvesting.[46] The pectoralis major muscle has two heads, the clavicular head and sternocostal head, each supplied by separate branches of the thoracoacromial artery, namely, the clavicular and pectoral branches, respectively. Given their distinct vascular supply, the two heads can be separated and only one head used as a flap to minimise excessive bulk as it restricts pedicle mobility.[46] The pectoralis major flap is most commonly raised as a pedicled myocutaneous flap with a skin island supplied by perforators within the flap.[46] In cases where only a small skin island is planned, preoperative Doppler mapping should be used to confirm the presence of an adequate perforator to supply that area of the skin.[46]

Although free flaps are often the method of choice in modern head and neck reconstruction, the pectoralis major flap has a role in certain clinical scenarios. It is particularly useful in salvage procedures after tumour resection, especially with extensive neck dissection in which microvascular free tissue transfer may be difficult given the lack of recipient vessels.[26] In such cases, the pectoralis major flap can provide soft tissue coverage for exposed vessels as well as adjuvant brachytherapy afterloading tubes, thus minimising the risk of vessel rupture and wound breakdown secondary to radiation.[26] Coverage with the pectoralis fascia flap has also been shown to prevent the development of pharyngocutaneous fistulas after pharyngeal repairs post salvage laryngectomy.[36] In developing countries, the pectoralis major flap is still being used for head and neck reconstruction in areas with insufficient health-care funding and resources to support microvascular surgery.[22]

18.4.2 Supraclavicular Flap

The supraclavicular flap is based on the supraclavicular artery, a branch of the transverse cervical artery, and was first described as an axial pedicled flap by Lamberty in 1979.[25] Harvested from the shoulder, the supraclavicular flap is a thin fasciocutaneous flap that is well matched in terms of colour and texture for reconstruction of the upper chest wall, neck, and face.[14] It has been shown to be useful in head and neck reconstructions for burn injuries[35] and post oncological resections, including oropharyngeal[2] and hypopharyngeal[7] defects.

When raising the flap, handheld Doppler is used to map the supraclavicular artery, which runs in the triangle bounded by the posterior edge of the SCM muscle, external jugular vein, and the medial part of the clavicle.[14] The flap is then elevated from lateral to medial via an incision extending from above the clavicle down to the deltoid in the subfascial plane, with the base of the supraclavicular artery as the pivot point.[37] Adams et al. have suggested the use of multislice detector CTA for preoperative flap planning to characterise the pedicle, resulting in increased surgical confidence and reduced operative time.[1] The multislice detector CTA is minimally invasive and can provide detailed characterisation of the pedicle, which cannot be achieved with the handheld Doppler as the intensity of the Doppler signal does not correspond to the vessel diameter or length.[1]

18.4.3 Sternocleidomastoid Flap

The SCM muscle has two heads originating from the manubrium and clavicle, which insert onto the lateral aspects of the mastoid process and superior nuchal line. It can be used to create a myocutaneous flap, as first described by Jianu in 1908, who used it for facial reanimation, or even a myo-osseous flap, with inclusion of a section of the clavicle, for mandibular reconstruction.[50] Other applications of the SCM flap include correction of pharyngocutaneous fistula post anterior cervical spine surgery[18] as well as post oncological oral reconstruction.[42] It is an unpopular flap choice, especially for post oncological reconstruction, given its proximity to nodal disease, susceptibility to damage from adjuvant radiotherapy, and tenuous supply to its skin island, resulting in higher failure rates.[23] In a large case series by Sebastian et al., the recorded incidences of total flap loss and skin loss were 7.5% and 22.7%, respectively.[38]

The SCM muscle has an unreliable pattern of blood supply with the superior third supplied by the occipital and posterior auricular arteries, middle third by the superior thyroid artery and branches of the external carotid artery, and lower third by inconsistent supply from the thyrocervical trunk.[23] As such, it is usually raised as a superiorly based flap with limited arc of rotation due to preservation of both the occipital and superior thyroid arteries to minimise the risk of ischaemia.[24] In a small case series, Avery suggested a superior thyroid artery-based perforator flap using predominantly the middle section of the muscle, thus allowing greater arc of rotation, for reconstruction of small- to medium-sized oral cavity defects in patients unsuitable for free-flap or pectoralis major flap reconstruction.[4] Preoperative CTA may help overcome this problem by allowing surgeons to clearly map the vascular supply and perforators to the SCM muscle to design flaps with more robust blood supply.

18.4.4 Trapezius Flap

The trapezius is a triangularly shaped muscle extending from the external occipital protuberance to the 12th thoracic vertebra and is composed of descending, transverse, and ascending parts. From a flap perspective, only the transverse and ascending parts are widely used, based on their blood supply from branches of the transverse cervical artery, namely, the superficial cervical artery (SCA) and dorsal scapular artery (DSA), respectively.[13]

First described as the lateral trapezius flap by Demergasso in 1978[11] the SCA-based trapezius flap can be raised as a myocutaneous flap for reconstructions of the hypopharynx, oropharynx, and upper oesophagus.[13] It can also be raised as an osteomyocutaneous flap for mandibular reconstructions but only with a small bony segment not exceeding 10 cm × 2 cm due to limitations in vascularisation.[13] The DSA-based trapezius flap was introduced by Baek et al. as the lower trapezius myocutaneous island flap in 1980 and is useful for lower face and anterior neck reconstructions.[50] When raising these as perforator flaps, a cuff of muscle usually needs to be taken given the small size of the perforators in these flaps.[13] Preoperative imaging could help surgeons identify available perforators and their size, allowing a more targeted approach to perforator dissection, hence minimising muscle loss and donor-site morbidity. From their experience, Hass et al. have found that Doppler ultrasound has not been effective in the identification of pedicle arteries.[13] As such, a more advanced imaging modality such as CTA may prove useful for the identification of pedicle arteries in the preoperative planning of trapezius flaps.

18.5 SUMMARY

The current trend of flap reconstruction has evolved through time due to the advancement in technology and better understanding of tissue flap pathophysiology expertise: from random-pattern flap to locoregional axial flap of McGregor and Morgan through to modern-day free tissue transfer with the use of imaging technology to identify blood vessels and use of microsurgical instrument to re-anastomose vessels to the defect site. The World Health Organization (WHO) has shown an increasing trend of life expectancy in the developing and developed world general population from the age of 76 in 1990 to 78 in 2000 and to 80 in 2009 with an increase in incidence of head and neck cancer.[49] Hence, there is an increasing need for tissue reconstruction.

The development of free tissue transfer and the use of microvascular anastomosis during the 1970s and 1980s has become a significant part in plastic and reconstructive surgery. As more and more free-flap reconstructions were performed, the specially trained surgeon has gained more confidence and experience with many reported increasing successful outcome with a more desirable aesthetic result. This has led to an increase in emphasis on the use of free-flap reconstruction as an approach to tissue reconstruction during the surgical training. However, the use of free-flap reconstruction still required a great deal of preoperative patient selection and intraoperative and post-operative care. McCrory et al. have conducted a study comparing free flap and locoregional flap in head and neck reconstruction. They have reported a similar immediate post-operative outcome (i.e. whilst the patient is still in the hospital) but an increase in operative time and ICU stay which in turn results in the increase of financial burden to the health fund. They have found a statistically significant difference for hospital cost between free flap and locoregional flap with an average of $USD 53585 vs. $USD 32984, respectively.[29] Due to this restriction, the reconstructive landscape has changed with more and more surgeons electing to perform locoregional reconstruction rather than a free-flap reconstruction based on reimbursement and operative time. The use of locoregional flap has provided an alternative for tissue defect reconstruction due to its simplicity and reliability, especially when free-flap reconstruction is not suitable. At that point, the flap evolution would have come full circle.

The use of preoperative planning with radiological imaging for locoregional flap reconstruction in the head and neck region is not always carried out. This procedure was viewed by many reconstructive surgeons as unnecessary. However, current literatures have shown potential benefit with decreasing surgical morbidity, operative time and assist in flap design. This could be due to an increasing population with a greater variation in vascular anatomy. There is also an increase in the ageing population and concurrently the incidence of co-morbid diseases. Patients may have undergone severe surgical intervention which can alter normal vascular anatomy. It is therefore necessary for preoperative imaging in order to avoid an unforeseen complication.

REFERENCES

1. AS Adams, MJ Wright, S Johnston, R Tandon, N Gupta, K Ward, C Hanemann, E Palacios, PL Friedlander, and ES Chiu, The use of multislice CT angiography preoperative study for supraclavicular artery island flap harvesting, *Ann Plast Surg*, 69(2012), 312–315.
2. AG Anand, EJ Tran, CP Hasney, PL Friedlander, and ES Chiu, Oropharyngeal reconstruction using the supraclavicular artery island flap: A new flap alternative, *Plast Reconstr Surg*, 129(2012), 438–441.
3. S Ariyan, The pectoralis major myocutaneous flap: A versatile flap for reconstruction in the head and neck, *Plast Reconstr Surg*, 63(1979), 73–81.
4. CME Avery, The sternocleidomastoid perforator flap, *Br J Oral Maxillofac Surg*, 49(2010), 573–575.
5. FC Behan, WM Rozen, J Wilson, S Kapila, A Sizeland, and MW Findlay, The cervico-submental keystone island flap for locoregional head and neck reconstruction, *J Plast Reconstr Aesthet Surg*, 66(2013), 23–28.
6. WL Chen, JT Ye, ZH Yang et al., Reverse facial artery-submental artery mandibular osteomuscular flap for the reconstruction of maxillary defects following the removal of benign tumours, *Head Neck*, 31(2009), 725–731.
7. ES Chiu, PH Liu, and PL Friedlander, Supraclavicular artery island flap for head and neck oncologic reconstruction: Indications, complications, and outcomes, *Plast Reconstr Surg*, 124(2009), 115–123.
8. AE Cicekcibasi, MT Yilmaz, D Kiresi, and M Seker, The mandibular landmarks about the facial artery and vein with multidetector computed tomography angiography (MDCTA): An anatomical and radiological morphometric study, *Int J Morphol*, 30(2012), 504–509.
9. RM Collar, D Zopf, D Brown, K Fung, and J Kim, The versatility of the temporoparietal fascia flap in head and neck reconstruction, *J Plast Reconstr Aesthet Surg*, 65(2012), 141–148.
10. A Cordova, S D'Arpa, R Pirrello, C Giambona, and F Moschella, Retroauricular skin: A flaps bank for ear reconstruction, *J Plast Reconstr Aesthet Surg*, 61(2008), S44–S51.
11. F Demergasso, The lateral trapezius flap, in *International Symposium of Plastic and Reconstructive Surgery* (New Orleans, LA, 1978).
12. Y Dusic, Hard palate reconstruction with a pedicled osteomyocutaneous mandible flap: Case report, *J Oral Maxillofac Surg*, 59(2001), 1355–1358.
13. F Haas and A Weiglein, Trapezius flap, in *Flaps and Reconstructive Surgery*, eds. FC Wei and S Mardini (Elsevier, 2009), pp. 249–269.
14. SOP Hofer and MAM Mureau, Pedicled perforator flaps in the head and neck, *Clin Plastic Surg*, 37(2010), 627–640.
15. SO Hofer, NA Posch, and X Smit, The facial artery perforator flap for reconstruction of perioral defects, *Plast Reconstr Surg*, 115(2005), 996–1003.
16. ND Houseman, GI Taylor, and WR Pan, The angiosomes of the head and neck: Anatomic study and clinical applications. *Plast Reconstr Surg*, 105(2000), 2287–2313.

17. DJ Hurwitz, JA Rabson, and Futrell JW, The anatomic basis for the platysma skin flap, *Plast Reconstr Surg*, 72(1983), 302–314.
18. VA Iyoob, Postoperative pharyngocutaneous fistula: Treated by sternocleidomastoid flap repair and cricopharyngeus myotomy, *Eur Spine J*, 22(2013), 107–112.
19. DA Janssen and DA Thimsen, The extended submental island lip flap: An alternative for esophageal repair, *Plast Reconstruct Surg*, 102(1998), 835–838.
20. RY Kannan and BS Mathur, Perforator flaps of the facial artery angiosome, *J Plast Reconstr Aesthet Surg*, 66(2012), 483–488.
21. N Karacal, O Ambarcioglu, U Topal et al., Reverse-flow submental artery flap for periorbital soft tissue and socket reconstruction, *Head Neck*, 28(2006), 40–45.
22. VD Kekatpure, NP Trivedi, BV Manjula, A Mathan Mohan, G Shetkar, and MA Kuriakose, Pectoralis major flap for head and neck reconstruction in era of free flaps, *Int J Oral Maxillofac Surg*, 41(2012), 453–457.
23. AC Kiemer, I Zelenka, and W Gstoettner, The sternocleidomastoid flap—Its indications and limitations, *Laryngoscope*, 111(2001), 2201–2204.
24. V Kumar, U Gaud, M Shukla, and M Pandey, Sternocleidomastoid island flap preserving the branch from superior thyroid artery for the reconstruction following resection of oral cancer, *Eur J Surg Oncol*, 35(2009), 1011–1015.
25. BG Lamberty, The supraclavicular axial patterned flap, *Br J Plast Surg*, 32(1979), 207–212.
26. HL Liu, JY Chan, and WI Wei, The changing role of pectoralis major flap in head and neck reconstruction, *Eur Arch Otorhinolaryngol*, 267(2010), 1759–1763.
27. D Martin, JF Pascal, J Baudet et al., The submental island flap: A new donor site. Anatomy and clinical applications as a free or pedicled flap, *Plast Reconstruct Surg*, 92(1993), 867–873.
28. JK Masson, A simple island flap for reconstruction of concha-helix defects, *Br J Plast Surg*, 25(1972), 399–403.
29. A McCrory, Free tissue transfer versus pedicled flap in head and neck reconstruction, *Laryngoscope*, 112(2002), 2161–2165.
30. SH Milton, Pedicled skin-flaps: The fallacy of the length:width ratio, *Br J Surg*, 57(1970), 502–508.
31. SL Moran, Temporoparietal fascia flap, in *Flaps and Reconstructive Surgery*, eds. FC Wei and S Mardini (Elsevier, 2009), pp. 159–173.
32. A Multinu, S Ferrari, B Bianchi et al., The submental island flap in head and neck reconstruction, *Int J Oral Maxillofac Surg*, 36(2007), 716–720.
33. PC Neligan and CB Novak, Head and neck, in *Flaps and Reconstructive Surgery*, eds. FC Wei and S Mardini (Elsevier, 2009), pp. 32–37.
34. NA Owens, A compound neck pedicle designed for repair of massive facial defects: Formation, development, and application, *Plast Reconstr Surg*, 15(1955), 369–374.
35. N Pallua and E Demir, Postburn head and neck reconstruction in children with the fasciocutaneous supraclavicular artery island flap, *Ann Plast Surg*, 60(2008), 276–282.
36. UA Patel and SP Keni, Pectoralis myofascial flap during salvage laryngectomy prevents pharyngocutaneous fistula, *Otolaryngol Head Neck Surg*, 141(2009), 190–195.
37. K Sandu, P Monnier, and P Pasche, Supraclavicular flap in head and neck reconstruction: Experience in 50 consecutive patients, *Eur Arch Otorhinolaryngol*, 269(2011), 1261–1267.
38. P Sebastian, T Cherian, MI Ahamed et al., The sternomastoid island myocutaneous flap for oral cancer reconstruction, *Arch Otolaryngol Head Neck Surg*, 120(1994), 629–632.
39. P Sebastian, S Thomas, BT Varghese et al., The submental island flap for reconstruction of intraoral defects in oral cancer patients, *Oral Oncol*, 44(2008), 1014–1018.
40. AH Taghinia, K Movassaghi, AX Wang et al., Reconstruction of the upper aerodigestive tract with the submental artery flap, *Plast Reconstr Surg*, 123(2009), 562–570.
41. BK Tan, YC Por, and HC Chen, Complications of head and neck reconstruction and their treatment, *Semin Plast Surg*, 24(2010), 288–298.
42. N Tanaka, A Yamaguchi, K Ogi, and G Kohama, Sternocleidomastoid myocutaneous flap for intraoral reconstruction after resection of oral squamous cell carcinoma, *J Oral Maxillofac Surg*, 61(2003), 1179–1183.
43. M Tang, M Ding, K Almutairi, and S Morris, Three-dimensional angiography of the submental artery perforator flap, *J Plast Reconstr Aesthet Surg*, 64(2010), 608–613.
44. M Uehara, JI Helman, JH Lillie et al., Blood supply to the platysma muscle flap: An anatomic study with clinical correlation, *J Oral Maxillofac Surg*, 59(2001), 642–646.

45. FC Wei and S Mardini, Free style flaps, in *Flaps and Reconstructive Surgery*, eds. FC Wei and S Mardini (Elsevier, 2009), pp. 617–624.
46. WI Wei and YW Chan, Pectoralis major flap, in *Flaps and Reconstructive Surgery*, eds. FC Wei and S Mardini (Elsevier, 2009), pp. 175–192.
47. IS Whitaker, RO Karoo, G Spyrou, and OM Fenton, The birth of plastic surgery: the story of nasal reconstruction from the edwin smith papyrus to the twenty-first century, *Plast Reconstr Surg*, 120(2007), 327.
48. J Wilson, WM Rozen, R Ross, MW Findlay, MW Ashton, and FC Behan, The superior thyroid artery perforator flap: Anatomical study and clinical series, *Plast Reconstr Surg*, 129(2012), 641–646.
49. World Health Organization (WHO). World health static 2011.
50. JY Yang, MR Rosen, and WM Keane, Flaps and grafts in the head and neck, in *Ballenger's Otorhinolaryngology*, ed. JB Snow, Jr. (PMPH, 2009).
51. S Youn, YH Kim, JT Kim, and SW Ng, Successful reconstruction of a large helical rim defect using retroauricular artery perforator-based island flap, *J Craniofac Surg*, 22(2011), 635–637.

19 Imaging for Recipient Vessels of the Head and Neck for Microvascular Transplantation

Gary Xia Vern Tan, Warren M. Rozen, Vachara Niumsawatt, Alberto Alonso-Burgos, and Edmund W. Ek

CONTENTS

19.1 OVERVIEW

Free microvascular tissue transfer has become the method of choice in head and neck reconstruction, particularly for significant defects post–tumour resection. A significant determinant of free-flap success is the status of the recipient vessels as revascularisation of the free flap is dependent on them. As such, preoperative evaluation of these vessels is crucial as it enables planning of the pedicle length, flap type, flap orientation to the recipient site, and requirement for a vein graft.[38] This is particularly important in head and neck cancer patients who have undergone previous neck dissection or chemoradiotherapy as well as those with cardiovascular co-morbidities, particularly tobacco smoking, as these may compromise the recipient vessels.[31] Radiotherapy has been shown to cause various injuries to blood vessels including endothelial damage, perivascular fibrosis, and microvascular occlusion,[4,7,35] but there is conflicting evidence in the literature about whether previous radiotherapy impairs flap survival and patency of the microvascular anastomosis.[1,5,29–31] The gold standard for imaging the head and neck vasculature is digital subtraction angiography (DSA). However, non-invasive imaging methods, such as ultrasonography (US), computed tomographic angiography (CTA), and magnetic resonance angiography (MRA), are preferred in current practice given their low-risk profile.

19.2 ANATOMY OF THE RECIPIENT VESSELS

Recipient vessels are selected based on the site of the defect and the proximity of the recipient vessels[31]. However, in the absence of healthy local vasculature, more distant vessels can be recruited, which may involve pedicle lengthening techniques such as vein grafting and formation of an

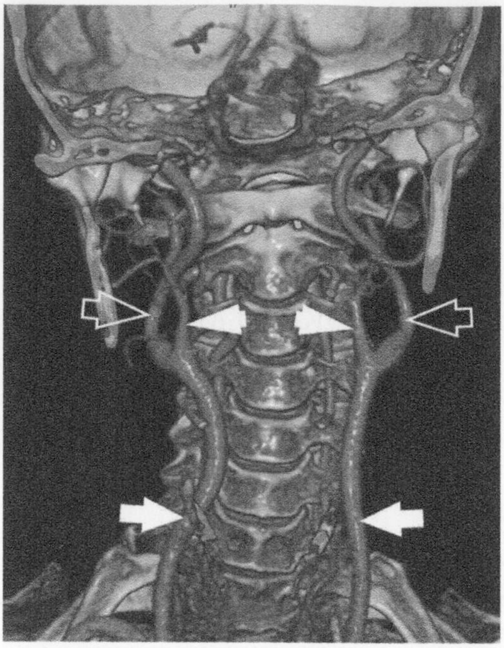

FIGURE 19.1 Carotid CTA and volume-rendered (VR) reformat from an anterior view. The common carotid artery (arrow) as well as the internal (open arrow) and external (arrowhead) carotid artery can be observed.

arteriovenous loop.[19,28,32] The calibre of the flap and recipient vessels should be similar (difference should not be more than a 3:1 ratio) to enable end-to-end anastomosis, although end-to-side anastomosis could be applied in cases with significant vessel calibre discrepancy.[18,31] There is ongoing debate in the literature about the benefits of end-to-end versus end-to-side venous anastomosis. Francis et al.[17] have suggested that this is dependent on surgeons' preferences because surgeons become more adept with their technique of choice that they use more often, thus leading to better outcomes (Figure 19.1).

19.2.1 Recipient Arteries

Recipient arteries in the head and neck are generally selected from the branches of the external carotid artery, which emerges from the common carotid, courses superiorly to run behind the neck of the mandible, and then divides within the parotid gland into the superficial temporal and maxillary arteries (Figure 19.2). For reconstructions in the upper third of the head, the ipsilateral superficial temporal artery is the primary choice, followed by the ipsilateral facial artery.[42] For mid- and lower face reconstructions, the ipsilateral facial artery is preferred with the second choice being the superior thyroid artery.[42] In lower face/neck reconstructions where the facial and superior thyroid vessels have been compromised by previous neck dissection or dense post-radiotherapy scarring, the ipsilateral superficial temporal or transverse cervical vessels can be utilised as they are usually not damaged.[42] Furthermore, Roche et al. have also described the use of internal mammary vessels as recipients in cases where bilateral neck vessels had been compromised, particularly in secondary or tertiary reconstructions required for radiation complications (e.g. fistulas and stenoses) or cancer recurrence.[11,13,14,34] In such cases where distant vascular access is necessitated, careful recipient and flap vessel selection is crucial to ensure adequate pedicle length and diameter, so as to avoid lengthening or salvage procedures (i.e. vein grafting and arteriovenous looping) that could compromise flap outcome (Figure 19.3).[31,42]

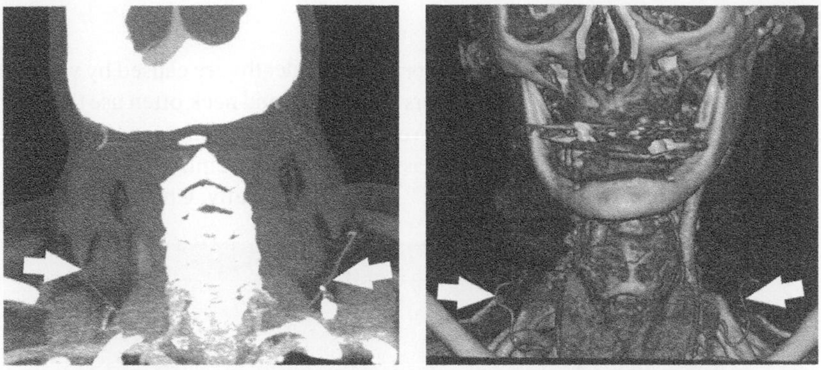

(a) (b)

FIGURE 19.2 Head and neck carotid CTA and maximum intensity projection (MIP) (a) and VR (b) reformats from an anterior view. Thyrocervical arteries can be observed (arrows).

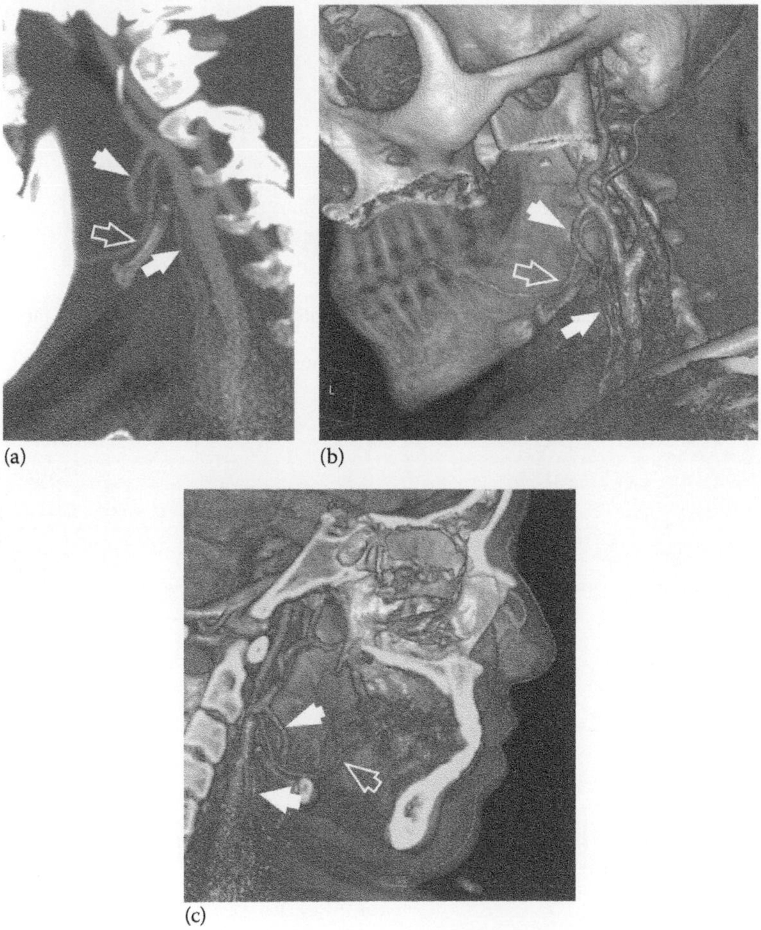

(a) (b) (c)

FIGURE 19.3 (a–c) Head and neck carotid CTA with MIP (a) and VR (b and c) reformats from external (a and b) and internal (c) views. The origin of the superior thyroid, lingual, and facial arteries from the external carotid artery can be observed (arrow, open arrow, and arrowhead in a, b, and c, respectively).

19.2.2 Recipient Veins

Careful recipient vein selection is crucial as a majority of flap deaths are caused by venous thrombosis (Figure 19.4).[9,26] Free microvascular tissue transfers to the head and neck often use the internal jugular vein (IJV), its tributaries, or the external jugular vein (EJV) as recipient veins (Figure 19.5).[42] Many studies have identified the IJV and its branches as the preferred recipient vessels, given their proximity to recipient arteries and easy accessibility.[30,31,37,42] Additionally, Chalian et al.[9] recommended

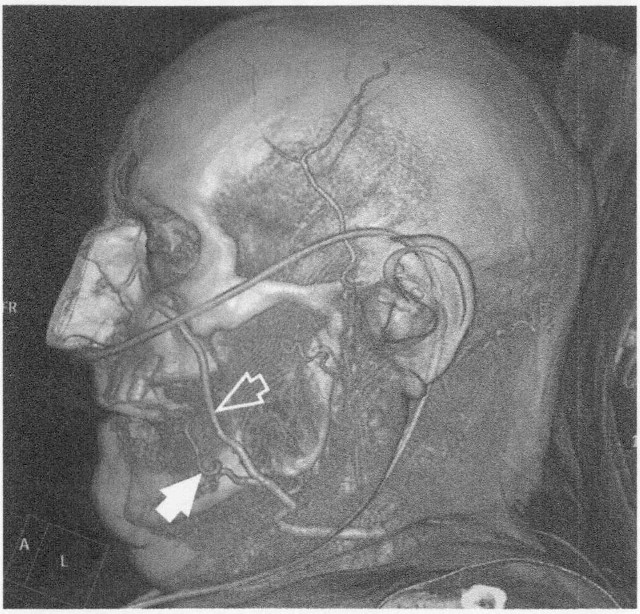

FIGURE 19.4 Head and neck carotid CTA with VR reformats from external view. The facial artery (arrow) and vein (open arrow) can be seen.

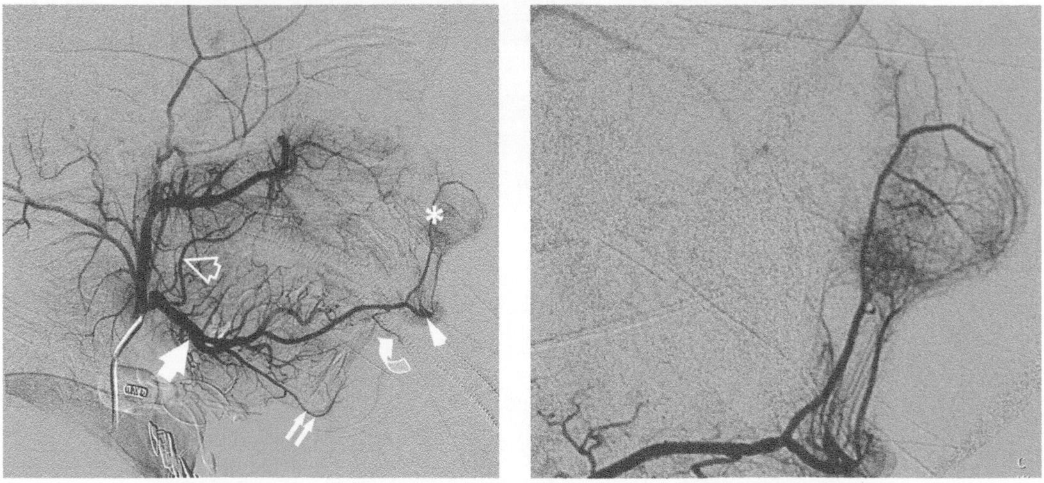

FIGURE 19.5 (a and b) Conventional head and neck angiography from the external carotid artery and right lateral view (a) and detail (b). The facial artery can be observed (arrow) as well as the ascending palatine artery (open arrow), tonsilar artery (double thin arrow), inferior labial artery (curved arrow), superior labial artery (arrowhead), and lateral nasal branch.

the IJV as the primary choice for recipient vein as they showed that anastomosis to the EJV failed at a significantly higher rate compared to the IJV. This was attributed to the small calibre and low flow through the EJV as well as likely serious intimal damage secondary to routine ligation during neck dissections.[9] The EJV is only used when the IJV is sacrificed during radical neck dissections, although this is becoming less common with the growing popularity of IJV-sparing modified neck dissections.[9] Interestingly, although the IJV has been shown to have thrombosis rates of 14%–33% after neck dissection, this does not seem to affect flap success and flap survival has been documented in the setting of IJV thrombosis.[2,8,16,39] As described with the neck arteries, veins can also be compromised by previous surgery or irradiation, resulting in the lack of suitable recipient veins in the neck.[36] The cephalic vein has been described as a salvage recipient vein in such cases with benefits including suitable size, potential for a long pedicle, ability to accommodate high venous outflow from the head and neck, as well as its location outside the field of neck irradiation and dissection.[21]

19.3 IMAGING TECHNIQUES

19.3.1 Ultrasonography

Handheld Doppler US has been widely used for preoperative identification of flap vessels as well as post-operative monitoring of flap pedicles (Figure 19.6). It is a convenient, quick, and easy method that can be readily performed at the bedside. It is completely non-invasive, does not pose any radiation risk, and can be used in patients with electronic implants. Although Doppler US can be used to identify and map blood vessels, it cannot give detailed information about vascular branching, particularly with smaller vessels in the head and neck, which may not be able to generate adequate Doppler signals.[20] Vessel US is also difficult in patients with thick subcutaneous adipose tissue, scarring from previous radiotherapy or surgery, and atherosclerotic vessels.[23] Furthermore, Doppler signals are difficult to quantify and its interpretation is highly operator dependent. Colour-coded duplex US can provide more information about flow dynamics within blood vessels, which is useful to identify occlusions. Colour-coded carotid duplex US has been shown to have a sensitivity of 86%–94% for near occlusions and 100% for total occlusions.[6,33] Overall, although US may be safe and convenient, it does not provide the surgeon with visualisation of complete vessel branching, which limits its use in preoperative planning of recipient vessels.

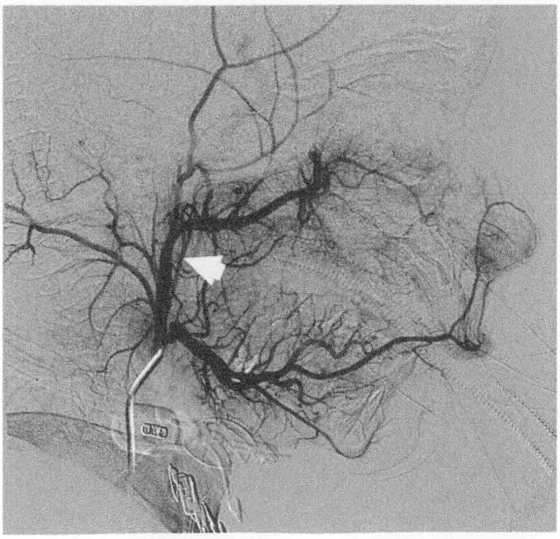

FIGURE 19.6 Conventional head and neck angiography from the external carotid artery and right lateral view. The ascending pharyngeal artery can be seen.

19.3.2 Digital Subtraction Angiography

DSA involves the injection of radio-opaque contrast into blood vessels via an intra-arterial catheter to allow visualisation of the vasculature via x-ray imaging (Figure 19.7). As it has been shown that non-selective angiography in supra-aortic vessels is ineffective for complete visualisation of the branches of the external carotid artery, selective catheter angiography was introduced as the gold standard for characterisation of head and neck vasculature.[3] Although DSA can provide detailed visualisation of head and neck vasculature, it is an invasive procedure with catheter-related risks including arterial bleeding, vessel laceration/dissection, and cerebral embolisation, which could result in permanent severe neurological deficits or even death.[12,15,40] In a large series of 2899 consecutive cerebral DSA examinations, Willinsky et al. found that neurological complications occurred more frequently in patients aged 55 years and older (1.8%) and those with cardiovascular disease (2.3%),[40] which correlates with the elderly patient population requiring post–oncological head and neck reconstruction. With the availability of non-invasive imaging modalities, such as CTA and MRA, it is difficult to justify the use of DSA for preoperative planning alone given its high risks (Figure 19.8).

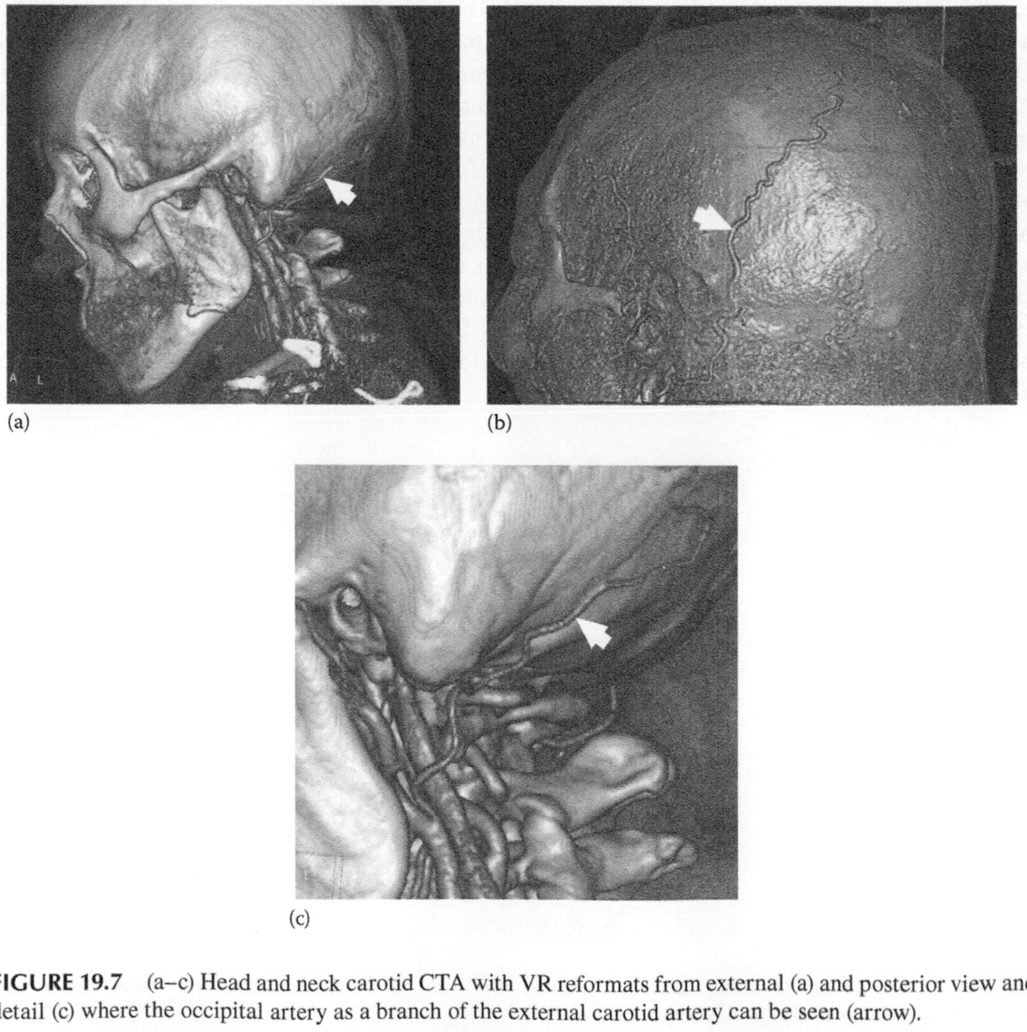

FIGURE 19.7 (a–c) Head and neck carotid CTA with VR reformats from external (a) and posterior view and detail (c) where the occipital artery as a branch of the external carotid artery can be seen (arrow).

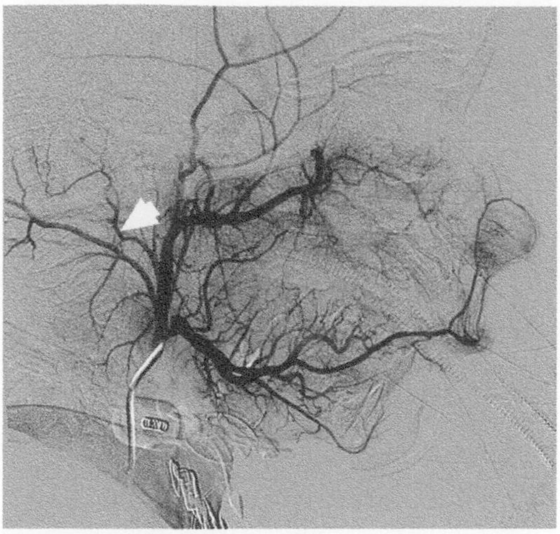

FIGURE 19.8 Conventional head and neck angiography from external carotid artery and right lateral view. The posterior auricular artery can be seen (arrow).

19.3.3 Magnetic Resonance Angiography

MRA is a non-invasive method of vessel imaging, which has been gaining popularity in the imaging of peripheral vascular disease (Figure 19.9).[25] Recent advances in MRA technology such as whole-body scanners, higher field strengths, and specialised surface coils have led to faster data acquisition speed and enhanced spatial resolution for whole-body MRA (WB MRA) protocols (Figure 19.10).[22] This has enabled non-invasive imaging of the entire vascular system without the high radiation dose and amount of iodine-based contrast that would be required in whole-body CTA.[23] With regard to preoperative planning of free-flap reconstruction in the head and neck, WB MRA would enable imaging of donor and recipient site vessels in a single session, such as for the planning of

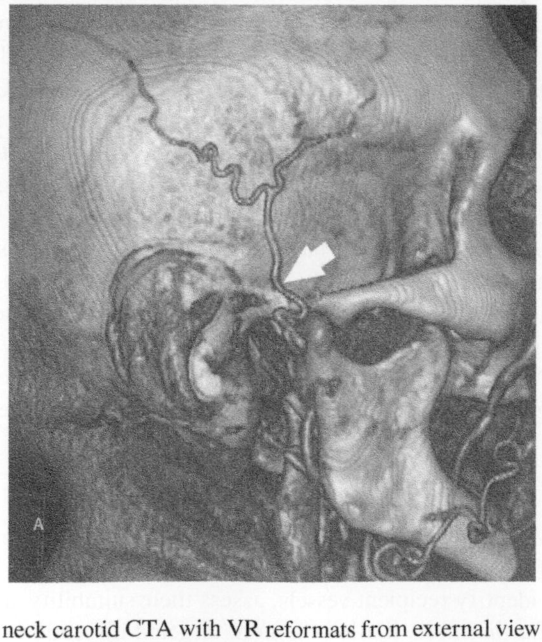

FIGURE 19.9 Head and neck carotid CTA with VR reformats from external view where the temporal artery as a branch of the external carotid artery can be seen (arrow).

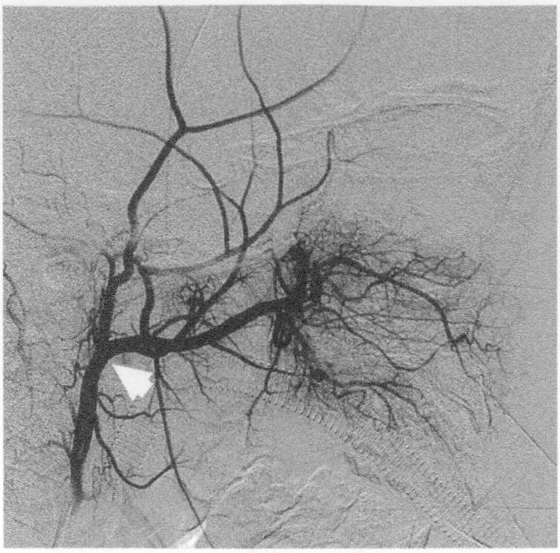

FIGURE 19.10 Conventional head and neck angiography from external carotid artery, lateral view, and selective catheterisation of the internal maxillary artery (arrow).

free fibular flap for mandibular reconstruction.[23] However, the routine use of MRA is limited by its cost as well as its contraindication in patients with internal metalware such as pacemakers.[38] Furthermore, MRA does not display vessel atherosclerosis as well as CTA, thus limiting its use in the assessment of occlusions in head and neck recipient vessels.[38]

19.3.4 Computed Tomographic Angiography

The development of multislice spiral CTA has made it a powerful tool for vessel imaging. CTA is now preferred over DSA as it is non-invasive, safer, and better tolerated by patients and requires less contrast agent, hence reducing the risk of nephrotoxicity.[38] CTA also requires shorter scanning time with associated less ionising radiation dose (1.1 mSv for women and 1.0 mSv for men) compared with the mean radiation dose of 4 mSv with DSA of the carotid artery, as evidenced by Kramer et al.[24] and the UNSCEAR 2000 Report,[10] respectively. Current spiral multisection CT scanners enable rapid data acquisition with high spatial resolution, which, combined with modern reconstruction and post-processing methods, allow detailed visualisation of recipient vessels, with external diameters as small as 0.6 mm in the head and neck.[38] CTA also provides volumetric data allowing 3D visualisation of vasculature from any angle, which cannot be achieved with conventional DSA.[41] The ability to produce easy-to-interpret 3D images has made CTA increasingly popular amongst surgeons, enabling them to identify any significant occlusions, stenoses, and variations in recipient vessels.[38] Furthermore, CTA provides information about the surrounding anatomical structures and their relationship with the recipient vessels, which can aid surgical planning of tumour resections whilst minimising recipient vessel compromise.[38] Furthermore, a biphasic CT protocol can be used to complete both vascular mapping and cancer staging in a single session, thus improving cost and time effectiveness.[27]

19.4 SUMMARY

With the increasingly widespread use of free tissue transfer for head and neck reconstruction, the importance of imaging for preoperative planning is gaining recognition. Its benefits are clear, in that it allows the surgeon to identify recipient vessels, assess their suitability, and tailor the flap to best reconstruct the defect. Furthermore, it allows a more targeted dissection of vessels, thus reducing morbidity at the surgical site and operating time, leading to overall risk minimisation for the patient. Various imaging modalities can be used for preoperative imaging of recipient vessels, each with their pros and cons. US is a quick and easy tool but is limited in its ability to fully characterise detailed vessel branching. DSA has been recognised as the gold standard for vessel imaging as it can characterise vascular architecture in detail, including branching and potential obstructions or stenoses. However, it is an invasive procedure which carries multiple risks, such as vessel dissection, arterial bleeding, and cerebral embolisation.[12,15,40] Consequently, less invasive imaging modalities are now preferred for preoperative planning, such as MRA and CTA. MRA enables whole-body vessel imaging, thus allowing imaging of both donor and recipient vessels within a single session, without the risks of irradiation carried by a similar procedure using CTA.[23] The drawbacks of MRA are its cost, limitations in characterising vessel atherosclerosis, and contraindication in patients with internal metalware.[38] CTA is increasingly recognised as the ideal modality for preoperative planning of free-flap reconstructions. Although it does carry some degree of radiation risk, recent advances in multislice spiral CTA have led to much shortened scanning times with associated less ionising radiation. With the use of CTA, the patency and location of recipient vessels can be characterised in great detail and displayed in easy-to-interpret 3D image reconstructions, making it a powerful tool for preoperative planning.[38] As such, the relative benefits of CTA compared to other imaging modalities make it the method of choice for preoperative characterisation of recipient vessels for microvascular tissue transfer in the head and neck.

REFERENCES

1. K Aitasalo, M Relander, and E Virolainen, The success rate of free tissue transfer after preoperative irradiation in head and neck reconstruction, *Ann Chir Gynaecol*, 86(1997), 311–317.
2. ML Amato, LR Rodriguez, and WL Lineaweaver, Survival of free tissue transfer following internal jugular venous thrombosis, *Plast Reconstr Surg*, 104(1999), 1406–1408.
3. F Barsekow, H Bach-Diesing, and H Becker, Superselective angiography—Possibilities and limitations in the pre-operative diagnosis of angiomas, *Fortschr Kiefer Gesichtschir*, 32(1987), 66–68.
4. JA Beckman, A Thakore, BH Kalinowski et al., Radiation therapy impairs endothelium-dependent vasodilation in humans, *J Am Coll Cardiol*, 37(2001), 761–765.
5. BP Bengstrom, MA Schusterman, BJ Baldwin et al., Influence of prior radiotherapy on the development of post-operative complications and success of free tissue transfers in the head and neck, *Am J Surg*, 166(1993), 326–330.
6. SS Berman, JJ Devine, LS Erdoes, and GC Hunter, Distinguishing carotid artery pseudo-occlusion with color-flow Doppler, *Stroke*, 26(1995), 434–438.
7. EF Bernstein, FJ Sullivan, JB Mitchell et al., Biology of chronic radiation effect on tissues and wound healing, *Clin Plast Surg*, 20(1993), 435–451.
8. DH Brown, S Mulholland, JH Yoo, PJ Gullane, JC Irish, P Neligan, and A Keller, Internal jugular vein thrombosis following modified neck dissection: Implications for the head and neck flap reconstruction, *Head Neck*, 20(1998), 169–174.
9. AA Chalian, TD Anderson, GS Weinstein, and RS Weber, Internal jugular vein versus external jugular vein anastomosis: Implications for successful free tissue transfer, *Head Neck*, 23(2001), 475–478.
10. M Charles, UNSCEAR report 2000: Sources and effects of ionizing radiation. United Nations Scientific Committee on the effects of atomic radiation, *J Radiol Prot*, 21(2001), 83.
11. JS Cooper, TF Pajak, AA Forastiere et al., Postoperative concurrent radiotherapy and chemotherapy for high-risk squamous cell carcinoma of the head and neck, *N Eng J Med*, 350(2004), 1937–1944.
12. KN Davies and PR Humphrey, Complications of cerebral angiography in patients with symptomatic carotid territory ischaemia screened by carotid ultrasound, *J Neurol Neurosurg Psychiatry*, 56(1993), 967–972.
13. F Demirkan, FC Wei, HC Chen, IH Chen, SP Hau, and CT Liau, Microsurgical reconstruction in recurrent oral cancer: Use of a second free flap in the same patient, *Plast Reconstr Surg*, 103(1999), 829–838.
14. F Demirkan, FC Wei, HC Chen, IH Chen, and CT Liao, Oromandibular reconstruction using a third free flap in sequence in recurrent carcinoma, *Br J Plast Surg*, 52(1999), 429–433.
15. JE Dion, PC Gates, AJ Fox, HJ Barnett, and RJ Blom, Clinical events following neuroangiography: A prospective study, *Stroke*, 18(1987), 997–1004.

16. CB Fisher, DE Mattox, and JS Zinreich, Patency of the internal jugular vein after functional neck dissection, *Laryngoscope*, 98(1988), 923–927.
17. DO Francis, RE Stern, D Zeitler, M Izzard, and ND Futran, Analysis of free flap viability based on recipient vein selection, *Head Neck*, 31(2009), 1354–1359.
18. GG Hallock, Flap selection, in *Flaps and Reconstructive Surgery*, eds. FC Wei and S Mardini (Elsevier, 2009), pp. 16–29.
19. C Head, JA Sercarz, E Abelmayor et al., Microvascular reconstruction after previous neck dissection, *Arch Otolaryngol Head Neck Surg*, 128(2002), 328–331.
20. RY Kannan and BS Mathur, Perforator flaps of the facial artery angiosome, *J Plast Reconstr Aesthet Surg*, 66(2012), 483–488.
21. KA Kim and BS Chandrasekhar, Cephalic vein in salvage microsurgical reconstruction in the head and neck, *Br J Plast Surg*, 51(1998), 2–7.
22. H Kramer, HH Quick, B Tombach, SO Schoenberg, and J Barkhausen, Whole-body MRA, *Eur Radiol*, 18(2008), 1925–1936.
23. M Kramer, E Nkenke, K Kikuchi, SA Schwab, R Janka, M Uder, and M Lell, Whole-body magnetic resonance angiography for presurgical planning of free flap head and neck reconstruction, *Eur Radiol*, 81(2010), 262–266.
24. M Kramer, E Vairaktaris, E Nkenke, KA Schlegel, FW Neukam, and M Lell, Vascular mapping of head and neck: Computed tomography angiography versus digital subtraction angiography, *J Oral Maxillofac Surg*, 66(2008), 302–307.
25. KF Kreitner, P Kalden, A Neufang et al., Diabetes and peripheral arterial occlusive disease: Prospective comparison of contrast-enhanced three-dimensional MR angiography with conventional digital subtraction angiography, *AJR Am J Roentgenol*, 174(2000), 171–179.
26. SS Kroll, MA Schusterman, GP Reece et al., Timing of pedicle thrombosis and flap loss after free tissue transfer, *Plast Reconstr Surg*, 98(1996), 1230–1233.
27. M Lell, BF Tomandl, K Anders, U Baum, and E Nkenke, Computed tomography angiography versus digital subtraction angiography in vascular mapping for planning of microsurgical reconstruction of the mandible, *Eur Radiol*, 15(2005), 1514–1520.
28. ML Miller, MA Schusterman, GP Reece et al., Interposition vein grafting in head and neck reconstructive microsurgery, *J Reconstr Microsurg*, 9(1993), 245–252.
29. A Momeni, RY Kim, A Kattan, J Tennefoss, TH Lee, and GK Lee, The effect of pre-operative radiotherapy on complication rate after microsurgical head and neck reconstruction, *J Plast Reconstr Aesthet Surg*, 64(2011), 1454–1459.
30. S Mulholland, JB Boyd, S McCabe et al., Recipient vessels in head and neck microsurgery: Radiation effect and vessel access, *Plast Reconstr Surg*, 92(1993), 628–632.
31. MY Nahabedian, N Singh, EG Deune, R Silverman, and AP Tufaro, Recipient vessel analysis for microvascular reconstruction of the head and neck, *Ann Plast Surg*, 52(2004), 148–155.
32. B Nakayama, Y Kamei, K Toriyama et al., Usefulness of a first transferred free flap vascular pedicle for secondary microvascular reconstruction in the head and neck, *Plast Reconstr Surg*, 109(2002), 1246–1253.
33. PJ Nederkoorn, Y van der Graaf, and MG Hunink, Duplex ultrasound and magnetic resonance angiography compared with digital subtraction angiography in carotid artery stenosis: A systematic review, *Stroke*, 34(2003), 1324–1332.
34. NA Roche, P Houtmeyers, HF Vermeersch, FB Stillaert, and PN Blondeel, The role of the internal mammary vessels as recipient vessels in secondary and tertiary head and neck reconstruction, *J Plast Reconstr Aesthet Surg*, 65(2012), 885–892.
35. S Schultz-Mosgau, GG Grabenbauer, F Wehrhan et al., Histomorphological structural changes of head and neck blood vessels after pre- or postoperative radiotherapy, *Strahlenther Onkol*, 178(2002), 299–306.
36. VK Shankhdhar, PS Yadav, J Dushyant, SS Seetharaman, and W Chinmay, Cephalic vein: Saviour in the microsurgical reconstruction of breast and head and neck cancers, *Ind J Plast Surg*, 45(2012), 485–493.
37. A Takamatsu, T Harashina, and T Inoue, Selection of appropriate recipient vessels in difficult, microsurgical head and neck reconstruction, *J Reconstr Microsurg*, 12(1996), 499–507.
38. O Tan, M Kantarci, D Parmaksizoglu, U Uyanik, and I Durur, Determination of the recipient vessels in the head and neck using multislice spiral computed tomography angiography before free flap surgery: A preliminary study, *J Craniofacl Surg*, 18(2007), 1284–1289.
39. MK Wax, H Quraishi, S Rodman, and K Granke, Internal jugular vein patency in patients undergoing micro-vascular reconstruction, *Laryngoscope*, 107(1997), 1245–1248.

40. RA Willinsky, SM Taylor, K TerBrugge, RI Farb, G Tomlinson, and W Montenera, Neurologic complications of cerebral angiography: Prospective analysis of 2,899 procedures and review of the literature, *Radiology*, 227(2003), 522–528.
41. M Wintermark, A Uske, M Chalaron et al., Multislice computerised tomography angiography in the evaluation of intracranial aneurysms: A comparison with intraarterial digital subtraction angiography, *J Neurosurg*, 98(2003), 828–836.
42. S Yazar, Selection of recipient vessels in microsurgical free tissue reconstruction of head and neck defects, *Microsurgery*, 27(2007), 588–594.

20 Imaging and Surgical Principles for TRAM (pTRAM) Flap

Diego Ribuffo, Matteo Atzeni, Maristella Guerra, and Luca Saba

CONTENTS

20.1 INTRODUCTION

The transverse rectus abdominis musculocutaneous (TRAM) flap had its introduction as a technique for breast reconstruction more than 20 years ago. Initially described by Holmstrom[1] as a free flap, it was later popularised by Hartrampf[2] as a pedicled flap, who independently conceived of its use as an abdominal island flap for breast reconstruction. Drawing on the work of Esser, Hartrampf theorised that the lower abdominal skin and fat could be transferred to the chest to create a breast mound based on circulation provided from the rectus abdominis muscle.

Both the pedicle and free TRAM procedures may be indicated for patients who desire immediate or delayed breast reconstruction.

Immediate breast reconstruction offers the patient improved cosmesis and reduces the psychological stress of losing a breast.[3–6] However, in patients requiring adjuvant radiation therapy after mastectomy, delayed reconstruction is often the preferred choice.[7,8]

Although there are no absolute indications for one type of flap over the other, several relative indications merit consideration. As a general rule, selection of one technique over the other must take into account the comfort level of the surgeon with either technique and is most commonly made by experience and comfort with microsurgical techniques and the availability of instrumentation and post-operative monitoring facilities. More specialised microsurgical flaps, such as perforator flaps and superficial inferior epigastric artery (SIEA) flaps, require even greater familiarity with microsurgical technique and close post-operative observation, with the ability to quickly return to the operating room for correction of acute microvascular complications. Using the pedicled flap will limit the vascularity as compared with a free TRAM flap but may have as much vascularity as a perforator flap if those vessels are not unusually large. Thus, the surgeon who chooses a pedicled TRAM flap is providing an autologous abdominal reconstruction with reduced technical and facility demands and a decreased risk of total flap loss as compared with free flap techniques. For these reasons, despite continued technical refinements, such as the free TRAM and deep inferior epigastric perforator (DIEP) flap, which limit the sacrifice of the rectus abdominis muscle and consequent abdominal wall morbidity, interest in the pedicle TRAM is ongoing, and since its first description, this flap is still one of the best choices for autologous breast reconstruction. Its advantages are well documented and include reliability, predictable blood supply, ease and speed of harvest, superior symmetry, contour, and aesthetic appearance of the breast mound, improved abdominal aesthetics with avoidance of microsurgical facilities, and favourable patient satisfaction.[2,9–12]

In general, patients requesting pedicled TRAM flap reconstruction must have enough abdominal soft tissue to allow for adequate flap harvest and donor-site closure. Highly motivated patients with limited co-morbidities are ideally suited for this reconstructive procedure. Several risk factors have been identified that place patients at higher risk for complications after pedicled TRAM flap reconstruction. These factors include cigarette smoking, obesity, post-operative radiation therapy, and extensive medical co-morbidities.[13–17] Despite an inherent increased risk, patients with the aforementioned risk factors may still choose to have a pedicled TRAM flap reconstruction. In this instance, any effort to increase flap blood supply should be considered to improve overall flap reliability. Commonly used techniques, which are discussed later, include flap *supercharging* and surgical delay. However, not all women are candidates for pedicled TRAM flap reconstruction, and there are a few absolute contraindications for this procedure: the presence of an old upper abdominal incision with previous division of the rectus abdominis muscles precludes a flap based on the superior pedicle from that side. A history of prior abdominoplasty likely indicates disruption of the perforating vessels to the abdominal skin and soft tissue, and a pedicled TRAM flap should not be performed.[18]

20.2 ANATOMY OF THE FLAP

This vertically oriented abdominal muscle extends between the costal margin and the pubic region. It is a long, flat muscle with three intersections located at the level of the umbilicus and the xiphoid process and midway between the xiphoid process and the umbilicus. The muscle is enclosed by the anterior and posterior rectus sheaths. Its size is about 25 × 6 cm. The muscle has two tendons of origin – the crest of the pubis and the symphysis pubis – and inserts in three fascicles into the cartilages of the fifth, sixth, and seventh ribs.

About the vascular anatomy, the vascular pedicles are the inferior epigastric artery and vein (originating from external iliac artery and vein) and the superior epigastric artery and vein (originating from internal mammary artery and vein). The minor pedicles are subcostal and six or seven intercostal arteries and venae comitantes. The motor nerve supply is based on intercostal nerves.

The rectus abdominis muscle flexes the vertebral column and tenses the abdominal wall.

20.3 SURGICAL PRINCIPLES AND TECHNIQUES

The pedicled TRAM flap procedure can be initiated concurrently with the mastectomy procedure to reduce overall operative time. The patient is ideally placed in the supine position for flap elevation. The patient is generally marked preoperatively and intraoperatively, with a tapering transverse ellipse with superior extensions above the umbilicus. These extensions capture the superior perforators, which emanate from the superior epigastric vessels. The position of the ellipse is an important aspect in overall flap design. If the superior skin incision is placed at or below the umbilicus, there is a risk of missing direct perforators from the superior epigastric vessels. Using a higher superior incision results in a more reliable pedicled flap.[19] The inferior margin is marked flexing the patient and pulling the upper flap taught over the proposed TRAM flap to check the location of the inferior incision. This ensures that the abdominal closure will not be too tight. After verification of appropriate positioning, the plastic surgeon start with the inferior incision and elevating the flap with its subcutaneous fat from lateral to medial, until reaching the lateral rectus perforators. In a unilateral reconstruction, the perforators are then divided on the side that will not be used, the umbilicus is cut free, and the dissection proceeds to the medial row of rectus perforators. It is usually possible to perform either an ipsilateral or a contralateral flap, according to surgeon's preference and experience.

The muscle is identified after incising the overlying anterior rectus sheath. When a skin island is used, it is essential to preserve the continuity of the skin island with the underlying anterior rectus sheath and the rectus abdominis muscle to preserve the musculocutaneous perforators.

When a skin island is used, it is preferable to expose the muscle proximal to the skin island for accurate location of muscle position. Then the skin island is incised and its edges elevated to the lateral and medial borders of the rectus sheath. Next, the skin island is elevated 1–3 cm off the lateral and medial surface of the anterior sheath to preserve adequate sheath for later direct closure or interposition of synthetic mesh.

At this point, various accepted techniques emerge, depending on the degree of rectus muscle harvest and/or preservation. In our experience, we believe that there is no advantage to leaving a medial or lateral strip of muscle; thus, we generally raise the entire muscle with both the medial and lateral row of perforators intact. Following that, generally, the surgeon looks for deep inferior epigastric arteries/veins (DIEAs/DIEVs) and identifies, dissects, ligates, and transfers them with the flap. The DIEVs may provide a backup blood supply in the event that the superior pedicle is inadequate in perfusing the flap. This may only be evident after the flap is tunnelled, folded, and inset within the mastectomy defect. If flap perfusion is in question or the flap appears threatened, the harvested (DIEA/DIEV) can then be anastomosed to the thoracodorsal system through the use of microsurgical techniques. This technique is referred to as supercharging the flap.[20]

The authors usually perform a surgical delay to increase flap reliability[21–27] when perfusion is a concern. The delay procedure most commonly involves the ligature of both superficial and deep inferior epigastric arteries 7 or 14 days before the flap transfer[28–30] to increase the blood flow to the flap from the superior epigastric arteries, although other more invasive delaying procedures have been reported.[31] It has been demonstrated that the selective delay manoeuvre causes a flow inversion in the abdominal area, with the superior epigastric artery becoming the only dominant pedicle. As a result, choke vessels are dilated, and cutaneous blood flow is more constant and more secure,[22,25,32,33] improving flap survival with beneficial long-term effects.[34–36] The muscle is separated from the posterior sheath at the distal aspect of the flap.

After the TRAM flap is elevated completely, it may be deepithelialised partly to assess blood flow and speed up the inset process. Next, it is passed through a subcutaneous tunnel and into the mastectomy defect. It is important during the tunnelling process to pay particular attention to the orientation of the pedicle, as excessive twisting, kinking, and/or tension can result in flap ischaemia. In its final resting state within the mastectomy defect, the abdominal skin island is typically rotated 180°, such that the inferior abdominal soft tissue provides the superior tissue within the new breast mound and vice versa and flap is trimmed and contoured to match the opposite breast mound.

Once the flap is inset, attention is turned to the abdominal wall. When closing the abdominal fascia, particular attention should be paid to incorporating the internal and external oblique fascia within the anterior rectus closure.

Zone IV is generally discarded in all cases because of its unreliable vascularisation and unpredictable viability. In patients requiring a large volume of abdominal soft tissue for unilateral reconstruction or seeking bilateral reconstruction, bipedicled or bilateral TRAM flaps can be used. The bipedicled TRAM flap uses both rectus muscles, providing increased blood flow at the expense of rectus muscle function. Because both rectus muscles are sacrificed during these procedures, trunk function during activities such as performing sit-ups or rising from a low chair may be impaired.

20.4 COMPLICATIONS

Pedicled TRAM flap procedure is generally a well-tolerated procedure. Complications are typically related to either donor-site or flap-related problems. Among flap complications, fat necrosis is the most common one, with a reported incidence of 10%–18%.[13,37–40] Several risk factors have been identified that place patients at greater risk for developing fat necrosis. These factors include active smoking, obesity,[15–17] and a history of prior[39] or post-reconstruction chest wall irradiation.[41,42]

Donor-site morbidity following pedicled TRAM flap reconstruction can be divided into early and late complications. Early complications can include delayed wound healing, haematoma, and/or seroma formation. The incidence of seroma formation is reportedly between 2% and 7% of cases.[43,44] The risk of seroma formation can be limited through the use of closed-suction drains. Late donor-site complications following pedicled TRAM flap reconstruction are related primarily to abdominal wall integrity. These complications can include contour abnormalities, such as abdominal bulging and hernia formation, and reduced trunk function. Abdominal bulging is the most common late complication following pedicled TRAM flap reconstruction, with some series reporting an incidence of nearly 44%.[45] Fortunately, the incidence of true hernia is much lower, approximately 1%–3% of cases.[13,45] Nahabedian and Manson established several important principles related to the preservation of abdominal wall integrity: First, muscle-sparing techniques do not significantly reduce the probability of contour abnormality. Second, mesh reinforcement is not necessary unless tension-free closure cannot be obtained. Third, the use of fascial plication superior and inferior to the harvest site, and incorporation of the oblique fascia within the anterior rectus sheath closure, can reduce the risk of contour abnormalities.[46–48]

20.5 IMAGING FOR pTRAM

There has been an increasing effort in modern autologous tissue reconstructive surgery to minimise donor-site morbidity and flap complications. As such, preoperative imaging has been taught as a means to predict individual vascular anatomy preoperatively and thus maximise flap vascularity and operative success.

The DIEA, a branch of the external iliac artery, uniformly originates as a single trunk but displays a variable course thereafter. Less than 15 anatomical studies in the literature directly describe the branching pattern of the DIEA, and among these, there is certainly much variation in the descriptions, with many patterns of branching depicted. The first such description, by Boyd et al. in 1983, described a general pattern of two or three major branches from the primary trunk.[49] Subsequently, studies have varied in their accounts of this branching pattern. Some pertain to a uniformly bifurcating pattern of the DIEA,[50–52] whereas others have described a third major branch occurring in a minority of cases.[53,54] Irrespective of other varying accounts, the first formal classification system for the branching pattern of the DIEA was described in 1988 by Moon and Taylor.[32] This described three branching *types*, with the DIEA comprising either a single trunk, a bifurcating trunk, or a trifurcating trunk. These were classified according to their size and anastomosis with branches of the superior epigastric artery above the umbilicus. Further study emphasised that this classification system was based on the size of an umbilical branch, which is ever present, and whether it arises as a lesser branch from the more medial trunk of a type I or type II artery or whether it is a dominant branch and forms a major trunk as is the case in a type III vessel.[55–57]

The concept of angiosomes, as described by Spear et al.,[15] Taylor et al.,[58] and Boyd et al.,[49] is also useful in illustrating the differences in blood supply between free TRAM and pedicled TRAM flaps. In any free TRAM flap, zone 1 is the primary angiosome, and zones 2 and 3 are considered to be the adjacent angiosomes. Zone 4, being two angiosomes away, is believed to be unreliable. By contrast, zone 1 in a pTRAM flap is separated from the primary angiosome (or vascular pedicle) by a choke system of vessels and, therefore, represents an adjacent angiosome. Therefore, according to these principles, it is suggested that zones 2 and 3 in a pTRAM flap are unreliable.

Although they are usually reliable, this explains why we occasionally observe intraoperative congestion and ischaemia and subsequent partial flap necrosis in zones 2 and 3 in pTRAM flaps, which may lead to the aforementioned complications described in previous studies and observed in clinical practice.[59] Complications can occur even when operating on carefully selected patients and using properly designed pTRAM flaps. Any clinically obvious intraoperative findings of ischaemia or congestion would naturally guide the surgeon to alter the flap design to include viable angiosomes and prevent complications.

The development of a technology capable of easy and reliable investigation of flap perfusion could be applied clinically in several ways. It would allow a preoperative planning and an objective post-operative flap monitoring, and it could be used to evaluate flap perfusion intraoperatively, thereby guiding the surgeon during planning and dissection of the flap.

20.5.1 Preoperative Imaging

20.5.1.1 Ecocolor Doppler and CT Angiography (MDCTA)

With the use of the pTRAM, to avoid complications as partial flap necrosis (average rate to 30%), occurring because of its unreliable cutaneous blood flow, and to increase flap reliability, some preoperative instrumental techniques have been suggested, including ecocolor Doppler (ECD), laser Doppler flowmetry,[31–35] and CT angiography.

ECD is a handy and inexpensive tool to analyse flow velocity, resistivity, and changes in diameter of the superior epigastric artery and to conduct an examination of the origin, course, and anatomic variations of perforator arteries and helps to improve knowledge of the haemodynamic changes occurring in the TRAM flap's vascular network after the delay manoeuvre.[31–34] Its results confirm that the selective delay manoeuvre causes a flow inversion in the abdominal area, with the superior epigastric artery becoming the only dominant pedicle. As a result, choke vessels are dilated and cutaneous blood flow is more constant and more secure.[22,25,32,33] Clinical studies indicate that delaying a TRAM flap reduces complications approximately to 5% to 10%, and this has been reported in several series.[22–24,60–62] Experimental studies have been based on in vivo and cadaver animal studies and helped to define the delay phenomenon and show why flap survival is improved with a delay procedure.[30,63,64] Increases in the area of flap survival in the rat model, as obtained by Ozgentas et al.[63] and Restifo et al.,[30] and increases in vascularity in the rabbit model have been shown. Perfusion in choke vessels crossing over from the nondelayed side to the delayed side in the rabbit model steadily increased from day 1 after the delay procedure and reached statistical significance by day 21.[64] What really happens after a selective delay has been demonstrated by Moon and Taylor.[32]

Rand et al.[65] stated that the preoperative ECD location of TRAM flap perforators improves the surgeon's ability to design and elevate the flap to capture the dominant vessels and maximise survival. In addition, preoperative knowledge of the number and flow velocity characteristics of the perforators allows for the selection of single-and double-pedicle and free TRAM flaps. Our group has shown in every patient an increase in the superior epigastric artery diameter and a decrease in resistivity index values. Furthermore, we showed that cutaneous blood flow in the delayed TRAM flap during the procedure is more stable.[33] Codner et al.[22] measured perfusion pressure in the region of midrectus perforators of TRAM flaps before and after delay. They noted a significant increase in perfusion pressure after delay procedure. However, some data about the use of ECD are debated. Operator dependence, false positives in detection of perforating vessels, and the amount of time that the study takes for the hospital staff and patient are reported in the literature.[66–69] Furthermore, the information cannot be reproduced so that the procedure must be repeated by the radiologist.

Moreover, although laser Doppler flowmetry has been applied for monitoring free and pedicled flaps in several studies, it has yielded conflicting results and has not gained general acceptance. It is very sensitive to various artefacts and does not distinguish between nutrient blood flow and random motion of cells in non-perfused tissue. Because laser Doppler flowmetry is expressed in arbitrary units that vary significantly between individuals and measurement sites, relevant information can only be gained by continuous or repeated measurements and comparison of recorded values to baseline values.

It has been postulated that the pTRAM's blood supply is based on the blood flow coming from the superior epigastric arteries through umbilical rectus muscle perforators.[21,32,49] Nevertheless, it is hard to tell which are the best perforators to use and also which side will benefit more of the selective delay procedure (e.g. the radiated internal mammary vessels may not increase their diameter sufficiently). Among last-generation angiographic diagnostic techniques, multidetector computed tomography (MDCT) has emerged as an outstanding non-invasive operator-independent option. MDCT offers thin-slice coverage of extended volumes, with an extremely high spatial resolution.[70–72] It has been postulated that MDCT angiography (MDCTA) scanning might give new information[70–72] about DIEA perforator location and size. Individual precise preoperative location andevaluation of perforating vessels and the origin, course, and variations of diameter of deep superior epigatric artery (DSEA) are highly desirable for improving our surgical strategy.

Rozen et al.[55] have recently documented by CT angiography the presence of either a single, bifurcating, or trifurcating major trunk of the DIEA, as classified by the system described by Moon and Taylor.[32]

The DIEA branching pattern was correlated with both the number of perforators and their intramuscular course. The branching pattern was not shown to have a relationship with the number of perforators traversing a rectus abdominis muscle. However, there was a significant relationship between the branching pattern and the course of the perforators. A bifurcating (type II) branching pattern demonstrated a reduced transverse distance traversed by each perforator, whereas a trifurcating (type III) branching pattern demonstrated perforators that traversed significantly greater transverse distances. Furthermore, perforators of the lateral branch of a type II artery demonstrated the shortest intramuscular course. A type I pattern demonstrated a distance intermediate to that of types II and III.

Preoperative knowledge of an individual's DIEA branching pattern can thus allow operative planning as to the side of choice for muscle dissection and the branch of choice in the case of a type II vessel.[55]

We have previously demonstrated the usefulness of MDCTA for preoperative planning in patients undergoing pTRAM flap breast reconstruction after selective vascular delay.[73] After written informed consent was obtained from all patients, a preoperative MDCTA can be performed for surgical planning. The volumetric data acquired are then used to reconstruct images with a slice width of 1.6 mm and a reconstruction interval of 0.6 mm. The resulting complete set of reconstructed images is automatically transferred to a computer workstation, which generates images in multiple planes and in 3D volume-rendered images. Data are stored in an interactive compact disc, which can easily be used and managed using a standard computer. After 5–7 days, selective vascular delay was carried out. Under local anaesthesia and IV sedation, the patient undergoes surgery with bilateral incision and ligation of both superficial and deep inferior epigastric arteries. A second MDCTA is then obtained after 15 days. A 3D reconstruction and axial images of the abdomen were obtained to locate precisely the points on the skin surface where the best perforators emerged from the fascia of the rectus abdominis muscles. All the information are transferred to a data form sheet so that the perforators are mapped in a format that allowed us to transpose their position preoperatively onto the abdominal skin of the patient. Finally, patients undergo breast reconstruction with a unipedicled TRAM flap. The left or right rectus muscle was selected, depending on the biggest increase found in DSEA.

In our studies,[73] MDCTA scanning showed an average increased diameter of the DSEA of 29.3% (Figure 20.1a,b). These results are comparable with ECD data.[24] Periumbilical perforator vessels emerging from rectus muscles are detected in every patient, and the best perforators emerging from the fascia are mapped in a data form sheet. The highest concentration of reliable perforators is found as expected in an area between 2 cm cranially and 4 cm caudally of the umbilicus and between 0.5 and 4.5 cm laterally from the linea alba. For these reasons, MDCTA allows a study of the donor area, which is very easy to interpret not only by the radiologist but also by the surgeon as it provides anatomic images. It also permits the option of having a virtual anatomic dissection of the patient on the computer because the pictures obtained are 3D anatomy reconstructions (Figures 20.2 and 20.3). It permits us to evaluate the increase in the diameter of DSEA without the theoretical errors of ECD.

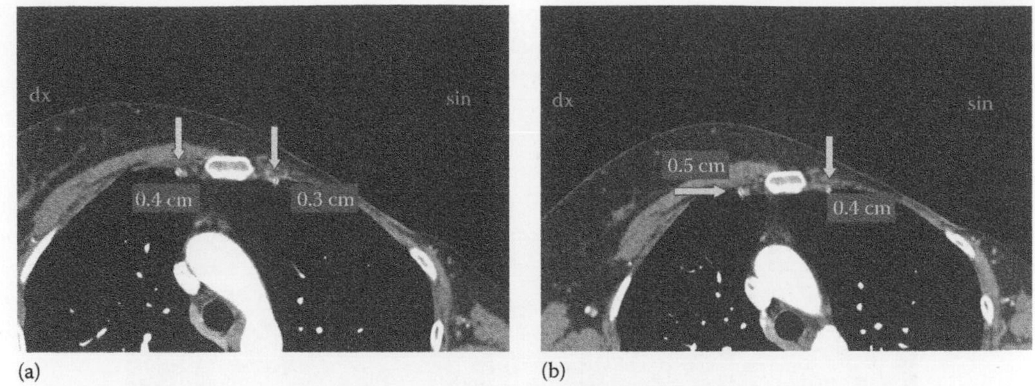

FIGURE 20.1 (a) Pre-operative axial angio-CT scan of DSEA at the level of the costomarginal artery. (b) Post-operative angio-CT scan, same patient. After the section of DIEA, diameters are increased after selective vascular delay.

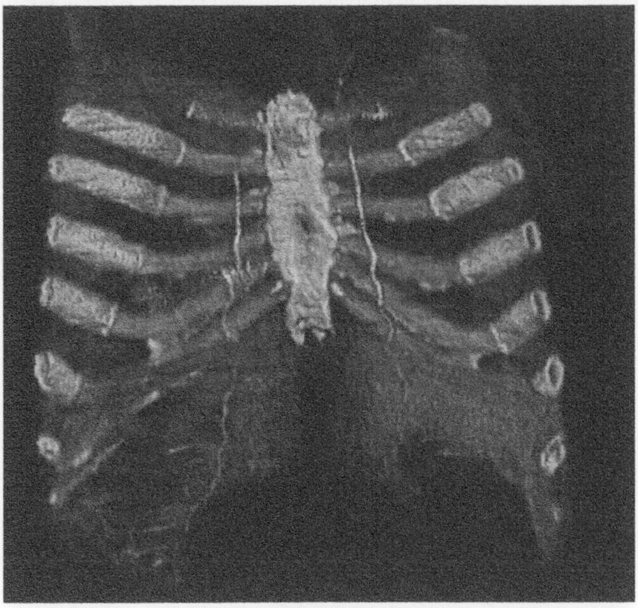

FIGURE 20.2 3D. Reconstruction with angio-CT of the internal chest wall showing DSEA bilaterally.

Furthermore, evaluation of the best perforator vessels in preoperative time allowed us to choose pre-operatively between the homolateral and contralateral side of the TRAM to plan the flap using the best vascularised tissue supplied by the dominant perforator with regard to its calibre and position (Figure 20.4). This method helps the surgeon to evaluate the best perforators, avoiding a possible intraoperative spasming effect. As a result of this, a lot of time is saved during surgery as it is no longer necessary to perform an extensive overview of all the perforators (Figures 20.5 and 20.6). Finally, the radiation rate is 10 mSv for each patient, which is three times the annual exposure to natural radiation. This technique is also well tolerated by patients because it is simple and speedy. Nowadays, the high sensitivity and specificity and the non-invasive, easy-to-interpret preoperative technique have made MDCTA the gold standard diagnostic tool for preoperative imaging of breast reconstruction with autologous abdominal tissues (Figure 20.7).

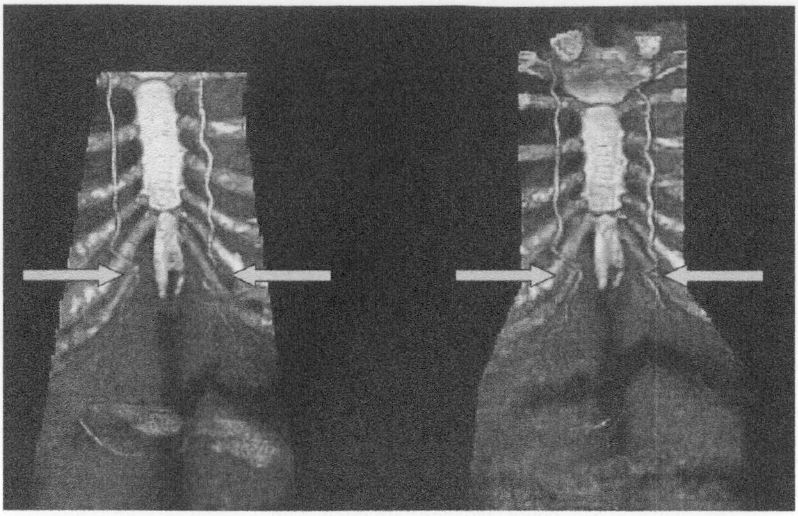

FIGURE 20.3 Pre-operative and post-operative scan focusing on DSEA. After delay, modifications in caliber are evident.

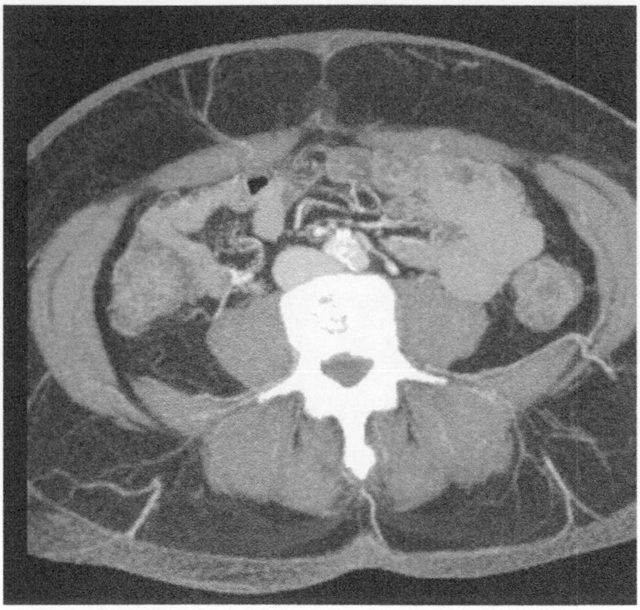

FIGURE 20.4 Axial angio-CT scan of the abdomen showing, in this case, perforator vessels on the right side, suggesting the surgeon the best side to harvest the pTRAM flap.

20.5.2 Intraoperative Imaging

20.5.2.1 Fluorescent Angiography

A variety of modalities have been used in an attempt to assist the surgeon intraoperatively in identifying potential sources of complication. These include fluorescein dye angiography, laser-assisted indocyanine green dye angiography (LA-ICGA), thermography, Doppler ultrasound, tissue oximetry, and various radioisotopes, among others.

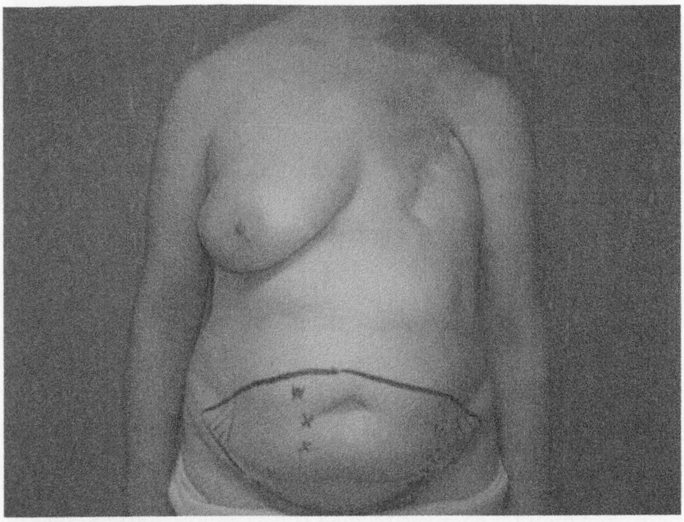

FIGURE 20.5 Pre-operative map of rectus muscle perforators skin markings.

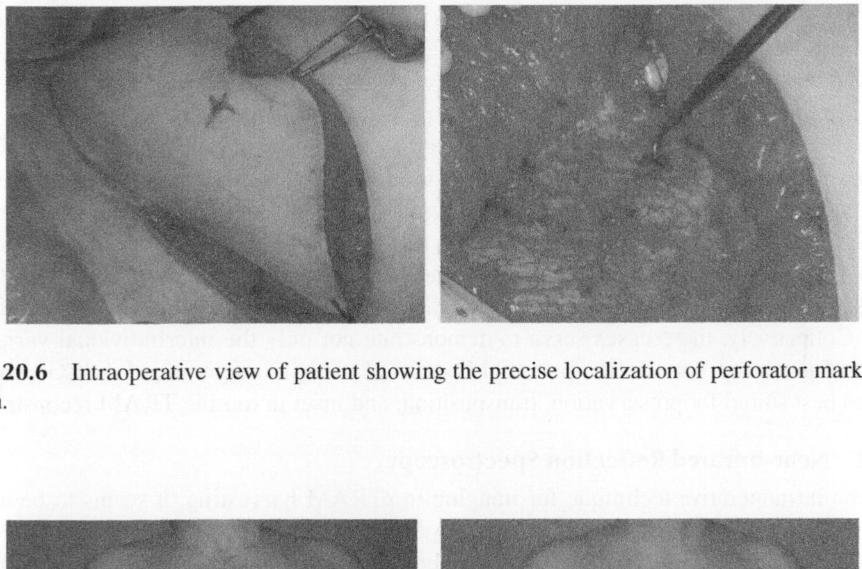

FIGURE 20.6 Intraoperative view of patient showing the precise localization of perforator marked before operation.

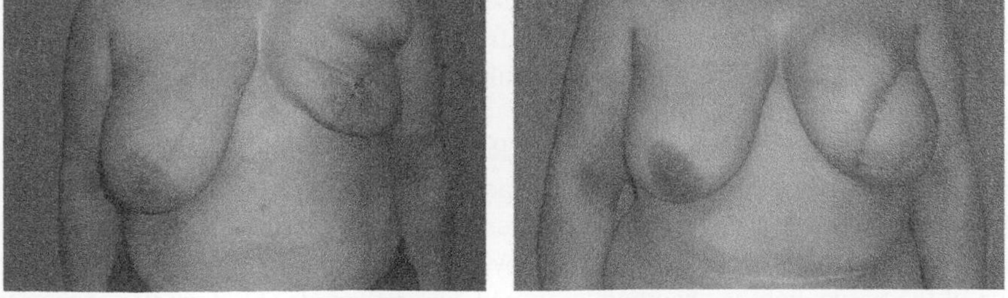

FIGURE 20.7 Pre-operative and post-operative view of a patient after breast reconstruction with the pTRAM flap.

Unfortunately, each has its own set of disadvantages, which has precluded their widespread clinical use for this purpose. The beneficial use of intraoperative fluorescent angiography was recently demonstrated in free tissue transfer reconstruction as an easy way of assessing flap perfusion and helping in surgical decision making[74–76] and more recently, laser-assisted indocyanine green dye angiography (LA-ICGA) has gained attention in plastic surgery. Lyophilised indocyanine green is injected through a peripheral or central intravenous line. This dye is excited by the laser camera, which results in a fluorescent image on the computer screen. Fluorescence intensity serves as a function of tissue perfusion and real-time information is recorded. Although the use of indocyanine green for flap analysis is not new, the ability to quantify flow over an entire zone is new, the result of newer technology and software. The benefits of LA-ICGA in microsurgical breast reconstruction have been demonstrated by Newman et al.,[74] and they recently reported first cases of these techniques applicable to pTRAM.[77] In the past, Yamaguchi et al.[78] have used indocyanine green imaging to correlate perfusion of the unipedicled TRAM flap and post-operative partial flap necrosis and presented an individual pattern of perfusion in which zone II was occasionally not as well perfused as zone III. Clinically, it has also been felt that there is an increase in fat necrosis in zone II compared with zone III.[79,80] This was well demonstrated clinically by Kim et al.[40] in 400 unilateral pedicled TRAM flaps, in which fat necrosis in zone II was significantly higher than in zone III.

This form of intraoperative angiography (LA-ICGA) begins with the intravenous injection of indocyanine green fluorescent dye, which may be administered via an existing central line or through peripheral access. The dye, which binds to plasma proteins, travels through the vascular system and courses through the microvasculature. As it does, the subdermal plexus can be visualised through the skin in real time. Images are dynamic and are captured in video format on a monitor in the operating room. The format is black and white – white represents the dye within the microvasculature (e.g. perfusion) and black represents the lack of dye (e.g. lack of perfusion). Varying shades of grey demonstrate gradients of perfusion throughout the imaged tissue.

In Newman's experience,[74,77] those images obtained and analysed with respect to cutaneous perfusion in real time at the operation helped to determine which tissues should be debrided before transfer and inset and which tissues should be preserved and included in the reconstruction. He has anticipated maturation of this technology shortly to a point in which the operating surgeon may be able to use objective numerical data to quantify the perfusion of different parts of the flap, thus adding to his armamentarium of tools by which to judge which portion of the flap to preserve for transposition. Collectively, these cases serve to demonstrate not only the interindividual variability of the zones of perfusion but also the potential benefits of using intraoperative LA-ICGA to identify the tissues best suited for preservation, transposition, and inset in routine TRAM reconstructions.

20.5.2.2 Near-Infrared Reflection Spectroscopy

Among the intraoperative technique for imaging in pTRAM harvesting, it seems to be a promising tool the near-infrared reflection spectroscopy.[81] Jöbsis[82] reported the first clinical use of near-infrared reflection spectroscopy to monitor cerebral oxygenation in neonates in 1977. Since then, near-infrared reflection spectroscopy has been used successfully in a variety of experimental and clinical situations.[83–88] Only recently has near-infrared reflection spectroscopy been discovered to be a promising new tool in plastic surgery to monitor dynamic changes in blood volume and tissue oxygen saturation in flaps non-invasively.[89]

Haemoglobin content and oxygenation of the TRAM flap skin island have been recently measured by Schuefler et al. by a new non-invasive near-infrared reflection spectroscopy device.[81] Light is emitted at 400–1200 nm wavelength with 0.3 nm intervals at a scan rate of up to 400 Hz in reflection mode and transmitted to a defined tissue volume by means of a special quartz fibre-optic cable. After penetration of the tissue, light is absorbed, scattered, and reflected. The diameter of the sensor fibre (1 mm) and the depth of light penetration (4 mm) define a cone-shaped volume of approximately 13 μL of tissue under investigation. The reflected light is detected by a sensor fibre and processed by an integrated computer performing a fingerprint analysis of the spectral data. During measurements, all data are continually displayed graphically and numerically on the monitor screen and simultaneously stored as a file on a hard disc. Data were transferred to a compatible desktop computer by means of interface for processing and analysis. A full set of near-infrared reflection spectroscopy measurements (15 positions) required approximately 30 min. Moreover, the regulation of cutaneous blood flow is subject to emotional states. Consequently, stable ambient and emotional conditions are mandatory during investigation of skin circulation by near-infrared reflection spectroscopy.

Several experimental studies have demonstrated the ability of near-infrared reflection spectroscopy to assess impaired perfusion in cutaneous and myocutaneous flaps and to differentiate between arterial and venous flap complications in the animal model.[90–92] The prospect of monitoring flaps buried deep to the skin was related to the penetrative capabilities of the near-infrared reflection spectroscopy systems used in some studies,[90,91] whereas others were designed for superficial skin measurements.[92] Moreover, near-infrared light penetration may differ between near-infrared reflection spectroscopy systems according to variations in the selected wavelengths, technical and geometrical factors, tissue characteristics, and chromophore concentrations. The near-infrared reflection spectroscopy system used is designed for superficial tissue measurements in reflection mode with a penetration depth of up to 4 mm. The near-infrared reflection spectroscopy system yields absolute values of total haemoglobin, deoxyhaemoglobin, and oxyhaemoglobin in milligrams per millilitre in addition to tissue oxygen saturation in percent in real-time mode, allowing direct comparison between different skin territories and individuals. It has been demonstrated that there are no significant differences among preoperative, early post-operative, and late post-operative values of tissue haemoglobin content and oxygenation in the mastectomy skin flap and contralateral breast. However, near-infrared reflection spectroscopy measurements of the TRAM flap reveal significant differences between preoperative and early post-operative values of tissue haemoglobin content and oxygenation and among zones I, II, and III early after surgery.

Limitations to the clinical use of near-infrared reflection spectroscopy are lack of an accepted standard, foremost because of the variety of spectrophotometers available today that have been developed and tested by different laboratories, using different numbers of wavelengths of near-infrared light and different algorithms for analysis of recovered light, and highly variable costs (approximately $25,000–$50,000).

Further experience is needed before near-infrared reflection spectroscopy can be advocated for routine clinical flap monitoring.

REFERENCES

1. Holmstrom H. The free abdominoplasty flap and its use in breast reconstruction. *Scand J Plast Reconstr Surg*. 1979;13:423–427.
2. Hartrampf CR, Scheflan M, Black PW. Breast reconstruction with a transverse abdominal island flap. *Plast Reconstr Surg*. 1982;69:341.
3. Kroll SS, Khoo A, Singletary SE et al. Local recurrence risk after skin-sparing and conventional mastectomy: A 6-year follow-up. *Plast Reconstr Surg*. 199;104:421–425.
4. Toth BA, Forley BG, Calabria R. Retrospective study of the skin-sparing mastectomy in breast reconstruction. *Plast Reconstr Surg*. 1999;104:77–84.
5. Al-Ghazal SK, Sully L, Fallowfield L, Blamey RW. The psychological impact of immediate rather than delayed breast reconstruction. *Eur J Surg Oncol*. 2000;26:17–19.
6. Miller MJ. Immediate breast reconstruction. *Clin Plast Surg*. 1998;25:145–156.
7. Kronowitz SJ, Robb GL. Breast reconstruction with postmastectomy radiation therapy: Current issues. *Plast Reconstr Surg*. 2004;114:950–960.
8. Spear SL, Ducic I, Low M, Cuoco F. The effect of radiation on pedicled TRAM flap breast reconstruction: Outcomes and implications. *Plast Reconstr Surg*. 2005;115:84–95.
9. Serletti JM. Breast reconstruction with the TRAM flap: Pedicled and free. *J Surg Oncol*. 2006;94:532–537.
10. Clough KB, O'Donoghue JM, Fitoussi AD, Vlastos G, Falcou MC. Prospective evaluation of late cosmetic results following breast reconstruction: II. TRAM flap reconstruction. *Plast Reconstr Surg*. 2001;107:1710–1716.

11. Moscona RA, Holander L, Or D, Fodor L. Patient satisfaction and aesthetic results after pedicled transverse rectus abdominis muscle flap for breast reconstruction. *Ann Surg Oncol.* 2006;13:1739–1746.
12. Alderman AK, Wilkins EG, Lowery JC, Kim M, Davis JA. Determinants of patient satisfaction in postmastectomy breast reconstruction. *Plast Reconstr Surg.* 2000;106:769–776.
13. Ducic I, Spear SL, Cuoco F, Hannan C. Safety and risk factors for breast reconstruction with pedicled transverse rectus abdominis musculocutaneous flaps: A 10-year analysis. *Ann Plast Surg.* 2005;55:559–564.
14. Namnoum JD. Breast reconstruction: TRAM flap techniques. In: *Grabb and Smith's Plastic Surgery.* Charles HT (Ed.) Philadelphia, PA: Wolters Kluwer Health/Lippincott Williams & Wilkins; 2007, pp. 641–647.
15. Spear SL, Ducic I, Cuoco F, Hannan C. The effect of smoking on flap and donor-site complications in pedicled TRAM breast reconstruction. *Plast Reconstr Surg.* 2005;116:1873–1880.
16. Spear SL, Ducic I, Cuoco F, Taylor N. Effect of obesity on flap and donor-site complications in pedicled TRAM flap breast reconstruction. *Plast Reconstr Surg.* 2007;119:788–795.
17. Moran SL, Serletti JM. Outcome comparison between free and pedicled TRAM flap breast reconstruction in the obese patient. *Plast Reconstr Surg.* 2001;108:1954–1960, discussion 1961–1962.
18. Chen L, Hartrampf CR, Bennet GK. Successful pregnancies following TRAM flap surgery. *Plast Reconstr Surg.* 1993;91:69–71.
19. Buck DW II, Fine NA. The pedicled transverse rectus abdominis myocutaneous flap: Indications, techniques, and outcomes. *Plast Reconstr Surg.* 2009;124:1047.
20. Marck KW, van der Biezen JJ, Dol JA. Internal mammary artery and vein supercharge in TRAM flap breast reconstruction. *Microsurgery* 1996;17:371–374.
21. Taylor GI, Corlett RJ, Caddy CM et al. An anatomic review of the delay phenomenon, II: Clinical applications. *Plast Reconstr Surg.* 1992;89:408.
22. Codner MA, Bostwick J III, Nahai F et al. TRAM flap vascular delay for high risk breast reconstruction. *Plast Reconstr Surg.* 1995;96:1615–1622.
23. Hudson DA. The surgically delayed unipedicled TRAM flap for breast reconstruction. *Ann Plast Surg.* 1996;36:238–242.
24. Restifo RJ, Ward BA, Scoutt LM. Timing, magnitude, and utility of surgical delay in the TRAM flap, II: Clinical studies. *Plast Reconstr Surg.* 1997;99:1217–1223.
25. Dhar SC, Taylor GI. The delay phenomenon: The story unfolds. *Plast Reconstr Surg.* 1999;104:2079–2091.
26. Taylor GI. Discussion of "The surgically delayed unipedicled TRAM flap for breast reconstruction". *Ann Plast Surg.* 1996;36:242–245.
27. Sano K, Hallock G, Rice DC. The relative importance of the deep and superficial vascular system for delay of the transverse rectus abdominis: Musculocutaneous flap as demonstrated in a rat model. *Plast Reconstr Surg.* 2002;109:1052–1057.
28. Ribuffo D, Scuderi N. TRAM flap delay: Which vessels should be ligated? *Plast Reconstr Surg.* 2003;111:948–949.
29. Restifo RJ, Ahmed SS, Ward BA et al. Surgical delay in TRAM flap breast reconstruction: A comparison of 7 and 14 day delay periods. *Ann Plast Surg.* 1997;38:330–333.
30. Restifo RJ, Ahmed SS, Isenberg JS et al. Timing, magnitude and utility of surgical delay in TRAM flap, I: Animal studies. *Plast Reconstr Surg.* 1997;99:1211–1216.
31. Restifo RJ, Ahmed SS, Rosser J et al. TRAM flap perforator ligation and the delay phenomenon: Development of an endoscopic/laparoscopic delay procedure. *Plast Reconstr Surg.* 1998;101:1503–1511.
32. Moon HK, Taylor GI. The vascular anatomy of rectus abdominis musculocutaneous flaps based on the deep superior epigastric system. *Plast Reconstr Surg.* 1988;82:815–832.
33. Ribuffo D, Muratori L, Antoniadou KA et al. A hemodynamic approach to clinical results in the TRAM flap after selective delay. *Plast Reconstr Surg.* 1997;99:1706–1714.
34. Hallock GG, Rice DC. Evidence for the efficacy of TRAM flap delay in a rat model. *Plast Reconstr Surg.* 1995;96:1351–1357.
35. Morrissey WM, Hallock GG. The increase in TRAM flap survival after delay does not diminish long term. *Ann Plast Surg.* 2000;44:486–490.
36. Hallock GG, Altobelli JA. The TRAM delay: Burning a lifeboat? *Plast Reconstr Surg.* 1998;102:1301–1303.
37. Johnson RM, Barney LM, King JC. Vaginal delivery of monozygotic twins after bilateral pedicle TRAM breast reconstruction. *Plast Reconstr Surg.* 2002;109:1653–1654.
38. Paige KT, Bostwick J III, Bried JT, Jones G. A comparison of morbidity from bilateral, unipedicled and unilateral, unipedicled TRAM flap breast reconstructions. *Plast Reconstr Surg.* 1998;101:1819–1827.
39. Watterson PA, Bostwick J, Hester R, Bried J, Taylor GI. TRAM flap anatomy correlated with a 10-year clinical experience with 556 patients. *Plast Reconstr Surg.* 1995;95:1185–1194.

40. Kim EK, Lee TJ, Eom JS. Comparison of fat necrosis between zone II and zone III in pedicled transverse rectus abdominis musculocutaneous flaps: A prospective study of 400 cases. *Ann Plast Surg.* 2007;59:256–259.
41. Halyard MY, McCombs KE, Wong WW et al. Acute and chronic results of adjuvant radiotherapy after mastectomy and transverse rectus abdominis myocutaneous (TRAM) flap reconstruction for breast cancer. *Am J Clin Oncol.* 2004;27:389–394.
42. Kronowitz SJ, Hunt KK, Kuerer HM et al. Delayed-immediate breast reconstruction. *Plast Reconstr Surg.* 2004;113:1617–1628.
43. Gabbay JS, Eby JB, Kulber DA. The midabdominal TRAM flap for breast reconstruction in morbidly obese patients. *Plast Reconstr Surg.* 2005;115:764–770.
44. Scevola S, Youssef A, Kroll SS. Drains and seromas in TRAM flap breast reconstruction. *Ann Plast Surg.* 2002;48:511–514.
45. Petit JY, Rietjens M, Garusi C et al. Abdominal complications and sequelae after breast reconstruction with pedicled TRAM flap: Is there still an indication for pedicled TRAM in the year 2003? *Plast Reconstr Surg.* 2003;112:1063–1065.
46. Nahabedian MY, Manson PM. Contour abnormalities of the abdomen after transverse rectus abdominis muscle flap breast reconstruction: A multifactorial analysis. *Plast Reconstr Surg.* 2002;109:81–87, discussion 88–90.
47. Kroll SS, Schusterman MA, Reece GP, Miller MJ, Robb G, Evans G. Abdominal wall strength, bulging, and hernia after TRAM flap breast reconstruction. *Plast Reconstr Surg.* 1995; 96:616–619.
48. Nahabedien MY, Dooley W, Singh N, Manson PN. Contour abnormalities of the abdomen after breast reconstruction with abdominal flaps: The role of muscle preservation. *Plast Reconstr Surg.* 2002;109:91–101.
49. Boyd JB, Taylor GI, and Corlett RJ. The vascular territories of the superior epigastric and deep inferior epigastric systems. *Plast Reconstr Surg.* 1984;73:1.
50. Ohjimi H, Era K, Tanahashi S, Kawano K, Manabe T, and Naitoh M. Ex vivo intraoperative angiography for rectus abdominis musculocutaneous free flaps. *Plast Reconstr Surg.* 2002;109:2247.
51. Ohjimi H, Era K, Fujita T, Tanaka T, and Yabuuchi R. Analyzing the vascular architecture of the free TRAM flap using intraoperative ex vivo angiography. *Plast Reconstr Surg.* 2005;116:106.
52. Tansatit T, Chokrungvaranont P, Sanguansit P, and Wanidchaphloi S. Neurovascular anatomy of the deep inferior epigastric perforator flap for breast reconstruction. *J Med Assoc Thai.* 2006;89:1630.
53. Itoh Y and Arai K. The deep inferior epigastric artery free skin flap: Anatomic study and clinical application. *Plast Reconstr Surg.* 1993;91:853.
54. El-Mrakby HH and Milner RH. The vascular anatomy of the lower anterior abdominal wall: A microdissection study on the deep inferior epigastric vessels and the perforator branches. *Plast Reconstr Surg.* 2002;109:539.
55. Rozen WM, Ashton MW, Pan WR, and Taylor GI. Raising perforator flaps for breast reconstruction: The intramuscular anatomy of the DIEA. *Plast Reconstr Surg.* 2007;120:1443.
56. Taylor GI, Hamdy H, El-Mrakby HH, and Milner RH. Vascular anatomy of the lower anterior abdominal wall: A microdissection study on the deep inferior epigastric vessels and the perforator branches. *Plast Reconstr Surg.* 2002;109:544.
57. Taylor GI, Watterson PA, and Zelt RG. The vascular anatomy of the anterior abdominal wall: The basis of flap design. *Perspect Plast Surg.* 1991;5:1.
58. Taylor GI, Palmer JH. The vascular territories (angiosomes) of the body: Experimental study and clinical applications. *Br J Plast Surg.* 1987;40:113.
59. Serletti J. Technical variations of the bipedicled TRAM flap in unilateral breast reconstruction: Effects of conventional versus microsurgical techniques of pedicle transfer on complications rates. *Plast Reconstr Surg.* 2004;114:385–388.
60. Codner MA, Bostwick J III. The delayed TRAM flap. *Clin Plast Surg.* 1998;25:183–189.
61. Rickard RF, Hudson DA. Influence of vascular delay on abdominal wall complications in unipedicled TRAM flap breast reconstruction. *Ann Plast Surg.* 2003;50:138–142.
62. Erdmann D, Sundin BM, Moquin KJ et al. Delay in unipedicled TRAM flap: Reconstruction of the breast, a review of 76 consecutive cases. *Plast Reconstr Surg.* 2002;110:762–767.
63. Ozgentas HE, Shenaq S, Spira M et al. Study of the delay phenomenon in the rat TRAM flap model. *Plast Reconstr Surg.* 1994;94:1018–1024.
64. Cederna PS, Chang P, Pittet-Cuenod BM et al. The effect of the delay phenomenon in the vascularity of rabbit rectus abdominis muscle. *Plast Reconstr Surg.* 1997;99:194–205.
65. Rand RP, Cramer MM, Strandness DE Jr. Color flow duplex scanning in the preoperative assessment of the TRAM flap perforators: A report of 32 consecutive patient. *Plast Reconstr Surg.* 1994;93:453–459.
66. Blondeel PN, Beyens G, Verghaege R et al. Doppler flowmetry in the planning of perforators flaps. *Br J Plast Surg.* 1998;51:202–209.

67. Masia J, Clavero JA, Larranaga JR et al. Multidetector-row computed tomography in the planning of abdominal perforator flaps. *J Plast Reconstr Aesthet Surg*. 2006;59:594–599.
68. Alonso-Burgos A, Garcia-Tutor E, Bastarrika G et al. Preoperative planning of deep inferior epigastric artery perforator flap reconstruction with multislice-CT angiography: Imaging findings and initial experience. *J Plast Reconstr Aesthet Surg*. 2006;59:585–593.
69. Giunta RE, Geisweid A, Feller AM. The value of preoperative Doppler sonography for planning free perforator flaps. *Plast Reconstr Surg*. 2000;105:2381–2386.
70. Kalra MK, Maher MM, Souza R et al. Multi-detector computed tomography technology: Current status and emerging developments. *J Comput Assist Tomogr*. 2004;28(Suppl. 1):S2–S6.
71. Lawler LP, Fishman EK. Multi-detector row computed tomography of the aorta and peripheral arteries. *Cardiol Clin*. 2003;21:607–629.
72. Schoepf UJ, Becker CR, Hofmann LK et al. Multislice CT angiography. *Eur Radiol*. 2003;13:1946–1961.
73. Ribuffo D, Atzeni M, Corrias F, Guerra M, Saba L, Sias A, Balestrieri A, Mallarini G. Preoperative angio-CT preliminary study of the TRAM flap after selective vascular delay. *Ann Plast Surg*. 2007;59(6):611–616.
74. Newman MI, Samson MC. The application of laser-assisted indocyanine green fluorescent dye angiography in microsurgical breast reconstruction. *J Reconstr Microsurg*. 2009;25:21–26.
75. Pestana IA, Coan B, Erdmann D, Marcus J, Levin LS, Zenn MR. Early experience with fluorescent angiography in free-tissue transfer reconstruction. *Plast Reconstr Surg*. 2009;123:1239–1244.
76. Losken A, Styblo TM, Schaefer TG, Carlson GW. The use of fluorescein dye as a predictor of mastectomy skin flap viability following autologous tissue reconstruction. *Ann Plast Surg*. 2008;61:24–29.
77. Newman MI, Samson MC, Tamburrino JF, Swartz KA, Brunworth L. An investigation of the application of laser-assisted indocyanine green fluorescent dye angiography in pedicle transverse rectus abdominis myocutaneous breast reconstruction. *Can J Plast Surg*. 2011;19(1):e1–e5.
78. Yamaguchi S, De Lorenzi F, Petit JY et al. The "perfusion map" of the unipedicled TRAM flap to reduce post-operative partial necrosis. *Ann Plast Surg*. 2004;53:205–209.
79. Jewell RP, Whitney TM. TRAM fat necrosis in a young surgeons practice: Is it experience, technique or blood flow? *Ann Plast Surg*. 1999;42:424–427.
80. Shestak KC. Breast reconstruction with a pedicled TRAM flap. *Clin Plast Surg*. 1998;25:167–187.
81. Scheufler O, Exner K, Andresen R Investigation of TRAM flap oxygenation and perfusion by near-infrared reflection spectroscopy and color-coded duplex sonography. *Plast Reconstr Surg*. 2004;113:141.
82. Jöbsis FF. Noninvasive, infrared monitoring of cerebral and myocardial oxygen sufficiency and circulatory parameters. *Science* 1977;198:1264.
83. Jöbsis-Vander Vliet FF, Piantadosi CA, Sylvia AL et al. Near infrared monitoring of cerebral oxygen sufficiency. *Neurol Res*. 1988;10:7.
84. Frank KH, Kessler M, Appelbaum K et al. The Erlangen micro-lightguide spectrophotometer EMPHO I. *Phys Med Biol*. 1989;34:1883.
85. Wilson JR, Mancini DM, McCully K et al. Noninvasive detection of skeletal muscle underperfusion with near-infrared-spectroscopy in patients with heart failure. *Circulation* 1989;80:1668.
86. Chance B, Wang NG, Maris M et al. Quantitation of tissue optical characteristics and hemoglobin desaturation by time- and frequency-resolved multiwavelength spectrophotometry. *Adv Exp Med Biol*. 1992;92:297.
87. Liu H and Chance B. Influence of blood vessels on the measurement of hemoglobin oxygenation as determined by time-resolved reflectance spectroscopy. *Med Phys*. 1995;22:1209.
88. Firbank M, Okada E, and Delpy DT. Investigation of the effect of discrete absorbers upon the measurement of blood volume with near-infrared spectroscopy. *Phys Med Biol*. 1997;42:465.
89. Hayden RE, Tavill MA, Nioka S et al. Oxygenation and blood volume changes in flaps according to near-infrared spectrophotometry. *Arch Otolaryngol Head Neck Surg*. 1996;122:1347.
90. Irwin MS, Thorniley MS, Dore CJ et al. Near infra-red spectroscopy: A non-invasive monitor of perfusion and oxygenation within the microcirculation of limbs and flaps. *Br J Plast Surg*. 1995;48:14.
91. Thorniley MS, Sinclair JS, Barnett NJ et al. The use of near-infrared spectroscopy for assessing flap viability during reconstructive surgery. *Br J Plast Surg*. 1998;51:218.
92. Stranc MF, Sowa MG, Abdulrauf B et al. Assessment of tissue viability using near-infrared spectroscopy. *Br J Plast Surg*. 1998;51:210.

21 Angio-CT Imaging of Deep Inferior Epigastric Artery and Deep Superior Epigastric Artery Perforators

Vachara Niumsawatt, Warren M. Rozen, Mark W. Ashton, Iain S. Whitaker, Emilio García-Tutor, and Alberto Alonso-Burgos

CONTENTS

21.1 OVERVIEW

Breast reconstruction with adipocutaneous free flaps from the abdominal wall combines the benefits of abdominoplasty with those of a prosthesis-free breast reconstruction.[1,2] The deep inferior epigastric perforator (DIEP) flap comprises the dissection of perforating branches of the deep inferior epigastric artery (DIEA) and deep inferior epigastric vein (DIEV) within the rectus abdominis muscle thus sparing both muscle and fascia.[3,4] This aims to reduce abdominal wall morbidity but results in more meticulous surgery and microsurgical revascularisation.[5–19]

Because of the numerous variations in the vascular anatomy of the DIEA, preoperative imaging is useful.[20–30] The ability to preoperatively define the location and diameter of perforating vessels has many advantages: reduced learning curve, operative time, and abdominal morbidity as well as increased flap reliability.[31–34]

21.2 VASCULAR ANATOMY OF DIEP FLAPS: OPTIMISING SUPPLY AND DRAINAGE

Perforating branches of the DIEA and DIEV arise together through the rectus abdominis superficial fascial compounding a vascular pedicle.[35–37] This vascular pedicle is used as vascular supply for DIEP flap. From this point, the main objective of any imaging technique performed for pre-surgical planning of DIEP flap is the identification of vascular pedicles with the widest calibre from those existing in each patient.

From pedicle to skin, the blood supply and drainage to the flap can be classified as having varying segments: the DIEA and DIEV, course deep to the rectus abdominis muscle, the intramuscular course of the DIEA and vein, the intramuscular course of the perforator branches (artery and vein), the pre-fascial course of the perforator branches, and the subcutaneous course.[20,38–40]

Two major philosophies are then followed in the raising of a DIEP flap, and these required different considerations when forming standards in preoperative imaging:

- Some groups routinely use a single vascular pedicle as the sole supply to the DIEP flap. These surgeons describe using only one perforator in up to 90% of the cases, with only the infrequent inclusion of a second perforator.
- Other groups describe the routine use of two or more perforators, with only the infrequent use of a single perforator (less than 20% of cases).

These fundamental differences in philosophy become important when considering the needs of preoperative imaging. When only a single perforator is likely to be used, the transverse intramuscular course is of little concern, as separation of muscle fibres precludes the need for muscle sacrifice. On the other hand, if two or more perforators are used, the transverse course of the perforators necessitates the dissection of the muscle intervening between the two perforators, and thus, preoperative awareness of the transverse course is essential. With these two techniques in mind, an evaluation of the most favourable anatomy for a DIEP flap can be discussed.

There are several factors for choosing a vascular pedicle for performing a DIEP flap, based upon maximising arterial supply and vein drainage as well as the ease and speed of operation and the clinical experience of complication in DIEP flap surgery:

- The size of the vascular pedicle and perforator is intuitive, in terms of optimising supply to the flap.
- Centrality of the perforator similarly maximises the supply to the peripheral parts of the flap (zones III and IV).[41–45]
- A short intramuscular course has several benefits. In all cases, a short, longitudinal, intramuscular course is associated with ease and speed of dissection and the likelihood of less muscular branches requiring ligation. In the case of more than one perforator being included in the flap, a short transverse distance is associated with reduced dissection time and a reduced need for muscle sacrifice.
- A perforating vein that communicates with the superficial system of veins is based on the broad experience that venous congestion is one of the more significant sequelae of DIEP flaps, and, in fact, there was general consensus that evaluation of the venous anatomy was just as, or more, important than evaluation of the arterial supply. This frequent observation was described where venous congestion occurred in cases where there was preferential superficial venous drainage of the flap and that wherever a communication between the deep and superficial venous systems was evident on preoperative angiography, problems with venous drainage were less likely to occur.
- A broad subcutaneous segment and ramification of perforators into the flap improved flap vascularity and flap design.

- A long subfascial segment was sought, as this was associated with a reduced intramuscular course, and tendinous intersections were avoided, as these were associated with difficult dissections.

Of all of these factors, the last two factors were considered the least important for perforator selection, although still worthy of consideration. Evaluation of these eight factors on preoperative imaging was thus considered essential to operative planning.

Then, the *vascular pedicle of my dreams* can thus be described in terms of these segments:[43,46,47]

1. Large-calibre DIEA and vascular pedicle
2. Large-calibre perforator (both artery and veins)
3. Central location within the flap
4. Short intramuscular course perforating veins that communicate with the superficial venous network
5. Broad subcutaneous branching, particularly into the flap
6. Longer subfascial course and avoids tendinous intersections

With this formal classification of the vascular anatomy of DIEP flaps and the requirements for optimal supply in DIEP flaps, the means to identifying these factors preoperatively can thus be easily determined.

21.3 MULTI-SLICES CTA FOR DIEP FLAPS

CTA is currently considered, both in the literature and among current practitioners, as the gold standard in preoperative imaging for DIEP flaps.[27,48–51] It can achieve all of the requirements for perforator mapping as described in this chapter and can do so with high accuracy, low cost, and low interobserver variability. Studies have shown CTA to be significantly more accurate than other imaging modalities, for both perforators mapping and demonstrating all the other vascular pedicle characteristics sought.

From those days when first cases were performed using a 4-row MDCT, limitation from the availability of the machine itself and the associated software is not an excuse to carry out this technique. Nowadays, any MDCT equipment present in any centre where DIEP flap procedures are performed can be used with this purpose. We do not need the latest technology for this exploration or even not the latest reformatting software. Having MDCT equipment with more than 16-row channels will not increase the spatial resolution desirable for this purpose (resulting slice width of less than 0.5 mm) but will decrease the exploration timing (apnoea). The image quality from angio-CT studies was obtained from the 4-row versus 64-row MDCT, and no subjective differences in the image quality were noticed (Figure 21.1). Thus, with a careful selection of the patient, range, flap procedure, and optimisation of the angio-CT scanning technique, the preoperative flap imaging is feasible by using a non-last-generation MDCT. Limitations of this technique refer mainly to limitations inherent to any MDCT angiographic study (radiation, iodinate contrast medium, and technical resources).

The highest spatial resolution and a Z-axis faster coverage of the 64-row MDCT or even the latest 256-row, compared with the first 4-row scanner, allowed a most easy and feasible range of exploration. This decisive advantage allows exploring the selected range in less time, avoiding motion artefacts and minimising the apnoea time needed (Figure 21.2). With the introduction of 64-row or beyond scanners, gantry rotation time is now less than 0.4 s; a slice thickness of 0.6 mm and a spatial resolution of 0.3 mm are now possible. Another important advantage is the ability to acquire data as isotropic voxels. This allows images in any plane or perspective with equally good spatial resolution. Isotropic resolution is critical to the management of large data sets. It is also known that using last-generation MDCT scans, radiation and contrast media needed are also optimised.

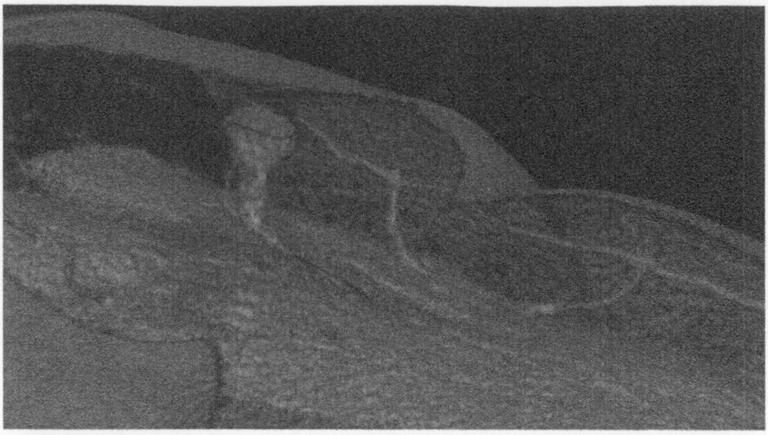

(a)

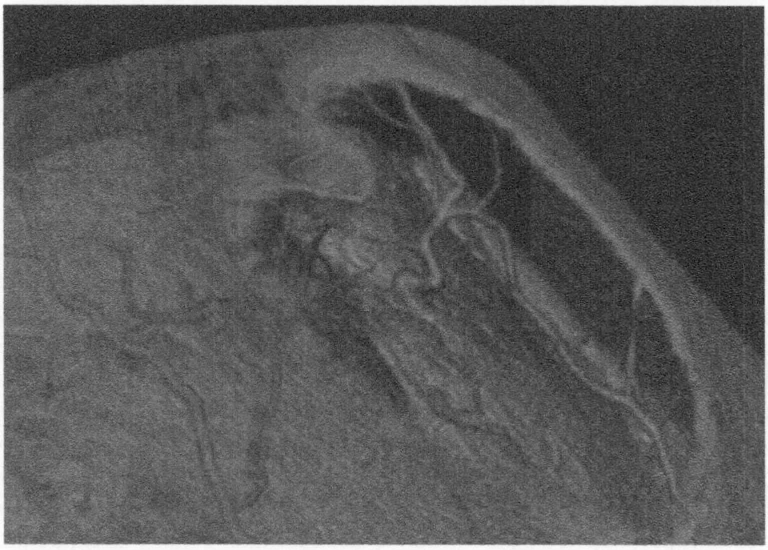

(b)

FIGURE 21.1 (a and b) CTA VR images taken from the first cases during the initial experience with CTA for DIEP flaps using a 4-row MDCT equipment. Image quality and information equal to those routinely carried out today with last-generation ones.

The radiation dose has been widely discussed and, although worthy of consideration, is not as significant as may have been initially thought. Studies of the radiation dosage have been performed across institutions, and when limited to the scanning range described earlier, the radiation dose is less than 6 mSV, which is considerably less than a standard abdominal CT scan and is the dose associated with four abdominal plain films. Considering the advantages of this technique referred to the planned surgery and also considering this exploration as a *one in a lifetime*, few would be concerned by this degree of radiation exposure. There are much more benefits than risks. In this sense, radiation dose reduction software and algorithms are however an interest and useful tool present only in the latest-generation equipments.[52,53]

The only relative contraindications for the use of CT is severe claustrophobia (although scan times are but a few seconds), a sensitivity to the intravenous contrast, or renal impairment.

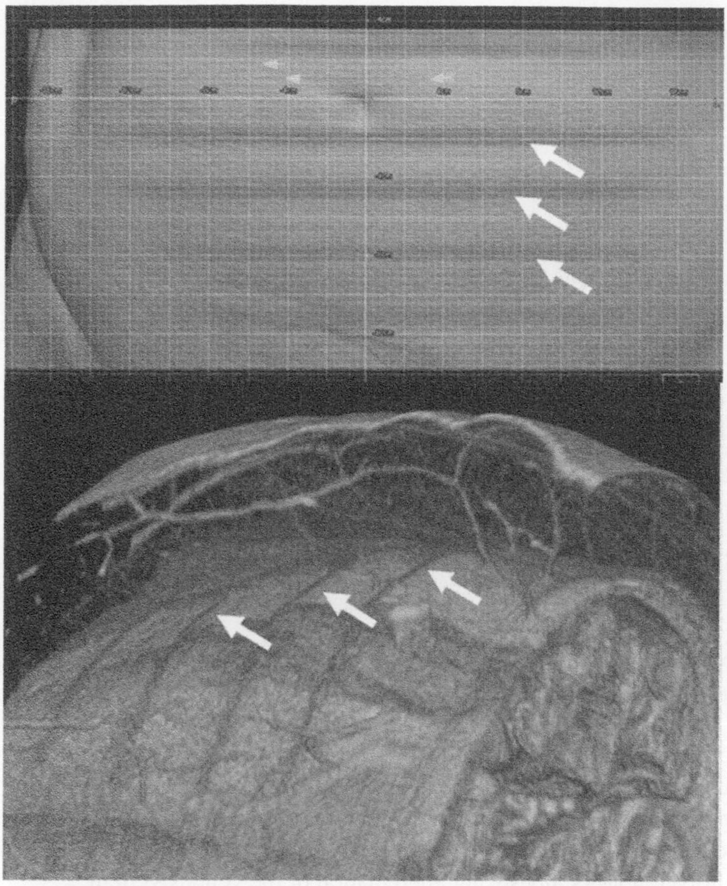

FIGURE 21.2 VR images taken from the first cases during the initial experience with angio-CT for DIEP flaps using a 4-row MDCT equipment where motion artefacts due to lack of apnoea capability.

21.4 SCANNING PROTOCOL

21.4.1 Scanning Timing

The scanning protocols are worthy of discussion, as two modes of scanning were described. Both methods used a bolus-tracking technique to identify filling of the appropriate vessels with contrast as a means to initiate scanning (Figure 21.3).

- The first technique, after identifying contrast filling, used an extensive delay before scanning, creating a venous-phase scan, which was able to achieve maximal filling of both arterial perforators and veins. When using a 64-row scanner, a 50 s delay was used. The benefit of this technique is a thorough examination of both arteries and veins, which is essential to complete preoperative planning. Although the DIEA and DIEV can be readily differentiated, the downside of such an approach is that there is very little ability to differentiate between the perforating arteries and veins and thus there is a risk of confounders. Similarly, the superficial inferior epigastric artery (SIEA) is difficult to assess with this method, both due to confounding by the superficial inferior epigastric veins (SIEVs) and by some inadequacy in filling by the timing of the scan. Haemodynamics of perforator vessels, compared with well-known haemodynamics in the intra-abdominal territories, would explain the delayed enhancement of the perforator vessels.

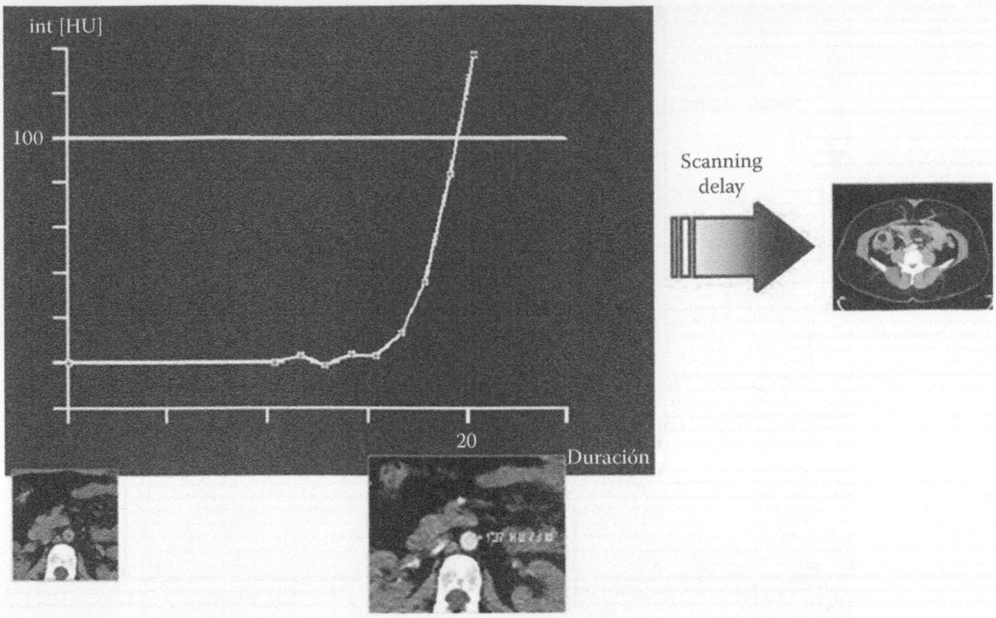

FIGURE 21.3 Bolus-tracking technique: after contrast injection and selected triggering threshold is reached, a preselected delay is awaited for the scanning.

- The second method of scanning does not use any delay in scanning after the contrast reaches the appropriate vessels, limited only by the minimal delay of the particular scanner (approximately 4 s). This is, therefore, a pure *arterial-phase* scan, which provides a presumed improved accuracy for perforating artery mapping and for demonstrating the SIEA; however, it lacks any strong appreciation of the venous system.

21.4.2 Study Range

One of the main steps in the scan protocol includes selecting the proper study range. In each patient, the scan range necessarily needs to include the surgical field, known for both the surgeon and radiologist. The position of the patient at the CT table should be equal to the final position adopted at the operating room. For a precise study of DIEP flaps, the range planned should include an upper limit 2–4 cm above the umbilicus and 12 cm below (origin of the DIEA and SIEA on the common femoral). Thus, the scanning protocol is focused and optimised only to explore the area of interest for the surgeon, avoiding unnecessary radiation and contrast media (Figure 21.4).

It is widely considered that CTA of internal mammary recipient vessels is not routinely indicated for several reasons. First, if patients have had any previous thoracic imaging with CT, these vessels can be well evaluated on these scans (Figure 21.5). Furthermore, ultrasonography is frequently available and is usually sufficient to identify and describe these vessels. However, where neither of these modalities is available, CTA may be an alternative option. The benefits of CTA must be balanced against its risks, which include contrast nephrotoxicity and allergic reactions, and radiation exposure. The radiation risk with thoracic imaging is substantially higher than that for donor sites, such as the abdominal wall, with reasons including exposure of the contralateral breast to radiation, as well as proximity to the thyroid gland. Current evidence suggests that although many cases may not warrant such imaging because of the risk, the benefits of preoperative CTA in selected patients may outweigh the risks of exposure, prompting an individualised approach.

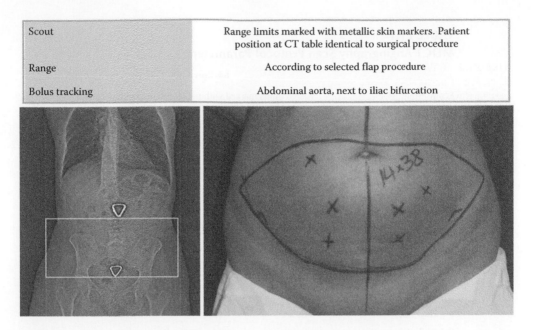

Scout	Range limits marked with metallic skin markers. Patient position at CT table identical to surgical procedure
Range	According to selected flap procedure
Bolus tracking	Abdominal aorta, next to iliac bifurcation

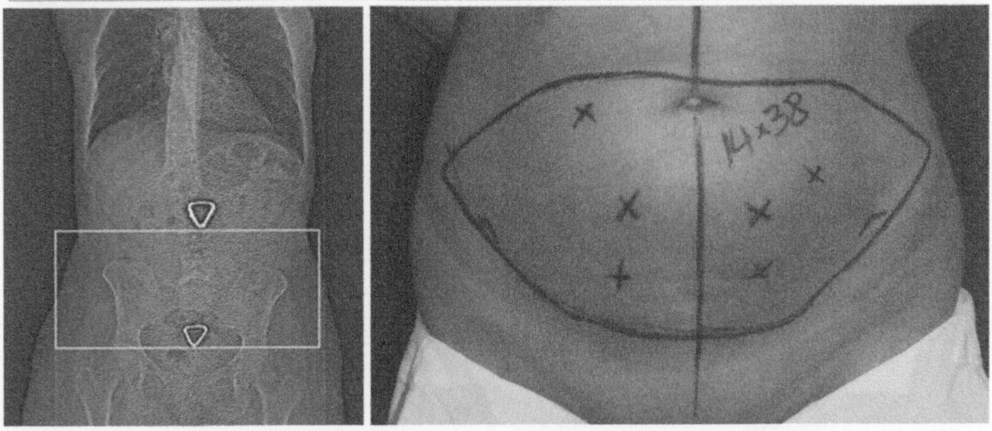

FIGURE 21.4 Scanning range selection. Scout and exploration are performed in the same position than surgery. Note metallic skin marks located during scout planning and after removed.

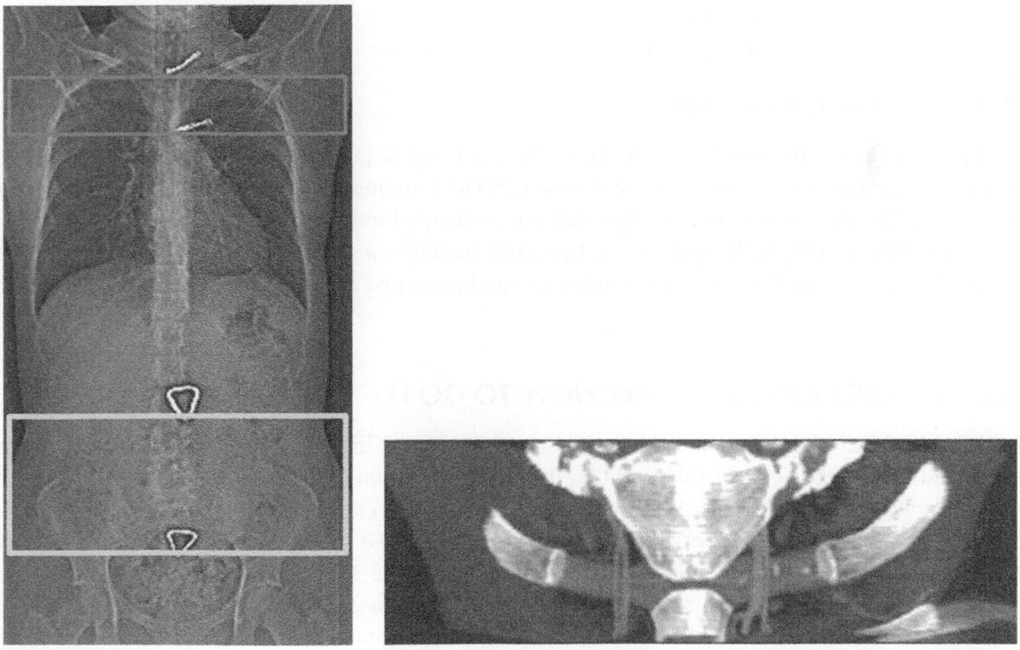

(a) (b)

FIGURE 21.5 (a) Scanning range selection in a patient where DIEP flap was planned. (b) Same patient as (a), planning of scan range where the internal mammary vessels are evaluated.

TABLE 21.1
MDCT Angiography Scan Protocol Parameters

	64-Row MDCT
Scout	Range limits marked with metallic skin markers. Patient position at CT table identical to surgical procedure
Range	According to selected flap procedure
Bolus tracking	Abdominal aorta, next to iliac bifurcation
Range acquisition parameters	
Triggering threshold	100 H.U.[a]
Collimation	0.6 mm
kV	120
mA s	200
Rotation time	0.5 s
Scan delay	60 s
Pitch	0.7
Contrast media	
Volume	120 cc
Flow rate	4 cc/s
Saline flush	
Volume	50 cc
Flow rate	4 cc/s
Reconstruction	
Slice thickness	0.75 mm
Reconstruction interval	0.4
Kernel	B10f

[a] H.U., Hounsfield units.

21.4.3 Technical Parameters

Scan protocol is summarised in Table 21.1. The scanning is performed in a breath-hold with the patient in supine position with arms-up position. MDCT angiography was performed following an injection of 120 mL of iodixanol contrast medium (320 mg of iodine per mL) at a flow rate of 4 mL/s by using bolus-tracking technique. No oral contrast medium is given. Patients did not wear clothes during the studies, so as to reproduce surgical conditions and to avoid artefacts in the images of postprocessing.

21.5 PREOPERATIVE IMAGING: HOW TO DO IT

Surgeons and radiologists must work together and as a team in the undertaking of thorough scan interpretation – there is a learning curve to the communication between teams, understanding the goals of imaging and surgery, and certainly in scan interpretation. Misunderstanding, breaking down of communication, or poor confidence will spoil any case as a bad selection criterion or a bad imaging technique. Co-interpretation of the imaging data in a 3D format, following the pedicle from its origin and through the soft tissues, is mandatory. That virtual surgery is indeed performed. This also saves time. We established this through lengthy international collaborations between radiological and surgical teams and in fact established an international meeting to discuss and clarify the aims and objectives of such a collaborative effort (Figure 21.6).

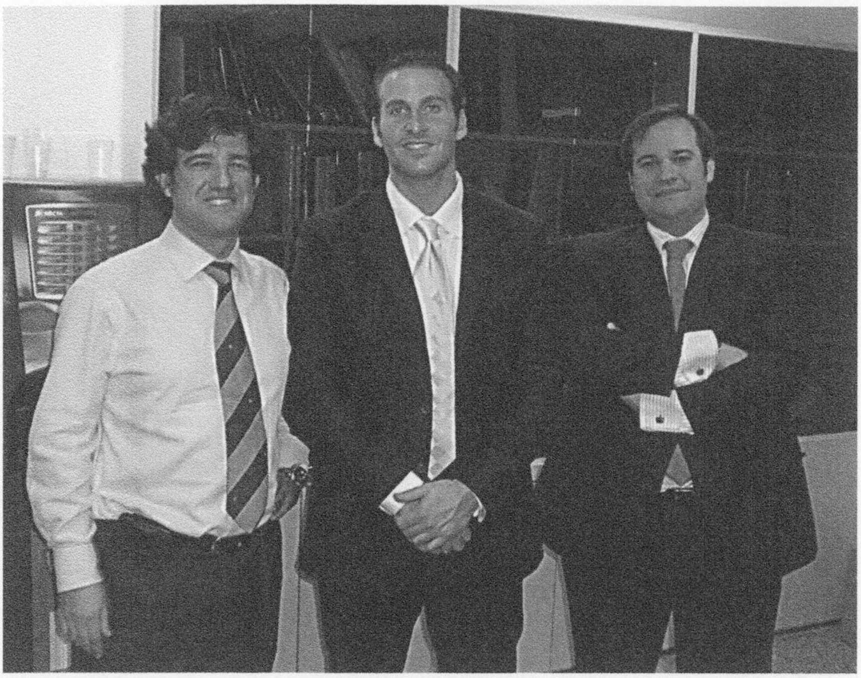

FIGURE 21.6 Working as a team is essential and the key point for this technique. From left to right, Dr. E. Garcia-Tutor, W. Rozen, and A. Alonso-Burgos during Navarra meeting in 2008; different perspectives from radiologist to surgeon, but a common interest in achieving optimal patient outcomes from imaging.

Three-dimensional reconstructions are essential in order to achieve the images discussed previously. These are achieved using computer software that performs multiplanar reconstructions. Volume-rendered technique (VRT) and maximum-intensity projection (MIP) reconstructions are widely used for this purpose and can be achieved with a wide variety of software programs from many software companies. MIP reconstructions are optimal for demonstrating vascular pedicles and intramuscular course. VRT reconstructions assign colour to data points which display a 2D representation of the 3D data set and are thus useful for representing the subcutaneous course of perforators and for generating perforator-location maps.

Selected images can be taken to the operating room in a portable USB stick in any feasible digital format. At the time of surgery, the surgeon marked the location previously described on the patient's skin with the aid of a metric rule.

Regardless, certain images are worth capturing in two dimensions for reference at subsequent stages, and these are as follows.

21.5.1 Location Maps

Two anterior views of the abdominal wall are preferred that demonstrate the location of perforators at the plane at which they emerge from the rectus sheath. Of these two views, the first should include a view that demonstrates the relative size of the perforators (with the locations shown) (Figure 21.7), and the second view should demonstrate the DIEA and its main branching pattern (with the location of perforators superimposed) (Figure 21.8). It is with these two views that the relative size of perforators and the location of perforators relative to their source vessels can be clearly seen.

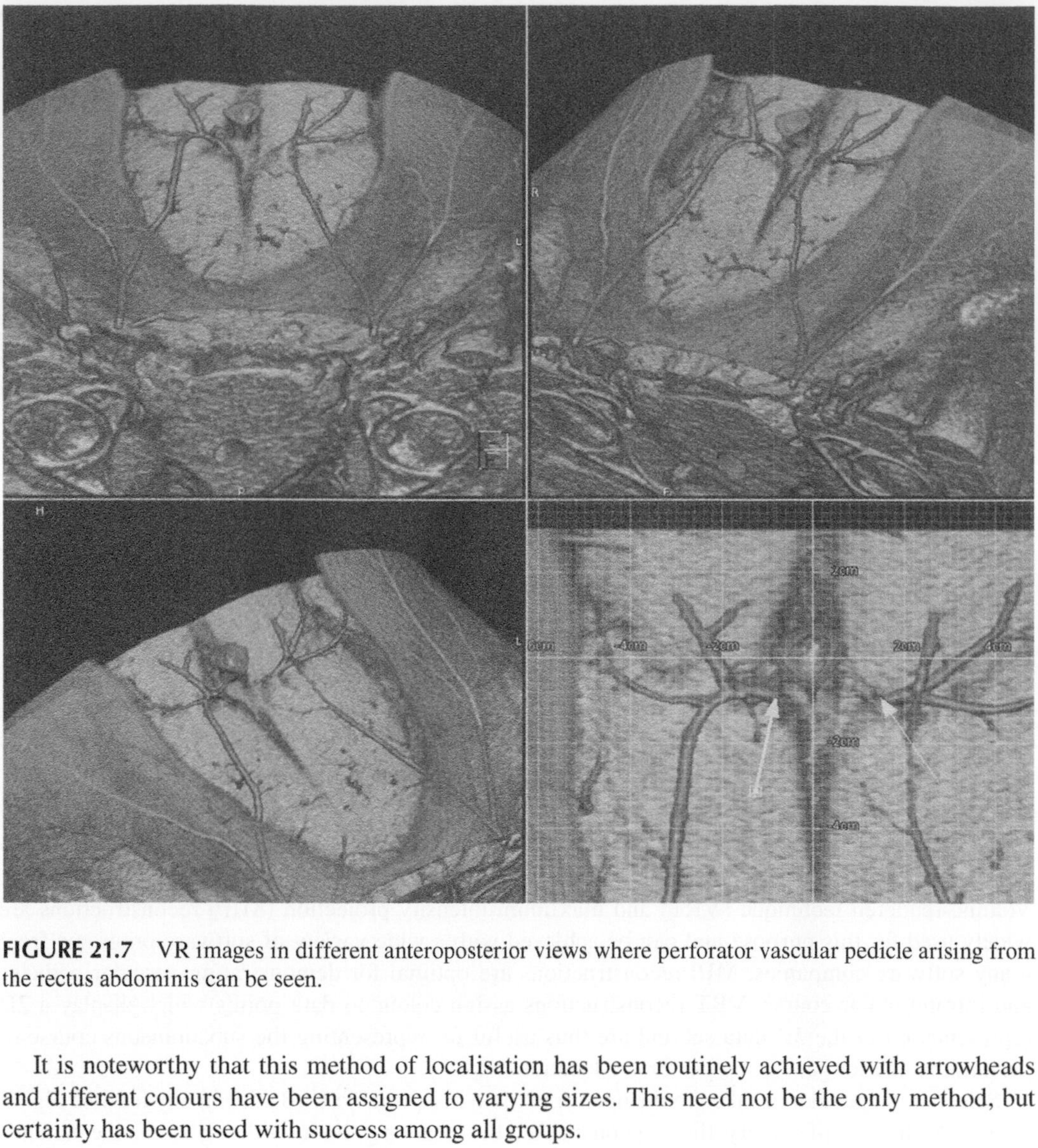

FIGURE 21.7 VR images in different anteroposterior views where perforator vascular pedicle arising from the rectus abdominis can be seen.

It is noteworthy that this method of localisation has been routinely achieved with arrowheads and different colours have been assigned to varying sizes. This need not be the only method, but certainly has been used with success among all groups.

The routine point of reference for localisation has been the umbilicus, and this has been achieved with success; however, other methods, such as skin-attached markers, have also been used successfully. Considering the umbilicus as an arbitrary central reference position (position X:0, Y:0), the exact location and course of the arterial perforators and the point at which they pierced the muscular fascia are pinpointed in the skin surface 3D-volume-rendered (VR) reconstruction with the aid of a grid (Figure 21.9).

21.5.2 Vascular Pedicle

A view of the pedicle and its branching pattern is essential in order to plan the branch of choice for inclusion as the vascular pedicle as well as to estimate its calibre. This is usually achieved in one of the location maps, but, where this is not possible, a separate image may be required. Perforator vessels with the widest diameters (parameter evaluated in the MIP reconstruction) and with a predicted easy dissection were reported and marked in each patient (Figure 21.10). Considering the fascia

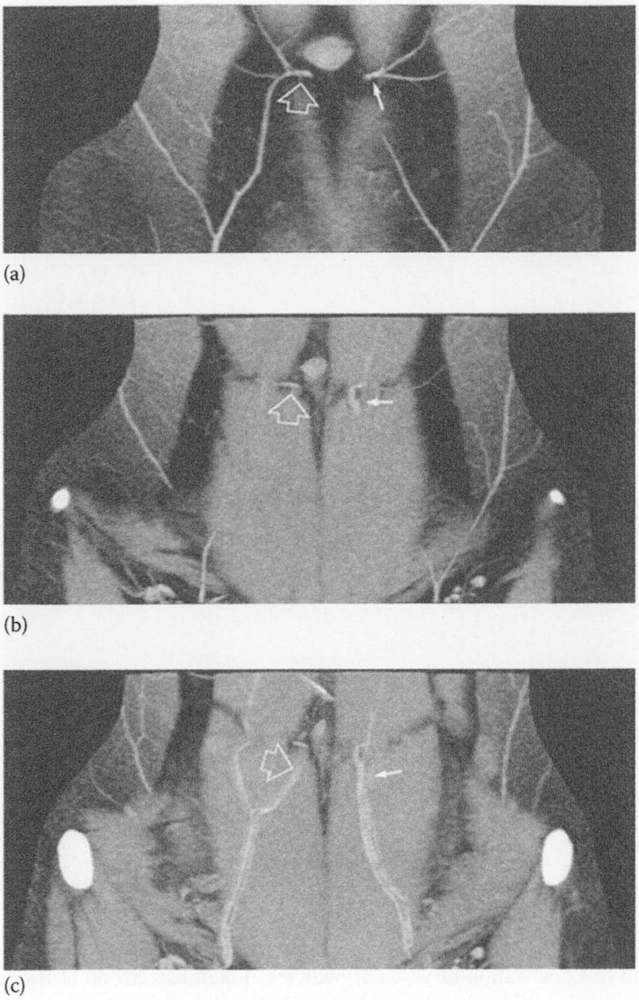

FIGURE 21.8 MIP consecutive coronal images where perforator vascular pedicle branching pattern from DIEA and vein can be seen.

penetration pattern, we considered as predicted easy dissection perforator vessels those in which a perpendicular fascia penetration pattern. Perforator vessels with a subfascial or epifascial course were considered as potential alternatives (Figure 21.11).

21.5.3 Intramuscular Course

The intramuscular course is highly important and needs to be demonstrated with imaging. As discussed, the longitudinal transverse distance is important in all cases as a means to predicting the extent of intramuscular dissection. This is best demonstrated with a curved, longitudinal MIP view on CTA (Figure 21.12).

The transverse distance is not highly important in the situation where a single perforator is used in the raising of a DIEP flap, and thus, a view demonstrating this transverse course is not routinely required for some institutions. However, for institutions where multiple perforators are routinely selected for the supply to flaps, visualisation of the transverse intramuscular distance is highly important. This is best demonstrated with axial MIP or curve-MIP views on CTA.

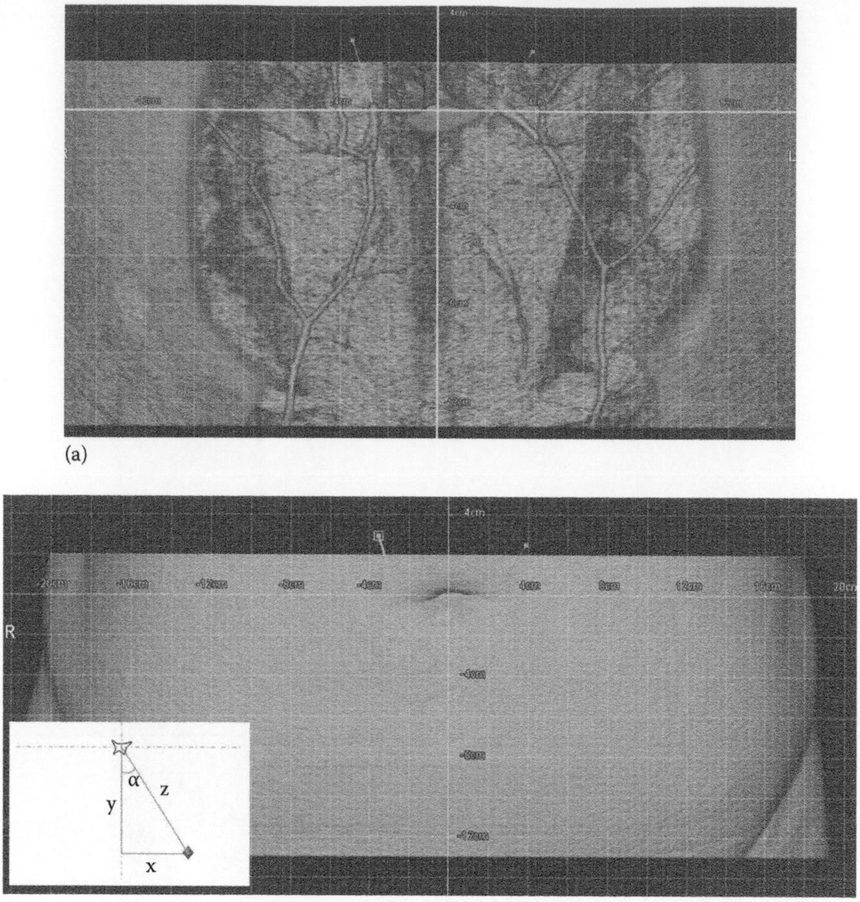

FIGURE 21.9 (a and b) Localisation of vascular pedicles. Taken as zero point the umbilicus, a Cartesian axes system can be applied for easy achieving with the aid of a grid.

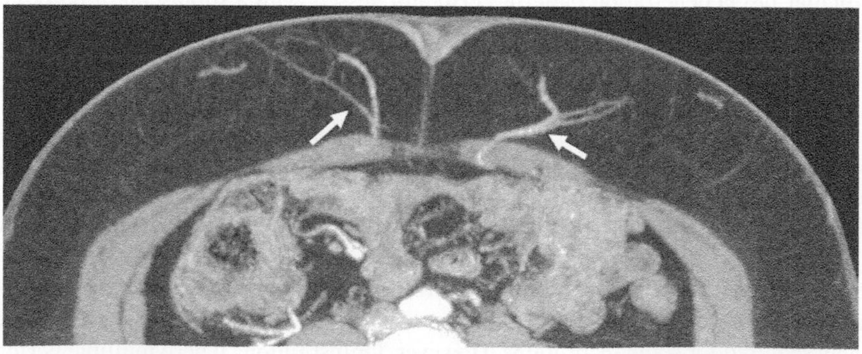

FIGURE 21.10 Axial MIP image where two main perforators vascular pedicles can be seen arising from the rectus abdominis and branching in the subcutaneous tissue (arrows).

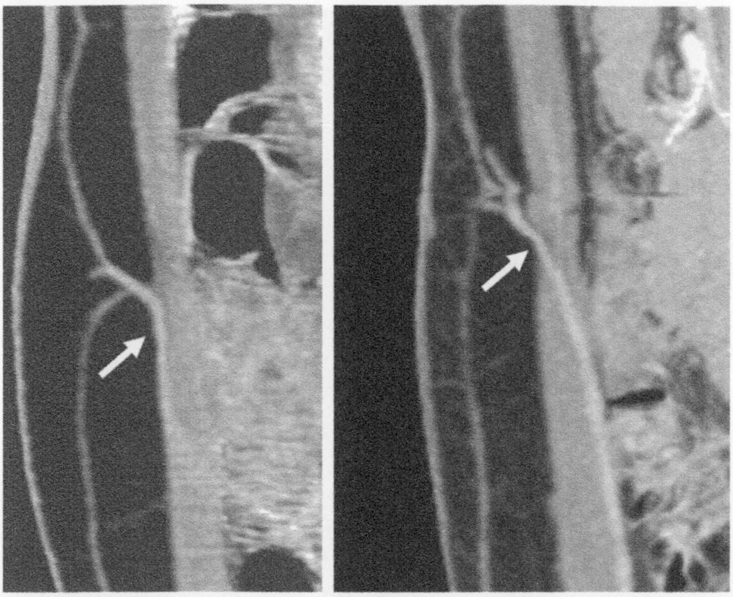

FIGURE 21.11 Sagittal MIP images where two fascial penetration patterns in two different main perforator vascular pedicles can be seen: subfascial (right) and direct (left).

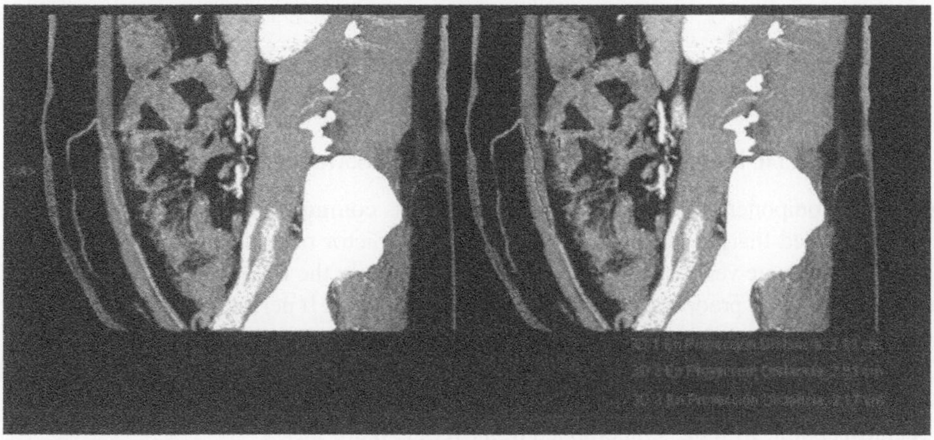

FIGURE 21.12 Curved MIP reformatted images where the intramuscular course of perforator vascular pedicles can be estimated.

21.5.4 Superficial Inferior Epigastric Artery and Vein

The views of the SIEA and superficial inferior epigastric vein (SIEV) are important for consideration of raising an SIEA flap.[44,54–57] An SIEA is only present with a calibre sufficient to raise an SIEA flap in up to 30% of patients, and this may certainly be predicted on preoperative imaging. Many surgeons routinely identify and preserve the SIEA intra-operatively for use as the major vascular pedicle or for preservation if the need for vascular augmentation is required.[44,54–69] More significantly, evaluation of the SIEV is highly important for predicting and planning the venous drainage of the flap, particularly as the SIEV and SIEA usually enter the abdominal wall pannus considerably distant from each other. Few authors would dispute that venous congestion is one of the more significant flap-related complications of DIEP flaps, and evaluation of the venous drainage on preoperative imaging is thus highly important (Figure 21.13).

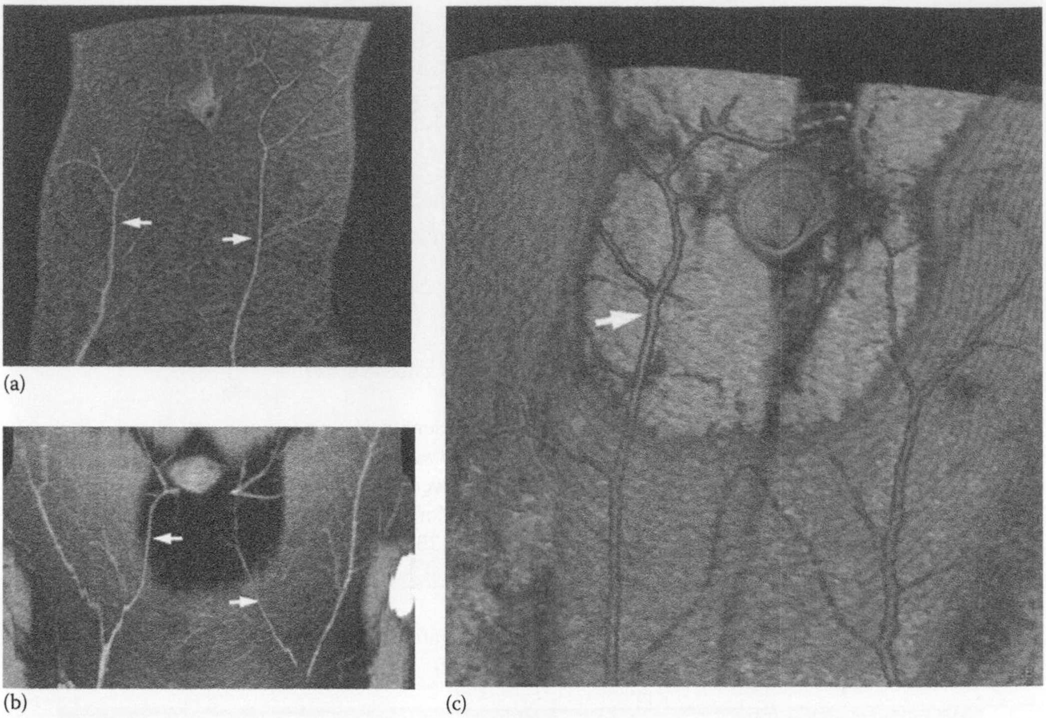

FIGURE 21.13 Preoperative CTA with VR images where the SIEV as drainage of perforator veins can be seen.

21.5.5 Superficial Inferior Epigastric Vein to Perforator Communication

An additional component of evaluation of the SIEV is its communication with the DIEV. Blondeel et al. demonstrated that a large SIEV system was a predictor of preferential superficial drainage and thus of inadequate venous drainage of the flap when only the DIEV was used in the flap. More recent experience with preoperative imaging has suggested that if perforating veins are clearly visualised as communicating with the SIEV, then adequate venous drainage can be predicted.

We suggest, per se, that a clear demonstration of this communication with the selected perforator(s) be demonstrated. In the case of CTA, this view is best achieved with a sagittal/oblique VRT reconstruction, with the skin cropped (removed) (Figure 21.13).

21.5.6 Abdominal Wall Competence and Contour

Often incorporated into one of the perforator-location maps, a view and evaluation of the deep fascial layers of the abdominal wall are required. This should include evaluation of the width and competence of the linea alba (for divarication of recti), assessment for any other scars or hernias, and an assessment of the thickness of rectus abdominis muscle. These factors can all help to predict abdominal wall complications and the need for greater attention to abdominal wall closure.

21.6 SUMMARY

Although there are generally low morbidity and in particular flap failure rate associated with DIEP flaps for autologous breast reconstruction, improvements in outcomes can still be achieved with an improvement in understanding of patients' anatomy.[29,30] Important information regarding perforators' location and characteristic are crucial in order to assist reconstructive surgeons in selection of an idea perforator to support the flap. Perforator selection is based on size, location, intramuscular, subcutaneous courses, and their association with motor nerves. With significant variability between individuals, a preoperative imaging has become an essential element of DIEP flap surgery. An accurate imaging can assist in patient selection, plan the operative technique, reduce operating time, and improve operative outcomes. Due to the ease, availability, high specificity, and sensitivity of CTA compared to other investigative modalities, it has become the current gold standard in preoperative DIEP flap reconstruction imaging.[48,50–53] Further improvement in computer software technology has allowed reconstructive surgeons to evaluate and manipulate digital images in 3D view or virtual reality. Thus, reconstructive surgeons can appreciate the viable anatomy of each individual patient and recognise any potential problem even before patients enter the operating theatre.

REFERENCES

1. Allen RJ, Treece P. Deep inferior epigastric perforator flap for breast reconstruction. *Ann Plast Surg* 1994;32(1):32–38.
2. Itoh Y, Arai K. The deep inferior epigastric artery free skin flap: Anatomic study and clinical application. *Plast Reconstr Surg* 1993;91(5):853–863.
3. Keller A. The deep inferior epigastric perforator free flap for breast reconstruction. *Ann Plast Surg* 2001;46(5):474–479.
4. Keller A. Fat necrosis in free rectus abdominis and deep inferior epigastric perforator flaps. *Plast Reconstr Surg* 2001;107:1611–1612.
5. Bajaj AK, Chevray PM, Chang DW. Comparison of donor site complications and functional outcomes in free muscle-sparing TRAM flap and free DIEP flap breast reconstruction. *Plast Reconstr Surg* 2006;117(3):737–746.
6. Blondeel N, Vanderstraeten GG, Monstrey SJ, Van Landuyt K, Tonnard P, Lysens R, Boeckx WD, Matton G. The donor site morbidity of free DIEP flaps and free TRAM flaps for breast reconstruction. *Br J Plast Surg* 1997;50(5):322–330.
7. Blondeel PN. One hundred free DIEP flap breast reconstructions: A personal experience. *Br J Plast Surg* 1999;52(2):104–111.
8. Bottero L, Lefaucheur JP, Fadhul S, Raulo Y, Collins ED, Lantieri L. Electromyographic assessment of rectus abdominis muscle function after deep inferior epigastric perforator flap surgery. *Plast Reconstr Surg* 2004;113(1):156–161.
9. Futter CM, Webster MH, Hagen S, Mitchell SL. A retrospective comparison of abdominal muscle strength following breast reconstruction with a free TRAM or DIEP flap. *Br J Plast Surg* 2000;53(7):578–583.
10. Garvey PB, Buchel EW, Pockaj BA, Casey W Jr, Gray RJ, Hernández JL, Samson TD. DIEP and pedicled TRAM flaps: A comparison of outcomes. *Plast Reconstr Surg* 2006;117(6):1711–1719.
11. Gill PS, Hunt JP, Guerra AB, Dellacroce FJ, Sullivan SK, Boraski J, Metzinger SE, Dupin CL, Allen RJ. A 10-year retrospective review of 758 DIEP flaps for breast reconstruction. *Plast Reconstr Surg* 2004;113(4):1153–1160.
12. Granzow JW, Levine JL, Chiu ES, Allen RJ. Breast reconstruction with the deep inferior epigastric perforator flap: History and an update on current technique. *J Plast Reconstr Aesthet Surg* 2006;69(6):571–579.
13. Hamdi M, Weiler-Mithoff EM, Webster MHC. Deep inferior epigastric perforator flap in breast reconstruction: Experience with the first 50 flaps. *Plast Reconstr Surg* 1999;103:86–95.
14. Hofer SO, Damen TH, Mureau MA, Rakhorst HA, Roche NA. A critical review of perioperative complications in 175 free deep inferior epigastric perforator flap breast reconstructions. *Ann Plast Surg* 2007;59(2):137–142.
15. Nahabedian MY. Secondary operations of the anterior abdominal wall following microvascular breast reconstruction with the TRAM and DIEP flaps. *Plast Reconstr Surg* 2007;120(2):365–372.
16. Nahabedian MY, Momen B. Lower abdominal bulge after deep inferior epigastric perforator flap (DIEP) breast reconstruction. *Ann Plast Surg* 2005;54(2):124–129.
17. Nahabedian MY, Momen B, Galdino G, Manson PN. Breast reconstruction with the free TRAM or DIEP flap: Patient selection, choice of flap, and outcome. *Plast Reconstr Surg* 2002;110(2):466–475.
18. Schaverien MV, Perks AGB, McCulley SJ. Comparison of outcomes and donor-site morbidity in unilateral free TRAM versus DIEP flap breast reconstruction. *J Plast Reconstr Aesthet Surg* 2007;60(11):1219–1224.
19. Tran NV, Buchel EW, Convery PA. Microvascular complications of DIEP flaps. *Plast Reconst Surg* 2007;119(5):1397–1405.

20. Heitmann C, Felmerer G, Durmus C, Matejic B, Ingianni G. Anatomical features of perforator blood vessels in the deep inferior epigastric perforator flap. *Br J Plast Surg* 2000;53(3):205–208.
21. Heo C, Yoo J, Minn K, Kim S. Circummuscular variant of the deep inferior epigastric perforator in breast reconstruction: Importance of preoperative multidetector computed tomographic angiography. *Aesthetic Plast Surg* 2008;32(5):817–819.
22. Lasso JM, Sancho M, Campo V, Jimenez E, Perez CR. Epiperitoneal vessels: More resources to perform DIEP flaps. *J Plast Reconstr Aesthet Surg* 2008;61(7):826–829.
23. Rozen WM, Houseman ND, Ashton MW. The circummuscular or paramuscular variants of deep inferior epigastric perforators detected with CTA: Should these be called variants at all? *Aesthetic Plast Surg* 2009;33(1):119–120.
24. Rozen WM, Houseman ND, Ashton MW. The absent inferior epigastric artery: A unique anomaly and implications for deep inferior epigastric artery perforator flaps. *J Reconstr Microsurg* 2009;25(5):289–293.
25. Whitaker IS, Rozen WM, Smit JM, Dimopoulou A, Ashton MW, Acosta R. Peritoneo-cutaneous perforators in deep inferior epigastric perforator flaps: A cadaveric dissection and computed tomographic angiography study. *Microsurgery* 2009;29(2):124–127.
26. Yano K, Hosokawa K, Nakai K, Kubo T. A rare variant of the deep inferior epigastric perforator: Importance of preoperative color-flow duplex scanning assessment. *Plast Reconstr Surg* 2003;111:1578–1579.
27. Alonso-Burgos A, Garcia-Tutor E, Bastarrika G, Cano D, Martinez-Cuesta A, Pina LJ. Preoperative planning of deep inferior epigastric artery perforator flap reconstruction with multi-slice-CT angiography: Imaging findings and initial experience. *J Plast Reconstr Aesthet Surg* 2006;59(6):585–593.
28. Rozen WM, Ashton MW. Modifying techniques in deep inferior epigastric artery perforator flap harvest with the use of preoperative imaging. *ANZ J Surg* 2009;79(9):598–603.
29. Rozen WM, Garcia-Tutor E, Alonso-Burgos A, Acosta R, Stillaert F, Zubieta JL, Hamdi M, Whitaker IS, Ashton MW. Planning and optimizing DIEP flaps with virtual surgery: The Navarra experience. *J Plast Reconst Aesth Surg* 2010;2010(63):2.
30. Rozen WM, Phillips TJ, Stella DL, Ashton MW. Preoperative CT angiography for DIEP flaps: 'must-have' lessons for the radiologist. *J Plast Reconstr Aesthet Surg* 2009;62(12): e650–e651.
31. Acosta R, Enajat M, Rozen WM, Smit JM, Wagstaff MJ, Whitaker IS, Audolfsson T. Performing two DIEP flaps in a working day: An achievable and reproducible practice. *J Plast Reconstr Aesthet Surg* 2010;63(4):648–654.
32. Ang GG, Rozen WM, Chauhan A, Acosta R. The pedicled 'propeller' deep inferior epigastric perforator (DIEP) flap for a large abdominal wall defect. *J Plast Reconstr Aesthet Surg* 2011;64(1):133–135.
33. Binder JP, Méria P, Desgrandchamps F, Revol M, Servant JM. Vaginal reconstruction after anterior pelvectomy by deep inferior epigastric perforator flap (DIEP). *Ann Urol (Paris)* 2006;40(3):192–202.
34. Zeng A, Xu J, Yan X, You L, Yang H. Pedicled deep inferior epigastric perforator flap: An alternative method to repair groin and scrotal defects. *Ann Plast Surg* 2006;57(3):285–288.
35. Boyd JB, Taylor GI, Corlett RJ. The vascular territories of the superior epigastric and deep inferior epigastric systems. *Plast Reconstr Surg* 1984;73(1):1–16.
36. Tansatit T, Chokrungvaranont P, Sanguansit P, Wanidchaphloi S. Neurovascular anatomy of the deep inferior epigastric perforator flap for breast reconstruction. *J Med Assoc Thai* 2006;89(10):1630–1640.
37. Taylor GI, Corlett RJ, Boyd JB. The versatile deep inferior epigastric (inferior rectus abdominis) flap. *Br J Plast Surg* 1984;37(3):330–350.
38. Kikuchi N, Murakami G, Kashiwa H, Homma K, Sato TJ, Ogino T. Morphometrical study of the arterial perforators of the deep inferior epigastric perforator flap. *Surg Radiol Anat* 2001;23(6):375–381.
39. Vandevoort M, Vranckx JJ, Fabre G. Perforator topography of the deep inferior epigastric perforator flap in 100 cases of breast reconstruction. *Plast Reconstr Surg* 2006;109(6):1912–1918.
40. Rozen WM, Murray ACA, Ashton MW, Bloom R, Stella DL, Phillips TJ, Taylor GI. The cutaneous course of deep inferior epigastric perforators: Implications for flap thinning. *J Plast Reconstr Aesth Surg* 2009;62(8):986–990.
41. Holm C, Mayr M, Hofter E, Ninkovic M. Perfusion zones of the DIEP flap revisited: A clinical study. *Plast Reconstr Surg* 2006;117(1):37–43.
42. Rahmanian-Schwarz A, Rothenberger J, Hirt B, Luz O, Schaller HE. A combined anatomical and clinical study for quantitative analysis of the microcirculation in the classic perfusion zones of the deep inferior epigastric artery perforator flap. *Plast Reconstr Surg* 2011;127(2):505–513.
43. Rozen WM, Ashton MW, Le Roux CM, Pan WR, Corlett RJ. The perforator angiosome: A new concept in the design of deep inferior epigastric artery perforator flaps for breast reconstruction. *Microsurgery* 2010;30(1):1–7. Epub July 6 2009.

44. Schaverien M, Saint-Cyr M, Arbique G, Brown SA. Arterial and venous anatomies of the deep inferior epigastric perforator and superficial inferior epigastric artery flaps. *Plast Reconstr Surg* 2008;121(6):1909–1919.
45. Wong C, Saint-Cyr M, Mojallal A, Schaub T, Bailey SH, Myers S, Brown S, Rohrich RJ. Perforasomes of the DIEP flap: Vascular anatomy of the lateral versus medial row perforators and clinical implications. *Plast Reconstr Surg* 2010;125(3):772–782.
46. Rozen WM, Ashton MW, Murray ACA, Taylor GI. Avoiding denervation of rectus abdominis during DIEP flap harvest: The importance of medial row perforators. *Plast Reconstr Surg* 2008;122(3):710–716.
47. Rozen WM, Kiil BJ, Ashton MW, Grinsell D, Seneviratne S, Taylor GI. Avoiding denervation of rectus abdominis during DIEP flap harvest II: An intraoperative assessment of the nerves to rectus. *Plast Reconstr Surg* 2008 November;122(5):1321–1325.
48. Casey W Jr, Chew RT, Rebecca AM, Smith AA, Collins JM, Pockaj BA. Advantages of preoperative computed tomography in deep inferior epigastric artery perforator flap breast reconstruction. *Plast Reconstr Surg* 2009;123(4):1148–1155.
49. Mah E, Temple F, Morrison WA. Value of pre-operative Doppler ultrasound assessment of deep inferior epigastric perforators in free flap breast reconstruction. *ANZ J Surg* 2005;75(Suppl.): A89–A97.
50. Masia J, Larranaga JR, Clavero JA, Vives L, Pons G, Pons JM. The value of the multidetector row computed tomography for the preoperative planning of deep inferior epigastric artery perforator flap. *Ann Plast Surg* 2008;60(1):29–36.
51. Mihara M, Nakanishi M, Nakashima M, Narushima M, Koshima I. Utility and anatomical examination of the DIEP flap's three dimensional image with multidetector computed tomography. *Plast Reconstr Surg* 2008;122:40–41e.
52. Rozen WM, Whitaker IS, Stella DL, Phillips TJ, Einsiedel PF, Acosta R, Ashton MW. The radiation exposure of computed tomographic angiography (CTA) in DIEP flap planning: Low dose but high impact. *J Plast Reconstr Aesthet Surg* 2009;62(12): e654–e655.
53. Rozen WM, Whitaker IS, Wagstaff MJD, Ashton MW, Acosta R. The financial implications of computed tomographic angiography (CTA) in DIEP flap surgery: A cost analysis. *Microsurgery* 2009;29(2):168–169.
54. Villafane O, Gahankari D, Webster M. Superficial inferior epigastric vein (SIEV): 'lifeboat' for DIEP/TRAM flaps. *Br J Plast Surg* 1999;52(7):599.
55. Rozen WM, Chubb D, Grinsell D, Ashton MW. The variability of the superficial inferior epigastric artery (SIEA) and its angiosome: A clinical anatomical study. *Microsurgery* 2010 January 7 [Epub ahead of print].
56. Rozen WM, Chubb D, Whitaker IS, Ashton MW. The importance of the superficial venous anatomy of the abdominal wall in planning a superficial inferior epigastric artery (SIEA) flap: Case report and clinical study. *Microsurgery* 2011;31(6):454–457.
57. Rozen WM, Grinsell D, Ashton MW. The perforating superficial inferior epigastric vein: A new anatomical variant detected with computed tomographic angiography. *Plast Reconstr Surg* 2010;125(3):119e–120e.
58. Allen RJ. In discussion of Chevray PM. Breast reconstruction with superficial inferior epigastric artery flaps: A prospective comparison with TRAM and DIEP flaps. *Plast Reconstr Surg* 2004 October;114(5):1077–1083. *Plast Reconstr Surg* 2004;114(5):1084–1085.
59. Arnez ZM, Khan U, Pogorelec D, Planinsek F. Breast reconstruction using the free superficial inferior epigastric artery (SIEA) flap. *Br J Plast Surg* 1999;52(4):276–279.
60. Chevray PM. Breast reconstruction with superficial inferior epigastric artery flaps: A prospective comparison with TRAM and DIEP flaps. *Plast Reconstr Surg* 2004;114(5):1077–1083.
61. Herrera FA, Antony AK, Selber JC, Buntic R, Brooks D, Buncke GM. How often is the superficial inferior epigastric artery adequate? An observational correlation. *J Plast Reconstr Aesthet Surg* 2009 [Epub ahead of print].
62. Hester TR, Nahai F, Beegle PE, J. B. Blood supply of the abdomen revisited, with emphasis of the superficial inferior epigastric artery. *Plast Reconstr Surg* 1984;74(5) 657–666.
63. Holm C, Mayr M, Hofter E, Ninkovic M. The versatility of the SIEA flap: A clinical assessment of the vascular territory of the superficial epigastric inferior artery. *J Plast Reconstr Aesthet Surg* 2007;60(8):946–951.
64. Koshima I. Short pedicle superficial inferior epigastric artery adiposal flap: New anatomical findings and the use of this flap for reconstruction of facial contour. *Plast Reconst Surg* 2005;116(4):1091–1097.
65. Reardon CM, O'Ceallaigh S, O'Sullivan ST. An anatomical study of the superficial inferior epigastric vessels in humans. *Br J Plast Surg* 2004;57(6):515–519.
66. Stern HS, Nahai F. The versatile superficial inferior epigastric artery free flap. *Br J Plast Surg* 1992;45(4):270–274.

67. Taylor GI. In discussion of Hester TR Jr, Nahai F, Beegle PE, Bostwick J III. Blood supply of the abdomen revisited, with emphasis of the superficial inferior epigastric artery. *Plast Reconstr Surg* 1984;74(5):667–670.
68. Ulusal BG, Cheng MH, Wei FC, Ho-Asjoe M, Song D. Breast reconstruction using the entire transverse abdominal adipocutaneous flap based on unilateral superficial or deep inferior epigastric vessels. *Plast Reconstr Surg* 2006;117(5):1395–1403.
69. Wolfram D, Schoeller T, Hussl H, Wechselberger G. The superficial inferior epigastric artery (SIEA) flap: Indications for breast reconstruction. *Ann Plast Surg* 2006;57(6):593–596.

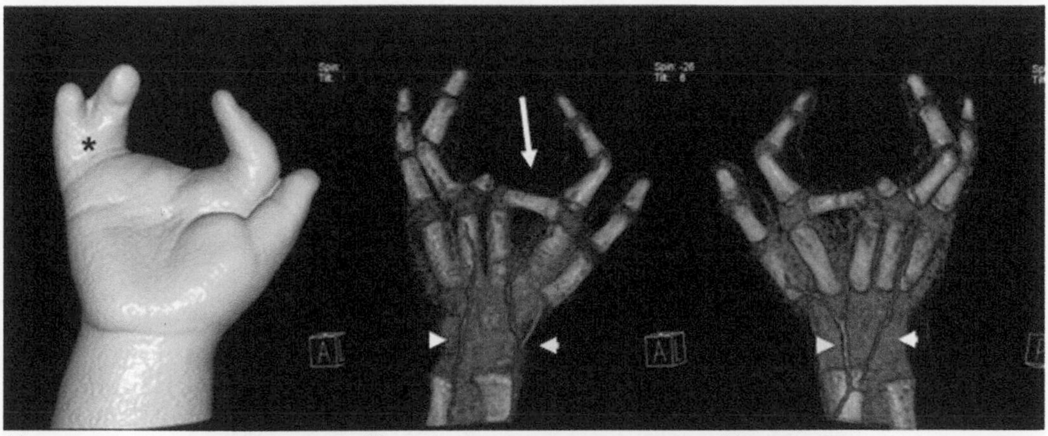

(a) (b) (c)

FIGURE 1.12 Right hand of patient affected by syndactytilies: VR reconstructions (a,b,c) show the fusion of the IV and V finger, absence of the III and fusion of the proximal phalange with the second interphalang (white arrow). Ulnar (white arrow head) and radial arteries (yellow arrow head).

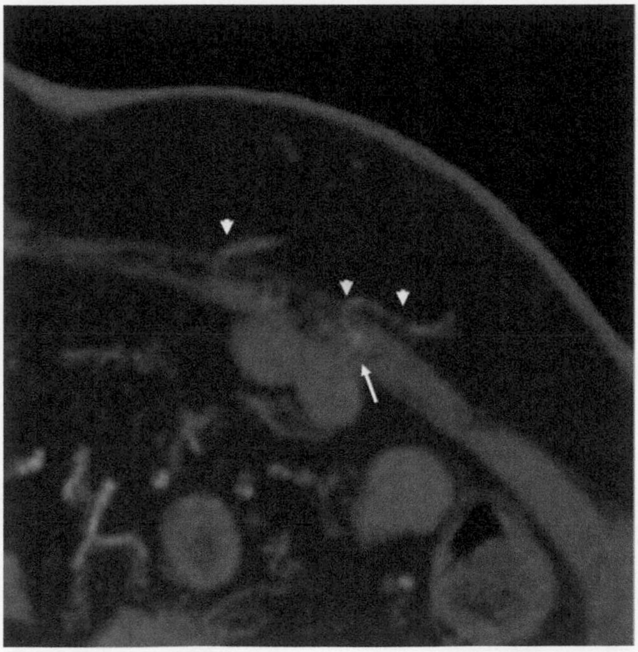

FIGURE 1.14 Axial MIP image shows intramuscular (white arrow), subfascial (yellow arrow head) and subcutaneous (white arrow head) segments of the left deep inferior epigastric perforating artery.

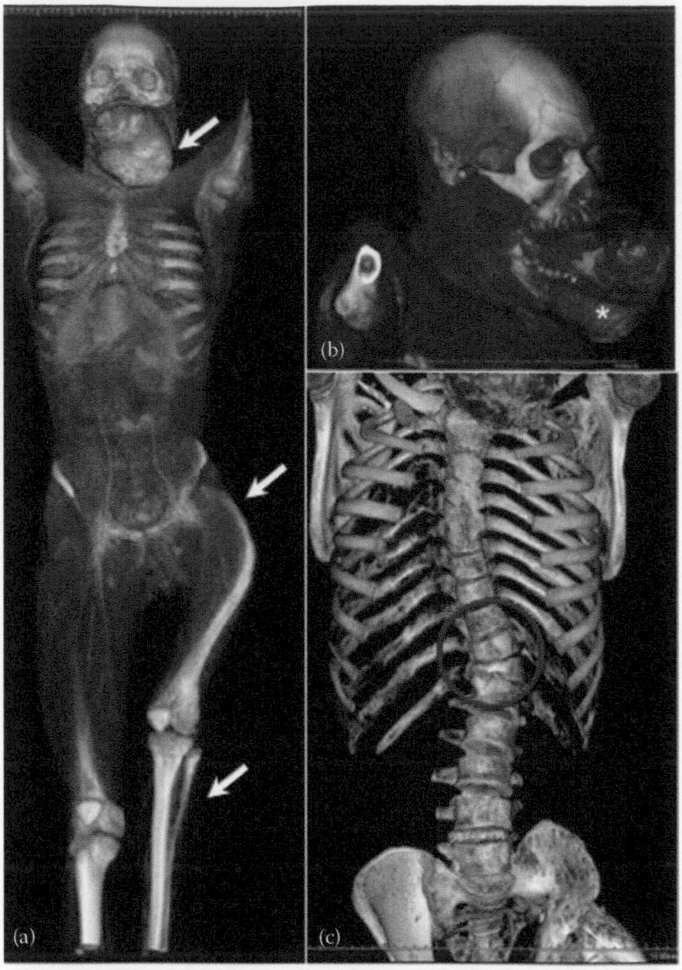

FIGURE 1.15 VR image of a patient affected by fibrous dysplasia with multiple bone deformities (a) (white arrows). (b) Mandibular localization (*); (c) vertebral fracture (red circle).

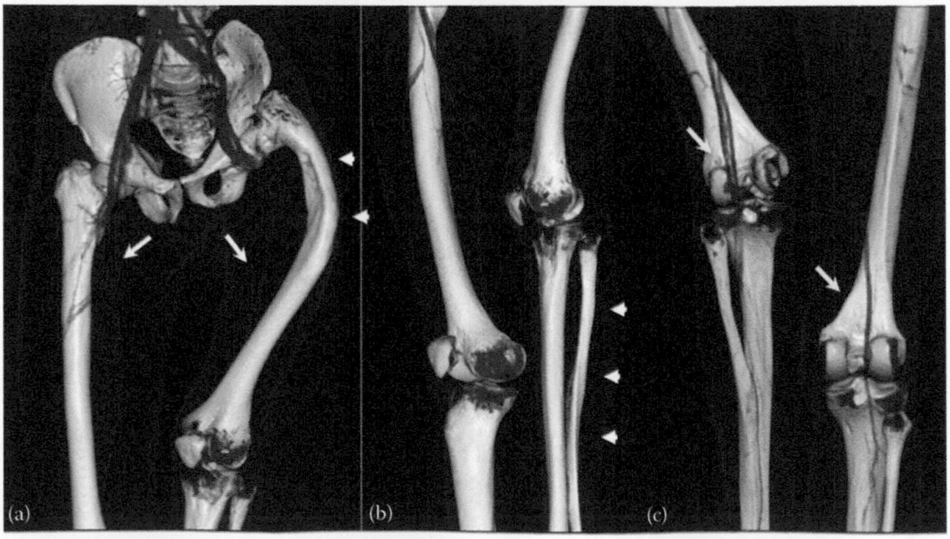

FIGURE 1.16 VR images of the same patient depict femural deformity (arrow head) and superficial femural artery (white arrow) in (a), fibular deformity in (b) and popliteal vessels in (c).

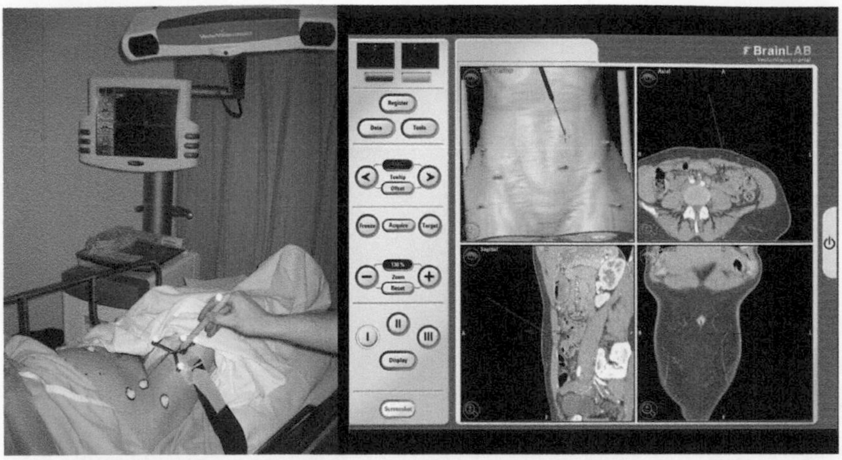

FIGURE 11.15 Left: Navigation station for registration and localisation of patient data, by means of fiducial-point registration, utilising a *stereotactic pointer*, *RS*, and FM for the abdominal wall donor site. Right: 3D multi-planar reconstruction images, as seen on BrainLAB *VectorVision Cranial* software, demonstrating coronal, sagittal, and axial planes during stereotactic navigation of a CTA of the abdominal wall vasculature. (Reproduced from Rozen, W.M. et al., *Surg. Radiol. Anat.*, July; 31(6), 401, 2009. With permission.)

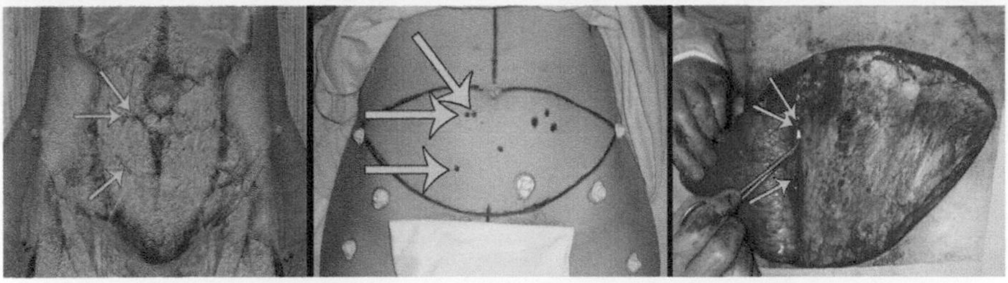

FIGURE 11.16 Correlation of CTA (left), CTA-guided stereotaxy (middle), and operative findings (right), demonstrating concordance for the three largest perforators selected preoperatively (blue arrows). (Reproduced from Rozen, W.M. et al., *Surg. Radiol. Anat.*, July; 31(6), 401, 2009. With permission.)

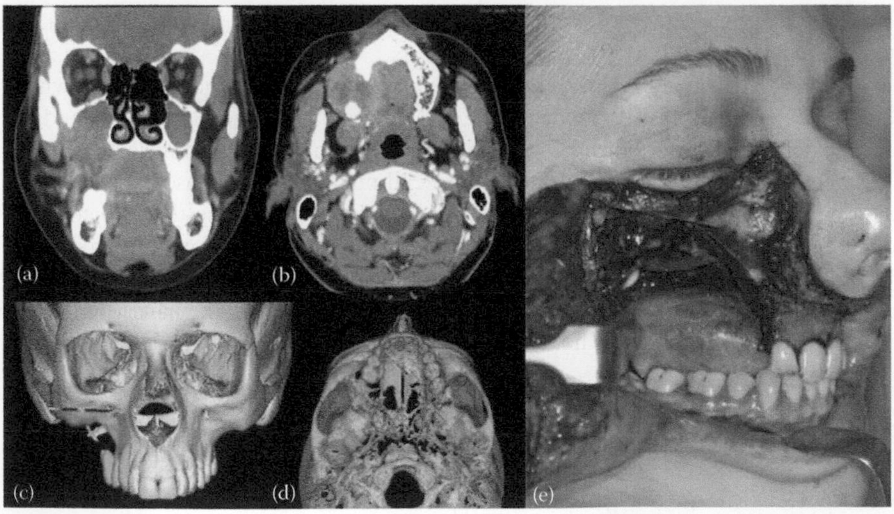

FIGURE 14.40 Axial (a) and coronal (b) view of an OSCC involving the alveolar bone, zygoma, and maxillary sinus (type IIb). The 3D surgical planning of resection is performed using 3D CT DICOM data in coronal (c) and palatal (d) view. Image (e) shows the surgical resection via Weber–Ferguson access.

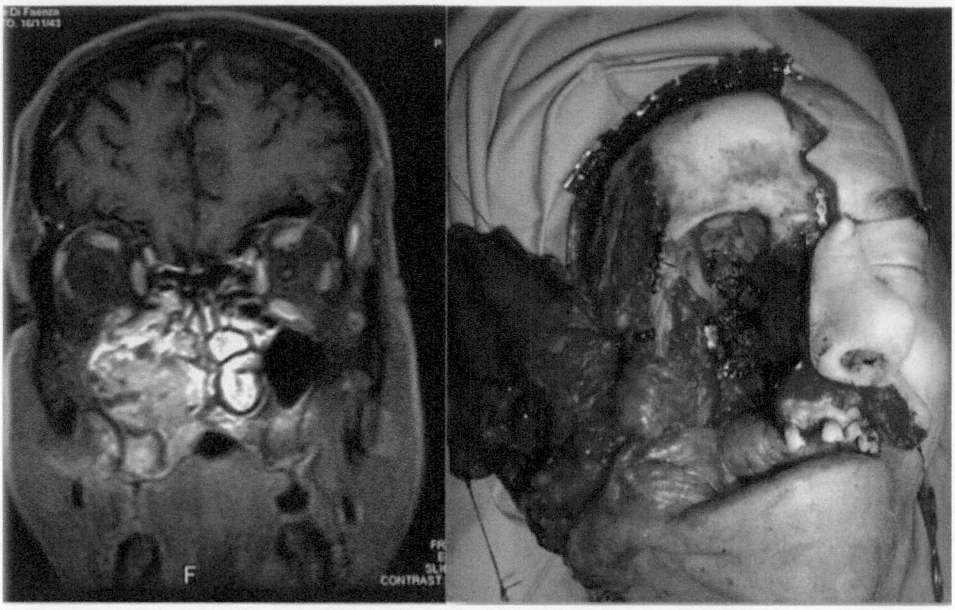

FIGURE 14.41 Radiological (MRI) and clinical images of a maxillary resection associated with an exenteratio orbitae (type IVb) for an adenoid cystic carcinoma originating from minor salivary glands of the palate.

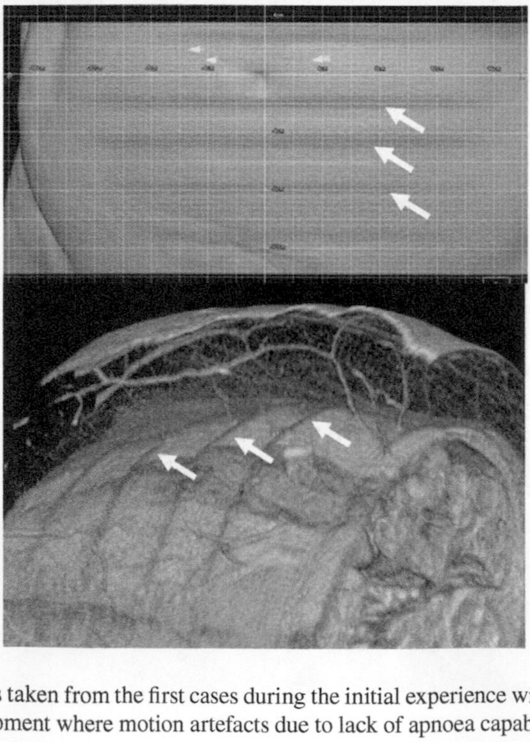

FIGURE 21.2 VR images taken from the first cases during the initial experience with angio-CT for DIEP flaps using a 4-row MDCT equipment where motion artefacts due to lack of apnoea capability.

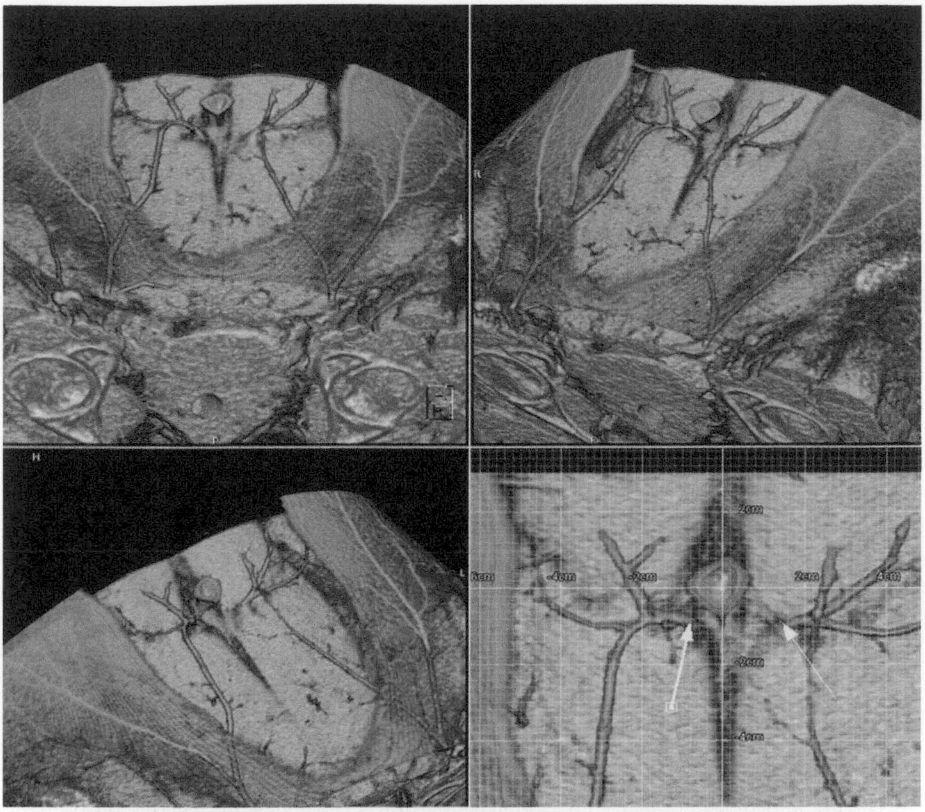

FIGURE 21.7 VR images in different anteroposterior views where perforator vascular pedicle arising from the rectus abdominis can be seen.

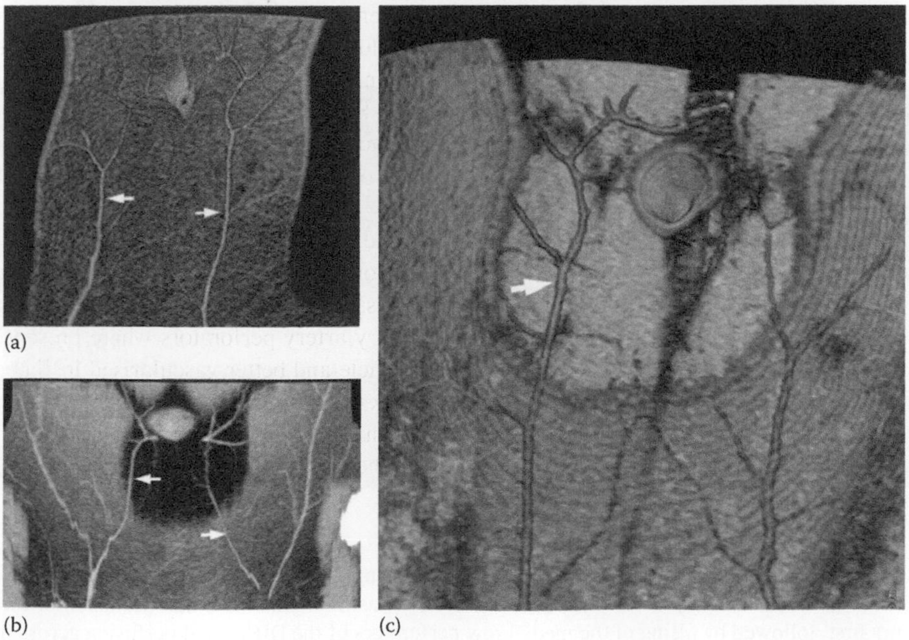

(a)

(b)

(c)

FIGURE 21.13 Preoperative CTA with VR images where the SIEV as drainage of perforator veins can be seen.

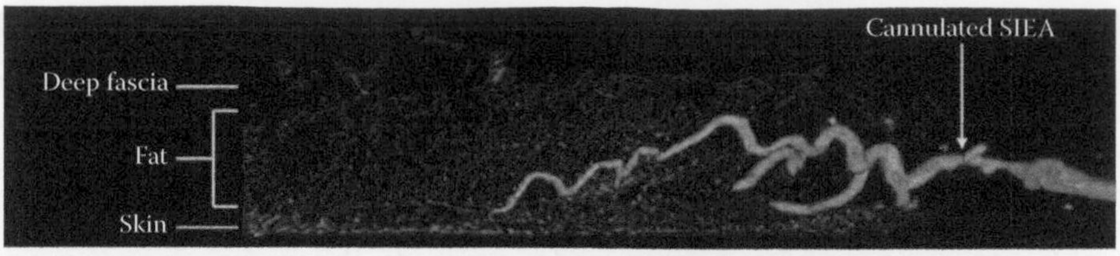

FIGURE 24.3 Lateral view of a CT angiogram of a SIEA flap, with the SIEA individually cannulated, during early injection with iodinated CT contrast medium. Note how the vessel becomes progressively more superficial within the flap as it courses the cephalad (Mark Schaverien and Michel Saint-Cyr, Department of Plastic Surgery, University of Texas Southwestern Medical Center).

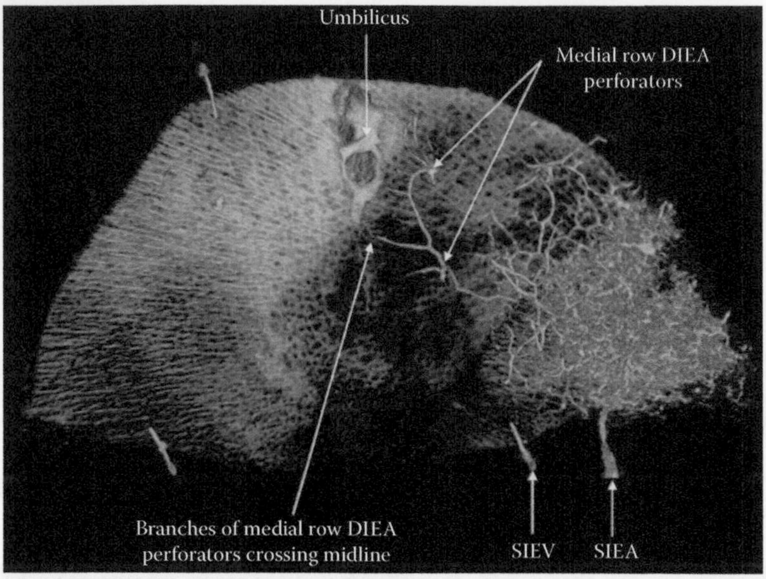

(a)

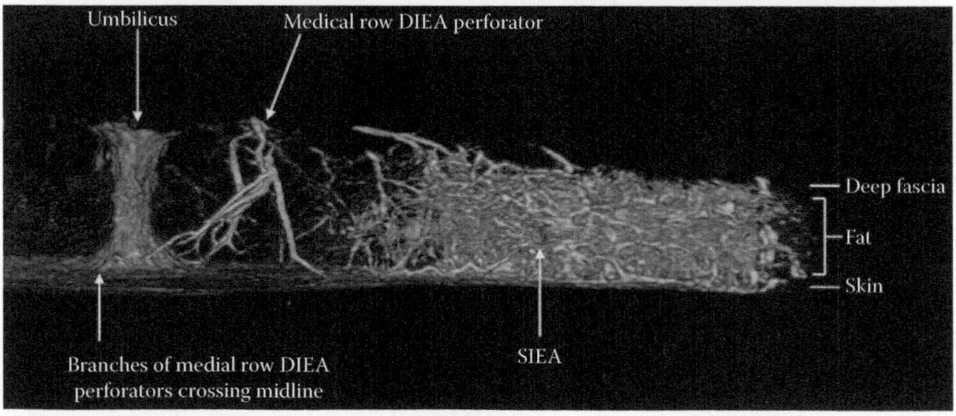

(b)

FIGURE 24.4 (a and b) Anterior and lateral views of a CT angiogram of a SIEA flap, with the SIEA individually cannulated, during injection with iodinated CT contrast medium. Note that perfusion of the lateral flap occurs first, followed by filling of the medial row perforators of the DIEA, and perfusion across the midline occurs via branches of these perforators (Mark Schaverien and Michel Saint-Cyr, Department of Plastic Surgery, University of Texas Southwestern Medical Center).

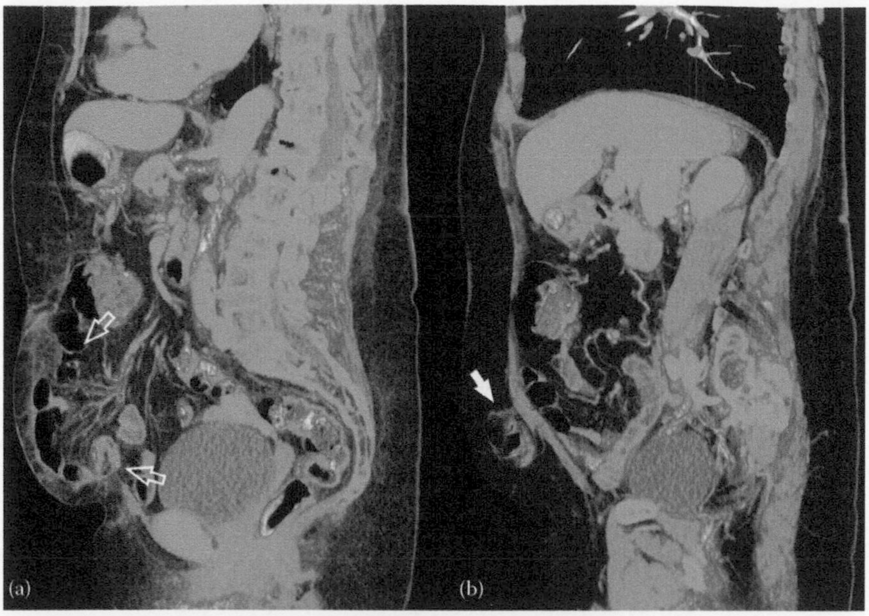

FIGURE 29.4 67-year-old female patient; volume rendering post-processed sagittal thick-slab CT images (panels a and b) show the hernia (arrows indicate the hernia).

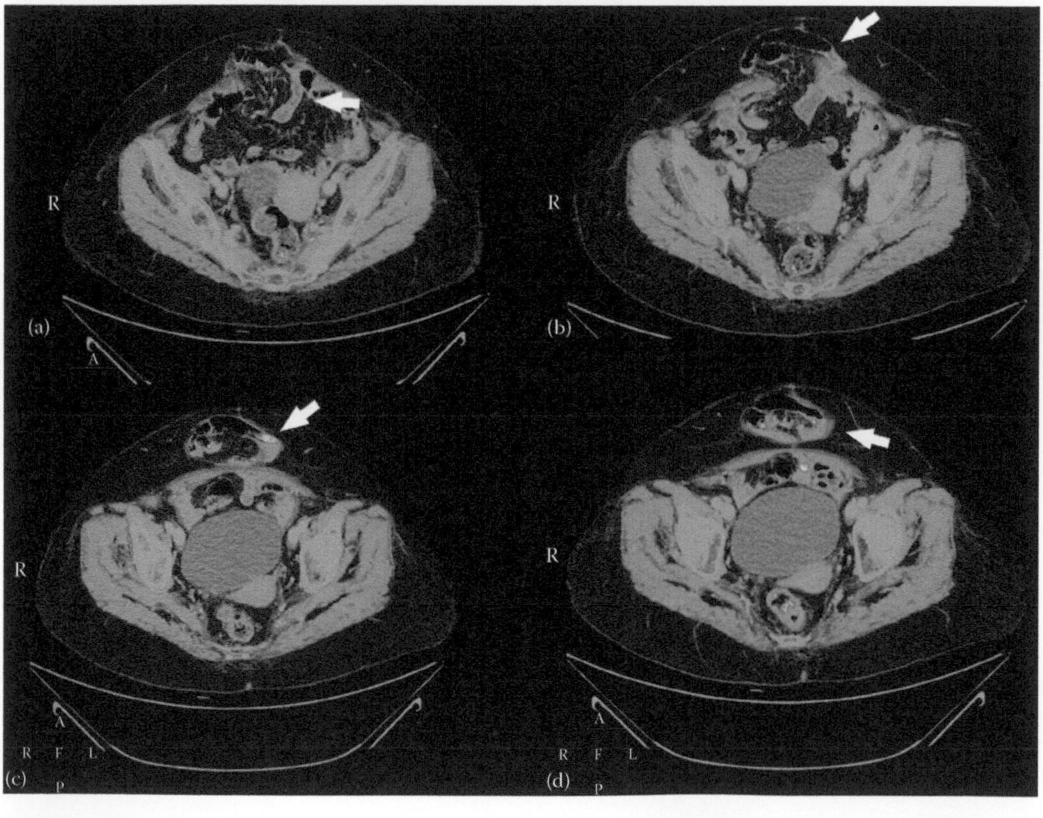

FIGURE 29.6 56-year-old female patient; volume rendering post-processed axial thick-slab CT images (panels a, b, c, and d) show the hernia (white arrows).

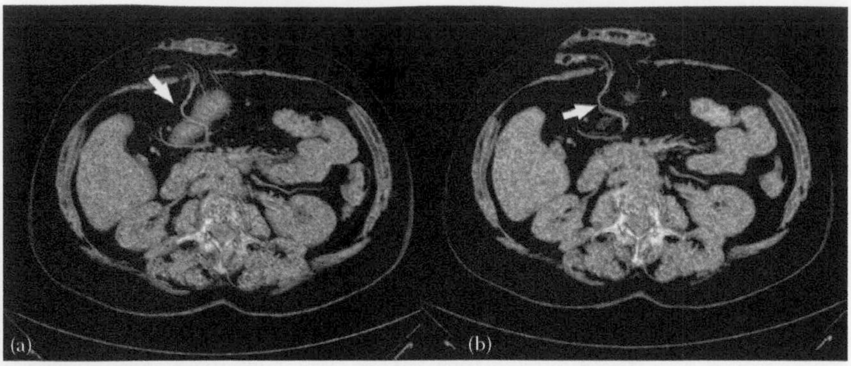

FIGURE 29.7 72-year-old male patient with hernia; volume rendering post-processed axial thick-slab CT images (panels a and b) show the arterial vessels from the superior mesenteric artery that penetrates into the hernia (white arrows).

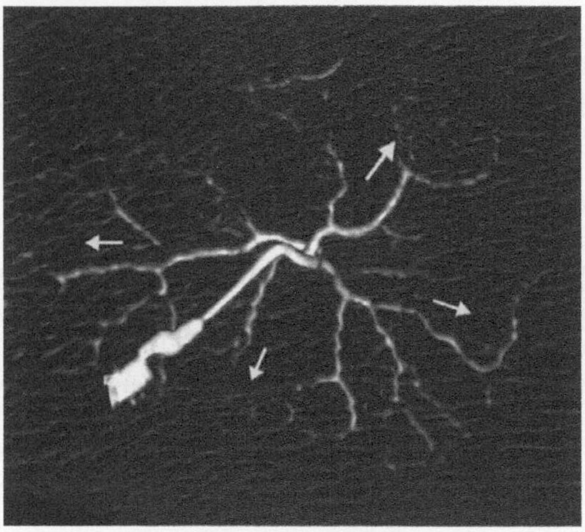

FIGURE 30.2 The perforasome.

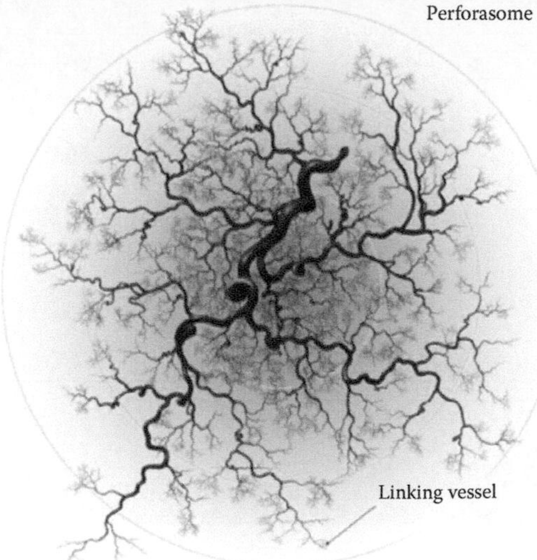

FIGURE 30.3 The perforasome.

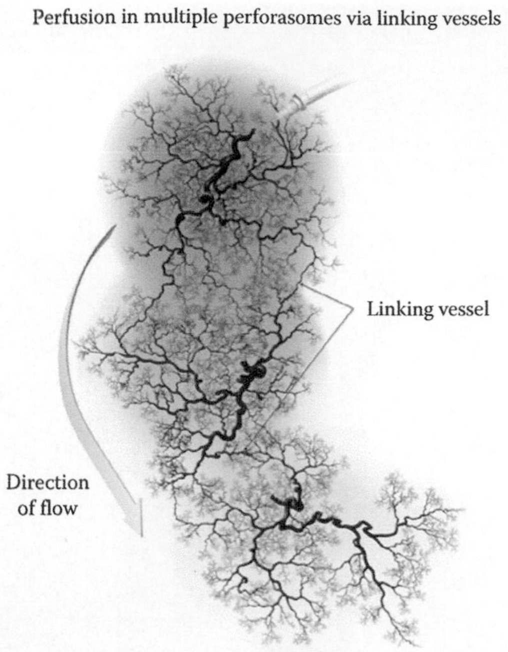

FIGURE 30.4 Linking vessels.

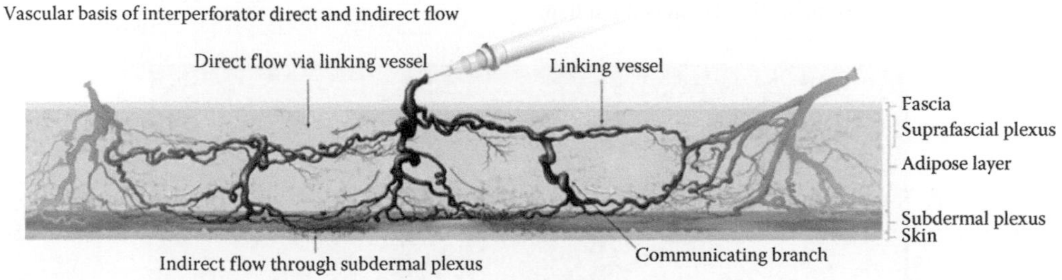

FIGURE 30.5 Direct and indirect linking vessels.

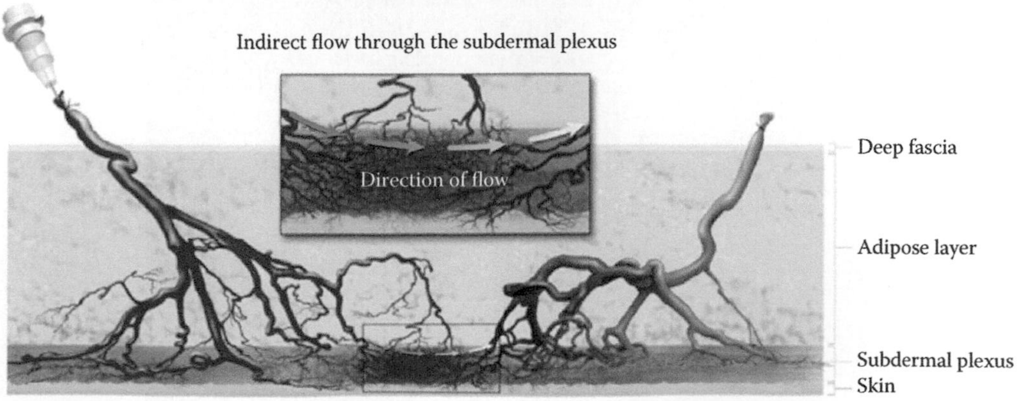

FIGURE 30.6 Indirect linking vessels: recurrent flow through the subdermal plexus.

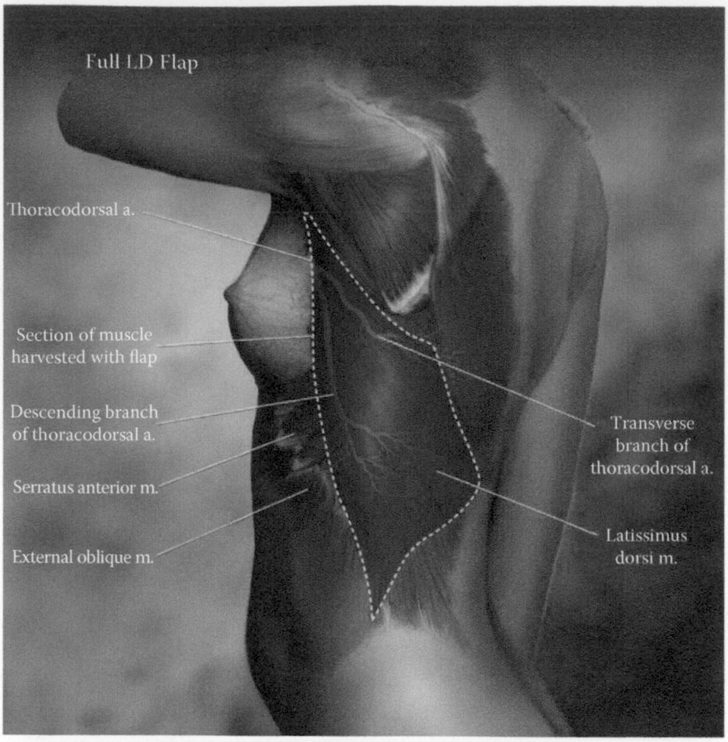

FIGURE 30.8 View of the full latissimus dorsi flap.

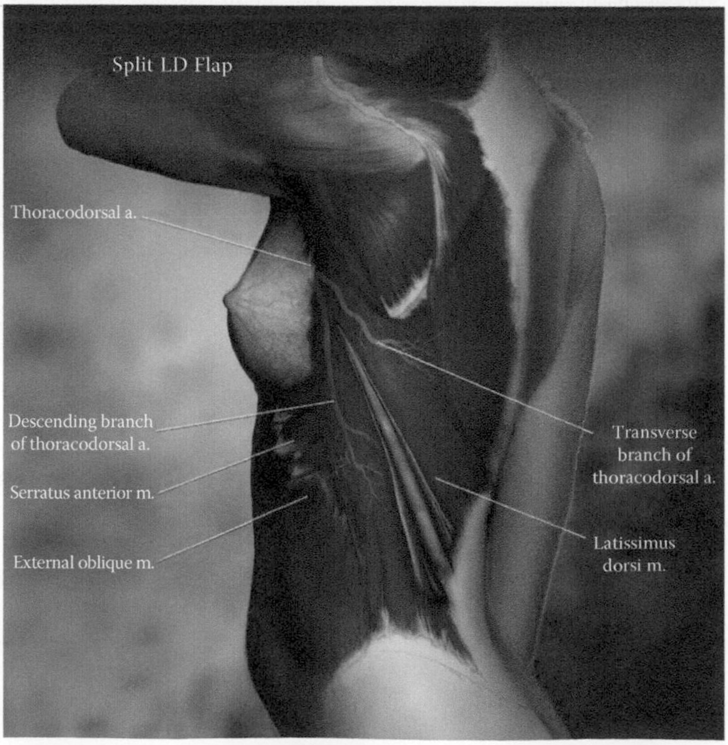

FIGURE 30.9 Split latissimus dorsi flap.

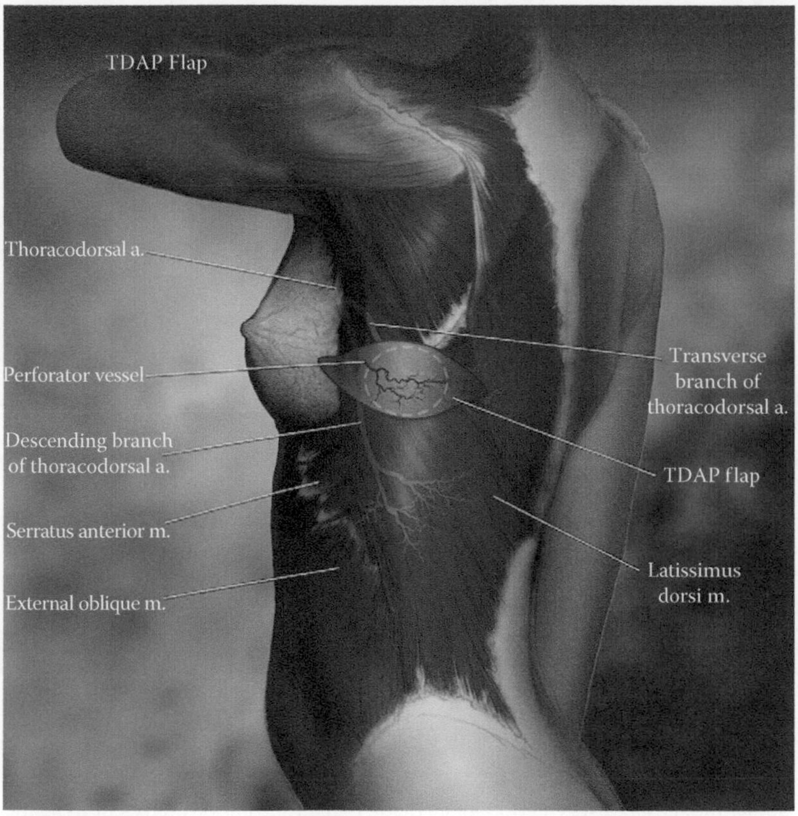

FIGURE 30.10 The TDAP flap.

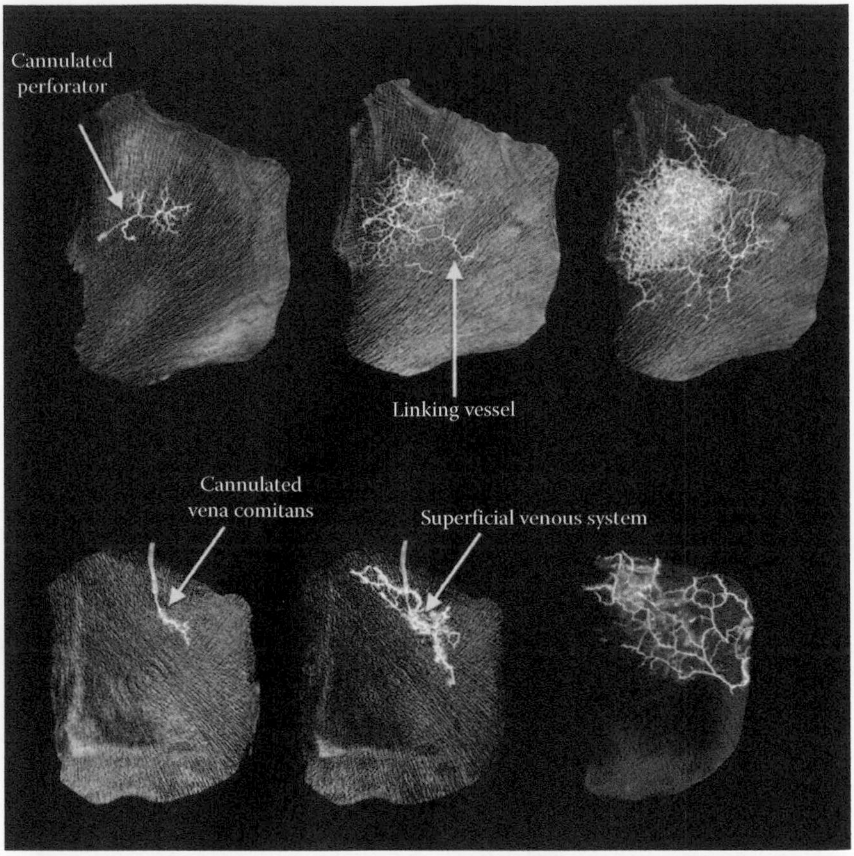

FIGURE 30.11 (Above) Anteroposterior dynamic CT angiograms of the most proximal perforator from the descending branch of the thoracodorsal artery at 0.5 mL filling increments. The flap is cut to follow the shape of the latissimus dorsi muscle. Note the large vascular territory and the dense network of linking vessels with the dorsal intercostal artery perforators. (Below) Anteroposterior images of dynamic filling of the venous system following cannulation of the vena comitans of the most proximal perforator from the descending branch of the thoracodorsal artery, with images acquired at 1 mL filling increments. The final image has been acquired following injection with a barium sulphate/gelatin mixture. The superficial venous system was arranged in a polygonal configuration at the level of the subdermal plexus, and flow into the deep venous system can be seen to occur through the venae comitantes of adjacent perforators within the same angiotome. Note that drainage in the superficial venous system occurred both superolaterally and inferomedially/medially towards the vertebral venous plexus, coursing progressively deeper within the flap as the veins approached the midline.

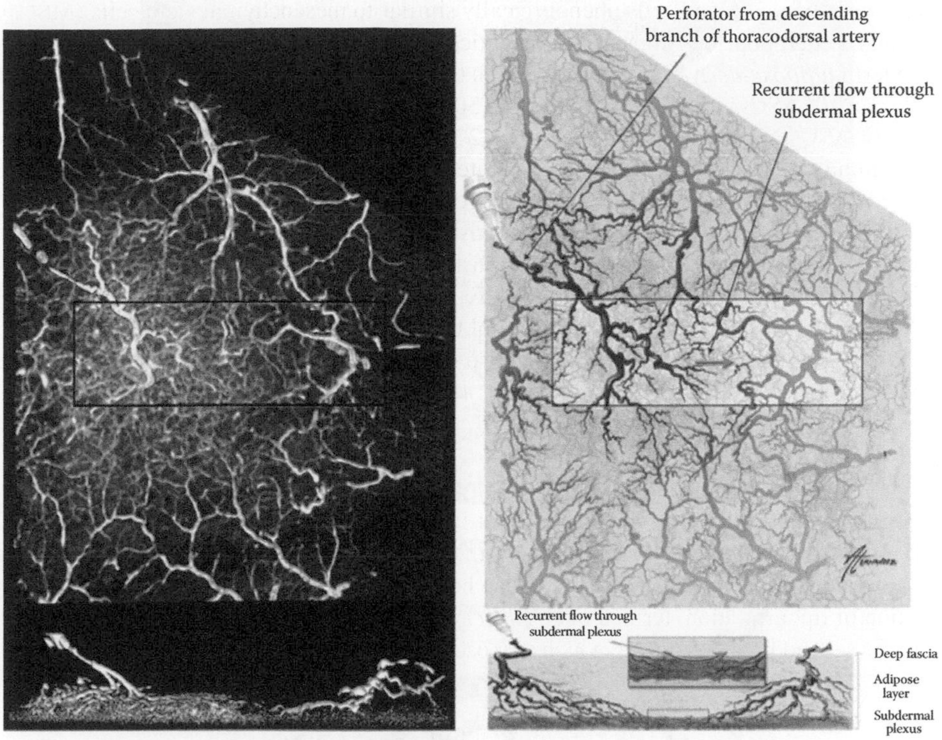

FIGURE 30.12 3D static image after cannulation of the most proximal perforator from the descending branch and injection with a barium sulphate/gelatin mixture, with illustration.

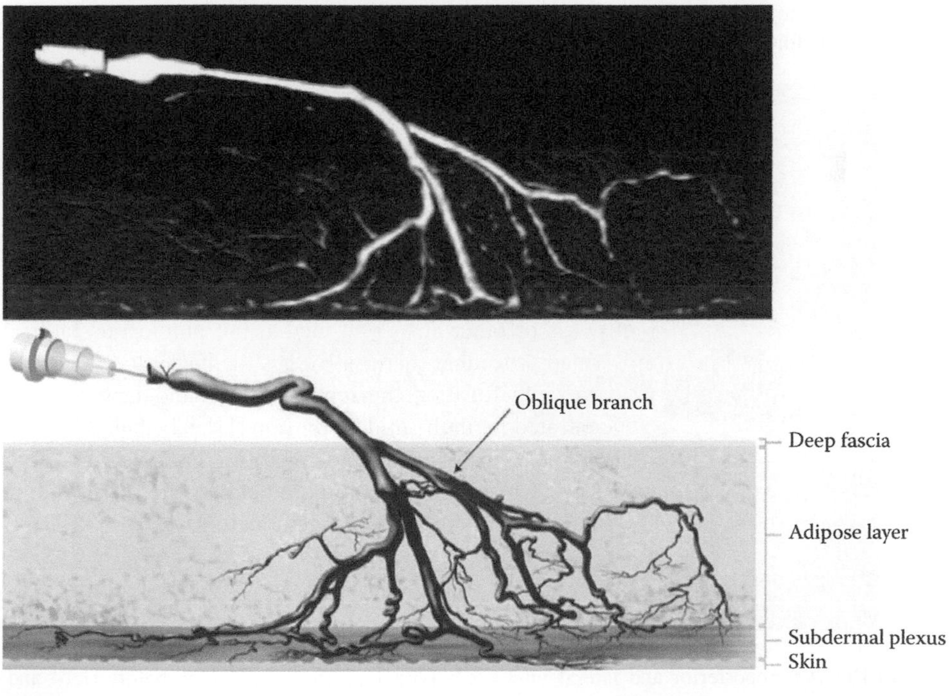

FIGURE 30.13 Type 1; the perforators enter the fascia directly and divide in several long oblique branches that course within the adipose layer down to the subdermal plexus.

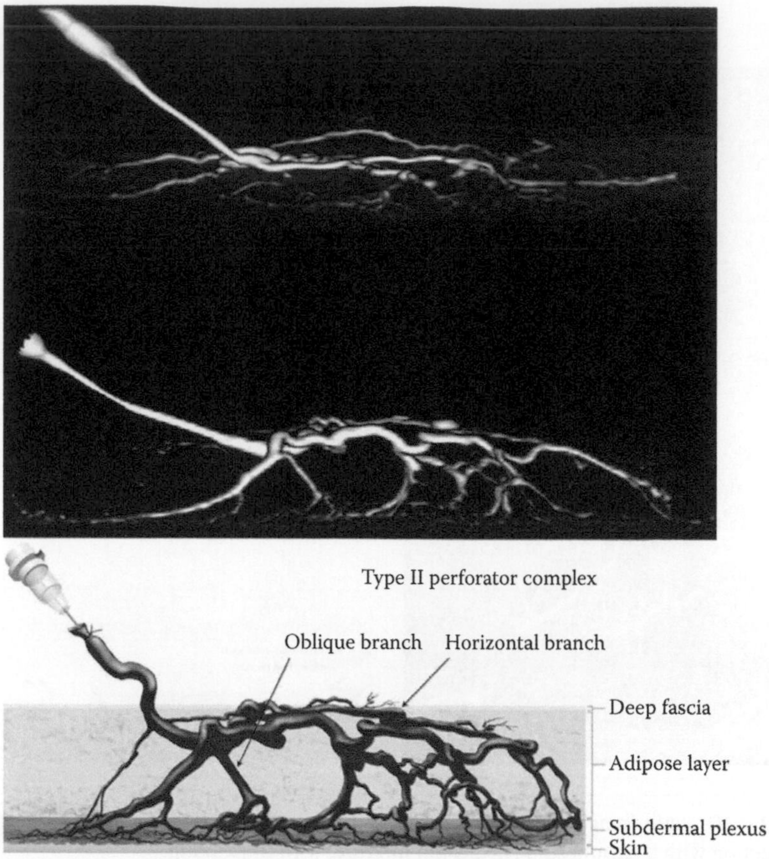

FIGURE 30.14 Type 2; the perforators give branches that run on a short distance (4.1 cm maximum) at a suprafascial level before entering obliquely in the flap and reaching the subdermal plexus.

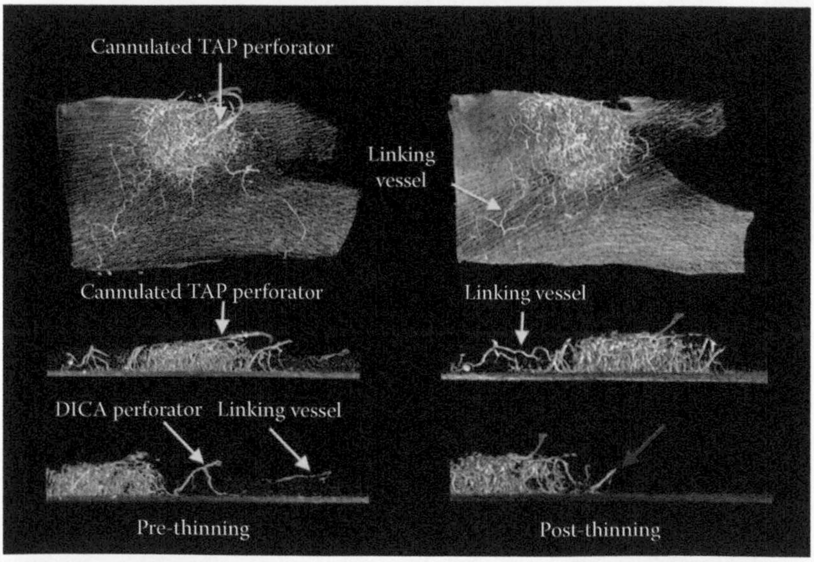

FIGURE 30.16 Anteroposterior and lateral views of a type 1 perforator complex before (left) and after (right) thinning between the deep and superficial adipose layers and injection of 1.5 mL of contrast. A 5 cm radius about the perforator has been preserved, and thinning has been performed at 90° to the horizontal, with washout of the contrast between successive stages.

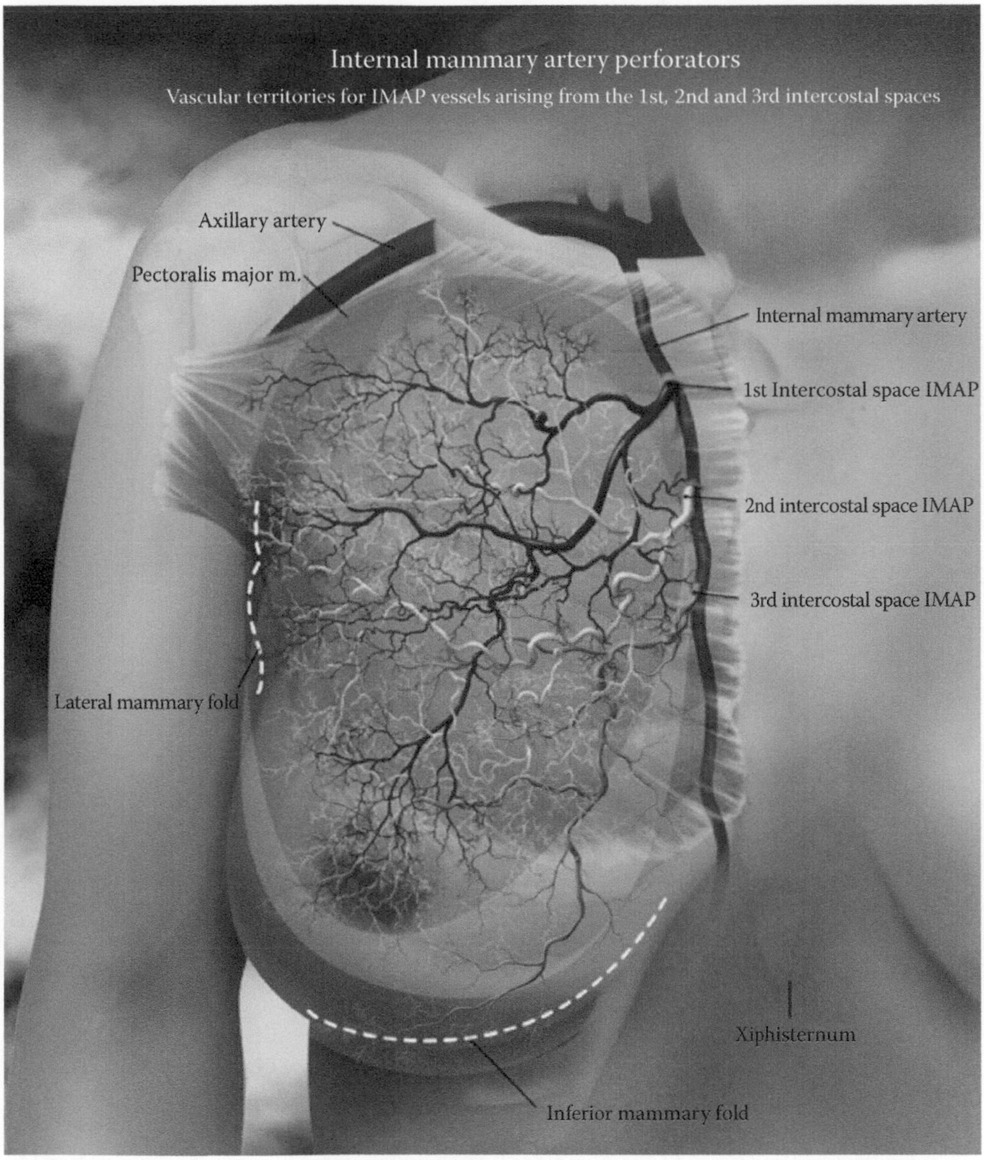

FIGURE 30.19 The IMAP arteries.

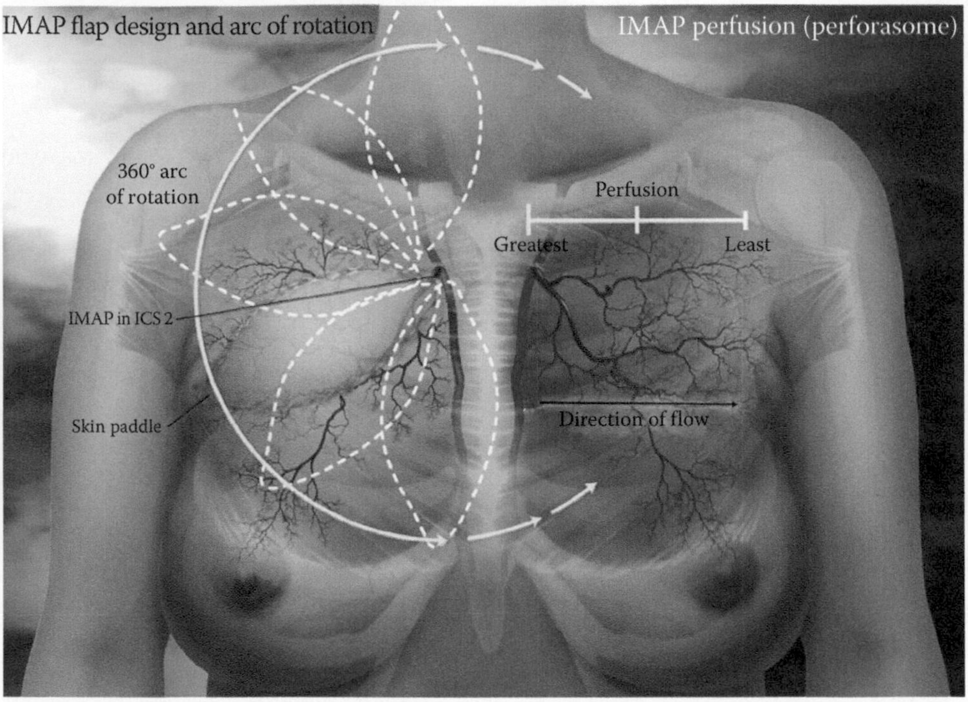

FIGURE 30.22 IMAP flap design and arc of rotation.

22 MR Imaging of Deep Inferior Epigastric Artery and Deep Superior Epigastric Artery Perforators

Vachara Niumsawatt, Alberto Alonso-Burgos, Iain S. Whitaker, and Warren M. Rozen

CONTENTS

22.1 OVERVIEW

Magnetic resonance imaging (MRI) uses a powerful magnetic field to align the nuclear magnetisation of hydrogen nuclei in the body. The technology then produces radio-frequency pulses which tip the alignment of the hydrogen nuclei away from the main magnetic field. This ultimately results in the hydrogen nuclei being able to produce a radio-frequency signal that is detectable by the scanner. The signals are then analysed by sophisticated computer software and produce digital information representing detailed pictures of organs, soft tissues, bone, and virtually all other internal body structures.[1] Further advances in the technology allow the use of injectable intravenous contrast agent (gadolinium) to enhance the vessels detection. This mode of investigation is termed *magnetic resonance angiography* (MRA).

MRA has progressed from an initial use for brain or solid organs to a feasible technique for vascular study. Even the very peripheral and small diameter vasculature can be evaluated by this radiation and iodinate contrast medium-free technique. Whole-body angio-MR permits rapid, non-invasive, and accurate evaluation of the entire vascular system and can be used for both diagnostic purposes and monitoring of vascular involvement of peripheral arterial disease, since it offers high enhanced contrast between blood and stationary tissue and fast acquisition times.

The development of MRI techniques using high-field equipments and blood-pool intravascular contrast agents has allowed to perform non-invasive and radiation-free MRA of very peripheral and small calibre territories. Perforator vessels could be feasibly evaluated using angio-MR technique, although there have until recently been very few published series evaluating this role.

22.2 USE OF MR IMAGING IN PERFORATOR FLAPS

Preoperative imaging of the abdominal wall vasculature prior to deep inferior epigastric artery (DIEA) perforator (DIEP) flaps and deep superior epigastric artery (DSEA) perforator (DSEP) flap have become a standard practice performed by most plastic and reconstructive surgeons. This procedure was done as a means to maximise operative success. In several literature, it has shown to significantly improve surgical outcome, decrease operating time, and reduce the incidence of flap complication.[3,4] Three most commonly used radiographic modalities in DIEP or DSEP are Doppler/colour duplex ultrasound (US), computed tomography angiography (CTA), and MRA. Each technique has its own unique characteristic with several literature describing their advantages and disadvantages.

MRA has been popularised and used in imaging larger vessels in many parts of the body such as the internal carotid arteries, intracerebral vessels, coronary vessels, aorta, and axial arteries of the upper and lower limbs.[5–9] It has a higher sensitivity and specificity in evaluating vessel course and size than other previously described techniques. There is also less risk profile as it does not emit ionising radiation with less toxic intravenous contrast compared with CTA. With increasing success in soft tissue and vascular imaging, this technique has then expanded into the field of reconstructive surgery. Preoperative MRA imaging of pedicles has been performed in flap reconstruction after trauma, head and neck.[10–16] Lorenze et al. have used MRA in fibular free flap planning for reconstruction of head and neck defects. In their study, bilateral lower vessel abnormalities were detected in 3 of 32 patients (9.4%) which allowed the reconstructive surgeon to alter the flap design prior to undertaking the operation. These abnormalities would have not been detected without the use of MRA. They were able to demonstrate that MRA has a high sensitivity and specificity in free fibular flap reconstruction as all vascular anatomies detected in vivo were seen with a similar characteristic. No complications arise from during both the imaging procedure or the operation.[10] Fukuyama et al. have performed a similar study which found not only a detailed course and characteristic of axial artery but also its associated perforators. Both intramuscular and septocutaneous perforator vessels as small as 1–2 mm in diameter can also be accurately detected with the use of MRA.[11,15,16]

Both Newman et al. and Vasile et al. studies used MRA to characterise the perforators of superior and inferior gluteal arteries. A detailed course and size of the perforators can be visualised accurately and helped in preoperative flap design.[17,18] They were able to demonstrate 132 perforator arteries located within 1 cm of the coordinates measured on MRA, all of which were surgically verified to be suitable for flap perfusion. During the operation, the arterial course and diameter through the gluteal muscles can be visualised accurately on MRA in 48 of 49 arteries (97.9%).[18] High-resolution MRA provided anatomic and clinical information of perforator vascular anatomy which conventionally has been impossible to obtain preoperatively or required multiple invasive natures. However, the high cost of the machine, setup of the facility, and requirement of specialist to operate and interpret the result have limited its use in free flap reconstruction.

22.3 MR IMAGING OF DIEA AND DSEA PERFORATORS

DIEP flap has become the workhorse in both immediate and delayed breast reconstruction. In the past, elevation of the DIEP flap was both demanding and difficult due to the vast anatomical variation of both DIEA and DSEA. It required a careful selection of a suitable perforator to support the flap. The operation is made more difficult as the retrograde dissection either intramuscular or around the rectus abdominis muscle during raising of the flap is needed. Challenges in DIEP flap preparation include knowledge of (1) DIEA and DSEA anatomy, (2) the positions of the perforator vessels on the branches artery, (3) their course in the intramuscular or intermuscular septum, and (4) the cutaneous distribution of the perforators. If a non-suitable perforator is selected, the flap could be compromised or may even need to be discarded. Currently, the most commonly used preoperative imaging modalities for preoperative planning included Doppler or colour duplex US, CTA, and MRA.

Doppler and colour duplex US has been extensively used in the past for preoperative planning of DIEP flaps. However, both techniques are operator dependent and thus have shown significant variability in terms of their accuracy.[19–24] CTA can be used in conjunction with 3D digital imaging reconstruction software which improved the diagnostic accuracy. In several international centres, it is considered to be the gold standard in preoperative imaging for DIEP flaps. Several literature have demonstrated a sensitivity and positive predictive value of 100% for perforators of greater than 1 mm in size. Philips et al. and Rozen et al. have demonstrated the use of CTA with an accurate description of the course of DIEA perforators as small as 0.3 mm in size. CTA is widely available, is cheaper to perform, uses less scanning times, is highly reproducible, and is less dependent on patient body habitus than that of MRA.[25,26] However, the risk profile of CTA includes radiation exposure, higher risk of nephrotoxicity, and allergy secondary to the intravenous contrast medium used.

The needs for a reliable, accurate, and lower rate of adverse effects imaging modality have pushed for the use of MRA in preoperative DIEP flap planning. In literature, the accuracy of identifying the perforators has been reported to be as high as 97%–100% with the perforators as small as 0.8 mm in diameter can be detected.[27,28] Neil-Dwyers study described the use of anatomical landmark (umbilicus) to describe the location of the DIEA perforators. This technique has greatly assisted reconstructive surgeon in preoperative designing and reduced operative time. However, they did not report its sensitivity or specificity in relation to its intra-operative finding.[29] Despite having a high degree of accuracy (high specificity) in identifying perforators of greater than 1 mm in size, it does not identify all perforators (low sensitivity). Rozen et al. found that MRA has a lower sensitivity in identifying the perforators when compared to CTA.[28] However, Hartung et al. have suggested that MRA sensitivity can be improved by increasing the field strength from 1.5 to 3.0 T.[30] This improvement is likely due to doubling of the signal-to-noise ratio (SNR). At 3.0 T, twice as many protons are aligned with the magnetic field, thus increasing the spatial resolution and decreasing acquisition time. Increased spatial resolution allows for improved visibility of the vessels and decreased acquisition time, thus decreasing breath-holding requirement which results in reduction of motion artefact.[30]

22.4 COMPARISON OF PREOPERATIVE IMAGING FOR DIEA PERFORATOR FLAPS

22.4.1 MRA Comparison to Doppler Ultrasound

One of the most inexpensive and common techniques for identifying and locating perforators is the use of unidirectional Doppler probe and colour duplex US (also known as *colour Doppler* US or Duplex in literature). This technique applies to the vascular flow in a colour code, depending on the direction and velocity, in the standard greyscale US image. It is simple and has an option of being a handheld device that can be used to mark the perforators just prior to the operation.[31,32] Duplex US can then provide information on both the perforator diameter and flow velocity. This innervation allows operator to detect the presence of an occlusion either by damaged vessel from atherosclerosis, trauma or previous surgery, or blood vessel disorders from peripheral vascular disease and thrombotic and embolic event.[33] After the examination, information obtained regarding the number of perforators and their courses can then be used to generate a perforator map to assist in flap planning. US device produced a cyclic sound pressure wave which is at a frequency greater than the upper limit of the human hearing range; thus, there is no discomfort or adverse reaction to patient. Patients are not required to undergo physical screening as there is no contraindication to perform Doppler US. Similar to MRA, there is no risk of radiation exposure to the patient.

Despite all the simplicity of the device, it is highly variable in terms of sensitivity and specificity. The device is operator dependent in both operation and interoperating the result. To our knowledge, there is no literature describing a direct comparison of MRA and Doppler US in preoperative DIEP flap imaging. However, Pratt et al. have performed a systemic review in the use of preoperative imaging modality between Doppler US and CTA in DEIP flap reconstruction. They have shown that Doppler US is less accurate and time consuming (20–120 min)[24,34] and provides less information regarding the intra-muscle course of the vessel. This accuracy seems to decrease with smaller and deeper vessels.[32] Furthermore, it does not provide information on other nearby vessels due to its narrow focus of US wave; thus, the superficial epigastric artery and branching pattern of the DSEA and DIEA cannot be identified.[24,32] This information is crucial during the dissection of the perforators in avoiding accidentally damaging the chosen perforator. Rozen et al. performed studies comparing CTA to MRA and Doppler US. They reported that US is the least reliable method of identifying DIEA perforator detection rate with a p-value of 0.0078 compared to the CTA, whereas MRA demonstrated a similar sensitivity (100%) but has a lower specificity (49%) than CTA.[24,28,35]

22.4.2 Comparison to CTA

CTA has been widely used and accepted in preoperative DIEP flap imaging. Several studies have suggested the beneficial role for CTA in the imaging of the abdominal wall vasculature.[24,35–37] CTA is cheaper and therefore is more widely available to be used than MRA. Procedural time, the need for computer software for digital reconstruction, and scanning protocol are similar in both modalities. Although reported by some literature that one of the benefits of MRA is that of no contrast reaction with intravenous gadolinium.[38] However, the development of nephrogenic systemic fibrosis in renal impairment patient has been described in literature by Hedley et al. and Perazella et al.[39–41] MRA does have the benefit of no radiation exposure to the patient when compared to CTA and is therefore considered by some to be safer. CTA is an ionising technique and delivers 6–8 mSv compared to 0.02 mSv in a conventional chest x-ray.[42] However, there are several absolute and relative contraindications for MRA as described in Section 22.4, 'MRI Protocol in DIEA and DSEA Perforators', while there are none for CTA.

Few studies are available on the value of MRA in preoperative perforator mapping of the DIEA. Most literature have found that MRA can accurately identify the presence of perforators of the DIEA (97%–100%) which is similar to that of CTA (see Figures 22.1 through 22.3).[18,28] However, MRA has a lower perforator detection rate compared to CTA. Rozen et al. study has shown that CTA is able to identify more perforates than MRA, in particular when the perforators are lesser than 1 mm in diameter. CTA can be used to accurately identify perforator as small as 0.3 mm in diameter, whereas the smallest perforator identified by MRA is 0.8 mm in literature.[28] Pauchot et al. have also found a similar result and hypothesis that this is likely because CTA has a better contrast differentiation in fat-surrounded vessels. Its analysis provided higher vessel contrast within the subcutaneous tissue, which improved perforator identification compared to MRA.[42] However, they have also found that MRA provides a better contrast between muscle and vessel; thus, it provided a better identification of the intramuscular course than that of CTA.

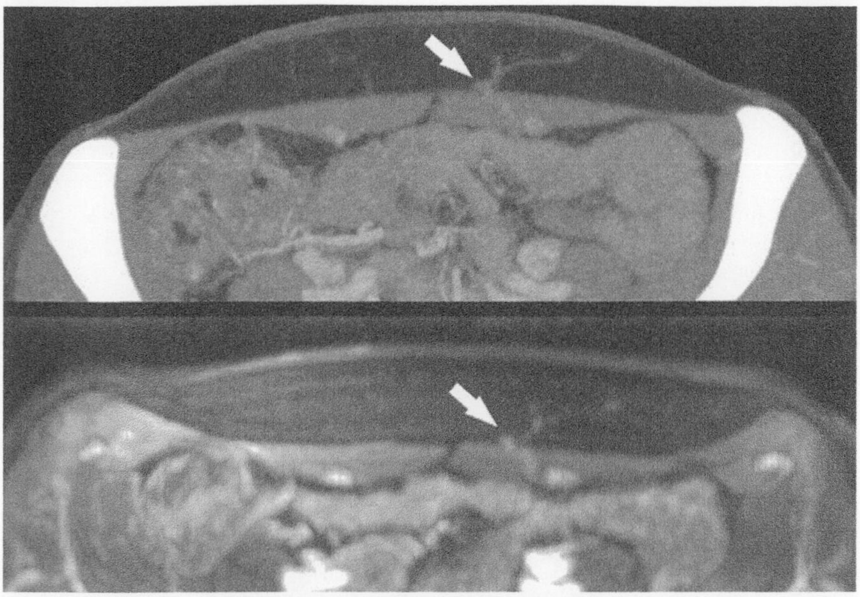

(a)

(b)

FIGURE 22.1 Comparative axial MIP images from CTA (a) and MRA (b) in the same patient where the main perforator vascular pedicle (arrow) can be seen.

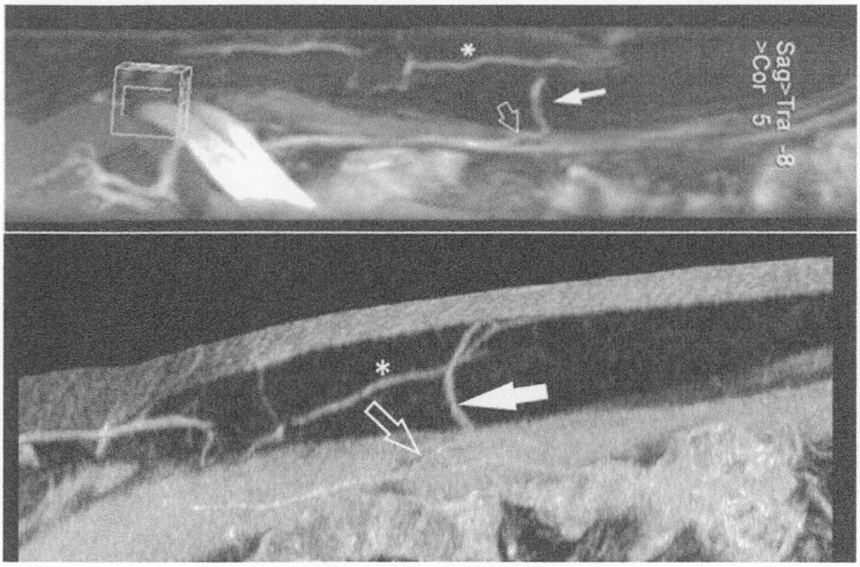

(a)

(b)

FIGURE 22.2 Comparative sagittal MIP images from MRA (a) and CTA (b) in the same patient where a main perforator vascular pedicle (arrow), intramuscular course (open arrow), and superficial venous plexus (asterisk) can be seen.

In order to improve the specificity of perforator identification, contrast-enhanced (CE) protocol was used. Neil-Dwyer et al. employed the use of CE-MRA in preoperative DIEP flap imaging compared to a conventional MRA. They were able to improve perforator identification and found a decreased need to convert DIEP free flap to free TRAM or MS TRAM with preoperative CE-MRA mapping.[29]

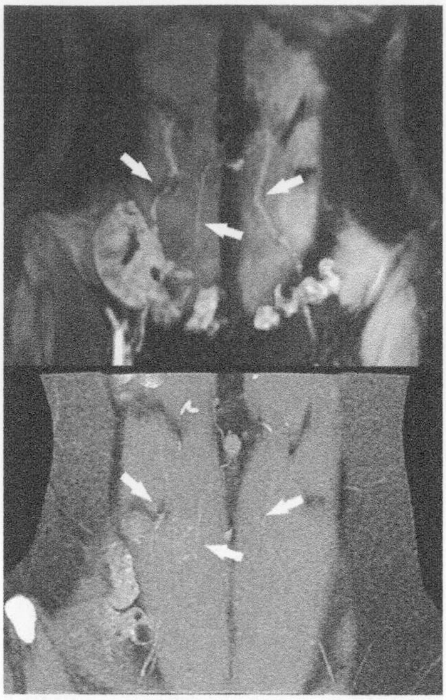

(a)

(b)

FIGURE 22.3 Comparative coronal MIP images from MRA (a) and CTA (b) in the same patient where branching pattern of DIEA (arrows) can be seen.

22.5 MRA PROTOCOL IN DIEA AND DSEA PERFORATORS

From our experience, we suggested the following protocol in performing MRA.

22.5.1 Pre-Imaging Preparation

Contraindications to MRA

- Severe obesity
- Implanted defibrillator or pacemaker
- Implanted ferromagnetic devices
- Cochlear implant

Relative contraindications

- Artificial heart valves
- Implanted drug infusion ports
- Implanted nerve stimulators
- Artificial limbs or metallic joint prostheses
- Metal pins, screws, plates, stents, or surgical staples

Considered limitations in performing any MRI study are as follows: if the patient is on continuous life-support devices, such as oxygen; pregnant (first trimester); claustrophobic; extremely anxious; confused; or unable to lie still.

22.5.2 Patient Preparation

- Patient is not required to fast prior to the procedure.
- Removal of all jewellery or metallic objects including hearing aids (may be affected by the magnetic field).
- Patient is asked to change into a gown that will have no metal such as zipper, hooks, buckles, or buttons.
- Patient needs to lie still during the procedure because motion can result in poor quality images.
- Inform radiographer of contrast allergy. However, MRA examination uses gadolinium which does not contain iodine and is less likely to cause an allergic reaction than iodine-containing contrast used for a CT scan.

22.5.3 Procedure

MRA scanning protocols follow the same philosophy as used and described for the CTA techniques for DIEP flaps. As a rule, the objectives of MRA are to identify the main perforators and related vascular pedicles and their main anatomical features:

- Location
- Intramuscular course
- Anastomosis with the superficial venous plexus

Having these in mind, CE-MRA is performed with a phased-array surface coil on a high-field unit. In this sense, the greatest advantage of 3-T high-field MR system, compared with 1.5-T or lower-field systems, is a higher spatial resolution, thus providing a more precise anatomical information, in less exploration time. In our experience, any aim to exploration in a 1.5-T or lower-field equipments only compounds to frustration.

As applied for the CTA, exploration range should always include the selected surgical field, and the patient position on the MR table during the scanning should be the same as in the surgical procedure.

22.5.4 Scanning Protocol

Initially, coronal, axial, and sagittal 2D true fast imaging with steady-state precession was performed to gain an overview of the major abdominal vessels and organs, and the resulting images were used as localisers. Next, CE-MRA of the anterior abdominal wall was performed using a high-resolution 3D T1-weighted volumetric interpolated breath-hold examination MR sequence. Since we consider the perforator vascular pedicle as a unit formed by perforator artery and vein as the goal of our study, scanning delay time after injection of contrast medium was fixed at 60 s, determined based on previous clinical experience with CTA.

- MRI setting as per Table 22.1.
- Field strength is set at 1.5 and 3.0 T.
- Study range is from 4 cm above the umbilicus to pubic symphysis in a caudo-cranial direction.
- Intravenous gadolinium-based contrast media (30 mL Magnevist [dimeglumine gadopentetate; Schering, Bergkamen, Germany]) is given at the rate of 2 mL/s with bolus trigger point from the common femoral artery (100 HU, minimum delay).
- The acquisition time ranges from 10 to 20 min.
- Image is reconstructed with 0.8 mm coronal acquisition slices.

TABLE 22.1
MRA DIEA and DSEA Scanning Protocol

Scan Type	MRA
Field strength	1.5 T and 3.0 T
Image acquisition	Total imaging matrix (TIM) technology
Slice resolution thickness	0.8 mm coronal acquisition slices
In-plane resolution	0.9 mm × 0.8 mm × 0.8 mm
IV contrast	Magnevist (dimeglumine gadopentetate, Schering) 30 mL IVI 2 mL/s
Contrast infusion	Care bolus technique
Contrast bolus tracking	From the common femoral artery no delay
Scanning range	Pubic symphysis – 4 cm above umbilicus
Body matrix coil	Overlying abdominal wall

Source: Rozen, W.M. et al., *Microsurgery*, 29(2), 119, 2009.

22.5.5 MRA Reporting

MRA images are transferred to a workstation. In the similar manner as for CTA native images as well as multiplanar reconstructions (MPR), maximum-intensity projection (MIP) and volume-rendered (VR) reconstructions, using commercially available software, are obtained and analysed.

The following information should be described when reporting an MRA preoperative DIEP flap imaging.

- DIEA branching pattern
  - Type (I–IV)
    - Type I: Single trunk
    - Type II: Bifurcation trunk
    - Type III: Trifurcation trunk
    - Type IV: Quadfurcation trunk
- Intramuscular course
  - Medial to the rectus abdominis muscle
  - Intramuscular through the rectus abdominis muscle
  - Lateral to the rectus abdominis muscle
- Size of perforators
  - Perforator which is greater or equal to 1 mm in diameter is classified as *dominant*.
  - Perforator which is lesser than 1 mm in diameter is classified as *minor*.
- Perforators origin
  - Originated from medial branch
  - Originated from lateral branch
- Perforator location
  - Distance and coordinate with reference point from the umbilicus
  - Horizontal and vertical plane

22.6 SUMMARY

MRA has been used in preoperative perforator imaging with high sensitivity and specificity. Its use in DIEP flap has been suggested and used in some centres. The result of the studies has shown some advantages over CTA which is currently considered the gold standard imaging modality in several centres.

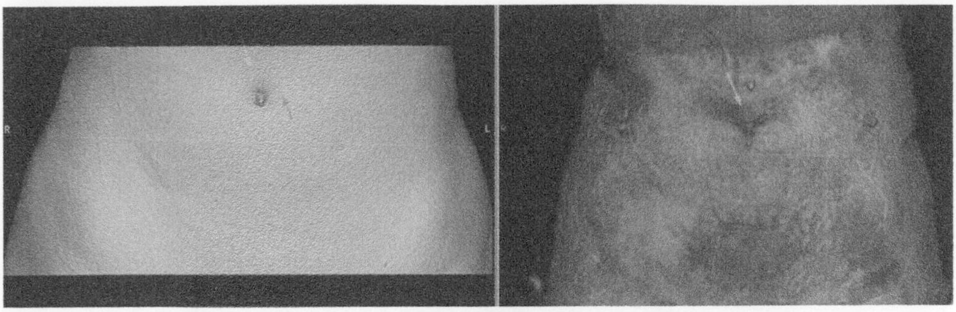

(a) (b)

FIGURE 22.4 Comparative VR reconstruction (anteroposterior view) from MRA (b) and CTA (a) in the same patient for location of main perforator vascular pedicles (arrows). Note the higher resolution and image quality from CTA reformatting.

The benefit of MRA includes better vessel contrast within the muscle, the nonionising nature of the technique, and better tolerance of the contrast media. However, its restriction of being expensive and time-consuming with various contraindications and having a lower sensitivity compared to CTA have hindered its uses in clinical practice. Rozen et al. reported that the financial cost of performing MRA is US$ 600 compared to US$ 400 for CTA.[28] It can provide a precise identification of intramuscular course but is less specific when locating the vessel surrounded by subcutaneous tissue compared to CTA. Both MRA and CTA have a similar accuracy in detecting perforator of greater than 1 mm in diameter. Our experience and the current studies seem to suggest that CTA is more superior in identifying perforator of lesser than 1 mm in diameter (see Figure 22.4).

From our experiences, MRA is an optimal non-invasive radiation-free technique for the location and identification of the main perforator vessels prior to performing DIEP and SGAP flap procedures (see Figures 22.5 and 22.6). MRA also provides an accurate identification of the

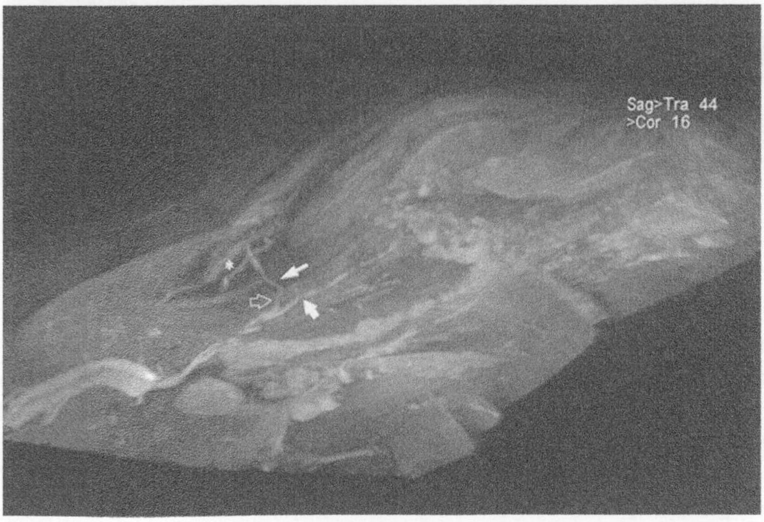

(a)

FIGURE 22.5 (a–c) Volume-rendered technique (VRT) MRI images, using a range of colour lookup table (CLUT) settings, to highlight the course of a DIEA perforator in the same patient. *(Continued)*

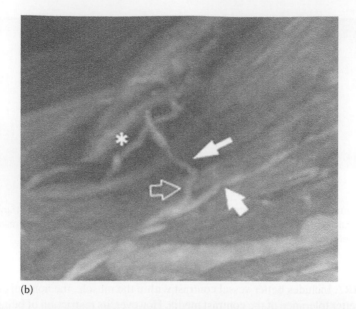

(b)

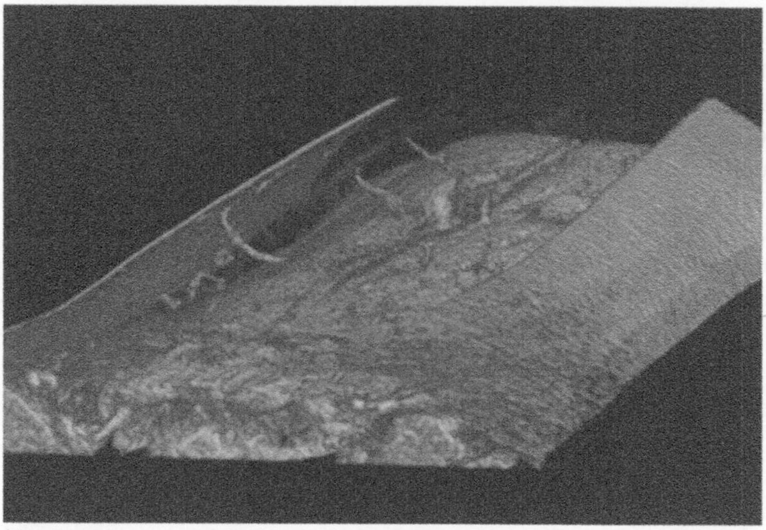

(c)

FIGURE 22.5 (*Continued*) (a–c) Volume-rendered technique (VRT) MRI images, using a range of colour lookup table (CLUT) settings, to highlight the course of a DIEA perforator in the same patient.

intramuscular course of the vessels and other anatomical parameters of interest for surgical procedure. MRA could be considered an alternative to CTA in patients that would be eligible for it, namely, those without metallic implants or claustrophobia, and in which Doppler or duplex studies could be insufficient. However, the opinion regarding the investigation of choice is still widely debated amongst reconstructive surgeons. The evaluation of images and co-working between radiologist and plastic surgeon is essential for preoperative planning, not only to evaluate, select, and mark the vessels but also to perform the 3D reconstructions more usefully and faster.

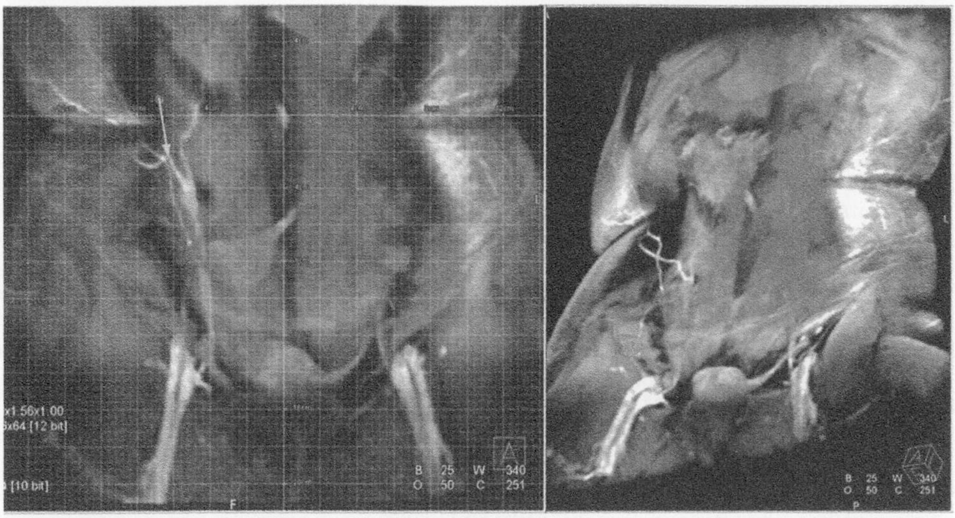

FIGURE 22.6 Location of the main vascular pedicle. Due to higher tissue resolution of MRA, the entire vascular pedicle can be seen, not only the subcutaneous but also the intramuscular course as well as the venous component.

REFERENCES

1. Hendee WR, Morgan CJ. Magnetic resonance imaging. Part I – Physical principles. *Western J Med* 1984;141(4):491–500.
2. Hartung MP, Grist TM, Francois CJ. Magnetic resonance angiography: Current status and future directions. *J Cardiov Magn Reson* 2011;13:19–30.
3. Rozen WM, Anavekar NS, Ashton MW, Stella DL, Grinsell D, Bloom R, Taylor GI. Does the preoperative imaging of perforators with CT angiography improve operative outcomes in breast reconstruction? *Microsurgery* 2008;28:516–523.
4. Rozen WM, Ashton MW, Grinsell D, Stella DL, Phillips TJ, Taylor GI. Establishing the case for CT angiography in the preoperative imaging of perforators for DIEA perforator flaps. *Microsurgery* 2008;28:227–232.
5. Law MW, Chung AC. Segmentation of intracranial vessels and aneurysms in phase contrast magnetic resonance angiography using multirange filters and local variances. *IEEE Trans Image Process* 2013;22(3):845–859.
6. Kramer JH, Arnoldi E, Francois CJ et al. Dynamic and static magnetic resonance angiography of the supra-aortic vessels at 3.0 T: Intraindividual comparison of gadobutrol, gadobenate dimeglumine, and gadoterate meglumine at equimolar dose. *Invest Radiol* 2013;48(3):121–128.
7. Galizia M, Ward E, Rodriguez H, Collins J, Carr J. Improved characterization of popliteal aneurysms using gadofosveset-enhanced equilibrium phase magnetic resonance angiography. *J Vasc Surg* 2013;57:837–841.
8. Chiribiri A, Botnar RM, Nagel E. Magnetic resonance coronary angiography: Where are we today? *Curr Cardiol Rep* 2013;15(2):328–334.
9. Ko SF, Sheu JJ, Lee CC et al. TRICKS magnetic resonance angiography at 3-tesla for assessing whole lower extremity vascular tree in patients with high-grade critical limb ischemia: DSA and TASC II guidelines correlations. *Sci World J* 2012;2012:1921–1950.
10. Lorenz RR, Esclamado R. Preoperative magnetic resonance angiography in fibular-free flap reconstruction of head and neck defects. *Head Neck* 2001;23(10):844–850.
11. Fukuyama H, Kameyama M, Nabatame H et al. Magnetic resonance images of neuro-Behcet syndrome show precise brain stem lesions. Report of a case. *Acta Neurol Scand* 1987;75(1):70–73.
12. Lohan DG, Tomasian A, Krishnam M et al. MR angiography of lower extremities at 3 T: Presurgical planning of fibular free flap transfer for facial reconstruction. *Am J Roentgenol* 2008;190:770–776.

13. Kelly AM, Cronin P, Hussain HK et al. Preoperative MR angiography in free fibula flap transfer for head and neck cancer: Clinical application and influence on surgical decision making. *Am J Roentgenol* 2007;188:268–274.
14. Hölzle F, Ristow O, Rau A et al. Evaluation of the vessels of the lower leg before microsurgical fibular transfer. Part II: Magnetic resonance angiography for standard preoperative assessment. *Br J Oral Maxillofac Surg* 2011;49(4):275–280.
15. Fukaya E, Grossman RF, Saloner D et al. Magnetic resonance angiography for free fibula flap transfer. *J Reconstr Microsurg* 2007;23:205–211.
16. Fukaya E, Saloner D, Leon P et al. Magnetic resonance angiography to evaluate septocutaneous perforators in free fibula flap transfer. *J Plast Reconstr Aesthet Surg* 2010;63:1099–1104.
17. Vasile JV, Newman T, Rusch DG et al. Anatomic imaging of gluteal perforator flaps without ionizing radiation: Seeing is believing with magnetic resonance angiography. *J Reconstr Microsurg* 2010;26(1):45–57.
18. Newman TM, Vasile J, Levine JL et al. Perforator flap magnetic resonance angiography for reconstructive breast surgery: A review of 25 deep inferior epigastric and gluteal perforator artery flap patients. *J Magn Reson* 2010;31(5):1176–1184.
19. Blondeel PN, Beyens G, Vergaeghe R, Van Landuyt K, Tonnard P, Monstrey SJ, Matton G. Doppler flowmetry in the planning of perforator flaps. *Br J Plast Surg* 1998;51:202–209.
20. Giunta RE, Geisweid A, Feller AM. The value of preoperative Doppler sonography for planning free perforator flaps. *Plast Reconstr Surg* 2000;105:2381–2386.
21. Hallock GG. Evaluation of fasciocutaneous perforators using color duplex imaging. *Plast Reconstr Surg* 1994;94:644–651.
22. Hallock GG. Doppler sonography and colour duplex imaging for planning a perforator flap. *Clin Plast Surg* 2003;30:347–357.
23. Mah E, Temple F, Morrison WA. Value of pre-operative Doppler ultrasound assessment of deep inferior epigastric perforators in free flap breast reconstruction. *ANZ J Surg* 2005;75(Suppl.):A89–A97.
24. Rozen WM, Phillips TJ, Ashton MW, Stella DL, Gibson RN, Taylor GI. Preoperative imaging for DIEA perforator flaps: A comparative study of computed tomographic angiography and Doppler ultrasound. *Plast Reconstr Surg* 2008;121:9–16.
25. Phillips TJ, Stella DL, Rozen WM, Ashton MW, Taylor GI. Abdominal wall CT angiography: A detailed account of a newly established preoperative imaging technique. *Radiology* 2008;249:1132–1144.
26. Rozen WM, Ashton MW, Stella DL, Phillips TJ, Taylor GI. The accuracy of CT angiography for mapping the perforators of the DIEA: A cadaveric study. *Plast Reconstr Surg* 2008;122:363–369.
27. Chernyak V, Rozenblit AM, Greenspun DT et al. Breast reconstruction with deep inferior epigastric artery perforator flap: 3.0-T gadolinium-enhanced MR imaging for preoperative localization of abdominal wall perforators. *Radiology* 2009;250(2):417–424.
28. Rozen WM, Stella DL, Bowden J, Taylor GI, Ashton MW. Advances in the pre-operative planning of deep inferior epigastric artery perforator flaps: Magnetic resonance angiography. *Microsurgery* 2009;29(2):119–123.
29. Neil-Dwyer JG, Ludman CN, Schaverien M, McCulley SJ, Perks AG. Magnetic resonance angiography in preoperative planning of deep inferior epigastric artery perforator flaps. *J Plast Reconstr* 2009;62(12):1661–1665.
30. Hartung MP, Grist TM, Francois CJ. Magnetic resonance angiography: Current status and future directions. *J Cardiov Magn Reson* 2011;13:19–25.
31. Mathes DW, Neligan PC. Preoperative imaging techniques for perforator selection in abdomen-based microsurgical breast reconstruction. *Clin Plast Surg* 2010;37(4):581–591.
32. Pratt GF, Rozen WM, Chubb D, Ashton MW, Alonso-Burgos A, Whitaker IS. Preoperative imaging for perforator flaps in reconstructive surgery: A systematic review of the evidence for current techniques. *Ann Plas Surg* 2012;69(1):3–9.
33. Heitland AS, Markowicz M, Koellensperger E, Schoth F, Feller AM, Pallua N. Duplex ultrasound imaging in free transverse rectus abdominis muscle, deep inferior epigastric artery perforator, and superior gluteal artery perforator flaps: Early and long-term comparison of perfusion changes in free flaps following breast reconstruction. *Ann Plas Surg* 2005;55(2):117–121.
34. Aubry S, Pauchot J, Kastler A, Laurent O, Tropet Y, Runge M. Preoperative imaging in the planning of deep inferior epigastric artery perforator flap surgery. *Skeletal Radiol* 2013;42(3):319–327.
35. Rozen WM, Phillips TJ, Ashton MW, Stella DL, Taylor GI. A new preoperative imaging modality for free flaps in breast reconstruction: Computed tomographic angiography. *Plast Reconstr Surg* 2008;122(1):38e–40e.

36. Alonso-Burgos A, Garcia-Tutor E, Bastarrika G, Cano D, Martinez-Cuesta A, Pina LJ. Preoperative planning of deep inferior epigastric artery perforator flap reconstruction with multislice-CT angiography: Imaging findings and initial experience. *J Plast Reconst Aesth Surg* 2006;59(6):585–593.
37. Masia J, Clavero JA, Larranaga JR, Alomar X, Pons G, Serret P. Multidetector-row computed tomography in the planning of abdominal perforator flaps. *J Plast Reconst Aesth Surg* 2006;59(6):594–599.
38. Schaverien MV, Ludman CN, Neil-Dwyer J, McCulley SJ. Contrast-enhanced magnetic resonance angiography for preoperative imaging of deep inferior epigastric artery perforator flaps: Advantages and disadvantages compared with computed tomography angiography: A United Kingdom perspective. *Ann Plas Surg* 2011;67(6):671–674.
39. Hedley AJ, Molan MP, Hare DL, Anavekar NS, Ierino FL. Nephrogenic systemic fibrosis associated with gadolinium-containing contrast media administration in patients with reduced glomerular filtration rate. *Australas Radio* 2007;51(3):300–308.
40. Perazella MA, Rodby RA. Gadolinium-induced nephrogenic systemic fibrosis in patients with kidney disease. *Am J Med* 2007;120(7):561–562.
41. Perazella MA, Reilly RF. Nephrogenic systemic fibrosis: Recommendations for gadolinium-based contrast use in patients with kidney disease. *Semin Dialysis* 2008;21(2):171–173.
42. Pauchot J, Aubry S, Kastler A, Laurent O, Kastler B, Tropet Y. Preoperative imaging for deep inferior epigastric perforator flaps: A comparative study of computed tomographic angiography and magnetic resonance angiography. *Eur J Plast Surg* 2012;35:795–801.

23 Surgical Principles of Deep Inferior Epigastric Artery and Deep Superior Epigastric Artery Perforator Flap

Vachara Niumsawatt, Mark W. Ashton, Warren M. Rozen, and Iain S. Whitaker

CONTENTS

23.1 OVERVIEW

The main blood supply of the anterior abdominal wall traditionally has been described as being supplied by a system of deep and superficial named arteries. The deep system is divided into the superior abdomen which has primary supplies by the deep superior epigastric artery (DSEA) and the inferior abdomen supplies by the deep inferior epigastric artery (DIEA). DSEA is a continuation course from the internal thoracic artery or internal mammary artery (IMA) and DIEA from external iliac artery. For the purpose of reducing confusion, the internal thoracic artery as used in the anatomical literature will be referred to as IMA as referred to by many clinicians. These vessels have an intramuscular course within the rectus abdominis (RA) muscle which they supply. They anastomose within the RA muscle midway between the xiphoid and the umbilicus. A flap can be raised as muscle, myocutaneous, or fasciocutaneous flap. Rectus muscle flap (transverse RA myocutaneous [TRAM] or vertical RA muscle [VRAM]) can be raised as superior pedicle based on the DSEA or inferior pedicle based on the DIEA. Better understanding of perforator flap and improvement in microsurgery has allowed plastic and reconstructive surgeons to harvest a flap based entirely on the perforator which allows the muscle to be spared, thus reducing the donor site morbidity. These flaps have become a work-horse flap in reconstructive surgery. DIEP flap has become widely accepted by both surgeons and patients in autologous breast reconstruction worldwide. Similarly, TRAM and VRAM flaps are commonly used in anterior thorax reconstruction.

23.2 DSEA AND DSEV ANATOMY

23.2.1 DSEA Anatomy

The DSEA originates as one of the two terminal branches of the IMA at the level of the sixth costal cartilage. The other terminal branch is the musculophrenic artery which perforates through the diaphragm at the eighth or ninth costal cartilage and ends considerably reduced in size opposite the last intercostal space. The DESA descends behind the lower costal cartilages to leave the thorax and enter the RA muscle. At the level of the seventh costal cartilages, the DSEA gives off a constant 'superficial' branch that pierces the RA fascia at 0.5–1.0 cm inferior to the xiphoid called the superficial superior epigastric artery (SSEA).[1,2] Within the rectus sheath, the DSEA has a variable branching pattern. It can remain as a single trunk, bifurcating, trifurcating, or in a rare circumstance four branches. It then descend to subsequently branch into a network of increasingly smaller calibre vessels which anastomose with a similar network arising from the DIEA system. In addition to inferior branches of the DSEA anastomosing with the DIEA, it also gives off lateral branches to anastomose with the intercostal arteries, branches deep to the RA to supply the posterior rectus sheath and peritoneum, muscular branches to supply the RA, and anterior perforating branches to supply skin and subcutaneous tissues.

Cutaneous perforators of the DSEA are located in the region bounded by the midline and the linea semilunaris. DSEA gives off perforators through its entire length from the xiphisternum in the plane midway between the xiphoid and the umbilicus. A multidetector computed tomography angiography (MDCTA) study performed by Mah et al. and Hamdi et al. has identified a mean of 3.1–3.9 anterior perforators with diameter greater than 0.5 mm, ranging from 2 to 7 perforators with no statistical differences between the left and the right side.[1,3] At least two perforators from the DSEA with a diameter of greater than 1 mm per hemiabdomen can constantly be identified in the study.[3] The highest concentration of the perforators is located between 1.5 and 6.5 cm lateral from the midline and 10–15 cm inferior to the xiphoid.[1] Bhatti et al. have also performed a cadaveric study to identify the perforators and location of the DSEA with similar result reported that the majority of the perforators were musculocutaneous (type C – Mathes and Nahai) and some perforators pass medial to the RA as septocutaneous (type B – Mathes and Nahai) in origin.[4]

23.2.2 DSEV Anatomy

The venous drainage of the anterior abdominal wall is highly variable and as such has been a minimal documented study in the literature. Carramenha e Costa et al. studied the venous anatomy of the TRAM flap which included the venous drainage of the RA and the anterior abdominal wall using cadaveric dye study. They were able to identify superficial epigastric and deep epigastric venous network. These two venous systems are interconnected with the superficial drains into the deep network. The superficial venous network (skin and subcutaneous tissue) communicated with deep epigastric veins by way of small venae comitantes accompanying the vertical perforators. The deep superior and inferior epigastric veins are the confluences of the venae comitantes of the deep superior and inferior epigastric arteries. At the upper third of the muscle, the deep superior epigastric vein (DSEV) extended longitudinally along the long axis of the muscle between the undersurface of the RA muscle and the posterior rectus sheath. It then veers off toward the medial border of the muscle just a few centimetres from the muscle origin and close to the costal border. In the middle third of the muscle, just above the umbilicus, the veins penetrated the muscle fibres and form a network of small branches. This network anastomoses with deep inferior epigastric vein (DIEV) network at the venule levels. Both of these networks then drain into the internal thoracic vein.[5]

23.3 DIEA AND DIEV ANATOMY

23.3.1 DIEA Anatomy

The DIEA is the dominant vascular supply to the anterior abdominal wall.[6,7] It arises from the external iliac artery directly opposite the origin of the deep circumflex iliac artery. The artery then encroaches upon the deep surface of RA from its lateral border 3–4 cm below the arcuate line. It pierces the transversalis fascia and enters the rectus sheath by passing anterior to the arcuate line. The artery variably gives off two large branches before ascending further, namely, a pubic branch that may represent an abnormal or accessory obturator artery and an early muscular branch to RA. The artery then ascends intramuscularly to anastomose with the DSEA as described in the previous section. Distinct branching pattern of the DIEA emerges above the arcuate line (described in Section 23.4).[8–10] Further branching of DIEA is similar to that of DSEA branches with lateral branches anastomosing with the intercostal, subcostal, and lumbar arteries and inferolateral branches with the ascending branch of the DCIA; deep branches supplying posterior rectus sheath and peritoneum; muscular branches supplying RA; and anterior branches supplying abdominal wall skin and subcutaneous tissues.

23.3.2 DIEV Anatomy

Rozen and Ashton studied the venous drain of the inferior abdominal wall which included a retrospective clinical study and cadaveric lead oxide dissection. They demonstrated the integrate network of venous drainage which is comprised of both superficial (skin and subcutaneous) and deep venous system (intramuscular) as described by Carramenha e Costa.[5,11] The superficial systems consist of superficial inferior epigastric vein (SIEV) which consistently lie superficial to Scarpa's fascia. It receives tributaries throughout its course, from superficial circumflex iliac vein (SCIV) to superficial pudendal vein. It also distributed multiple deep branches throughout its course via the venae comitantes accompanying the DIEA. The deep venous system is comprised of two venae comitantes of the DIEA which accompany the major branches of the DIEA within or deep to the RA muscle. Venous communications between these two venae comitantes were identified throughout the RA muscle. Caudal to the arcuate line, the venae comitantes follow the DIEA course which turned laterally and encroach upon the femoral vein. The two venae comitantes then constitute and form a single DIEV. From their study, DIEV has a mean diameter of 3.2 mm (2.3–3.9 mm) and the mean distance between DIEA and DIEV throughout their course was <5.0 mm.[11] A presence of intravascular valves orientated toward a caudal venous flow of the DIEV system was also noted. The DIEV then anastomoses with DSEV intramuscularly as described in the DSEV section.

23.4 DSEA AND DIEA NETWORK AND VARIATION

23.4.1 DSEA and DIEA Anastomosis Pattern

Main branches of the DSEA run intramuscularly, descending down from coronal to caudal and the main branches of DIEA ascending up from caudal to coronal in the same plain (as described in the DSEA and DIEA anatomy section). They then anastomose midway between the xiphoid and the umbilicus. However, there are several anastomosis patterns described in the literature. In 1988, Moon and Taylor have developed a formal classification system for the branching pattern of the DIEA and it is corresponding DSEA into three types. This classification is based on the quantifying number of branching (type) with the DIEA comprising either as a single trunk (type 1), a bifurcating trunk (type 2), or a trifurcating trunk (type 3) at the arcuate line. Moon and Taylor also noted in their study that only 2% had the anatomy symmetrical on both sides.[8]

Further study by Rozen et al. has found 27% of specimens displaying single trunk, 58% showing bifurcate pattern, and 16% trifurcate pattern. There was no correlation between the number of perforators and the type of DIEA. However, they were able to identify the relationship between the branching pattern and their intramuscular course. A bifurcating (type 2) branching pattern demonstrated a reduced transverse distance traversed by each perforators, whereas a trifurcating (type 3) branching pattern demonstrated perforators that traversed significantly at greater transverse distances. Furthermore, the bifurcating branching pattern demonstrated a shortest intramuscular course, the single trunk has an intermediate course, and the trifurcate trunk has the longest course of all three.[9] The significance of such findings lies with the preoperative planning of DIEA perforator flaps. Muscle preservation plays an important role in reducing donor site morbidity in both DIEA and muscle sparing (MS) TRAM flap reconstruction. Shorter transverse distances traversed by perforators correlate with less RA muscle sacrificed in the raising of a perforator flap. Rozen et al.[10] have also reported a rare case of DIEA which has four major branches above the arcuate line which they have added as a type 4 pattern to the Moon and Taylor's classification.

23.4.2 DIEA Lateral and Medial Role Perforators

Development of DIEA perforators and MS-TRAM free flap has become increasingly utilised in autologous breast reconstruction. Unlike TRAM flap, these flaps rely on dissecting of one or several musculocutaneous perforators and leaving the RA muscle intact. DIEA can form a single trunk, bifurcate, trifurcate, or even have a fourth branch as described in the previous section. During dissection of deep inferior epigastric perforator (DIEP) free flap, it was found that the perforators that emerged from the muscle can be classified as medial role, lateral role, or both. This classification is most commonly described as bifurcating trunk and single trunk were found to be the most frequent and provide the most relevant information in flap reconstruction. Rozen et al.[12] had performed both cadaveric and CTA studies to characterise the property of these perforators as shown in Table 23.1. From this study, the medial row perforators have a greater diameter and shorter and directed course toward the skin. In the superficial adipose layer (above Scarpa's fascia), all perforators were found to branch extensively. However, medial row perforators distributed a greater number of branches and branches of a larger diameter than lateral row perforators. In terms of distribution, medial row perforators uniformly distributed branches that reached the midline or across it in which the lateral row perforators do not. The lateral row perforators branch toward the lateral abdominal wall and away from the midline.[13] This pattern of branching greatly affected the perfusion zones of the flap (see Figures 23.1 and 23.2).

TABLE 23.1
DIEA Perforator Characteristics for Medial and Lateral Row

	Medial Row Perforator	Lateral Row Perforator
Mean diameter	1.3–1.4 mm	1 mm
Course in deep adipose layers[a]	Direct superficial	Lateral
Course in superficial adipose layers[a]	Extensive branching	Limited branching
Midline-crossing branch	98%–100%	0%–2%

[a] The deep adipose and superficial adipose layers are separated by Scarpa's fascia.

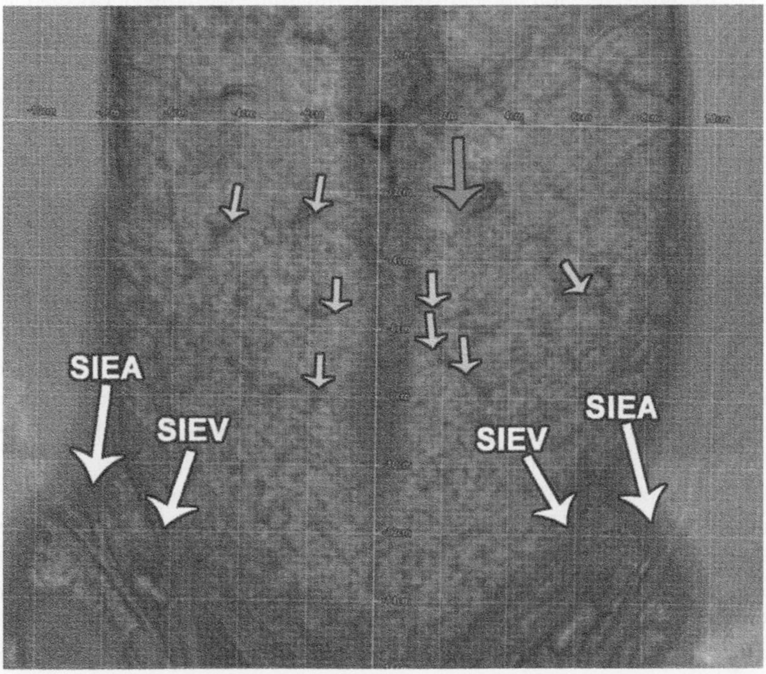

FIGURE 23.1 CTA with volume-rendered technique (VRT) reformat, demonstrating a large 1.5 mm perforator (blue arrow) and multiple smaller perforators (yellow arrows) at the point at which they pierce the anterior rectus sheath. A numbered grid is centred at the umbilicus for localisation. The superficial inferior epigastric artery (SIEA) and vein (SIEV) on each side is demonstrated. (Reproduced from Rozen, W.M. and Ashton, M.W., *ANZ J. Surg.*, 79, 598, 2009. With permission.)

The anterior abdominal wall skin and subcutaneous tissue had been shown to be sequentially perfused in zones. They are divided into four zones of perfusion spanning the abdominal wall flap, filling sequentially from the entry of vascular pedicle. The zone of greatest vascularity has been described as zone I (where the DIEA directly emerges from the RA), the ipsilateral lateral abdominal wall is zone II, contralateral midline abdominal wall is zone III, and contralateral lateral abdominal wall is zone IV.[14–16] Further study into the zone of perfusion of the DIEA perforators cannot be described in the same manner as the angiosome of DIEA in the myocutaneous flap (i.e. TRAM flap). This is due to the fact that perforator flap has a single perforator source and an axial artery has multiple perforators.[13,17] Rozen et al. have termed this concept *perforator angiosome*. In the medial row perforator, zone I which has the most abundant blood supply is located midline, and in the lateral row it is located lateral to the abdominal wall. The medial row zones are

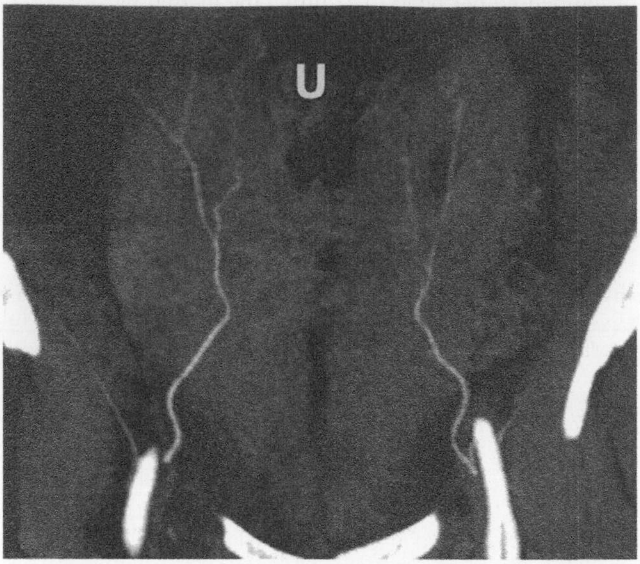

FIGURE 23.2 CTA with VRT reformat, demonstrating the branching pattern of the deep inferior epigastric arteries (DIEAs). The left side is a type 2 (bifurcating) pattern and the right is a type 3 (trifurcating) pattern. U, Umbilicus. (Reproduced from Rozen, W.M. and Ashton, M.W., *ANZ J. Surg.*, 79, 598, 2009. With permission.)

centred mid-abdominal line as it is over the position of perforators as they emerge from the anterior rectus sheath. However, in lateral row, perforators do not centre over the point of emergence but rather are course lateral to the location RA. This is due to a lengthy lateral course traversed by lateral row perforators before reaching Scarpa's fascia and branches.

The primary zones (zones I and II) of medial row perforators routinely cross the midline to perfuse the medial parts of the contralateral hemiabdominal wall. Lateral row perforators do not primarily communicate with branches that cross the midline. This results in primary zones of the medial row perforator to lie within the majority of the DIEP flap (central to the abdomen), whereas the lateral row is concentrated over the lateral edge of the flap. From these studies, it can be concluded that medial row perforators are more advantageous in terms of more extensive branching and greater calibre branches in a more central volume of the abdominal wall flap. These perforators are therefore preferable due to the ease of dissection with less trauma to the RA muscle tissue, and more tissue volume can be recruited in the flap design.

23.5 NERVE SUPPLY OF THE ANTERIOR ABDOMINAL AND POTENTIAL IN FLAP RECONSTRUCTION

23.5.1 Nerve Anatomy

Nerves to the anterior abdomen wall supply both sensory and motor function (see Figure 23.3). The anterior and lateral cutaneous branches of the ventral rami of the seventh–twelfth intercostal nerves and the ventral rami of the first and second lumbar nerves have important sensory and motor functions. T7 passes to the area just below the infrasternal notch, T10 toward the umbilicus, and T12 to an area just below the umbilicus. For the remaining nerves, they course in between each segments of the abdomen. The nerves emerge from the costal margin as a mixed sensory and motor nerve transverses the neurovascular plane between the internal oblique and transversus abdominis muscle. The nerves form a plexus running with the most lateral branch of the DIEA before running between the RA muscle and posterior rectus sheath.

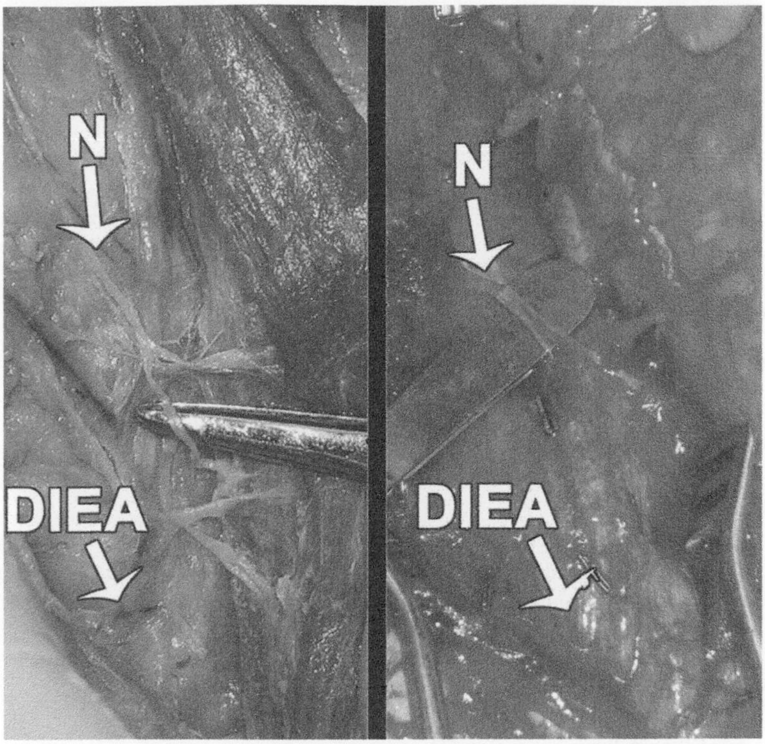

FIGURE 23.3 Photographs of the nerves innervating RA muscle, shown to approach the rectus muscle from its lateral border and be intimately associated with the lateral row perforators. Left = cadaveric dissection, Right = intraoperative photograph. (Reproduced from Rozen, W.M. and Ashton, M.W., *ANZ J. Surg.*, 79, 598, 2009. With permission.)

They entered the rectus sheath from its lateral and posterior margin. Rozen et al. have noted in the study that the nerve plexus is not associated with the medial branch of DIEA when present (i.e. in types 2, 3, and 4). The deep (motor) branches run intramuscularly to the RA which they supply and run corresponding to the line of the DSEA and DIEA.[8] Superficial (sensory) branches accompany the perforator of the DSEA and DIEA toward the skin to supply the sensation of the anterior abdominal wall. There are no midline crossovers of the nerve fibres.[18–20] Due to the relationship of DSEA, DIEA, and its perforators and innervated nerves to the RA, these nerves are at risk during the raising of a DIEA perforator flap. The nerve can easily be damaged or resected during flap elevation especially from the lateral row DIEA. Damage to these nerves may lead to denervation of the RA muscle resulting in muscular atrophy and contribute to donor site morbidity.

23.6 SURGICAL APPROACHES

23.6.1 Muscle and Myocutaneous Flap

23.6.1.1 TRAM/VRAM Flap

The RA myocutaneous flap, first reported by Mathes and Bostwick,[21] is an axial transposition flap based on the superior epigastric artery. It has become popular through its variants such as the pedicle muscle, pedicle myocutaneous, and myocutaneous free flaps.[7] Holmstrom[22] was the first to publish the use of the TRAM transposition flap in breast reconstruction showing that a large abdominal skin paddle based transversely across the midline can survive on a single pedicle.

Flap type: Pedicle or free muscle/myocutaneous flap

Flap classification: Type 3 (Mathes/Nahai).

Application

Superior pedicle flap: Anterior and lateral thorax, breast, abdomen, and posterior trunk.

Inferior pedicle flap: Perineum, vagina, groin, and lower extremity

Microvascular free flap: Breast, posterior trunk, upper extremity, lower extremity, head, and neck (functional muscle).

Vascular supply of the flap

Arterial supply.

Dominant pedicle: DSEA.
Length: 3 cm (range 2–4 cm).
Diameter: 1.5 mm (range 1–2.5 mm).
Origin: Internal thoracic artery.
Course: It runs deep to the sixth intercostal space. The DSEA then runs superficially to the transversus thoracis muscle passing laterally to the xiphoid process. It then runs between the RA and posterior rectus sheath. It anastomoses with the DIEA midline between the xiphoid and umbilicus.

Dominant pedicle: DIEA.
Length: 7 cm (range 6–8 cm).
Diameter: 3.5 mm (range 3–5 mm).
Origin: External iliac artery.
Course: DIEA arises superior to the inguinal ligament and passes superomedially between the peritoneum and the transversalis fascia. It then runs intramuscularly and can form a single, bifurcate, or trifurcate trunk. The medial row gives vertical perforators toward the skin and lateral row perforators run laterally around the rectus sheath.

Minor pedicle: Subcostal and intercostal arteries.
Length: 2 cm.
Diameter: 0.5–1 mm.
Origin: Thoracic aorta.
Course: They run below each corresponding rib. At the anterior portion of each costal arch, the vascular pedicles associate with the intercostal nerves and perforate the transversalis fascia in its lateral aspect. These pedicles anastomose with the DSEA within the deep surface of the RA. They also accompany by the venae comitantes which drain into the inferior vena cava.

Venous drainage

Dominant venous drainage: DSEV.
Length: 3 cm (range 2–4 cm).
Diameter: 2.5 mm (range 1.5–3 mm).
Course: Vein accompanying the perforating pedicles drain into the venae comitantes of the DSEA.

Dominant venous drainage: DIEV.
Length: 6 cm (range 4–8 cm).
Diameter: 4 mm (range 2–5 mm).
Course: Vein accompanying the perforating pedicles drain into the venae comitantes of the DIEA.

Minor venous drainage: SIEV.
Length: 6.4 cm (range 3.5–10 cm).
Diameter: 2.1 mm (range 1–3 mm).

Course: This drains to the saphenous blub and cooperates in skin drainage of the anterior abdomen.

Flap design

Anatomical landmarks: RA muscle is located in the anterior abdomen with their medial limits situated in the midline, except in multiparous women who may have diastasis of the RA muscles. The superior limit is the rib cage with the muscle arising from the fifth, sixth, and seventh costal cartilages. The inferior limit is its insertions at the pubic symphysis and crest. In thin patients, this muscle is easily palpable by getting the patient to crunch.

Flap marking: The standard skin island is located directly over the RA muscle in the vertical orientation. This skin island may extend across the midline or beyond the lateral aspect of the muscle. The limitation of the flap is primarily related to achieving direct donor site closure. A skin island may also be designed transversely across the abdomen. This is usually done and located opposite or distal to the flap base. Thus, if the pedicle is superiorly based, the skin island is between the umbilical and pubic hairline. In inferiorly based flap, the skin island is designed just inferior to the costal margin. Although the skin island can be designed from across the entire abdomen between the two mid-axillaries lines, the perfusion is less reliable in zones III and IV (contralateral abdomen). Xiphoid and pubic symphysis are marked as a reference point of vertical midline to the abdominal wall and allowing for positioning of the umbilicus. This is crucial in the case where skin island flap extends above the umbilicus.

Skin flap dimensions

Upper abdominal skin flap:
Length: 12–14 cm.
Maximum width for primary closure: 5–6 cm.
Thickness: 2.5 cm (range 1–6 cm – depending on body habitus).
Lower abdominal skin flap:
Length: 13 cm (range 10–20 cm).
Maximum width for primary closure: 20 cm (depending on the amount of skin laxity).
Width: 25 cm (range 20–40 cm).
Thickness: 2.5 cm (range 1–6 cm – depending on body habitus).

Muscle dimensions

Length: 25 cm (range 23–29 cm).
Width: 6 cm (range 4–8 cm).
Thickness: 1.5 cm (range 0.7–2 cm); in athletic patient, 2–3.5 cm.

Flap elevation

Myocutaneous flap: After skin marking, the patient is placed in the supine position. If skin flap is taken involving the umbilicus, then incision is made around it. Care is taken not to injure the umbilicus and its stalk. The dissection begins with a superior incision followed by undermining of the upper abdomen. Above the level of the superior incision, extensive undermining laterally to the rectus muscle should not be performed in order to protect the nourishment of the abdominal native skin flap. The lower skin incision is made and the skin of the flap is undermined from lateral to medial above the plane of the external oblique and its anterior sheath. Skin flap is dissected to the lateral and medial border of the ipsilateral rectus sheath. The anterior rectus sheath is then incised on its lateral and medial aspect to expose underlying muscle. Temporary suture is placed around the skin island flap between the skin island, anterior sheath and muscle to avoid disruption or shearing of tissue layers, and musculocutaneous perforating vessels during the remaining flap elevation. The muscle is then separated from the posterior sheath at the distal aspect of the flap beyond the skin island. If pyramidalis muscle (small triangular muscle located between the pubis and linea alba) is identified, it should be preserved by bluntly dissecting off the RA muscle. During the dissection of the muscle, careful dissection is needed to avoid damaging the posterior rectus sheath especially caudal to the arcuate line (semicircular line or arch of Douglas). This arcuate line is located approximately at the level of the anterosuperior iliac spines (ASIS). After the dissection of the muscle off the rectus sheath, the distal muscle is then divided.

Superiorly based pedicle TRAM flap

In superiorly based rectus flap, the DIEA and accompanying veins can be traced at its inferior portion where it is located at the lateral edge of the sheath and divided. If further pedicle length is needed, DIEA can be dissected to the level of the inguinal ligament and divided. In patient whose IMA has been ligated (i.e. in coronary artery bypass graft), preservation of the minor pedicle T8 subcostal artery and associated motor nerve is recommended to provide retrograde flow from the superior epigastric artery.

Inferiorly based pedicle TRAM flap

In inferiorly based rectus flap, the DSEA and accompanying veins are located at the deep medial surface of the muscle. The superior muscle is then divided at the costal margin.

Muscle flap: An incision is performed by a median, paramedian, or even a low transverse incision with the abdominal flap undermined to expose the muscle. The anterior rectus sheath is incised to provide an adequate exposure for muscle elevation. The anterior rectus sheath is then dissected off the muscle. Dissection is then carried out to separate the muscle from the medial and lateral aspect of the rectus sheath. Care is taken not to injure the rectus sheath and muscle at each tendinous intersection. These are located at the xiphoid, umbilicus, and midway between the two. The pedicle is then dissected according to previous description in myocutaneous flap elevation.

Arch of rotation: There are two standard arch of rotation. In superiorly based pedicle flap (DSEA), the point of rotation occurs at the costal margin, and the muscle will provide coverage to the anterior thorax including mediastinum and lateral hemithorax. When the muscle is based on its inferior vascular pedicle (DIEA), the rotation occurs at the pubis and the muscle reaching the groin, perineum, and inferior trunk.

23.6.2 Fasciocutaneous Flap

23.6.2.1 DSEA Flap

Flap type: Pedicle fasciocutaneous flap

Flap classification: Type C (Mathes/Nahai)

Application

Pedicle flap: Anterior thorax and upper abdomen.

Vascular anatomy

Arterial supply.
Dominant pedicle: DSEA.
Length: 6 cm (range 4–8 cm).
Diameter: 1.5 mm (range 1–2.5 mm).
Origin: Internal thoracic artery.

Course: DSEA runs deep to the sixth intercostal space. It passes superficially to the transversus thoracis muscle running laterally to the xiphoid process. It then courses between the RA and posterior rectus sheath and, eventually, anastomoses with the DIEA midline between the xiphoid and umbilicus.

Venous drainage

Dominant venous drainage: DSEV.
Length: 6 cm (range 4–8 cm).
Diameter: 2.5 mm (range 1.5–3 mm).

Course: Vein accompanying the DSEA and its perforator which then drain into the internal mammary vein.

Flap design/elevation technique: A fasciocutaneous pedicle flap is designed as a transverse skin paddle. In the pedicle flap, the edges are from the midline at the lower edge of the wound, based over the DSEA perforators. Flap width is measured to match the height of the defect, and the height of the flap is designed to match the width of the flap. The width of the flap is designed not to go beyond the anterior auxiliary line as in this location, the skin island is no longer supplied by the DSEA perforators but the adjacent territory.[3] The flap was raised from lateral to medial, above the level of the anterior rectus sheath. The anterior rectus sheath can be included with skin island flap to provide additional vascular supply. Further dissection of fine perforators is necessary only for greater mobility and reach. The flap can rotate 180° (propeller flap) on its pivot point.[23]

23.6.2.2 DIEP Flap

Flap type: Free fasciocutaneous flap.

Application

Microvascular free flap: Breast, posterior trunk, upper extremity, lower extremity, head, and neck (tongue reconstruction and facial contour defect).

Vascular anatomy

Arterial supply.
Dominant pedicle: DIEA.
Length: 16 cm (range 14–18 cm).
Diameter: 3.5 mm (range 3–4 mm).
Origin: External iliac artery.
Course: DIEA arises superior to the inguinal ligament and passes superomedially between the peritoneum and the transversalis fascia. It then runs intramuscularly and can form a single, bifurcate, or trifurcate trunk. The medial row gives vertical perforators toward the skin and lateral row perforators run laterally around the rectus sheath.

Venous drainage

Dominant venous drainage: DIEV.
Length: 16 cm (range 14–18 cm).
Diameter: 4 mm (range 2–5 mm).
Course: Vein accompanying the perforating pedicles and drain into the venae comitantes of the DIEA.

Minor venous drainage: SIEV.
Length: 5 cm (range 4–7 cm).
Diameter: 4 mm (range 3–5 mm).
Course: It is a large, superficially located, vertically orientated vein draining the lower abdomen. The SIEV accompanies the superficial inferior epigastric artery (SIEA) located medially and more superficially than SIEA.

Flap design: The flap is designed basing on the preoperative CTA imaging to locate appropriate perforators (see Figures 23.1 through 23.6). Careful selection of side of the abdomen is crucial with consideration of tissue amount, intramuscular course, DIEA row (lateral or medial), perforator size, and the need for bilateral or unilateral reconstruction. Patient is placed in the supine position. The anatomical landmarks are the umbilicus, both ASIS and pubic symphysis. The major perforators are marked on the skin. A handheld Doppler can be used to confirm and locate these perforates once the patient has undergone general anaesthetic. Lines are drawn in a curve shape from one side of the ASIS to the other capturing perforates within the flap. Usually, the superior line is drawn 4–5 cm above the umbilicus and across the pubic hair line.

Flap elevation: After induction with general anaesthetic and flap marking, the lower abdominal incision is made first. The subcutaneous fat is dissected using electrocautery diathermy. The SIEV

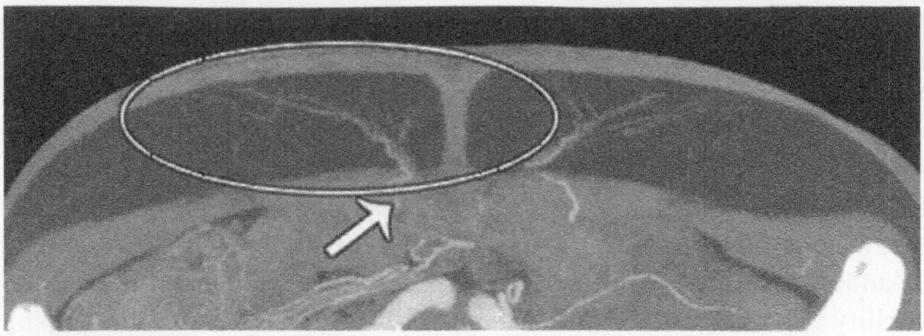

FIGURE 23.4 CTA with axial maximum intensity projection (MIP) reformat, demonstrating the subcutaneous course of perforators. Based on the subcutaneous distribution and branching pattern of the perforator selected (arrow), a preoperative estimate of well-vascularised flap volume can be achieved. (Reproduced from Rozen, W.M. and Ashton, M.W., *ANZ J. Surg.*, 79, 598, 2009. With permission.)

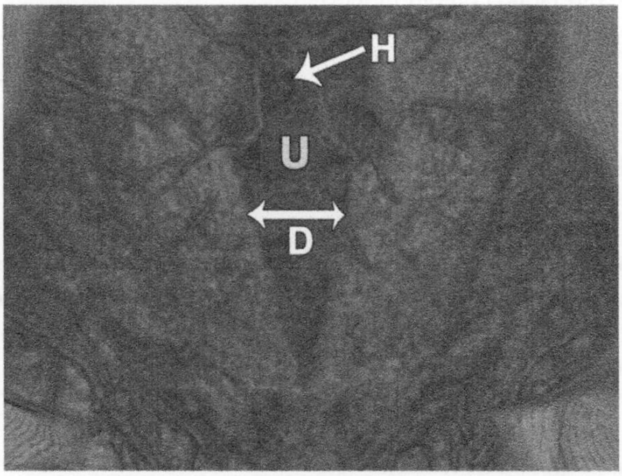

FIGURE 23.5 CTA images with VRT reformat, demonstrating the abdominal wall contour. A supra-umbilical hernia (H) is demonstrated, and substantial rectus divarication (D) can be seen. U, Umbilicus. (Reproduced from Rozen, W.M. and Ashton, M.W., *ANZ J. Surg.*, 79, 598, 2009. With permission.)

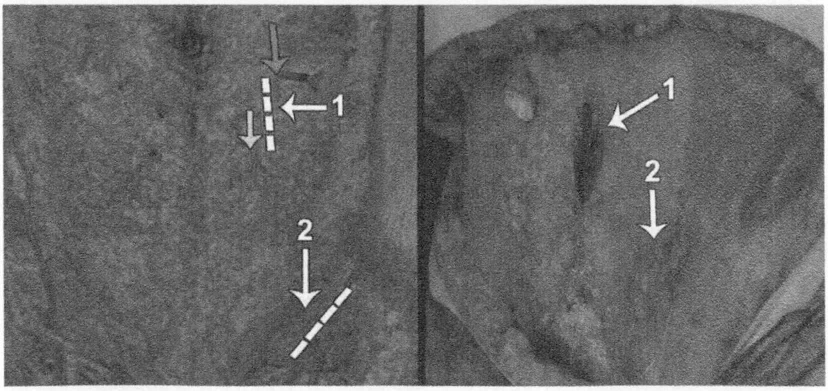

FIGURE 23.6 Technique to minimally open rectus sheath is demonstrated, with a small periumbilical incision to follow the perforators included in the flap (arrow 1), and an oblique lower abdominal incision to access the pedicle (arrow 2). Left = CTA; Right = intraoperative photograph. (Reproduced from Rozen, W.M. and Ashton, M.W., *ANZ J. Surg.*, 79, 598, 2009. With permission.)

is identified on both sides in the superficial subcutaneous tissue (above Scarpa's fascia) proximally 4–5 cm from midline laterally. This vessel can be used for anastomosis if an additional venous drainage is required. The dissection can then proceed through the Camper and Scarpa's fascia. When dissected laterally, SIEA can be identified which is usually located at the midpoint of the inguinal ligament, 2–3 cm lateral to the SIEV and deep to Scarpa's fascia. In DIEP flap, the SIEA can be ligated and flap can be undermined from one lateral edge to the midline superior to the anterior sheath. This technique allows for preservation of the contralateral side as a lifeboat. If medial row perforators are chosen, the flap can be dissected rapidly until reaching the semilunar line, where a careful dissection is needed to locate and preserve the perforators. Once one or two suitable musculocutaneous perforators (preferably with diameter >1 mm) from the RA muscle is identified which are corresponding to the peroperative imaging. The periumbilical and superior incisions are made according to the preoperative marking. The incision is performed in the similar fashion as the inferior portion of the flap. Again, suitable musculocutaneous perforators preserved without scarification of any vessels prior to a final perforator are chosen. Once the best perforator has been chosen, it is then skeletonised above the anterior rectus sheath. A longitudinal incision over the anterior rectus sheath is then made starting from the emergences of the perforator toward the pubis. DIEV can be found adjacent to the DIEA forming a deep inferior epigastric pedicle (DIEP). The DIEP course is then traced with fasciotomy and intramuscular dissection. At this point, the patient should be put in a paralysis state by the anaesthetist as activation of muscle contraction during dissection could damage the pedicle.

For intramuscular dissection, sagittal splitting of the muscle between its fibres is performed thereby minimising muscular damage. Continuing with blunt dissection, the pedicle is separated from the muscle tissue with side branches that are carefully ligated and cut. The inferior portion of DIEP usually lies on the posterior side of the RA. The dissection is continued until they reached the lower lateral border of the rectus muscle. During dissection, one or more segmental intercostal nerves can be identified. They split into sensory and motor branches. The sensory branches usually follow the perforators which can be sacrifices. The motor branches however travel transversely within the muscle layer and should be preserved (more detail in Section 23.5). Once the dissection is completed, contralateral side of the flap can then be detached off the anterior rectus sheath in a similar manner. Flaps can be transferred with large skin islands where needed (particularly in the delayed breast reconstruction setting) or de-epithelialised for large adipofascial flaps, such as for skin-sparing mastectomies (see Figures 23.7 and 23.8).

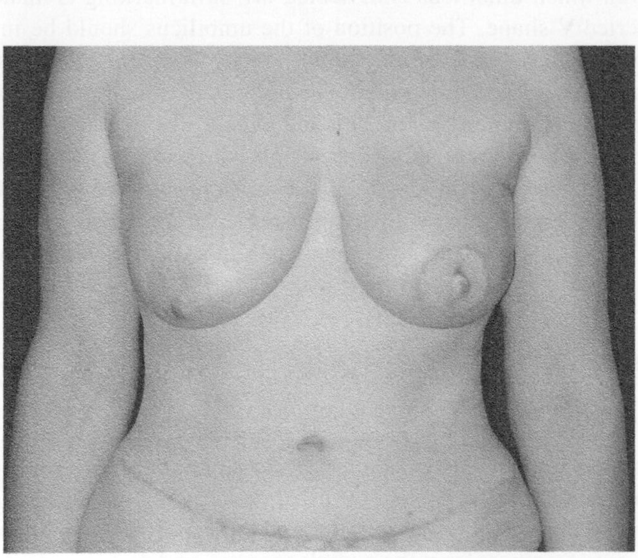

FIGURE 23.7 Post-operative photograph of a DIEA perforator (DIEP) flap breast reconstruction following skin-sparing mastectomy. (Reproduced from Rozen, W.M. and Ashton, M.W., *Aesthet. Plast. Surg.*, 33, 327, 2009. With permission.)

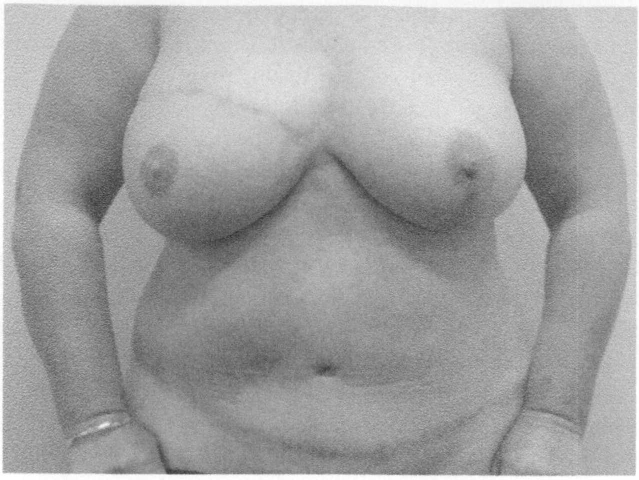

FIGURE 23.8 Post-operative photograph of a DIEA perforator (DIEP) flap breast reconstruction following traditional skin-losing mastectomy. (Reproduced from Rozen, W.M. and Ashton, M.W., *Aesthet. Plast. Surg.*, 33, 327, 2009. With permission.)

23.7 DONOR SITE CLOSURE

The donor site closure is performed as standard direct closure. An onlay mesh is placed on top of the posterior rectus sheath to help prevent abdominal hernia due to the disruption of the muscle and rectus sheath. The rectus sheath is then closed with a continuous 0 polydioxanone (PDS) (Ethicon) suture. Two drain tubes are placed under the skin flap with one located in the superior portion and the other in the inferior portion. In the lower abdominal myocutaneous (superior pedicle base) or free perforator flap (DIEP), the patient is placed in a V-shape or beach-chair position where both head and legs are elevated to decrease tension over the lower abdomen. In the skin island flap in which umbilicus is dissected off, skin marking is made over the superior skin flap in an inverted V shape. The position of the umbilicus should be in the midline using the reference marking from the xiphoid and pubic symphysis. It should be positioned at approximately 12–15 cm from the pubic symphysis.[24] The umbilicus is then passed through the superior abdominal flap. Once the umbilicus is repositioned, a careful inspection of the perfusion to the umbilicus is performed. An exsanguinating of the umbilicus can result from the skin tunnel being too tight. Once the umbilicus is secured with 3/0 absorbable suture, Scarpa's facia is then closed with 2/0 Vicryl. A deep dermal stitch with an absorbable suture running in a continuous fashion across the incision line. The superficial layer can then be closed with either a subcuticular running or and interrupted suture.

23.8 FLAP MODIFICATION TECHNIQUE

23.8.1 Supercharged

In a thin patient who has an inadequate abdominal tissue or patient with midline abdominal scar, in which perfusion is limited to the ipsilateral hemi-flap, raising of the flap can be restricted by perfusion zone. The DIE vessels are the dominant blood supply and perfusion of the flap is the least reliable in the zones farthest from the pedicle (zones 3 and 4).[14] In order to increase this perfusion zone, an additional vessel can be included in the flap. This *charged technique* improves the blood supply to add additional volume of tissue included in the flap. In the *supercharged* procedure, superficial epigastric vessels (for inferior base pedicle), DIE vessels, or superficial circumflex iliac vessels (for superior base pedicle) can be anastomosed to recipient vessels providing additional vascular flap through the flap.

23.8.2 Muscle Sparing TRAM

The principal disadvantage of the transverse RA musculocutaneous (TRAM) flap is abdominal morbidity such as bulge, hernia, and weakness secondary to the scarification of the RA muscle.[25–29] This has led to the development of various modifications of TRAM flap, revolving around the concept for MS-TRAM flap and eventually perforator flaps (DSEP and DIEP). It is possible to split the muscle between the medial and lateral row vessels where only one segment of muscle is required for reconstruction. However, the preserved muscle must retain its vascularisation and innervation; therefore, it is not suitable when the DSEA or DIEA is of a single trunk.[30] A non-vascularised muscle will not be innervated which lacks the ability to contract and subsequently leads to atrophy. For this purpose, it is important to detect the course of the DIEA or DSEA through preoperative imaging (i.e. CTA) in order to maintain the vascularisation. MS-TRAM is usually used if the abdominal wall perforators are insufficient in size; therefore, more than two perforators should be selected to supply the flap. Performing three or more perforator dissections is risky and causes damage to the muscle, thus defeating the purpose of the operation. In this situation, the multiple smaller perforators can be safely harvested with a small cuff of muscle. In 2002, Nahabedian et al. described a classification system for the free MS-TRAM flap as follows: MS0, no RA muscle is spared; MS1, lateral muscle is spared; MS2, both lateral and medial strips of muscle are spared; and MS3, no muscle is harvested and all muscle is spared (deep inferior epigastric perforator DIEP flap).[30] In a study comparing MSO to MS1 and MS2, the incidence of abdominal bulges seems to have decreased. However, a partial flap loss and incidence of fat necrosis have increased, which is likely due to the less perforator vessel recruited in the MS group.[31,32]

23.8.3 Stacked DIEP Flaps

Another option to maximise the use of available tissue in DIEP flap is to combine both sides of the DIEP flap via a microvascular anastomosis which allows for flow, through of blood. This technique allows the patient who has inadequate amount of hemiabdominal tissue to reconstruct a larger breast to match the contralateral side. In 2008, DellaCroce et al. first described this technique which they called *stacked DIEP* in autologous breast reconstruction and presented at the annual meeting of the American society for reconstructive microsurgery, California. The DIEP flap is raised in a normal manner starting with the primary hemiabdomen flap. In this flap, all large branches including the distal extent of the DIE vessels are dissected for at least 2 cm. It is then ligated and clipped off to be used for anastomosis to the second flap. The second flap is then raised in a similar manner as the primary flap. Once the DIE vessels of the second flap is identified and harvested as a single composite with ligation of the pedicels at their dissection point. During the dissection, if SIEA is large enough, it can be used as a backup for anastomosis point for connecting the primary flap. However, DellaCroce found it is easier to use DIEA due to flap orientation and inset. The flaps can either be folded or separated into two separate flaps near the midline. The anastomosis is performed between the primary flap's distal pedicle and the recipient vessels (IMA). The primary flap is then connected to the secondary flap by anastomosis of selected branch point from primary flap and the pedicle of the secondary flap. These anastomoses allow for a flow through of arterial blood and drainage of the venous blood. The secondary flap is then de-epithelised and buried, while the primary flap sits on top. From DellaCroce's experience, they have found no flap failure or returns to surgery from any flap-related problems.[33] All patients were reported to have a high satisfaction cosmetic result, making this technique a reproducible, safe, but technically demanding solution for patients with inadequate abdominal fatty tissue.

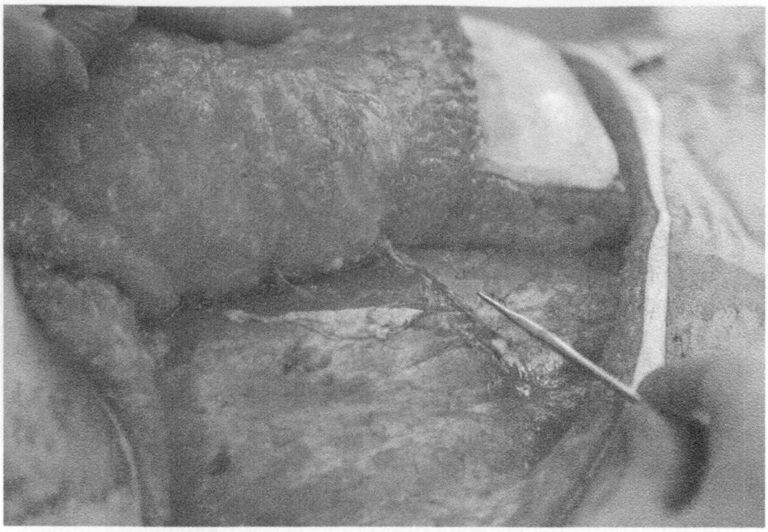

FIGURE 23.9 Intraoperative photograph of a DIEA perforator (DIEP) flap being performed for breast reconstruction, demonstrating perforators (green arrow) traversing the RA muscle to supply the overlying integument of the anterior abdominal wall. (Reproduced from Rozen, W.M. and Ashton, M.W., *Aesthet. Plast. Surg.*, 33, 327, 2009. With permission.)

23.8.4 Sensory Innervation

DIEP flap can also be harvested as a sensate flap. A pure sensory branch of the intercostal nerve usually accompanied the selected perforator on its way to the skin, in its suprafascial course (see Figure 23.9). They are the nerves which branch from the mixed segmental nerve with both motor and sensory nerve running intramuscularly. This sensory branch can be harvested by epineural splitting of the mixed nerve up to the lateral edge of the rectus sheath. It has a length of 3–9 cm which can be used to anastomose the nerve at the recipient site.[34,35] A study by Blondeel et al. showed statistically significantly better pressure sensation in the central region of innervated DIEP flaps compared with DIEP flaps which did not have neural anastomosis.[34] However, sensated DIEP flaps were significantly less sensitive than normal breasts. Erogenous sensation was reported in only 30% of the innervated DIEP flaps. Yap et al. have shown that breasts reconstructed with innervated free MS TRAM flaps have statistically significantly better fine touch and temperature sensation than do breasts reconstructed with nonsensate free MS-TRAM flaps. Interestingly, fine touch sensitivity was better throughout the breasts reconstructed with reinnervated flaps, not just in the central zone.[35] Even though the innervation of DIEP can improve the quality and reliability and provide sensation to the reconstructed breast, the harvest of these nerves typically results in additional dissection through the RA muscle. The division of some motor nerve fibres of the rectus muscle may be needed. Therefore, surgeons and patients must weigh the advantages of increased sensation of the reconstructed breast against the potential disadvantages at the abdominal donor site morbidity.

23.8.5 DSEA Perforator Flaps

The superior abdominal wall has also been used in DSEA perforator flaps and/or thoraco-epigastric flaps, for loco-regional reconstruction. These are based on the perforators of the DSEA as they emerge in the region between the xiphisternum and the umbilicus (see Figures 23.10 and 23.11). One particular application is for sternal reconstruction (see Figure 23.12), where preoperative imaging with either Doppler ultrasound, Duplex, CTA, or MRA can be used to localise one or more perforators and to create a *freestyle* flap to transpose into the chest-wall defect. Such flaps can be raised for a range of trunk defects.

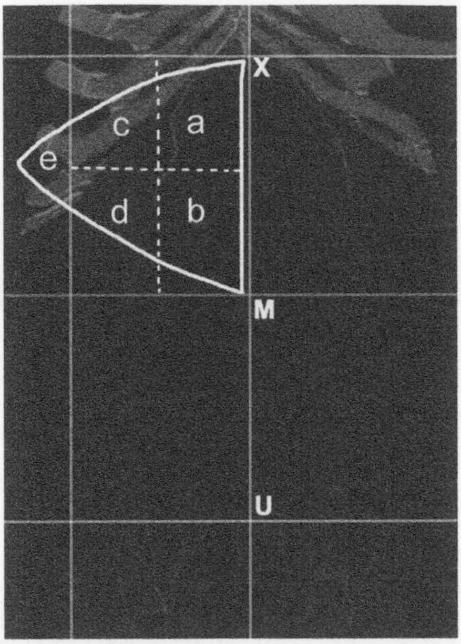

FIGURE 23.10 Schematic of the anterior abdominal wall, demonstrating the orientation a flap based on DSEA perforators. The DSEA perforators lie in the area between the midline and linea semilunaris and between the xiphisternum (X) and the plane midway (M) between the xiphisternum and the umbilicus (U). Zones a–d are depicted for the analysis of perforator location. Zone e is supplied by intercostal artery perforators. (Reproduced from Mah, E. et al., *Plast. Reconstr. Surg.*, 123, 1719, 2009. With permission.)

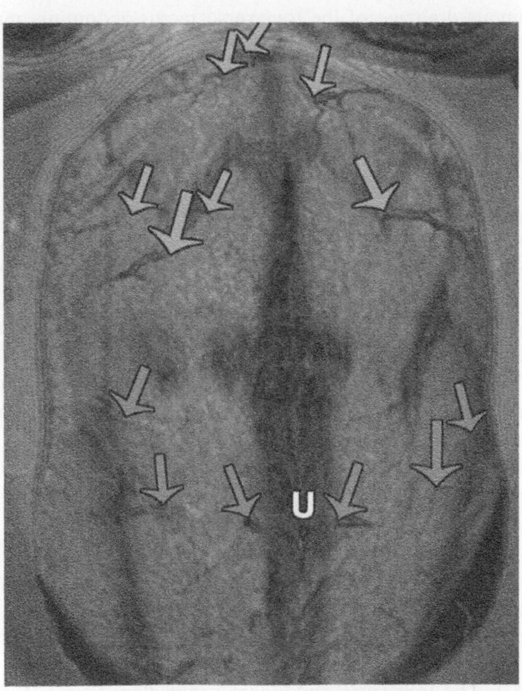

FIGURE 23.11 CTA of the anterior abdominal wall, demonstrating the supra-umbilical cutaneous perforators. Periumbilical perforators originate from the DIEA while peri-xiphisternal perforators originate from the DSEA. U, Umbilicus. (Reproduced from Mah, E. et al., *Plast. Reconstr. Surg.*, 123, 1719, 2009. With permission.)

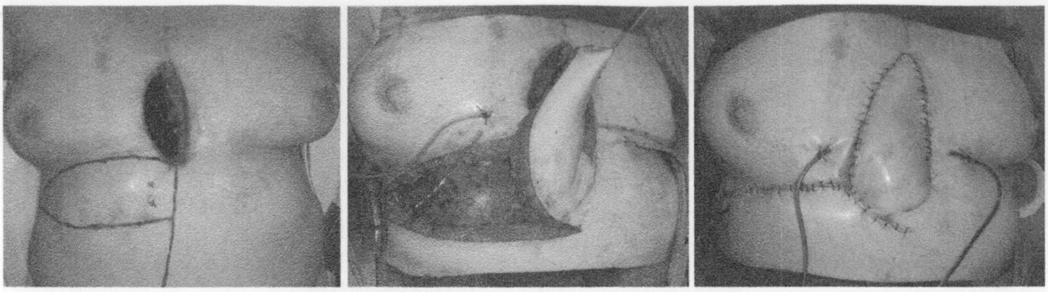

FIGURE 23.12 Sternal reconstruction with the DSEA perforator or thoraco-epigastric flap. Left: Flap design and preoperative perforator localisation. Middle: Flap harvest, with rectus sheath incision noted. Right: Flap inset and direct donor site closure. (Reproduced from Mah, E. et al., *Plast. Reconstr. Surg.*, 123, 1719, 2009. With permission.)

REFERENCES

1. Hamdi M, Van Landuyt K, Ulens S, Van Hedent E, Roche N, Monstrey S. Clinical applications of the superior epigastric artery perforator (SEAP) flap: Anatomical studies and preoperative perforator mapping with multidetector CT. *J Plast Reconstr Aesthet Surg* 2009;62;1127–1134.
2. Rozen WM, Ashton MW, Taylor GI. Reviewing the vascular supply of the anterior abdominal wall: Redefining anatomy for increasingly refined surgery. *Clin Anat* 2008;21(2):89–98.
3. Mah E, Rozen WM, Ashton MW, Flood S. Deep superior epigastric artery perforators: Anatomical study and clinical application in sternal reconstruction. *Plast Reconstr Surg* 2009;123(6):1719–1723.
4. Bhatti AF, Iqbal S, Lee TC. Variation in surface marking of superior epigastric vessels. A guide to safe laparoscopic port insertion. *Surgeon* 2008;6(1):50–52.
5. Carramenha e Costa MA, Carriquiry C, Vasconez LO, Grotting JC, Herrera RH, Windle BH. An anatomic study of the venous drainage of the transverse rectus abdominis musculocutaneous flap. *Plast Reconstr Surg* 1987;79(2):208–213.
6. Taylor GI, Daniel RK. The anatomy of several free flap donor sites. *Plast Reconstr Surg* 1975;56(3):243–253.
7. Taylor GI, Corlett RJ, Boyd JB. The versatile deep inferior epigastric (inferior rectus abdominis) flap. *Br J Plast Surg* 1984;37:330–350.
8. Moon HK, Taylor GI. The vascular anatomy of rectus abdominis musculocutaneous flaps based on the deep superior epigastric system. *Plast Reconstr Surg* 1988;82(5):815–832.
9. Rozen WM, Palmer KP, Suami H et al. The DIEA branching pattern and its relationship to perforators: The importance of preoperative computed tomographic angiography for DIEA perforator flaps. *Plast Reconstr Surg* 2008;121(2):367–373.
10. Rozen WM, Ashton MW, Grinsell D. The type 4 DIEA: A newly identified branching pattern of the deep inferior epigastric artery. *Plast Reconstr Surg* 2010;126(2):86e–87e.
11. Rozen WM, Chubb D, Whitaker IS, Ashton MW. The importance of the superficial venous anatomy of the abdominal wall in planning a superficial inferior epigastric artery (SIEA) flap: Case report and clinical study. *Microsurgery* 2011;31(6):454–457.
12. Rozen WM, Ashton MW, Le Roux CM, Pan WR, Corlett RJ. The perforator angiosome: A new concept in the design of deep inferior epigastric artery perforator flaps for breast reconstruction. *Microsurgery* 2010;30(1):1–7.
13. Rozen WM, Kapila S, Donahoe S. Why there are two rows of deep inferior epigastric artery perforators despite variability in the number of deep inferior epigastric artery trunks: An anatomical and embryological argument. *Clin Anat* 2011;24(6):786–788.
14. Hartrampf CRJ, Scheflan M, Black PW. Breast reconstruction with a transverse abdominal island flap. *Plast Reconstr Surg* 1982;69:216–225.
15. Scheflan M, Dinner MI. The transverse abdominal island flap, Part 1. Indications, contraindications, results, and complications. *Ann Plast Surg* 1983;10:24–35.
16. Scheflan M, Dinner MI. The transverse abdominal island flap, Part 2. Surgical technique. *Ann Plast Surg* 1983;10:120–129.

17. Tregaskiss AP. Re: Perfusion zones of the DIEP flap revisited – A clinical study. *Plast Reconstr Surg* 2006;118:816.
18. Rozen WM, Ashton MW, Murray AC, Taylor GI. Avoiding denervation of rectus abdominis in DIEP flap harvest: The importance of medial row perforators. *Plast Reconstr Surg* 2008;122(3):710–716.
19. Rozen WM, Ashton MW, Kiil BJ et al. Avoiding denervation of rectus abdominis in DIEP flap harvest II: An intraoperative assessment of the nerves to rectus. *Plast Reconstr Surg* 2008;122(5):1321–1325.
20. Rozen WM, Tran TM, Barrington MJ, Ashton MW. Avoiding denervation of the rectus abdominis muscle in DIEP flap harvest III: A functional study of the nerves to the rectus using anesthetic blockade. *Plast Reconstr Surg* 2009;124(2):519–522.
21. Mathes SJ, Bostwick J. A rectus abdominis myocutaneous flap to reconstruct abdominal wall defects. *Br J Plast Surg* 1977;30:282–287.
22. Holmstrom H. The free abdominoplasty flap and its use in breast reconstruction: An experimental study and clinical case report. *Scand J Plast Reconstr Surg* 1974;13:423–427.
23. Woo KJ, Pyon JK, Lim SY, Mun GH, Bang SI, Oh KS. Deep superior epigastric artery perforator 'propeller' flap for abdominal wall reconstruction: A case report. *J Plast Reconstr Aesthet Surg* 2010;63(7):1223–1226.
24. Rodriguez-Feliz JR, Makhijani S, Przybyla A, Hill D, Chao J. Intraoperative assessment of the umbilicopubic distance: A reliable anatomic landmark for transposition of the umbilicus. *Aesthe Plast Surg* 2012;36(1):8–17.
25. Gill PS, Hunt JP, Guerra AB et al. A 10-year retrospective review of 758 DIEP flaps for breast reconstruction. *Plast Reconstr Surg* 2004;113(4):1153–1160.
26. Lejour M, Dome M. Abdominal wall function after rectus abdominis transfer. *Plast Reconstr Surg* 1991;87:1054–1061.
27. Kroll SS, Schusterman MA, Reece GP, Miller MJ, Robb G, Evans G. Abdominal wall strength, bulging, and hernia after TRAM flap breast reconstruction. *Plast Reconstr Surg* 1995;96:616–619.
28. Hartrampf CR Jr. Abdominal wall competence in transverse abdominal island flap operations. *Ann Plast Surg* 1984;12(2):139–146.
29. Nahabedian MY, Dooley W, Singh N et al. Contour abnormalities of the abdomen following breast reconstruction with abdominal flaps: The role of muscle preservation. *Plast Reconstr Surg* 2002;109:91–101.
30. Nahabedian MY, Tsangaris T, Momen B. Breast reconstruction with the DIEP flap or the muscle-sparing (MS-2) free TRAM flap: Is there a difference? *Plast Reconstr Surg* 2005;115(2):436–444.
31. Kroll SS, Marchi M. Comparison of strategies for preventing abdominal-wall weakness after TRAM flap breast reconstruction. *Plast Reconstr Surg* 1992;89(6):1045–1051.
32. Adamthwaite J, Wilson ADH, James S, Searle A, Harris P. A safe approach to sparing the rectus muscle in abdominal-based microvascular breast reconstruction – TRAM, MS-TRAM, DIEP or SIEA? *Eur J Plast Surg* 2012;35:653–661.
33. DellaCroce FJ, Sullivan SK, Trahan C. Stacked deep inferior epigastric perforator flap breast reconstruction: A review of 110 flaps in 55 cases over 3 years. *Plast Reconstr Surg* 2011;127(3):1093–1099.
34. Blondeel PN, Demuynck M, Mete D, Monstrey SJ, Landuyt KV, Matton G. Sensory nerve repair in perforator flaps for autologous breast reconstruction: Sensational or senseless? *Br J Plast Surg* 1999;52:37–44.
35. Yap LH, Whiten SC, Forster A, Stevenson JH. The anatomical and neurophysiological basis of the sensate free TRAM and DIEP flaps. *Br J Plast Surg* 2002;55:35–45.
36. Rozen WM, Ashton MW. Modifying techniques in deep inferior epigastric artery perforator flap harvest with the use of preoperative imaging. *ANZ J Surg* 2009;79(9):598–603.
37. Rozen WM, Ashton MW. Improving outcomes in autologous breast reconstruction. *Aesthetic Plast Surg* 2009;33(3):327–335.

24 Imaging and Surgical Principles of the Superficial Inferior Epigastric Artery Flap

Mark Schaverien

CONTENTS

24.1 BACKGROUND

The superficial inferior epigastric artery (SIEA) flap is based on the SIEA and the superficial inferior epigastric vein (SIEV). Use of the flap was first described by Wood (1863) as a pedicled flap for reconstruction following the release of a burns contracture to the wrist in an 8-year-old child. Antia and Buch first described the use of the free deepithelialised flap for soft tissue reconstruction of the face (1971). Its use in breast reconstruction was introduced by Grotting (1991) and popularised by Arnez et al. (1999a,b).

The principal advantage over other flaps harvested from the lower abdomen is reduced donor-site morbidity as the rectus sheath is left fully intact, avoiding the risk of postoperative bulge or hernia and leading to reduced postoperative pain. The limitations of the flap, however, include variable vascular anatomy and vascular territory and a shorter, smaller calibre pedicle than that of flaps based on deep inferior epigastric artery (DIEA) (Reardon et al. 2004; Taylor and Daniel 1975). For these reasons, presurgical and intraoperative imaging are valuable modalities for flap planning and intraoperative flap design.

24.2 INDICATIONS

The SIEA flap is versatile with widespread applications including reconstruction of the breast, upper and lower extremities, head and neck, trunk, and penile reconstruction (Cheng et al. 1995; Chevray 2004a; Granzow et al. 2006; Koshima 2005; Koshima et al. 1996; Lipa 2007; Liu et al. 2010; Longaker et al. 1996; Raab et al. 2009; Siebert et al. 1996; Stern and Nahai 1992; Stevenson et al. 1984; Woodworth et al. 2006). Although the entire abdominal pannus can be reliably perfused by the superficial inferior epigastric pedicle in selected cases, flap perfusion is usually limited to 1–2 cm beyond the midline (Chevray 2004a; Granzow et al. 2006; Hester et al. 1984; Lipa 2007; Taylor and Daniel 1975; Wolfram et al. 2006). The most popular indication for the SIEA flap is breast reconstruction and the flap is therefore most ideal for bilateral breast reconstruction or unilateral reconstruction of small- or moderately sized breasts (Figures 24.1a,b and 24.2a,b). The SIEA

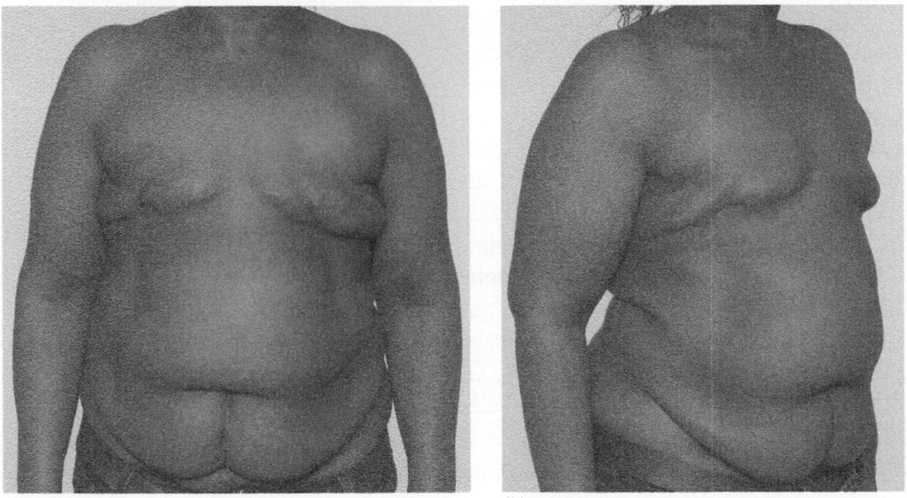

(a) (b)

FIGURE 24.1 Preoperative anterior (a) and right oblique (b) photographs of a patient undergoing bilateral delayed breast reconstruction. Note the presence of low midline abdominal scar.

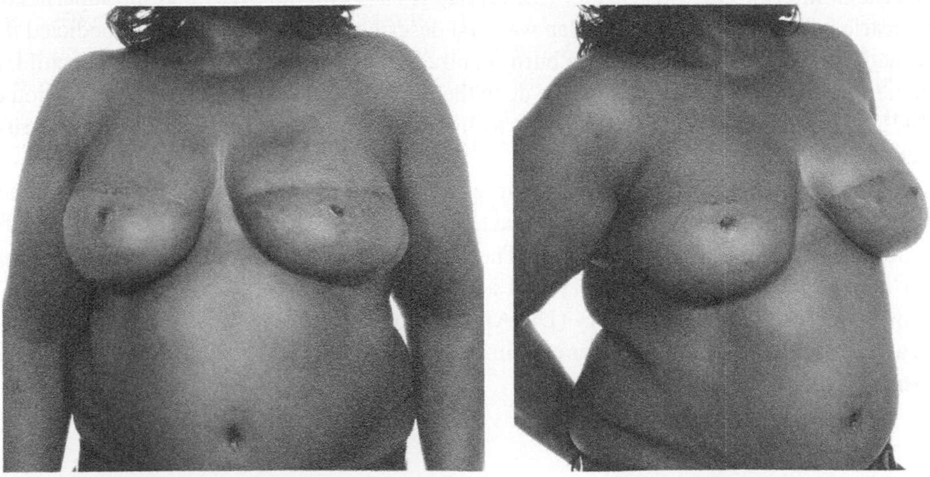

(a) (b)

FIGURE 24.2 Six-month postoperative anterior (a) and right oblique (b) photographs following bilateral breast reconstruction using SIEA flaps. There were no postoperative complications.

flap is best considered an alternative to the DIEA perforator (DIEP) flap in patients with suitable anatomy to decrease donor-site morbidity compared with other flap techniques from the lower abdomen (Selber et al. 2010; Wu et al. 2008). The flap also has utility in reconstruction of partial breast defects (Rizzuto and Allen 2004).

The thickness of the flap is directly related to body habitus and in selected cases may provide a thin pliable flap for head and neck and extremity reconstruction. The SIEA and SIEV lie superficial to Scarpa's fascia within the flap, and therefore flap thinning deep into Scarpa's fascia can be performed if a thin flap is required primarily (Hester et al. 1984).

24.3 CONTRAINDICATIONS

The only absolute contraindication to SIEA flap harvest is previous abdominoplasty. Relative contraindications include previous abdominal liposuction and the presence of abdominal scars, particularly following a Pfannenstiel incision (Mahajan et al. 2012). A low midline abdominal incision usually precludes flap harvest across the midline and may require bipedicled flap designs if large flaps are required. Where abdominal scars are present, preoperative imaging is necessary.

24.4 ANATOMY

The SIEA is a direct cutaneous vessel that has a common origin with the superficial circumflex iliac artery in 79% of cases, and a separate origin in the remainder, approximately 2 cm caudal to the inguinal ligament (Taylor and Daniel 1975). It pierces the cribriform fascia and crosses the inguinal ligament before continuing in a superior course through the subcutaneous tissue of the abdominal wall superficially or just deep to Scarpa's fascia, becoming progressively more superficial as it courses the cephalad within the flap (Figure 24.3). There is considerable variation in the source of drainage of the SIEV, usually draining into the saphenous bulb but also variably draining into the deep inferior epigastric vein, the great saphenous vein, or a common trunk with the superficial circumflex iliac vein (Rozen et al. 2011). It crosses the inguinal ligament at the midpoint or medially within 1 cm of the midpoint, close to the SIEA, coursing through the subcutaneous tissue in a more superficial plane than the artery. Taylor and Daniel (1975) found the SIEA to be present in 65% of 46 cadaver dissections. Allen and Heitland (2002) found the SIEA to be present in 72% of 100 cadaver dissections and in 58% of dissections bilaterally. Herrera et al. (2010) found the SIEA to be present in 80% (51 of 64) of dissections and of adequate calibre in 44% (28 of 64) of all cases. Reardon et al. (2004) noted a patent SIEA in 20/22 (91%) of their dissections. Rozen et al. (2010a), in a clinical anatomical study of CT angiograms in 250 patients, identified the SIEA in 94% of hemiabdomens, with a diameter greater than 1.5 mm in only 24% of cases. These findings were similar to those of Chevray (2004a), where the vessel presence and calibre were only sufficient for SIEA transfer in 30% of 47 consecutive abdominal breast reconstructions. Reardon et al. (2004) found that the SIEA was located within 1 cm of the midpoint of the inguinal ligament in 68% of cases and within 2 cm

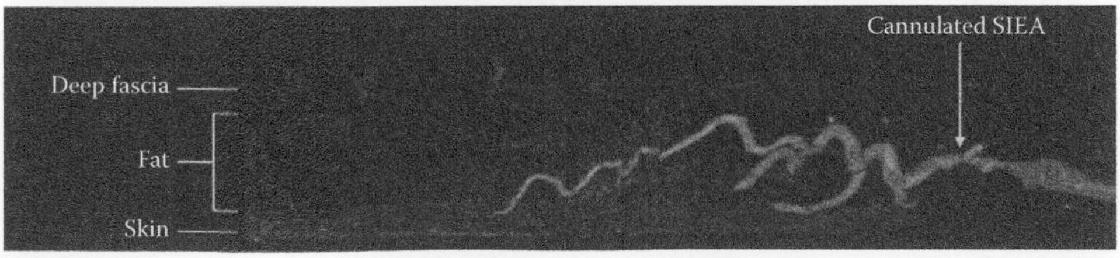

FIGURE 24.3 Lateral view of a CT angiogram of a SIEA flap, with the SIEA individually cannulated, during early injection with iodinated CT contrast medium. Note how the vessel becomes progressively more superficial within the flap as it courses the cephalad (Mark Schaverien and Michel Saint-Cyr, Department of Plastic Surgery, University of Texas Southwestern Medical Center).

of the midpoint in 77% of cases. The pedicle length ranged from 3 to 7 cm (mean 5.2 cm) and the vessel calibre from 1.2 to 2.5 mm (mean 1.9 mm).

The SIEA predominantly perfuses the lateral zone of the lower abdomen where the pedicle enters (Holm et al. 2007), typically perfusing the ipsilateral medial zone of the flap via recurrent flow through the subdermal plexus into the medial row of DIEPs, and perfusion across the midline is possible via the connections across the midline between the medial row perforators (Figure 24.4a,b; Schaverien et al. 2008). Reliable flap harvest is therefore usually limited to the ipsilateral hemiflap (Holm et al. 2007). There is however significant variability in the anatomical course and branching pattern of the SIEA, with branches crossing the midline in approximately 5% of cases (Rozen et al. 2010a), leading to significant variability in its angiosome (Holm et al. 2008). Laser-induced fluorescence of indocyanine green studies by Holm et al. (2008) have demonstrated that the perfused vascular territory of the SIEA is highly variable, with perfusion of the entire abdominal ellipse seen in only 20% of patients.

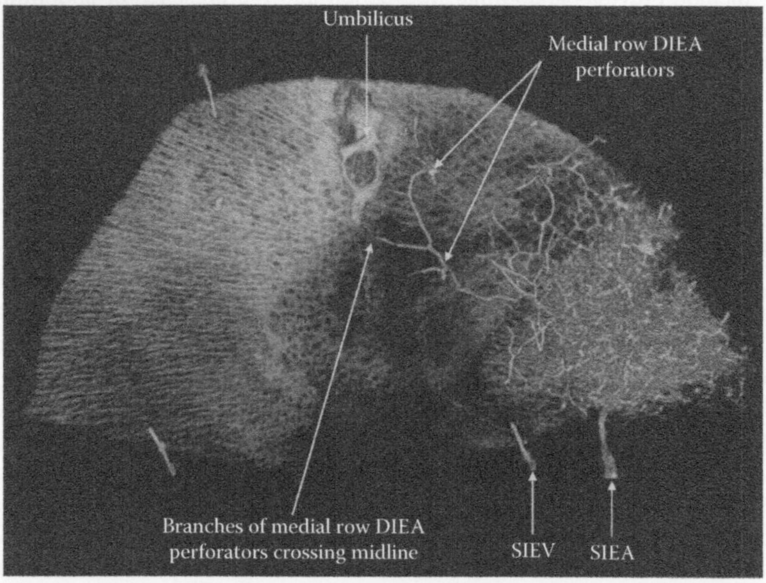

(a)

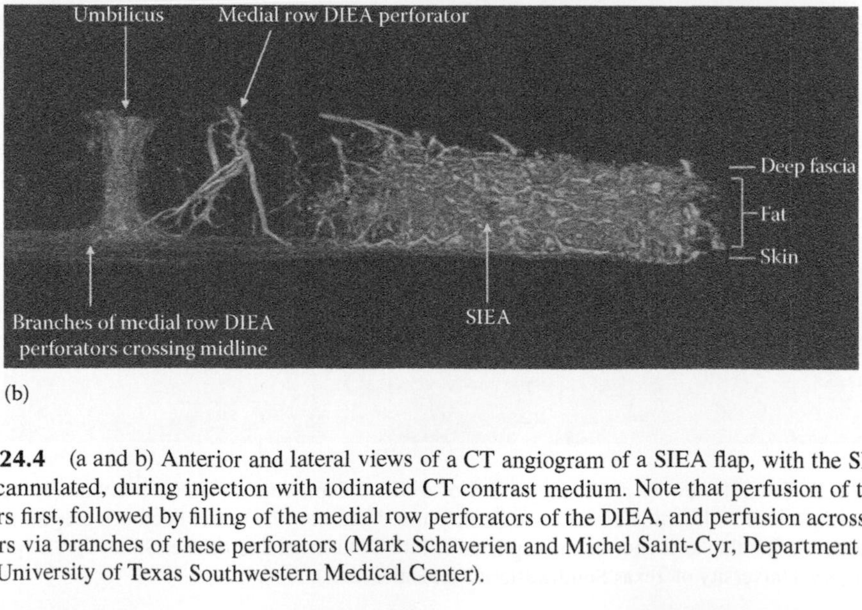

(b)

FIGURE 24.4 (a and b) Anterior and lateral views of a CT angiogram of a SIEA flap, with the SIEA individually cannulated, during injection with iodinated CT contrast medium. Note that perfusion of the lateral flap occurs first, followed by filling of the medial row perforators of the DIEA, and perfusion across the midline occurs via branches of these perforators (Mark Schaverien and Michel Saint-Cyr, Department of Plastic Surgery, University of Texas Southwestern Medical Center).

Ulusal et al. (2006), however, using intraoperative laser Doppler measurement of SIEA flap perfusion in 14 patients, found no statistically significant difference between the different perfusion zones of the flap. They reported successful use of a mean of 92.3% of the original flap by weight, with fat necrosis occurring in only one flap. Lateral extension of the flap design is also possible via perforators of the deep circumflex iliac artery and the lateral intercostal perforators (Allen and Heitland 2002; Hester et al. 1984; Taylor et al. 2011). The angiosome of the SIEA demonstrates an inverse relationship with that of the DIEA (Holm et al. 2008; Rozen et al. 2010a), suggesting that pre- and intraoperative imaging are valuable for determining when the conditions for SIEA flap harvest are most favourable.

There is increasing emphasis on the importance of consideration of the anatomy of the SIEV in flap harvest, which like the SIEA demonstrates significant anatomical variability (Rozen et al. 2009a, 2011; Schaverien et al. 2008, 2010). Rozen et al. (2011) in a clinical anatomical study of 200 hemiabdominal walls with preoperative computed tomographic angiography (CTA) imaging, found that the presence of more than a single major SIEV trunk was present in 80 hemiabdominal walls (40% of overall sides) and reported a clinical case with two SIEVs draining into separate venous trunks, where well-demarcated venous congestion occurred within the flap following use of only one of these trunks. Anatomical studies have found that the SIEV does not cross the midline in between 8 and 36 percent of cases (Blondeel et al. 2000; Rozen et al. 2009; Schaverien et al. 2008), although the importance of this anatomical variation to SIEA flap design has yet to be established.

24.5 IMAGING

24.5.1 Duplex Ultrasound

Although handheld acoustic Doppler ultrasound can be a useful modality for locating the SIEA and SIEV vessels and DIEP flap perforators, this technique only provides information on the presence of blood vessels and may be unreliable due to its high sensitivity and low specificity (Hallock 2011; Lipa 2007; Taylor et al. 1990). Colour duplex ultrasound gives much more information due to its ability to image the vessels, including the flow velocity of the blood within them, and does not require intravenous contrast. It is, however, a time-consuming modality that is significantly operator dependent and which does not provide a *roadmap* of the vascular anatomy that can be re-reviewed (Blondeel et al. 1998).

Rozen et al. (2008a) compared duplex ultrasound with CTA in eight patients undergoing both modalities prior to DIEP flap breast reconstruction and found that whereas CTA clearly displayed the SIEA system, duplex ultrasound was unable to highlight the SIEA. Scott et al. (2010) performed a prospective study comparing preoperative duplex ultrasound with CTA in 22 consecutive patients undergoing 30 abdomen-based microsurgical breast reconstructions. The SIEA and SIEV were not detected by colour duplex ultrasound in any of the patients; however, in all eight SIEA flap breast reconstructions, the SIEAs were identified preoperatively using CTA. The results of these studies suggest that colour duplex ultrasound is an unsuitable method for preoperative SIEA flap planning.

24.5.2 Computed Tomographic Angiography

The use of CTA for presurgical imaging for the DIEP flap has gained widespread acceptance. Multi-slice CT enables angiograms of the anterior abdominal wall to be performed in less than 20 s, and various volume-rendering functions enable visualisation of the vascular anatomy in three dimensions with elimination of superimposition of structures outside the area of interest. These images provide a surgical roadmap that can be analysed preoperatively and also referred to in the surgical theatre. The modality enables preoperative evaluation of the perforators of the DIEA, including their calibre and course within the muscle and flap, facilitating flap harvest and leading to reduced operating times and complications (Rozen et al. 2008b; Smit et al. 2009). The SIEA can be imaged using a standard arterial phase CTA scan protocol for preoperative imaging of the DIEP flap, and therefore all of the abdominal vessels can be imaged simultaneously (Figure 24.5; Rozen et al. 2009b).

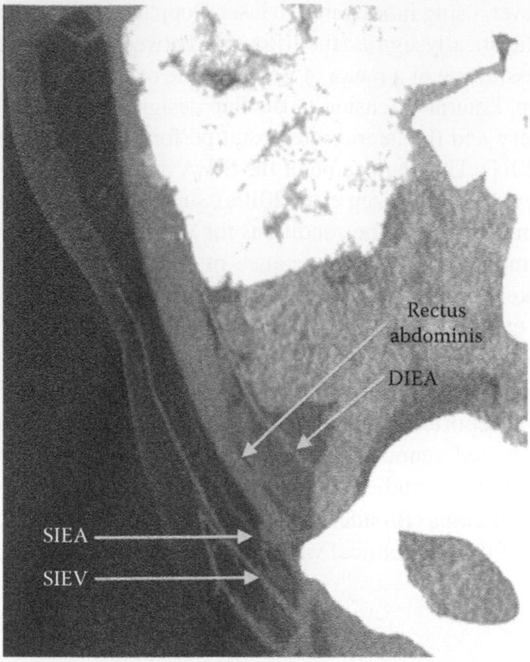

FIGURE 24.5 Sagittal view of a CT angiogram in mixed arterial and venous phase demonstrating the SIEA, SIEV, and DIEA. Note that the SIEV is consistently located more superficially within the flap than the SIEA.

Fukaya et al. (2011) investigated 17 patients who had preoperative CTA in preparation for a free abdominal flap procedure and found that detailed appraisal of the SIEA and SIEV calibre and course was possible in all cases. The authors concluded that CTA should be performed routinely in SIEA flap planning. Piorkowski et al. (2011) performed a retrospective single surgeon analysis of preoperative CT angiograms for 177 free flaps in 113 patients undergoing breast reconstruction with free abdominal flaps. Forty-nine patients (43%) were noted to have at least one visible SIEA, of which only 24 of those patients (21%) were felt to have a SIEA of adequate calibre. Twelve SIEA flaps (10.6%) were performed in 12 patients, and therefore overall 50% of patients found to have at least one adequate SIEA on CT angiogram had a single breast reconstructed with a SIEA flap. In no cases was a usable SIEA that had not been visualised on CTA found during surgery, indicating that CTA was very accurate for SIEA flap planning. Rozen et al. (2010a), in a large clinical anatomical study in 250 patients, found CTA to be a very accurate modality for imaging of the SIEA and noted significant variability in the presence, calibre, and degree of branching of the SIEA. A 100% concordance was found with intraoperative findings, suggesting that presurgical imaging may therefore be useful in SIEA flap planning.

CTA has the advantage of availability in most centres; although CTA will always have the disadvantage compared with other modalities of an inherent exposure to ionising radiation, the dose may be reduced compared with standard abdominal CTA using specialised protocols (Rozen et al. 2009b). In addition, the nephrotoxic effects of iodinated contrast media used in CTA also may pose a risk of further reduction of renal function in compromised patients as well as acute contrast-induced renal failure and hypersensitivity reactions (ten Dam and Wetzels 2008).

24.5.3 Magnetic Resonance Angiography

Like CTA, contrast-enhanced MRA (CE-MRA) provides accurate anatomical information on the SIEA (Rozen et al. 2009c; Schaverien et al. 2011a). The SIEA can be imaged using a standard CE-MRA protocol for presurgical imaging of the DIEP flap (Figure 24.6; Schaverien et al. 2011a).

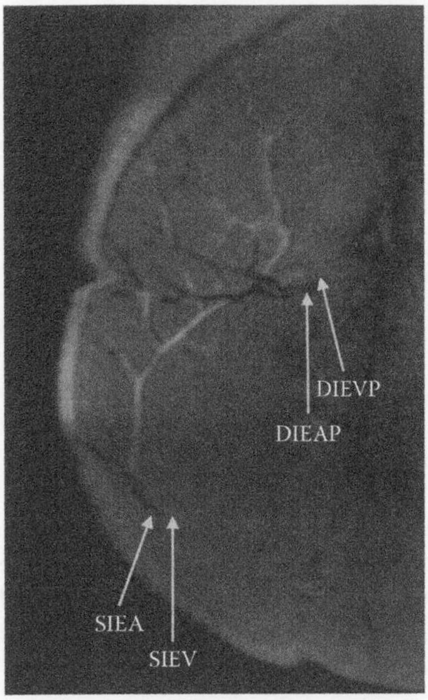

FIGURE 24.6 Sagittal oblique minimum intensity projection MR angiogram in the early arterial phase demonstrating the SIEA, SIEV, and a DIEA arterial perforator with its venae comitantes and the anatomical relationship between them. (Modified from Schaverien, M.V. et al., *Ann. Plast. Surg.*, 67, 671, 2011.)

Rozen et al. (2009c) performed a pilot study comparing CTA and CE-MRA with operative findings in six patients undergoing DIEP flap breast reconstruction and found that the SIEA was accurately imaged in all cases.

The principal advantages of MRA are the avoidance of ionising radiation and the inherent ability to image the superficial venous system of the anterior abdominal wall as flow voids and during early contrast enhancement (Schaverien et al. 2011b). Although CTA may also allow evaluation of the venous system, this either necessitates simultaneous enhancement of the arterial and venous systems or two separate scans (Rozen et al. 2009a, 2010b; Schaverien et al. 2010). The scanning time is similar to CTA at around 17 s with breath-hold image acquisition. MRA is less available than CTA and is more operator dependent. It is contraindicated in patients with certain cardiac pacemakers and metal implants. The gadolinium-based contrast agent is associated with a rare syndrome of nephrogenic systemic fibrosis in patients with severe renal impairment (Ledneva et al. 2009); however non-contrast MR using fresh blood imaging is a very promising advancement that needs to be further investigated (Masia et al. 2010).

24.5.4 Laser Fluorescence

Laser-induced indocyanine green imaging is becoming increasingly utilised for intraoperative, real-time assessment of flap circulation. Intravenous indocyanine green fluoresces under illumination with a laser light source, and this is recorded by a digital video camera, followed by quantitative analysis of the sequences using special software compared with a control region outwith the surgical field. Holm et al. (2007) performed a study of the SIEA angiosome in 10 patients and found a statistically significant reduction in flap perfusion across the midline and cautioned against inclusion of the portion of the flap lateral to the border of the contralateral rectus sheath. In a later study, Holm et al. (2008) performed a study of the vascular territory of the SIEA in 25 patients using the modality and found that it did not cross the midline in 64% of patients, did not perfuse the flap at all in 8%, and perfused the entire abdominal ellipse in 20% of patients. As a SIEA flap was originally intended in all patients, intraoperative perfusion measurements changed the surgical plan in 44% of patients, suggesting that this is a very valuable imaging modality, particularly if the contralateral flap zones are needed for reconstruction. Partial flap necrosis was seen in only one case. The findings of these and other studies using dynamic laser-fluorescence videoangiography suggest that its use may lead to a decreased rate of complications (Komorowska-Timek and Gurtner 2010).

24.6 FLAP MARKINGS

Standard abdominoplasty horizontal elliptical flap markings are made as for a transverse rectus abdominis myocutaneous (TRAM) or DIEP when used for breast reconstruction, although oblique or vertical designs may be used for reconstruction of other regions or for pedicled flaps. The SIEA flap is best utilised for unilateral reconstruction of small- to medium-sized breasts where the whole abdominal pannus is not required or for bilateral reconstruction. Where a large flap is required, a DIEP or TRAM flap may be a better choice (Lipa 2007). The flap is marked with the patient standing, with the lower marking following coursing just above the pubic hairline in the suprapubic crease and extending laterally to the anterior superior iliac spines. The upper marking skirts just above the umbilicus to complete the ellipse. The flap markings may be extended laterally to the midaxillary line if more tissue is required (Granzow et al. 2006; Lipa 2007). Closure is checked with patient lying down, and the upper marking adjusted if necessary.

24.7 SURGICAL PRINCIPLES

The patient is positioned supine and the lower incision is made first. Care is taken to preserve the SIEV which is found superficial to Scarpa's fascia and medial to the midpoint of the inguinal ligament, as this can be a lifeboat for secondary anastomosis in case of venous congestion of a DIEP or rarely a TRAM flap, as well as the pedicle for the SIEA flap. Where present, the SIEA is found lateral to the midpoint of the inguinal ligament and deep to the SIEV, either just superficial or deep to Scarpa's fascia, and its calibre and pulsation are carefully assessed. An artery pedicle diameter of 1 mm or greater at the level of the inguinal ligament is generally considered adequate to support the flap, although some authors have reported that the presence of a palpable pulse is sufficient for successful flap harvest, irrespective of the diameter of the artery (Dorafshar et al. 2010). The pedicle contralateral to the recipient vessels is usually preferred due to easier flap inset, although the vessels on both sides are inspected. If the SIEA vessels are inadequate, then a DIEP or TRAM flap is raised instead.

If potentially suitable for SIEA flap harvest, the chosen SIEA and SIEV are dissected to their origins to provide adequate pedicle length, with care not to cause disruption to the delicate lymphatics that surround the vein as this may lead to a seroma. The remaining incisions are completed and may be beveled outwards to increase the volume of tissue included, and the flap is then raised from the anterior rectus sheath. Where the DIEA perforators are encountered, these are preserved, and once the flap is islanded on these perforators and the SIEA and SIEV, the perforators can be clamped and perfusion within the flap assessed clinically or with intraoperative fluorescence videoangiography. If the flap volume perfused is found to be inadequate, options include conversion to a DIEP or TRAM flap or harvest of a bipedicled SIEA flap.

The location of the pedicle at the side of the flap and the short pedicle length creates special considerations for flap inset compared with other free abdominal flaps, and the contralateral internal mammary artery and vein are the preferred recipient vessels. The calibre of the vessels also well suits anastomosis to the second or third internal mammary artery perforators where present and of sufficient calibre. The flap is rotated 90° to allow the pedicle and better vascularised ipsilateral flap portions to be positioned superomedially, reducing the risk of flap-related complications occurring in the more aesthetically important central chest area. The inferior portion of the flap is usually folded on itself and may be deepithelialised for 2–3 cm to direct the pedicle towards the recipient vessels and avoid kinking (Zenn 2006). Removal of rib cartilage and muscle must be performed sufficiently to avoid compression of the pedicle, and the flap is then shaped and inset over closed suction drains. The abdominal flap is undermined superiorly to the xiphisternum and laterally to the costal margins to allow closure as for an aesthetic abdominoplasty over closed suction drains, the umbilicus is reinset.

24.8 OUTCOMES

The largest series reported by Granzow et al. (2006) included 210 breast reconstructions with SIEA flaps in 174 patients with no flap losses. Fat necrosis occurred in 13% of flaps and donor-site seromas occurred in 4%. There were no hernias or abdominal bulges. Selber et al. (2008) reported results of 72 consecutive SIEA flaps, with two total flap losses (2.9%) and no abdominal hernias or bulges. When compared with 569 consecutive muscle-sparing free TRAM flaps (one total flap loss; 0.18%), the rate of complete flap loss was approximately 16-fold higher. There was also a higher incidence of vessel thrombosis requiring anastomotic revision in the SIEA group (17.4%) compared with the free TRAM group (6.0%). Cheng et al. (2006) compared outcomes in 30 DIEP with 12 SIEA flaps for immediate and delayed breast reconstruction performed by a single surgeon and reported no complete flap losses but one partial flap loss in the SIEA group (8.3%), suggesting similar outcomes between the groups. Ulusal et al. (2006) compared 30 DIEP with 14 SIEA flaps and found a flap loss rate of 0% in the DIEP group and 7% in the SIEA group. Fat necrosis occurred in 3.3% of DIEP and 7.1% of SIEA flaps. Baumann et al. (2010) in a prospective series specifically reporting the outcome of fat necrosis found a 14% rate in 57 SIEA flaps, associated with smoking and inclusion of the contralateral zone of the flap. Chevray (2004a) in a prospective study of 47 free abdominal flaps including 14 SIEA flaps found that the average hospital stay was significantly shorter for patients who underwent unilateral breast reconstruction with SIEA flaps than it was for those who underwent reconstruction with TRAM or DIEP flaps. The SIEA flap loss rate was 7.1% (one flap) due to arterial thrombosis, and the partial flap loss rate was 14.3% (two flaps).

Spiegel and Khan (2007) performed a comparative study of 99 SIEA flap reconstructions in 82 patients. In the first 72 flaps, there was a 6.9% rate of flap loss because of arterial thrombosis, and in the remaining 27 flaps, in which all had a SIEA diameter of 1.5 mm or greater at the level of the lower abdominal incision, there were no losses. The overall rate of fat necrosis was 1% and the partial flap failure rate was 5.1%, with smoking at the time of surgery associated with increased donor-site complications. Dorafshar et al. (2010) used an algorithm of SIEA vessel selection based on the presence of a palpable pulse rather than vessel calibre, with a mean SIEA diameter of 0.96 mm. They reported a complete flap loss rate of 1.9% (one flap) and fat necrosis or partial flap loss in 5.7% (three flaps), suggesting that the presence of a palpable arterial pulse may be sufficient to permit successful utilisation of this flap (Table 24.1).

TABLE 24.1
Summary of Outcomes from Published Studies

Study	No. Flaps	Complete Flap Loss (%)	Partial Flap Loss (%)	Fat Necrosis (%)	Donor-Site Bulges or Hernias (%)
Granzow et al. (2006)	210	0		13	0
Selber et al. (2008)	72	2.9			0
Cheng et al. (2006)	12	0	8.3		
Ulusal et al. (2006)	14	7		7.1	
Baumann et al. (2010)	57			14	
Chevray (2004a)	14	7.1	14.3		
Spiegel and Khan (2007)	99	5.1	5.1	1	
Dorafshar et al. (2010)	53	1.9	5.7		

Wu et al. (2008) used a patient survey evaluating donor-site morbidity following free-flap breast reconstruction and found that SIEA flaps resulted in significantly less abdominal donor-site morbidity than DIEP flaps in bilateral cases and muscle-sparing free TRAM flaps in unilateral and bilateral cases. Selber et al. (2010) demonstrated in a study of bilateral SIEA, DIEP, and MS-TRAM flap breast reconstructions that abdominal wall strength following various combinations of bilateral free-flap breast reconstruction techniques closely adhered to the degree of surgical muscle sacrifice.

24.9 DISCUSSION

The SIEA flap is versatile and has most popularly found application in free-flap breast reconstruction. It is most ideal for small- to medium-sized breast reconstructions or for bilateral breast reconstruction (Cheng et al. 1995; Chevray 2004a; Granzow et al. 2006; Koshima 2005; Koshima et al. 1996; Lipa 2007; Liu et al. 2010; Longaker et al. 1996; Raab et al. 2009; Siebert et al. 1996; Stern and Nahai 1992; Stevenson et al. 1984; Woodworth et al. 2006). In a bilateral reconstruction, even if only one side is harvested as a SIEA flap, the donor-site morbidity is still reduced to virtually that of a unilateral DIEP or TRAM flap (Selber et al. 2010; Wu et al. 2008). The flap has significant advantages compared with other abdominal flaps in terms of virtually absent donor-site morbidity, faster flap harvest, and shorter hospital stay (Chevray 2004a,b; Granzow et al. 2006; Selber et al. 2010; Wu et al. 2008). The utility of the flap is limited by significant anatomical variability, with the anatomy permitting flap harvest in only approximately 30% of patients (Chevray 2004a). A SIEA diameter of at least 1 mm at the lower abdominal incision is required for flap harvest, although some authors have suggested that the presence of a palpable arterial pulse within the vessel is sufficient regardless of vessel calibre (Dorafshar et al. 2010), whilst others have provided outcomes evidence for selecting a pedicle of 1.5 mm or greater in diameter (Spiegel and Khan 2007). One solution to inadequate SIEA calibre may be the use of vascular delay. Gregorič et al. (2011) have demonstrated an increase in the diameter of the SIEA vessels by a mean of 0.37 mm (29% increase) in patients with SIEAs present but of inadequate calibre for microvascular transfer using selective delay via ligation of the DIEA.

The variability of the presence, calibre, and angiosome of the SIEA suggests that imaging with CTA or MRA is extremely valuable prior to flap harvest (Fukaya et al. 2011; Piorkowski et al. 2011; Rozen et al. 2008a, 2009c, 2010a; Scott et al. 2010). Intraoperative dynamic fluorescence videoangiography has demonstrated great success for assessing intraoperative flap circulation and guiding flap design and may reduce the incidence of flap-related complications (Holm et al. 2007, 2008; Komorowska-Timek and Gurtner 2010).

Studies have reported a complete flap failure rate of 0%–7.1%, which is mainly due to arterial thrombosis. Selber et al. (2008) reported an approximately 16-fold higher complete flap loss rate overall when compared with the muscle-sparing TRAM flap. The rate of partial loss ranged from 5.1% to 14.3%, and the rate of fat necrosis from 1% to 14% (Baumann et al. 2010; Cheng et al. 2006; Chevray 2004a; Dorafshar et al. 2010; Granzow et al. 2006; Selber et al. 2008; Spiegel and Khan 2007; Ulusal et al. 2006). Although the rate of donor-site seroma may be high due to the increased dissection around the inguinal lymphatics (Granzow et al. 2006), no studies have reported donor-site hernia or bulge (Selber et al. 2010; Wu et al. 2008).

24.10 CONCLUSIONS

The SIEA flap enables flap harvest with donor-site morbidity similar to an aesthetic abdominoplasty. The main limitations of the flap are variable presence, calibre, anatomy, and vascular territory of the SIEA and SIEV. CTA, MRA, and dynamic laser-fluorescence videoangiography are invaluable pre- and intraoperative imaging modalities for flap planning and intraoperative flap design, with the potential to lead to faster procedures with reduced flap-related complications.

REFERENCES

Allen, R.J., Heitland, A.S. 2002. Superficial inferior epigastric artery flap for breast reconstruction. *Semin Plast Surg* 16:35.

Antia, N.H., Buch, V.I. 1971. Transfer of an abdominal dermo-fat graft by direct anastomosis of blood vessels. *Br J Plast Surg* 24(1):15–19.

Arnez, Z.M., Khan, U., Pogorelec, D., Planinsek, F. 1999a. Breast reconstruction using the free superficial inferior epigastric artery (SIEA) flap. *Br J Plast Surg* 52(4):276–279.

Arnez, Z.M., Khan, U., Pogorelec, D., Planinsek, F. 1999b. Rational selection of flaps from the abdomen in breast reconstruction to reduce donor site morbidity. *Br J Plast Surg* 52(5):351–354.

Baumann, D.P., Lin, H.Y., Chevray, P.M. 2010. Perforator number predicts fat necrosis in a prospective analysis of breast reconstruction with free TRAM, DIEP, and SIEA flaps. *Plast Reconstr Surg* 125(5):1335–1341.

Blondeel, P.N., Arnstein, M., Verstraete, K. et al. 2000. Venous congestion and blood flow in free transverse rectus abdominis myocutaneous and deep inferior epigastric perforator flaps. *Plast Reconstr Surg* 106:1295–1299.

Blondeel, P.N., Beyens, G., Verhaeghe, R. et al. 1998. Doppler flowmetry in the planning of perforator flaps. *Br J Plast Surg* 51(3):202–209.

Cheng, K.X., Hwang, W.Y., Eid, A.E., Wang, S.L., Chang, T.S., Fu, K.D. 1995. Analysis of 136 cases of reconstructed penis using various methods. *Plast Reconstr Surg* 95(6):1070–1080.

Cheng, M.H., Lin, J.Y., Ulusal, B.G., Wei, F.C. 2006. Comparisons of resource costs and success rates between immediate and delayed breast reconstruction using DIEP or SIEA flaps under a well-controlled clinical trial. *Plast Reconstr Surg* 117(7):2139–2142.

Chevray, P.M. 2004a. Breast reconstruction with superficial inferior epigastric artery flaps: A prospective comparison with TRAM and DIEP flaps. *Plast Reconstr Surg* 114:1077–1083.

Chevray, P.M. 2004b. Update on breast reconstruction using free TRAM, DIEP, and SIEA flaps. *Semin Plast Surg* 18(2):97–104.

Dorafshar, A.H., Januszyk, M., Song, D.H. 2010. Anatomical and technical tips for use of the superficial inferior epigastric artery (SIEA) flap in breast reconstructive surgery. *J Reconstr Microsurg* 26(6):381–389.

Fukaya, E., Kuwatsuru, R., Iimura, H., Ihara, K., Sakurai, H. 2011. Imaging of the superficial inferior epigastric vascular anatomy and preoperative planning for the SIEA flap using MDCTA. *J Plast Reconstr Aesthet Surg* 64(1):63–68.

Granzow, J.W., Levine, J.L., Chiu, E.S., Allen, R.J. 2006. Breast reconstruction using perforator flaps. *J Surg Oncol* 94(6):441–454.

Gregorič, M., Flis, V., Milotić, F., Mrđa, B., Stirn, B., Arnež, Z.M. 2011. Delaying the superficial inferior epigastric artery flap: A solution to the problem of the small calibre of the donor artery. *J Plast Reconstr Aesthet Surg* 64(9):1181–1186.

Grotting, J.C. 1991. The free abdominoplasty flap for immediate breast reconstruction. *Ann Plast Surg* 27(4):351–354.

Hallock, G.G. 2011. Acoustic Doppler sonography, color duplex ultrasound, and laser Doppler flowmetry as tools for successful autologous breast reconstruction. *Clin Plast Surg* 38(2):203–211.

Herrera, F.A., Selber, J.C., Buntic, R., Brooks, D., Buncke, G.M., Antony, A.K. 2010. How often is the superficial inferior epigastric artery adequate? An observational correlation. *J Plast Reconstr Aesthet Surg* 63(3):e310–e311.

Hester, T.R. Jr., Nahai, F., Beegle, P.E., Bostwick, J. III. 1984. Blood supply of the abdomen revisited, with emphasis on the superficial inferior epigastric artery. *Plast Reconstr Surg* 74:657–670.

Holm, C., Mayr, M., Höfter, E., Ninkovic, M. 2007. The versatility of the SIEA flap: A clinical assessment of the vascular territory of the superficial epigastric inferior artery. *J Plast Reconstr Aesthet Surg* 60(8):946–951.

Holm, C., Mayr, M., Höfter, E., Raab, N., Ninkovic, M. 2008. Interindividual variability of the SIEA Angiosome: Effects on operative strategies in breast reconstruction. *Plast Reconstr Surg* 122(6):1612–1620.

Komorowska-Timek, E., Gurtner, G.C. 2010. Intraoperative perfusion mapping with laser-assisted indocyanine green imaging can predict and prevent complications in immediate breast reconstruction. *Plast Reconstr Surg* 125(4):1065–1073.

Koshima, I. 2005. Short pedicle superficial inferior epigastric artery adiposal flap: New anatomical findings and the use of this flap for reconstruction of facial contour. *Plast Reconstr Surg* 116(4):1091–1097.

Koshima, I., Inagawa, K., Jitsuiki, Y., Tsuda, K., Moriguchi, T., Watanabe, A. 1996. Scarpa's adipofascial flap for repair of wide scalp defects. *Ann Plast Surg* 36(1):88–92.

Ledneva, E., Karie, S., Launay-Vacher, V. et al. 2009. Renal safety of gadolinium-based contrast media in patients with chronic renal insufficiency. *Radiology* 250:618.

Lipa, J.E. 2007. Breast reconstruction with free flaps from the abdominal donor site: TRAM, DIEAP, and SIEA flaps. *Clin Plast Surg* 34(1):105–121.

Liu, Y., Song, B., Zhu, S., Jin, J. 2010. Reconstruction of the burned hand using a super-thin abdominal flap, with donor-site closure by an island deep inferior epigastric perforator flap. *J Plast Reconstr Aesthet Surg* 63(3):e265–e268.

Longaker, M.T., Flynn, A., Siebert, J.W. 1996. Microsurgical correction of bilateral facial contour deformities. *Plast Reconstr Surg* 98(6):951–957.

Mahajan, A.L., Zeltzer, A., Claes, K.E., Van Landuyt, K., Hamdi, M. 2012. Are Pfannenstiel scars a boon or a curse for DIEP flap breast reconstructions? *Plast Reconstr Surg* 129(4):797–805.

Masia, J., Kosutic, D., Cervelli, D., Clavero, J.A., Monill, J.M., Pons, G. 2010. In search of the ideal method in perforator mapping: Noncontrast magnetic resonance imaging. *J Reconstr Microsurg* 26(1):29–35.

Piorkowski, J.R., DeRosier, L.C., Nickerson, P., Fix, R.J. 2011. Preoperative computed tomography angiogram to predict patients with favorable anatomy for superficial inferior epigastric artery flap breast reconstruction. *Ann Plast Surg* 66(5):534–536.

Raab, N., Holm-Muehlbauer, C., Ninkovic, M. 2009. Free superficial inferior epigastric artery flap for aesthetic correction of mild pectus excavatum. *Plast Reconstr Surg* 123(6):209e–211e.

Reardon, C.M., O'Ceallaigh, S., O'Sullivan, S.T. 2004. An anatomical study of the superficial inferior epigastric vessels in humans. *Br J Plast Surg* 57(6):515–519.

Rizzuto, R.P., Allen, R.J. 2004. Reconstruction of a partial mastectomy defect with the superficial inferior epigastric artery (SIEA) flap. *J Reconstr Microsurg* 20(6):441–445.

Rozen, W.M., Anavekar, N.S., Ashton, M.W. et al. 2008b. Does the preoperative imaging of perforators with CT angiography improve operative outcomes in breast reconstruction? *Microsurgery* 28:516.

Rozen, W.M., Chubb, D., Grinsell, D., Ashton, M.W. 2010a. The variability of the Superficial Inferior Epigastric Artery (SIEA) and its angiosome: A clinical anatomical study. *Microsurgery* 30(5):386–391.

Rozen, W.M., Chubb, D., Whitaker, I.S., Ashton, M.W. 2011. The importance of the superficial venous anatomy of the abdominal wall in planning a superficial inferior epigastric artery (SIEA) flap: Case report and clinical study. *Microsurgery* 31(6):454–457.

Rozen, W.M., Garcia-Tutor, E., Alonso-Burgos, A. et al. 2010b. Planning and optimising DIEP flaps with virtual surgery: The Navarra experience. *J Plast Reconstr Aesthet Surg* 63(2):289–297.

Rozen, W.M., Pan, W.R., Le Roux, C.M., Taylor, G.I., Ashton, M.W. 2009a. The venous anatomy of the anterior abdominal wall: An anatomical and clinical study. *Plast Reconstr Surg* 124(3):848–853.

Rozen, W.M., Phillips, T.J., Ashton, M.W., Stella, D.L., Gibson, R.N., Taylor, G.I. 2008a. Preoperative imaging for DIEA perforator flaps: A comparative study of computed tomographic angiography and Doppler ultrasound. *Plast Reconstr Surg* 121(1 Suppl):9–16.

Rozen, W.M., Stella, D.L., Bowden, J., Taylor, G.I., Ashton, M.W. 2009c. Advances in the pre-operative planning of deep inferior epigastric artery perforator flaps: Magnetic resonance angiography. *Microsurgery* 29(2):119–123.

Rozen, W.M., Whitaker, I.S., Stella, D.L. et al. 2009b. The radiation exposure of Computed Tomographic Angiography (CTA) in DIEP flap planning: Low dose but high impact. *J Plast Reconstr Aesthet Surg* 62(12):e654–e655.

Schaverien, M., Saint-Cyr, M., Arbique, G., Brown, S.A. 2008. Arterial and venous anatomies of the deep inferior epigastric perforator and superficial inferior epigastric artery flaps. *Plast Reconstr Surg* 121(6):1909–1919.

Schaverien, M.V., Ludman, C.N., Neil-Dwyer, J. et al. 2010. Relationship between venous congestion and intraflap venous anatomy in DIEP flaps using contrast-enhanced magnetic resonance angiography. *Plast Reconstr Surg* 126(2):385–392.

Schaverien, M.V., Ludman, C.N., Neil-Dwyer, J. et al. 2011a. Contrast-enhanced magnetic resonance angiography for preoperative imaging in DIEP flap breast reconstruction. *Plast Reconstr Surg* 128(1):56–62.

Schaverien, M.V., Ludman, C.N., Neil-Dwyer, J., McCulley, S.J. 2011b. Contrast-enhanced magnetic resonance angiography for preoperative imaging of deep inferior epigastric artery perforator flaps: Advantages and disadvantages compared with computed tomography angiography: A United Kingdom perspective. *Ann Plast Surg* 67(6):671–674.

Scott, J.R., Liu, D., Said, H., Neligan, P.C., Mathes, D.W. 2010. Computed tomographic angiography in planning abdomen-based microsurgical breast reconstruction: A comparison with color duplex ultrasound. *Plast Reconstr Surg* 125(2):446–453.

Selber, J.C., Fosnot, J., Nelson, J. et al. 2010. A prospective study comparing the functional impact of SIEA, DIEP, and muscle-sparing free TRAM flaps on the abdominal wall: Part II. Bilateral reconstruction. *Plast Reconstr Surg* 126(5):1438–1453.

Selber, J.C., Samra, F., Bristol, M. et al. 2008. A head-to-head comparison between the muscle-sparing free TRAM and the SIEA flaps: is the rate of flap loss worth the gain in abdominal wall function? *Plast Reconstr Surg* 122(2):348–355.

Siebert, J.W., Anson, G., Longaker, M.T. 1996. Microsurgical correction of facial asymmetry in 60 consecutive cases. *Plast Reconstr Surg* 97(2):354–363.

Smit, J.M., Dimopoulou, A., Liss, A.G. et al. 2009. Preoperative CT angiography reduces surgery time in perforator flap reconstruction. *J Plast Reconstr Aesthet Surg* 62:1112.

Spiegel, A.J., Khan, F.N. 2007. An Intraoperative algorithm for use of the SIEA flap for breast reconstruction. *Plast Reconstr Surg* 120(6):1450–1459.

Stern, H.S., Nahai, F. 1992. The versatile superficial inferior epigastric artery free flap. *Br J Plast Surg* 45(4):270–274.

Stevenson, T.R., Hester, T.R., Duus, E.C., Dingman, R.O. 1984. The superficial inferior epigastric artery flap for coverage of hand and forearm defects. *Ann Plast Surg* 12(4):333–339.

Taylor, G.I., Corlett, R.J., Dhar, S.C., Ashton, M.W. 2011. The anatomical (angiosome) and clinical territories of cutaneous perforating arteries: Development of the concept and designing safe flaps. *Plast Reconstr Surg* 127(4):1447–1459.

Taylor, G.I., Daniel, R.K. 1975. The anatomy of several free flap donor sites. *Plast Reconstr Surg* 56: 243–253.

Taylor, G.I., Doyle, M., McCarten, G. 1990.The Doppler probe for planning flaps: Anatomical study and clinical applications. *Br J Plast Surg* 43(1):1–16.

ten Dam, M.A., Wetzels, J.F. 2008. Toxicity of contrast media: An update. *Neth J Med* 66:416.

Ulusal, B.G., Cheng, M.H., Wei, F.C., Ho-Asjoe, M., Song, D. 2006. Breast reconstruction using the entire transverse abdominal adipocutaneous flap based on unilateral superficial or deep inferior epigastric vessels. *Plast Reconstr Surg* 117(5):1395–1403.

Wolfram, D., Schoeller, T., Hussl, H., Wechselberger, G. 2006. The superficial inferior epigastric artery (SIEA) flap: Indications for breast reconstruction. *Ann Plast Surg* 57(6):593–596.

Wood, J. 1863. Extreme deformity of the neck and forearm. *Med Chir Trans* 46:151.

Woodworth, B.A., Gillespie, M.B., Day, T., Kline, R.M. 2006. Muscle-sparing abdominal free flaps in head and neck reconstruction. *Head Neck* 28(9):802–807.

Wu, L.C., Bajaj, A., Chang, D.W., Chevray, P.M. 2008. Comparison of donor-site morbidity of SIEA, DIEP, and muscle-sparing TRAM flaps for breast reconstruction. *Plast Reconstr Surg* 122(3):702–709.

Zenn, M.R. 2006. Insetting of the superficial inferior epigastric artery flap in breast reconstruction. *Plast Reconstr Surg* 117(5):1407–1411.

25 Surgical Principles and Breast Imaging and Monitoring after Autologous Fat Transfer

Paolo Persichetti, Barbara Cagli, Tiziano Pallara, Donata Maria Antonia Assunta Vaccaro, Carlo Augusto Mallio, and Bruno Beomonte Zobel

CONTENTS

25.1 AUTOLOGOUS FAT TRANFER

25.1.1 About Adipose Tissue

Adipose tissue is a highly specialised connective tissue, composed of a major lipid-filled cell type, the adipocyte that is surrounded by stromal vascular cells (SVCs) such as fibroblasts, immune cells, collagen fibres, and blood vessels. Adipocytes are connected by a highly organised extracellular matrix (ECM) thus forming the fat lobules. There are two forms of adipose tissue: brown and white. In humans, brown adipose tissue, so called because of its colour, attributed to its high vascularisation, is predominantly found during the neonatal period and is responsible for producing heat from triglycerides. During the ageing process, brown fat is progressively replaced by white adipose tissue [6]. The latter, composed of adipocytes with a single large lipid inclusion and a large peripherally located nucleus, represents thus the predominant type of fat in humans. It is specialised in a variety of physiological processes including the storage of energy-rich triglycerides, cushioning of vital structures and organs, metabolic homeostasis, immunity, regulation of proliferation, and angiogenesis [4,41], as well as it serves to impart a normal appearance. Hence, fat tissue influences metabolic homeostasis by producing a variety of hormones, cytokines, growth factors, and other peptides termed adipokines, such as TNF-α, IL-6, and leptin, which exert their effects in an endocrine, paracrine, and autocrine manner. With this in mind, while adipose tissue has historically been considered a semi-inert tissue, now it is being considered an out-and-out organ. Like bone marrow, adipose tissue is thought to originate from multipotent stem cells within the embryonic mesoderm. As the stem cells proliferate, some of them differentiate step by step until forming mature adipocytes. Furthermore, the proteolytic digestion of intact human adipose tissue yields a *fibroblast-like* population of cells, known as stromal vascular fraction (SVF) that collects lineage-committed preadipocytes and cells phenotypically similar to mesenchymal stem cells (MSCs). The International Federation for Adipose Therapeutics and Science (IFATS) reached a consensus to adopt the term *adipose-derived stem cells* (ASCs) to identify this multipotent cell population [5,49]. Routinely, 1×10^7 ASCs have been isolated from 300 ml of *lipoaspirato*; in other words, the average frequency of ASCs in processed *lipoaspirato* is 2% of nucleated cells [3,30]. Found their towering plasticity, human ASCs are known to differentiate into several cell lineages including adipogenic, osteogenic, chondrogenic, myogenic, cardiomyogenic, and neurogenic-like cell types. Also ASCs have been shown to possess angiogenic characteristics and to differentiate into vascular endothelial cells. Furthermore, numerous studies have demonstrated that ASCs express/secrete multiple growth factors including IGF, HGF, TGF-β1, and VEGF. Because of these biological characteristics, adipose tissue has recently proven to be a potent tool for cell-based therapies, and ASCs are one of the most promising stem cell populations identified so far, since human adipose tissue is ubiquitous and easily obtained in large quantities with little donor site morbidity or patient discomfort.

25.1.2 History of Lipofilling

Autologous fat transfer, first introduced by Neuer in 1893, has become nowadays a well-established method of soft-tissue augmentation for both aesthetic and reconstructive indications [33]. The history of adipose tissue transplant or lipofilling can be divided into three periods: the first is before the introduction of lipoaspiration, termed *open surgery*, when adipose tissue was harvested by surgical excision; the second period is during which adipose tissue was obtained by aspiration and reinjected as such; the last period is where the adipose tissue undergoes non-traumatic refinements before grafting [31]. Autologous fat grafting was primarily used to correct body defects after trauma, cancer surgery, or congenital defects but has been widened to include treatment of many other problems, such as burns, scars, and wrinkles. However, in the last 20 years, although several different techniques of lipoinjection have been developed and have allowed for more widespread use of clinical fat grafting, a standardised methodology has not been adopted by all practitioners yet. Variables that remain to be settled include (1) the ideal cannula and technique for harvesting, (2) the ideal donor site, (3) the best way of processing the fat to ensure maximal take and viability of the graft, and (4) the best technique for reinjecting the fat. The most common harvesting approach is lipoaspiration, first introduced by Illouz in 1983 [21]. Commonly used donor sites are abdominal, thigh, flank, or knee fat. Results from several studies about the ideal donor site remain unchallenged, and thus, at present, there are no indications that one donor site is superior to another one [42]. However, Schipper's research showed that ASCs harvested from superficial abdominal regions are significantly more resistant to apoptosis than those harvested from other adipose tissue depots [37]. Once the fat is harvested, it is often prepared for injection through the use of several methods, including washing with physiologic buffers, centrifugation for separation of cells from debris, decantation, or by concentrating it using cotton towels or other absorbent media. For autologous fat grafting, the Coleman technique is a well-described procedure that centrifuges the harvested lipoaspirato at approximately 3000 rpm for 3 min. After centrifugation, the upper (oil) level and the bottom (liquid) layer are decanted, resulting in a concentrated fat in the middle portion [11]. The fat is subsequently injected into the subcutaneous tissues with an assortment of delivery methods using either sharp or blunt needles. The transplanted fat graft, however, has an unpredictable and often high rate of resorption, ranging from 25% to 80%, and which is why investigators are looking to discover new ways of increasing its viability [28]. Therefore, variations of the Coleman technique and many other ASC isolation and purification methodologies have been described. In an effort to use ASCs to improve fat grafting outcomes, cell-assisted lipotransfer (CAL) was popularised by K. Yoshimura. In short, this technique admixes SVF, isolated from adipose tissue, with fat graft material from the same patient for breast augmentation and facial lipoatrophy correction [46]. Another technology that has received considerable attention for fat grafting is the concept of external tissue expansion of the recipient bed before fat grafting. Mainly for breast enhancement applications, recipient site pre-expansion is believed to be beneficial for several reasons including enhancement of parenchymal space and increased angiogenesis. Some studies showed promising results with patients who wore the BRAVA prior surgery, having more retention of the injected fat at 6 months [15,48]. At present, lack of consensus on the best fat grafting technique still remains, which stems in large part from equivocal results obtained when multiple methodologies were compared.

25.1.3 Fat Grafting–Related Events

Soft-tissue volume loss acquired through ageing, traumatic injury, tumour resection, pathologies, or congenital malformation is a common and sometimes very challenging problem that is frequently presented to plastic surgeons. Fat naturally fulfils many of the characteristics required of a soft-tissue filler. It is autologous, non-immunogenic, biocompatible, natural-appearing, easily available in most patients, inexpensive, and potentially removable and long lasting. However, it has not been well documented yet how adipose grafts survive after lipofilling. It has been suggested that in response to local bleeding from the injured recipient tissue, PDGF, EGF, and TGF-β are released from activated platelets. At the same time, grafted adipose tissue is placed under severe ischemia until direct vascular supply is formed. Furthermore, primary injury factors (such as bFGF, TNF-α, TGF-β, EGF, damage-associated molecular pattern molecules, and some proteases) are released from the injured host tissue (ECM disrupted) and dying grafted tissue. These soluble factors, in turn, activate resident dormant stem cells. Inflammatory cells as well as endothelial progenitor cells are recruited from bone marrow to the injured tissue. ASCs are likely to stay functional for up to 72 h even under severe ischemia and to play main roles in the repairing and regenerating processes detected up to 3 months, when adipogenesis and angiogenesis are completed. Animal experiments indicated that almost all adipocytes die within a few days after fat grafting. Some of the dead adipocytes are replaced with new adipocytes of next generation during the first 3 months, while others are not. Left lipid droplets are absorbed by macrophage phagocytosis, but the process is very slow and dependent on the diameter of the lipid droplets; the larger the diameter, the faster the absorption. Hence, the final volume retention is established by the rate of successful replacement of adipocytes [45].

Nowadays, literature regarding fat grafting applications consists mostly of case series and a few small, lesser-quality experimental studies. However, preliminary results are positive and encourage further study in this field.

25.1.4 Diagnostic Imaging of Subcutaneous Fat Tissue

Subcutaneous adipose tissue, like all the fat present in the body, shows distinctive appearance in the diagnostic imaging techniques and is usually recognised without any doubt (Figure 25.1).

The subcutaneous fat has a low attenuation on x-rays and thus appears as hypodense on computed tomography (CT) and radiolucent on conventional radiography.

CT scan Hounsfield unit (HU) values, considered as the reference standard to define the fat tissue, typically range from −190 to −30 HU.

On ultrasound, subcutaneous fat tissue is characterised by low amplitude echoes. Ultrasound appearance of subcutaneous fat is hypoechoic lobules with hyperechoic branches which represent connective tissue fibres.

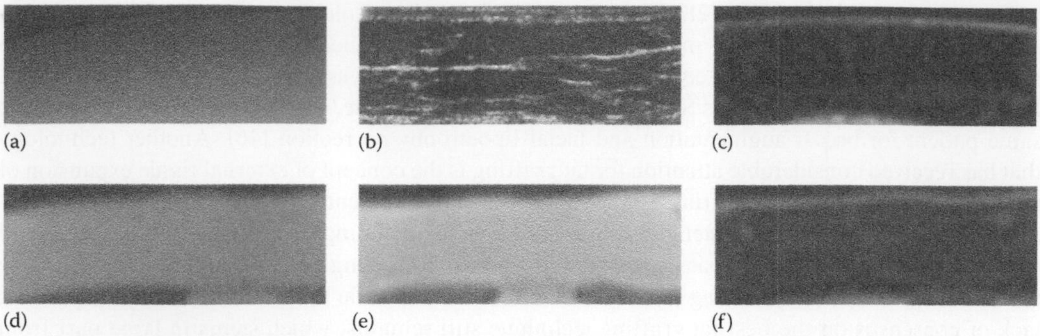

FIGURE 25.1 Typical appearance of subcutaneous adipose tissue in diagnostic imaging such as x-ray radiolucent (a), hypoechoic with hyperechoic thin branches in ultrasound (b), hypodense in CT (c), and hyperintense in both T2- (d) and T1- (e) weighted sequences with signal dropout in fat-saturated T1-weighted sequences (f) in MRI.

At magnetic resonance imaging (MRI), there are two main parameters to vary the contrast in the images: repetition time (TR) and echo time (TE). Fat recovers longitudinal magnetization faster (shorter T1) and is characterised by transverse relaxation more rapid than water (shorter T2). By selecting a short TR sequence, the fat recovers longitudinal magnetization more quickly than water; thus, difference in relaxation time between fat and water can be detected; conversely with long TR sequence, this does not occur. Therefore, in T1-*weighted* sequences (short TR and TE), the subcutaneous fat appears hyperintense and water hypointense. In T2-*weighted* sequences (long TR and TE), both subcutaneous fat and water appear hyperintense, but the water has a higher signal intensity.

To suppress the signal from fat tissue, MRI fat suppression techniques are currently used.

Fat suppression can be performed with three methods: fat saturation, inversion recovery imaging, and opposed-phase imaging.

The choice of one of the three techniques depends on the amount of fat in the tissue to be analysed and the result to be achieved that are related to both tissue characterization and contrast enhancement.

Fat saturation is used for signal suppression for large quantities of fat and for post-contrast acquisition. However, this technique is more sensitive to magnetic field inhomogeneity and movement artefacts.

Inversion recovery enables a homogeneous and complete fat suppression also with low-field-strength magnets, but it is not specific for fat, and the signal intensities, from tissues with long and short T1, are not always clear.

Opposed-phase imaging is usually performed to characterise tissues containing low fat quantity.

25.2 FAT GRAFTING IN BREAST RECONSTRUCTION

Although fat injection has been used since 1990s to correct both congenital and iatrogenic contour deformities of the face, trunk, and extremities, its use in the breast has gone largely unreported and is still controversial. At present, breast indications for lipofilling include micromastia, post-augmentation deformity (with and without removal of implant), tuberous breasts, Poland's syndrome, postlumpectomy deformity, post-mastectomy deformities, damaged tissue resulting from radiotherapy, and nipple reconstruction [18,35].

Aesthetic results deriving from conservative surgery of breast cancer, especially when associated with radiotherapy, are challenging for plastic surgeons. Natural volume re-establishment of irradiated breast, through pedicled or free flaps or prostheses, may be difficult in this particular case, and the aforementioned approaches give poor-quality cosmetic results. Therefore, the mini-invasive aspect of fat grafting led plastic surgeons to introduce this technique in this field with good outcomes, permitting a direct and definitive correction of glandular deformities, skin retraction, and scars [1].

Recent advances in breast reconstruction techniques have led to crucial improvements in aesthetic outcomes also for patients undergoing radical mastectomy. Patient's expectations for a natural-appearing reconstructed breast become increasingly high. Therefore, plastic surgeons are performing more secondary procedures to perfect contour deformities and asymmetry (Figure 25.2). Contour breast deformities can occur between the native chest wall and the reconstructed breast (*step-off deformities*); they are considered intrinsic as a result of an irregularity within the flap or implant or extrinsic which include defects caused by radiation or capsule contracture [23]. The latter contour deformities of the reconstructed breast are relatively common and are independent of the type of reconstruction used, thereby presenting also a frequent therapeutic challenge to reconstructive surgeons. During the expansion process, the cutaneous and subcutaneous tissues become extremely thin and tense. Then once the prosthesis is put in place, the capsule may tighten around it, causing contracture and producing highly unaesthetic results. For these reasons, fat grafting is now being inserted in several protocols for breast reconstruction (autologous and/or with expander and prostheses) and formation of new and better subcutaneous tissue, at each stage of surgery. Contour irregularities are often in the upper quadrants and axillary fold, the areas most likely to be visible in low-cut clothing or in a bathing suit and therefore the most socially relevant. Fat transplantation improves the aesthetic results, adds volume, and contrasts capsular contraction especially in patients who have received radiotherapy. Superficial tissues become more elastic and natural appearing [13,14,38,39] (Figure 25.3).

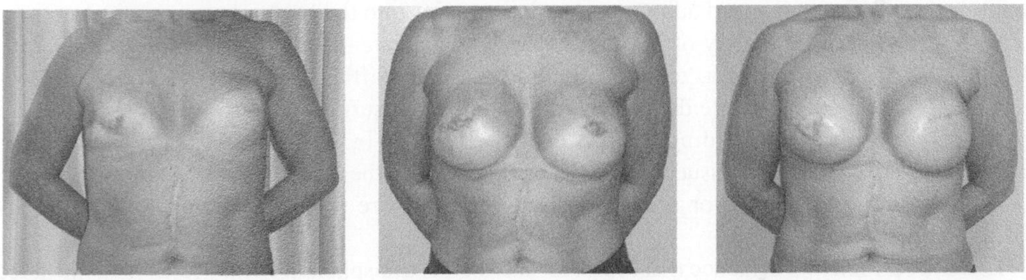

(a) (b) (c)

FIGURE 25.2 Patient with bilateral breast reconstruction with implants after mastectomy and upper quadrant contouring lipofilling. Preoperative condition (a). Three months after bilateral implant breast reconstruction and one lipofilling session (b). One year after two lipofilling sessions and nipple-areola complex reconstruction (c).

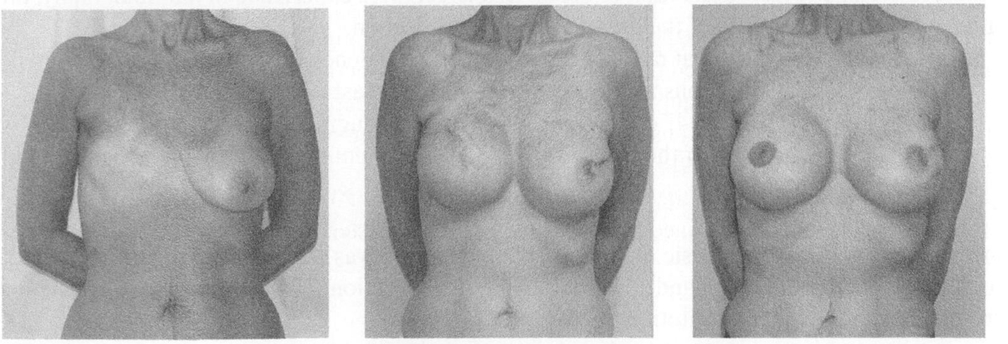

(a) (b) (c)

FIGURE 25.3 Patient with right breast mastectomy (a). Right breast reconstruction with implants and left additive mastoplasty (b). Bilateral nipple–areola complex reconstruction and contouring lipostructure (c).

25.2.1 Fat Grafting in Breast Augmentation

Breast augmentation with liposuctioned fat has been performed in the last years, highlighting two crucial limitations: the small volume of fat that can be transferred in a single session and the uncertain and often too little percentage graft survival. In response to overcome these limits, it was postulated that preparation of the recipient breast by external expansion is the 'key missing ingredient to preserve the graft-to-recipient interface' [25]. Khouri et al. studies showed that the pre-expansion of the recipient breast with BRAVA device, an external breast soft-tissue expander worn for 10 h/day for 4 weeks before the procedure of lipofilling, causes a marked temporary increase in breast size and generates a larger and more fertile recipient matrix that will allow more fat graft droplets to be diffusely dispersed. In this way, the aforementioned approach ensures a very high adipose tissue survival rate, with augmentation volumes comparable to implants.

25.2.2 Diagnostic Imaging in Breast Fat Autologous Transplantation

The use of fat transplantation in breast augmentation was first officially criticised by the American Society of Plastic and Reconstructive Surgeons (ASPRS) in 1987. They asserted that fat grafting would hinder breast cancer detection in subsequent radiological examinations and, consequently, that it should no longer be used [2]. The doubt was tied to the fact that breast tissue changes, after fat injection, with formation of high density nodules and calcifications, could potentially interfere with breast cancer detection in mammography.

Actually, it is impossible to predict the entity of reabsorption and any standardised techniques to quantify the volume of injected adipose tissue that remains into the breast do not exist yet.

Later, the American Society of Plastic Surgeons (ASPS) created the Fat Graft Task Force and, after analysing additional data, reported in 2009 that fat grafting may be considered for breast augmentation and outcomes are dependent on technique and surgeon expertise [18]. However, different opinions still exist regarding this procedure [47] so that in 2007 a public warning against fat injection into the breast was issued jointly by the ASPS and the ASPRS for similar reasons; both societies strongly support the ongoing research efforts that are trying to establish the safety and efficacy of the procedure.

There is currently no evidence that breast fat autologous transplantation interferes with the detection of breast cancer.

However, we need further work to refine and standardise the technique of fat drawing, preparation, and injection, to facilitate the reproducibility of best results.

Today, beyond the simple mammography, the use of other diagnostic imaging techniques makes easier to do a differential diagnosis between benign post-necrotic breast tissue changes and cancer.

Nevertheless, a correct evaluation of breast lesions requires experience in mammography, ultrasound, and MRI appearance of the breast after the fat injection.

Several papers suggested that radiologists have good confidence in differentiating between post-surgery fat necrosis calcifications and those suspicious for breast cancer [29].

Moreover, another study [34] confirmed that breast lipoaugmentation does not interfere with post-operative follow-up, and if there is any doubt, a percutaneous biopsy should be performed.

25.2.2.1 Findings

In the majority of the cases, basic mammographic follow-up was carried out, with or without ultrasound and/or MRI, 6 months and 1 year after the first injection; however, different protocols are currently used in different institutions.

In a suspected breast lesion, less than 1 year after the final intervention, careful evaluation is mandatory because the lesion could be both a primary breast cancer and a locoregional recurrence. It has been observed [22] that most of the breast lesions, after lipofilling of the breast, are detected during the first 6 months after each session. If breast lesions are not evident in the first year after

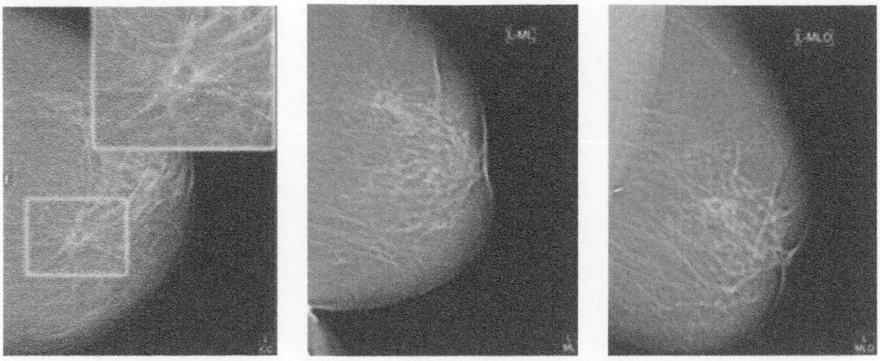

(a) (b) (c)

FIGURE 25.4 Mammogram of left breast: C-C (a), M-L (b), and M-L-O (c) projections. In the supero-internal quadrant, an architectural distortion area with central radiolucency attributable to post-surgery steatonecrosis was found; minute calcifications were also present.

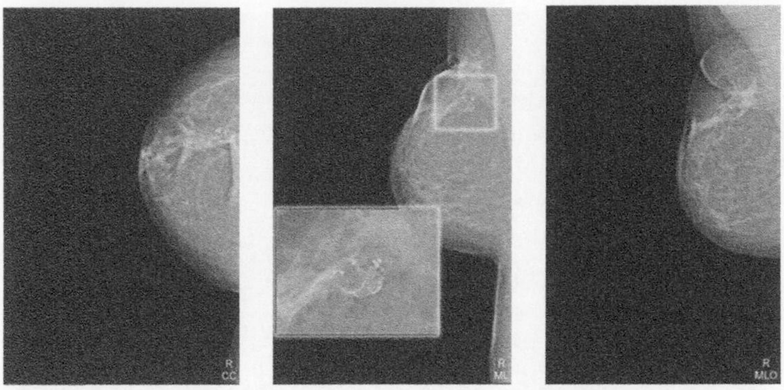

(a) (b) (c)

FIGURE 25.5 Mammogram of right breast: C-C (a), M-L (b), and M-L-O (c) projections. Presence of an architectural distortion area with central oval radiolucency surrounded by a partially calcified shell, which was attributed to post-surgical steatonecrosis. Deformation of the cutaneous plane was also documented.

the final procedure of lipofilling, they are not likely to be directly associated with the procedure. This assumption is supported by a long-term follow-up series of 230 patients (range = 2–25 years, mean = 11.3 years) studied with mammographic and ultrasonographic examinations [22].

The early post-operative mammograms should be similar to those obtained after breast reduction surgery. The main mammographic findings that can be expected at a later phase are fibrotic reaction with parenchymal asymmetrical densities and heterogeneity of the subcutaneous tissues, radiolucent round mass with a thin-walled calcification, known as *eggshell* appearance (Figures 25.4 through 25.6). Greasy fluid collection named *oil cyst* or gross irregular calcifications could also be found in case of fat necrosis.

Ultrasound evaluations usually show mixed (Figure 25.7) and/or solid (Figures 25.8 and 25.9), slightly hyperechoic oval, lobular, or irregularly shaped fatty mass or anechoic lesions (Figure 25.10), with posterior acoustic enhancement or shadowing and cystic lesions with internal echo.

Distortion of the normal parenchymal architecture, inhomogeneity and increased echogenicity of the subcutaneous mammary tissues, could also be detected (Figure 25.11).

MRI is a reliable technique for the follow-up of patients treated with autologous fat grafting (Figures 25.12 through 25.14).

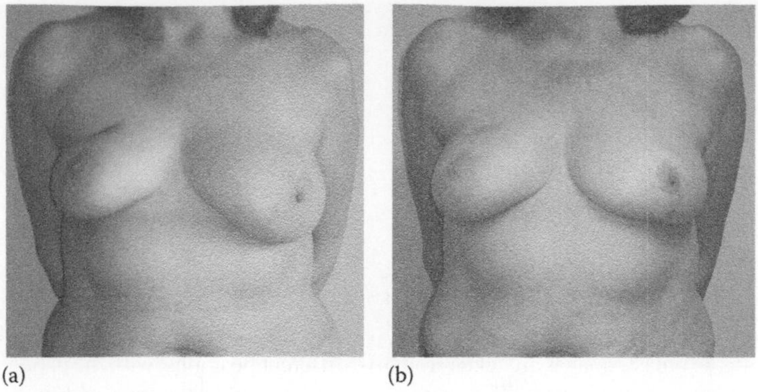

FIGURE 25.6 Clinical view of the patient in Figure 25.5 who presented a nodule in the upper external quadrant of the right breast. She underwent a lumpectomy (a) and multiple lipofilling sessions on the same side (b).

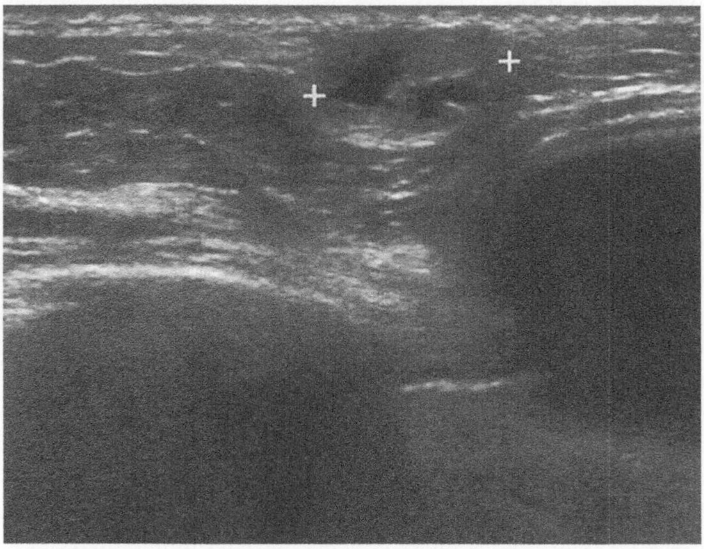

FIGURE 25.7 Breast ultrasound image: in the subcutaneous adipose tissue, near a breast prosthetic device, a round lump with mixed content was detected and classified as a possible expression of liponecrosis. Due to its appearance, the lesion was subjected to cytological examination which confirmed its liponecrotic nature.

The native fat tissue in MRI is characterised by signal hyperintensity in both T1- and T2-*weighted* sequences.

Transplanted fat tissue is not always distinguishable from native; sometimes it could show a slightly different signal intensity from the native fat tissue: T1 signal intensity lower and T2 signal intensity higher than that of native fat tissue.

In T1 sequences obtained after gadolinium, the enhancement pattern depends on the intensity of the associated inflammatory tissue reaction and on the time elapsed from the procedure. However, transplanted fat tissue tends to show slightly higher enhancement than native fat tissue that could be explained by a lower fat content and/or fibrosis of the injected areas or higher tissue perfusion [16].

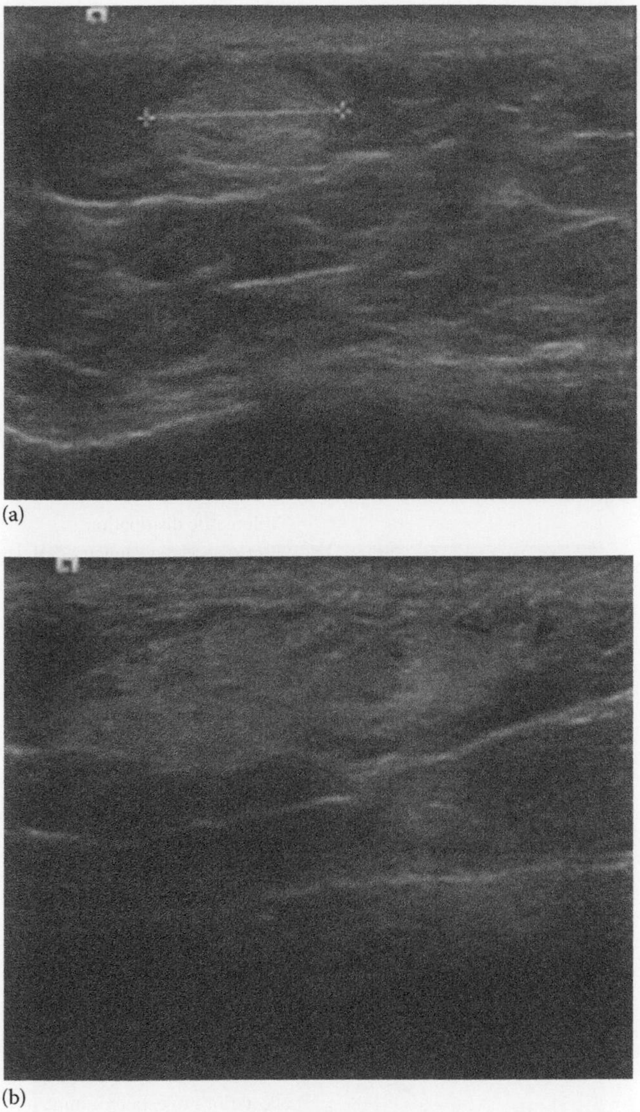

FIGURE 25.8 Breast ultrasound images: in the subcutaneous adipose tissue, in a patient who underwent lipografting treatment on the right upper (a) and lower (b) quadrants of the right breast, two solid nodular areas predominantly hyperechoic, consistent with focal steatonecrosis, were found.

25.2.2.2 MRI Perspectives

The quantification of fat survivability and reabsorption after lipografting is a key point.

Reports based on patient satisfaction after procedure have been published [10,17,24].

MRI volumetric evaluation of fat volume survival after gluteal fat grafts [32,44] has been considered a feasible technique to integrate with clinical indicators of fat reabsorption.

The interest of many authors, regarding the use of serial volumetric MRI measurements to quantify the breast volume and the percentage of fat reabsorption after breast fat grafting, has increased in recent years. The results of published studies have shown that the volumetric MRI technique allows a quantitative evaluation of breast volume and thus the grafted fat tissue survival quantification after breast autologous fat transplantation [15,19,25].

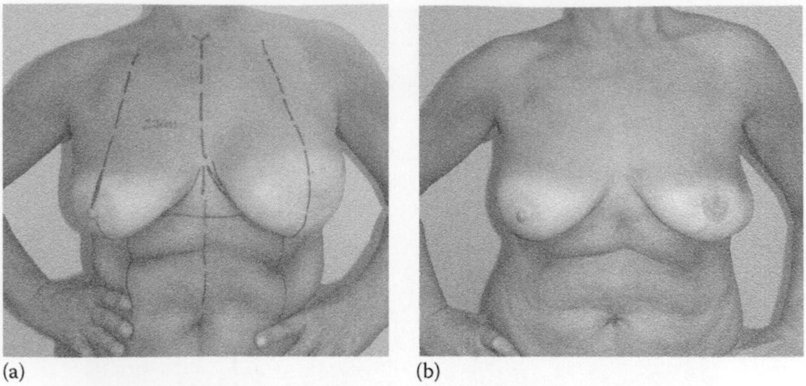

FIGURE 25.9 Clinical view of the patient in Figure 25.8. Patient with severe left breast capsular contracture (a) who underwent breast reconstruction with autologous latissimus dorsi pedicled flap, nipple reconstruction, areola tattoo, and subsequent breast lipostructure (b).

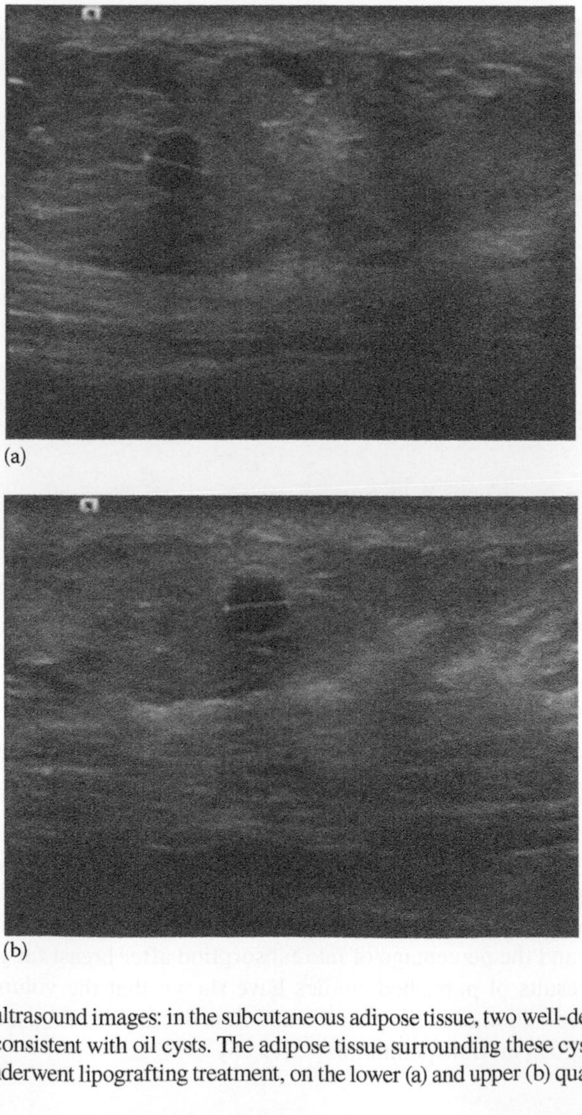

FIGURE 25.10 Breast ultrasound images: in the subcutaneous adipose tissue, two well-demarcated, anechoic lacunar areas were detected, consistent with oil cysts. The adipose tissue surrounding these cysts is diffusely inhomogeneous, in a patient who underwent lipografting treatment, on the lower (a) and upper (b) quadrants of her right breast.

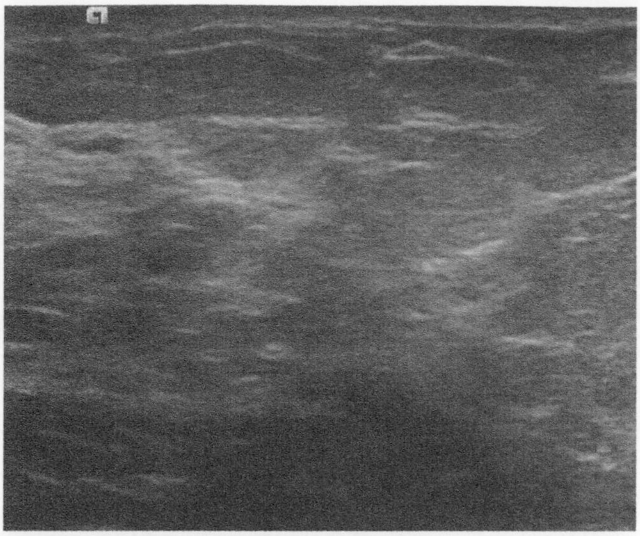

FIGURE 25.11 Breast ultrasound image: diffuse inhomogeneity and hyperechogenicity of subcutaneous adipose tissue in a patient who underwent lipografting treatment.

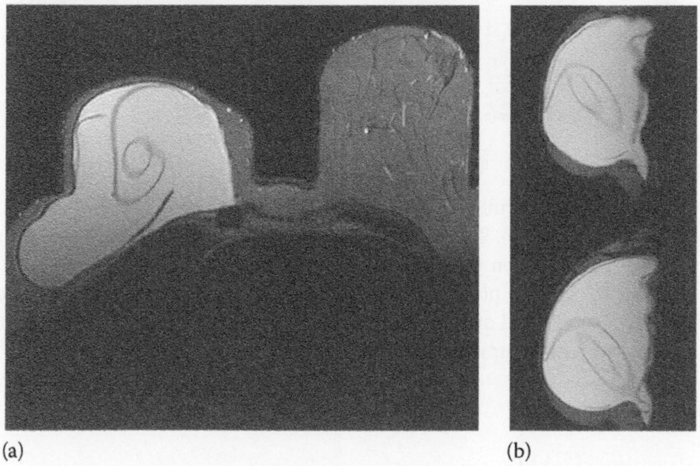

(a) (b)

FIGURE 25.12 MRI images T2-weighted TIRM sequence: axial (a) and sagittal water sat (b) scans. Presence of right silicone breast implant. The *linguine sign* led to the diagnosis of prosthetic intracapsular rupture.

However, a standardised volumetric MRI protocol does not exist, for the timing of execution or the technique used. Similarly, surgical techniques of autologous adipose tissue are not standardised. Additional efforts are critical to achieve shared surgical and imaging protocols and to refine techniques with a more objective results comparison.

25.3 FAT GRAFTING FOR BURN OUTCOMES AND CHRONIC ULCERS

During the past 20 years, acute burn therapy had considerable advancements. Despite this, the same improvement in long-term burn outcomes, which are still a social, economical, and psychological problem in terms of both functional and aesthetic aspects, was not found. Mature scars resulting from severe burns are challenging in their treatment because of abnormal fibrodysplasia, hypertrophy, and keloids secondary to infections and inflammation activity. Recent researches in this field,

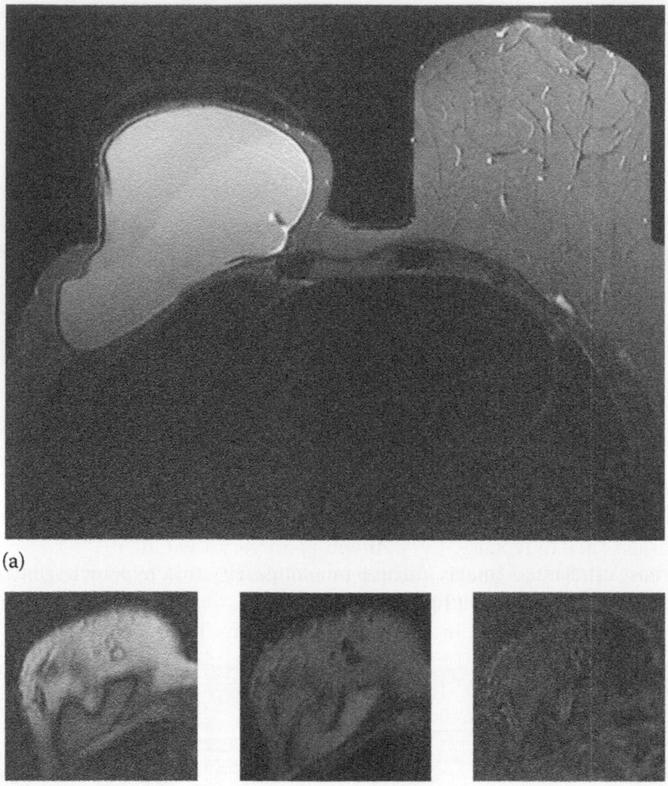

(a) (b) (c) (d)

FIGURE 25.13 Same case shown in Figure 25.12. MRI images of T2-weighted TIRM axial scan (a), T1-weighted FLASH3D axial scan (b), T2-weighted TIRM axial scan (c), and post-gadolinium T1-weighted axial FLASH3D scan with subtraction technique (d). The patient was treated with right prosthetic device replacement (a) and ipsilateral breast lipografting. As an outcome of the lipografting procedure, in the subcutaneous adipose tissue, two small oval areas separated by thin fibrous wall were found, with typical adipose tissue signal intensity and no post-contrast enhancement (b–d).

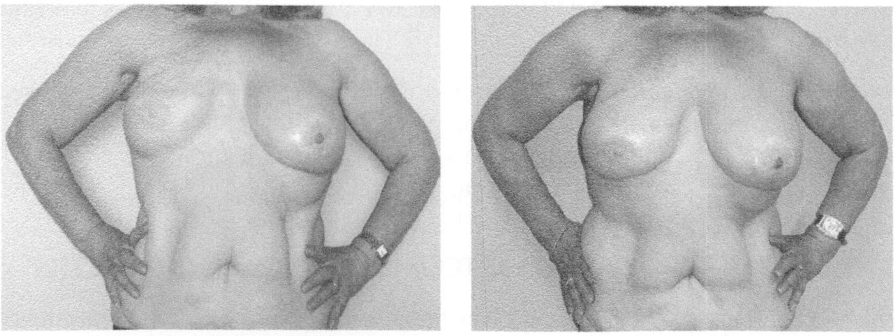

(a) (b)

FIGURE 25.14 Clinical view of the patient in Figures 25.12 and 25.13. (a) Preoperative view. (b) Postoperative view.

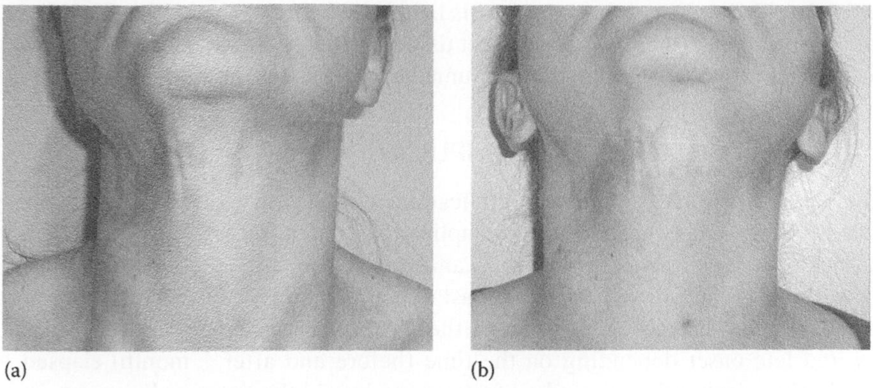

FIGURE 25.15 Patient with burn outcomes under her lower jaw (a). Results after two lipofilling sessions (b).

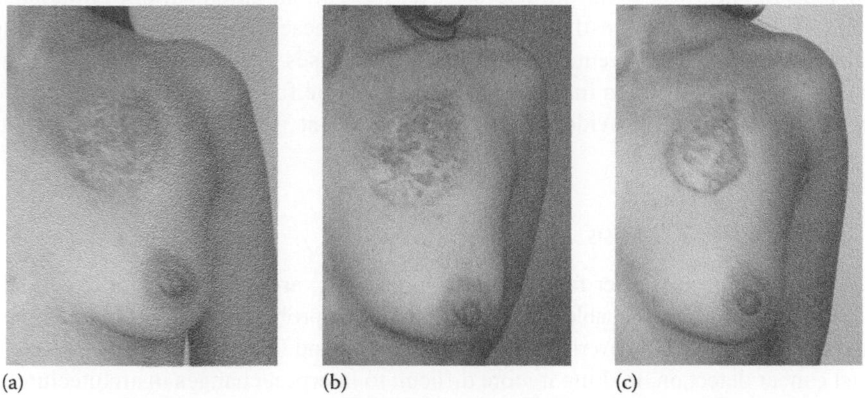

FIGURE 25.16 Patient with history of dermatofibrosarcoma protuberans excision on her left breast (a). Multiple lipofilling sessions showed scar improvement and reduction (b and c).

supported by clinical, instrumental, and histological findings, showed favourable results from the treatment of both mature and *evolving* scar tissue in the case of severe, old burn outcomes using fat grafting. Lipostructure at the dermohypodermal junction seems to increase the adipose layer widely destroyed by burn trauma and poorly regenerated during the reparative process and to improve the structural features of the ECM, increasing its production [27] (Figure 25.15).

Among wounds, post-traumatic ones are very common and often result in retracted, painful scars (Figure 25.16). Within these scars, some ulcerated areas tend to become chronic, significantly affecting the patient's quality of life. Scar remodelling by lipofilling showed complete closure of these lesions, just 2 weeks after the procedure. Results from these studies widened fat grafting application in all types of ulcers (i.e. post-traumatic, vascular, and pressure ulcers), as an additional or alternative procedure, with low morbidity [26].

25.4 FAT GRAFTING IN THE MANAGEMENT OF CONTOUR IRREGULARITIES FOLLOWING AESTHETIC PROCEDURES

Fat grafting is considered a potential tool also for refinements derived from iatrogenic skin irregularities and depressions, appearing after aesthetic procedures such as liposuction. Visible skin irregularities, such as severe depressions and retractions caused by excessive fat removal, could be fully appreciated only after the healing process, including also areas that are insufficiently reduced by lipoaspiration. Refinement procedures in this field include both approaching false depression by resuctioning and overcorrected regions with fat tissue transfer, because areas of excessive or insufficient fat removal can yield an asymmetrical, unnatural, or otherwise disappointing result [8].

25.5 FAT GRAFTING–RELATED COMPLICATIONS

Beside the several benefits, risks and complications associated with fat grafting emerged and are listed as follows: anaesthesia-related complications, infection, bleeding, less than expected beneficial outcome, interference with breast cancer detection, and others (fat embolism, strokes, lipoid meningitis). Some calcifications in breast tissues should be expected after breast fat injection, due to the partial necrotic reaction of the fat implanted. Complications can be divided into early and late onset depending on the time (before and after 1 month) elapsed from the procedure. Early complications include infections, such as both superficial surgery-site and deep tissue abscess formation; ecchymosis; striae; and hematomas of the treated site. Cases matching sepsis criteria, observed 1–3 weeks after surgery, have also been reported [40,43]. Late complications include liponecrotic cysts, fat necrosis, fat resorption, calcification, granuloma, nipple retraction, and unsatisfactory aesthetic results. Overall, these events are not unduly high, considering the low level of invasiveness of the procedure. Cases of severe complications appear to be extremely rare, and causation in these cases could not be fully determined. Therefore, actual studies found no compelling evidence that would warrant a strong recommendation against autologous fat grafting.

25.5.1 Differential Diagnosis

The most frequent sequelae, after fat injection and necrosis, are fibrotic reaction, variable degree of tissue calcifications, and palpable lumps; therefore, the problem of differential diagnosis with cancer has been discussed. The overlapping of breast tissue and fat transplantation may compromise early breast cancer detection, making it more difficult to interpret changes in architectural patterns. Slow and progressive microcalcifications and non-calcified lesions can occur after necrotic reaction in the treated areas; thus, imaging findings can lead to suspicion regarding the presence of cancer. Careful follow-up, by experienced clinicians and radiologists, is mandatory to choose appropriate diagnostic procedures and minimise unnecessary biopsies, avoiding delays and misdiagnosis of breast cancer.

The most common imaging findings, after breast lipografting, are the liponecrotic cysts (Figure 25.17) that do not present, usually, problem diagnosis, due to their characteristically benign appearances in ultrasonography, mammography, and MRI [9,20].

In a review of 12 articles, mammographic findings after fat injection were reported by Rosing et al. [36]. A benign-appearing eggshell calcification pattern, easily discernable from the microcalcifications suspicious for breast cancer, was found in nine articles. Microcalcification findings were reported by 3 of the 12 authors; however, no biopsy-proven diagnosis was documented. The most recent study considered by Rosing et al. involved 20 patients followed after fat grafting with mammographic examination [7]. According to the BI-RADS classification (Breast Imaging-Reporting and Data System), 85% of the patients had BI-RADS 2 benign lesions, and 15% were considered to have BI-RADS 3 lesions (probably benign). After further evaluations with digital mammography, three of these patients were downgraded to BI-RAD 2 lesions.

Another study, which included 30 patients who had undergone fat grafting after breast reconstruction surgery, was published [34]. Ultrasound, mammogram, MRI diagnostic imaging follow-up was able to detect four patients with benign microcalcifications.

In a retrospective examination of 17 breast fat grafting procedures, one case of cancer detection in a potentially grafted area and another in a non-grafted site were also reported without any delay in diagnosis [12].

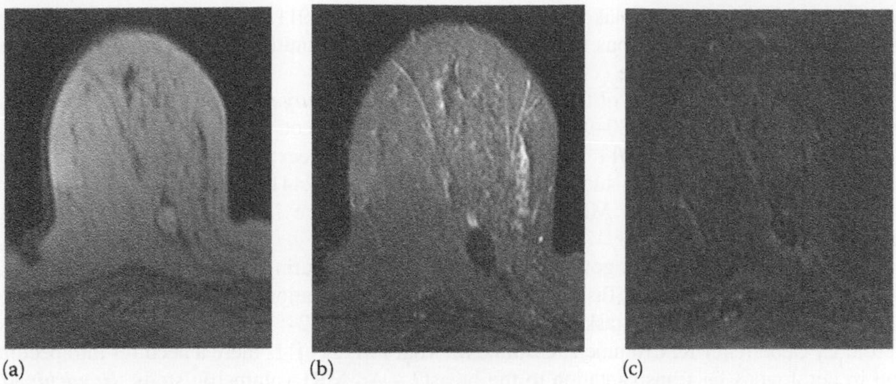

FIGURE 25.17 Left breast MRI images of T1-weighted FLASH3D axial scan (a), T2-weighted TIRM axial scan (b), and post-gadolinium T1-weighted axial FLASH3D scan with subtraction technique (c). In the infero-external quadrant of the left breast, an oval area characterised by the signal intensity of adipose tissue, delineated by a thin fibrous wall and without post-contrast enhancement, was observed (a–c). The imaging findings were suggestive of post-surgical liponecrosis.

So, according to the recent literature, there is currently no evidence of delay or misdiagnosis of malignancy after breast fat grafting procedure.

Diagnostic imaging examinations should be able to differentiate normal appearance from those associated with risk of breast cancer, and in case of any doubt, percutaneous biopsy is performed.

The experience and accuracy, in the clinical–radiological follow-up assessment, is essential after autologous fat transplantation, as well as after any surgical procedure, since any type of invasive breast procedure can lead to fat necrosis and to some degree of consequent calcifications.

REFERENCES

1. Amar O, Bruant-Rodier C, Lehmann S, Bolecker V, Wilk A. 2008. Greffe de tissue adipeux: Restauration du volume mammaire après traitement conservateur des cancers du sein, aspect Clinique et radiologique. *Ann Chir Plast Esthet* 53: 169–177.
2. American Society of Plastic and Reconstructive Surgeons (ASPRS). 1987. Report on autologous fat transplantation. Ad-Hoc Committee on New Procedures. *Plast Surg Nurs* 7: 140–141.
3. Boquest AC, Shahdadfar A, Brinchmann JE et al. 2006. Isolation of stromal stem cells from human adipose tissue. *Methods Mol Biol* 325: 35–46.
4. Bucky LP, Percec I. 2008. The science of autologous fat grafting: Views on current and future approaches to neoadipogenesis. *Aesthet Surg J* 28: 313–321.
5. Bunnel BA, Flaat M, Gagliardi C, Patel B, Ripoll C. 2008. Adipose-derived stem cells: Isolation, expansion and differentiation. *Methods* 45: 115–120.
6. Cannon B, Nedergaard J. 2004. Brown adipose tissue: Function and physiological significance. *Physiol Rev* 84: 277–359.
7. Carvajal J, Patino JH. 2008. Mammographic findings after breast augmentation with autologous fat injection. *Aesthet Surg J* 28: 153–162.
8. Castello MF, Lazzeri D, Agostini T, Silvestri A, Gasparotti M, D'Aniello C. 2011. Management of contour irregularities following superficial liposuction. *Plast Reconstr Surg* 128: 601–602.
9. Castelló JR, Barros J, Vázquez R. 1999. Giant liponecrotic pseudocyst after breast augmentation by fat injection. *Plast Reconstr Surg* 103: 291–293.
10. Coleman SR. 1995. Long-term survival of fat transplants: Controlled demonstrations. *Aesthetic Plast Surg* 19: 421–425.
11. Coleman SR. 2006. Structural fat graft: More than a permanent filler? *Plast Reconstr Surg* 118: 108S–120S.
12. Coleman SR, Saboeiro AP. 2007. Fat grafting to the breast revisited: Safety and efficacy. *Plast Reconstr Surg* 119: 775–785.

13. De Blacam C, Momoh AO, Colakoglu S, Tobias AM, Lee BT. 2011. Evaluation of clinical outcomes and aesthetic results after autologous fat grafting for contour deformities of the reconstructed breast. *Plast Reconstr Surg* 128: 411e–418e.
14. Delay E. 2006. Lipomodeling of the reconstructed breast. In *Surgery of the Breast: Principles and Art*, 2nd edn., Spear SE, ed., pp. 930–946. Philadelphia, PA: Lippincott Williams and Williams.
15. Del Vecchio DA, Bucky LP. 2011. Breast augmentation using preexpansion and autologous fat transplantation: A clinical radiographic study. *Plast Reconstr Surg* 127: 2441–2450.
16. Goehde SC, Kuehl H, Ladd ME. 2005. Magnetic resonance imaging of autologous fat grafting. *Eur Radiol* 15: 2423–2426.
17. Guerrerosantos J. 1996. Autologous fat grafting for body contouring. *Clin Plast Surg* 23: 619–631.
18. Gutowski KA, ASPS Fat Graft Task Force. 2009. Current applications and safety of autologous fat grafts: A report of the ASPS fat graft task force. *Plast Reconstr Surg* 124: 272–280.
19. Herold C, Ueberreiter K, Cromme F, Grimme M, Vogt PM. 2011. Is there a need for intrapectoral injection in autologous fat transplantation to the breast? – An MRI volumetric study. *Handchir Mikrochir Plast Chir* 43: 119–124.
20. Hyakusoku H, Ogawa R, Ono S, Ishii N, Hirakawa K. 2009. Complications after autologous fat injection to the breast. *Plast Reconstr Surg* 123: 360–370.
21. Illouz YG. 1986. The fat cell "graft": A new technique to fill depressions. *Plast Reconstr Surg* 78: 122–123.
22. Illouz YG, Sterodimas A. 2009. Autologous fat transplantation to the breast: A personal technique with 25 years of experience. *Aesthetic Plast Surg* 33: 706–715.
23. Kanchwala SK, Glatt BS, Conant EF, Bucky LP. 2009. Autologous fat grafting to the reconstructed breast: The management of acquired contour deformities. *Plast Reconstr Surg* 124: 409–418.
24. Kaufman MR, Miller TA, Huang C et al. 2007. Autologous fat transfer for facial recontouring: Is there science behind the art? *Plast Reconstr Surg* 119: 2287–2296.
25. Khouri RK, Eisenmann-Klein M, Cardoso E et al. 2012. Brava and autologous fat transfer is a safe and effective breast augmentation alternative: Results of a 6-year, 81-patient, prospective multicenter study. *Plast Reconstr Surg* 129: 1173–1187.
26. Klinger M, Caviggioli F, Vinci V, Salval A, Villani F. 2010. Treatment of chronic posttraumatic ulcers using autologous fat graft. *Plast Reconstr Surg* 126: 154e–155e.
27. Klinger M, Marazzi M, Vigo D, Torre M. 2008. Fat injection for cases of severe burn outcomes: A new perspective of scar remodeling and reduction. *Aesthetic Plast Surg* 32: 465–469.
28. Kølle ST, Oliveri RS, Glovinski PV, Elberg JJ, Nielsen AF, Drzewiecki KT. 2012. Importance of mesenchymal stem cells in autologous fat grafting: A systematic review of existing studies. *J Plast Surg Hand Surg* 46: 59–68.
29. Kneeshaw PJ, Lowry M, Manton D, Hubbard A, Drew PJ, Turnbull LW. 2006. Differentiation of benign from malignant breast disease associated with screening detected micro calcifications using dynamic contrast enhanced MRI. *Breast* 15: 29–38.
30. Mizuno H, Tobita M, Uysal AC. 2012. Concise review: Adipose-derived stem cells as a novel tool for regenerative medicine. *Stem Cells* 30: 804–810.
31. Mojallal A, Foyatier JL. 2004. Historical review of the use of adipose tissue transfer in plastic and reconstructive surgery. *Chir Plast Esthétique* 49: 419–425.
32. Murillo WL. 2004. Buttock augmentation: Case studies of fat injection monitored by magnetic resonance imaging. *Plast Reconstr Surg* 114:1606–1614.
33. Neuber GA. 1893. Fettrasplantation. *Bericht uber die Verhandlungen der Deutscht Gesellsch Chir* 22: 66.
34. Pierrefeu-Lagrange AC, Delay E, Guerin N, Chekaroua K, Delaporte T. 2005. Radiological evaluation of breasts reconstructed with lipomodeling. *Ann Chir Plast Esthet* 51: 18–28.
35. Rigotti G, Marchi A, Galiè M et al. 2007. Clinical treatment of radiotherapy tissue damage by lipoaspirate transplant: A healing process mediated by adipose-derived adult stem cells. *Plast Reconstr Surg* 119: 1409–1422.
36. Rosing JH, Wong G, Wong MS, Sahar D, Stevenson TR, Pu LL. 2011. Autologous fat grafting for primary breast augmentation: A systematic review. *Aesthetic Plast Surg* 35: 882–890.
37. Schipper BM, Marra KG, Zhang W et al. 2008. Regional anatomic and age effects on cell function of human adipose-derived stem cells. *Ann Plast Surg* 60: 538–544.
38. Serra-Renom JM, Muñoz-Olmo JJ, Serra-Mestre JM. 2010. Fat grafting in postmastectomy breast reconstruction with expanders and prostheses in patients who have received radiotherapy: Formation of new subcutaneous tissue. *Plast Reconstr Surg* 125: 12–18.

39. Spear SL, Wilson HB, Lockwood MD. 2005. Fat injection to correct contour deformities in the reconstructed breast. *Plast Reconstr Surg* 116: 1300–1305.
40. Talbot SG, Parrett BM, Yaremchuk MJ. 2010. Sepsis after autologous fat grafting. *Plast Reconstr Surg* 126: 162e–164e.
41. Tanzi MC, Farè S. 2009. Adipose tissue engineering: State of the art, recent advances and innovative approaches. *Expert Rev Med Devices* 6: 533–551.
42. Ullmann Y, Shoshani O, Fodor A et al. 2005. Searching for the favorable donor site for fat injection: In vivo study using the nude mouse model. *Dermatol Surg* 31: 1304–1307.
43. Valdatta L, Thione A, Buoro M, Tuinder S. 2001. A case of life-threatening sepsis after breast augmentation by fat injection. *Aesthetic Plast Surg* 25: 347–349.
44. Wolf GA, Gallego S, Patron AS et al. 2006. Magnetic resonance imaging assessment of gluteal fat grafts. *Aesthetic Plast Surg* 30: 460–468.
45. Yoshimura K, Eto H, Kato H, Doi K, Aoi N. 2011. In vivo manipulation of stem cells for adipose tissue repair/reconstruction. *Regen Med* 6: 33–41.
46. Yoshimura K, Sato K, Aoi N et al. 2008. Cell-assisted lipotransfer for cosmetic breast augmentation: Supportive use of adipose-derived stem/stromal cells. *Aesthetic Plast Surg* 32: 48–55.
47. Zheng DN, Li QF, Lei H et al. 2008. Autologous fat grafting to the breast for cosmetic enhancement: Experience in 66 patients with long-term follow up. *J Plast Reconstr Aesthet Surg* 61: 792–798.
48. Zocchi ML, Zuliani F. 2008. Bicompartmental breast lipostructuring. *Aesthetic Plast Surg* 32: 313–328.
49. Zuk PA, Zhu M, Ashjian P et al. 2002. Human adipose tissue is a source of multipotent stem cells. *Mol Biol Cell* 13: 4279–4295.

26 Surgical Principles and Imaging of Breast Implants and Their Follow-Up

Luca Andrea Dessy, Nefer Fallico, Gloria Pasqua Fanelli, Carlo De Masi, Luca Saba, Diego Ribuffo, and Nicolò Scuderi

CONTENTS

26.1 INTRODUCTION

Placement of an implant is the most common form of breast augmentation and an increasing number of women with breast prosthesis presents for mammographic screening or implant evaluation.

The main role of imaging breast implants is to provide essential information about tissue and implant integrity and to detect implant abnormalities as well as breast diseases unrelated to implants. In fact, an accurate study of breast parenchyma and of peri-prosthetic regions is always mandatory to detect either breast cancer or cancer recurrence.

It is important that radiologists are able to recognise the normal appearance of the more commonly used implants on different imaging modalities and to detect possible breast implant complications.

Currently, the most common forms of augmentation seen on imaging are silicone and saline implants and are single lumen. The radiological report of breast implants should include number (unilateral or bilateral), type (single/multiple lumen), and location (subglandular or subpectoral) of implants, and any complication, if present. Complications that can be observed when imaging breast implants are peri-implant fluid collection, which can be due to seroma, hematoma, or infection; implant rupture; gel bleed; and capsular contraction (Table 26.1).

First-level examinations in breast imaging are breast ultrasound and, in case of appropriate age, mammography. However, the physician should be aware of the limits of these techniques and all doubtful cases should be investigated with breast magnetic resonance imaging (MRI).[38,46,49] Computed tomography (CT) is reserved for patients in whom breast MRI is contraindicated because of severe claustrophobia or indwelling metallic devices that are not compatible with magnetic resonance.

In this chapter, the imaging appearance of breast implants on various imaging modalities is reviewed and commonly encountered complications are presented.

26.2 MAMMOGRAPHY

The usefulness of mammography in the assessment of implant integrity is scarce; however, it is important for the assessment of the surrounding breast tissue.[17] In fact, detection of breast cancer is the first indication to mammography in elder women. The radiologist is able to evaluate the breast implant on a yearly basis and to detect possible complications. The screening mammogram should be performed with standard and implant-displaced (Eklund technique) craniocaudal and mediolateral oblique views.[14,16]

26.2.1 Appearance of Normal Implants

On mammography, silicone implants appear as dense oval masses in either a subglandular or subpectoral position (Figures 26.1 through 26.3).[47] Because of the density of the silicone, a discernable envelope and its accompanying folds are not visualised on mammography[33] (Table 26.2). Mammographically, saline implants are seen as oval masses with a dense peripheral envelope and a valve with a more lucent centre (Table 26.2). Folds in the implant envelope, the valve, glandular

TABLE 26.1
Breast Implant Complications

Presence of peri-implant fluid collection (seroma, hematoma, or infection)
Implant rupture (intra- or extracapsular)
Gel bleed
Capsular contraction
Breast implant-associated lymphoma

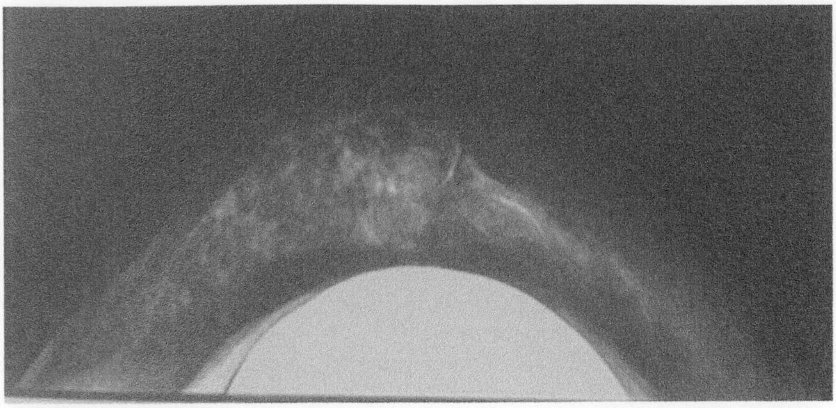

FIGURE 26.1 Mammographic imaging of a regular subpectoral implant. The silicone implant appears as a dense oval mass in a subpectoral position.

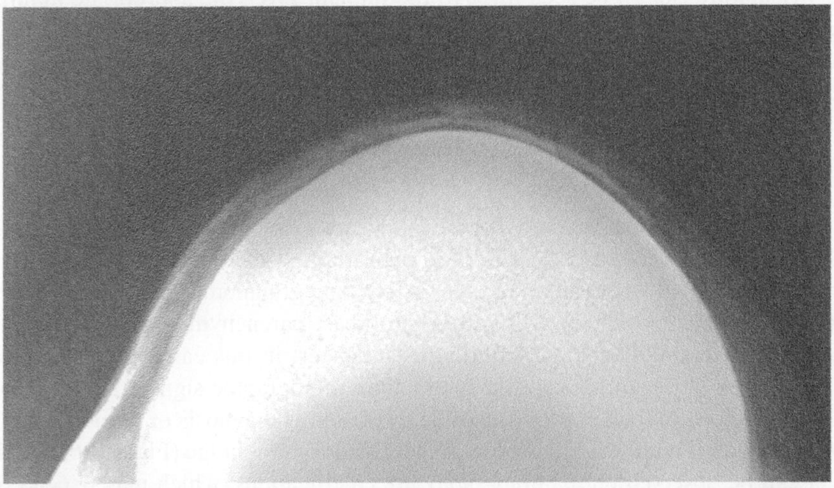

FIGURE 26.2 Mammographic imaging of a subpectoral silicone implant in breast reconstruction after mastectomy.

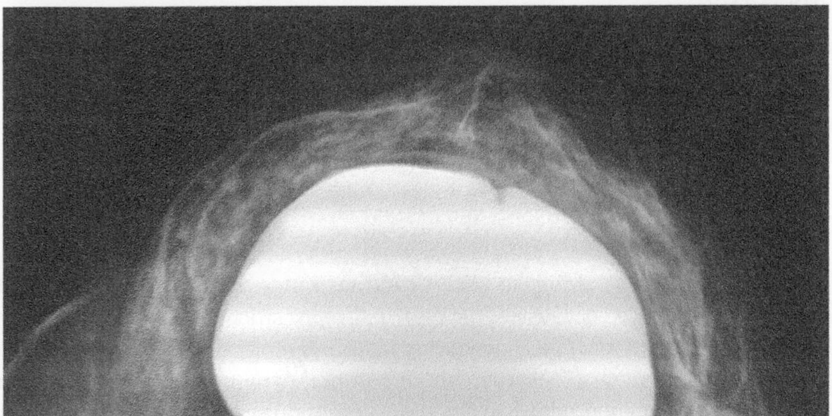

FIGURE 26.3 Mammographic imaging of a subglandular silicone implant with a contour bulge. This is a suspect sign of rupture of the silicone implant.

TABLE 26.2
Imaging Appearance of Breast Implant on Four Imaging Modalities

	Implant Type	
Imaging Modality	**Silicone**	**Saline**
Mammography	Dense oval masses	Oval masses with dense peripheral envelope and visible valve
Ultrasound	Anechoic with echogenic envelope	Anechoic with echogenic envelope
Magnetic resonance imaging	T2, high signal; T1, low signal; silicone sensitive, high signal with low signal envelope on all sequences	T2, high signal; T1, low signal; silicone sensitive, low signal with low signal envelope and valve on all sequences
Computed tomography	Dense oval masses with surrounding high-density ring	Hypodense oval mass with hyperdense peripheral ring and valve

tissue, and vasculature can all be seen through the implant given the appropriate mammographic technique.[35] Double-lumen implants are less commonly used and may be seen with an inner silicone-gel-filled envelope surrounded by an outer adjustable saline-filled envelope or an inner adjustable saline-filled envelope surrounded by an outer silicone envelope.

26.2.2 Alterations Detected by Mammography

Alterations most commonly detected by this technique are extracapsular rupture and capsular contraction. Specific mammographic evidence of implant rupture is extravasation of silicone outside the implant shell with radiopaque material, that is, silicone granulomas composed of free silicone and surrounding fibrous tissue reaction, within the breast parenchyma or further in the axilla.[19] Sometimes, extracapsular silicone can mimic breast cancer; in this case, implant rupture should always be considered.[33] Regarding capsule contraction, radiographic signs may not be present but the typical appearance is a thicker profile capsule.[16,33] Usually, diagnosis of intracapsular rupture is not possible, although sometimes, it can be suggested by a contour bulge (Figure 26.3). Other abnormalities that can be observed on mammography are calcifications, which may depend on chronic inflammatory response, and seroma.

26.2.3 Advantages

Mammography is relatively inexpensive, and many women older than 50 years, including women with breast implants, receive yearly screening examinations provided by national health systems or personal health insurances. This technique can provide some information about implants integrity, showing alterations such as capsule deformity and extracapsular rupture.

26.2.4 Limitations

Mammography is limited in its ability to identify intracapsular ruptures, which account for up to 80%–90% of implant failures,[40] because of the high density of silicone that hides internal structures of implants to the x-rays used for typical screening mammography.[12]

Moreover, several case reports describe silicone implant rupture from compression during a mammogram, mainly in women who had intracapsular ruptures before the examination. Thus, mammographic compression can potentially convert an intracapsular rupture to an extracapsular rupture.[26]

26.3 ULTRASONOGRAPHY

In breast implants, ultrasound imaging has to be regarded as a first-level examination; in fact it is a non-invasive, inexpensive, and easily available technique and it is usually well accepted by patients. Breast ultrasound can often be a valid means to diagnose problems concerning breast implants. Nevertheless, its performance requires an accurate knowledge of breast diseases as well as of breast implants imaging features. It is performed with the patient in supine position with her ipsilateral arm raised behind her head to examine the medial part of the breast, while the lateral part of the breast is studied by using oblique position of the patient.[2] Ultrasonography (US) breast implant examination involves evaluation of morphology, contour and contents, peri-implant tissues, and axillae. Thus, the transversal-to-longitudinal ratio of the implants is calculated, the regularity of implant margins (radial folds) and the homogeneity of the implant lumen are checked, and signs of free silicone or granulomas in the breast or in the axillary lymph nodes are sought.[9]

26.3.1 Appearance of Normal Implants

The most reliable sign of an intact implant is an anechoic interior (Figure 26.4).[19] The posterior interface may be difficult to visualise because of its depth. Reverberation artefacts are commonly encountered in the anterior aspect of the implant and should not be confused with abnormalities. The implant membrane, sometimes visualised as a thin echogenic line, should be continuous and intact. Radial folds present as echogenic lines that extend from the periphery to the interior of the implant. These folds are normal infoldings of the implant membrane into the silicone gel. On ultrasound, both saline and silicone implants appear internally anechoic with triangular shape, surrounded by a linear echogenic envelope (Table 26.2). The envelope is variable in appearance, consisting of a single echogenic line or parallel echogenic lines. The fibrous capsule may also be visualised sonographically as two parallel echogenic lines superficial to the implant surface (Figure 26.4). If calcification of the fibrous capsule is present, echogenic foci with posterior shadowing may be seen

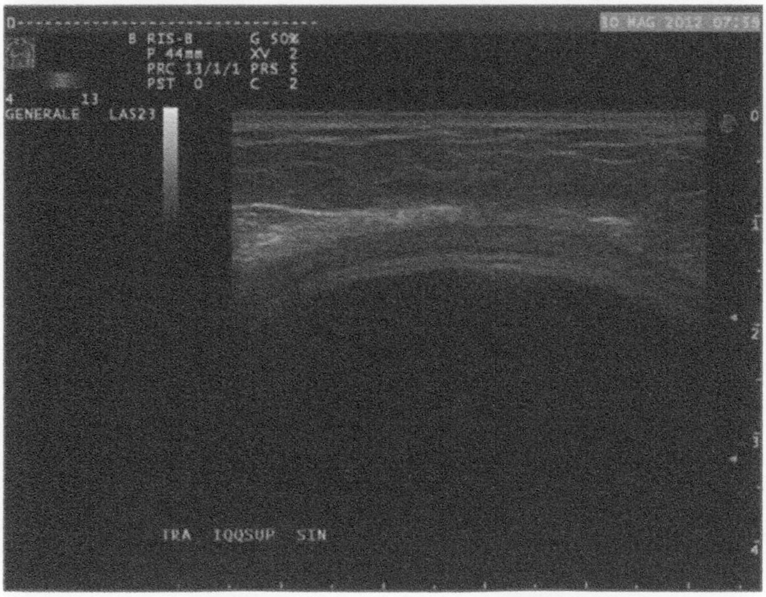

FIGURE 26.4 Ultrasound imaging of the breast showing the presence of an intact silicone implant. An anechoic interior is visible.

within the fibrous capsule.[3] Undulations and folds in the envelope are seen as waves and extension of the envelope into the implant without intervening fluid. The valve of saline implants may be seen as a focal disruption or separation in the parallel lines of the capsule. The second chamber of a double-lumen implant can be visualised and should not be confused for a rupture.[21]

26.3.2 Alterations Detected by US

Breast ultrasound can identify implants integrity and abnormalities as capsular contraction, peri-implant fluid collection, and implant rupture.

US can easily detect extracapsular rupture because of the echogenic appearance of silicone among soft tissue. In fact, extracapsular rupture is characterised by hyperechoic nodules, which represent silicone granulomas, outside the fibrous capsule (Figure 26.5). This pattern is usually called as *snow-storm* and it is the most reliable sign of extracapsular rupture at US.[13,50] The granulomas should be differentiated from breast tumours through correlation of clinical, mammographic, and sonographic findings. As many silicone granulomas are located in the axilla (Figure 26.6), in case of extracapsular rupture, axilla evaluation is recommended to detect either adenopathy or free silicone.

US can also detect intracapsular rupture by identifying a series of parallel echogenic lines inside the implant, which represent the layers of the collapsed implant shell.[11] This sign is commonly known as the *stepladder sign*[7,48] and it is the most reliable sign of intracapsular rupture.[15,50] It is important not to confuse the stepladder sign with normal prominent radial folds. Further sign of intracapsular rupture is accumulation of low-level homogeneous echoes in the silicone gel probably due to influx of body fluids that mix with silicone producing a change in echotexture. Anyway, central internal echoes can be caused even by implants infolding and they should be differentiated from intracapsular rupture, although this is not always easy especially in case of double-lumen implants or implants with textured coatings. As sonographic signs of intracapsular rupture can accompany extracapsular rupture, a careful search for extracapsular rupture should be performed, including a search for silicone nodules in the axilla.

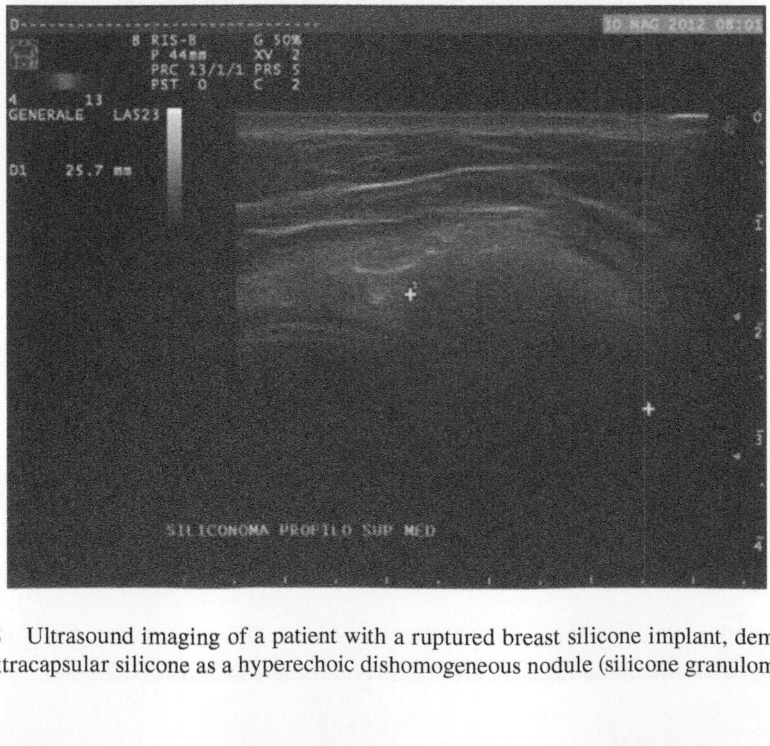

FIGURE 26.5 Ultrasound imaging of a patient with a ruptured breast silicone implant, demonstrating the presence of extracapsular silicone as a hyperechoic dishomogeneous nodule (silicone granuloma).

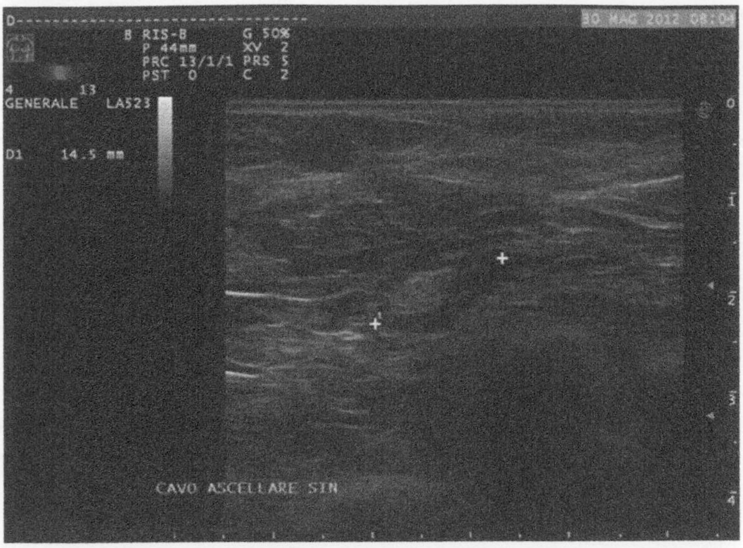

FIGURE 26.6 Ultrasound imaging of the same patient of Figure 26.5. The presence of silicone granuloma is evident in the axilla near to a reactive lymph node (image with calipers). Il siliconoma è in basso a destra dell'immagine, si potrebbe evidenziare posizionando un asterisco.

26.3.3 Advantages

US is relatively inexpensive when compared with MRI or CT, and no ionising radiation is used. US can detect both extracapsular (snowstorm) and intracapsular (stepladder) rupture.[24,48] A completely negative US examination strongly supports implant integrity, limiting the application of MRI to cases suspicious at US.[15,17] Moreover, US is very useful in patients who are claustrophobic or have a contraindication for MRI.

26.3.4 Limitations

One limitation of US is that the evaluation of the posterior wall of a silicone implant is impeded by the marked attenuation of the ultrasound beam. Similarly, residual silicone granulomas from extracapsular rupture or from previous direct silicone injections compromise the evaluation of a new implant.

Moreover, there are conflicting reports on the usefulness of US for detecting implant ruptures depending on the experience of the operator, type of equipment used, and technical factors.[9,11,21,30,34,36] US is operator dependent and proficiency in ultrasonographic evaluation of implants requires a steep learning curve. Finally, in order to accomplish the best results, on-site evaluation is recommended.

26.4 MRI

MRI is the most reliable imaging method for the evaluation of silicone implant integrity, with sensitivity of 74%–100% and specificity of 63%–100%,[23] while it does not have a role in evaluating saline implant integrity in view of the clear clinical appearance of a ruptured saline implant. Despite this fact, when MRI is performed to evaluate the breast tissue, all types of breast augmentation may be encountered.

Breast MRI is performed with the patient in the prone position. In order to avoid diagnostic inaccuracy, a field strength of at least 1 T is needed. Multiplanar dedicated T1- and T2-weighted MRI techniques are used for evaluating implant integrity.[37] Silicone-sensitive inversion recovery sequences or a modified 3-point Dixon technique is also used to detect high-signal silicone in the evaluation of implant rupture.[41] The use of contrast agents in MRI studies for the assessment of breast implant integrity is not recommended. However, when the priority is the detection of recurrence or residual tumours, contrast-enhanced MRI of the breast is useful for characterising parenchymal lesions. Contrast agent administration (0.2 mmol/kg bodyweight) is via antecubital venous access at standard flow rate of 2/mL/s followed by a 10 mL saline flush.

26.4.1 Appearance of Normal Implants

Silicone gel within an implant has homogeneously high signal intensity on T2-weighted images and low signal intensity on T1-weighted images surrounded by a low-signal envelope and fibrous capsule on all sequences (Figure 26.7, Table 26.2).[19,23,31] Saline implants follow fluid signal on all sequences, high signal intensity on T2- weighted images, and low signal intensity on T1-weighted images (Table 26.2). The envelope and fibrous capsule have low signal on all sequences, as is the valve, which is seen as a low-signal mural nodule on all sequences.[1] Folds in the envelope are seen as low-signal linear and curvilinear lines extending from the envelope into the silicone gel or saline. Folds are frequently seen in both saline and silicone implants and should not be mistaken for rupture.

26.4.2 Alterations Detected by MRI

Intracapsular rupture is determined by the rupture of the implant shell with the capsule remaining intact (Figure 26.8). The collapsed implant shell is visualised on MRI as curvilinear hypointense lines, which are referred to as the *linguine sign* (Figures 26.9 and 26.10).[10,18] Other signs of intracapsular rupture are hypointense, subcapsular lines which are generated by minimal displacement of shell and are parallel to fibrous capsule and the *teardrop sign* and *keyhole sign*, which depend on focal silicone invagination between the inner shell and fibrous capsule.[24] These more subtle findings are typical of uncollapsed silicone implant ruptures, which count for up to 52% of implant ruptures.[4] These signs should always be differentiated from normal findings in intact implants such as radial folds, which are thicker than linguine sign and always connect to the periphery of the implant (Figure 26.7).[17,19]

Rarely, intracapsular rupture can show multiple hyperintense foci on T2-weighted images or multiple hypointense foci on water-suppression images within the implant lumen resulting from the mixing of the fluid around the implant and the internal silicone. These findings are referred to as the *salad oil sign* or *droplet sign*. Without other MRI evidence of implant rupture, water droplets

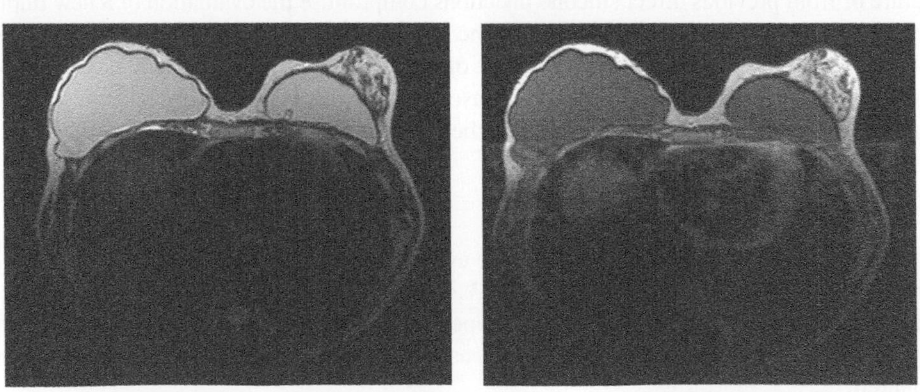

(a) (b)

FIGURE 26.7 MRI of a patient with breast silicone implants. The T2-weighted (a) and T1-weighted (b) images demonstrate the regular morphology of the implants.

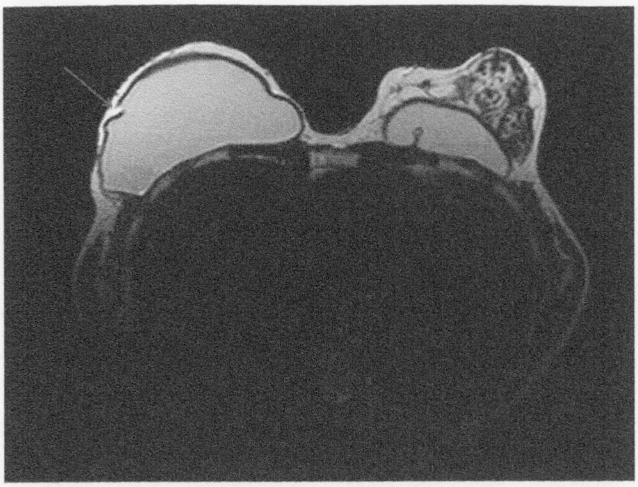

FIGURE 26.8 MRI of the same patient in Figure 26.7. The T2-weighted image demonstrates the intracapsular rupture of the right breast implant.

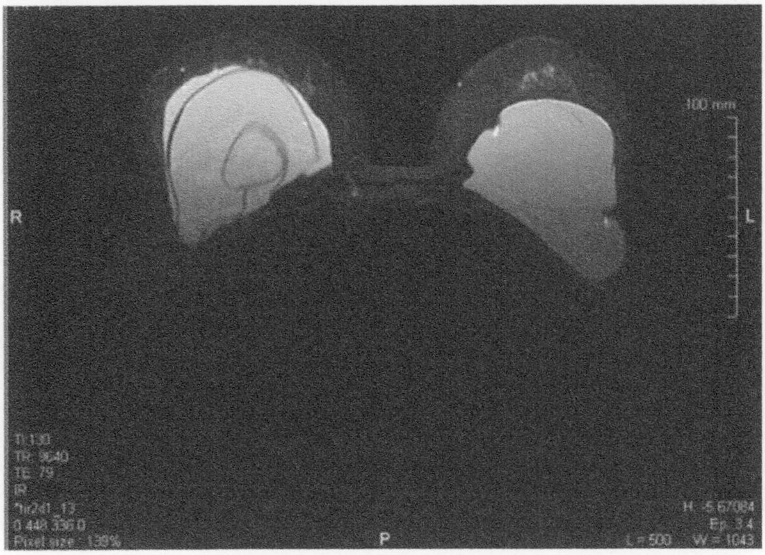

FIGURE 26.9 MRI of a patient with breast silicone implants. The T2-weighted image demonstrates the typical linguine sign on the right implant.

or small amounts of air within a silicone implant are not reliable signs of implant rupture.[13,17,19] However, this sign should prompt the search for subtle signs of intracapsular rupture.[13]

Extracapsular rupture can be suggested by the presence of silicone outside the capsule, which can be best and easily seen with silicone only sequences.[17,27,43]

Unlike rupture, gel bleed is a microscopic silicone leakage through an intact implant shell.[50] For this reason, the presence of silicone gel in regional lymph nodes can be due to gel bleed and not be always indicative of an implant rupture (Figure 26.11). However, with the introduction of new cohesive gel implants, the phenomenon of gel bleeding has notably reduced.[10] Most normal transudation of microscopic amounts of silicone gel cannot be detected by MRI. Only when a gel bleed is

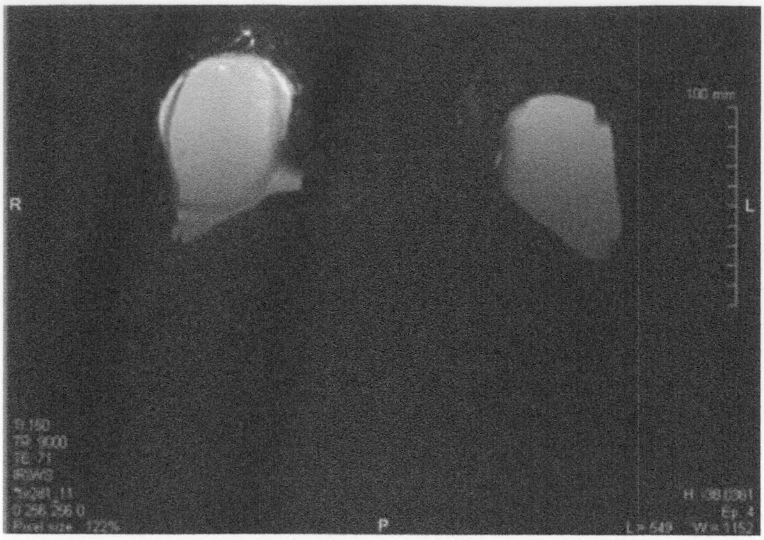

FIGURE 26.10 MRI of a patient with breast silicone implants. The silicone-sensitive inversion recovery axial sequences demonstrate the right implant: linguine sign and subareolar high signal intensity are due to intra- and extracapsular rupture.

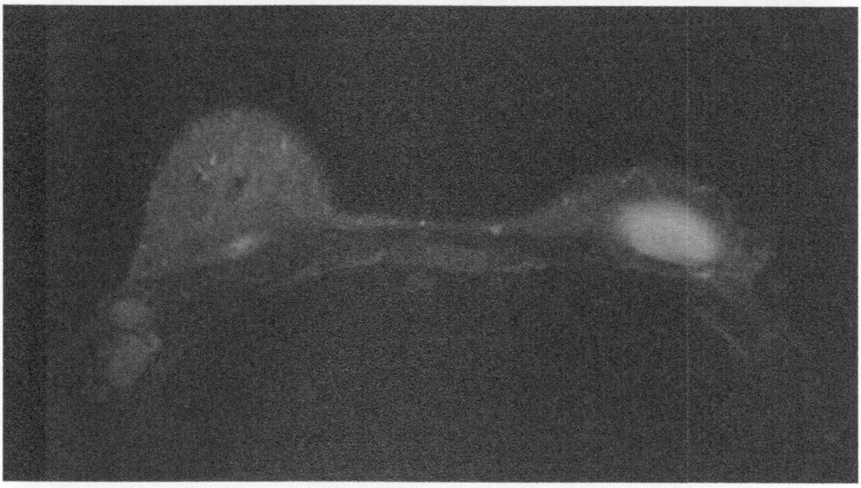

FIGURE 26.11 MRI of a patient with breast silicone implants. The T2-weighted image demonstrates the presence of silicone in the axillary lymph nodes.

extensive, the silicone gel can be detected outside the implant shell forming the *inverted teardrop sign*. An uncollapsed implant rupture can have a similar or identical magnetic resonance appearance to a large gel bleed.

26.4.3 Advantages

Magnetic resonance is the most accurate method for the evaluation of breast implants because of its high spatial and soft-tissue resolutions.[51] The usefulness of MRI derives from its ability to suppress or emphasise the signal from water, fat, or especially silicone, which makes it ideal for the characterisation of breast implants. Breast MRI might resolve diagnostic doubt especially in cases where with US it is difficult to distinguish between radial folds and intracapsular rupture.

Other advantages of MRI are that no ionising radiation is used and many different magnetic resonance pulse sequences can be used to optimise the silicone image, allowing optimal visualisation of the silicone implants. Furthermore, MRI has multiplanar capability, allowing visualisation of the silicone implant in any plane.

26.4.4 Limitations

Magnetic resonance is the most expensive imaging modality for the evaluation of silicone breast implants. Moreover, MRI often shows radial folds or normal infoldings of the implant shell, which can be confused with implant rupture or leak. This is one of the major pitfalls and causes of false positives on MRI, mimicking the total collapse of the implant shell.[10,13]

Finally, not all patients are able to undergo MRI because of cardiac pacemakers, aneurysm clips, or metallic foreign bodies which are not compatible with MRI. Notably, some kind of breast tissue expanders should be considered a contraindication to MRI because of the magnetic marker of the filling valve: expander manufacturers list possible consequences such as overheating, possible expander displacement, and possible reduction of magnetisation of the marker.[37] Also, some patients are very claustrophobic and unable to complete an MRI examination. Size and weight restrictions will also prevent some patients from having an MRI examination of the breast.

26.5 CT

CT is not the study of choice in breast implant evaluation because of its low sensitivity and specificity in detecting implant rupture. Therefore, it should be reserved for patients in whom MRI is contraindicated.

26.5.1 Appearance of Normal Implants

At CT, an intact silicone implant is characterised by an oval shape and homogeneous grey density within a surrounding high-density ring (Table 26.2). The implant often has contour deformities or implant bulges or hernias.

26.5.2 Alterations Detected by CT

The computed tomographic findings of intracapsular silicone implant rupture are similar to the MRI findings. The collapsed implant shell can usually be easily identified on the CT images consisting of collapse of the white ring into the silicone gel to form the linguine sign.[8] Extracapsular rupture can be difficult to identify because of silicone and soft tissues have similar radiodensities on CT imaging. However, in most cases, the collapsed implant shell can be identified, so that the implant failure is not missed.

As with MRI, it is important to differentiate normal prominent radial folds from an actual collapsed implant shell.[32]

26.5.3 Advantages

CT is widely available and can be used in the evaluation of breast implant rupture. CT is accurate in detecting intracapsular silicone breast implant ruptures and is capable of depicting the linguine sign. Many patients who are unable to complete a magnetic resonance examination because of claustrophobia or size or weight restrictions can complete a computed tomographic examination. Most CT scanners have higher weight limits and larger bores than most MRI units.

26.5.4 Limitations

CT does use ionising radiation to obtain images; therefore, this modality should not be the study of choice, especially in young women in the evaluation of breast implants. Actually, most CT images of ruptured breast implants are incidental findings in asymptomatic patients or in already known failed implants. Also, the ability of CT to detect extracapsular silicone is limited because of the similar radiodensity between silicone and soft tissues.

26.6 IMPLANT COMPLICATIONS

Breast implant complications are seroma, hematoma, and infection, which result as a peri-implant fluid collection; capsular contraction; implant rupture; and, less commonly, gel bleed and breast-implant-associated lymphoma.

26.6.1 Peri-Implant Fluid Collection

Fluid collections surrounding breast implants result from the foreign body reaction generated by the implant capsule. The presence of peri-prosthetic liquid is a common and nonspecific finding and does not necessarily warrant intervention.[4,33] On ultrasound imaging, the fluid can present multiple internal echoes or be anechoic (Figure 26.12). On MRI, the fluid collection presents with homogeneous increased T2 signal surrounding an intact implant (Figure 26.13).

26.6.2 Capsular Contraction

Capsular contraction is the most common implant complication and is more commonly seen with silicone implants as a result of foreign body reaction.[22,25] The fibrous capsule around the implant contracts, resulting in hardening and deformity of the implant, which leads to alteration in breast shape and discomfort.[17] Capsular contraction is a clinical diagnosis and often is not appreciated on imaging. Mammographically, the implant may appear spherical rather than elliptical in shape or it may develop unusual areas of bulging.[4] Capsular contraction may not always have findings sonographically or on MRI; however, thickening of the echogenic fibrous capsule

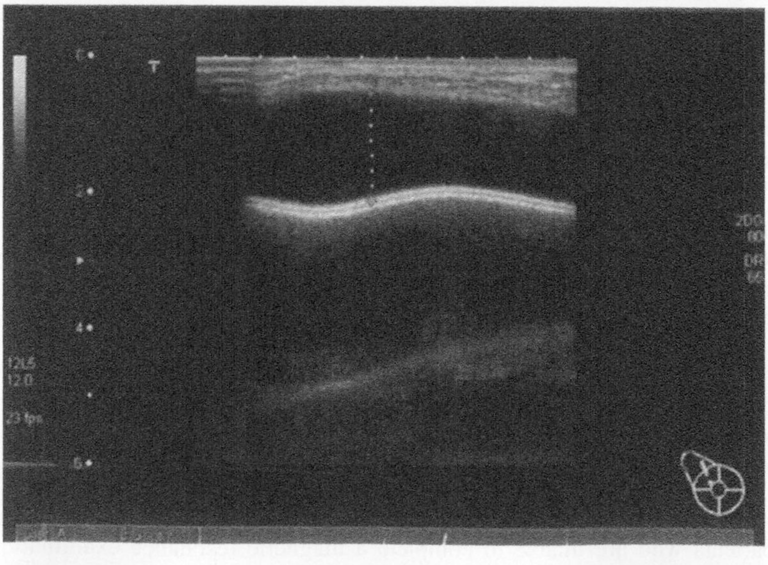

FIGURE 26.12 Ultrasound imaging of the breast showing the presence of peri-prosthetic fluid.

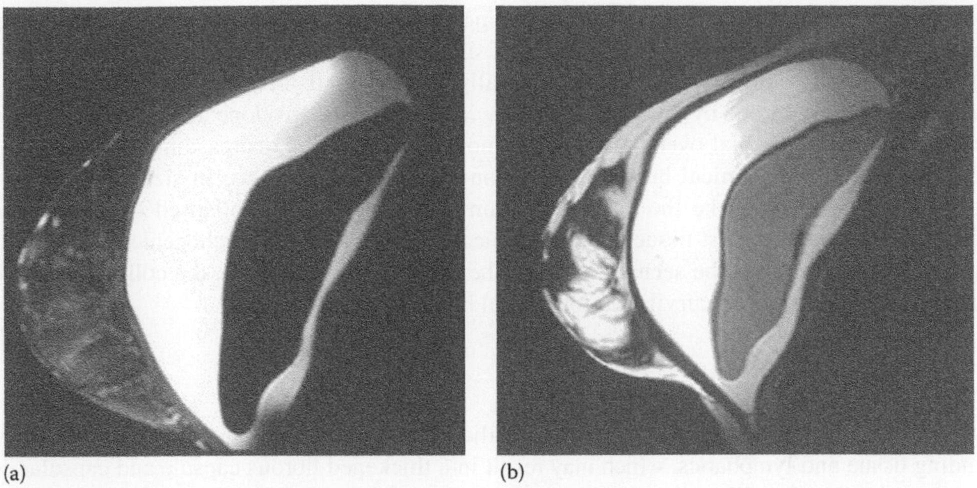

FIGURE 26.13 MRI of the breast. The T1-weighted (a) and T2-weighted (b) images demonstrate the presence of peri-prosthetic fluid.

with an increased number of radial folds and an increased anterior–posterior diameter may be seen.[33] If it is symptomatic, treatment consists of capsulectomy or capsulotomy.[25]

26.6.3 Rupture

Rupture is the most common indication for breast implant removal.[13,25,33] For silicone breast implants, there are two types of rupture: intracapsular and extracapsular. Intracapsular rupture is defined as rupture of the polyurethane envelope with silicone contained within the surrounding fibrous capsule.[6] This type of rupture may not be detectable mammographically, because the density of the silicone prevents visualisation of the implant envelope. The shape of the implant is generally maintained; however, the implant may appear expanded compared to the contralateral implant. On ultrasound, the presence of horizontal echogenic lines corresponding to the collapsed envelope within the anechoic silicone gel, that is, the *stepladder sign*, may be seen, which is in contrast to the normal vertical extension of radial folds.[48] The silicone gel between the fibrous capsule and the collapsed envelope may be slightly increased in echogenicity, although this is a less reliable sign. The most sensitive and specific imaging test for intracapsular rupture is MRI. The ruptured envelope is seen as multiple low-signal curvilinear lines within the high-signal silicone gel on T2-weighted and silicone-sensitive sequences, the so-called linguine sign.[18,19] More subtle areas of focal separation of the envelope from the fibrous capsule forming teardrop-shaped involutions of the envelope or subcapsular lines with intervening silicone are early signs of intracapsular rupture, referred to as the *teardrop or keyhole sign.*[19] Silicone signal does not extend beyond the low-signal fibrous capsule.

Extracapsular rupture may be diagnosed mammographically, sonographically, or on MRI. Free silicone is seen as dense lobulated masses outside the implant margins. Extremely dense axillary lymph nodes may be present because silicone gel is cleared by the lymphatics of the breast. Less-specific mammographic signs of extracapsular rupture include implant asymmetry or irregularity of the implant contour. Sonographic evaluation may reveal masses with a well-defined echogenic anterior surface and dirty shadowing (snowstorm sign).[33] Hypoechoic or anechoic masses with or without posterior shadowing may also be seen.[39] MRI is useful for the evaluation of mammographically occult extracapsular rupture and can evaluate the extent of free silicone. The contour of the implant may be irregular, with globular masses or linear collections of high signal intensity free silicone separate from the implant in the breast tissue or within the axilla on T2-weighted and silicone-selective sequences. There is no enhancement with gadolinium administration, unless there is active inflammation related to the formation of silicone granulomas.

Rupture of saline implants is evident clinically and with all forms of imaging because the extruded saline is resorbed by the lymphatics, leaving a collapsed envelope and capsule.[3] The leakage can be acute or gradual over a few days or months, resulting in decrease in size or change of shape of the implant. Clinical breast examination to evaluate difference in size of shape of the implant is sufficient to make the diagnosis. Mammographically, the collapsed envelope is seen folded posterior to the breast tissue.[33] Sonographically, multiple stacked echogenic linear and curvilinear parallel lines may be seen posterior to the breast tissue. On MRI, the collapsed envelope appears as multiple stacked curvilinear low-signal bands.

26.6.4 Gel Bleed

A gel bleed is the transudation of microscopic silicone gel across an intact envelope into the surrounding tissue and lymphatics, which may result in a thickened fibrous capsule and capsular contraction. Additionally, silicone may be visualised in axillary lymph nodes mammographically, sonographically, and on MRI.

26.6.5 Breast-Implant-Associated Lymphoma

Breast implant-associated anaplastic large-cell lymphoma (ALCL) is a rare, but likely underreported entity, which most commonly presents with an effusion developing between the breast implant and the host fibrous capsule that surrounds it.[45] More than 100 cases are reported in the literature.[44] Recently, after expert consultation, a review confirmed *a positive association between breast implants and ALCL development.*[28] It has been described in association with breast implants used for post-cancer reconstructive surgery and when implanted for purely cosmetic reasons. It is a clinically indolent disease with a favorable prognosis that is distinct from systemic anaplastic lymphoma kinase–negative ALCL. Generically, these cases have presented in three ways: most commonly, as late seromas; next, as a mass attached to the implant capsule; and a few that have been serendipitously discovered during surgery for significant capsular contracture.[29] Metastases have been rare, but the axillary nodes should be physically examined and submitted to biopsy if palpable. Radiological imaging can remark these signs but do not allow to obtain a precise diagnostic data. Ultrasound examination can reveal large fluid collection surrounding the implant. Mammography can reveal an effusion and exclude parenchymal abnormality. MRI can confirm these signs, evidencing an intact implant and the presence of fluid collection between the primary silicone implant and the pseudo-capsule.[42] Recurrent, clinically evident seroma occurring 6 months or more after breast implantation should be aspirated and sent for cytological analysis. A capsular contracture occurring years after the implantation should alarm surgeons, and ALCL should be included by pathologists in the differential diagnosis. A contracture that behaves as refractory to several surgical revisions during which the prosthesis is reimplanted should be further investigated and always sent for all pathological examinations.[20] Management should consist of removal of the involved implant and capsule, which is likely to prevent recurrence, and evaluation for other sites of disease. A total capsulectomy should be performed. Multiple biopsy sites should be marked for the pathologist to include adherent and nonadherent areas. There have been several cases of bilateral disease, so if a diagnosis is made in one breast, it would seem prudent to remove the other implant and capsule.[5]

REFERENCES

1. Azavedo, E. and Bone, B. 1999. Imaging breasts with silicone implants. *Eur Radiol* 9: 349–355.
2. Bassetti, E., Pediconi, F., Luciani, M. L., Santucci, E., Miglio, E., and Candreva, R. 2011. Breast prosthesis: Management of patients after plastic surgery. *J Ultrasound* 14: 113–121.

3. Berg, W. A., Caskey, C. I., Hamper, U. M. et al. 1993. Diagnosing breast implant rupture with MR imaging, US, and mammography. *Radiographics* 13: 1323–1336.
4. Berg, W. A., Nguyen T. K., Middleton M. S., Soo, M. S., Pennello, G., and Brown, S. L. 2002. MR imaging of extracapsular silicone from breast implants: Diagnostic pitfalls. *AJR Am J Roentgen* 178: 465–472.
5. Brody, G. S. 2012. Brief recommendations for dealing with a new case of anaplastic large T-cell lymphoma. *Plast Reconstr Surg* 129: 871–872.
6. Brown, S. L., Silverman, B. G., and Berg, W. A. 1997. Rupture of silicone-gel breast implants: Causes, sequelae, and diagnosis. *Lancet* 350: 1531–1537.
7. Caskey, C. I., Berg, W. A., Anderson, N. D., Sheth, S., Chang, B. W., and Hamper, U. M. 1994. Breast implant rupture: Diagnosis with US. *Radiology* 190: 819–823.
8. Chul, T. K., Sun, J. H., Suk, R. T., and Choi, J. W. 2005. Analysis of 30 breast implant rupture cases. *Aesthetic Plast Surg* 29: 460–469.
9. Cilotti, A., Marini, C., Iacconi, C. et al. 2006. Ultrasonographic appearance of breast implant complications. *Ann Plast Surg* 56: 243–247.
10. Colombo, G., Ruvolo, V., Stifanese, R., Perillo, M., and Garlaschi, A. 2011. Prosthetic breast implant rupture: Imaging–pictorial essay. *Aesthetic Plast Surg* 35: 891–900.
11. DeBruhl, N. D., Gorczyca, D. P., Ahn, C. Y., Shaw, W. W., and Bassett, L. W. 1993. Silicone breast implants: US evaluation. *Radiology* 189: 95–98.
12. Destouet, J. M., Monsees, B. S., Oser, R. F., Nemecek, J. R., Young, V. L., and Pilgram, T. K. 1992. Screening mammography in 350 women with breast implants: Prevalence and findings of implant complications. *AJR Am J Roentgenol* 159: 973–978.
13. Di Benedetto, G., Cecchini S., Grassetti, L. et al. 2008. Comparative study of breast implant rupture using mammography, sonography, and magnetic resonance imaging: Correlation with surgical findings. *Breast J* 14: 532–537.
14. Eklund, G. W., Busby, R. C., Miller, S. H., and Job, J. S. 1988. Improved imaging of the augmented breast. *AJR Am J Roentgenol* 151: 469–473.
15. Frank, S., Mahdi, R., and Sherko, K. 2010. Imaging in patients with breast implants—Results of the First International Breast (Implant) Conference 2009. *Insights Imaging* 1: 93–97.
16. Gannot, M. A., Harris, K. M., Ilkhanipour, Z. S., and Costa-Greco, M. A. 1992. Augmentation mammoplasty; normal and abnormal findings with mammography and US. *Radiographics* 12: 281–295.
17. Glynn, C. and Litherland, J. 2008. Imaging breast augmentation and reconstruction. *Br J Radiol* 81: 587–595.
18. Gorczyca, D. P., DeBruhl, N. D., Mund, D. F., and Bassett, L. W. 1994. Linguine sign at MR imaging: Does it represent the collapsed silicone implant shell? *Radiology* 191: 576–577.
19. Gorczyca, D. P., Gorczyca, S. M., and Gorczyca, K. 2007. The diagnosis of silicone breast implant rupture. *Plast Reconstr Surg* 120(Suppl. 1):49S–61S.
20. Handel, N., Cordray, T., Gutierrez, J., and Jensen J. A. 2006. A long-term study of outcomes, complications, and patient satisfaction with breast implants. *Plast Reconstr Surg* 117: 757–767.
21. Harris, K. M., Ganott, M. A., Shestak, K. C., Losken, H. W., and Tobon, H. 1993. Silicone implant rupture: Detection with US. *Radiology* 187: 761–768.
22. Henriksen, T. F., Fryzek, J. P., Hölmich, L. R. et al. 2005. Surgical intervention and capsular contracture after breast augmentation: A prospective study of risk factors. *Ann Plast Surg* 54: 343–351.
23. Hölmich, L. R., Fryzek, J. P., Kjøller, K. et al. 2005. The diagnosis of silicone breast-implant rupture: Clinical findings compared with findings at magnetic resonance imaging. *Ann Plast Surg* 54: 583–589.
24. Hölmich, L. R., Vejborg, I. M., Conrad, C., Sletting, S., and McLaughlin, J. K. 2005. The diagnosis of breast implant rupture: MRI findings compared with findings at explantation. *Eur J Radiol* 53: 213–225.
25. Hvilsom, G. B., Holmich, L. R., Henriksen, T. F., Lipworth, L., McLaughlin, J. K., and Friis, S. 2009. Local complications after cosmetic breast augmentation: Results from the Danish Registry for Plastic Surgery of the breast. *Plast Reconstr Surg* 124: 919–925.
26. Juanpere, S., Perez, E., Huc, O., Motos, N., Pont, J., and Pedraza, S. 2011. Imaging of breast implants—A pictorial review. *Insights Imaging* 2: 653–670.
27. Kaiser, W. A. 2007. *Signs in MR-Mammography*. Springer, Berlin, Heidelberg.
28. Kim, B., Roth, C., Young, V. L. et al. 2011. Anaplastic large cell lymphoma and breast implants. *Plast Reconstr Surg* 128: 629–639.
29. Lazzeri, D., Zhang, Y. X., Huemer, G. M., Larcher, L., and Agostini, T. 2012. Capsular contracture as a further presenting symptom of implant-related anaplastic large cell lymphoma. *Am J Surg Pathol* 36: 1735–1736.

30. Levine, R. A. and Collins, T. L. 1991. Definitive diagnosis of breast implant rupture by ultrasonography. *Plast Reconstr Surg* 87: 1126–1128.
31. Middleton, M. S. 1998. Magnetic resonance evaluation of breast implants and soft-tissue silicone. *Top Magn Reson Imaging* 9: 92–137.
32. Middleton, M. S. and McNamara, M. P. 2003. *Breast Implant Imaging*. Philadelphia, PA: Lippincott Williams & Wilkins.
33. O'Toole, M. and Caskey, C. I. 2000. Imaging spectrum of breast implant complications: Mammography, ultrasound, and magnetic resonance imaging. *Semin Ultrasound CT MR* 21: 351–361.
34. Palmon, L. U., Foshager, M. C., Parantainen, H., Everson, L. I., and Cunningham, B. 1997. Ruptured or intact: What can linear echoes within silicone breast implants tell us? *AJR Am J Roentgenol* 168: 1595–1598.
35. Reynolds, H. E. 1995. Evaluation of the augmented breast. *Radiol Clin North Am* 33: 1131–1145.
36. Rosculet, K. A., Ikeda, D. M., Forrest, M. E. et al. 1992. Ruptured gel-filled silicone breast implants: Sonographic findings in 19 cases. *AJR Am J Roentgenol* 159: 711–716.
37. Sardanelli, F., Boetes, C., Borisch, B. et al. 2010. Magnetic resonance imaging of the breast: Recommendations from the EUSOMA working group. *Eur J Cancer* 46: 1296–1316.
38. Sardanelli, F., Giuseppetti, G. M., Panizza, P. et al. 2004. Sensitivity of MRI versus mammography for detecting foci of multifocal, multicentric breast cancer in fatty and dense breasts using the whole-breast pathologic examination as a gold standard. *AJR Am J Roentgenol* 183: 1149–1157.
39. Scaranelo, A. M. and de Fatima Ribeiro Maia, M. 2006. Sonographic and mammographic findings of breast liquid silicone injection. *J Clin Ultrasound* 34: 273–277.
40. Scaranelo, A. M., Marques, A. F., Smialowski, E. B., and Lederman, H. M. 2004. Evaluation of the rupture of silicone breast implants by mammography, ultrasonography and magnetic resonance imaging in asymptomatic patients: Correlation with surgical findings. *Sao Paulo Med J* 122: 41–47.
41. Schneider, E. and Chan, T. W. 1993. Selective MR imaging of silicone with the three-point Dixon technique. *Radiology* 187: 89–93.
42. Smith, T. J. and Ramsaroop, R. 2012. Breast implant related anaplastic large cell lymphoma presenting as late onset peri-implant effusion. *Breast* 21: 102–104.
43. Soo, M. S., Kornguth, P. J., Walsh, R., Elenberger, C. D., and Georgiade, G. S. 1996. Complex radial folds versus subtle signs of intracapsular rupture of breast implants: MR findings with surgical correlation. *AJR Am J Roentgenol* 166: 1421–1427.
44. Taylor, C. R., Siddiqi, I. N., and Brody, G. S. 2013. Anaplastic large cell lymphoma occurring in association with breast implants: Review of pathologic and immunohistochemical features in 103 cases. *Appl Immunohistochem Mol Morphol* 21: 13–20.
45. Thompson, P. A. and Prince, H. M. 2013. Breast implant-associated anaplastic large cell lymphoma: A systematic review of the literature and mini-meta analysis. *Curr Hematol Malig Rep* 8: 196–210.
46. Van Goethem, M., Schelfout, K., Dijckmans, L. et al. 2004. MR mammography in the pre-operative staging of breast cancer in patients with dense breast tissue: Comparison with mammography and ultrasound. *Eur Radiol* 14: 809–816.
47. Venkataraman, S., Hines, N., and Slanetz, P. J. 2011. Challenges in mammography: Part 2, multimodality review of breast augmentation—Imaging findings and complications. *AJR Am J Roentgenol* 197: 1031–1045.
48. Venta, L. A., Salomon, C. G., Flisak, M. E., Venta, E. R., Izquierdo, R., and Angelats, J. 1996. Sonographic signs of breast implant rupture. *AJR Am J Roentgenol* 166: 1413–1419.
49. Warner, E., Plewes, D. B., Shumak, R. S. et al. 2001. Comparison of breast magnetic resonance imaging, mammography, and ultrasound for surveillance of women at high risk for hereditary breast cancer. *J Clin Oncol* 19: 3524–3531.
50. Yang, N. and Muradali, D. 2011. The augmented breast: A pictorial review of the abnormal and unusual. *AJR Am J Roentgenol* 196: 451–460.
51. Yasuo, A., Ritsu, A., Shinichiro, K., and Kumazaki, T. 2007. Silicone-selective multishot echo-planar imaging for rapid MRI survey of breast implants. *Eur Radiol* 17: 1875–1878.

27 Lymphatic Imaging of the Breast
Evolving Technologies and the Future

Jaume Masia, Gemma Pons, Maria Luisa Nardulli, Juan Angel Clavero, Xavier Alomar, and Joan Duch

CONTENTS

27.1 INTRODUCTION

Breast cancer is the most frequent malignant cancer in women, its incidence is raising up to 1%–2% every year, and the estimated risk of breast cancer in women is approximately one every eight women.[1]

Despite these fearsome data, the preventive measurements adopted and the early detection and treatment are decreasing cancer-associated mortality. But on the other hand, as a consequence of the increased survival of these patients, there is an augmentation of morbidities associated with breast cancer. Several studies on the quality of life demonstrate that the most disabling sequela after breast cancer is the lymphoedema and not the amastia or breast asymmetry. This is due to the fact that the functional limitation, the aesthetic defect, and the risk of serious infections caused by the lymphoedema face the patients to deal with serious problems after breast cancer.[2,3]

Halsted[4] first described chronic oedema of the upper limb following mastectomy for breast cancer. Since then, lymphoedema has become a well-known post-operative side effect in breast cancer.

According to the International Society of Lymphedema (ISL),[5] lymphoedema is the result of accumulation of fluid and other elements (e.g. protein) in the tissue spaces due to an imbalance between interstitial fluid production and transport (usually low output failure).

Two main types of lymphoedema are recognised: primary, in which the cause is unknown but often presumed to be due to congenital lymphatic dysplasia, and secondary, in which there is an apparent underlying cause such as inflammation, malignancy, or surgery. However, even though the literature often categorises lymphoedema as primary or secondary, the division can be a bit artificial. In fact, we are becoming more and more conscious that genetic variations can explain the anatomical susceptibility of some individuals to the development of lymphoedema, even if the exact cause is unknown.[6] According to the classification earlier, breast-cancer-related lymphoedema (BCRL) is a common type of secondary lymphoedema that leads to pain, recurrent infections, disability, and an overall reduced quality of life.

Nowadays, post-mastectomy lymphoedema affects an estimated 6%–30% of survivors.[7] It is reported that 20%–30% of patients with breast cancer undergone axillary lymphadenectomy developed superior ipsilateral limb lymphoedema.[8] This rate seems to increase (35%–40%) if radiotherapy is associated. But it is interesting to point out that also if more conservative procedures, such as the sentinel lymph node (LN) biopsy (SLNB), are performed, the reported rate of lymphoedema in these patients varies from 4%–10% to 3%–22%.[9,10] In contrast, a recent study[7] has demonstrated the benefit of immediate breast reconstruction in diminishing the incidence and delaying the onset of BCRL, compared to patients who had undergone mastectomy without reconstruction, with or without axillary RT, and axillary dissection. Both autologous tissue and impalant-based immediate breast reconstruction have a positive effect to prevent lymphoedema. It is known that vascularised tissue has the potential to restore lymphatic flow by promoting angiogenesis and lymphatic regeneration, but on the other hand, there is also the evidence that the process of tissue expansion and capsule formation reduces the incidence of lymphoedema due to the increased expression of vascular endothelial growth factor (VEGF).[11]

For a long time, lymphoedema has been considered an incurable pathology and as a consequence has been undervalued. Complex physical therapy (CPT) has been the treatment of choice for lymphoedema during many years. Only in refractory cases not responding to CPT, surgical palliative procedures as excision or liposuction had been undertaken. The aim of these techniques is to reduce the subcutaneous tissue in order to limit the excess bulk and weight of the affected limb. Among these techniques, the Charles procedure,[12] which consists of the excision of all the subcutaneous tissue and posterior grafting over the muscular fascia of the affected limb, has been popular during many years. This aggressive technique has been only indicated in cases of extreme functional limitation because of the poor aesthetic and functional result. An evolution of this technique is the vibroliposuction based on the Håkan Brorson technique.[13,14] This surgical procedure allows the reduction of hypertrophic adipose tissue in organised non-pitting lymphoedema and it is considered a valuable surgical option in selected cases.

Although lymphatic system is known since the early years, its particular anatomical characteristics have made very difficult the study and knowledge of the physiopathology of this vascular system. The high anatomical variability (about number and location of lymph vessels and nodes) between the different individuals and the small calibre (0.2–0.6 mm diameter) and high fragility of the lymph vessels have made almost impossible to work with these ultra-fine lymph structures during many years.

Nevertheless, nowadays, thanks to the improvement of microsurgical dissection techniques, the development of ultra-fine microsurgical instruments and high-magnification microscopes, and the evolution of imaging techniques, the possibility of reconstructing the lymphatic system has become a reality. By means of microlymphatic surgery (supermicrosurgery[15]), in well-selected cases, the lymphatic system can be restored and regenerated.

Several reconstructive techniques have been described during the last decades and all of them aim to restore a normal lymphatic flow. These surgical procedures include: lymphaticovenular end-to-end or end-to-side anastomosis (LVA),[16] microsurgical multiple lymphaticovenular anastomoses (LVAs) by introducing lymphatics together into the vein by a U-shaped stitch,[17] microsurgical lymphatic grafting,[18] or microsurgical LN transfer techniques.[19] According to the respective authors, microsurgical techniques described up to now lead to good results. However, the long-term outcomes are not clear.

As there is no consensus on the most effective surgical procedure nor on the right surgical indication between the experts,[20] with the aim of looking for the ideal treatment, we finally decided to assess the potential of combining microsurgical autologous LN transplantation (ALNT) and LVA, which offered more reliable reproducibility and minimised the donor site sequelae with respect to other techniques described till now. We used the LVA and ALNT, with the necessary modifications with respect to the original ones, combined one with each other whenever possible and we loved to name this cocktail of techniques *Barcelona Cocktail* or *Combined Surgical Treatment* for breast-cancer-related lymphoedema (*Combined Surgical Treatment for Breast Cancer related Lymphedema, Journal of Reconstructive Microsurgery,* article accepted for publication).

It must be stressed that the development of these ultra-refined surgical techniques was possible partly thanks to the development and improvement of equally sophisticated imaging techniques, which allow to study the lymphatic system from both a morphological and functional point of view and contribute to the proper planning of surgery.

Now, we will focus a little more on the techniques we currently use.

27.1.1 Surgical Technique

27.1.1.1 Microsurgical Autologous Lymph Node Transplantation

The concept is based on replacing the axillary LNs, which have been surgically resected or damaged by adjuvant radiotherapy, for a lympho-adipo-cutaneous flap that contains 3–6 nodes (Figure 27.1a and b). ALNT combines high microsurgical expertise with current advances in the research on lymphangiogenesis. As LNs produce VEGF-C, which is considered the main promoter of lymphangiogenesis, lymphatic connections are expected to form spontaneously within the approximately 6-month period.[21]

C. Becker[19] was the first to popularise an inguinal fatty flap containing LNs for arm lymphoedema treatment. Although multiple LNs flaps from different locations as submental, cervical/supraclavicular, contralateral toracodorsal axis, or axillary donor sites have been recently described, an evolution of C. Becker's flap based on LNs vascularised from superficial inferior epigastric or superficial circumflex iliac vessels is the most widely used (Figure 27.2a through c). We consider this flap the best option, not only for the best aesthetic result achieved but also because as superficial inferior epigastric nodes are responsible for lower abdominal lymphatic drainage, no donor site/inferior limb

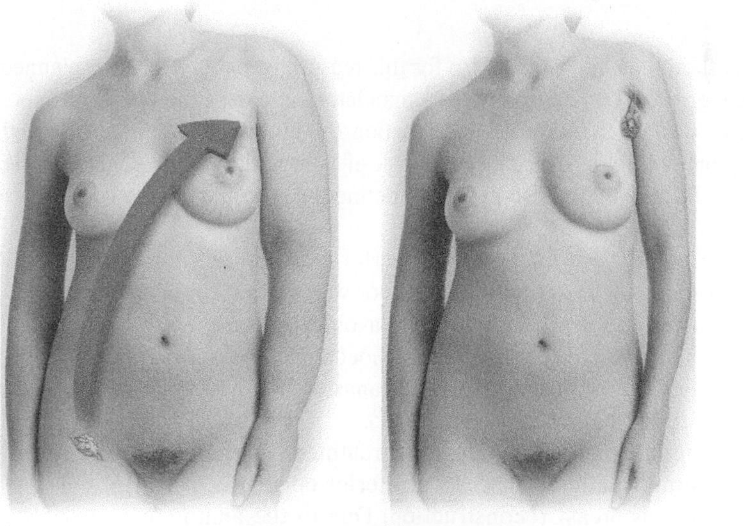

(a) (b)

FIGURE 27.1 (a and b) The concept of ALNT is based on replacing the axillary LNs that have been surgically resected or damaged by adjuvant radiotherapy, for a lympho-adipo-cutaneous flap that contains 3–6 nodes.

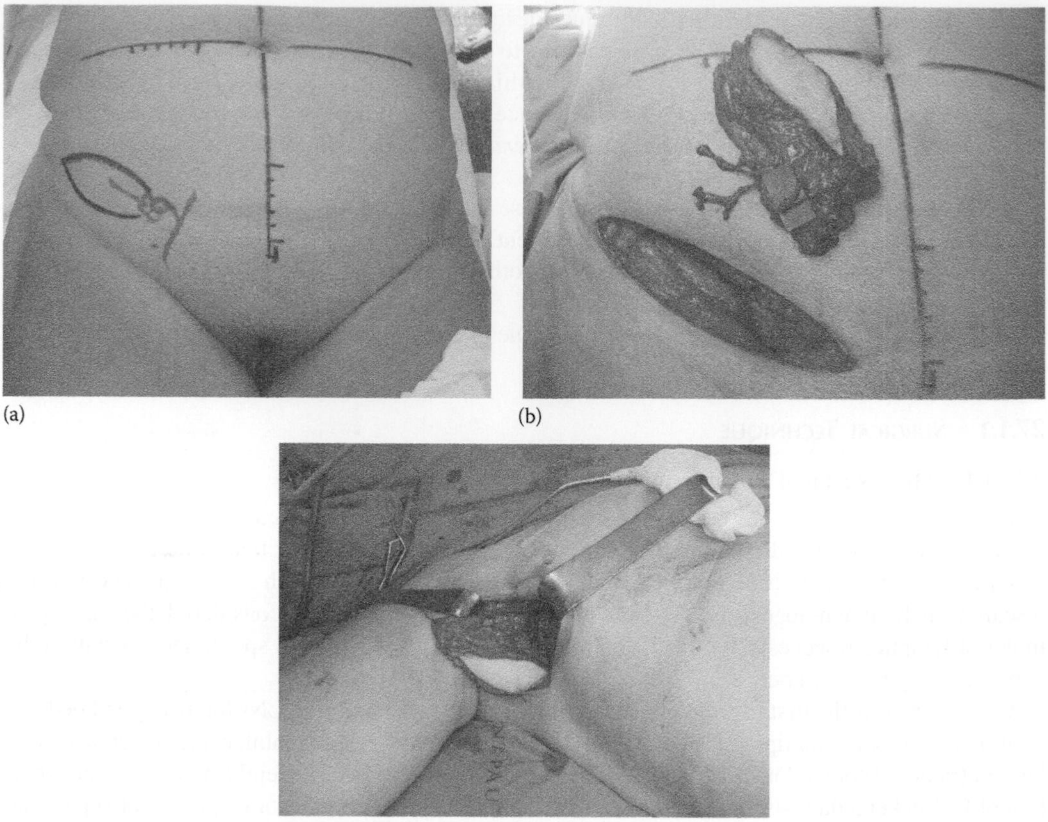

(a) (b) (c)

FIGURE 27.2 Preoperative drawing of (a) the LN flap containing the superficial inferior epigastric nodes, (b) the LN flap with its superficial circumflex iliac pedicle and the superficial inferior epigastric vein, and (c) the anastomosis with the thoracodorsal vessels in axilla.

lymphoedema should be induced.[22] Also for this reason, when an ALNT is planned, in our practice, computed tomography (CT) angiography is mandatory to assess the prevalent superficial circumflex iliac system, as well as the number and location of superficial inguinal LNs and the relationship with the deep ones, in order to reduce the risk of iatrogenic lymphoedema of the donor site/limb. Multidetector CT angiograms also permit to define the size and course of the vessels which supply the harvesting LN[23] (Figure 27.3).

On the same basis, we intraoperatively perform an indirect lymphography after indocyanine green dye (ICG) injection into the II and IV foot web spaces, in order to localise LNs draining the inferior limb. This is of crucial importance to avoid harvesting a flap containing these LNs, which would induce an iatrogenic inferior limb lymphoedema.

At the recipient area, we normally perform anastomosis between the vessels of the flap and thoracodorsal system or its branches (Figure 27.2c).

We should emphasise that lymphoedema treatment and autologous breast reconstruction can be approached simultaneously. The deep inferior epigastric perforator (DIEP) flap is the first choice for autologous breast reconstruction. Due to the anatomical proximity, DIEP flap and inguinal LN transfer can be performed as a single flap (LN-DIEP flap) (Figure 27.4a and b), but LNs in these cases have their own vascularisation, independent from the abdominal flap.

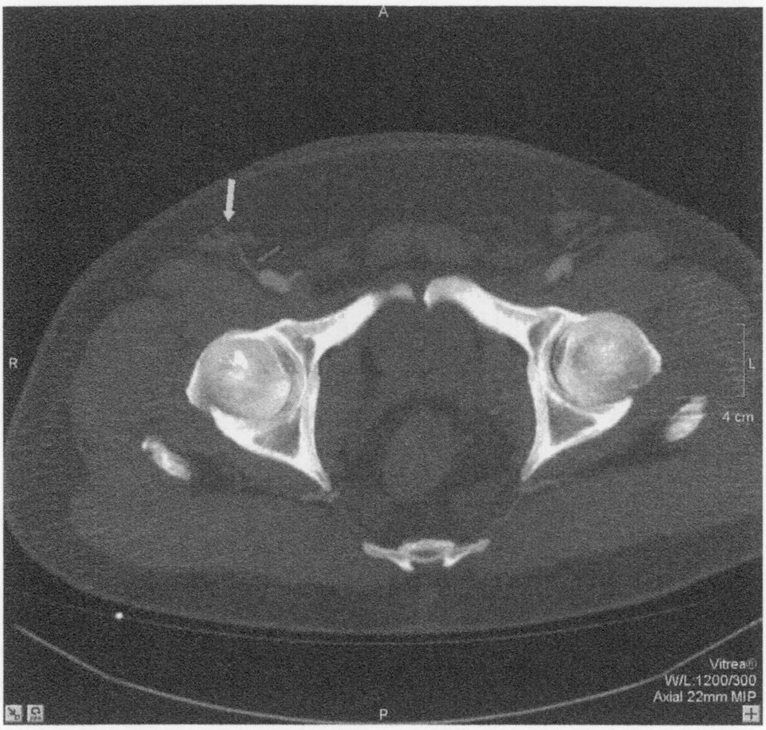

FIGURE 27.3 When an ALNT is planned, in our practice, CT angiography is mandatory to assess the prevalent superficial circumflex iliac system (small grey arrow), as number and location of superficial inguinal LNs (big white arrow) and the relationship with the deep ones, in order to reduce the risk of iatrogenic lymphoedema of the donor site/limb. Multidetector CT angiograms also permit to define the size and course of the vessels which supply the harvesting LN.[23]

Moreover, in certain cases of mastectomy with immediate reconstruction accompanied by a nodal dissection, with the purpose of a lymphoedema prophylactic surgery, LN transplantation would be accompanied by lymph–lymphatic anastomosis (total breast restoration anatomy: T-BAR) (Figure 27.4c).

27.1.1.2 Lymphaticovenular Anastomosis

This surgical technique is based on the supermicrosurgery concept.[15] That means it requires specific surgical instrumentation and an expertise in handling very small (less than 0.6 mm calibre) and fragile structures (lymph vessels and venules). The technique consists in small cutaneous incisions placed in the lymphoedematous limb in order to find functional lymphatic vessels, which are anastomosed to subdermal venules (Figure 27.5a through e). This procedure has the aim to redirect excess lymph fluid from the lymphoedematous limb into the venous system.[15,16] The main challenge of this surgery is the localisation of the functional lymph vessels and its posterior dissection and anastomosis. Because of these difficulties, diagnostic imaging techniques are essential to proceed to an individual preoperative assessment of the lymphatic system, in order to locate the functional lymphatic vessels. Intraoperatively, we also inject intradermally 0.1–0.2 mL of patent blue dye, which is a lymphotrophic dye, about 2 cm distally to the point where we have planned the cutaneous incision. This simple manoeuvre is very helpful to identify and dissect the lymphatic vessels.

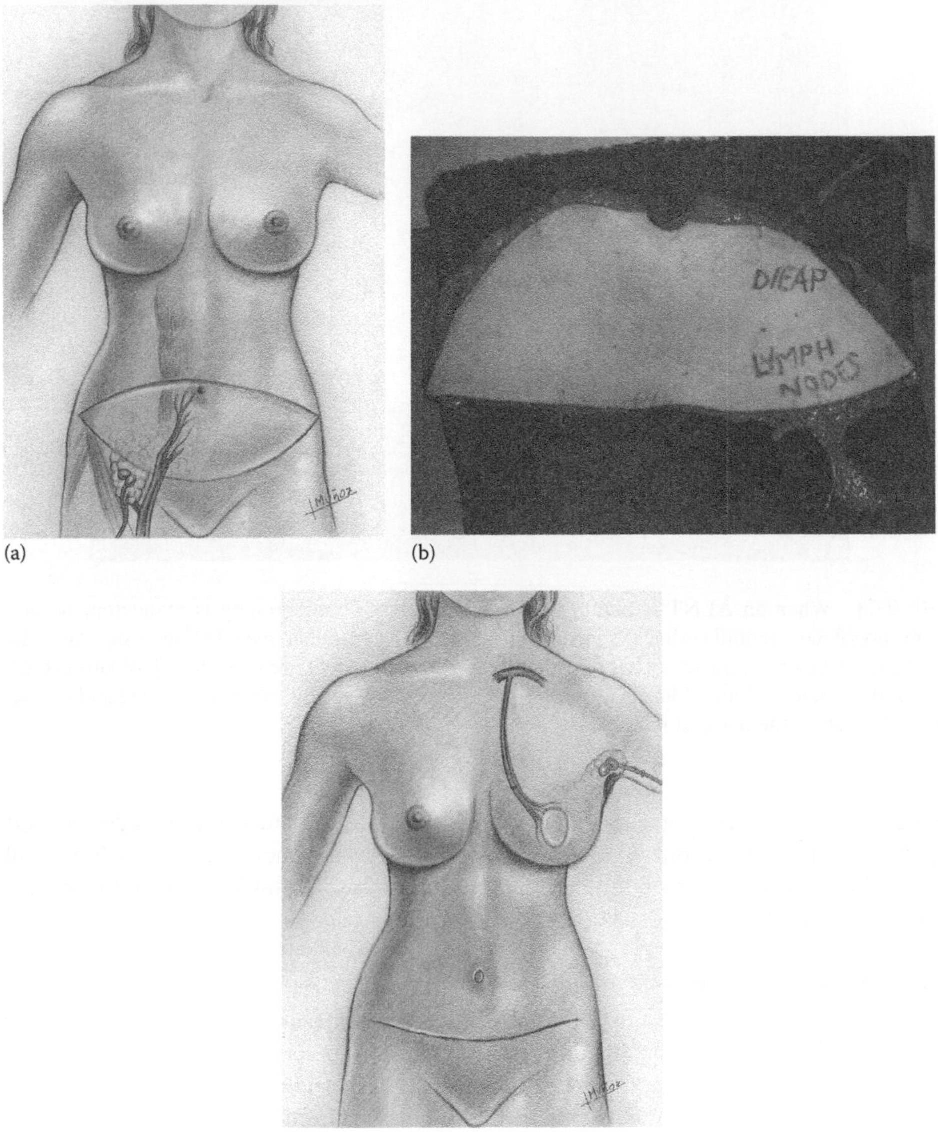

FIGURE 27.4 (a–c) Lymphoedema treatment and autologous breast reconstruction can be approached simultaneously. Due to the anatomical proximity, DIEP flap and inguinal LN transfer can be performed as a single flap (LN-DIEP flap) (a and b). T-BAR concept is performed when also a lymph–lymphatic anastomosis is carried out in axilla between lymphatics of the flap and those draining the superior limb.

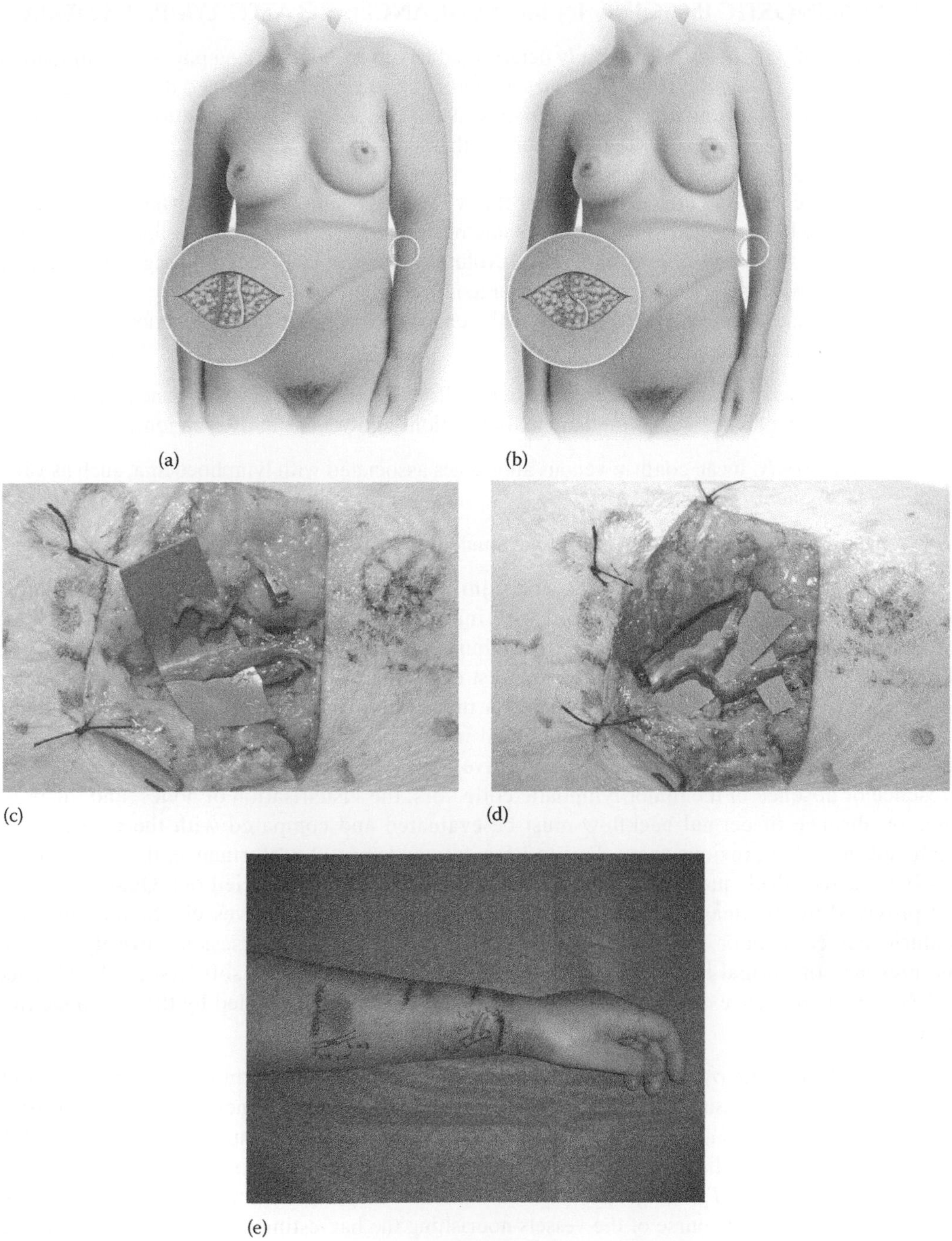

FIGURE 27.5 (a–e) LVA consists of performing small cutaneous incisions placed in the lymphoedematous limb in order to anastomose functional lymphatic vessels with subdermal venules, with the aim of redirecting excess lymph fluid from the lymphoedematous limb into the venous system.[15,16] Intraoperatively, we inject intradermally 0.1–0.2 mL of patent blue dye, which is a lymphotrophic dye, about 2 cm distally to the point where we have planned the cutaneous incision. This simple manoeuvre is very helpful to identify and dissect the lymphatic vessels.

27.2 DIAGNOSTIC IMAGING IN BREAST-CANCER-RELATED LYMPHOEDEMA

The diagnosis of lymphoedema is mainly determined by clinical history and physical examination. Nevertheless, diagnostic imaging techniques are essential to confirm suspected diagnosis, to study the morphological and functional characteristics of the lymphatic system, and to perform a right preoperative assessment in order to plan a correct therapeutic strategy.

The complexity of the morphological and functional features of the lymphatic system makes very difficult the study and understanding of this vascular system. Although different exploratory techniques have been applied along history, some of them have been abandoned for their potential adverse effects. Currently, the technological evolution has provided specific diagnostic imaging techniques that help us in the diagnosis and therapeutic strategy.

In order to make a differential diagnostic with venous pathologies that can contribute to oedema, two exams can be considered:

X-rays of bones. Radiographs of bones may identify limb-length discrepancies, bone abnormalities, and phleboliths in patients with lymphatic malformations and venous malformations.

Venous duplex study. It can confirm venous anomalies associated with lymphoedema, such as valve incompetence, aneurysm, and ectasia.[24]

Other specific diagnostic imaging exams to evaluate lymphatic system are:

Lymphoscintigraphy (*LS*). It is a simple and minimal invasive functional test for the evaluation of the lymphatic system. It is performed with injection of 37 MBq (1 mCi) of 99 mTc-labeled human serum albumin or 99 mTc-labeled sulphur colloid into the first and second webspace of the fingers. This technique still remains the test of choice to exclude or confirm lymphoedema as the cause of a chronic limb swelling. It is mainly useful for the evaluation of lymphatic function, but it also gives some morphological information about lymphatic system, although the latter is quite coarse and merely orientative. Anyway, the appearance time at axilla, the presence or absence of the major lymphatic collectors, the visualisation of nodes, and the presence or absence of dermal backflow must be evaluated and compared with the contralateral limb and/or with a previous exam. Due to LS safety and ease of performance, the exam can be easily repeated. Both qualitative and quantitative analyses can be carried out. Qualitative data are provided by the image of the radioactive tracer in the lymphatic vessels. Some lymphatic patterns can confirm or exclude the diagnosis of lymphoedema and assess its severity, such as the presence of dermal backflow (accumulation of radiotracer in the soft tissue), the absence of LNs, or the presence of abnormal LNs. Quantitative data are provided by the clearance rate of the tracer.

CT scan and magnetic resonance imaging (*MRI*). They permit to confirm the presence of a limb oedema and the soft tissue hypertrophy, to exclude underlying malignancy or causes of obstruction of the main venous axis. After a liposuction for late-stage limb lymphoedema, CT and MRI axial sections show the limb circumference reduction achieved with the surgery. Moreover, when an ALNT is planned, *CT angiography* permits to assess the prevalent superficial circumflex iliac system and the size and course of the vessels nourishing the harvesting LN, as well as the number and location of superficial inguinal LNs.[23]

High-resolution echography. Similar to CT and MRI, it permits to evaluate the suprafascial and subfascial thickness of oedematous tissue and can allow a periodic assessment of the response to the treatment with no morbidity for the patient.

Bioimpedance spectroscopy. It uses electric current to measure the degree of tissue fluid retention. As the volume of fluid in an upper limb increases, the impedance of electric flow decreases. This technique is useful in detecting early-stage lymphoedema.

Oil contrast lymphangiography. Oil-based contrast medium is injected directly into lymphatic vessels so that they can be viewed on radiographs. It is able to delineate precisely the courses of the lymphatic vessels. However, lymphangiography lost popularity because it can damage the lymphatic vessels and worsen lymphoedema. Its use is indicated in selected patients with chylous dysplasia and gravitational reflux disorders when it permits a clearer definition of the extension of the pathological alterations.[24]

ICG indirect lymphography and MR lymphangiography. We will detail these topics in the succeeding text.

Sometimes other kind of exams can be useful, such as:

Skin biopsy. It is indicated in cases of suspected sarcoma skin cancer or differential diagnosis of warty lesions.

Genetic tests. They are essential for the detection of specific hereditary syndromes (i.e. FOXC2 for lymphoedema-distichiasis syndrome and VEGF receptor 3 for Milroy disease).

27.2.1 Diagnostic and Assessment Approach of the Authors

Clinical evaluation is certainly the first step in our assessment algorithm. In all patients, we follow the *Protocol for Lymphedema Evaluation* (created from the members of *International Framework for Lymphedema Surgical Treatment*). After recording a detailed personal history and careful clinical exploration, we classify the lymphoedema as primary or secondary, and according to the *ISL*, we define a lymphoedema stage. In order to get objective data of the lymphoedema, we take photographic documentation and measurements of the affected and contralateral limb circumferences. In case the patient is accepted as a surgical candidate, circumferential measurements will be taken periodically at 3, 6, 12, 24, and 36 months post-operatively.

As we already pointed out, the anatomy and physiopathology of lymphatic system is very difficult to understand, but on the other hand, we need as much information as possible about the lymphatic system in order to clarify the mechanisms of the lymphoedema and to decide what therapeutic option we can offer to the patient.

For this reason diagnostic imaging techniques are considered indispensable tools to perform an adequate diagnostic and therapeutic strategy.

27.2.1.1 Preoperative Diagnostic Imaging Techniques

Systematically, the imaging techniques we perform are

- LS
- Magnetic resonance lymphography (MRL)
- ICG indirect lymphography
- CT angiography: in case LN transfer is planned

27.2.1.1.1 Lymphoscintigraphy

After the subcutaneous injection of a 37 MBq (1 mCi) of 99 mTc-labeled human serum albumin or 99 mTc-labeled sulphur colloid into the first and second webspace of the fingers of each hand using a 27G needle, we ask the patient to make a fist repetitively during a fixed period of time, in order to standardise the mobilisation. The images are obtained with the patient in a supine position, with a low-energy collimator with parallel holes, and using a 20% window centred on the photopeak of 99 mTc (140 keV).

During the first 40 min following the injection, dynamic images are taken, including the entire arm, the axilla, and the liver.

Then images are captured 60, 120 and 180 min after the injection and interpreted. Theoretically, the images can be evaluated in three different ways:

1. Visual (qualitative) interpretation
2. Semi-quantitative interpretation using the transport index
3. Quantitative interpretation through calculation of the liver fraction

1. Visual (qualitative) interpretation is the method most often used, as it is easy to perform; however, small differences between pre- and post-operative studies may be difficult to identify.
   It allows the visualisation and assessment of the following:
   a. Dermal backflow: It is an increased tracer activity in the dermis, probably as a consequence of lymphatic valve insufficiency, related to an increased pressure gradient and obstruction in the deeper lymphatic system. The inversion of lymph flow towards the superficial lymphatic network and the visualisation of tracer in the dermis are defined as dermal backflow.
   b. The extent and type of distribution of dermal backflow (no dermal backflow; small, localised, dermal backflow; circumferential dermal backflow involving one segment of the limb; circumferential dermal backflow involving more than one limb segment) bring important information about the extent and location of the lymphatic obstruction.
   c. Lymph vessels: Their features (normal, hypoplastic, absent, diffuse, dilatation of lymphatic vessels, existence of collateral lymphatic vessels) and position must be evaluated. Anyway, it must be stressed that, differently from its functional importance, the morphological information proved by LS is coarse and merely orientative.
   d. Lymph nodes (cubital, axillary, supra- and infraclavicular): We have to evaluate and describe aspects such as symmetrical bilateral LN visualisation, asymmetrical axillary LNs, other LN visible, any LN on the affected side visible only on the late images, and no LN visible on the affected side.
   e. Criteria for lymphatic dysfunction include delayed (>30 min), asymmetric, or absent visualisation of regional LNs and the presence of *dermal backflow*. Additional findings include asymmetric visualisation of lymphatic channels and collateral lymphatic channels. All of these parameters are correlated with a clinical diagnosis of lymphoedema (Figure 27.6a and b).
2. Semi-quantitative interpretation using the transport index, by Kleinhans et al.[25] In this index, five parameters (temporal and spatial distribution of the radionuclide, appearance time of LNs, and graded visualisation of LNs and vessels) are evaluated and scored from 0 to 9, where 0 means no abnormalities and 9 indicates that the condition for a given parameter could not be worse. The five scores are then added, resulting in the transport index, which can vary from 0 (normal) to 45 (most abnormal).
3. Quantitative interpretation through calculation of the liver fraction. LS is performed with focus on the liver uptake and the results would be useful once compared to post-operative ones. In the case of correct subcutaneous administration of the radioactive tracer, the liver can be visualised after some time through uptake via blood vessels. The radioactive tracer reaches the blood stream either via the thoracic duct or, in the case of a functioning lymphatic venous anastomosis, via this shunt.[26]

Preoperative limb LS is performed mainly to assess lymphatic function of the limb and to perform a good surgical planning. If the result of the image shows us functional deficiency because LNs are completely absent in the axillary region, we plan LN transfer to that anatomical area. In case the patient is affected by lymphoedema, but the LS show remaining LNs functioning at the axillary region, we plan to inset the LN flap at the cubital fossa.

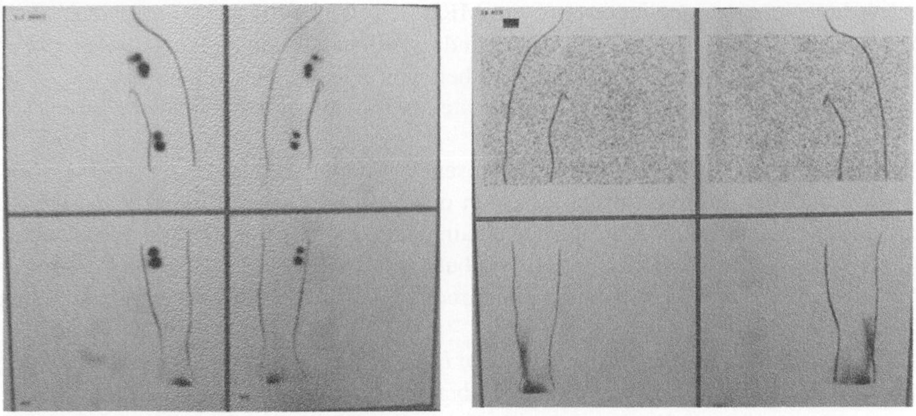

(a) (b)

FIGURE 27.6 (a and b) LS in a patient with right superior lymphoedema post-nodal dissection and radiotherapy. In the immediate images, the radiotracer migration is not observed in both limbs. In the left upper extremity (healthy), after 180 min, we can observe the presence of the radiotracer in the elbow and armpit LNs, indicating good lymphatic drainage (a). In the right upper extremity, the elbow nodal stations are not displayed, with a very mild presence of the tracer at the armpit; some lymphatic vessels are represented in the forearm (b). These findings indicate a significant impairment of the right arm lymphatic drainage.

Post-operatively, we perform a second LS 12 months after surgery in order to evaluate the grade of improvement in the lymphatic drainage and to assess transplanted LNs and LVA viability.

LS can demonstrate the effectiveness of vascularised LN transplantation because transplanted nodes can be visualised and new lymph drainage pathways can appear. LS qualitative method is also useful to verify the long-term patency of LVA after by direct findings like reduction of dermal backflow together with the appearance of preferential lymphatic pathways not visible before microsurgery or the disappearance of the tracer at the site of LVA due to direct tracer passage into the blood stream.

Occasionally, LS can be also indicated when there is a suspicion of donor site damage after LNs flap transfer. In these cases, LS can demonstrate diminished lymph transport at the donor site lower limb, comparing the images to the non-operated limb.[22]

27.2.1.1.2 Magnetic Resonance Lymphography

Since many years, the role of MRI to improve diagnosis of lymphoedema is well known.[27] Normally, fluid retention in fat tissue on T2-weighted or STIR imaging can indicate lymphoedema.[28]

The use of MRI in order to visualise lymphatic vessels (MRI lymphography: MRL) is considerably more recent. In the last few years, MRL has specially been described as a valid diagnostic method that provides valuable information about the main functional features of peripheric lymphatic system; that means that it permits to study and visualise lymphatic vessels and sometimes LNs and proceed to plan a therapeutic strategy. It has also been considered as a safe method because it is a minimally invasive and a radiation-free technique.[29–37]

MRL has been used by Lohrmann et al.[34] to evaluate lymphatic system in patients undergoing microsurgical reconstruction of lymphatic vessels. Their study evaluates post-operative improvements of epifascial oedema and other issues indirectly related to lymphatic drainage in patients who underwent lymphatic microsurgery.

Also, MRL performed without contrast medium[36,38] has been described as heavily T2-weighted sequences that permit the visualisation of static fluid signal in the fluid-containing structures such as lymphatic vessels, whereas solid tissues and flowing blood have no signal.

Besides these previous applications of the MRL described earlier, our main interest that has brought us to start using this exam is to get an individual map of the lymphatic system in order to analyse it and plan our surgery (LVA surgery) when indicated.

So routinely in our clinical practice, we indicate MRL in all our lymphoedema patients to

- Visualise oedema, so as to confirm the presence of lymphoedema
- Visualise and evaluate lymphatic vessels in order to have an overall idea of the lymphatic drainage of the limb; this allows also to obtain, indirectly, functional information about lymphatic system in the affected limb and contributes to select the most suitable surgical treatment
- Visualise and evaluate other findings indirectly related to abnormal lymphatic drainage, such as *dermal backflow*
- And finally for the *preoperative planning of LVA surgery*: According to the morphological, functional, and topographic information obtained from images, MRL permits to obtain a map with specific coordinates system that gives us information about the exact location of the lymphatic channels that are suitable for LVA. This is of extreme importance because, before the increasing diffusion of photodynamic eye (PDE) indirect lymphography of the last years, in most of the centres, LVA surgery has been carried out without definite criteria for the selection of the most appropriate LVA site (Figure 27.7a through c).

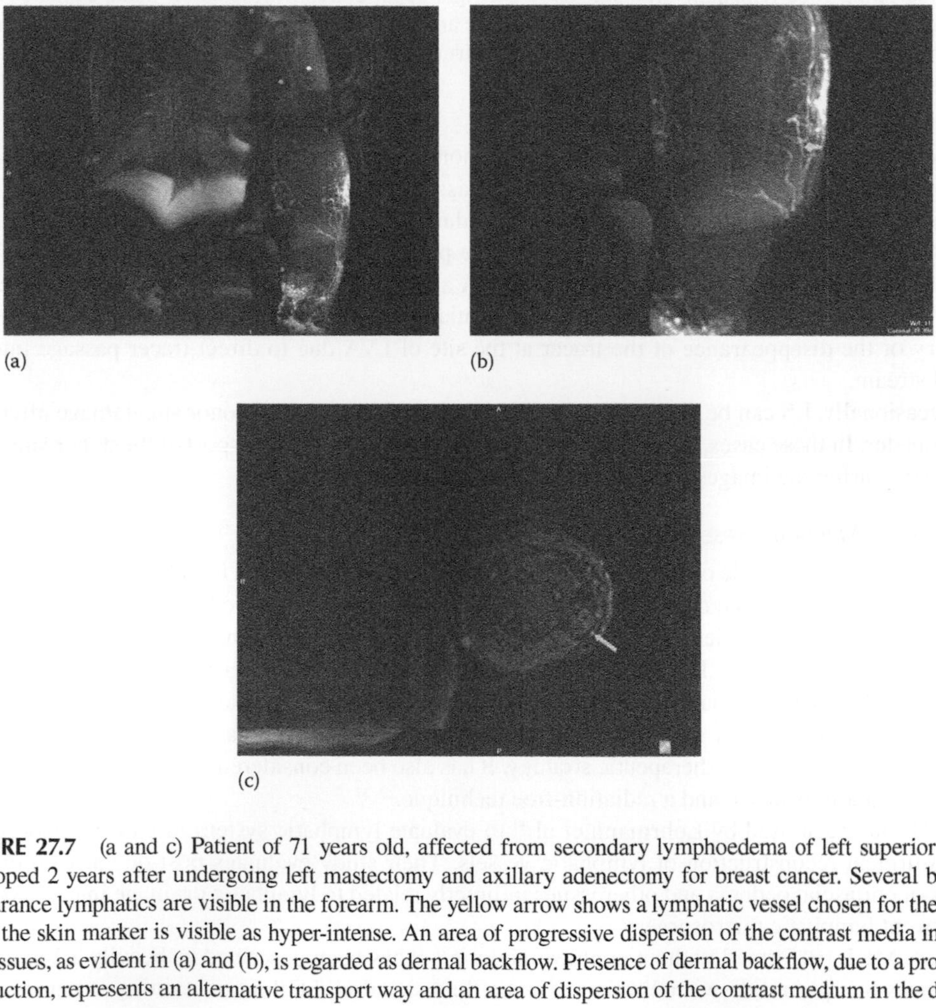

(a) (b) (c)

FIGURE 27.7 (a and c) Patient of 71 years old, affected from secondary lymphoedema of left superior limb, developed 2 years after undergoing left mastectomy and axillary adenectomy for breast cancer. Several beaded appearance lymphatics are visible in the forearm. The yellow arrow shows a lymphatic vessel chosen for the LVA. Also, the skin marker is visible as hyper-intense. An area of progressive dispersion of the contrast media into the soft tissues, as evident in (a) and (b), is regarded as dermal backflow. Presence of dermal backflow, due to a proximal obstruction, represents an alternative transport way and an area of dispersion of the contrast medium in the derma.

An ideal diagnostic imaging technique for preoperative planning of LVA should be able to allow a global evaluation of lymphoedematous limb and to localise lymphatic channels, in order to choose the most suitable ones for the anastomosis.

LS, although still represents the most common technique for pre- and post-operative lymphatic system evaluation, does not satisfy these requirements, because, while enabling the display of the main lymphatic trunks and LNs, it is characterised by a rather low resolution of images obtained, providing mostly functional information. Moreover, it is *time consuming* and requires exposure to ionising radiations.[39]

On the other hand, in the last years, a novel indirect lymphographic method based on fluorometric sensing using indocyanine green (ICG) dye has been described. An ICG fluorescence high-sensitivity near-infrared video camera system (PDE) enables non-invasive detection of the fluorescence of the dye (ICG) in the lymphatic channels. From 2007, we performed this preliminary lymphography on patients undergoing LVA. The fluorescence lymphography is almost non-invasive and can be performed easily. The method can be repeated in the same patient. Nevertheless, this technology enables only the visualization of superficial subdermal and subcutaneous lymphatic vessels, till a maximum deep of 1.5–2 cm in subcutaneous tissue, so that the detection of lymphatic vessels may be difficult in a fat subject or in a fat-rich region. Moreover, it allows the visualisation of a very limited area at one image (10 cm × 10 cm), while it is not able to provide a dynamic picture of the whole limb.

In contrast, MRL provides a number of distinct advantages over LS and the ICG lymphography. Its resolution is 30×–100× greater than LS, has excellent temporal resolution, and does not use ionising radiation. Unlike ICG lymphography, it allows to enhance both deep and superficial lymphatic vessels and to visualise the whole limb, so as to furnish a global evaluation of the lymphatic system.

Despite its many benefits, MRL is impractical to provide intraoperative guidance, as can be done with ICG lymphography using a near-infrared video camera system (PDE).

Our technique is based on T1-weighted sequences, obtained after intradermal injection of contrast medium, that permit a more clear visualisation of lymphatic vessels, allowing to get more information about their morphology and localisation. To get the right information, the medium contrast injection is crucial because we look not only for morphological and topographic information (lymphatic vessels size, appearance, localisation and depth in subcutaneous tissue, etc.) but also for functional data that we get when there is contrast medium uptake from the working lymphatics channels. This information is of paramount importance in our decisional treatment protocol, as the presence of functioning lymphatic vessels permits us to predict a satisfactory response to LVA surgery.

According to our protocol, MRL is performed approximately 1–4 weeks before surgery, as the following:

- *Skin markers*: With the aim of mapping the lymph channels and transferring the information obtained from MRL to the patient, we use a simple system that consists in placing hyper-intense markers on the skin surface at predetermined fixed points located along a reference line. In the upper limb, this line goes from acromion to the nail of the thumb, passing through the central point of the cubital fossa. Then, beginning from the central point of the cubital fossa (point 0), we place hyper-intense markers along the reference line every 10 cm, below the *point 0* for 30 cm (–10, –20, –30 cm), and above it for 10 cm (+10 cm) (Figure 27.8).
- *Contrast medium*: A mixture of gadobenate dimeglumine (MultiHance®, Bracco, Italy – 668 Da) (9 mL) and lidocaine (1 mL) is prepared. Using 24-gauge cannulae, 1 mL sample of this mixture is injected strictly intracutaneously in each interdigital space and at the base of radial aspect of thumb of the lymphoedematous limb.

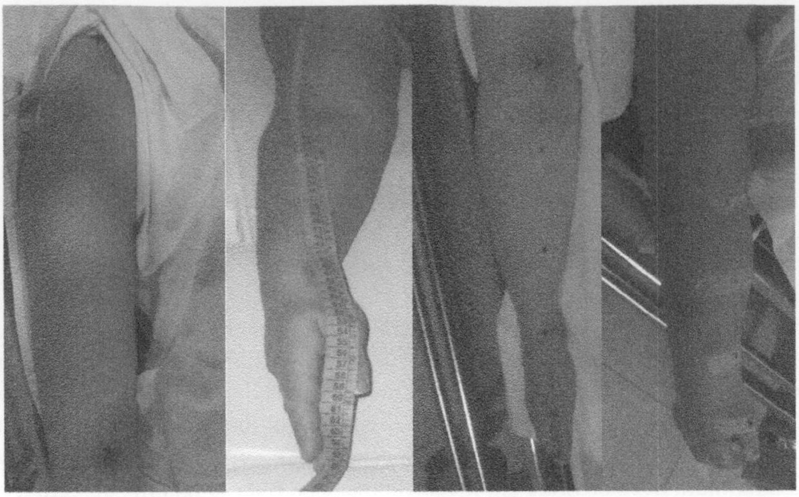

FIGURE 27.8 In order to localise the most suitable lymphatics for LVA and map them with respect to the skin, we collocate hyper-intense markers on skin surface, at predetermined fixed points, located along a reference line. In the upper limb, this line goes from acromion to the nail of the thumb, passing through the central point of the cubital fossa. Then, beginning from the central point of the cubital fossa (point 0), we place hyper-intense markers along the reference line every 10 cm, below the *point 0* for 30 cm (–10, –20, –30 cm), and above it for 10 cm (+10 cm).

- *MRI*: MRL is performed on a 3.0 T MR system (MAGNETOM VERIO, Siemens Medical Solutions) with a maximum gradient strength of 45 mT/m, a minimum rise time of 225 μs, and 32 receiver channels. For signal reception, we use 2 four channels upper extremity coils. MRL is performed using a coronal T1-weighted 3DGRE sequence (FLASH) with spectral-fat saturation and sequence parameters as follows: repetition time (TR) 5.65 ms, echo time (TE) 2.5 ms, flip angle (FA) 24, slices 192, slice thickness (SL) 1 mm, interslice gap 0.20 mm, bandwidth (BW) 390 Hz/pixel, field of view (FOV) 450 mm, matrix 302 × 384, in-plane resolution 1.3 × 1.3 mm^2, and acquisition time (TA) 160 s. Parallel imaging using GRAPPA algorithm is applied at an acceleration factor of R = 2, with 24 reference lines and auto-matrix coil mode. Two locations are examined, the first from the carpal to the elbow and the second from the elbow to the axillary region. An axial STIR sequence (TR 3770 ms, TE 29 ms, inversion time [TI] 200 ms, FA 130°, SL 6 mm, in-plane resolution 1.6 × 1.3 mm^2, FOV 430 mm, GRAPPA, R = 2) is performed. The 3D MRI images are reconstructed from the postcontrast coronal images at each time point using a MIP technique. The examination time for one patient is approximately 1 h. As MRL is not as time critical as MRI, the high signal gain at 3.0 T can be used to increase spatial resolution. The voxel size obtained in our study is approximately ½ of the minimum voxel size achieved at 1.5 T (1 vs. 2 mm^3). Because of technical reasons, it is not possible to examine both upper limbs in the patients suffering from upper limb lymphoedema. We have never observed systemic complications during or after the examination. Some patiens have reported temporary local pain, increased oedema, or appearance of blisters in the site of contrast injection.
- *Data (image) interpretation*. Images analysis and interpretation are carried out by a constant team formed by two radiologists and two plastic surgeons. The use of MIP generated from the high-resolution isotropic 3D data sets facilitates the assessment of the images.
- Systematically, the team analyses the images obtained (software Vitrea®) and special attention is put to get the following information:
  - 3D assessment of the whole extremity
  - Enhancement of superficial lymphatics (*epifascial*)

- Enhancement of deep lymphatics (*subfascial*)
- Course of lymphatic vessels (*continuous or not*)
- Calibre of lymphatic vessels
- Depth of lymphatic channels in subcutaneous tissue
- Qualitative appearance of lymphatic vessels: *beaded appearance*, distended as *a column*, and tortuous
- Presence of contractile units (*lymphangions*), due to still patent valves
- Presence of *dermal backflow*, due to a proximal obstruction, which represents an alternative transport way and an area of dispersion of the contrast medium at the dermis
- Presence of *perforators* between the deep and superficial lymphatic system
- Enhancement of nodes

- In accordance to the literature, we have found that healthy lymphatic channels have a typically beaded appearance, undulating outer borders and changing calibre. In contrast, lymphatic vessels in oedematous limbs are often irregularly shaped, have irregular diameter, or are twisted.
- Anyway, as some superficial and deep lymphatic vessels can have a different appearance, that is, a smooth appearance and straight course,[31,33] it is not always easy to distinguish lymphatics from veins and this can lead to have some false positives in the information obtained.
- *Mapping of lymphatics.* After the analysis of MRL images, the surgeons select the most suitable lymphatics for LVA surgery. The lymphatics considered the best options to be anastomosed are those located more proximally, with a bigger calibre and beaded appearance.

Beginning with a 3D image and then passing at an axial projection, the radiologist is able to mark both the reference skin markers (Figure 27.9) and the reference central line. This line represents also the *Y*-axis in a system of Cartesian axes, where the *X*-axis is a virtual line, perpendicular to Y, passing through the point 0 (central point of cubital fossa). By using these axes, the radiologist is able to give us the exact *coordinates* of the chosen lymphatic, measuring their distance in mm from the point 0. Every point (so every lymphatic, marked with a pink arrow) located above the point 0 was considered positive (+) as regards the *Y*-axis and negative (–) if located below it. With respect to the

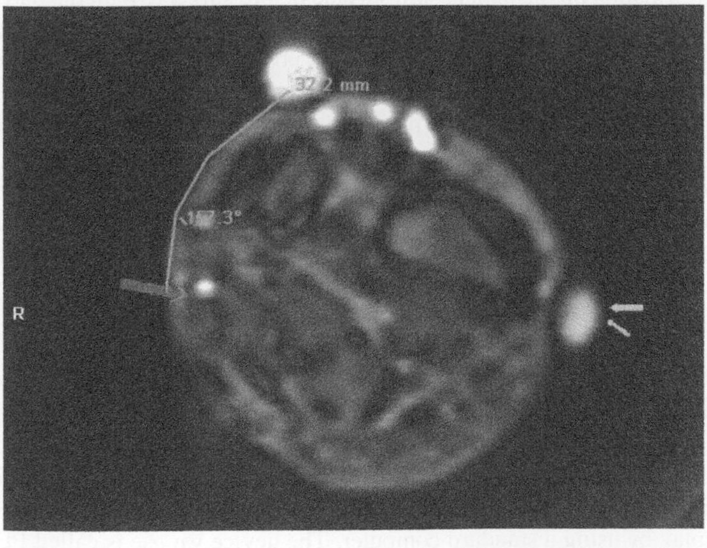

FIGURE 27.9 The couple of arrows on the right indicate a skin hyper-intense, while the arrow on the left indicates a lymphatic vessel marker.

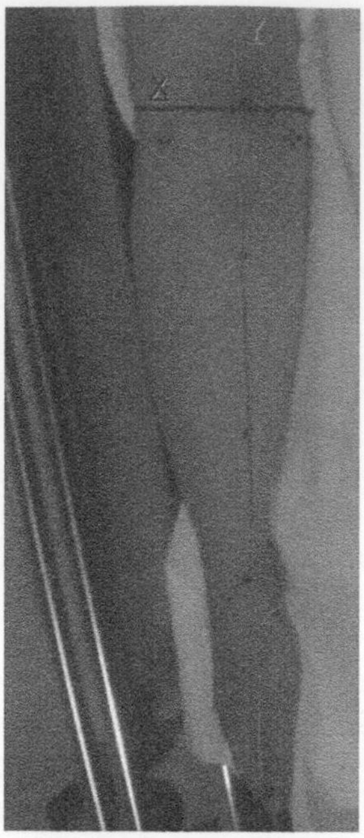

FIGURE 27.10 The reference central line represents the *Y*-axis in a system of Cartesian axes, where the *X*-axis is a virtual line, perpendicular to *Y*, passing through the point 0 (central point of cubital fossa). This system enables to obtain the exact *coordinates* of the chosen lymphatic, measuring their distance in millimetre from the point 0.

X-axis, every point is considered positive if located at the right side of *X*, with the limb patient visualised in a frontal view, and negative if it is located at the other side (Figure 27.10). In the axial view, it is also possible to measure the depth of the chosen lymphatic in the subcutaneous tissue (*Z*-axis).

Also, the calibre of lymphatics is measured, although this value is not exact because the contrast increases temporarily the calibre of the lymph vessel.

All these data are transcribed in a table and stored in a conventional CD, so the surgeon can transfer all the information on the patient skin surface before surgery. With the patient in the supine position and upper limbs at 90°, the surgeon marks the same reference line on the limb and, along it, the points corresponding to the hyper-intense markers position. By this way, after marking point 0, it is possible to transfer the coordinates data of every chosen lymphatic on the skin surface. All the dots marked on the skin will represent the precise points to perform the skin incision and look for the lymphatic and the vein in order to anastomose them.

The process of transferring the information obtained by the images to the cutaneous surface of the patient can be subject to human error; that means that the mark of the skin could not correspond with the real location of the lymph vessel. Nevertheless, these small discrepancies are completely compensated thanks to the fact that the area that we explore with the cutaneous incision correspond to 2–4 cm, which provides an ample margin to locate the lymph channel.

27.2.1.1.3 Indocyanine Green Dye Indirect Lymphography by Photodynamic Eye

This procedure consists in injecting ICG, subcutaneously at second and fourth or second and third webspace of the affected and contralateral limb, with a 27-G needle (0.1 mL of ICG for each injection) (Figure 27.11a). The uptake of ICG from the lymphatic channels permits to visualise them as fluorescent images collected by an infrared camera system. The fluorescent images are digitalised for real-time display by using a standard computer. The device we use is called PDE (Hamamatsu Photonics K.K., Hamamatsu, Japan), which has been also described for the non-invasive identification of sentinel LNs in sentinel node biopsy.[40]

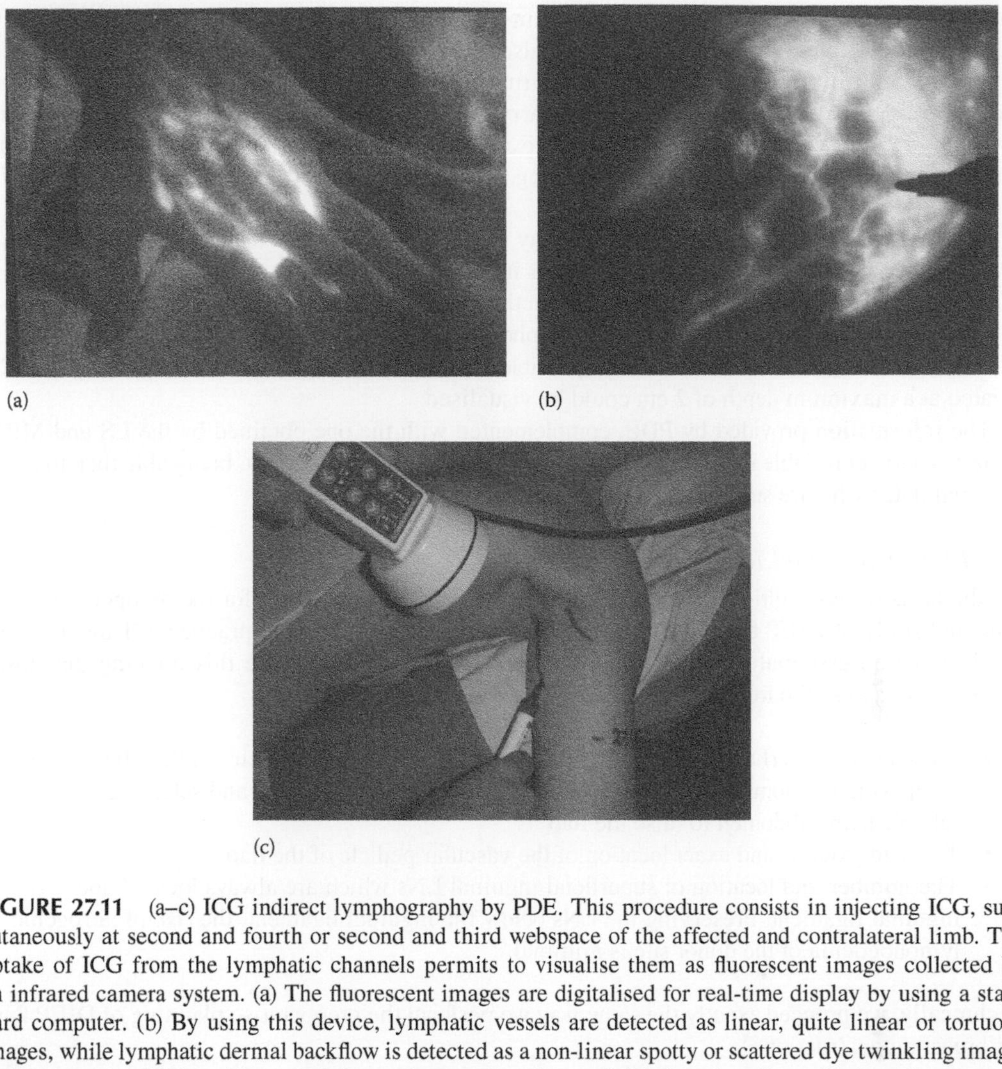

(a) (b) (c)

FIGURE 27.11 (a–c) ICG indirect lymphography by PDE. This procedure consists in injecting ICG, subcutaneously at second and fourth or second and third webspace of the affected and contralateral limb. The uptake of ICG from the lymphatic channels permits to visualise them as fluorescent images collected by an infrared camera system. (a) The fluorescent images are digitalised for real-time display by using a standard computer. (b) By using this device, lymphatic vessels are detected as linear, quite linear or tortuous images, while lymphatic dermal backflow is detected as a non-linear spotty or scattered dye twinkling image. (c) Preoperative PDE enables a real-time enhancement of superficial (less than 2 cm depth with respect to skin surface) and functional lymphatics, giving information about the morphological features and presence or absence of functional lymph channels with a patent lumen.

By using this device, lymphatic vessels are detected as linear, quite linear, or tortuous images, while lymphatic dermal backflow is detected as a non-linear spotty or scattered dye twinkling image (Figure 27.11b). Interestingly, the PDE fluorescent pattern has been used also to stage limb lymphoedema.[41] Preoperative PDE enables a real-time enhancement of superficial (less than 2 cm depth respect skin surface) and functional lymphatics, giving information about the morphological features and presence or absence of functional lymph channels with a patent lumen (Figure 27.11c). This information is crucial, because, similarly to what we already pointed out about MRL, it is very important to locate the functioning lymph vessels. The uptake of ICG in a lymphatic channel and its transport distally to proximally means that the channel is still working and maintains its contractile features. A patient with lymphatics functioning is a potential candidate to LVA surgery.

The exam is performed for the first time to select the patients who are candidates for surgery, it is repeated the immediate day before surgery, and finally, on the exact day of the surgery, the PDE lymphography is performed again without injecting more ICG dye. This last exam permits a real-time visualisation of the lymphatic system giving new information in case ICG dye had progressed along the hours. All the exams are recorded in a hard disk in order to have all the preoperative information collected. PDE lymphography is also of paramount importance for the correct planification of ALNT. In fact, it allows, most of the times, to visualise the LNs. So, just before, to begin the harvesting of an LN flap for ALNT, we carry out PDE lymphography after ICG injection into the II and IV foot webspaces, in order to localise LNs draining the inferior limb. This is of crucial importance to avoid harvesting a flap containing these LNs, which would induce an iatrogenic inferior limb lymphoedema.

Post-operatively, we use PDE lymphography to get an overall view of the lymphatic system to evaluate if modifications have been produced in relation to preoperative images. We also use it to assess LVA patency and to select new functional lymphatic channels in case secondary revision surgery is planned. Finally, the PDE lymphography can confirm the presence and viability of autotransplanted LNs. This is not always possible because of the limitations of PDE; only the LNs located at a maximum depth of 2 cm could be visualised.

The information provided by PDE, complemented with the one obtained by the LS and MRL, permits us to get reliable information about the patient's lymphatic system, being able then to select the candidates who are suitable to perform surgical treatment.

27.2.1.1.4 Computed Tomography Angiography

On the basis of our multi-year experience in the use of CT angiography for the preoperative planning and study of DIEP flap[23] and other perforator flaps, in our clinical practice, CT angiography has become an essential tool to plan also ALNT (Figure 27.3). We use this imaging diagnostic technique to assess the following:

- Presence of superficial inferior epigastric system/superficial iliac circumflex iliac system comparing the dominancy of one side with respect to the other one and selecting the most reliable hemi-abdomen to raise the flap
- The size, course, and exact location of the vascular pedicle of the flap
- The number and location of superficial inguinal LNs which are always located above the inguinal ligament. Preserving the LNs below the inguinal ligament, the risk of iatrogenic lymphoedema of the donor site is minimal.

Technically, we proceed exactly the same way we perform the preoperative planning of DIEP flaps for breast reconstruction.[23]

27.3 CONCLUSIONS

Summarising, we can state that

LS plays an important role in lymphoedema diagnosis and assessment. It represents the gold standard to detect the viability of the nodes and the donor site impairment after nodes harvesting. However, it has significant drawbacks, that is, it is an expensive and time-consuming procedure and involves the use of a radioisotope as tracer. Furthermore, the rather low resolution of images obtained makes it not useful to determine the exact localisation of lymphatics in LVA planning.

MRL provides a number of distinct advantages over LS, that is, the higher resolution of the images obtained and the lack of exposure to ionising radiation, while similar to LS, gives also functional information about lymphatic system.

Unlike ICG lymphography, it allows to enhance both deep and superficial lymphatic vessels and to visualise the whole limb, as to furnish a global evaluation of the lymphatic system. Furthermore, MR images can easily be obtained in 3D providing robust visualisation of the lymph flow.

As it enables the preoperative mapping of lymphatic vessels through a system of coordinates, MRL is extremely useful to plan LVA, reducing significantly the false positives when combined with

ICG lymphography. Anyway, differently to the latter, MRL is impractical to provide intraoperative guidance.

ICG lymphography with PDE system is a simple technique, easily repeatable, and is an almost complication-free procedure. Moreover, it is performed by a portable device and can be carried out pre- and intraoperatively to identify lymphatic vessels. Anyway, unlike MRL, it enables only the identification of the superficial lymphatic network, till a maximum depth of 1.5–2 cm in subcutaneous tissue, so that the detection of lymphatic vessels may be difficult in a fat subject or in a fat-rich region. Moreover, it allows the visualisation of a very limited area at one image (10 cm × 10 cm), while it is not able to provide a dynamic picture of the whole limb.

As each of these imaging procedures plays an important role in lymphoedema diagnosis and assessment but also involves drawbacks and limits, none represents the ideal one. However, when combined together, these techniques allow an appropriate pre- and post-operative assessment of patients suffering from lymphoedema and enable in vivo to gain a deeper insight into a system that until not so long ago is almost unknown.

REFERENCES

1. Ferlay J, Shin HR, Bray F et al. 2010. Estimates of worldwide burden of cancer in 2008: GLOBOCAN 2008. *Int J Cancer* 127(12):2893–2917.
2. Crosby M, Card A, Liu J et al. 2012. Immediate breast reconstruction and lymphedema incidence. *Plast Reconstr Surg* 129(5):789–795.
3. Chachaj A, Malyszczak K, Pyszel K et al. 2010. Physical and psychological impairments of women with upper limb lymphedema following breast cancer treatment. *Psychooncology* 19:299–305.
4. Halsted WS. 1921. The swelling of the arm after operation for cancer of the breast—Elephantiasis chirurgica: Its causes and prevention. *Bull Johns Hopkins Hosp* 32:309.
5. International Society of Lymphology. 2003. The diagnosis and treatment of peripheral lymphedema. Consensus document of the International Society of Lymphology. *Lymphology* 36(2):84–91.
6. Hurlbert M, Hutchison, NA, McGarve CL et al. Avon Foundation for Women White Paper. 2011. Recent advances in breast cancer-related lymphedema detection and treatment, Lymphedema Research Foundation, http://www.avonfoundation.org/assets/le-meeting/le-white-paper.pdf.
7. Card A, Crosby MA, Liu J et al. 2012. Reduced incidence of breast cancer-related lymphedema following mastectomy and breast reconstruction versus mastectomy alone. *Plast Reconstr Surg* 130(6):1169–1178. doi:10.1097/PRS.0b013e31826d0faa.
8. Rockson SG. 2008. Secondary lymphedema: Is it a primary disease? *Lymphat Res Biol* 6(2):63–64.
9. Armer J, Fu MR, Wainstock JM et al. 2004. Lymphedema following breast cancer treatment, including sentinel lymph node biopsy. *Lymphology* 37:73–91.
10. Ashikaga T, Krag DN, Land SR et al. 2010. National Surgical Adjuvant Breast, Bowel Project. Morbidity results from the NSABP B-32 trial comparing sentinel lymph node dissection vs axillary dissection. *J Surg Oncol* 102(2):111–118. Abstract.
11. Lantieri LA, Martin-Garcia N, Wechsler J et al. 1998. Vascular endothelial growth factor expression in expanded tissue: A possible mechanism of angiogenesis in tissue expansion. *Plast Reconstr Surg* 101(2):392–398.
12. Charles RH. 1912. *Elephantiasis Scroti*. London, U.K.: Churchill.
13. Brorson H, Svensson H. 1998. Liposuction combined with controlled compression therapy reduces arm lymphedema more effectively then controlled compression therapy alone. *Plast Reconstr Surg* 102:1058–1067.
14. Brorson H. 2000. Liposuction gives complete reduction of chronic large arm lymphedema after breast cancer. *Acta Oncol* 39:407.
15. Koshima I, Inagawa K, Urushibara K et al. 2000. Supermicrosurgical lymphaticovenular anastomosis for the treatment of lymphedema in the upper extremities. *J Reconstr Microsurg* 16:437–442.
16. Koshima I, Nanba Y, Tsutsi T et al. 2004. Minimal invasive lymphaticovenular anastomosis under local anesthesia for leg lymphedema. *Ann Plast Surg* 53(3):261–266.
17. Campisi C, Boccardo F. 2002. Lymphedema and microsurgery. *Microsurgery* 22:74–80.
18. Baumeister R, Siuda S. 1990. Treatment of lymphedemas by microsurgical lymphatic grafting: What is proved? *Plast Reconstr Surg* 85(1):64–74.

19. Becker C, Assouad J, Riquet M, Hidden G. 2006. Postmastectomy lymphedema: Long-term results following microsurgical lymph node transplantation. *Ann Surg* 243:313–315.
20. Rausky J, Robert N, Binder JP et al. 2012. In search of an ideal surgical treatment for lymphedema. Report of 2nd European Conference on Supermicrosurgery (Barcelona—March 2012). *Ann Chir Plast Esthét* 57(6):594–599.
21. Lähteenvuo M, Honkonen K, Tervala T et al. 2011. Growth factor therapy after autologous lymph node transfer in lymphedema. *Circulation* 123(6):613–620.
22. Viitanen TP, Mäki MT, Seppänen MP et al. 2012. Donor site lymphatic function after microvascular lymph node transfer. *Plast Reconstr Surg* 130(6):1246–1253.
23. Masia J, Clavero JA, Larrañaga JR et al. 2006. Multidetector-row computed tomography in the planning of abdominal perforator flaps. *J Plast Reconstr Aesthet Surg* 59(6):594–599.
24. Bergan J, Bunke N. 2011. In *Lymphedema: A Concise Compendium of Theory and Practise*, Lee BB, Bergan J, Rockson SG (Eds.). Springer-Verlag, London, p. 7.
25. Kleinhans E, Baumeister RG, Hahn D et al. 1985. Evaluation of transport kinetics in lymphoscintigraphy: Follow-up study in patients with transplanted lymphatic vessels. *Eur J Nucl Med* 10(7–8):349–352.
26. Damstra RJ, Voesten HG, van Schelven WD et al. 2009. Lymphatic venous anastomosis (LVA) for treatment of secondary arm lymphedema. A prospective study of 11 LVA procedures in 10 patients with breast cancer related lymphedema and a critical review of the literature. *Breast Cancer Res Treat* 113:199–206.
27. Duewell S, Hagspiel KD, Zuber J et al. 1992. Swollen lower extremity: Role of MR imaging. *Radiology* 184: 227–231.
28. Mihara M, Hara H, Araki J et al. Indocyanine green (ICG) lymphography is superior to lymphoscintigraphy for diagnostic imaging of early lymphedema of the upper limbs. *PLoS One* 7(6):e38182. doi:10.1371/journal.pone.0038182.
29. Liu NF, Lu Q, Jiang ZH et al. 2009. Anatomic and functional evaluation of the lymphatics and lymph nodes in diagnosis of lymphatic circulation disorders with contrast magnetic resonance lymphangiography. *J Vasc Surg* 49:980–987.
30. Lohrmann C, Foeldi E, Langer M. 2006. Indirect magnetic resonance lymphangiography in patients with lymphedema: Preliminary results in humans. *Eur J Radiol* 59(3):401–406.
31. Lohrmann C, Foeldi E, Speck O, Langer M. 2006. High-resolution MR lymphangiography in patients with primary and secondary lymphedema. *AJR Am J Roentgenol* 187:556–561.
32. Lohrmann C. 2007. Magnetic resonance imaging of lymphatic vessels without image subtraction: A practicable imaging method for routine clinical practice? *J Comput Assist Tomogr* 31(2):303–308.
33. Lohrmann C, Foeldi E, Bartholoma JP et al. 2007. Interstitial MR lymphangiography. A diagnostic imaging method for the evaluation of patients with clinically advanced stages of lymphedema. *Acta Tropica* 104:8–15.
34. Lohrmann C, Felmerer G, Foeldi E et al. 2008. MR lymphangiography for the assessment of the lymphatic system in patients undergoing microsurgical reconstructions of lymphatic vessels. *Microvasc Res* 76(1):42–45.
35. Lohrmann C, Foeldi E, Langer M. 2009. MR imaging of the lymphatic system in patients with lipedema and lipo-lymphedema. *Microvasc Res* 77:335–339.
36. Liu NF, Wang C, Sun M. 2005. Noncontrast three-dimensional magnetic resonance imaging vs lymphoscintigraphy in the evaluation of lymph circulation disorders: A comparative study. *J Vasc Surg* 41:69–75.
37. Liu NF, Lu Q, Liu PA et al. 2010. Comparison of radionuclide lymphoscintigraphy and dynamic magnetic resonance lymphangiography for investigating extremity lymphoedema. *Br J Surg* 97:359–365.
38. Arrìve L, Azizi L, Lewin M et al. 2007. MR lymphography of abdominal an retroperitoneal lymphatic vessels. *Am J Roentgenol* 189(5):189.
39. Unno N, Inuzuka K, Suzuki M et al. 2007. Preliminary experience with a novel fluorescence lymphography using indocyanine green in patients with secondary lymphedema. *J Vasc Surg* 45:1016–1021.
40. Tagaya N, Yamazaki R, Nakagawa A et al. 2008. Intraoperative identification of sentinel lymph nodes by near-infrared fluorescence imaging in patients with breast cancer. *Am J Surg* 195(6):850–853.
41. Yamamoto T, Yamamoto N, Doi K et al. 2011. Indocyanine green-enhanced lymphography for upper extremity lymphedema: A novel severity staging system using dermal backflow patterns. *Plast Reconstr Surg* 128:941.

28 Breast Imaging for Aesthetic and Reconstructive Plastic Surgery

Jeremy Nickfarjam, Oren Tepper, and Nolan Karp

CONTENTS

28.1 BACKGROUND

Surgery of the breast was first described around 3000 BCE by ancient Egyptian physicians who extirpated tumours [1]. In the late nineteenth century, radical mastectomy became the standard of care for breast cancer after Halsted reported en bloc resection of the breast tumour, breast tissue, pectoralis muscles, and ipsilateral axillary contents [2]. As the field of breast oncology continued to evolve, less invasive techniques were employed including preservation of pectoralis muscle [3] and skin sparing mastectomy, which further improved the overall aesthetic result with preservation of the inframammary fold [4]. With greater concern for breast aesthetics and breast conservation therapy, plastic surgeons now play an integral role in breast reconstruction.

Aesthetic breast surgery dates back to the sixteenth century, when reduction mammoplasty procedures were first described [5]. Breast augmentation, however, did not become an essential component of aesthetic breast surgery until the 1960s. Despite hurdles created by concern for leakage, and an FDA moratorium for 14 years in the United States, breast augmentation with either saline or silicone breast implants is now commonly performed worldwide. According to the American Society of Plastic Surgeons, approximately 300,000 breast augmentations and 40,000 reduction mammoplasties are performed in the United States per year. The variety of different surgical techniques for breast reduction and augmentation is a testament to the great evolution that has occurred over the last 50 years. Consumer-driven demand for safer, more reliable, and less invasive techniques has led the plastic surgery community to further refine the field of breast surgery. As a result, various methods to aid in preoperative planning have been reported in our literature.

28.1.1 Early Breast Measurements

While surface measurements have always been possible on the breast, surgeons have made significant advancements in creating algorithms to guide surgical planning. For instance, the TEPID system, described by John Tebbetts, serves as a system for evaluating breast and uses quantitative tissue assessment with a systematic approach in selecting the proper breast implant given the tissue parameters present [6,7]. Another is the Biodynamics system devised by Allergan. It is a computerised system in which the surgeon enters a series of measurements and the software computes a best fit implant. However, this system relies on external sizers tried on by patients which can be variable in application and lacking complete objectivity.

Perhaps the most valuable preoperative measurement to obtain in breast surgery is breast volume. Prior to the advent of imaging techniques, surgeons relied only on imprecise methods to estimate breast volume. For instance, breast dimensions were first expressed with the advent of the bra, which included band size, bust circumference, and cup size. Although many surgeons have used these measurements in reporting data for insurance reimbursement, bra sizes have been found to correlate poorly with actual breast volume, especially with respect to quantifying breast hypertrophy [8,9]. Other methods focused mainly on surface measurement, such as that described by Smith et al. In a study of 55 female patients, distances from the axilla, lateral fold, sternal notch, bottom of the breast, and inframammary fold to the nipple were quantified. Using anthropometric formulas, one can geometrically derive breast volume based on the shape of a cone [10,11]. Another study used sternal-notch-to-nipple distance to predict weight of resection, with distance of 25.5–28 cm to have a predicted weight of 400–600 g and distance of 28.5 cm or greater to have a predicted weight of resection more than 600 g [12].

Other creative methods for direct measurements of the breast volume have been described [13], such as adjustable geometric cones called the Grossman–Roudner device [14]. However, this device is limited by its inability to assess breast volumes exceeding 425 cc or account for tissue lateral to the pectoral fold [15,16]. Water displacement techniques and mathematical equations have been used based on the Archimedes' principle of buoyancy. Tezel and Numanoglu described a homemade water displacement device that successfully measured breast volume using a simple intraoperative technique [17,18]. However, this technique is limited by patients who have both rib cage and breast asymmetry and does not appear to be practical for the average physician. Thermoplastic casts have also been described to assess breast volume and asymmetry [19], but similar to the other techniques described, it is felt to be cumbersome to perform, subject to user variability, and limited in the data generated by the method.

With the advent of CT, 3D reconstructions made volumetric measurements more accurate and easier to perform. Computed tomography (CT) has made it possible to register curved images using a rotating x-ray beam with detectors. Three-dimensional images can be reconstructed using computer software of the images obtained from various axes [20,21]. Advantages of 3D imaging using CT include the ability to register cross sections of the body and the ability to analyse the morphology quantitatively [22]. One disadvantage is that accuracy is dependent on the thickness of the original slices and orientation of the object during registration. Furthermore, metal objects, such as dental restorations, may cause artefacts and distort images of the nearby anatomy. Lastly, CT involves the use of relatively high doses of radiation and the full cooperation of the subject.

28.1.2 3D Breast Imaging and Mammometrics

With the advent of 3D imaging technology, surgeons now have the ability to analyse the breast in a way that was never possible before. In 2010, Tepper et al. introduced the concept of mammometrics, which is a system used to define true breast parameters [23]. This concept has reflected in many ways what craniofacial/maxillofacial surgeons have used with cephalometrics in studying true movements that they would like to achieve in orthognathic surgery. Mammometrics offers a means of transforming breast surgery to a more objective specialty.

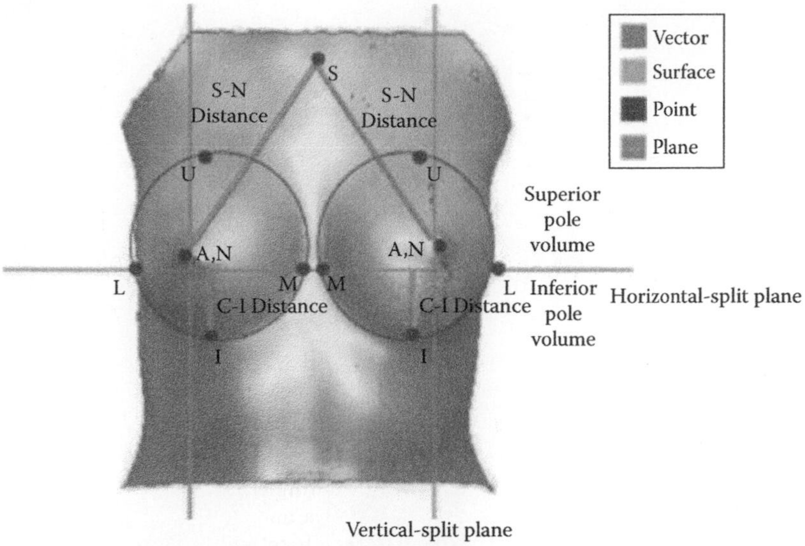

FIGURE 28.1 Overview of a single 3D image summarising standard mammometric points, planes, distances and volumes. S, sternal notch; N, nipple point; A, anterior most point; M, medial inframammary fold point; L, lateral inframammary fold point; C, chest wall; I, inferior most point; U, uppermost point.

With this concept, fixed planes and points on the breast and torso can be used to quantify not only breast volume but also breast shape, contour, AP projection, volumetric distribution, and position of the breast relative to the chest (Figure 28.1). Various anatomical *mammometric points* are marked on an anteroposterior view: nipple, sternal notch, inferior-most point of the breast, lateral inframammary fold, and medial inframammary fold. Using a sagittal view, the following points are identified: the anterior-most point of the breast and upper point at which the breast takes off from the chest wall. Mammometric planes are then created based on the 3D image of the patient. These planes include a chest wall plane, a horizontal-split plane, a vertical-split plane, and an inframammary fold plane (Figure 28.2). Based on these data points and planes, the total volume of each breast can be calculated as well as the volumes of the medial, lateral, superior, or inferior poles. Overall, these 3D-based breast measurements can be used to help guide operative planning, objectively analyse surgical results, and document post-operative changes that occur over time.

28.1.3 3D Hardware: Photography

Several 3D imaging systems are available today. Most are based on stereophotogrammetry, laser scanning, or both, and each provides advantages and disadvantages specific to their use. The methodology of stereophotogrammetry resembles that of human eye physiology, in which depth perception is made with binary vision focusing on an object from slightly different views. Similarly, stereophotogrammetry makes use of two pictures of the same object taken simultaneously from different angles. These images are then matched in space to create a 3D image of the object [24–26]. Advantages of stereophotogrammetry include the ability to objectify distances based on fixed landmarks, which are done relatively quickly. Disadvantages include a relative inferiority of the quality of the image compared to laser systems.

Laser systems use triangulation and measure the reflection of light off of the object's surface to create an image. The laser scanner then captures the scanned area in approximately 2 seconds and converts the surface shape into a polygon lattice of approximately 300,000 points [27]. Advantages of the laser system include ease of use, speed of obtaining data, and special accuracy. Disadvantages include that the laser systems may not be able to create a 360° view of the object. In addition, the object must be still to obtain an accurate image and use of infrared scanners may carry concern over optical safety.

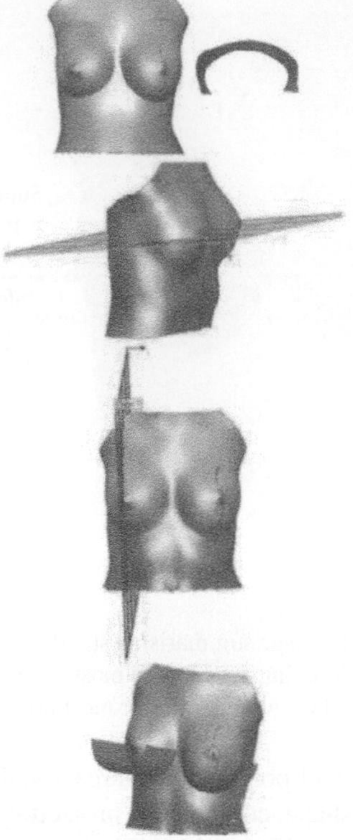

FIGURE 28.2 Mammometric planes. Shown here are multiple angles of the curved chest wall plane with and without a breast overlay. This curvature is based on the individual's torso. The horizontal-split plane is an xy plane that intersects the lateral borders of the inframammary fold. The vertical split place is a yz plane, or sagittal plane, through the midpoint of the breast width. The inframammary plane is a plane though the patient's natural inframammary fold.

Regardless of technique, one needs to obtain pictures from multiple angles to create a 3D picture with multiple cameras placed at various distances circumferentially of the subject. The 3D scanner is attached to a tripod head that can be adjusted in height. While the camera is level with the breast, patients are asked to stand with their arms at their sides in five different positions for a scan: +90°, +45°, 0°, −45°, and −90° relative to the lens of the camera (Figure 28.3). The camera is lowered to the floor and five additional inferior views are obtained at the same angles.

Practical differences among these imaging modalities also must be taken into consideration. The size of 3D scanners varies greatly, ranging from a single handheld portable device to machines that serve as rooms to accommodate/scan large equipment or the entire human body [28]. Cost may also play a significant role in the use of 3D imaging with 3D systems ranging from $20,000 to $100,000 [29]. However, more affordable systems are currently being developed.

28.2 CLINICAL APPLICATIONS

Galdino and Nahabedian in 2002 first reported uses of 3D imaging using photographic techniques. Analysis of 100 patients revealed that 3D photography was effective in analysing breast asymmetry, evaluating patients for breast augmentation with respect to implant distribution, assessing breast volume in breast reconstruction using implants, and examining breast volume in patients undergoing reduction mammoplasty [29].

In 2005, Losken was among the first to perform an analysis of 3D imaging of the breast. His group had compared the volume obtained from 3D images in pre-mastectomy patients and compared them

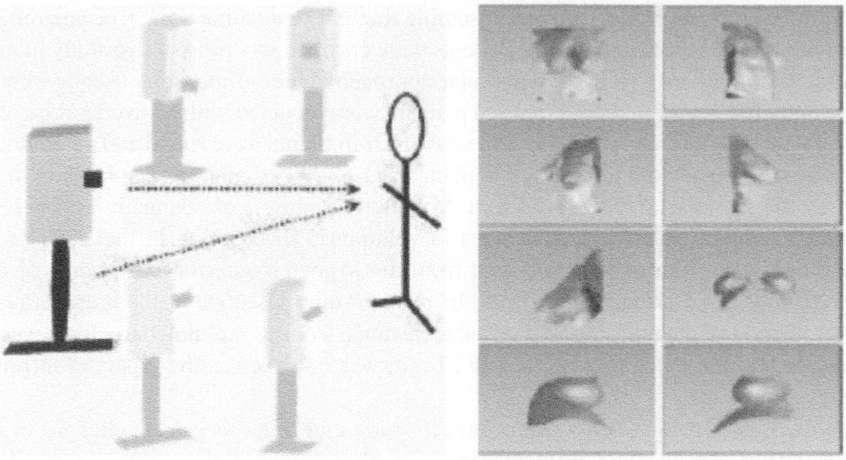

(a) (b)

FIGURE 28.3 (a) The 3D laser scanner is attached to a tripod head that can be adjusted in height. While the camera is level with the breast, images are taken from five different positions: with the patient +90, +45, 0, −45 and −90 relative to the camera's source. The camera is then lowered to the floor and five additional inferior views are obtained at the same angles. (b) Representative breast images of scans taken from various angles.

to the volume of the mastectomy specimens using water displacement techniques. Anthropometric values were also evaluated in comparing sternal-notch-to-nipple distances to distances obtained using 3D images. Independent raters had found a relative difference in measured volume to be −2% with a level of agreement at 0.975 and a relative difference in sternal-notch-to-nipple distance to be −6% with a level of agreement at 0.975. The authors had found that breast volume and surface measurements using 3D imaging technology are consistent with reproducible accuracy [30]. Since these early reports, numerous authors have now reported their experience with 3D breast imaging in aesthetic and reconstructive breast surgery.

28.3 3D IMAGING FOR BREAST AUGMENTATION

Three-dimensional imaging technology serves as a useful tool in preoperative planning for breast augmentation. Assessment of breast symmetry can be made based on breast volume and mammometrics. For example, breast volume analysis and volumetric distribution can be performed as described earlier. These measurements can offer a useful compliment to the existing systems for implant selection including the TEPID system, the High Five System, and the Body Logic System. The TEPID system, based on patient's tissue characteristics, addresses tissue (T), tissue envelope (E), parenchyma (P), implant (I), and tissue dynamics (D) [21]. The High Five System assesses implant coverage/pocket planning, implant size/volume, implant type, inframammary fold position, and incision [22]. The Body Logic System, developed by Mentor (Santa Barbara, CA), includes base diameter, projection, and volume measurements for determining the correct implant. Three-dimensional imaging offers a complete objective evaluation of the breast prior to breast augmentation which is not offered in any of these systems.

Post-operative analysis can help objectively characterise the morphological changes that occur with augmentation. Breast volume can be calculated and compared to the actual volume of the implant used, and volume of distribution can determine any changes that occur with round versus anatomic implants in the superior and inferior breast poles. Breast projection and internal angle can be determined and may vary depending on the technique and type of implant used. Surface distances, such as the distance from the sternal notch to the nipple and the distance of the nipple to inframammary fold, may also vary depending on the implant size and type.

In 2009, our group reported a study representing the first to document the true anatomic changes that occur with breast augmentation [31]. Patients were enrolled in a prospective study in undergoing augmentation mammoplasty using a periareolar approach. Three-dimensional scans were obtained both before and after augmentation. Fourteen patients were included with an average age of 32 years. Fourteen implants were silicone and 14 were saline. All implants were round and smooth and placed in the submuscular plane with an average implant size of 304 cc's and average implant documented projection by the manufacturer was 37.3 mm. Volumetric analysis of change in breast volume was consistent with implant size without changes in volumetric distribution in the superior and inferior poles. There was about a 20% decrease from the expected anterior–posterior projection with both types of implants. Furthermore, a 13.6° increase in internal angle of the breast was seen with increased projection of the breast. Lastly, a stable distance from sternal notch to nipple was observed after augmentation, but an increase of nearly 27 mm was observed in the nipple to inframammary fold length.

3D imaging may also serve as a useful tool to study and track long-term changes in the breast after augmentation. For instance, implant migration, changes in nipple position, and redistribution of soft tissue are all thought to occur clinically, however, none of these have been well studied to date. Such analysis may have potential practical applications including the choice of pocket, incision techniques, implant selection, and other variables.

28.4 3D IMAGING FOR REDUCTION MAMMOPLASTY

The use of 3D imaging can have a substantial impact on the preoperative and post-operative planning and management of patients undergoing reduction mammoplasty. Preoperative assessment of breast volume and symmetry has traditionally been based on surgeon and patient perspectives, both of which carry a degree of inherent bias [32]. Standard digital photography has become the mainstream in the assessment of the breasts before and after surgery but fails to objectively document true anatomic changes that occur [33]. Three-dimensional imaging can objectively assess multiple useful breast parameters in planning for reduction.

For example, surface measurements and volumetric analysis may aid in quantifying the degree of breast asymmetry and differential resection volumes. Such information may help refute or support the commonly held thought that medial pedicle technique should be reserved for smaller breasts [34,35] compared to inferior pedicle technique thought to be ideal for larger breasts [36–39].

Three-dimensional imaging may also play a valuable role in post-operative evaluation of the breast after reduction mammoplasty. In 2008, we reported for the first time, the anatomical changes that occur immediately following medial pedicle short scar reduction. Thirty patients underwent reduction mammoplasty with 3D analyses done at a mean of 80 days after surgery. The overall change in breast anatomy was outlined in colour map comparison (Figure 28.4). (Breast shape analysis showed a 4.8 cm elevation in the height of point of maximal projection with a corresponding elevation in the lowest point of the breast and a 1.8 cm decrease in the anteroposterior distance following surgery.) Sternal-notch-to-nipple distance was reduced by 6.1 cm and internipple distance was reduced by 2.9 cm. Average preoperative and post-operative volume in the patient group was 1040 and 677 cm^3, respectively. Preoperatively, 45% of breast volume was above the inframammary fold and 55% below the inframammary fold. Post-operatively, 76% was above the inframammary fold and 24% below the inframammary fold (Figure 28.5). Three-dimensional imaging identified a 31% increase in percentage volumetric tissue in the upper pole of the breast.

Also of interest, 3D imaging affords the ability to assess long-term changes following reduction mammoplasty. For instance, Choi et al. studied the development of pseudoptosis in medial pedicle breast reduction and found that anterior–posterior projection, sternal-notch-to-nipple distance, internipple distance, total breast volume, and percent tissue distribution in the upper pole of the breast remain stable nearly 2 years following reduction mammoplasty [40].

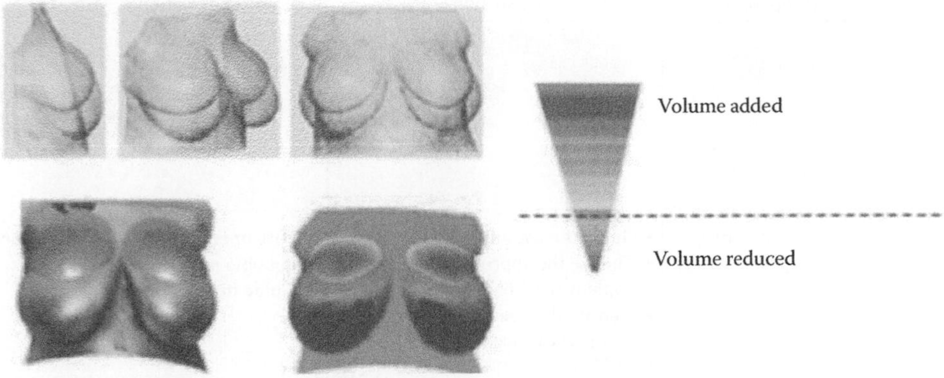

FIGURE 28.4 A relative colour map was generated between preoperative and postoperative three-dimensional images. A depiction of colour map analysis is shown; preoperative and postoperative images are demonstrated on the top row, whereas the bottom row shows the preoperative image with the postoperative changes represented by a spectrum of colour (red, volume added; blue, volume subtracted).

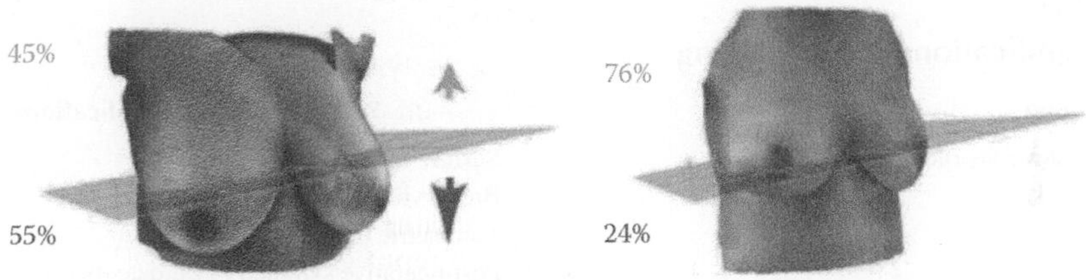

FIGURE 28.5 Percentage volumetric distribution. Each breast was divided into an upper and lower pole in order to determine the percentage of volumetric distribution. An identical plan was used on preoperative and postoperative images, and an example of volumetric distribution in right breast is shown for a representative patient (left) preoperatively and (right) postoperatively.

28.5 3D IMAGING AND BREAST RECONSTRUCTION

Preoperative assessment of the breasts before mastectomy with reconstruction may serve as a useful tool for surgical planning. At present, most surgeons base their reconstruction on physical examination and visual size estimates of breast size. For instance, in the case of tissue expander–implant reconstruction, surgeons have few standard measurements to assist them in their choice of optimal tissue expander size, total expansion volume, and permanent implant size/shape. Rather, these decisions are based on one's clinical intuition and experience. Unfortunately, this instinctual approach may result in suboptimal outcomes and need for revision or symmetry procedures [41–44].

Three-dimensional imaging offers an accurate measure of the baseline breast volume of both the unaffected and pre-mastectomy breast as a guide for sizing the new breast and target volume of expansion. Furthermore, volumetric studies of the breasts can help in choosing the appropriate tissue expander size, taking into account some degree of overexpansion and possibility of contralateral symmetry procedure. Three-dimensional imaging may also be useful during the expansion process. The final expansion volume can be measured and help direct the exchange procedure. This can be especially useful in determining the final implant size for exchange, which will also aid in determining the type of matching procedure needed with respect to volume (augmentation, reduction, or mastopexy).

Post-operative assessment of the breasts after reconstruction using 3D imaging can also be done. Degree of symmetry with respect to volume, shape, and tissue distribution can be quantified. In addition, anterior–posterior projection, surface curvature, distances, and direct vectors can be calculated. Such data can be used to study the success of various reconstructive techniques.

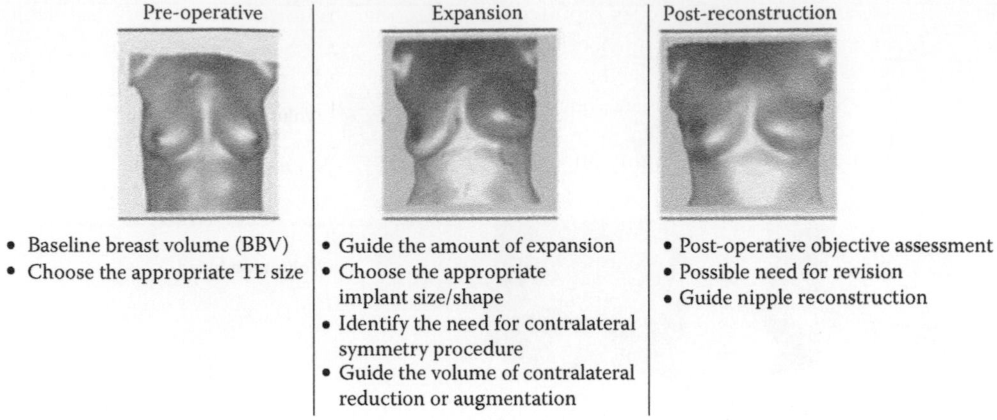

Pre-operative
Expansion
Post-reconstruction
• Baseline breast volume (BBV)
• Choose the appropriate TE size
• Guide the amount of expansion
• Choose the appropriate implant size/shape
• Identify the need for contralateral symmetry procedure
• Guide the volume of contralateral reduction or augmentation
• Post-operative objective assessment
• Possible need for revision
• Guide nipple reconstruction

FIGURE 28.6 A summary of how 3D volumetric data can provide clinical data at various stages of TE-implant reconstruction.

TABLE 28.1
Clinical applications of 3D imaging

Clinical Setting	Potential Clinical Applications
Implant breast reconstruction	Surface measurements
	Breast volume
	Volumetric distribution
	Post-operative symmetry (validate revision procedure)
	Implant size/shape
	Outlines surgical procedure
	Posterior projection of implant
	Postmastectomy residual breast volume
	Post-operative oedema
	Implant migration/contracture
Autogenous (flap) breast reconstruction	Surface measurements
	Breast volume
	Volumetric distribution
	Post-operative symmetry (validate revision procedure)
	Outlines surgical procedure
	Postmastectomy residual breast volume
	Post-operative oedema
Breast augmentation	Surface measurements
	Breast volume
	Volumetric distribution
	Preoperative asymmetry
	Implant size/shape
	Posterior projection of implant
	Post-operative oedema
	Implant migration/retracture
Breast reduction	Surface measurements
	Breast volume
	Volumetric distribution
	Preoperative asymmetry
	Post-operative symmetry (validate revision procedure)
	Outlines surgical procedure
	Post-operative oedema

In 2008, Karp, Choi, and colleagues reported a study to determine the potential of 3D imaging to serve as a guide for surgical management [45]. Patients scheduled for unilateral mastectomy were enrolled, and 3D scans were taken using the same technique described. Tissue expanders were selected based on preoperative base width measurements as well as 3D volumetric data. Three-dimensional volumes taken at the time of final expansion were used as a guide for the final implant size/shape. Contralateral symmetry procedure was also performed according to patient's desires, clinical judgement, and 3D measurements (Figure 28.6). Using 3D imaging as an adjunct, an average of 2.08 operations were performed to complete reconstruction, including mastectomy. The average post-operative volume was 395 cc with an average post-operative symmetry of 95% compared to 88% preoperatively.

28.6 SUMMARY

We are currently experiencing a paradigm shift in breast surgery, as we can more accurately assess our patients. At present, 3D surface imaging has proven to be a valuable adjunct for breast reduction, augmentation, and reconstruction (Table 28.1). As 3D breast imaging continues to evolve, so will our approach and understanding of breast surgery procedures. Given the relative ease of this technology, along with decreasing costs, 3D breast photography is likely to become the standard of care in the coming years.

REFERENCES

1. Breasted J. *The Edwin Smith Surgical Papyrus*. Chicago, IL: The University of Chicago Press, 1930.
2. Halstead WS. The results of operations for the cure of cancer of the breast performed at the Johns Hopkins Hospital from June 1889 to January, 1894. *Annals of Surgery* 1894;20:497–555.
3. Patey DH, Dyson WH. The prognosis of carcinoma of the breast in relation to the type of operation performed. *British Journal of Cancer* 1948;2:7–13.
4. Toth BA, Lappert P. Modified skin incisions for mastectomy: The need for plastic surgical input in preoperative planning. *Plastic and Reconstructive Surgery* 1991;87:1048–1053.
5. Biesenberger H. *Deformitaten und Kosmetische Operationen der weiblichen Brust*. Vienna, Austria: Wilhem Maudich, 1931.
6. Tebbetts JB. Breast implant selection based on patient tissue characteristics and dynamics: The TEPID approach. *Plastic and Reconstructive Surgery* 2002;190:1396.
7. Tebbetts JB, Adams WP. Five critical decisions in breast augmentation using five measurements in 5 minutes: The high five decision support process. *Plastic and Reconstructive Surgery* 2005;116:2005–2016.
8. Pechter, EA. A new method for determining bra size and predicting postaugmentation breast size. *Plastic and Reconstructive Surgery* 1998;102:1259.
9. Sigurdson LJ, Kirkland SA. Breast volume determination in breast hypertrophy: An accurate method using two anthropomorphic measurements. *Plastic and Reconstructive Surgery* 2006;118(2):313–320.
10. Smith DJ, Palin WE, Katch VL, Bennett JE. Breast volume and anthropometric measurements: Normal values. *Plastic and Reconstructive Surgery* 1986;78(3):331–335.
11. Qiao Q, Zhou G, Ling Y. Breast volume measurement in young Chinese women and clinical application. *Aesthetic Plastic Surgery* 1997; 21:362.
12. Sommer NZ, Zook EG, Verhulst SJ. The prediction of breast reduction weight. *Plastic and Reconstructive Surgery* 2002;109(2):506–511.
13. Sigurdson LJ, Kirkland SA. Breast volume determination in breast hypertrophy: An accurate method using two anthropomorphic measurements. *Plastic and Reconstructive Surgery* 2006;118(2):313–320.
14. Grossman AJ, Roudner LA. Measurement of breast volume: comparison of techniques, Palin WE, Jr., et al. *Plast. Reconstr. Surg*. 1986;77:253.
15. Grossman AJ, Roudner LA. A simple means of accurate breast volume determination. *Plastic and Reconstructive Surgery* 1980;66:851–852.
16. Palin WE, Von Fraunhofer JA, Smith DJ. Measurement of breast volume: Comparison of techniques. *Annals of Human Biology* 1979;6:363.

17. Westreich M. Anthropomorphic breast measurement: Protocol and results in 50 women with aesthetically perfect breasts and clinical application. *Plastic and Reconstructive Surgery* 1997;100:468–479.
18. Tezel E, Numanoglu A. Practical do-it-yourself device for accurate volume measurement of breast. *Plastic and Reconstructive Surgery* 2000;105:1019–1023.
19. Edsander-Nord A, Wickman M, Jurell G. Measurement of breast volume with thermoplastic casts. *Scandinavian Journal of Plastic and Reconstructive Surgery Hand Surgery* 1996;30:129–132.
20. Zonneveld FW, Lobregt S, Muelen JCH, van der, Vaandrager JM. Three-dimensional imaging in craniofacial surgery. *World Journal of Surgery* 1989;13:328–342.
21. Vannier MW, Hildebolt CF, Gayou DE, Marsh JL. Introduction to 3D imaging. In: Udupa JK, Herman GT (eds.), *3D Imaging in Medicine*. Boca Raton, FL: CRC Press, 1991.
22. Herman GT. Quantitation using 3D images. In: Udupa JK, Herman GT (eds.), *3D Imaging in Medicine*. Boca Raton, FL: CRC Press, 1991.
23. Tepper OM, Unger JG, Small K, Feldman D, Kumar N, Choi M, Karp NS. Mammometrics: The standardization of aesthetic and reconstructive breast surgery. *Plastic and Reconstructive Surgery* 2010;125(1):393–400.
24. Ras F, Habets L, van Ginkel FC et al. Quantification of facial morphology using stereophotogrammetry—Demonstration of a new concept. *Journal of Dentistry* 1996;24(5):369–374.
25. Burke PH, Beard LFH. Stereophotogrammetry of the face. A preliminary investigation into the accuracy of a simplified system evolved for contour mapping by photography. *American Journal of Orthodontics* 1967;53:769–782.
26. Seibert JP. Human body 3D imaging by speckle texture projection photogrammetry. *Sensor Review* 2000;3:218–226.
27. Tepper OM, Small K, Rudolph L, Choi M, Karp N. Virtual 3-dimensional modeling as a valuable adjunct to aesthetic and reconstructive breast surgery. *The American Journal of Surgery* 2006;192:548–551.
28. Avis NJ, McClure J, Kleinermann F. Surface scanning soft tissues. *Study Health Technology Information* 2005;111:29–32.
29. Galdino GM, Nahabedian M, Chiaramonte M, Geng JZ, Klatsky S, Manson P. Clinical applications of three-dimensional photography in breast surgery. *Plastic and Reconstructive Surgery* 2002;110:58–70.
30. Losken A, Seify H, Denson DD, Paredes AA JR, Carlson GW. Validating three-dimensional imaging of the breast. *Annals of Plastic Surgery* 2005;54(5):477–478.
31. Tepper OM, Small KH, Unger JG, Feldman DL, Kumar N, Choi M, Karp NS. 3D analysis of breast augmentation defines operative changes and their relationships to implant dimensions. *Annals of Plastic Surgery* 2009;62(5):570–575.
32. Anderson RC, Cunningham B, Tafesse E, Lenderking WR. Validation of the breast evaluation questionnaire for use with breast surgery patients. *Plastic and Reconstructive Surgery* 2006;118(3):597–602.
33. Eadie C, Herd A, Stallard S. An investigation into digital imaging in assessing cosmetic outcome after breast surgery. *Journal of Audiovisual Media in Medicine* 2000;23(1):12–16.
34. Karp NS. Medial pedicle/vertical breast reduction made easy: The importance of complete inferior glandular resection. *Annals of Plastic Surgery* 2004;52(2):458–464.
35. Hall-Findlay EJ. A simplified vertical reduction mammaplasty: Shortening the learning curve. *Plastic and Reconstructive Surgery* 1999;104(3):748–759.
36. Weiner DL, Aiache AE, Silver L, Tittiranonda T. A single dermal pedicle for nipple transposition in subcutaneous mastectomy, reduction mammaplasty, or mastopexy. *Plastic and Reconstructive Surgery* 1973;51(2):115–120.
37. Courtiss EG, Goldwyn RM. Reduction mammaplasty by the inferior pedicle technique: An alternative to free nipple and areolar grafting for severe macromastia or extreme ptosis. *Plastic and Reconstructive Surgery* 1977;59(4):500–507.
38. Georgiade NG, Serafin D, Morris R, Georgiade G. Reduction mammaplasty utilizing an inferior pedicle nipple-areolar flap. *Annals of Plastic Surgery* 1979;3(3):211–218.
39. Robbins TH. A reduction mammaplasty with the areola-nipple based on an inferior dermal pedicle. *Plastic and Reconstructive Surgery* 1977;59(1):64–67.
40. Choi M, Unger J, Small K, Tepper O, Kumar N, Feldman D, Karp N. Defining the kinetics of breast pseudoptosis after reduction mammaplasty. *Annals of Plastic Surgery* 2009;62(5):518–522.
41. Losken A, Carlson GW, Schoemann MP, Jones GE, Culbertson JH, Hester TR. Factors that influence the completion of breast reconstruction. *Annals of Plastic Surgery* 2004;52:258–261.
42. Nahabedian MY. Symmetrical breast reconstruction: Analysis of secondary procedures after reconstruction with implants and autologous tissue. *Plastic and Reconstructive Surgery* 2005;115:257–260.

43. Losken A, Carlson GW, Bostwick J III, Jones GE, Culbertson JH, Schoemann M. Trends in unilateral breast reconstruction and management of the contralateral breast: The Emory experience. *Plastic and Reconstructive Surgery* 2002;110:89–97.
44. Lee S. Three-dimensional photography and its application to facial plastic surgery. *Archives of Facial Plastic Surgery* 2004;6:410–414.
45. Tepper OM, Karp NS, Small K, Unger J, Rudolph L, Pritchard A, Choi M. Three-dimensional imaging provides valuable clinical data to aid in unilateral tissue expandor-implant breast reconstruction. *The Breast Journal* 2008;14(6):543–550.

29 Imaging for Incisional Median Abdominal Wall Hernias

Pietro Giorgio Calò, Giuseppe Pisano, Luca Saba, Matteo Atzeni, Fabio Medas, and Angelo Nicolosi

CONTENTS

29.1 INTRODUCTION

Incisional hernias (IHs), which are hernias that occur through a surgical scar in the anterior abdominal wall, are serious and common complications of abdominal surgery [4,5]. IHs occur in 0.5%–23% of patients after abdominal surgery [1,2,4,5,7]; their reported prevalence may be as high as 41% after aortic surgery [2]. IHs can give rise to serious morbidity, such as strangulation and incarceration, in 6%–14.6% of cases [4].

Post-operative hernias appear in the first years after surgery, usually a few months after the operation, and are usually a complication of laparotomic operations [16]. They are more common in obese and elderly patients and are associated with persistent post-operative coughing and abdominal distension [19]; pre-existing diseases such as diabetes, cirrhosis, chronic obstructive bronchial disease, malignant tumour, and malnutrition are general risk factors [1,18]. Local risk factors are post-operative infections of the wound, especially if caused by anaerobic germs [18]. Hernias occur more commonly through midline incisions in the hypovascular linea alba and are relatively less common following transverse incisions, especially where muscle-splitting approaches have been used [19,20]. The abdominal wall closure is particularly prone to dehiscence after peritonitis [19]. In 5%–10%, IHs may remain clinically silent for up to 5 years until detection [1].

Typically, properitoneal fat or the greater omentum protrudes through the hernia defect. If the hernia is left untreated, bowel loops may be incorporated into the hernia and become incarcerated or strangulated [16].

29.1.1 Incisional Hernias at Port Sites

IHs at port sites after laparoscopic surgery occur at a reported frequency of between 0.1% and 3% of all laparoscopic procedures. About one-quarter occur at the umbilicus, with the incidence higher in aponeurotic than in muscular approaches and when cutting rather than radially expanding (blunt) trocars are used [19].

29.1.2 Parastomal Hernias

Parastomal hernias are considered a form of IH. Parastomal hernias are common, with an incidence of between 6% and 36% in reported series. They are more common in transverse loop colostomies and tend to occur lateral to the stoma. The incidence of parastomal hernias is not related to the underlying gastrointestinal disease and is probably not related to the position of the stoma with respect to the rectus abdominis muscle [19]. They are aggravated by factors such as obesity, malnutrition, chronic cough, or abdominal distention [1]. The surgical revision rate has been reported to be between 10% and 20% of all stomas. Up to 20% of parastomal hernias shown by computed tomography (CT) are not detectable clinically [19].

29.2 PATHOGENESIS

The pathogenic mechanism differs from other types of abdominal wall hernias, that is, those involving orifices or anatomic canals. In order to strengthen the abdominal wall after laparotomy, its three layers (peritoneum, muscular fascia, and skin) are sutured separately. However, the muscular fascia may be rebuilt by an inadequate surgical technique or may be involved in an infection that develops post-operatively. In both cases, the consequence is weakening of the muscular structure or, even, failure of the sutures at several sites. Consequently, the support provided by the rebuilt abdominal wall gives way, and one or more initially small holes develop [8]. The first consequence of this particular anatomic situation is that, in the sites in which the described process has developed, wall resistance to abdominal effort is much reduced and its capacity is guaranteed exclusively by the skin externally and the peritoneum internally. Over time, as a result of pressure inside the abdominal cavity, a part of the moving viscera (generally, small-bowel loops but, more seldom, large-bowel loop) can escape into the subcutaneous space through the openings that have developed. This results in a hernia that, owing to factors determining a sudden increase of abdominal pressure (cough, vomiting, and muscular efforts), eventually becomes larger. IH can easily become worse, above all because of the visceral–visceral and visceral–parietal adhesions that may develop or due to obstructions, incarceration, and strangulation of the bowel. Owing to these fearful complications, surgical therapy of IH, even when asymptomatic, is mandatory [8].

29.3 SURGICAL TREATMENT

Many different operation techniques have been introduced for IH repair: either an abdomino-plastic surgery with direct suture or, recently preferred because of the lower recurrence rates, the implantation of synthetic mesh material via an open or laparoscopic approach [7,14].

For IH repair, synthetic prosthetic material is used on a regular basis, successfully reducing the rate of recurrence. The currently preferred material is the polypropylene (PP) mesh because of its low costs, easy handling, and a good long-term stability (Figure 29.1); it induces a local inflammatory reaction that may promote the formation of intra-abdominal adhesions [14]. With the introduction of coated prosthetic material (e.g. expanded polytetrafluoroethylene [ePTFE], coated PP), the incidence of adhesions after mesh implantation was reduced (Figure 29.2).

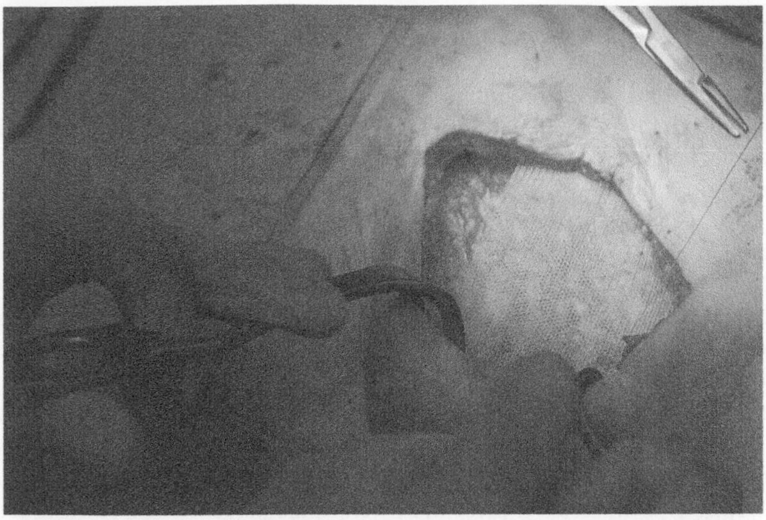

FIGURE 29.1 IH repair with PP mesh.

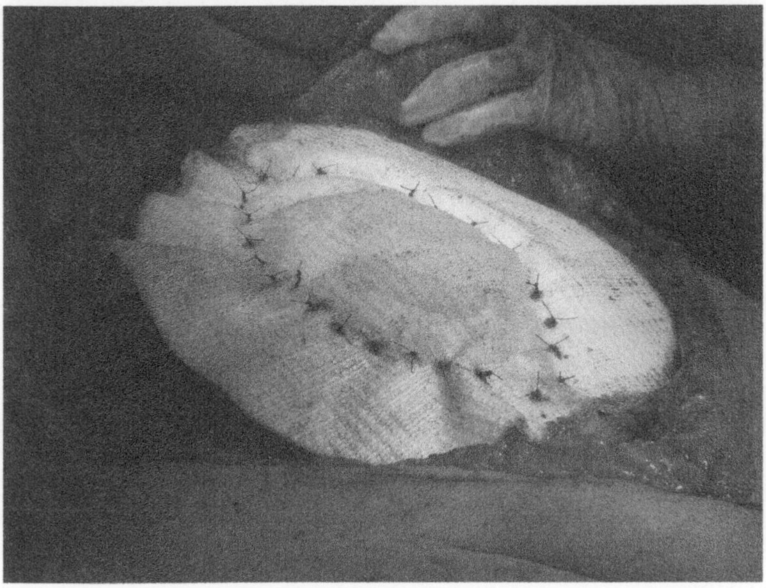

FIGURE 29.2 IH repair with coated PP.

But still a number of patients with continuing or recurrent abdominal complaints remain after IH repair [14]. The mesh is usually placed preperitoneally (open repair) or intraperitoneally (laparoscopic repair) at the backside of the anterior abdominal wall, respectively, the rectus muscle, often causing typical complications like seroma, intra-abdominal adhesions, reduced abdominal wall mobility, or muscle atrophy [7,14]. Open surgical repair of ventral hernias has the disadvantage of the patient having to spend several post-operative days in the hospital, with the frequent abdominal drains and a long recovery period at home. Moreover, the recurrence rate is high at 18%–41% after the initial repair [10].

29.4 DIAGNOSIS

Clinical diagnosis of an IH is often difficult, especially in obese patients, those with significant abdominal pain and distension, or those in whom the hernia has been dissected along muscle layers [1].

Various imaging techniques are required to confirm the presence of IH, especially in subjects in whom particular clinical conditions, such as obesity, make clinical diagnosis of small hernias difficult or uncertain. In addition, it is necessary to locate precisely the site of the abdominal hole, the volume of the hernia sac, its contents, the width of the muscular diastasis, and the muscular thickness surrounding it. Correct evaluation of these elements is prerequisite for correct surgical planning [8].

In the past years, the first diagnostic approach to IH was planar abdominal x-ray in two projections. If the patient can be placed in the upright position, P-A and L-L projections are obtained. In supine patients, A-P and L-L projections are taken, the latter by horizontal x-ray. Nonetheless, in spite of the information it supplies, planar abdominal x-ray only partially answers the surgeon's questions. In fact, this technique, although easily carried out, convenient, and inexpensive, is only able to determine the presence of bowel loops inside the hernia sac, pointing out both centrally and peripherally occlusive phenomena, if present, as well as the presence of free air as a sign of bowel perforation. Planar x-ray is not able to supply all the necessary morphostructural information about the abdominal wall, the site of the lesion, and the possible complications that can develop inside the hernia sac due to occlusion [8].

In the presence of IH complicated by intestinal occlusion, the first clinical problem consists of differentiating those bowel loops at risk merely due to the occlusive problem from those also at vascular risk of gangrene and perforation. In the latter case, emergency surgery is required. However, planar abdominal x-ray supplies adequate answers only through a series of indirect radiographic signs that may differ between patients and which are interpreted controversially. Moreover, with this imaging technique, optical problems arise that are related to the magnification of structures examined in relation to their distance from the film, such that the real volume of the IH cannot be determined accurately [8].

Radiography performed with orally administered barium and frequent fluoroscopic inspection is useful in detecting IHs. Areas of surgical scarring should be imaged in profile during performance of the Valsalva manoeuvre [16].

Diagnostic tools such as ultrasonography (US) and CT are commonly used for imaging hernias, whereas the use of magnetic resonance imaging (MRI) is still debated [5].

Of the first-level imaging techniques, US has consolidated its diagnostic role in the study of the abdominal wall (Figure 29.3). This non-invasive, inexpensive, easily practicable, and repeatable technique supplies important diagnostic information in the evaluation of IH. In fact, US of the abdominal wall allows the identification of small, occult IHs and in larger-sized formations to study their contents as both the width of the abdominal hole and the thickness of the adjacent musculature can be measured [8].

The limitations of US in uncomplicated conditions depend on the presence of adiposus panniculus, which, if too thick, prohibits correct execution of this technique. In complicated IH, in which mechanical occlusion of the herniated bowel develops, the diagnostic obstacle is sonographic obstruction, which is a consequence of meteorism of the involved bowel loops and does not allow a complete abdominal study. However, in these cases, it is always possible to evaluate the parietal thickness of the bowel loops, the degree of dilatation, the presence of interposed fluid, and possible associated solid lesions. Moreover, if Doppler technology is also available, information can be obtained about parietal blood flow in the hidden loops, while *real-time* visualisation allows an evaluation of their peristaltic movement [8].

US imaging has a moderate sensitivity and negative predictive value, but the specificity and positive predictive value are very high [5].

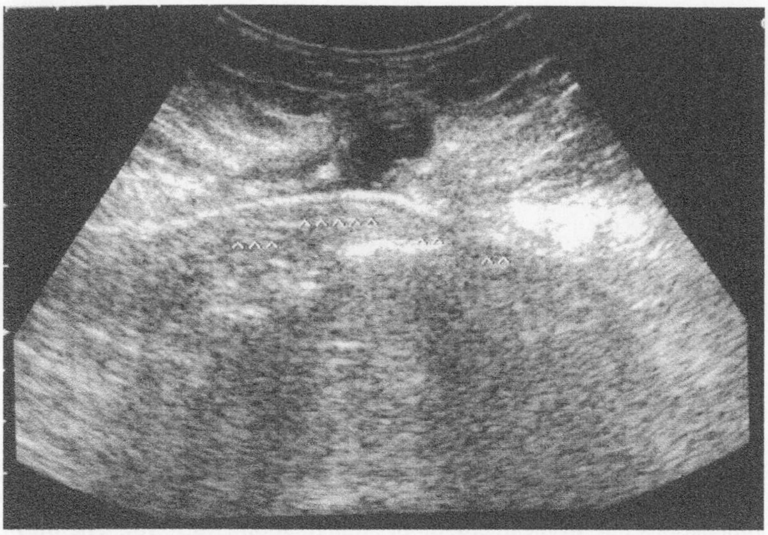

FIGURE 29.3 Ultrasonogram of a female patient with IH (the peritoneum is marked with short arrows).

CT and MRI can provide useful preoperative information about patients with long-standing symptomatic IHs [11]. Cross-sectional imaging depicting the volume of the hernia sac, the contents, and the size of the defect allows the surgeon to assess the technical difficulties and estimate the chances of a successful repair [19].

Currently, the imaging technique able to supply the very accurate information necessary for a correct surgical approach is CT (Figure 29.4) that nowadays represents an accurate method of identifying the various types of abdominal wall hernias, especially if they are clinically occult, and of

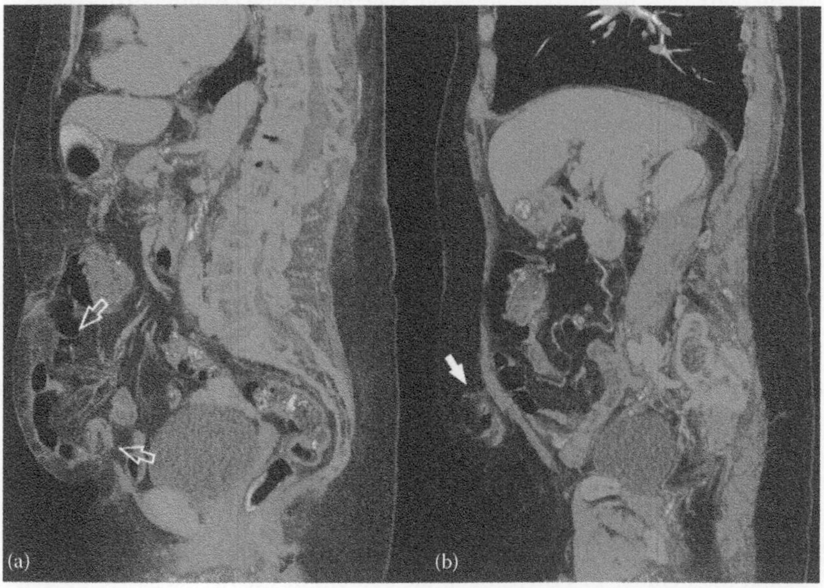

FIGURE 29.4 67-year-old female patient; volume rendering post-processed sagittal thick-slab CT images (panels a and b) show the hernia (arrows indicate the hernia).

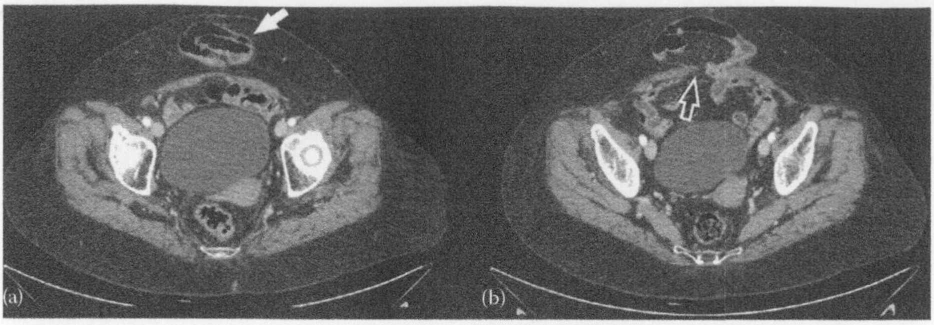

FIGURE 29.5 62-year-old female patient; CT images (panels a and b) show the hernia (white arrow) as well as its origin (white open arrow).

distinguishing them from other diseases such as hematomas, abscesses, and neoplasms [1,8]. CT clearly demonstrates the anatomical site of the hernia sac (Figure 29.5), the content, and any occlusive bowel complications due to incarceration or strangulation [1,8,16,18]. The intrinsic characteristics of CT make it well suited for examining the particular anatomic features of IH, especially in those cases involving complex structural conditions. CT is non-invasive, easily practicable, and has a high diagnostic accuracy [8]. Advantages of CT include more accurate identification of abdominal wall hernias and their content differentiation of hernias from other abdominal masses (tumours, hematomas, abscesses, and aneurysms) and detection of complications (incarceration, bowel obstruction, volvulus, and strangulation) [1,8]. Furthermore, the recent introduction into routine use of multi-detector CT (MDCT) has further improved diagnostic confidence regarding pathologies of the abdominal wall, thus enhancing the relevance of CT in this particular diagnostic field and in resultant therapeutic choices [7].

MDCT has the potential to further advance the preoperative assessment of these hernias. By permitting rapid acquisition of 3D image data sets and exquisite multiplanar (MPR) informations, MDCT precisely delineates hernia type, location, size, and shape (Figure 29.6) [1].

The study technique consists of initial scans without intravenous (IV) contrast perfusion [8]. IV administration of contrast material is necessary for the characterisation of the vascular supply [2]. Positive oral contrast material or water may be used to better visualise bowel loop, but most radiologists perform this type of examination without oral contrast material [2]. Supine images were acquired from the diaphragm to the pubic region during a single breath hold and reconstructed at 2 mm intervals or less. MPR informations are analysed by using dedicated workstations. Postural manoeuvres and manoeuvres to increase intra-abdominal pressure (e.g. straining or Valsalva manoeuvre) were not routinely performed, although they may help depict subtle anterior hernias [1].

These are acquired in order to anatomically locate the site of hernia formation, define its relations with adjacent structures, and, inside the hernia sac, evaluate the presence of free air or possible spontaneously hyperdense formations that might raise interpretative doubts in subsequent contrast studies. The latter almost never implies administration of oral contrast, which completely opacifies the visceral lumen, making evaluation of parietal perfusion of the bowel loops very difficult. Instead, the administration of IV contrast is better as it yields a series of data regarding intestinal vascularisation (Figure 29.7), particularly useful in emergency cases. By simple axial reconstruction, CT overcomes the diagnostic limits of traditional radiology and US, above all in obese patients and in those with hidden IH (Figure 29.8). Axial images allow the site of the hernia, the number of orifices, and the content of the hernia sac to be determined and accurately point out structures related to density, air or fluid content, and their degree of enhancement [8]. Consequently, IH can be differentiated from other abdominal masses, such as haematomas, abscess, or tumours [8,18]. Based on the panoramic quality of CT and its ability to provide superior anatomic detail, abdominal and retroperitoneal parenchymatous organs, the state of the

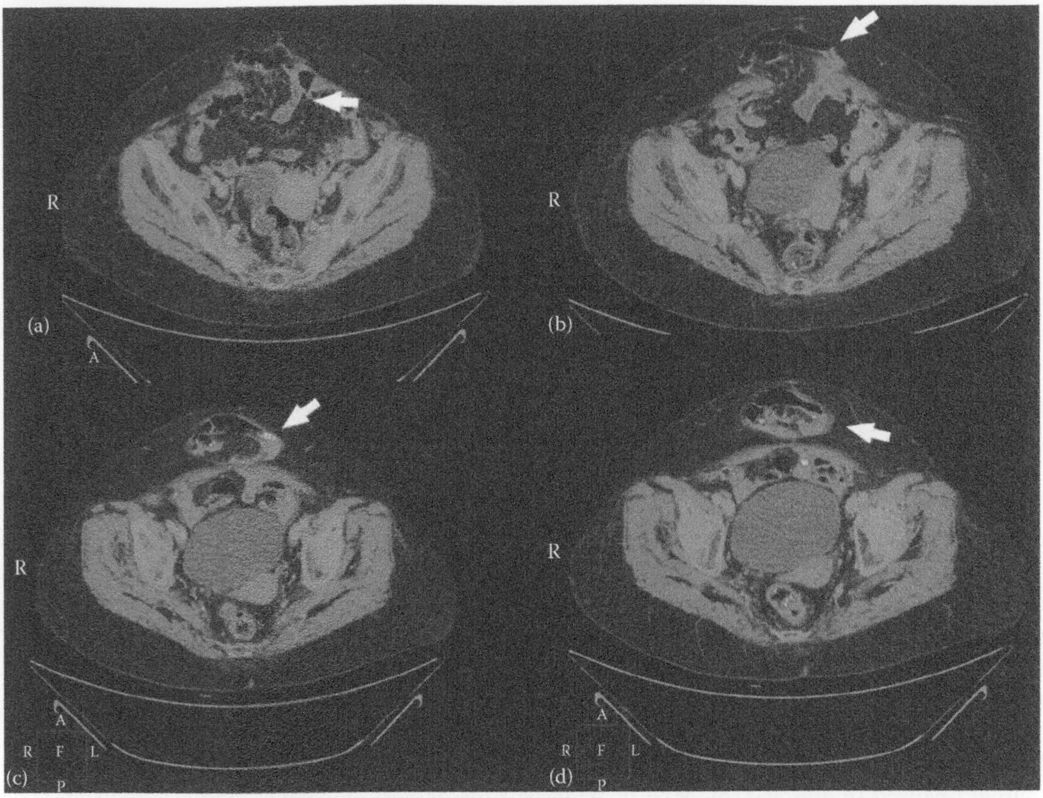

FIGURE 29.6 56-year-old female patient; volume rendering post-processed axial thick-slab CT images (panels a, b, c, and d) show the hernia (white arrows).

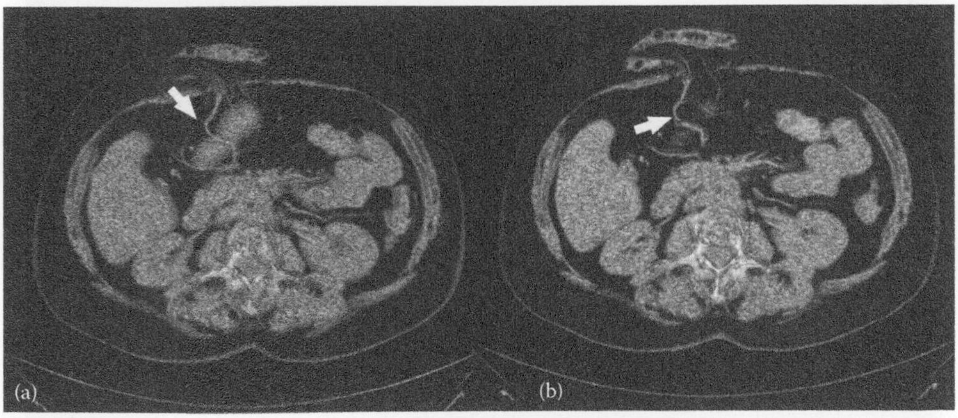

FIGURE 29.7 72-year-old male patient with hernia; volume rendering post-processed axial thick-slab CT images (panels a and b) show the arterial vessels from the superior mesenteric artery that penetrates into the hernia (white arrows).

bowel at the bottom and forward hernia sites, possible anomalies, and the presence of occlusive pathologies, even in their initial phases, can be determined [8].

MDCT allows the acquisition of a wide study volume within extremely short times, and with the application of particularly advanced software, axial reconstructions with a thickness of less than 1 mm as well as MPR and volumetric reconstructions are obtained [8].

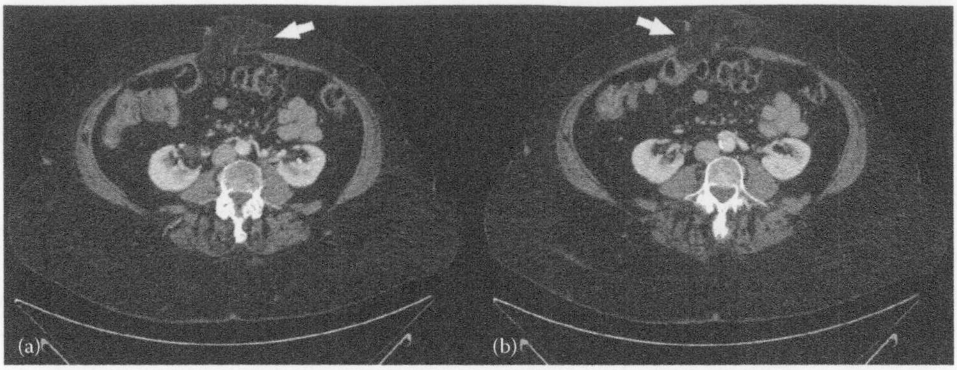

FIGURE 29.8 62-year-old female patient; CT axial images (panels a and b) show the hernia with fat involvement (white arrows).

In diagnoses of IH, the advantages deriving from MDCT depend on the possibility to acquire extensive information about the size of the hernia relative to its surface extension (expressed in mm^2) and total volume (expressed in mm^3). With MPR reconstructions, it is also possible to accurately measure muscular diastasis (Figure 29.9), not only in relation to the distance between flaps, but also to the total surface of the hole. For the surgeon, the latter is more important than the measurement of the maximum transverse diameter of the hernia sac and yields a suggestive and useful virtual reconstruction of the wall as well as an evaluation, in the planning phase, of the possibility of a plastic approach or, alternatively, the most suitable type of support yielding correct surgical reconstruction. In this type of evaluation, the possibility of accurately measuring the thickness of the abdominal muscle involved in diastasis, by MDCT reconstruction, is very important, and it is indispensable

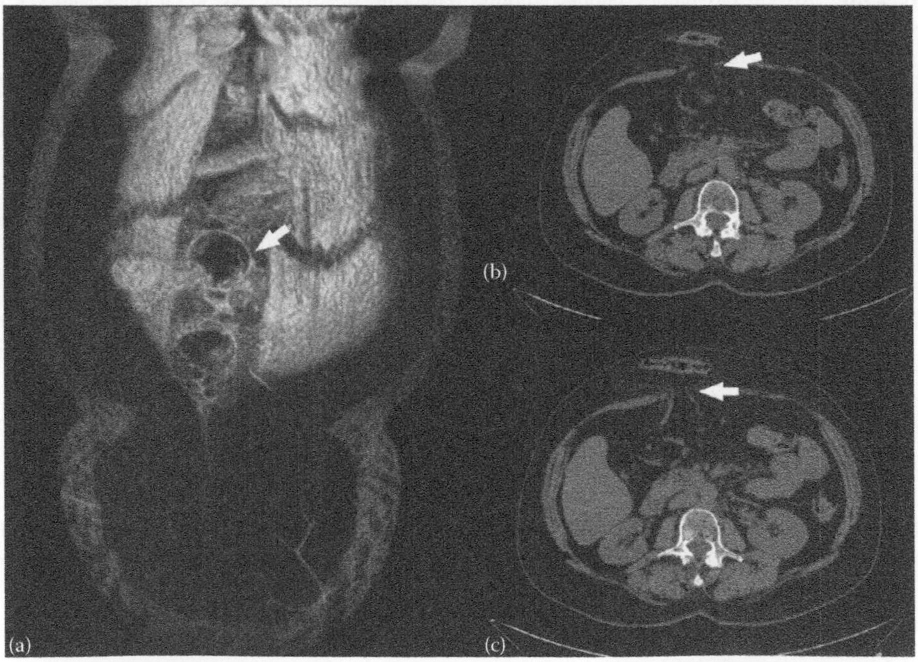

FIGURE 29.9 73-year-old female patient; volume rendering post-processed coronal thick-slab CT images (panel a); the CT axial images (panels b and c) confirm the hernia and the vessel involvement.

in deciding the most favourable technique. MDCT is also an invaluable method in diagnosing the acute complications of IH, mainly occlusive and ischaemic ones. It is a frequently recurring event that bowel involved in IH is choked or forms a volvulus, with the consequent appearance of a clear occlusive symptomatology owing to excessive angulation and adhesion inside the visceral sac [8].

Precise evaluation of hernia content by MDCT also allows identification of the occlusion and, in most cases, the event that generated it by characterising the underlying case. Additionally, the true extent of the bowel dilatation at the bottom of the obstacle, the hernia content, the abdominal wall thickness, and the possible presence of a fluid collection can be distinguished. Thus, MDCT provides a broad range of important information to the surgeon [8].

The technical characteristics of MDCT particularly suit the evaluation of the ischaemic complications frequently occurring to the detriment of choked bowel loops. Moreover, in complicated IHs, the high speed of data acquisition enabled by MDCT, with the consequent ability to examine wide body zones in very short times, allows evaluation of the contrast-enhanced bowel walls during various phases of the CT study, thus generating important information about blood flow in the involved bowel [8].

Abdominal wall defects may not be visible on supine CT scans. As a substitute for examination in the erect position, Emby et al. [6] propose to perform CT examination in the left or right lateral decubitus position, while increasing intra-abdominal pressure, by having patients perform a Valsalva manoeuvre.

The technique is of particular value in obese patients in whom clinical assessment is difficult and in patients with atypical or unexplained abdominal pain in whom other investigations have had negative findings [6].

A few studies suggest that MRI may permit detection of abdominal wall hernias, but it is not possible to adequately perform the exams using the Valsalva manoeuvre because the movement artefacts reduce in most of the exams the image quality [2].

29.5 POST-OPERATIVE EVALUATION AND FOLLOW-UP

In the acute post-operative phase, CT is able to distinguish between wound hematoma and early wound dehiscence with an intact skin closure, which may be difficult to assess by clinical examination [19]. In addition, because of its superior anatomic detail, MDCT may potentially detect subtle signs of strangulation, such as mesenteric stranding, poor bowel wall enhancement, wall thickening, free air, or fluid in the hernia sac [1].

US can be a useful tool for evaluating hernias repaired with mesh implants, including potential complications that may occur. Precise anatomic delineation of a mesh implant and a recurrent hernia is important for surgeons considering revision operations. Dynamic imaging offers advantages over other cross-sectional techniques because recurrent hernias may be transient with the Valsalva manoeuvre [13].

CT is a useful imaging tool for postsurgical follow-up [1,10]. CT is able to precisely demonstrate the site of the mesh and its fixation to the abdominal wall, and it can show fluid collections at the repair site of the ventral hernia even when they are not palpable. Moreover, a recurrent hernia can be detected clearly on CT [10].

CT visualisation of the mesh in the repair of ventral hernia depends on the thickness of the mesh and the composition of high-density material. The Gore-Tex Dual Mesh is visualised clearly on CT. PP mesh is not visible at CT because it is isoattenuating relative to surrounding tissues. ePTFE mesh is a strong, inert, 1 mm thick macrofilament that rapidly becomes fixated within the tissues. Its thickness and high attenuation allow visualisation at CT as a linear hyperattenuating structure [2]. CT is limited in the detection of adhesions and associated with radiation exposure. CT is also useful in the assessment of post-operative complications such as bowel obstruction and ischaemia [14].

In patients with laparoscopic repair of incisional ventral hernia, the best imaging technique should be considered the CT because it can show the correct site of the mesh, subclinical fluid collection in the abdominal wall, and recurrent hernia [10].

Functional MRI is a promising method to evaluate the post-operative situation of the abdomen after hernia repair, providing an overall view not only of the typical complications, particularly adhesions, but also of the mesh itself [14]. Functional cine MRI is the non-invasive method to evaluate implanted ePTFE mesh used for laparoscopic hernia repair without radiation exposure. Although other mesh materials like PP mesh could not directly be visualised, functional cine MRI provides an excellent and comprehensive evaluation of the typical complications related to all kinds of IH repair [14]. Functional cine MRI is suitable for follow-up studies in patients after hernia repair to detect and evaluate the implanted meshes, ePTFE meshes can be visualised directly, and typical complications like intestinal adhesions and abdominal wall dysmotility can be assessed reliably [7].

In the experiences of Fischer et al. [7] and Kirchhoff et al. [14], only one of the used mesh types, the PTFE mesh, was clearly visible in MRI images, allowing an accurate assessment of the mesh and its fixation. A reason for this might be that the ePTFE mesh is microporous and hydrophobic, and therefore, it is not going to be infiltrated by collagen tissue. Moreover, this material is not absorbable, and the fixing titanium tackers are easily identified due to the discrete susceptibility artefacts. In contrast, the PP mesh, fixated by resolvable sutures, is most likely incorporated by fibrous connective tissue in-growth forming an enduring tissue layer adjacent to the anterior abdominal wall [7,14]. Presumably due to this, it could not be identified on MRI images several months after the operation [7].

Functional cine MRI is the first non-invasive method to evaluate implanted ePTFE mesh used for laparoscopic hernia repair without radiation exposure. Although other mesh materials like PP mesh could not be visualised directly, functional cine MRI provides an excellent and comprehensive evaluation of the typical complications related to all kinds of IH repair. Functional MRI may contribute to the understanding of the complex problems in this large patient group with IHs [7].

29.6 DIAGNOSIS OF COMPLICATIONS

Complications after surgical hernia repair may occur in up to 50% of cases, depending on surgical technique and the status of the hernia sac vasculature. Approximately one-half of these complications may require surgical re-intervention, and accurate diagnosis at multi-detector row CT is necessary for optimal patient treatment [2].

The most common complications of abdominal wall hernias are bowel obstruction secondary to intra-abdominal adhesions, incarceration, and strangulation [2].

These complications can often be detected at clinical evaluation. Presenting symptoms may include abdominal pain, vomiting, and distention. Physical examination may reveal a firm, tender abdominal wall mass. Abdominal distention, dehydratation, or peritoneal signs eventually can become manifest [2].

29.6.1 Adhesions

The formation of adhesions after mesh implantation for IH repair is observed frequently in 20%–55% of the patients, depending on the mesh type. Intra-abdominal adhesions often result in chronic abdominal complaints, and they are the cause for 40%–75% of all re-operations required for intestinal obstruction [7,14]. In patients who underwent abdominal surgery, hospital readmissions for disorders directly or possibly related to adhesions were necessary in 35% over the following 10 years, causing considerable costs for the health-care system. For these patients, a reliable non-invasive diagnostic method is desirable, because the only other alternative would be a repeated operation, causing an additional risk of new adhesions [7].

Animal studies reported adhesions in 20%–55% of the cases, depending on the implanted mesh type [14].

The results of Kirchhoff et al. [14] show a higher incidence of adhesions in the laparoscopically treated group. The most common adhesion type was found between small-bowel loops and the anterior abdominal wall and between bowel loops as described in the literature.

Imaging studies are required when the clinical manifestation is misleading or inconclusive or preoperative assessment of the hernia or secondary obstruction is required. Early diagnosis of hernia complications is feasible with multi-detector row CT, potentially improving patient outcome by preserving bowel viability [2].

High-resolution ultrasound for the detection of abdominal wall adhesions is based on the visceral slide produced by either respiratory movement or manual compression. Abdominal wall adhesions can be detected according to the restricted slide of the bowel loops along the anterior abdominal wall with a high sensitivity and specificity. To achieve these good results, an experienced and well-trained investigator is mandatory. This method is limited to the assessment of adhesions at the anterior abdominal wall; the whole abdominal and pelvic cavity cannot be investigated, and the thin prosthetic mesh material itself cannot be assessed at all because of the lack of echogenic properties [3,7].

On static (contrast-enhanced) CT images, adhesions cannot be detected directly in most cases but can only be assumed due to indirect signs like scar tissue, sudden changes of the diameter of the bowel lumen, or bowel conglomerations. CT can demonstrate typical adhesion-related complications like hernia recurrence, seroma or strangulated obstruction, or bowel ischaemia. But dynamic imaging of visceral slide should not be performed with CT due to the repeated considerable radiation exposure [7].

In the study of Lienemann et al. [15], functional cine MRI allowed detection and mapping of intra-abdominal adhesions with a sensitivity and specificity of 87.5% and 92.5%, respectively, with intraoperative findings as standard of reference. In the experience of Kirchhoff et al. [14], for the detection of adhesions, MRI reached an overall accuracy of 86% with the highest detection rate in the mid-centre segments.

29.6.2 Bowel Obstruction

After adhesions, abdominal wall hernias are the second leading cause of small-bowel obstruction (10%–15% of cases). Colonic obstruction caused by abdominal wall hernia is uncommon [2].

Most cases of bowel obstruction secondary to abdominal wall hernia occur after incarceration and strangulation. In these cases, bowel obstruction occurs with the transition point at the level of the hernia. Key CT findings include dilated bowel proximal to the hernia and normal-calibre, reduced-calibre, or collapsed bowel distal to the obstruction. The degree of change in calibre helps to predict the grade of obstruction. Other findings may include tapering of the afferent and efferent limbs at the hernia defect, dilatation of the herniated bowel loops, and fecalisation of small-bowel contents proximal to the obstruction. Findings of strangulation may also be observed [2].

Incarceration refers to an irreducible hernia and is diagnosed clinically when a hernia cannot be reduced or pushed back manually. The diagnosis of incarceration cannot be made with imaging alone but can be suggested when herniation occurs through a small defect and the hernia sac has a narrow neck. Detection is important because incarceration predisposes to complications such as obstruction, inflammation, or ischaemia. Impending strangulation of these hernias should be suspected when there is free fluid within the hernia sac, bowel wall thickening, or luminal dilatation [2].

In strangulation, multi-detector row CT findings include closed-loop obstruction and ischaemia. Findings in closed-loop obstruction include dilated, fluid-filled U- or C-shaped loops of bowel entrapped within the hernia sac and proximal obstruction. Findings in ischaemia include wall thickening, abnormal mural hypo- or hyperattenuation and enhancement, mesenteric vessel engorgement, fat obliteration, mesenteric haziness, and ascites. Strangulated abdominal wall hernias are associated with a high surgical fatality rate (6%–23%) secondary to the strangulated viscus [2].

29.6.3 Seromas

Fluid collection occurs frequently in the immediate post-operative period after hernia repair (up to 17% of cases). These collections usually contain serous fluid (seromas) or blood products (hematomas), and their formation is related to both the surgical technique and the properties of the mesh used [2].

The hernia sac is left in situ and creates a space that has accumulated fluid in approximately 16% of laparoscopic repairs. Fluid collection also can be visualised on CT subcutaneously around the hernia sac. The fluid collection usually is a seroma (sterile fluid accumulation). A seroma is considered a complication if it persists for more than 6 weeks, steadily grows, or produces symptoms. On CT, the seroma has a globular, tubular, or multilobular appearance; if it contains air–fluid levels, it closely resembles a bowel loop or a recurrent ventral hernia. The rim of the collection may enhance because of the recent surgical procedure [10].

Most seromas resolve without manipulation within 30 days; aspiration may be indicated if the collection persists for more than 6 weeks, steadily grows, produces symptoms, or it is suspected to be infected. Imaging-guide aspiration or drainage may be problematic for large collections located under the mesh due to infolding of the mesh layers. In such cases, an oblique approach with use of small-diameter catheters may be necessary [2].

CT helps to identify fluid collections, to differentiate them from hernia recurrence (which may be difficult at physical examination, especially in obese patients), and to confirm their resolution. At CT, post-operative fluid collections can have a globular, tubular, or multilobular appearance. Some collections may be loculated with enhancing rims, reflecting recent surgical intervention, whereas others may contain air–fluid levels, resemble bowel loops, or be mistaken for recurrent hernias [2].

Infected post-operative fluid collections occur in 1%–5% of patients after hernia repair, depending on the surgical technique used and whether the surgery was delayed. These complications tend to occur more frequently in older female patients, especially after surgical repair of strangulated and incarcerated hernias. They tend to manifest early in the post-operative period (<2 weeks after surgery) and constitute an important risk factor for hernia recurrence [2].

Infected fluid collection may involve subcutaneous (superficial) or mesh-surrounding (deep) tissues. Differentiation is important because superficial infections are managed conservatively, whereas deep infections require intervention such as percutaneous drainage or prosthesis removal [2].

Diagnosis is usually based on clinical criteria such as the presence of fever or leucocytosis and the amount of time elapsed since surgery. Imaging is used to confirm the presence and define the location and volume of collection, to guide aspiration, and to monitor treatment [2].

Findings that are suspicious for infected fluid collection vary and include the development of gas or thick septa in a previously *simple* collection, an enhancing rim, fat stranding in surrounding tissues, or the development of a new collection one or more weeks after surgical repair. Imaging findings alone do not adequately help to predict the nature of a fluid collection, and imaging-guide aspiration is often necessary to establish the diagnosis [2].

Inflammatory reactions may lead to fibrosis of tissues surrounding the mesh. This condition may be suspected if the mesh has an asymmetric or irregular shape at CT. Mesh shrinkage may also occur. Less frequently, meshes may detach from supporting tissues and migrate within the abdominal wall [2].

Finally, it should be noted that CT is indicated for evaluation and, in several cases, for percutaneous treatment of the complications of IH [8,10]. Above all, when a fluid collection forms, following suturing or prosthetic implant, CT identifies the site of collection, its volume, and density; differentiates seromas from haematomas; and precociously locates the appearance of overlying infective phenomena [8,12]. This allows the establishment of drainage by percutaneous catheters, which can be left in situ until the infective process resolves [8].

29.7 DIAGNOSIS OF RECURRENCE

Hernia recurrence constitutes the most common complication after hernia repair, usually occurring generally 2–3 years after surgery. A small proportion of recurrent hernias occur 5 or more years after surgery, usually related to the ageing of tissues and the weakening of muscles [2].

The recurrence rates after IH repair are widespread throughout the literature ranging from 1% to 25% for open mesh repair and 0%–9% for laparoscopic repair. The prevalence of hernia recurrence varies with the type of repair: it may be seen in up to 30%–54% of cases after open surgery without mesh placement, up to 10%–32% after open surgery with mesh placement, and up to 7.5% after laparoscopic surgery [2,4,7,10,14,17]. Recurrence rate for laparoscopic repair is comparable with those obtained with the open mesh procedure, but laparoscopic repair offers a shorter hospital stay [4,10]. High incidence of recurrent IHs makes the selection of the imaging modality very important for this condition [4].

The diagnosis of this new hernia relapse is usually easy using abdominal inspection and palpation, although between 5% and 10% are not detected at physical examination [12,16]. After a hernioplasty, the existence of the non-resorbable mesh and the fibrosis that accompanies it may complicate its clinical diagnosis or render it impossible [12]. Obesity, abdominal distension, and a spontaneous contraction of the abdominal wall are factors which may make its detection difficult during physical examination [2,12]. In these circumstances, evaluation of the abdominal wall by a CT may provide a correct diagnosis of the hernia relapse (Figure 29.10). The existence of the mesh and the intense fibrosis may complicate its diagnosis. Even when the injury is palpable in the abdominal wall, the diagnosis may not always be clear. The hernia tumour can be confused with a haematoma, lipoma, or with a liquid build-up located on the mesh [9,12].

The post-operative assessment by CT of symptomatic patients who have been operated on for an intraperitoneal hernioplasty with unabsorbable mesh facilitates carrying out a correct diagnosis in the detection or exclusion of hernia relapse [12].

Although CT is a widely used technique in the assessment of IH, because it enables viewing of the herniated intestinal loop, the defect in the abdominal wall, and the width of the hernia ring, its diagnostic value in detection of a hernia relapse after repair of an IH with prosthetic material is insufficiently defined. The existence of the intraperitoneal mesh, the possible adherence of an

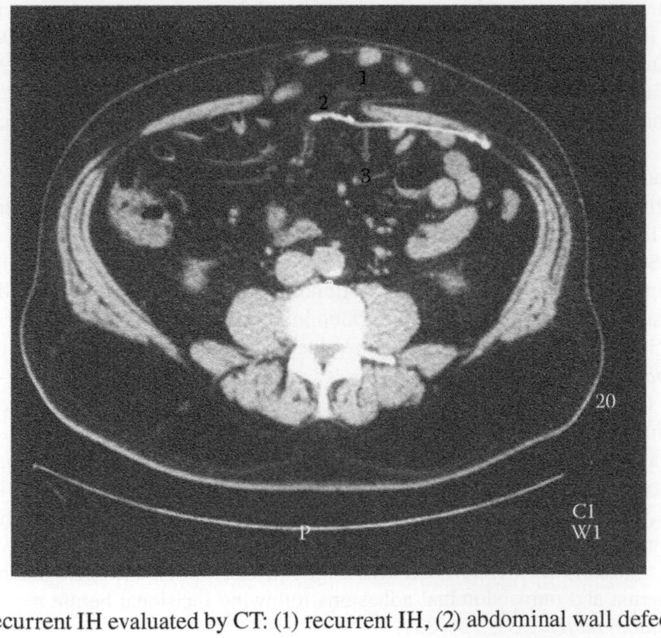

FIGURE 29.10 Recurrent IH evaluated by CT: (1) recurrent IH, (2) abdominal wall defect, and (3) displaced mesh.

intestinal loop to the mesh, and the relatively frequent formation of a subcutaneous collection of liquid due to the porosity of the mesh could lead to an error occurring in the radiological interpretation, in particular when using CT technology from 1 to 16 detector row [11,12].

In the experience of Gutierrez de la Peña [12], the hernia relapse was correctly diagnosed in 98% of cases by CT and in 88% of cases in the physical examination; the sensitivity was 1 in the examination by CT and 0.75 in the physical examination, and the specificity was 0.97 and 0.90, respectively; the positive predictive value in the CT exam was 0.88, whereas in the physical examination, it was 0.60; the negative predictive values were 1 and 0.95, respectively. Comparing both methods, CT shows a greater diagnostic reliability in the detection of hernia relapses after repair of IHs with prosthetic material. A negative predictive value of 1 and a positive predictive value of 0.88 convert it into an instrument of great use in the diagnosis of hernia relapses [12].

With regard to the symmetry of the rectus abdominis muscle, MRI provides valuable information. For planning surgery in case of recurrent hernia, the surgeon needs this information to plan the side of the surgical approach [14].

29.8 CONCLUSIONS

In summary, current imaging techniques, and in particular the CT and MRI, allow many if not all of the diagnostic questions related to IH to be answered rapidly and accurately. The integrated use of these techniques is therefore indispensable to choose the correct therapeutic approach.

REFERENCES

1. Aguirre, D.A., Casola, G., and Sirlin C. 2004. Abdominal wall hernias: MDCT findings. *AJR* 183: 681–690.
2. Aguirre, D.A., Santosa, A.C., Casola, G., and Sirlin, C.B. 2005. Abdominal wall hernias: Imaging features, complications, and diagnostic pitfalls at multi-detector row CT. *RadioGraphics* 25: 1501–1520.
3. Bingener, J., Kazantsev, G.B., Chopra, S., and Schwesinger, W.H. 2004. Adhesion formation after laparoscopic ventral incisional hernia repair with polypropilene mesh: A study using abdominal ultrasound. *JSLS* 8: 127–131.
4. Den Hartog, D., Dur, A.H.M., Kamphuis, A.G.A., Tuinebreijer, W.E., Hermans, J.J., and Kreis, R.W. 2009. Pre-, intra-, and postoperative sonography of the abdominal wall in patients with incisional hernias repaired via a three-layered operative suture method. *J Clin Ultrasound* 37: 394–398.
5. Den Hartog, D., Dur, A.H.M., Kamphuis, A.G.A., Tuinebreijer, W.E., and Kreis, R.W. 2009. Comparison of ultrasonography with computed tomography in the diagnosis of incisional hernias. *Hernia* 13: 45–48.
6. Emby, D.J and Aoun, G. 2003. CT technique for suspected anterior abdominal wall hernia. *AJR* 181: 431–433.
7. Fischer, T., Ladurner, R., Gangkofer, A., Mussack, T., Reiser, M., and Lienemann, A. 2007. Functional cine MRI of the abdomen for the assessment of implanted synthetic mesh in patients after incisional hernia repair: Initial results. *Eur Radiol* 17: 3123–3129.
8. Gagliardi, N, Stavolo C., Nicotra, S., Russo, G., and Galasso, R. 2008. Diagnostic imaging of incisional hernia. In *Incisional Hernia*, F. Crovella, G. Bartone, and L. Fei (eds.), pp. 79–86. Milan, Italy: Springer.
9. Goodman, P. and Raval, B. 1990. CT of the abdominal wall. *AJR* 154: 1207–1211.
10. Gossios, K., Zikou, A., Vazakas, P. et al. 2003. Value of CT after laparoscopic repair of postsurgical ventral hernia. *Abdom Imaging* 28: 99–102.
11. Grolleau, J.L, Otal, P., Micheau, P., Chavoin, J.P., and Costagliola, M. 1997. Imagerie de la paroi éventrée: Place et intérêt de la tomodensitométrie. *Ann Chir* 51: 327–332.
12. Gutiérrez de la Peña, C., Vargas Romero, J., and Diéguez García, J.A. 2001. The value of CT diagnosis of hernia recurrence after prosthetic repair of ventral incisional hernia. *Eur Radiol* 11: 1161–1164.
13. Jamadar, D.A., Jacobson, J.A., Girish, G. et al. 2008. Abdominal wall hernia mesh repair. Sonography of mesh and common complications. *J Ultrasound Med* 27: 907–917.
14. Kirchoff, S., Ladurner, R., Kirchhoff, C., Mussack, T., Reiser, M.F., and Lienemann, A. 2010. Detection of recurrent hernia and intraabdominal adhesions following incisional hernia repair: A functional cine MRI-study. *Abdom Imaging* 35: 224–231.

15. Lienemann, A., Sprenger, D., Steitz, H.O., Korell, M., and Reiser, M. 2000. Detection and mapping of intraabdominal adhesions by using functional cine MR imaging: Preliminary results. *Radiology* 217: 421–425.
16. Miller, P.A., Mezwa, D.G., Feczko, P.J., Jafri, Z.H., and Madrazo, B.L. 1995. Imaging of abdominal hernias. *RadioGraphics* 15: 333–347.
17. Paajanen, H. and Hermunen, H. 2004. Long-term pain and recurrence after repair of ventral incisional hernias by open mesh: Clinical and MRI study. *Langenbecks Arch Surg* 389: 366–370.
18. Stabile Ianora, A.A., Midiri, M., Vinci, R., Rotondo, A., and Angelelli, G. 2000. Abdominal wall hernias: Imaging with spiral CT. *Eur Radiol* 10: 914–919.
19. Toms, A.P., Cash, C.C., Fernando, B., and Freeman, A.H. 2002. Abdominal wall hernias: A cross-sectional pictorial review. *Semin Ultrasound CT MR* 23: 143–155.
20. Toms, A.P., Dixon, A.K., Murphy, M.P., and Jamieson, N.V. 1999. Illustrated review of new imaging techniques in the diagnosis of abdominal wall hernias. *Br J Surg* 86: 1243–1249.

30 Imaging and Surgical Principles of Perforator Flaps of the Trunk

Michel Saint-Cyr

CONTENTS

The Hippocrates' aphorism of *Primum Non Nocere* has dictated the ultimate goals of a reconstructive procedure: to restore the normal while achieving both excellent cosmetic and functional outcomes. Despite promising results in bioengineering and vascularised composite allografts,[1–6] reconstruction of common defects using autologous tissue remains amongst the most performed procedures.

As Sir Harold Gillies stated, 'Plastic surgery is a constant battle between vascular supply and beauty'. It is therefore impossible to discuss a flap design without a good knowledge of the vascular anatomy of a specific region. Despite a common *vascular skeleton*, many anatomical variations have been described in different regions of the body.[7–10] Several authors have therefore emphasised the need of a good preoperative planning, using imaging as a guiding tool, in order to harvest more predictable, reliable, and safer flaps.[11–17] Nevertheless, those techniques will never replace the knowledge of anatomy and clinical judgment. Indeed, these two elements tend to be even more critical when it comes to the planning of freestyle flaps, where the flap is designed based only on the Doppler signal marking the presence of a perforator in a specific region and for a specific patient.[18,19]

Modern investigating techniques as well as perfusion studies have led to an increased knowledge in the vascular anatomy and physiology of flaps.[20–35] When taken into account during flap design, these new information help perform safer procedures and potentially decrease complication rates.

In this chapter, we will first develop the current vascular considerations relative to perforator flaps in order to better understand the critical role of imaging in the preoperative planning as well as during the follow-up.

Perforator flaps present several advantages and have replaced standard flaps in many indications.[36–38] Harvested on the trunk, perforator flaps have found an indication in breast oncoplasty as well as in head and neck reconstruction and chest wall reconstruction. In the second part of the chapter, the thoracodorsal artery perforator (TDAP) flap, the supraclavicular artery flap, and the internal mammary artery perforator (IMAP) flap will be reviewed with an emphasis on the vascular supply.

30.1 VASCULAR CONSIDERATIONS LEADING TO A SAFER FLAP DESIGN

The transfer of tissue, under the form of a flap, relies on adequate blood supply. Manchot, Salmon, Cormack, Lamberty, Taylor, Palmer, and other pioneers have largely contributed to the knowledge of vascular anatomy of flaps. Based on these previous studies, Koshima and Soeda described in 1989 the first perforator flap ever described, the *deep inferior epigastric perforator* (DIEP) flap.[39] This revolutionary concept means that a flap could be harvested without the underlying muscle that was thought to be indispensable until then. The preservation of the function of the donor site represents one of the main advantages of perforator-based reconstructive procedures. On the other hand, certain unpredictability can occur, due to anatomic variations in the size and repartition of perforators. Many studies have defined the topography of these perforators and their related flaps[40–52] (Figure 30.1).

Nevertheless, some questions regarding the physiology of perforator flaps remain unanswered. Most notably, the amount of tissue being vascularised by a single perforator still needs to be clearly defined.

In 1987, Taylor and Palmer defined the vasculature of the human body as organised in *angiosomes*.[53] Each angiosome is a block of tissue supplied by source vessels and linked to each other via *choke vessels* (named as is because of their relatively small calibre).

Two decades later, with an increasing use of perforator flaps and a critical need of a better assessment of their vascular architecture, Saint-Cyr et al. focused on the perforator itself, and not the source vessel anymore. They conducted several anatomical studies[21,24–31,33,34] during which the largest perforator of a specific flap was injected with contrast agent and scanned through a 32- or 64-slice CT scanner. In an original article entitled *The Perforasome Theory*, Saint-Cyr et al. defined the *perforasome* (Figures 30.2 and 30.3) as the vascular territory of a single perforator.[34] This amount of tissue was also coined *perforator angiosome* by Rozen et al.[54] and *cutaneous angiosome* by Taylor and Palmer.[55]

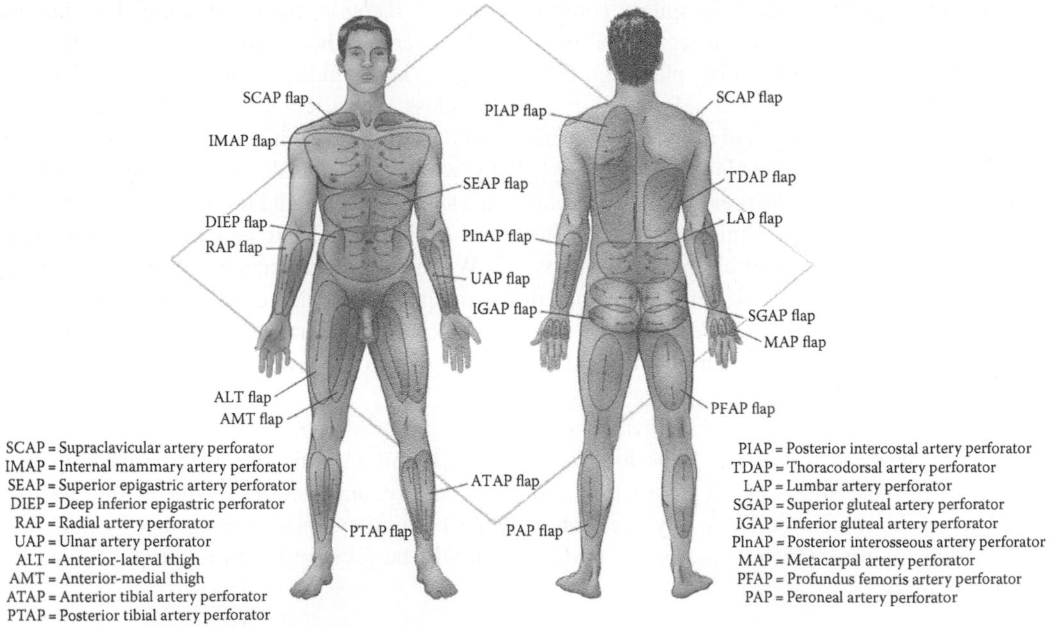

FIGURE 30.1 Perforators of the human body.

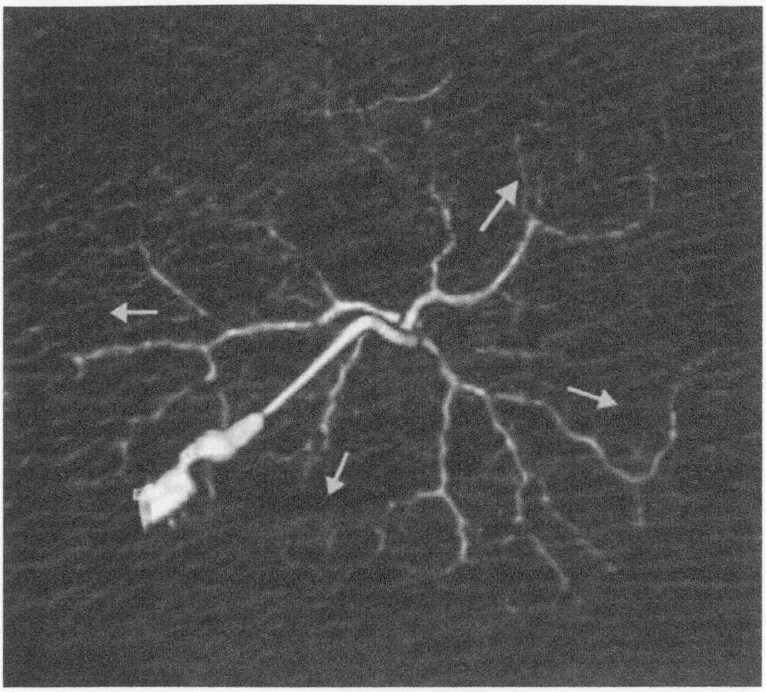

FIGURE 30.2 The perforasome.

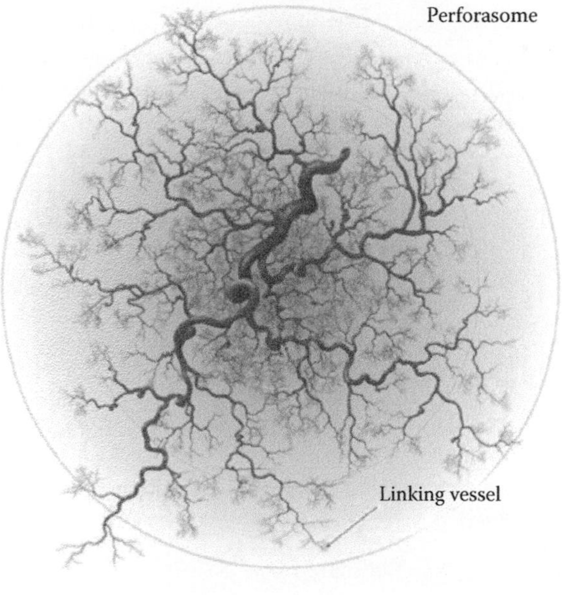

FIGURE 30.3 The perforasome.

Based on the perforasome theory,[34] four principles were found to be clinically relevant:

1. The perforasomes are connected to one another by means of linking vessels, both direct and indirect (Figure 30.4).
   a. The direct linking vessels are macroscopic vessels establishing a direct *bridge* between two branches of adjacent perforators (Figure 30.5).
   b. The indirect linking vessels refer to what Taylor and Palmer[53,55,56] called the *choke vessels* and constitute the microscopic subdermal network (Figure 30.6).
2. The orientation of linking vessels dictates the design of the flap: axial in the extremities and perpendicular to the midline in the trunk. The organisation of vessels in the trunk will be extensively developed in the next section of this chapter.
3. Perforators from a specific source pedicle have perforasomes that will be preferentially filled before filling perforasomes from adjacent source vessels.
4. The location of a perforator is critical for the interperforasome blood flow: the blood flood in linking vessels is distal from joints or non-mobile skin. On the contrary, when a perforator is relatively centrally located in between two articulations, the flow is multidirectional (Figure 30.7).

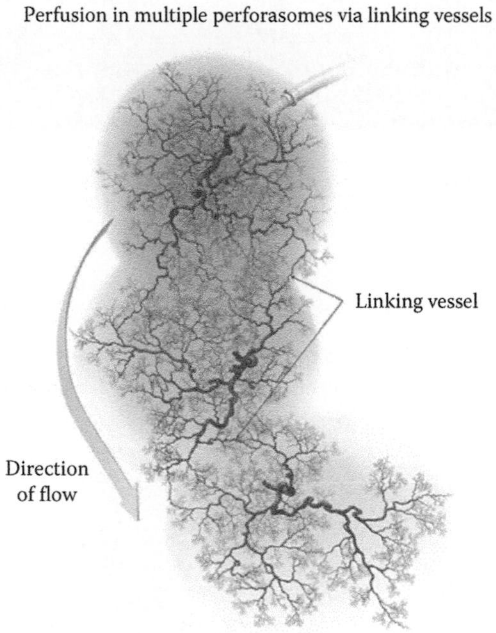

FIGURE 30.4 Linking vessels.

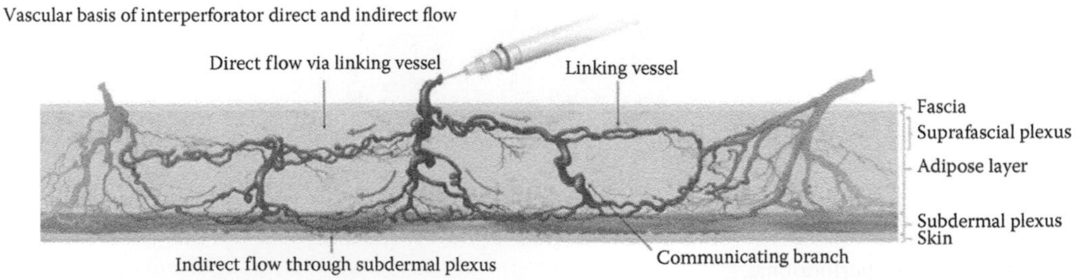

FIGURE 30.5 Direct and indirect linking vessels.

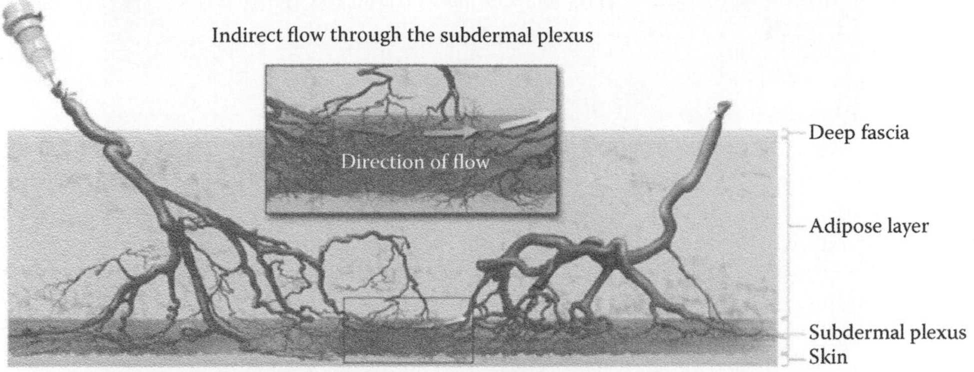

FIGURE 30.6 Indirect linking vessels: recurrent flow through the subdermal plexus.

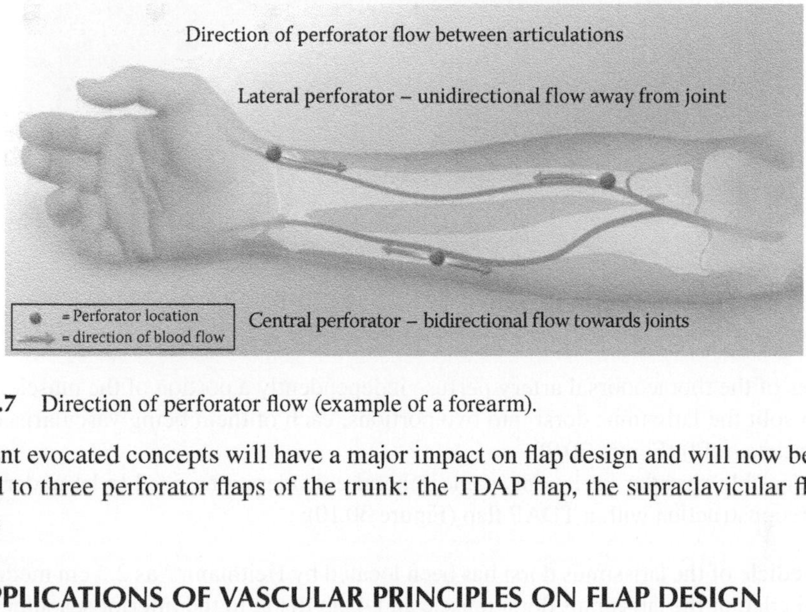

FIGURE 30.7 Direction of perforator flow (example of a forearm).

The different evocated concepts will have a major impact on flap design and will now be developed with regard to three perforator flaps of the trunk: the TDAP flap, the supraclavicular flap, and the IMAP flap.

30.2 APPLICATIONS OF VASCULAR PRINCIPLES ON FLAP DESIGN

30.2.1 Thoracodorsal Artery Perforator Flap

It was first described by Angrigiani[57] as a 'latissimus dorsi musculocutaneous flap without the muscle' as compared to the latissimus dorsi muscle flap described by Tansini[58] (Figure 30.8).

The TDAP flap was then rebaptised according to the origin of its source pedicle. The TDAP flap is a thin and pliable flap, with a potentially long pedicle. As a perforator flap, it preserves the function of the underlying latissimus dorsi flap and has been rapidly known as a very versatile flap for the coverage of soft tissue defects.[59] Nevertheless, its harvest is often associated to a tedious dissection and most of the published clinical series are small. A technical complexity is often mentioned, which to our knowledge is mostly due to anatomical variations in the size and location of the perforators.[60]

The distribution pattern of the TDAPs has been described both on cadavers and during reconstructive procedures.[28,30,44,57,60–64] The thoracodorsal artery is a branch of the subscapular artery and vascularises the latissimus dorsi and overlying skin. After reaching the deep surface of the latissimus dorsi, the artery gives rise to a bifurcation into a transverse branch (or horizontal branch) running 3.5 cm from the flap edge and a descending branch (also called lateral branch or vertical branch in the literature) parallel to the free border of the muscle, 2 cm from the margin.[44] Since the

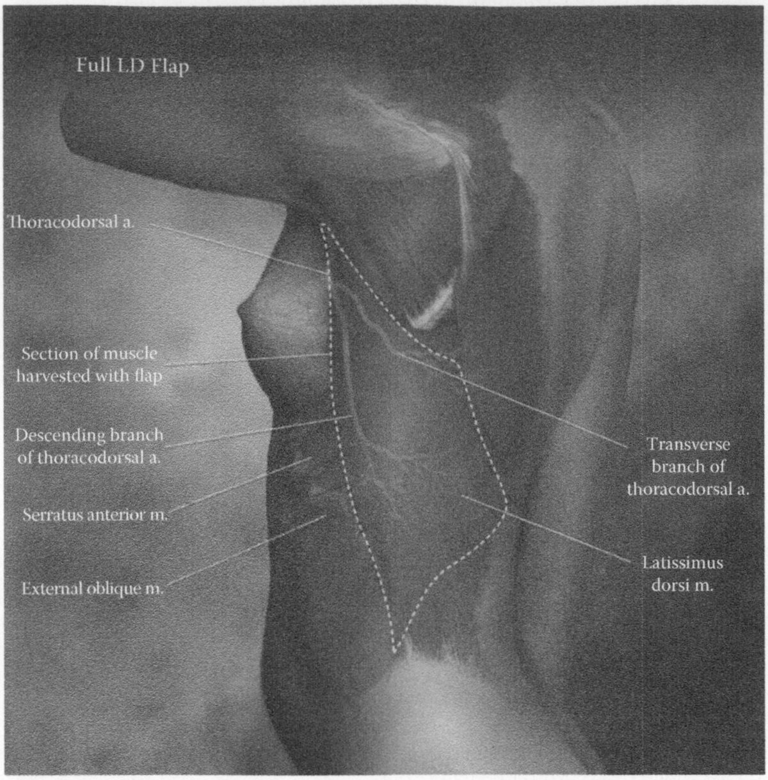

FIGURE 30.8 View of the full latissimus dorsi flap.

two branches of the thoracodorsal artery perfuse independently a portion of the muscle, it has been proposed to split the latissimus dorsi into two portions, each of them being vascularised by one of the two branches (ref?) (Figure 30.9).

Despite possible vascular variations, some general considerations need to be understood when planning a reconstruction with a TDAP flap (Figure 30.10):

- The pedicle of the latissimus dorsi has been located by Heitmann[44] as 2.5 cm medial to the lateral edge of the latissimus dorsi muscle and 4 cm distal to the inferior scapular border.
- Although most of the perforators are musculocutaneous, some septocutaneous perforators have been described as contouring the anterior edge of the latissimus dorsi muscle towards the skin. They may be found on average in 56% cases, according to three different studies. By avoiding the intramuscular dissection, harvesting a TDAP flap based on a septocutaneous perforator is easier and takes less time. Nevertheless, Mun et al.[49] relate the main drawbacks of the technique (variation of the perforator course, shorter pedicle length, and relatively inferior perforator size). According to their experience, there is a tendency to design the skin paddle more proximal and lateral as compared to a musculocutaneous perforator. When dealing with reconstruction of a breast defect, the consequence would be a lateral shift of the breast mound.
- There is an average of 3.28 (range 1–5.5) perforators with a diameter superior to 0.5 mm,[28,30,44,49,61] and a majority of these vessels are originating from the descending branch of the thoracodorsal artery.[57,62] Heitmann[44] reports a ratio of 56% from the descending branch versus 44% from the transverse branch, whereas Schaverien[30] found a ratio as high as 70% versus 30%, respectively.
- There is always at least one perforator (>0.5 mm) from the descending branch for many authors,[28,30,49,61] whereas others[63] have described it in only 85% cases.

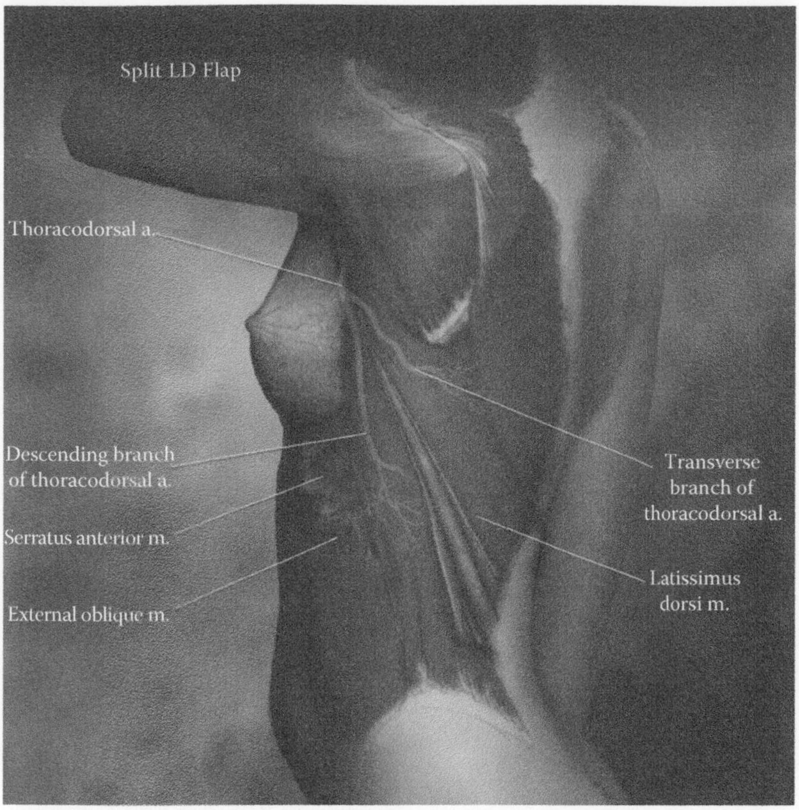

FIGURE 30.9 Split latissimus dorsi flap.

- The first perforator is found proximal and is described as having the largest diameter in many series. Although there are some slight differences in the literature in regard to the location of the first and largest perforator, it is safe to consider this proximal perforator to exit 8 cm below the posterior axillary fold and within 0–5 cm from the lateral edge of the latissimus dorsi muscle.[28,30,44,49,57,60–63]
- In his initial description of the TDAP flap, Angrigiani[57] mentioned that the size of the flap is related to the diameter of the perforator. Besides, there seems to be an inverse relationship between the size and number of musculocutaneous perforators.[61] The mean vascular territory of a perforator from thoracodorsal artery was evaluated at 255 cm^2 by Thomas et al.[61] and only 141.1 cm^2 by Schaverien et al.[28] These areas were calculated on static cadaveric models.
- Based on the previous work of Saint-Cyr[33] and on the perforasome theory[34] summarised in this chapter, Schaverien[28] added a comprehensive description of the vascular dynamics and physiology of the flap (Figures 30.11 and 30.12).
- The axiality of the arterial vascular is oriented inferomedially (Figure 30.15).
- Two patterns of perforators were described within the flap, and there was no predominance of one type over the other (Figures 30.13 and 30.14).
- Flaps as large as 25 × 15 cm[60] can be harvested safely, as long as the skin paddle follows the inferomedial orientation of the linking vessels and the skin paddle is placed over the perforators (Figure 30.15).
- Although the viability of the skin paddle is not a concern when the underlying latissimus dorsi is harvested, the situation is different when a fasciocutaneous perforator flap is considered. In those cases, the necessity to design the skin paddle over the region with the highest density of perforators has been emphasised.[30]

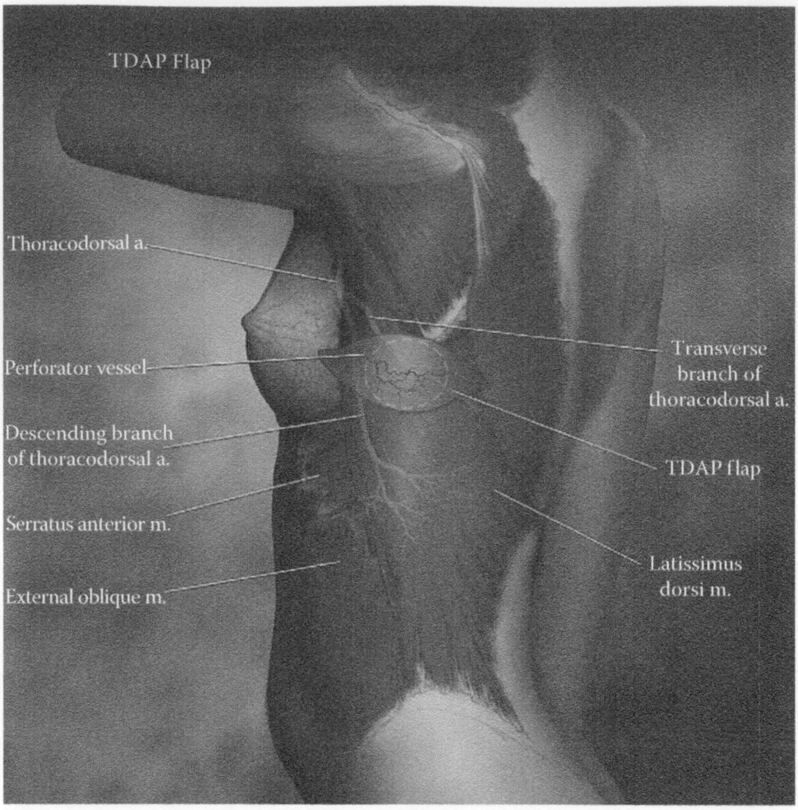

FIGURE 30.10 The TDAP flap.

- If the skin paddle needs to be located elsewhere in the flap or for the need of pedicle length, it is still possible to harvest a descending branch muscle-sparing latissimus dorsi flap. Unlike the TDAP flap, the descending branch muscle-sparing latissimus dorsi flap is not dependent on a specific perforator. Besides, with a transversely oriented skin paddle following the natural adipose tissue rolls, it gives an aesthetically pleasing donor site. The descending branch muscle-sparing latissimus dorsi flap can therefore be used whether as a salvage of a TDAP flap if no suitable perforator was found, or to avoid the intramuscular dissection of the TDAP flap.[23]
- Despite the original thinness of the flap, there has been an interest in additional thinning of the TDAP flap.[65,66] With perfusion studies and scanning of the flaps, Schaverien[28] demonstrated that there was no change in the vascular territory of the thoracodorsal artery after an additional 27% thinning since the linking vessels are located superficially, at the level of the subdermal plexus (Figures 30.16 and 30.17). Besides, when taking into account the two patterns of perforators previously described, thinning of the flap should only be avoided in a radius of 4.1 cm around a type 2 perforator in order to prevent any branch disruption.
- In a cadaveric model, Guerra[63] described the range of motion of the TDAP flap as less important than a latissimus dorsi flap. Nevertheless, the flap could easily reach the anterior chest wall, the clavicle area, the axilla, and even beyond the elbow and base of the neck with an additional dissection.
- When considering preoperative Doppler marking, it is important to note that when marking the patient in a sitting position and operating in decubitus, there is a shift in the location of the marked perforators.[63,64] Schwabegger et al.[64] justified the high-resolution power Doppler imaging as the optimal procedure in the planning of TDAP flaps.

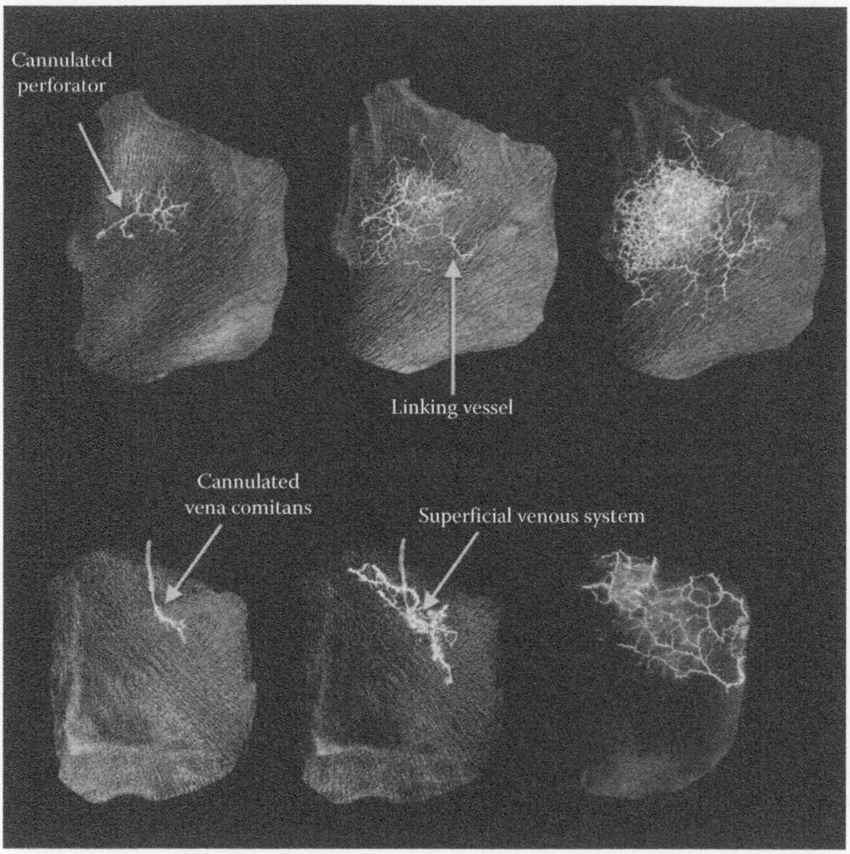

FIGURE 30.11 (Above) Anteroposterior dynamic CT angiograms of the most proximal perforator from the descending branch of the thoracodorsal artery at 0.5 mL filling increments. The flap is cut to follow the shape of the latissimus dorsi muscle. Note the large vascular territory and the dense network of linking vessels with the dorsal intercostal artery perforators. (Below) Anteroposterior images of dynamic filling of the venous system following cannulation of the vena comitans of the most proximal perforator from the descending branch of the thoracodorsal artery, with images acquired at 1 mL filling increments. The final image has been acquired following injection with a barium sulphate/gelatin mixture. The superficial venous system was arranged in a polygonal configuration at the level of the subdermal plexus, and flow into the deep venous system can be seen to occur through the venae comitantes of adjacent perforators within the same angiotome. Note that drainage in the superficial venous system occurred both superolaterally and inferomedially/medially towards the vertebral venous plexus, coursing progressively deeper within the flap as the veins approached the midline.

In conclusion, whatever preoperative imaging, the surgeon should know the anatomical landmarks relative to the perforator's location. Three systems can be used as summarised by Guerra:

1. The perforators are located 8 cm below the posterior axillary fold and 2–3 cm from the anterior border of the latissimus dorsi muscle.
2. The hilus can be located 2.5 cm medial to the lateral edge of the latissimus dorsi and 4 cm distal to the inferior scapula border.
3. A line of cleavage can be located between the muscle bundles. It has a white aspect on the descending branch since the pedicle is accompanied by the nerve. Perforators can be found following this line.

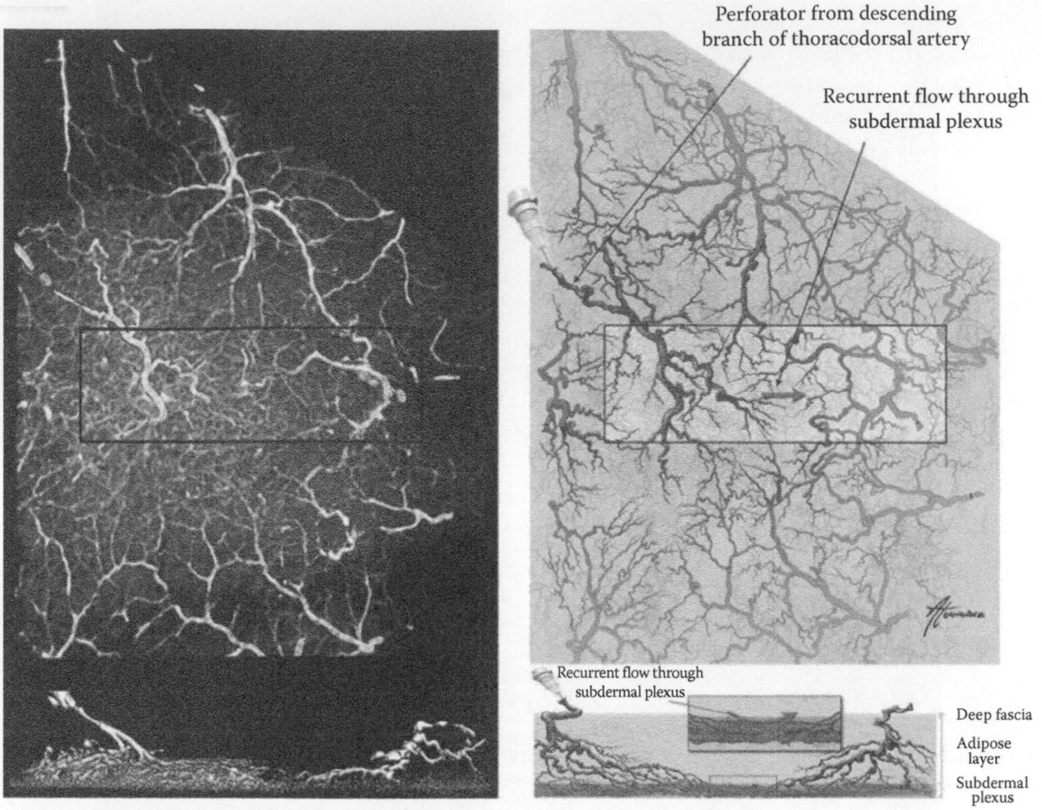

FIGURE 30.12 3D static image after cannulation of the most proximal perforator from the descending branch and injection with a barium sulphate/gelatin mixture, with illustration.

30.2.2 Supraclavicular Artery Flap (Island and Perforator Flap)

Free autologous tissue transfers under the form of fasciocutaneous flaps are the actual gold standard for head and neck reconstructions. Nevertheless, they require a technical expertise, an increased operative time, the presence of recipient vessels, and an adequate monitoring post-operatively.[67–69] Most of the local flaps are not adequate in size, and regional flaps have been associated with an increased morbidity.[69]

Because its skin properties are close to the facial skin, the supraclavicular artery flap has gained in popularity since its first description by Pallua in 1997.[70] Interestingly, the vascular supply of the supraclavicular artery flap was discovered in several steps throughout time, emphasising again the contribution of many pioneer authors.

Toldt, an anatomist who also described the so-called fascia well known by gastrointestinal surgeons, first described the *arteria cervicalis superficialis.* Based on this work, Kazajian performed the *shoulder flap* as the first clinical application. It is only 30 years later that Lamberty found the consistency, a branch that he named the *superficial transverse cervical artery.*[71]

Unfortunately, a high incidence of necrosis of the tip of the flap was reported in the literature.[72] In an attempt to find the anatomic basis of this high failure rate, Cormack and Lamberty published an article called *Misconceptions regarding the cervico-humeral flap.* They described for the first time the supraclavicular artery as the 'fasciocutaneous vessel that supplies a proximally based shoulder flap'. These pioneers of our current vascular knowledge also stated that a division of this vessel could occur during the proximal mobilisation of the cervico-humeral flap, explaining high necrosis rates.[73] Finally, Pallua rediscovered this flap and enlarged progressively its use and its indications.[70,74,75]

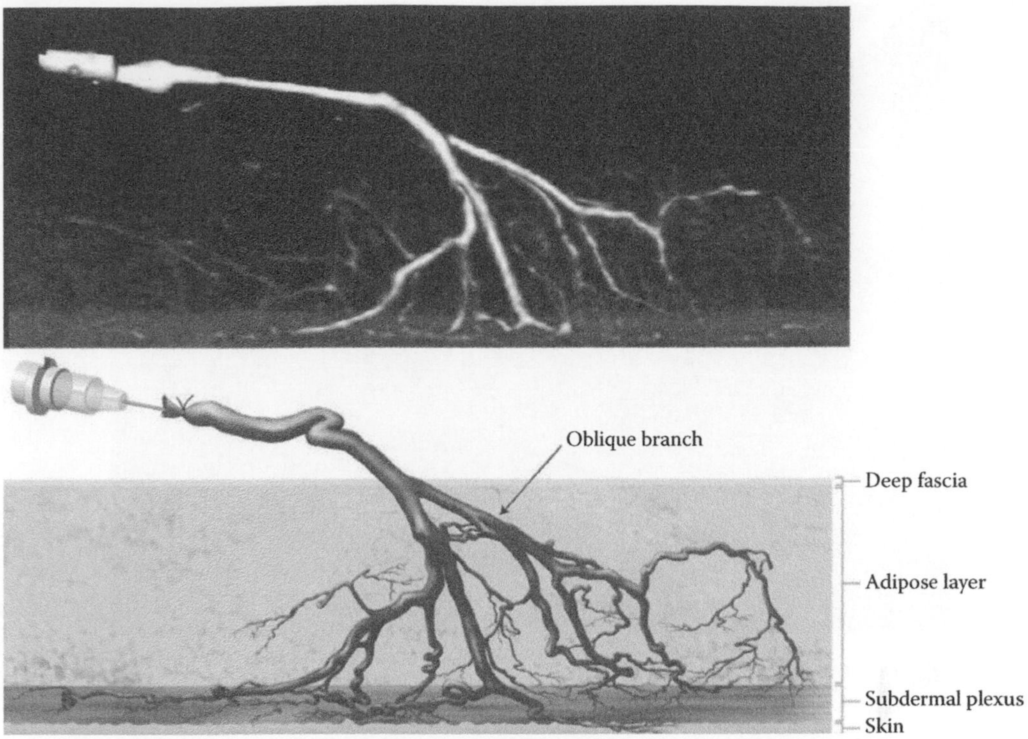

FIGURE 30.13 Type 1; the perforators enter the fascia directly and divide in several long oblique branches that course within the adipose layer down to the subdermal plexus.

The supraclavicular artery island flap is a thin, pliable, and axial flap that presents a good colour match with head and neck and a wide arc of rotation.[76] Although considered non-reliable in the past, it has now gained the rank of workhorse flap in the reconstruction of defects of the non–previously irradiated lower third of the face and neck.[69]

Although most commonly harvested as an axial island flap, the supraclavicular flap has been shown reliable as a true perforator flap, based on perforators arising from the transverse cervical artery.[77]

The vascular supply to the flap comes from the supraclavicular vessels which branch off of the transverse cervical vessels. The transverse cervical artery has been shown to arise from the thyrocervical trunk in 54.2% of cases and from the subclavian artery in 45.8%. The transverse cervical artery runs posteriorly and laterally towards the trapezius muscle and travels beneath the omohyoid muscle and superficial to the scalene muscles and brachial plexus within the fibrofatty tissue of the supraclavicular fossa. After passing underneath the omohyoid muscle, it branches to the supraclavicular artery and an average of four perforators to the supraclavicular skin.[77,78] Although a Japanese study[79] described inframillimetric supraclavicular arteries in some specimens, the size of the pedicle has been found to be consistent in our population with a mean length at 5 cm and a mean diameter of 1.5 mm. Liu et al.[80] hypothesised that those differences may be explained by the differences between the Western and Asian populations.

Based on the previous work of Saint-Cyr,[33] Chan et al. performed CT injection studies in order to refine the microvascular architecture of the supraclavicular artery flap. While scanning in a timely manner, the authors have noticed the important contribution of the linking vessels in the overall flap perfusion, by perfusing adjacent perforasomes. The linking vessels were found to follow the axiality of the upper limb, which correlates with the perforasome theory (Figure 30.18).

They concluded that adequately sized flaps were perfused to the tip of the flap due to the contribution of direct linking vessels as well as recurrent flow through the subdermal plexus.

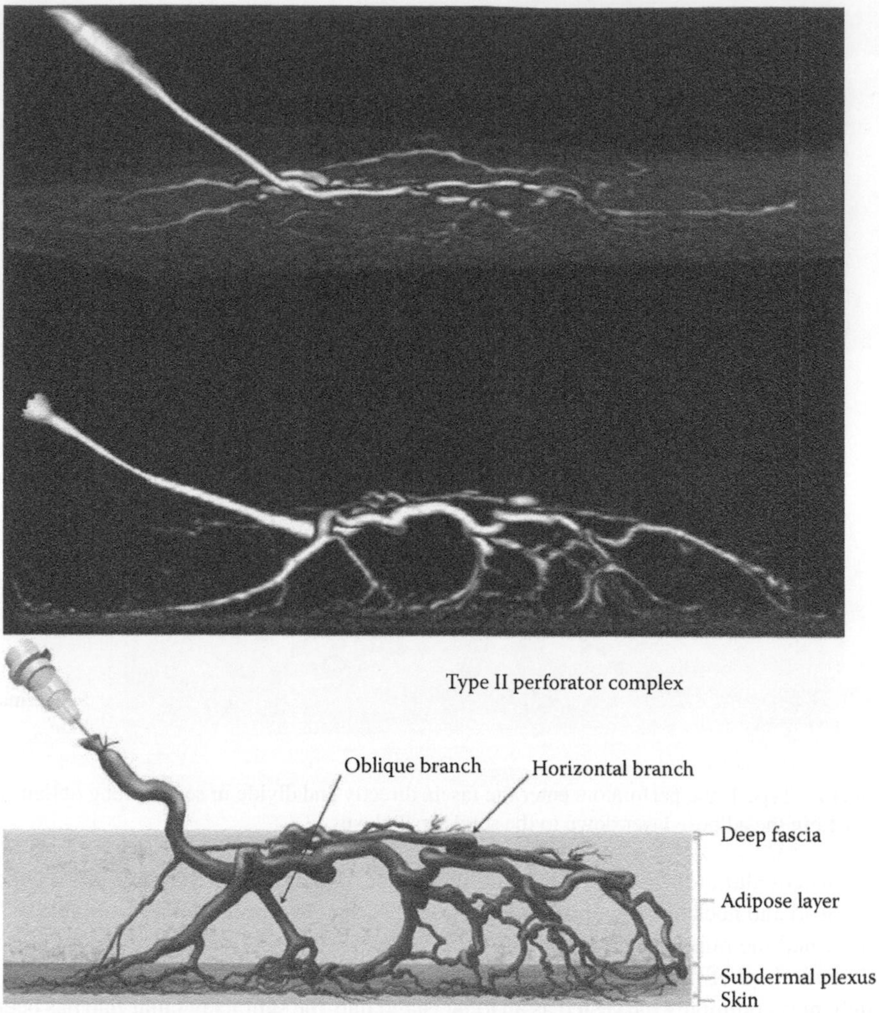

FIGURE 30.14 Type 2; the perforators give branches that run on a short distance (4.1 cm maximum) at a suprafascial level before entering obliquely in the flap and reaching the subdermal plexus.

This maximal size was found to be at a mean of 24.2 cm in length and 8.7 cm in width for an average surface of 152.8 cm^2. As mentioned in this cadaveric study, the surface of the flap may be underestimated, and flaps as long as 35 cm have been successfully harvested in the past.[72]

Although the previous studies confirmed a reliable and consistent pedicle, the course of the vessel may be a concern in some patients. Adam et al.[76] perform head and neck reconstructions with supraclavicular flap on a routine basis. They have found the Doppler signal not to correlate with the clinical findings in some patients, explaining their decision to perform commonly a CT angiography preoperatively.

In summary, it is possible to harvest the flap only with preoperative Doppler marking as described by Wei and Mardini.[19] Nevertheless, the surgeon level of confidence may preoperatively be increased by the use of CT angiography that will provide useful information such as location, approximate vessel diameter, and pedicle length.

In conclusion, with the work of several authors mentioned in this chapter, the supraclavicular flap has become a safe and reliable flap, which is now considered as full part of the reconstructive armamentarium and useful in patients with tumour ablation, burn contractures, and radiation injuries.[76]

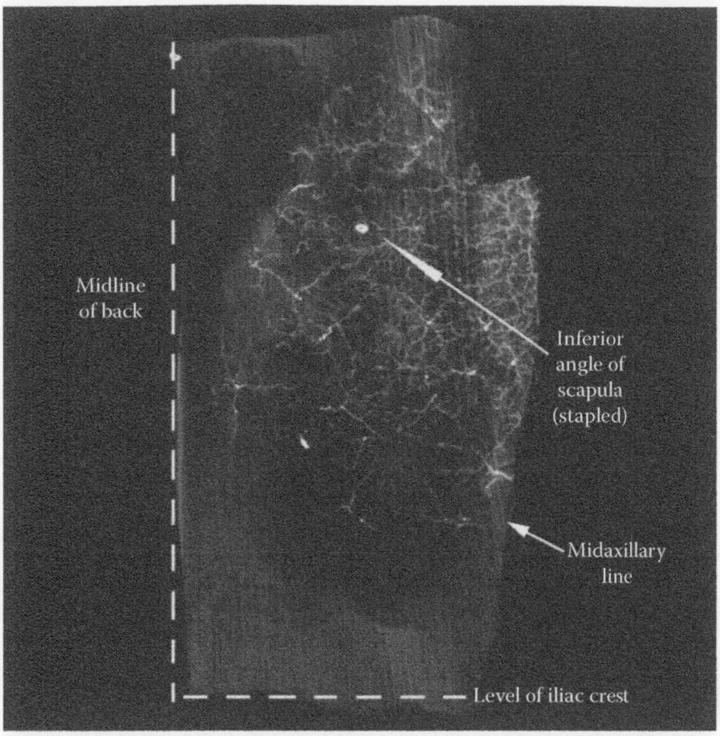

FIGURE 30.15 CT angiography of the hemi-back skin only without underlying latissimus dorsi muscle and following injection of the thoracodorsal artery with iodine contrast. Note the inferomedial orientation of the linking vessels.

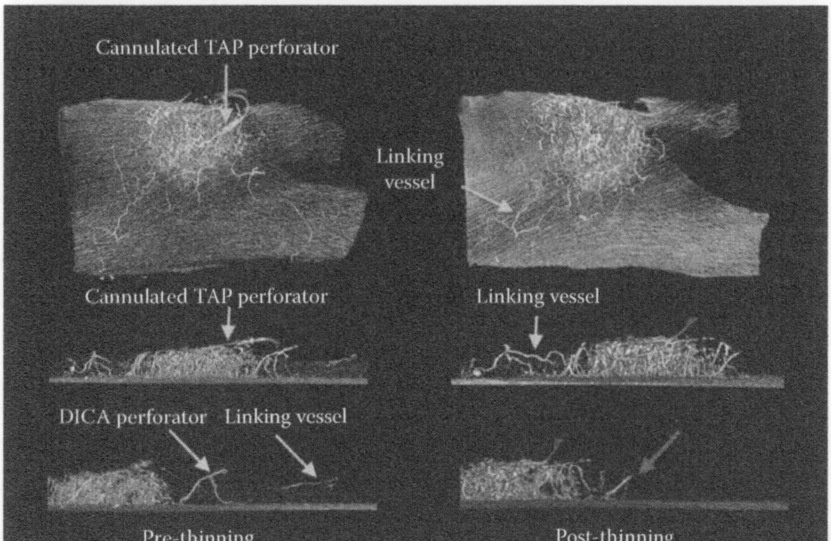

FIGURE 30.16 Anteroposterior and lateral views of a type 1 perforator complex before (left) and after (right) thinning between the deep and superficial adipose layers and injection of 1.5 mL of contrast. A 5 cm radius about the perforator has been preserved, and thinning has been performed at 90° to the horizontal, with washout of the contrast between successive stages.

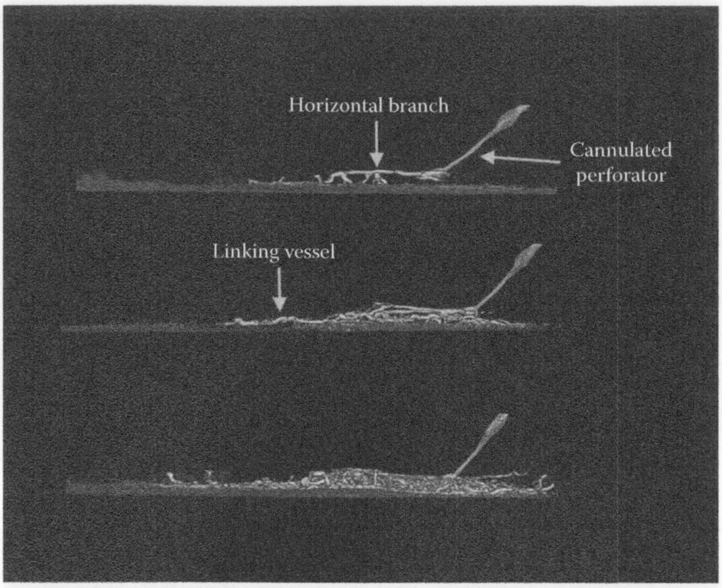

FIGURE 30.17 The linking vessels are found at the level of subdermal plexus, allowing safe thinning of the flap.

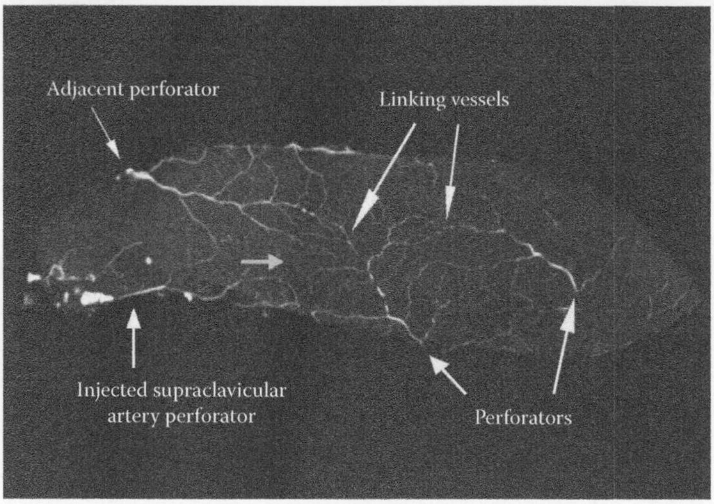

FIGURE 30.18 CT angiography of a supraclavicular flap after injection of iodine contrast (note the presence of linking vessels in perfusion of the flap to the tip).

30.2.3 Internal Mammary Artery Perforator Flap

For the same reasons as previously mentioned, island flaps have always had an important place in the head and neck reconstructive armamentarium, and the deltopectoral flap, described in 1965 by Bakamjian, is a good example. The deltopectoral flap was a workhorse flap for many years despite its known drawbacks such as the necessity to skin graft the donor site, the formation of a dog ear after rotation of the flap, the necessity of a delay procedure, and a high rate of necrosis.[26,81,82] For those reasons, the deltopectoral flap was replaced by the pectoralis major flap described in 1979 by Ariyan.[83] Still used in many indications, the pectoralis major flap has the main disadvantage to be bulky.[26]

It is only after the internal mammary vessels were considered as recipient vessels in breast reconstruction that they were considered potentially donor vessels on which a flap could be based.[84]

In 2006, Yu[85] reported two cases of tracheostoma and anterior neck reconstruction using an IMAP flap. Vesely and Neligan thereafter published cases of anterior neck reconstructions using the IMAP flap.[81,86]

The internal mammary artery (IMA) usually arises from the lower aspect of the subclavian artery. It passes downward, forward, and medially, behind the sternocleidomastoid muscle, the clavicle, and the subclavian and internal jugular veins. It ends at the sixth intercostal space by dividing into its terminal branches, the superior epigastric and musculophrenic arteries.[82] The mean diameter of the IMA was measured at 3.2 mm.[87]

The IMAPs branch off the IMA laterodorsal to the lateral border of the sternum (Figure 30.19). They then pass through the intercostal space, pierce the pectoralis major muscle at its medial border, and penetrate the overlying fascia, subcutaneous tissue, and skin of the ventromedial thorax.[84] Wong described an average of three IMAPs, whereas Morris has found up to five perforators (>0.5 mm) on a hemi-chest.[26,87] The mean length of the IMAPs was measured at 47 mm. All the perforators

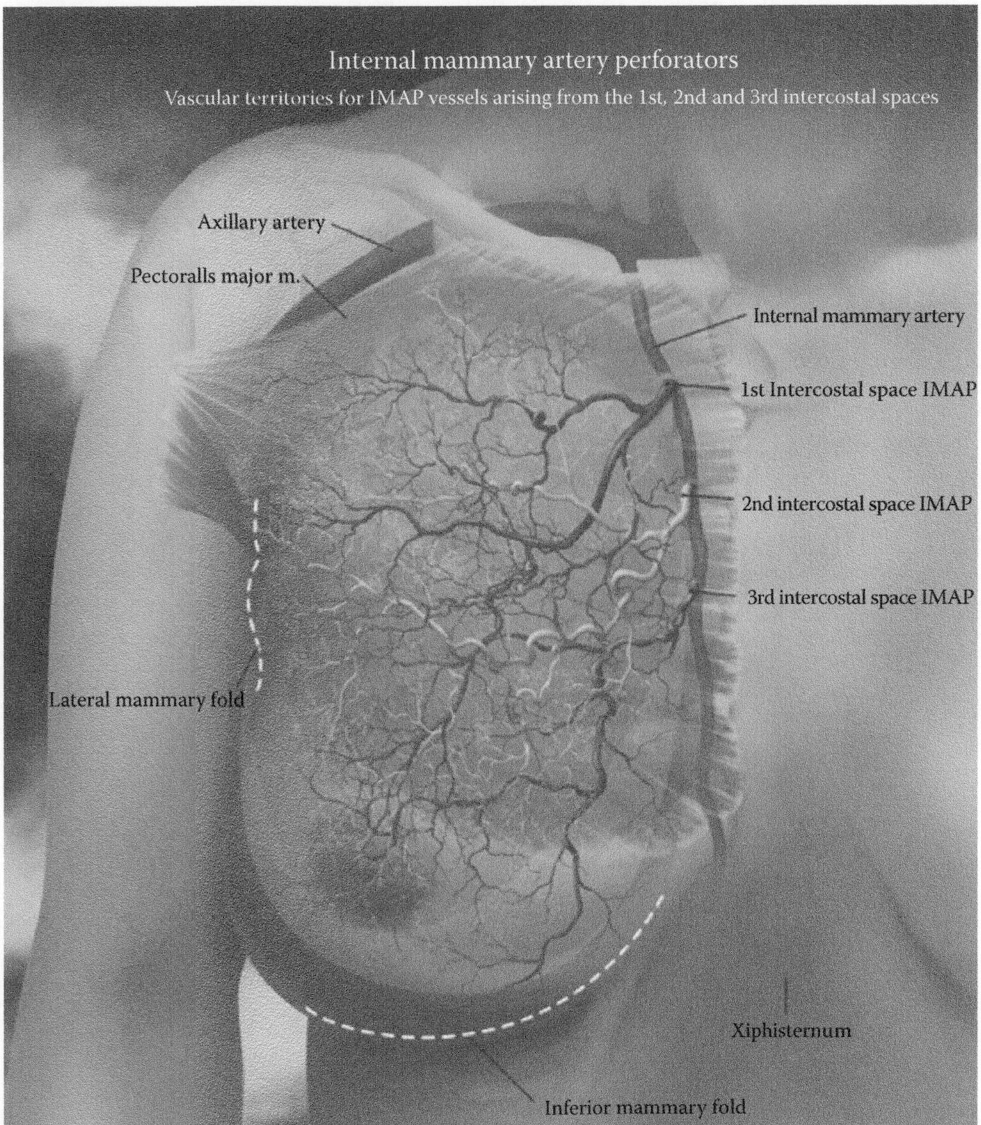

FIGURE 30.19 The IMAP arteries.

were accompanied by the anterior branch of the intercostal nerve,[88] which offers the possibility to harvest sensate IMAP flaps.[89]

The topographic repartition of the IMAP flaps has been described by several authors, consequently to cadaveric dissections and injection studies. All the anatomic studies have confirmed the presence of a dominant IMAP, located in the second intercostal space in more than two-thirds of the population.[26,82,84,87–91] The dominance of one perforator in the perfusion of the chest wall confirms the concept developed by Palmer and Taylor who also found that the largest perforator was at least twice the diameter of the second largest vessel in about 85% cases.[91] There seems to be a symmetric number of perforators on the two hemithorax, but their relative location may vary.[26,82] Two perforators may be found in the same intercostal space. Schmidt relates that this duplication always correlates with a missing perforator on the ipsilateral side, most often in the adjacent territory.[84]

Although there is no physiologic argument for this specific attitude, it is common to include the IMA largest perforator and one or two non-dominant vessels in the flap design.[82,88] Moreover, in a study conducted by Paes et al., it was shown that there was no influence on the size of the flap when including an additional perforator to the largest one. Furthermore, it was even thought to be a main disadvantage since the inclusion of two perforators would require the removal of an extra rib cartilage to obtain the same rotation capacity.[82] There has been no complications relative to the rib cartilage resection reported in the literature but is known to be associated with pneumothorax, contour deformity of the thorax, and intercostal neuralgia.[88]

Based on a previously described technique,[33] Saint-Cyr and Wong have performed injection studies and imaging using a CT scanner. Their findings correlate with the previously described perforasome theory.[34] The flap perfusion was enhanced by the presence of linking vessels establishing a contact between two IMAPs (Figure 30.20) but also between the IMAPs and the lateral thoracic artery (Figure 30.21).

As a consequence of the presence of the linking vessels:

- The distribution pattern of the linking vessels gives a substantial physiologic explanation for the survival of extensive flaps in both superoinferior and mediolateral dimensions. It also gives an additional argument for the collateral flow in the pectoral region, thus preventing devastating effects from ischaemia.
- The linking vessels were found at the level of the subdermal plexus (indirect linking vessels) and between the dermis and the fascia (direct linking vessels), making safe the harvest of the flap in a plane superficial to the pectoralis fascia. Besides, if a thinning of the flap is needed, it can be performed safely until halfway through the thickness of the flap.

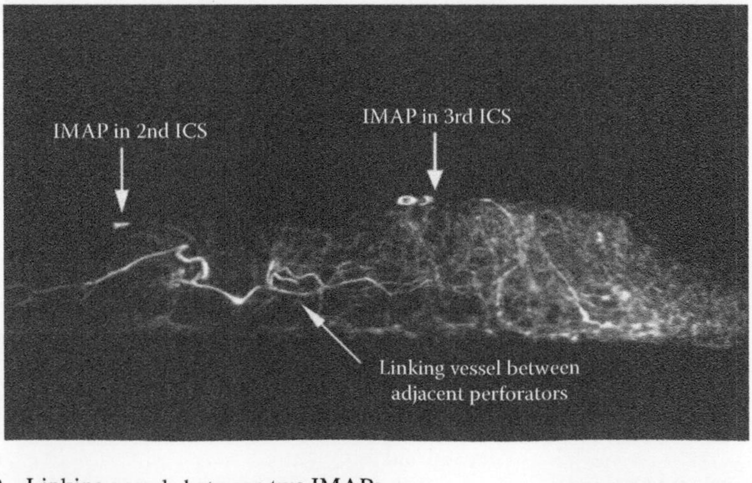

FIGURE 30.20 Linking vessels between two IMAPs.

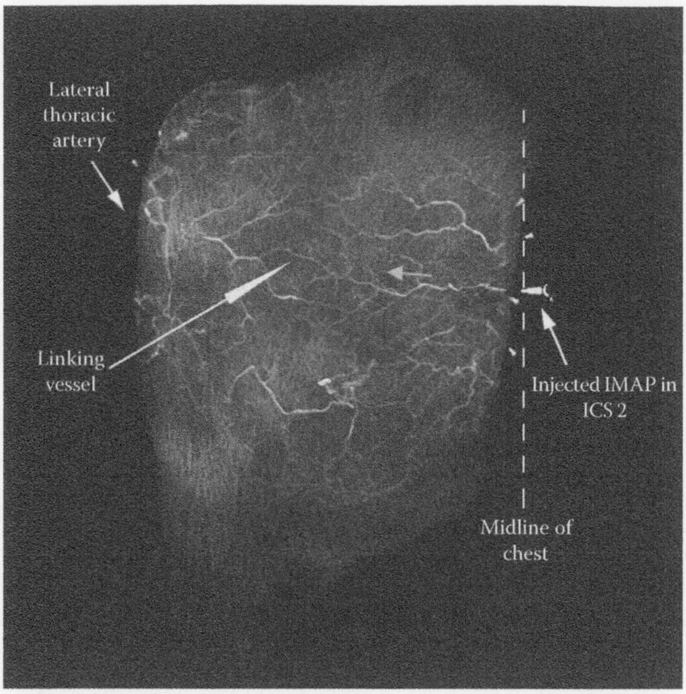

FIGURE 30.21 Linking vessels between an IMAP and the lateral thoracic artery.

- The linking vessels were seen to be transversally oriented at the first and second intercostal spaces, whereas they were inferolaterally oriented for the third intercostal space and below. Based on the perforasome theory, the skin paddle should be designed following the orientations of the linking vessels, transverse above the third intercostal space and oblique inferolateral below the third intercostal space.

The methylene blue injection study performed by Schmidt[84] in which he described flaps as large as 20 × 13 cm correlates with Saint-Cyr and Wong's findings.[26,89] Finally, it has also been used as pre-expanded, enabling the harvest of larger skin paddles while still achieving primary closure. Besides, this pre-expansion led to a thinning of the flap, providing a better match for the thin skin of the neck.[89]

The IMAP flap is most commonly used as a pedicled flap in head and neck reconstruction and has a great arc of rotation (Figure 30.22).

Schellekens[88] defines the *enhanced* vascular pedicle as

Enhanced vascular pedicle = Length of perforator + length of included portion of IMA

The mean length of an IMAP being 47 mm in average, the pedicle can measure 92 mm if the largest perforator is located in the second intercostal space, 104 mm if it is located in the third intercostal space, and 61 mm if it is located in the first intercostal space.

Some authors recommended the use of preoperative imaging under the form of duplex Doppler investigation or 3D CT angiography. With the variations described amongst the internal mammary vessels from a patient to another but also in the contralateral side of the same patient, it is useful to identify the largest perforator preoperatively.[87,88] Particularly, the CT angiography preoperative assessment is now popular in this indication. Despite the common drawbacks of this technique (use of iodine contrast, radiation), it is widely used and allows direct measurement of the perforator diameter. With regard to health-care expenses as well as potential harmful radiations, Schellekens et al.[92]

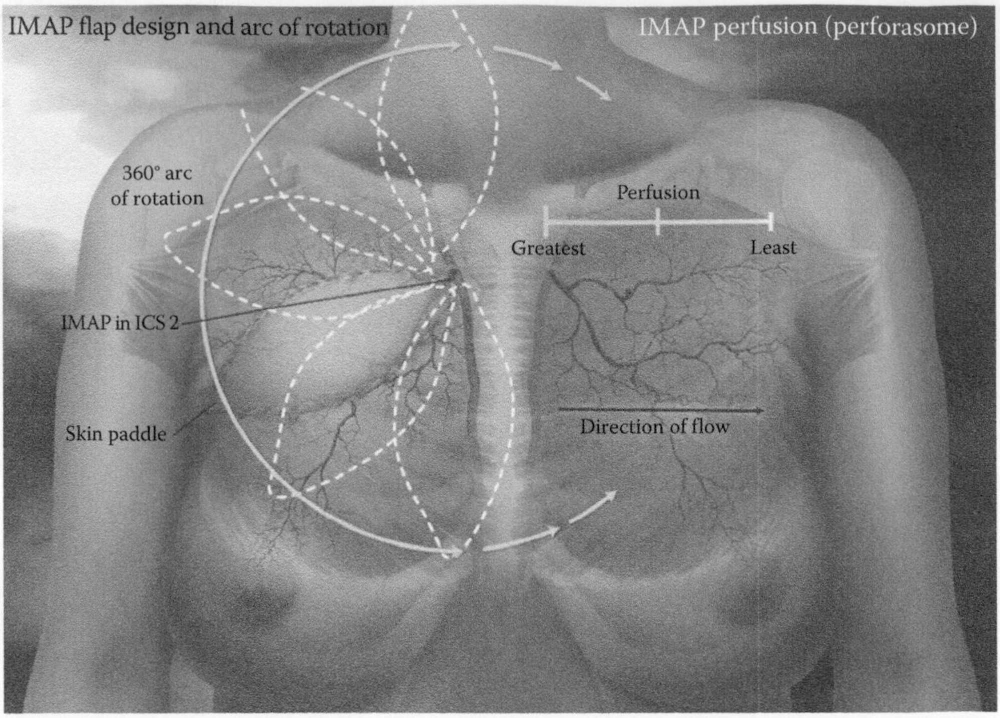

FIGURE 30.22 IMAP flap design and arc of rotation.

proposed to assess first the previous examinations that a patient may have had for any other indication in the past. They have shown that this information is available for a majority of patients, thus avoiding the extra cost and side effects.

In conclusion, the internal mammary perforator flap is a pliable, thin, and reliable flap with a larger arc of rotation when compared to the deltopectoral flap. This flap possesses a good texture and colour match for facial reconstructions but is also useful in breast and thorax reconstructive procedures.[84,87]

30.3 CONCLUSION

In conclusion, we want to emphasise again the benefits of a good vascular knowledge with regard to reconstructive procedures. Anatomy is everything to plastic surgery, and it is just a matter of discovering and understanding it. This chapter summarises several research studies on vascular supply of the flaps in application to perforator flaps of the trunk.

Both functional and cosmetic outcomes must be achieved, and we therefore need to *customise* our reconstructive procedures. This can only be done with a good preoperative planning during imaging, which has a certain role to play.

When both a good knowledge of the anatomy and a wise use of imaging technologies are paired, the surgeon *knows what he is looking for* and will ultimately achieve better results for an increased patient satisfaction.

REFERENCES

1. Devauchelle B, Badet L, Lengele B et al. First human face allograft: Early report. *Lancet* 2006;368(9531):203–209.
2. Petruzzo P, Badet L, Gazarian A et al. Bilateral hand transplantation: Six years after the first case. *Am J Transplant* 2006;6(7):1718–1724.

3. Petit F, Minns AB, Dubernard JM, Hettiaratchy S, Lee WP. Composite tissue allotransplantation and reconstructive surgery: First clinical applications. *Ann Surg* 2003;237(1):19–25.
4. Dubernard JM, Owen E, Herzberg G et al. Human hand allograft: Report on first 6 months. *Lancet* 1999;353(9161):1315–1320.
5. Delaere PR. Tracheal transplantation. *Curr Opin Pulm Med* 2012;18(4):313–320.
6. Siemionow M, Ozturk C. An update on facial transplantation cases performed between 2005 and 2010. *Plast Reconstr Surg* 2011;128(6):707e–720e.
7. Hallock GG. Muscle perforator flaps: The name game. *Ann Plast Surg* 2003;51(6):630–632.
8. Kleintjes WG. Forehead anatomy: Arterial variations and venous link of the midline forehead flap. *J Plast Reconstr Aesthet Surg* 2007;60(6):593–606.
9. Lakhiani C, Lee MR, Saint-Cyr M. Vascular anatomy of the anterolateral thigh flap: A systematic review. *Plast Reconstr Surg* 2012;130(6):1254–1268.
10. Ramirez AR, Gonzalez SM. Arteries of the thumb: Description of anatomical variations and review of the literature. *Plast Reconstr Surg* 2012;129(3):468e–476e.
11. Nahabedian MY. Overview of perforator imaging and flap perfusion technologies. *Clin Plast Surg* 2011;38(2):165–174.
12. Saba L, Atzeni M, Rozen WM et al. Non-invasive vascular imaging in perforator flap surgery. *Acta Radiol* 2013;54(1):89–98.
13. Rozen WM, Paddle AM, Chubb D, Wilson J, Grinsell D, Ashton MW. Guiding local perforator flaps with preoperative imaging: Revealing perforator anatomy to improve flap design. *Plast Reconstr Surg* 2012;130(1):130–134.
14. Haddock NT, Greaney P, Otterburn D, Levine S, Allen RJ. Predicting perforator location on preoperative imaging for the profunda artery perforator flap. *Microsurgery* 2012;32(7):507–511.
15. Tong WM, Dixon R, Ekis H, Halvorson EG. The impact of preoperative CT angiography on breast reconstruction with abdominal perforator flaps. *Ann Plast Surg* 2012;68(5):525–530.
16. Masia J, Kosutic D, Cervelli D, Clavero JA, Monill JM, Pons G. In search of the ideal method in perforator mapping: Noncontrast magnetic resonance imaging. *J Reconstr Microsurg* 2010;26(1):29–35.
17. Masia J, Navarro C, Clavero JA, Alomar X. Noncontrast magnetic resonance imaging for preoperative perforator mapping. *Clin Plast Surg* 2011;38(2):253–261.
18. Lecours C, Saint-Cyr M, Wong C et al. Freestyle pedicle perforator flaps: Clinical results and vascular anatomy. *Plast Reconstr Surg* 2010;126(5):1589–1603.
19. Wei FC, Mardini S. Free-style free flaps. *Plast Reconstr Surg* 2004;114(4):910–916.
20. Wong C, Maia M, Saint-Cyr M. Lateral intercostal artery perforator flap in combination with thoracoabdominal advancement flap for correction of contour deformities following autologous breast reconstruction. *Plast Reconstr Surg* 2011;127(6):156e–158e.
21. Wong C, Mojallal A, Bailey SH, Trussler A, Saint-Cyr M. The extended transverse musculocutaneous gracilis flap: Vascular anatomy and clinical implications. *Ann Plast Surg* 2011;67(2):170–177.
22. Wong C, Saint-Cyr M. Increasing the versatility of the latissimus dorsi skin paddle in breast reconstruction. *Plast Reconstr Surg* 2010;125(1):16e–17e.
23. Wong C, Saint-Cyr M. The pedicled descending branch muscle-sparing latissimus dorsi flap for trunk and upper extremity reconstruction. *J Plast Reconstr Aesthet Surg* 2010;63(4):623–632.
24. Wong C, Saint-Cyr M, Arbique G et al. Three- and four-dimensional computed tomography angiographic studies of commonly used abdominal flaps in breast reconstruction. *Plast Reconstr Surg* 2009;124(1):18–27.
25. Wong C, Saint-Cyr M, Mojallal A et al. Perforasomes of the DIEP flap: Vascular anatomy of the lateral versus medial row perforators and clinical implications. *Plast Reconstr Surg* 2010;125(3):772–782.
26. Wong C, Saint-Cyr M, Rasko Y et al. Three- and four-dimensional arterial and venous perforasomes of the internal mammary artery perforator flap. *Plast Reconstr Surg* 2009;124(6):1759–1769.
27. Schaverien M, Saint-Cyr M, Arbique G, Brown SA. Arterial and venous anatomies of the deep inferior epigastric perforator and superficial inferior epigastric artery flaps. *Plast Reconstr Surg* 2008;121(6):1909–1919.
28. Schaverien M, Saint-Cyr M, Arbique G, Brown SA, Rohrich RJ. Three- and four-dimensional arterial and venous anatomies of the thoracodorsal artery perforator flap. *Plast Reconstr Surg* 2008;121(5):1578–1587.
29. Schaverien M, Saint-Cyr M, Arbique G, Hatef D, Brown SA, Rohrich RJ. Three- and four-dimensional computed tomographic angiography and venography of the anterolateral thigh perforator flap. *Plast Reconstr Surg* 2008;121(5):1685–1696.
30. Schaverien M, Wong C, Bailey S, Saint-Cyr M. Thoracodorsal artery perforator flap and Latissimus dorsi myocutaneous flap—Anatomical study of the constant skin paddle perforator locations. *J Plast Reconstr Aesthet Surg* 2010;63(12):2123–2127.

31. Schaverien M, Saint-Cyr M. Perforators of the lower leg: Analysis of perforator locations and clinical application for pedicled perforator flaps. *Plast Reconstr Surg* 2008;122(1):161–170.
32. Saint-Cyr M, Mujadzic M, Wong C, Hatef D, Lajoie AS, Rohrich RJ. The radial artery pedicle perforator flap: Vascular analysis and clinical implications. *Plast Reconstr Surg* 2010;125(5):1469–1478.
33. Saint-Cyr M, Schaverien M, Arbique G, Hatef D, Brown SA, Rohrich RJ. Three- and four-dimensional computed tomographic angiography and venography for the investigation of the vascular anatomy and perfusion of perforator flaps. *Plast Reconstr Surg* 2008;121(3):772–780.
34. Saint-Cyr M, Wong C, Schaverien M, Mojallal A, Rohrich RJ. The perforasome theory: Vascular anatomy and clinical implications. *Plast Reconstr Surg* 2009;124(5):1529–1544.
35. Bergeron L, Tang M, Morris SF. A review of vascular injection techniques for the study of perforator flaps. *Plast Reconstr Surg* 2006;117(6):2050–2057.
36. Geddes CR, Morris SF, Neligan PC. Perforator flaps: Evolution, classification, and applications. *Ann Plast Surg* 2003;50(1):90–99.
37. Saint-Cyr M, Schaverien MV, Rohrich RJ. Perforator flaps: History, controversies, physiology, anatomy, and use in reconstruction. *Plast Reconstr Surg* 2009;123(4):132e–145e.
38. Sinna R, Qassemyar Q, Perignon D, Benhaim T, Robbe M. About perforator flaps…20 years later. *Ann Chir Plast Esthet* 2011;56(2):128–133.
39. Koshima I, Soeda S. Inferior epigastric artery skin flaps without rectus abdominis muscle. *Br J Plast Surg* 1989;42(6):645–648.
40. Atik B, Tan O, Mutaf M, Senel B, Yilmaz N, Kiymaz N. Skin perforators of back region: Anatomical study and clinical applications. *Ann Plast Surg* 2008;60(1):70–75.
41. Hallock GG. Anatomic basis of the gastrocnemius perforator-based flap. *Ann Plast Surg* 2001;47(5):517–522.
42. Hamdi M, Spano A, Van Landuyt K, D'Herde K, Blondeel P, Monstrey S. The lateral intercostal artery perforators: Anatomical study and clinical application in breast surgery. *Plast Reconstr Surg* 2008;121(2):389–396.
43. Hamdi M, Van Landuyt K, de Frene B, Roche N, Blondeel P, Monstrey S. The versatility of the intercostal artery perforator (ICAP) flaps. *J Plast Reconstr Aesthet Surg* 2006;59(6):644–652.
44. Heitmann C, Guerra A, Metzinger SW, Levin LS, Allen RJ. The thoracodorsal artery perforator flap: Anatomic basis and clinical application. *Ann Plast Surg* 2003;51(1):23–29.
45. Koshima I, Moriguchi T, Soeda S, Kawata S, Ohta S, Ikeda A. The gluteal perforator-based flap for repair of sacral pressure sores. *Plast Reconstr Surg* 1993;91(4):678–683.
46. Kato H, Hasegawa M, Takada T, Torii S. The lumbar artery perforator based island flap: Anatomical study and case reports. *Br J Plast Surg* 1999;52(7):541–546.
47. Minabe T, Harii K. Dorsal intercostal artery perforator flap: Anatomical study and clinical applications. *Plast Reconstr Surg* 2007;120(3):681–689.
48. Moscatiello F, Masia J, Carrera A, Clavero JA, Larranaga JR, Pons G. The 'propeller' distal anteromedial thigh perforator flap. Anatomic study and clinical applications. *J Plast Reconstr Aesthet Surg* 2007;60(12):1323–1330.
49. Mun GH, Lee SJ, Jeon BJ. Perforator topography of the thoracodorsal artery perforator flap. *Plast Reconstr Surg* 2008;121(2):497–504.
50. Ogawa R, Hyakusoku H, Murakami M, Aoki R, Tanuma K, Pennington DG. An anatomical and clinical study of the dorsal intercostal cutaneous perforators, and application to free microvascular augmented subdermal vascular network (ma-SVN) flaps. *Br J Plast Surg* 2002;55(5):396–401.
51. Rad AN, Singh NK, Rosson GD. Peroneal artery perforator-based propeller flap reconstruction of the lateral distal lower extremity after tumor extirpation: Case report and literature review. *Microsurgery* 2008;28(8):663–670.
52. Thione A, Valdatta L, Buoro M, Tuinder S, Mortarino C, Putz R. The medial sural artery perforators: Anatomic basis for a surgical plan. *Ann Plast Surg* 2004;53(3):250–255.
53. Taylor GI, Palmer JH. The vascular territories (angiosomes) of the body: Experimental study and clinical applications. *Br J Plast Surg* 1987;40(2):113–141.
54. Rozen WM, Ashton MW, Le Roux CM, Pan WR, Corlett RJ. The perforator angiosome: A new concept in the design of deep inferior epigastric artery perforator flaps for breast reconstruction. *Microsurgery* 2010;30(1):1–7.
55. Taylor GI, Corlett RJ, Dhar SC, Ashton MW. The anatomical (angiosome) and clinical territories of cutaneous perforating arteries: Development of the concept and designing safe flaps. *Plast Reconstr Surg* 2011;127(4):1447–1459.

56. Taylor GI. The angiosomes of the body and their supply to perforator flaps. *Clin Plast Surg* 2003;30(3):331–342, v.
57. Angrigiani C, Grilli D, Siebert J. Latissimus dorsi musculocutaneous flap without muscle. *Plast Reconstr Surg* 1995;96(7):1608–1614.
58. Maxwell GP. Iginio Tansini and the origin of the latissimus dorsi musculocutaneous flap. *Plast Reconstr Surg* 1980;65(5):686–692.
59. Sever C, Uygur F, Kulahci Y, Karagoz H, Sahin C. Thoracodorsal artery perforator fasciocutaneous flap: A versatile alternative for coverage of various soft tissue defects. *Indian J Plast Surg* 2012;45(3):478–484.
60. Hamdi M, Van Landuyt K, Hijjawi JB, Roche N, Blondeel P, Monstrey S. Surgical technique in pedicled thoracodorsal artery perforator flaps: A clinical experience with 99 patients. *Plast Reconstr Surg* 2008;121(5):1632–1641.
61. Thomas BP, Geddes CR, Tang M, Williams J, Morris SF. The vascular basis of the thoracodorsal artery perforator flap. *Plast Reconstr Surg* 2005;116(3):818–822.
62. Spinelli HM, Fink JA, Muzaffar AR. The latissimus dorsi perforator-based fasciocutaneous flap. *Ann Plast Surg* 1996;37(5):500–506.
63. Guerra AB, Metzinger SE, Lund KM, Cooper MM, Allen RJ, Dupin CL. The thoracodorsal artery perforator flap: Clinical experience and anatomic study with emphasis on harvest techniques. *Plast Reconstr Surg* 2004;114(1):32–41; discussion 42–33.
64. Schwabegger AH, Bodner G, Ninkovic M, Piza-Katzer H. Thoracodorsal artery perforator (TAP) flap: Report of our experience and review of the literature. *Br J Plast Surg* 2002;55(5):390–395.
65. Kim JT, Kim SK. Hand resurfacing with the superthin latissimus dorsi perforator-based free flap. *Plast Reconstr Surg* 2003;111(1):366–370.
66. Kim JT, Koo BS, Kim SK. The thin latissimus dorsi perforator-based free flap for resurfacing. *Plast Reconstr Surg* 2001;107(2):374–382.
67. Lyons AJ. Perforator flaps in head and neck surgery. *Int J Oral Maxillofac Surg* 2006;35(3):199–207.
68. Granzow JW, Suliman A, Roostaeian J, Perry A, Boyd JB. The supraclavicular artery island flap (SCAIF) for head and neck reconstruction: Surgical technique and refinements. *Otolaryngol Head Neck Surg* 2013;148(6):933–940.
69. Chiu ES, Liu PH, Friedlander PL. Supraclavicular artery island flap for head and neck oncologic reconstruction: Indications, complications, and outcomes. *Plast Reconstr Surg* 2009;124(1):115–123.
70. Pallua N, Machens HG, Rennekampff O, Becker M, Berger A. The fasciocutaneous supraclavicular artery island flap for releasing postburn mentosternal contractures. *Plast Reconstr Surg* 1997;99(7):1878–1884; discussion 1885–1876.
71. Lamberty BG. The supra-clavicular axial patterned flap. *Br J Plast Surg* 1979;32(3):207–212.
72. Di Benedetto G, Aquinati A, Pierangeli M, Scalise A, Bertani A. From the "charretera" to the supraclavicular fascial island flap: Revisitation and further evolution of a controversial flap. *Plast Reconstr Surg* 2005;115(1):70–76.
73. Lamberty BG, Cormack GC. Misconceptions regarding the cervico-humeral flap. *Br J Plast Surg* 1983;36(1):60–63.
74. Pallua N, Magnus Noah E. The tunneled supraclavicular island flap: An optimized technique for head and neck reconstruction. *Plast Reconstr Surg* 2000;105(3):842–851; discussion 852–844.
75. Pallua N, Demir E. Postburn head and neck reconstruction in children with the fasciocutaneous supraclavicular artery island flap. *Ann Plast Surg* 2008;60(3):276–282.
76. Adams AS, Wright MJ, Johnston S et al. The use of multislice CT angiography preoperative study for supraclavicular artery island flap harvesting. *Ann Plast Surg* 2012;69(3):312–315.
77. Cordova A, D'Arpa S, Pirrello R, Brenner E, Jeschke J, Moschella F. Anatomic study on the transverse cervical vessels perforators in the lateral triangle of the neck and harvest of a new flap: The free supraclavicular transverse cervical artery perforator flap. *Surg Radiol Anat* 2009;31(2):93–100.
78. Chen WL, Zhang DM, Yang ZH et al. Extended supraclavicular fasciocutaneous island flap based on the transverse cervical artery for head and neck reconstruction after cancer ablation. *J Oral Maxillofac Surg* 2010;68(10):2422–2430.
79. Abe M, Murakami G, Abe S, Sakakura Y, Yajima T. Supraclavicular artery in Japanese: An anatomical basis for the flap using a pedicle containing a cervical, non-perforating cutaneous branch of the superficial cervical artery. *Okajimas Folia Anat Jpn* 2000;77(5):149–154.
80. Liu PH, Chiu ES. Supraclavicular artery flap: A new option for pharyngeal reconstruction. *Ann Plast Surg* 2009;62(5):497–501.

81. Neligan PC, Gullane PJ, Vesely M, Murray D. The internal mammary artery perforator flap: New variation on an old theme. *Plast Reconstr Surg* 2007;119(3):891–893.
82. Paes EC, Schellekens PP, Hage JJ, van der Wal MB, Bleys RL, Kon M. A cadaver study of the vascular territories of dominant and nondominant internal mammary artery perforators. *Ann Plast Surg* 2011;67(1):68–72.
83. Ariyan S. The pectoralis major myocutaneous flap. A versatile flap for reconstruction in the head and neck. *Plast Reconstr Surg* 1979;63(1):73–81.
84. Schmidt M, Aszmann OC, Beck H, Frey M. The anatomic basis of the internal mammary artery perforator flap: A cadaver study. *J Plast Reconstr Aesthet Surg* 2010;63(2):191–196.
85. Yu P, Roblin P, Chevray P. Internal mammary artery perforator (IMAP) flap for tracheostoma reconstruction. *Head Neck* 2006;28(8):723–729.
86. Vesely MJ, Murray DJ, Novak CB, Gullane PJ, Neligan PC. The internal mammary artery perforator flap: An anatomical study and a case report. *Ann Plast Surg* 2007;58(2):156–161.
87. Gillis JA, Prasad V, Morris SF. Three-dimensional analysis of the internal mammary artery perforator flap. *Plast Reconstr Surg* 2011;128(5):419e–426e.
88. Schellekens PP, Paes EC, Hage JJ, van der Wal MB, Bleys RL, Kon M. Anatomy of the vascular pedicle of the internal mammary artery perforator (IMAP) flap as applied for head and neck reconstruction. *J Plast Reconstr Aesthet Surg* 2011;64(1):53–57.
89. Saint-Cyr M, Schaverien M, Rohrich RJ. Preexpanded second intercostal space internal mammary artery pedicle perforator flap: Case report and anatomical study. *Plast Reconstr Surg* 2009;123(6):1659–1664.
90. Rosson GD, Holton LH, Silverman RP, Singh NK, Nahabedian MY. Internal mammary perforators: A cadaver study. *J Reconstr Microsurg* 2005;21(4):239–242.
91. Palmer JH, Taylor GI. The vascular territories of the anterior chest wall. *Br J Plast Surg* 1986;39(3):287–299.
92. Schellekens PP, Aukema TS, Hage JJ, Prevoo W, Kon M. Can previous diagnostic examinations prevent preoperative angiographic assessment of the internal mammary perforators for (micro)surgical use? *Ann Plast Surg* 2014;72(5):560–565.

31 Phalloplasty in Female-to-Male Sex Reassignment Surgery

Zdeněk Dvořák and Jiří Veselý

CONTENTS

31.1 INTRODUCTION

The goals of penile reconstruction are an aesthetic acceptable penis and its triple function:

1. To have 'something more in pants'
2. To enable urination in the standing position
3. To allow penetration during sexual intercourse

These conditions make the desired result particularly challenging.

There were two schools of penis and urethra reconstruction – the classic reconstruction using tubed flaps (Gillies and Harrison 1948, Hester 1978, Hentz et al. 1987, Laub et al. 1989, Exner 1992) requiring a multistage operation and a one-stage microsurgical reconstruction (Chang and Hwang 1984, Gilbert 1986, Gilbert et al. 1987, Biemer 1988, Hage 1992, Veselý et al. 1992). Followers of the classic school emphasise the size of the reconstructed penis, which can be, at least in some cases, really huge (Veselý et al. 2002). A really difficult step in this case is to form a functional urethra, as healing is often complicated by stenosis or fistulas. Urethral strictures are more common especially in cases where a skin graft is used.

On the other hand, microsurgical reconstructions are usually one-stage procedures. The size of the constructed phallus depends on the kind of flap employed and the thickness of the subcutaneous tissue. The most significant advantage of Chang's microsurgical reconstruction technique of the urethra (Chang and Hwang 1984) is the good supply of the urethra, and in our experience, this is ensured by Biemer's flap with a longer urethral part inserted to the middle of the flap where the forearm is out of hair zones (Biemer 1988).

Nowadays, one-stage microsurgical reconstruction is usually preferred.

The development of procedures for phalloplasty has followed those of the reconstructive surgery. The principal phalloplasty techniques are reviewed from a historical point of view, but many of them are still commonly employed.

31.1.1 Tubulised Flap

Bogoras (1936) first reported a total penile reconstruction in 1936. After him, several different procedures with local flaps have been described and published by different authors (Gillies and Harrison 1948, Orticochea 1972, Matti et al. 1988, Santi et al. 1988, Cheng et al. 1995, Petrovic 1995). Results of these techniques, often requiring multiple procedures, frequently dissatisfied the patients. An important role was played by the Maltz–Gillies technique of penile and urethra reconstruction by means of a tubed abdominal bipedicled flap to construct the urethra by the so-called 'tube within a tube' technique (Maltz 1946, Gillies and Harrison 1948, Gillies and Millard 1957). This method of phalloplasty has been applied for decades up to the present. Its principal concept consists of raising a narrow skin strip in the mesogastrium up to the hypogastrium, creating the urethra by suturing the flap over a catheter and by mobilising another skin flap from the side of the previous one, thus creating two tubes – inside the urethra and outside the penis. Gillies also made this technique popular by implanting a costal graft inside the penis.

Another widespread phalloplasty technique was Stanford bipedicled infra-umbilical skin flap 'reported by a surgery team from Stanford, Palo Alto, California. The flap was raised in the vertical line between the navel and the pubic area in such a way that the penis could be formed only by dissection of a proximal pedicle. Thus, the number of transfers to the definitive site was reduced. The flap is predominantly supplied by blood from the inferior pedicle from the superficial external pudendal vessels (Laub et al. 1989). Another part of Laub's concept was the modelling of a blind pocket from a part of the flap to create a cavity for temporary insertion of a stiffener. An improvement on this reconstruction method was the incorporation of a microsurgical sensitive forearm flap (FF) on the radial vessels – the Chinese flap – to form the urethra and glans (Hentz et al. 1987, Laub et al. 1989).

Hester et al. (1978) performed a single-stage penile reconstruction with the infra-umbilical flap using a vertically located branch of superficial inferior epigastric vessels in a subcutaneous pedicle. The name of this surgical technique is the single subcutaneous pedicled infra-umbilical flap. As opposed to the previous infra-umbilical flaps, the pedicle was not formed by the cutaneous tissue of the flap, but only by the subcutaneous tissue, incorporating the vessels running laterally from the midline. Thus, the pedicle base was located laterally on the pubic area and not in the midline as in the previous methods. Bouman (1987) reported using these pedicles on both sides of the infra-umbilical flap. The midline flap had two subcutaneous pedicles including superficial inferior epigastric vessels.

The pedicled groin flap belongs to the other classic methods as the method of choice for phallus reconstruction (Puckett and Montie 1978). Currently, it is one of the most frequently used classical techniques. Exner (1992) used bilateral groin flaps to cover a rectus abdominis muscular flap, which incorporated a prosthesis. Puckett (1978) reported the use of the groin flap and a hydraulic prosthesis.

Morales and co-workers (1956) and later Julian et al. (1969) used a single tubed skin flap from the thigh in oncological patients with a scarred abdomen or patients after radiotherapy. Kaplan and Wesser used a proximally pedicled thigh flap to reconstruct a sensitive phallus (Kaplan and Wesser 1971). The tubed scapular flap as inner 'tube in tube within tube' was reported by Veselý et al. (1992).

Pedicled musculocutaneous flap (m. gracilis [Orticochea 1972, Horton et al. 1977], m. rectus abdominis [Santi et al. 1988]) did not provide the expected results because of denervating atrophy of the muscles.

31.1.2 Microsurgical Penile Reconstruction

In the 1980s, microsurgery has created dramatic changes in many fields. The introductions of microvascular free flap transfer have started a new era for reconstructive surgery with a great impact in phalloplasty. Microsurgery now represents the conditio sine qua non (ultimate condition) to obtain the best result in this procedure (Pucket 1982, Chang and Hwang 1984, Upton et al. 1987, Biemer 1988, Harashina et al. 1990, Sadove and McRoberts 1992, Hage et al. 1993b). Recently, some authors have described useful techniques with local flaps for those cases of neophalloplasty where microsurgery is not possible (Hage 1996, Mutaf 2001).

Microsurgical penile reconstruction provides a one-stage method of creating the phallus and the urethra usually at the same time. But the urethra can be formed secondarily too. The preferred and most frequently used flap is the forearm fasciocutaneous flap (Chang and Hwang 1984). Biemer (1988) devised a method using the long part of the flap to form the urethra – pars fixa urethrae – so that it could span the width between the external orifice and the urethra in the phallus. Biemer also used a flap with a radial bone graft.

Nowadays, authors prefer to build functional penis using free latissimus dorsi musculocutaneous flap with motoric nerve suture.

31.2 PHALLOPLASTY BY MICROVASCULAR RECONSTRUCTION

31.2.1 Standard Techniques

Currently, two standard types of free flaps are used for neophalloplasties: latissimus dorsi musculocutaneous free flap and radial forearm free flap. Both methods are offered to the patients and pros and cons are discussed in detail. Majority of them prefer reconstruction with latissimus dorsi free flap. All patients know risks of complications in the case of urethra reconstruction, and many of them prefer single-stage procedure without subsequent urethra reconstruction.

The ideal goal of total penile reconstruction makes this surgery particularly challenging. A natural looking and functioning man's phallus does not seem to be achievable yet. All actual methods of reconstruction are associated with multitude of problems. The cosmetic result is remarkably demanding but it might be easier to obtain appearance rather than to fulfil functional requirements of this organ. An ideal neophallus should permit the patient to urinate in a standing position and to engage in sexual intercourse with erogenous sensations. The complications joined with these two functions are fistula formation and loss of rigidity.

31.2.1.1 Forearm Flap

One of the standard techniques is to create the penis, glans, and urethra from one fasciocutaneous sensitive FF with a microsurgical transfer to the pubic area and a primary anastomosis to the urethral orifice. The basic principle, on which the design of shape and location of the flap on the forearm are based, is the fact that the urethra must be constructed from the hairless part of the forearm, that is, on the ventral side along the longitudinal axis. The urethra is sutured over a catheter Chapter 18. The length of the flap, forming the neourethra, is as a rule 16–20 cm. This length is made up of three parts:

1. Pars fixa urethrae – approx. 4–7 cm long
2. Pars pendularis urethrae incorporated in the shaft of the neophallus – 9–10 cm long
3. Another flap part, forming the glans and the urethra inside – 3 cm long

On both sides of the pars pendularis urethrae, there are two de-epithelialised skin strips 0.5 cm wide, and the lateral parts of the flap form the shaft of the penis after suturing. These parts of the flap have dimensions of 10 × 5–7 cm.

The most distal part of the flap, forming the glans, is also separated from the lateral parts of the flap by a strip of de-epithelialised skin of the same width as around the urethra.

The flap is situated on the forearm in such a way that the radial vascular bundle is placed approximately on the radial border of the urinary conduit along with the radial cutaneous nerve. The flap is circumcised in ischaemia of forearm and the marked skin strips are de-epithelialised. Then it is isolated over the whole area and raised, and the individual structures are sutured together around a catheter.

The neophallus and the urethra are transferred to the pubic region over the clitoris, where a second surgical team has prepared the recipient vessels and nerve – deep inferior epigastric vessels and ilioinguinal nerve. All three vessels, that is, radial artery and both venae commitantes, are anastomosed subcutaneously, using an end-to-end technique. Further, the greater saphenous vein is prepared in the left groin from the isolated incision and is anastomosed to a cephalic or basilic vein of the flap.

With the patient in the gynaecological position, the outer orifice of the female urethra is circumcised, and the reconstructed pars fixa of the urethrae along with a ball catheter are inserted through a subcutaneous tunnel in the labium major. The ball catheter is inserted into the urinary bladder. Anastomosis of both orifices is performed with absorbable suture 5/0.

When using the fascial FF, the size of the penis is limited by the forearm length, its circumference, and the quantity of subcutaneous fat. It is the author's opinion that it is possible to use the fasciocutaneous FF with the radial vessels and another two large venous sinuses, v. cephalica and v. basilica, taking almost the entire circumference of the forearm, thus including the territory of skin supplied by the ulnar artery.

Using standard FF technique, no inner stiffener of the phallus is used. The patients are usually advised to employ a removable PVC splint in the shape of the eaves of a roof attached to the penis by means of two condoms (Trengove-Jones 1993). Since its first report (Chang and Hwang 1984, Biemer 1988), the radial forearm free flap represented for many years the gold standard procedure in phallus reconstruction, allowing to achieve the result also in a *one-stage* procedure. Despite the anatomic and clinical advantages of this technique for phalloplasty, the outcome of reconstruction is still far from an optimal result. The limits in sexual function became more evident after several years of the application of this and similar procedures. The use of transplants and implants in order to obtain sufficient rigidity for penetration has often led to complications and failures of different free and pedicle flaps (Koshima et al. 1986, Jordan et al. 1994, Hage 1997). Autologous cartilage and bone transplants, used to avoid these complications, cause a permanent rigidity which is embarrassing to the patient. Moreover, these tissues tend to resorb, curve, or fracture (Jordan et al. 1994). Conversely, alloplastic prostheses have the possibility to give an erection to the neophallus, although they are expensive and have a tendency to infection, tissue erosion, and extrusion. These frequent complications led the surgeons to modify the techniques (Upton et al. 1987, Sasaki et al. 1999) and to adopt new ones (Tobin et al. 1981, Sun and Huang 1985, Gilbert et al. 1987, 1995, Davies and Matti 1993, Hage et al. 1993a, Petrovic 1995, Hage 1996, Mutaf 2000, Akoz and Kargi 2002).

Also, the forearm donor site scars represent nowadays stigmata (sign of recognition) for female-to-male transsexual patients and motivate surgeons to search for different donor areas.

31.2.1.2 Latissimus Dorsi Flap

The second standard technique is the use of a free latissimus dorsi flap.

Since Tansini first described the use of the latissimus dorsi flap, the latissimus is widely used in reconstructive surgery. Its neural anatomy has been extensively described (Hallock 2004), and its employ to restore muscular function continuously shows new horizons particularly as a free newly innervated flap (Adamian 1996). Adamian was the first to use latissimus dorsi flap for total phalloplasty (Veselý et al. 1992).

The autors used the following procedure during the reconstruction of the penis. The surgical technique starts with a longitudinal lazy *S* or transverse incision along the medial region of the thigh to expose the recipient neurovascular pedicle of gracilis muscle (medial circumflex femoral vessels and motoric branch of the obturator nerve). A myocutaneous latissimus dorsi free flap (average 16 × 12.5 cm paddle of skin and 14 × 4 cm calf of muscle) is planned on the back (Figure 31.1). The flap is harvested protecting carefully the musculocutaneous perforators of lateral branch of the thoracodorsal vessels that nourish the skin paddle (Figure 31.2). The flap is then rolled into a cylinder to obtain the desired shape and sutured together (Figures 31.1 through 31.3).

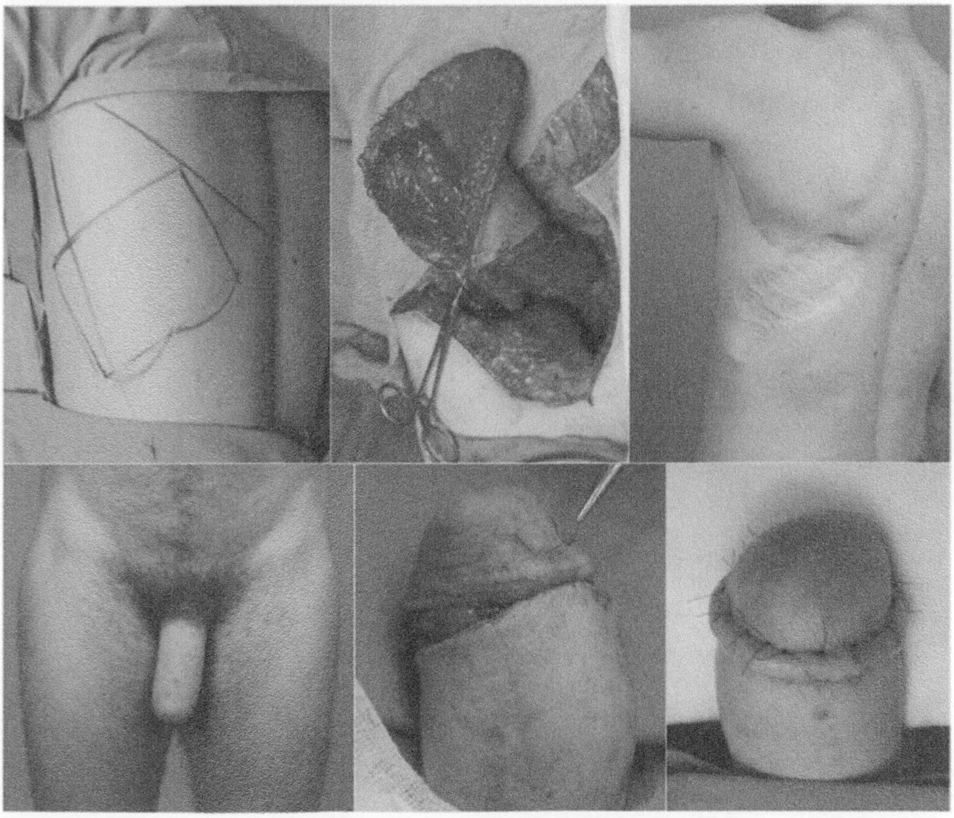

FIGURE 31.1 Above left – Preoperative drawing of latissimus dorsi myocutaneous flap. Above centre – The flap is harvested, rolled into a cylinder, and sutured. Above right – Donor site scar 1 year after surgery. Below left – Clinical result 6 months after surgery. Below centre and right – Intraoperative view of second-stage glans plasty.

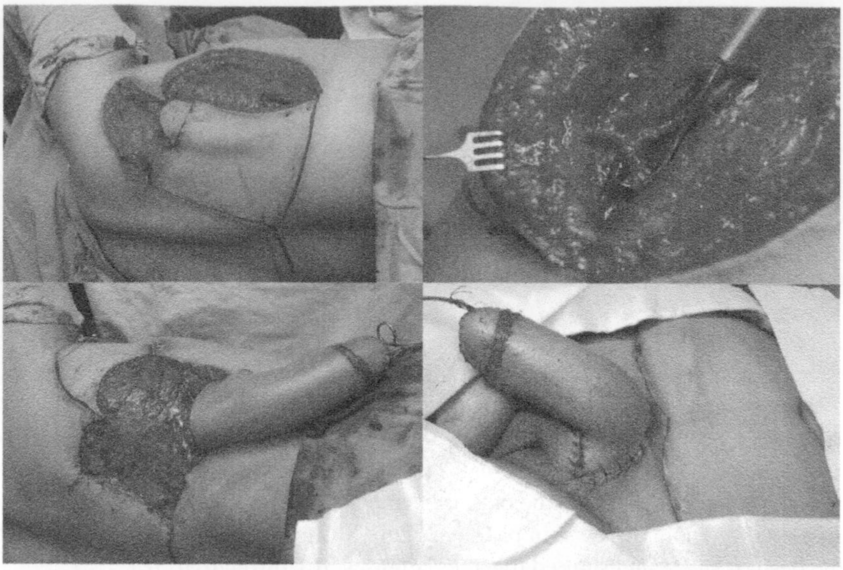

FIGURE 31.2 Above left – Intraoperative view of latissimus dorsi harvesting. Above right – Flap pedicle dissection. Below left – The flap is rolled into a cylinder and sutured. Below right – Pedicle vessel anastomoses are completed and the flap is sutured to the recipient area; glans plasty is performed at the same stage.

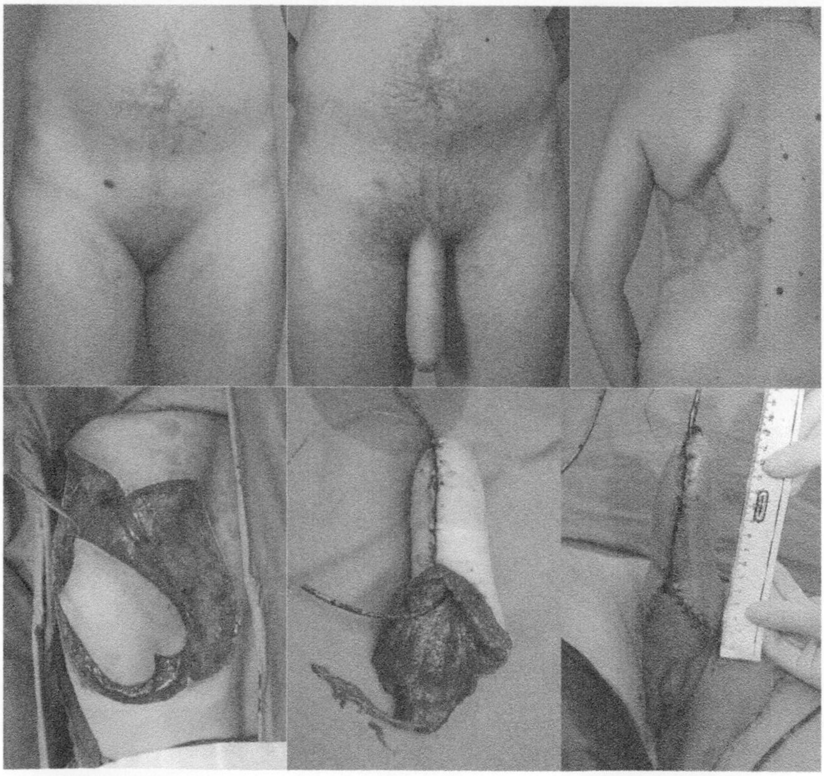

FIGURE 31.3 Above left – Preoperative view. Above centre – Clinical result 1 year after phalloplasty with a latissimus dorsi myocutaneous flap. Above right – Donor site scar 1 year after surgery. Below left – Latissimus dorsi myocutaneous flap harvesting. Below centre – The flap is rolled into a cylinder and sutured. Below right – Pedicle vessel anastomoses are completed and the flap is sutured to the recipient area.

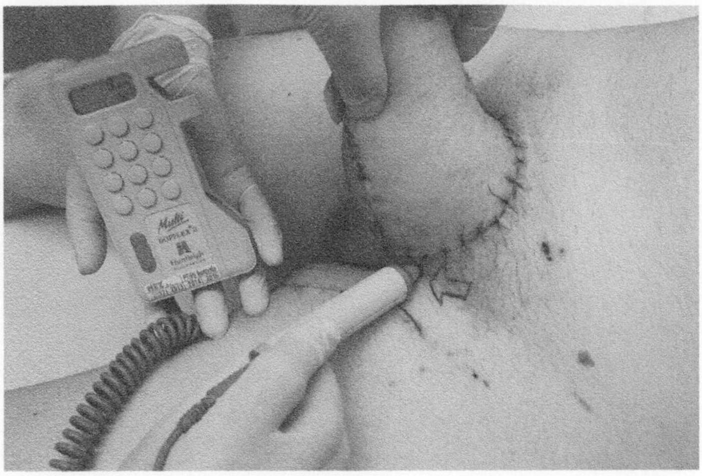

FIGURE 31.4 Monitoring of the flap ensured by Doppler.

The neurovascular thoracodorsal pedicle is divided at its origin. The flap is then transferred and sutured to the recipient area (Figures 31.2 and 31.3).

The thoracodorsal pedicle is passed through a subcutaneous tunnel to the thigh and then sutured end to end to the medial circumflex femoral artery and one comitant vein. End-to-end motor nerve coaptation is achieved with the anterior branch of the obturator nerve to the gracilis muscle. On the back, the donor site is partly sutured directly and an area of average 5 × 8 cm is skin mesh grafted (Figures 31.1 and 31.3).

Postoperatively, the monitoring of the flap is ensured by Doppler in A mode on the radix of a neopenis. The site of monitoring is marked with an indelible marker (Figure 31.4). The electrostimulation of sutured motor nerve and muscle of penis flap is performed 2–4 times a week until satisfactory voluntary movement of the muscle is obtained (Figures 31.5 and 31.6).

The first function in female-to-male transsexuals frequently follows the urine passage in the neourethra (Jordan et al. 1987, Biemer 1988, Hage and Bloem 1993, Byun et al. 1994). Some patient required subsequent reconstruction of the urethra even if they were aware of the theoretical disadvantage of a three-stage reconstruction and risk of fistula formation. The advantage of using a full-thickness skin grafting of the main flap or vascularised portion of a separate flap remains theoretical (Tamai et al. 1970). These previous experiences convinced the authors to use a separate free flap to reconstruct the urethra. Radial forearm free flap for urethral reconstruction achieved this objective with minimal donor site morbidity and high overall satisfaction in our previous studies (Hage et al. 1993b, Veselý 1996,

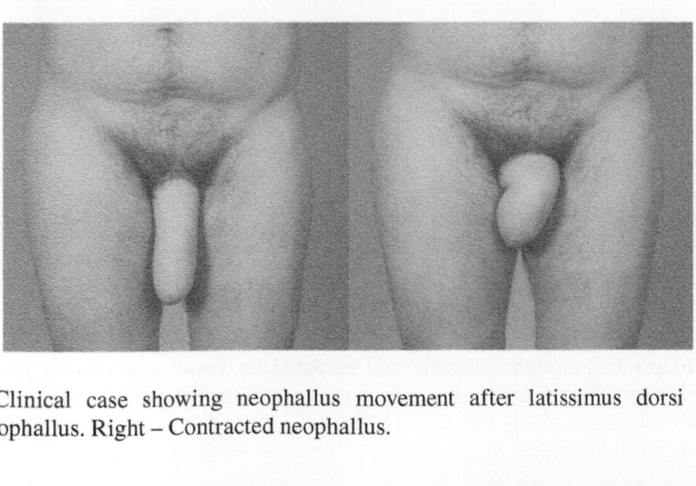

FIGURE 31.5 Clinical case showing neophallus movement after latissimus dorsi flap phalloplasty. Left – Relaxed neophallus. Right – Contracted neophallus.

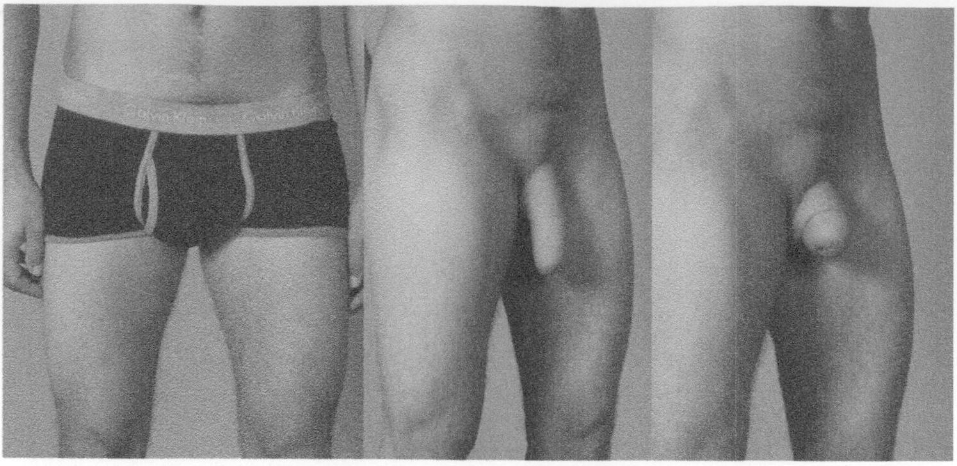

FIGURE 31.6 Clinical case showing neophallus movement after latissimus dorsi flap phalloplasty. Left – Relaxed neophallus. Right – Contracted neophallus.

Veselý et al. 1999, Veselý and Haage 1999). In the author's opinion, thinner and less hairy radial forearm free flap is more advantageous for urethral reconstruction despite lesser donor site morbidity of lateral arm free flap. If the patient desires urethra reconstruction, it is reconstructed in a second-stage procedure about 6 months later with a radial forearm free flap (15–17 cm length, 3 cm width). The flap is tubed around the catheter Ch. 18 and placed inside the anterior side of the neophallus into the subcutaneous tissue (Figure 31.7). The suture of the tube is buried in proximity to the surface of the latissimus muscle. The radial artery and vein are usually sutured to the deep inferior epigastric vessels. The forearm donor site is then closed with a skin graft. The neourethra can usually reach about 3 cm distally from the radix of penis. In the third stage, it is further elongated by the reconstruction of the missing part of the urethra with local flaps and anastomosed to urethral opening (Figure 31.7).

The second function, the need of a proper penile stiffness for sexual intercourse, has been managed by surgeons in two ways: penile implants or autologous stiffener materials. The prosthesis has the possibility to give a voluntary erection to the penis, and so permitting to engage in sexual intercourse, although they are expensive and have a high tendency to erosion and infection of the surrounded tissues and later extrusion. Autologous materials such as cartilage and bone transplants, used to avoid these complications, tend to resorb, curve, or fracture (Jordan et al. 1994). Furthermore, they present a permanent rigidity that makes the patient uncomfortable or embarrassed. In the author's opinion, the best reconstruction should be done with an autologous material able to change in stiffness if necessary. The muscle tissue largely answered to these requirements.

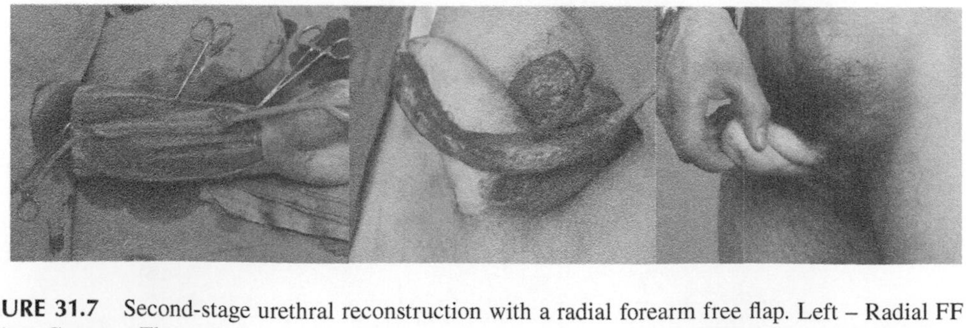

FIGURE 31.7 Second-stage urethral reconstruction with a radial forearm free flap. Left – Radial FF harvesting. Centre – Flap rolled around a catheter and prepared for vessel anastomoses in the recipient area. Right – Clinical result showing the urethral meatus at the apex of the neophallus.

The first successful functional muscle transplantation was reported in 1970 (Harii et al. 1976). Since then, neurovascular muscle transplantation has been used in different areas to restore facial expression (Manktelow and Zuker 1989), improve limb motion (Ninkovic 1994, Blanc et al. 1993), increase cardiac function (Ninkovic et al. 1997), and restore sphincter function (McKee and Kuzon 1989).

The most critical part of the functional muscle transfer is the nerve selection and adjustment (Blanc et al. 1993, Ninkovic et al. 1994). In order to minimise the time of muscle denervation, the nerve coaptation was placed as closely as possible to the neuromuscular junction. Also, electrostimulation began soon after the surgery and continued until satisfactory voluntary contraction was achieved (Figures 31.5 and 31.6).

The author selected the latissimus dorsi free flap for the amount of the skin and muscular paddle, as well as for the length of the pedicle. Besides, the skin grafting on the back was better accepted by the patients in comparison to traditional method of reconstruction with radial forearm free flap (Figures 31.1 and 31.3). As recipient nerve, the anterior branch of the obturator nerve proved to be the best for its proximity. Moreover, the contraction of the adductors and gracilis muscles bring the patient in possibility to sexual penetration with the deliberate contraction of the transplanted muscle and cause negligible involuntary movements during walking.

Only few disadvantages of this procedure were noted. Some difficulties can arise in overweight patients when the skin envelope of the penis is wrapped around the strip of latissimus dorsi muscle even if the subcutaneous tissue of the flap was thinned. Therefore, the procedure may not be advised in obese patients. On the other hand, the latissimus dorsi musculocutaneous free flap offers option of bigger penis construction.

31.2.2 Non-Typical Microvascular Techniques of Reconstructions

Non-typical reconstructions of microvascular techniques include using other free flaps such as the rectus abdominis flap and the groin flap, lateral arm flap (LAF) (Upton et al. 1987), and the peroneal flap.

31.2.2.1 Rectus Abdominis Muscle as the Corpus of the Penis

1. The rectus abdominis muscle isolated on the inferior pedicle running subcutaneously to the mons pubis was covered by a fasciocutaneous FF. The urethra was formed by a free skin transplant harvested from the skin of the breasts that were amputated in a one-stage operation. The flat rectus abdominis muscle was rolled around the urethra. The recipient vessels were the lateral circumflex femoral artery using a venous graft from the greater saphenous vein. A sensory nerve was sutured in the left groin. The glans was not primarily reconstructed (Santi et al. 1992).
2. The penis and urethra were reconstructed from three flaps – the pedicled rectus abdominis and two microsurgical ones – the LAF and the fasciocutaneous FF. The penile body was formed by a reduced, distally pedicled rectus abdominis flap, to which the urinary conduit from the LAF was fixed. Both flaps were covered by the FF. A sensory nerve of the penis was sutured to the pudendal nerve and the vascular pedicle to the deep epigastric vessels of the contralateral rectus abdominis. The vascular pedicle LAF was anastomosed at the distal end of the phallus to radial vessels, the artery end to side, and the vein end to end (Veselý et al. 1994).
3. The penis was created from a pedicled musculocutaneous flap rectus abdominis with a vertically oriented skin island to reconstruct the urinary conduit. This was sutured over a catheter Chapter 18, and the flap complex was covered by a forearm fasciocutaneous flap. The nerve was sutured to the ilioinguinal nerve and the vascular pedicle of the FF to deep inferior epigastric vessels in a usual fashion.

31.2.2.2 Flap within a Flap

The method was previously described by Laub (1995). In this procedure, a standard tubed flap is complemented with a microsurgical FF, reconstructing the urinary conduit and the glans, while the penile part is formed by the tubed flap. Simultaneously with the urethra, the glans was reconstructed and the microsurgical flap was inserted into the previous flap after tunnelling. Since the flap for the urethra raised from the forearm is only 3–4 cm wide, the scarred area in the forearm is small. This technique can be used in patients to correct the small size of his penis which had been created previously.

A flap within a flap in the author's modification provided the patient with a sufficiently rigid penis, and he was capable of sexual intercourse without a stiffener. All scars or scarring processes during healing contribute to the rigidity.

31.2.2.3 Penis with a Tunnel for a Temporary Inner Stiffener

This reconstructive technique requires two microsurgical flaps and represents the original method of the author. The technique always combines the forearm fasciocutaneous flap and the lateral forearm fasciocutaneous flap.

In the first case, a tunnel for a temporary stiffener, so-called baculum, was preformed from the cavity of a part of the FF, created by suturing de-epithelialised parts as in the construction of the urethra. The LAF reconstructed the urethra itself. The vascular pedicle of the LAF is always a parasite on the radial vessels of FF with the arterial anastomosis end to side and the venous end to end.

In other cases, both the penis and the urethra were reconstructed in the typical manner, with the exception of lateral parts of FF expanded to a base width of 8–10 cm, the width at the glans being 7–9 cm according to the thickness of the subcutaneous fat of both the FF and the LAF. The venous supply of the flap is enhanced by using vena basilica. The baculum was created from the LAF and it was always transferred to the dorsum of the penis. A blind distal pocket of the tunnel for a temporary stiffener was fixed by suturing it to the distal end of the phallus at the base of the glans. The proximal end of the baculum was sutured on the dorsum of the penis base in a fan-like manner. The authors prefer to locate the baculum on the dorsal side of the penis to allow easy hygiene of the blind pocket. The flap located in this site can be followed postoperatively without any difficulties. The patient will support a stiffener in the form of a strong but elastic rod on the symphysis.

The primary suture of urethral conduits is not always done because of the length of duration of the entire operation. While a typical reconstruction is a two-team effort which lasts 5–6 h, a more complex technique using two microsurgical flaps is accomplished in 7–8 h.

In this technique combining two microsurgical flaps, a significant higher risk of partial necrosis of both flaps was encountered. Examination showed that it was caused by excessive congestion, tissue compression, and microvascular stream in pasty patients. The Doppler monitoring of patency of vascular anastomoses can prevent the loss of the flaps.

The author's experience has shown that the LAF is suitable for forming a tunnel and the urethra should be reconstructed from the FF.

31.3 LOCATION OF THE URETHRA

The location of the urethra in the centre of the flap according to Biemer's design (Biemer 1988) is preferred both in standard reconstruction techniques and in two-flap transfer. Reasons for placing the urethra flap on the forearm are the hairless skin and better supply of the urethral flap thanks to proximity of the vascular pedicle of vasa radialis. If the skin on the forearm in the location of the designed urethra is hairy, it is necessary to obtain permanent depilation prior to performing the reconstruction.

31.4 CREATING GLANS PENIS

When creating the glans in the author's group of patients, the primary reconstruction from the FF using a modification of the Norfolk technique is the best. In reconstruction technique, the author does not suture skin to skin but the subcutaneous tissue of the glans to the skin of the penile shaft (Figure 31.1). It ensures gradual and longer healing in the region of the sulcus of the glans, and the final scar provides a good reconstruction. Only in a few cases, sulcus formation using a skin graft was employed; this led to a good result (Figure 31.2). Sculpting the glans on the reconstructed penis is considered to be a very important factor that makes the appearance of the neophallus closer to reality, even though the shapes of the created glans and the natural glans differ substantially.

31.5 SCROTAL RECONSTRUCTION

Creating an adequate scrotum is possible only after colpectomy and closure of the vaginal introitus; two techniques are used for this:

1. The labia majora combined with a distally pedicled rectus abdominis musculocutaneous flap with primary placement of silicone testicular prostheses
2. V-Y flap advancement of the labia majora distally with the primary placement of silicone testicular prostheses

31.6 CONCLUSION

The basis of the author's current phallus reconstructions is the typical technique described and the non-typical one using two microsurgical flaps. Recently, functional muscle transfers of myocutaneous latissimus dorsi free flap have been used for neophalloplasties.

Although the method enables reconstruction of urethra with radial forearm free flap, the majority of patients were satisfied even without the urethral reconstruction. High percentage of motor reinnervation gives some patients the ability to use the penis for sexual intercourse. Nowadays, nearly all authors' patients request the penile reconstruction with motor-innervated latissimus dorsi free flap, because the penis is more voluminous with lesser donor site morbidity and able to move and stiffen with no need for penile prosthesis.

Following the complications of two-flap one-stage transfers due to the tissue congestions, which appeared to be a specific phenomenon of the microsurgical transfers, preventive factors of tissue compression in using two-flap reconstruction have been considered:

1. Strict selection of patients excluding obese patients and preferring thin patients
2. Locating the LAF as distally as possible on the upper part of the arm – as far as the external part of the elbow and forearm
3. Expanding the lateral parts of the FF
4. Necessity of deriving venous blood from the ulnar edge of the flap via v. basilica

REFERENCES

Akoz T. and Kargi E. Phalloplasty in a female-to-male transsexual using a double-pedicle composite groin flap. *Ann Plast Surg*. 48: 423, 2002.

Biemer E. Penile reconstruction by the radial arm flap. *Clin Plast Surg*. 15: 425–430, 1988.

Blanc P., Girard C., Vedrinne C., Mikaeloff P., and Estanove, S. Latissimus dorsi cardiomyoplasty: Perioperative management and postoperative evolution. *Chest*. 103: 214, 1993.

Bogoras N. Uber die volle plastische Wiederherstellung eines zum Koitus fahigen Penis (Peni plastica totalis). *Zentralbl Chir*. 22: 1271, 1936.

Bouman F.G. The first step in phalloplasty in female transsexuals. *Plast Reconstr Surg*. 79: 662–664, 1987.
Byun J.S., Cho B.C., and Baik B.S. Result of one-stage penile reconstruction using an innervated radial osteocutaneous flap. *J Reconstr Microsurg*. 10: 321, 1994.
Chang T.S. and Hwang W.Y. Forearm flap in one-stage reconstruction of the penis. *Plast Reconstr Surg*. 74: 251–258, 1984.
Chen Y.B. and Chen H.C. Penile reconstruction for a victim of electrical injury with bilateral below-elbow amputations. *Plast Reconstr Surg*. 87: 771, 1991.
Cheng K.X., Hwang W.Y., Eid A.E. et al. Analysis of 136 cases of reconstructed penis using various methods. *Plast Reconstr Surg*. 95: 1070, 1995.
Davies D.M. and Matti B.A. A method of phalloplasty using the deep inferior epigastric flap. *Br J Plast Surg*. 41: 165, 1988.
Exner K. Penile reconstruction in female to male transsexualism: A new method of phalloplasty, *X. IPRAS Congress*, Madrid, Spain, 1992.
Gilbert D.A. One-stage reconstruction of the penis using an innervated radial forearm osteocutaneous flap. *J Reconstr Microsurg*. 3: 25–26, 1986.
Gilbert D.A., Horton C.E., Terzis J.K. et al. New concepts in phallic reconstruction. *Ann Plast Surg*. 18: 128, 1987.
Gilbert D.A., Schlossberg S.M., and Jordan G.H. Ulnar forearm phallic construction and penile reconstruction. *Microsurgery*. 16: 314, 1995.
Gillies H. and Harrison R.J. Congenital absence of the penis. *Br J Plast Surg*. 15: 471–487, 1948.
Gillies H. and Millard D.R. Jr. *The Principles and Art of Plastic Surgery,* vol. 2. London, U.K.: Butterworth, pp. 368–384, 1957.
Hage J.J. *From Peniplastica Totalis to Reassignment Surgery of the External Genitalia in Female-to-Male Transsexuals*. VU University Press, Amsterdam, the Netherlands, pp. 62–63, 1992.
Hage J.J. Metaidoioplasty: An alternative phalloplasty technique in transsexuals. *Plast Reconstr Surg*. 97: 161, 1996.
Hage J.J. Dynaflex prosthesis in total phalloplasty. *Plast Reconstr Surg*. 99: 479, 1997.
Hage J.J. and Bloem J.J.A.M. Review of the literature on construction of a neourethra in female-to-male transsexuals. *Ann Plast Surg*. 30: 278, 1993.
Hage J.J., Bloem J.J.A.M, and Bouman F.G. Obtaining rigidity in the neophallus of female-to-male transsexuals: A review of the literature. *Ann Plast Surg*. 30: 327, 1993a.
Hage J.J., Bouman F.G., de Graaf F.H. et al. Construction of the neophallus in female-to-male transsexuals: The Amsterdam experience. *J Urol*. 149: 1463, 1993b.
Hallock, G. Restoration of quadriceps femoris function with a dynamic microsurgical free latissimus dorsi muscle transfer. *Ann Plast Surg*. 52: 89, 2004.
Harashina T., Inoue T., Tanaka I. et al. Reconstruction of the penis with free deltoid flap. *Br J Plast Surg*. 43: 217, 1990.
Harii K., Ohmori K., and Torii S. Free gracilis muscle transplantation, with microneurovascular anastomoses for the treatment of facial paralysis. *Plast Reconstr Surg*. 57: 133, 1976.
Hentz V.R., Pearl R.M., Grossman J.A.I, Wood M.B., and CooneyW.P. The radial forearm flap: A versatile source of composite tissue. *Ann Plast Surg*. 19: 485–453, 1987.
Hester T.R., Hill H.L. and Jurkiewicz M.J. One-stage reconstruction of the penis. *Br J Plast Surg*. 31: 279–285, 1978.
Horton C.E., McCraw J.B., Devine C.J., and Devine P.C. Secondary reconstruction of the genital area. *Urol Clin N Am*. 4: 133–141, 1977.
Jordan G.H., Alter G.J. and Gilbert D.A. et al. Penile prosthesis implantation in total phalloplasty. *J Urol*. 152: 410, 1994.
Jordan G.H., Gilbert D.A., Winslow B.H. et al. Single-stage phallic reconstruction. *World J Urol*. 5: 14, 1987.
Kaplan I. and Wesser D. A rapid method for reconstructing a functional sensitive penis. *Br J Plast Surg*. 24: 342–344, 1971.
Koshima I., Tai T., and Yamasaki M. One-stage reconstruction of the penis using an innervated radial forearm osteocutaneous flap. *J Reconstr Microsurg*. 3: 19, 1986.
Laub D.R., Eicher W., Laub D.R. Jr., and Hentz V.R. In Eicher W. (ed.), *Plastic Surgery in the Sexually Handicapped*. Berlin, Germany: Springer, pp. 113–128, 1989.
Maltz M. Maltz reparative technique for the penis. In Maltz M. (ed.), *Evolution of Plastic Surgery*. New York: Froben Press, 278–279, 1946.
Manktelow R.T. and Zuker R.M. The principles of functioning muscle transplantation: Applications to the upper arm. *Ann Plast Surg*. 22: 275, 1989.
Matti B.A., Matthews R.N., and Davies D.M. Phalloplasty using the free radial forearm flap. *Br J Plast Surg*. 41: 160, 1988.

McKee N.H. and Kuzon M.W. Jr. Functioning free muscle transplantation: Making it work? What is known? *Ann Plast Surg*. 23: 249, 1989.

Morales P.A., OĆonnor J.J. Jr, and Hotchkiss R.S. Plastic reconstructive surgery after total loss of penis. *Am J Surg*. 92: 403–408, 1956.

Mutaf M.A. New surgical procedure for phallic reconstruction: Istanbul flap. *Plast Reconstr Surg*. 105: 1361, 2000.

Mutaf M.A. Nonmicrosurgical use of the radial forearm flap for penile reconstruction. *Plast Reconstr Surg*. 107: 80, 2001.

Ninkovic M., Stenzl A., Hess M. et al. Functional urinary bladder wall substitute using free innervated latissimus dorsi muscle flap. *Plast Reconstr Surg*. 100: 402, 1997.

Ninkovic M., Sucur D., Starovic B., and Markovic S. A new approach to persistent traumatic peroneal nerve palsy. *Br J Plast Surg*. 47: 185, 1994.

Orticochea M. A new method of total reconstruction of the penis. *Br J Plast Surg*. 25: 347–366, 1972.

Petrovic S. Phalloplasty in children and adolescents using the extended pedicle island groin flap. *J Urol*. 154: 848, 1995.

Puckett C.L. and Montie J.E. Construction of male genitalia in the transsexual, using a tubed groin flap for the penis and a hydraulic inflation device. *Plast Reconstr Surg*. 61: 523–530, 1978.

Sadove R.C. and McRoberts J.W. Total phallic reconstruction with the free fibula osteocutaneous flap. *Plast Reconstr Surg*. 89: 1001, 1992.

Sadove R.C., Sengezer M., McRoberts J.W., and Wells M.D. One-stage total penile reconstruction with a free sensate osteocutaneous fibula flap. *Plast Reconstr Surg*. 92: 1314, 1993.

Santi P., Adami M., Berrino P., Galli A., Muggianu M., and Veselý J. Neophalloplasty using a rectus abdominis muscle flap and a radial forearm free flap. *Eur J Plast Surg*. 15, 94–97, 1992.

Santi P., Berrino P., Canavese G., Galli A., Rainero M.L., and Badellino F. Immediate reconstruction of the penis using an inferiorly based rectus abdominis myocutaneous flap. *Plast Reconstr Surg*. 81: 961–964, 1988.

Sasaki K., Nozaki M., Morioka K. et al. Penile reconstruction: Combined use of an innervated forearm osteocutaneous flap and big toe pulp. *Plast Reconstr Surg*. 104: 1054, 1999.

Semple J.L., Boyd J.B., Farrow G.A., and Robinette M.A. The "cricket bat" flap: A one-stage free forearm flap phalloplasty. *Plast Reconstr Surg*. 88: 514, 1991.

Shenaq S.M. and Dinh T.A. Total penile and urethral reconstruction with an expanded sensate lateral arm flap: Case report. *J Reconstr Microsurg*. 5: 245, 1989.

Sun G.C. and Huang J.J. One-stage reconstruction of the penis with composite iliac crest and lateral groin skin flap. *Ann Plast Surg*. 15: 519, 1985.

Tamai S., Komatsu S., Sakamoto H. et al. Free muscle transplants in dogs, with microsurgical neurovascular anastomoses. *Plast Reconstr Surg*. 46: 219, 1970.

Tobin G.R., Schusterman B.A., Peterson G.H., Nichols G., and Bland K.I. The intramuscular neurovascular anatomy of the latissimus dorsi muscle: The basis for splitting the flap. *Plast Reconstr Surg*. 67: 637, 1981.

Upton J., Mutimer K.L., Loughlin K., and Ritchie J. Penile reconstruction using the lateral arm flap. *J Royal Coll Surg*. Edinburgh 32: 97–101, 1987.

Veselý J. Technika rekonstrukce penisu a močové roury u transformace female-to-male. *Prakt Lék*. 76 (Suppl. 1): 18, 1996.

Veselý J., Bařinka L., Santi P., Berrino P., and Mugianu M. Reconstruction of the penis in transsexual patients. *Acta Chir Plast*. 34 (1): 44–54, 1992.

Veselý J. and Haage J. From the history of penis reconstruction. *Acta Chir Plast*. 41: 43, 1999.

Veselý J., Kučera J., Hrbatý J. et al. Our standard method of reconstruction of the penis and urethra in female to male transsexuals. *Acta Chir Plast*. 41: 39, 1999.

Veselý J., Procházka V., Válka J., Mrázek T., Santi P., and Berrino P. Use of two microsurgical flaps in one stage reconstructive surgery. *Acta Chir Plast*. 36 (4): 99–103, 1994.

Veselý J., Stupka, I., Molitor, M., and Hýža, P. A variety of methods for penile reconstruction. *Eur J Plast Surg*. 25: 292, 2002.

32 Imaging and Surgical Principles of the Gluteal Arteries and Perforator Flaps

Julie Vasile, Maria M. Lotempio, and Robert J. Allen

CONTENTS

The tremendous anatomic variability of the vascular system can make perforator flap reconstruction challenging for surgeons at all experience levels. Accurate preoperative anatomic imaging of vasculature greatly enhances the ability of devising a surgical strategy before going to the operating room. Preoperative knowledge of the best or dominant perforating vessels for each donor site shifts the brunt of the perforator selection process preoperatively, which can reduce operating time and general anaesthesia requirements and potentially increase flap success. In addition, the best donor site for a flap can be chosen based on patient preference, adequate tissue adiposity, and location of the best vessels.

Gluteal artery perforator (GAP) flaps frequently provide adequate tissue for flap reconstruction, even in thin patients. It is an excellent alternative for patients with insufficient abdominal and thigh tissue. Common indications for gluteal flaps in breast reconstruction are insufficient abdominal tissue, prior abdominoplasty, extensive abdominal liposuction, failed abdominal flap, pear-shaped habitus (greatest volume of fat distributed on the buttocks), and patient preference. Gluteal flaps result in a scar that a patient does not have to see in the mirror daily and can be psychologically more acceptable for certain patients.

32.1 PERTINENT ANATOMY

GAP flaps can be harvested from the superior or inferior buttock and are usually based on branches from the superior gluteal artery or inferior gluteal artery, respectively. Occasionally, we have based gluteal flaps on branches from the deep femoral artery. GAP flaps are based on arterial branches that *perforate* through or around the gluteal muscles, and are harvested with preservation of gluteal muscle and function.[1–4] The superior gluteal artery exits the pelvis superior to the piriformis muscle, and its branches perforate through the gluteus maximus and gluteus medius muscles. The superior GAPs are located in a large territory extending along the superior two-thirds of a line from the posterior superior iliac spine to the greater trochanter.[5] The inferior gluteal artery exits the pelvis inferior to the piriformis muscle, and its branches perforate through the gluteus maximus muscle.[3–5] The inferior GAPs are located in a large territory extending along the middle third of the lower buttock.[5]

32.2 SUPERIOR VERSUS INFERIOR GAP FLAPS

The superior gluteal artery perforator (SGAP) flap harvests the upper buttock tissue, while the inferior gluteal artery perforator (IGAP) flap harvests the inferior buttock tissue. The decision to choose a superior or inferior gluteal flap is based on patient preference and anatomy.

The trade-offs of each gluteal flap influence patient preference. An advantage of superior gluteal flaps is that the scar can be covered by a bathing suit; however, the scar is located on a more prominent position on the buttock. An additional disadvantage is harvesting a superior gluteal flap can disturb the superior fullness of the buttock, considered the aesthetic unit of the buttock, which may cause unfavourable flattening of this area. Conversely, the scar from an inferior gluteal flap can be located in a less prominent area of the buttock in the inferior gluteal crease. An additional advantage is an inferior gluteal flap may remove the *saddle bags*, a common area of fat deposition in women, without disturbing the aesthetic unit of the buttock.[3,4] A disadvantage of the inferior gluteal flap is the lateral portion of the scar can be visible in a bathing suit and sometimes the inferior gluteal crease can be distorted or shifted cephalad or caudal. Contrary to previous reports, the sciatic nerve has never been injured with an inferior gluteal flap in our experience and is never exposed during dissection of the flap.[4] Rarely, temporary paresthesias can occur if the posterior femoral cutaneous nerve is stretched during harvest of an inferior gluteal flap.[6]

Anatomic considerations on the surgeon's decision to choose a superior or inferior gluteal flap are based on the distribution of fat on the buttock and location of the best perforators in the buttock. As the location of the best perforators from the superior and inferior gluteal artery covers a large territory, cross-sectional anatomic gluteal imaging with intravenous contrast has been immensely helpful for viewing the anatomy. We typically use magnetic resonance angiography (MRA) preoperatively to view the gluteal vessels because of the lack of radiation exposure and iodinated contrast.[7] With our colleagues in radiology, we have developed an MRA protocol for high-resolution cross-sectional anatomic imaging of the vasculature. Over the years, the protocol has been fine-tuned to consistently yield reliable information of multiple donor sites in one study that guides the preoperative plan, flap design, and dissection.[7–10]

32.3 MRA PROTOCOL

The current MRA protocol is detailed in the following. Patients are instructed to remove clothing that causes compression of the tissue, such as tight undergarments. A vitamin E capsule is placed on surface landmarks to serve as a reference point for perforator location. On the buttock, the surface landmark is the superior point of the gluteal crease. A 1.5 T MR machine is currently used to achieve homogenous fat suppression over a wide field of view. Patients are imaged in the prone position to avoid distortion of the tissue and perforator location and to decrease motion artefact. Gadofosveset trisodium (Lantheus Medical Imaging, Billerica, MA), a blood pool contrast agent that binds to albumin with a longer half-life of 48 min, and the lack of radiation allow multiple acquisitions of multiple donor sites in one examination.[11]

An initial T2-weighted sequence is acquired to aid in localization of the areas of interest. Then transverse pre- and post-contrast 3D liver acquisition volume accelerator (LAVA) sequence is acquired with the following parameters: TR/TE/flip = 3.9/1.9/15, bandwidth = 125 kHz, slice thickness = 3 mm reconstructed at 1.5 mm using twofold zero interpolation, matrix = 512 × 128–256,

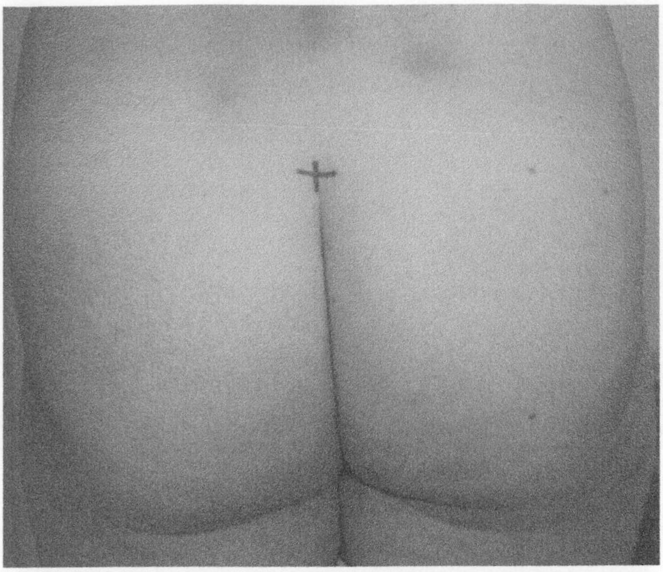

FIGURE 32.1 Photograph of buttock with marker at superior point of gluteal crease. (Printed from Vasile, J.V. et al., *J. Reconstr. Microsurg.*, 26(1), 45, 2010. With permission.)

flip angle = 15°, and parallel acceleration factor = 2. Central frequency and shim field of view are adjusted to maximise fat suppression over areas of interest in the pre-contrast images. Ten millilitres of gadofosveset trisodium is injected and followed by a 20 mL flush of normal saline at 1 mL/s. Arterial phase scanning is started at the time of contrast seen in abdominal aorta with automated triggering. K space is mapped sequentially, so the absolute centre of k space is collected in the middle of the scan (20 s after contrast detection). Phase coding is set right to left. Then equilibrium phase transverse 3D LAVA at higher resolution without parallel imaging sequence is acquired with the following parameters: TR/TE/flip = 4/1.9/15, bandwidth = 125 kHz, and matrix = 512 × 512 (172–240). Lower-resolution coronal and sagittal sequences are acquired to evaluate internal organs.

Post-processing is performed on a computer workstation, and 3D surface-rendered images are generated. The diameter, location, and course of all large gluteal perforators are identified by the radiologist. The landmark reference point is at the top of the gluteal crease. Figure 32.1 illustrates the reference point. The locations of the vessels at the superficial gluteal fascia level are determined at a perpendicular point on the skin surface in relation to the reference point. The locations of the perforators in relation to the reference point are measured along the curved skin surface of the prone buttock to yield the most accurate information. The distance of a perforator from the reference point is calculated in the longitudinal and transverse dimensions to yield coordinate locations for the perforators. The locations of the perforators are superimposed on surface-rendered 3D-reconstructed images to assist the surgeon with the preoperative markings. Figure 32.2 shows how a gluteal perforator coordinate location is measured. Vessel calibre measurements are calculated just above the anterior rectus fascia level. The course of each perforator is described in terms of intramuscular course or septocutaneous course.

32.4 OPTIMAL PERFORATOR SELECTION

From the radiology report and by reviewing the MRA images, the optimal vessels are chosen. The foremost factors in determining the optimal vessel upon which to base a flap in order of importance are vessel diameter, length of pedicle, location at which a vessel enters the planned flap, and vessel

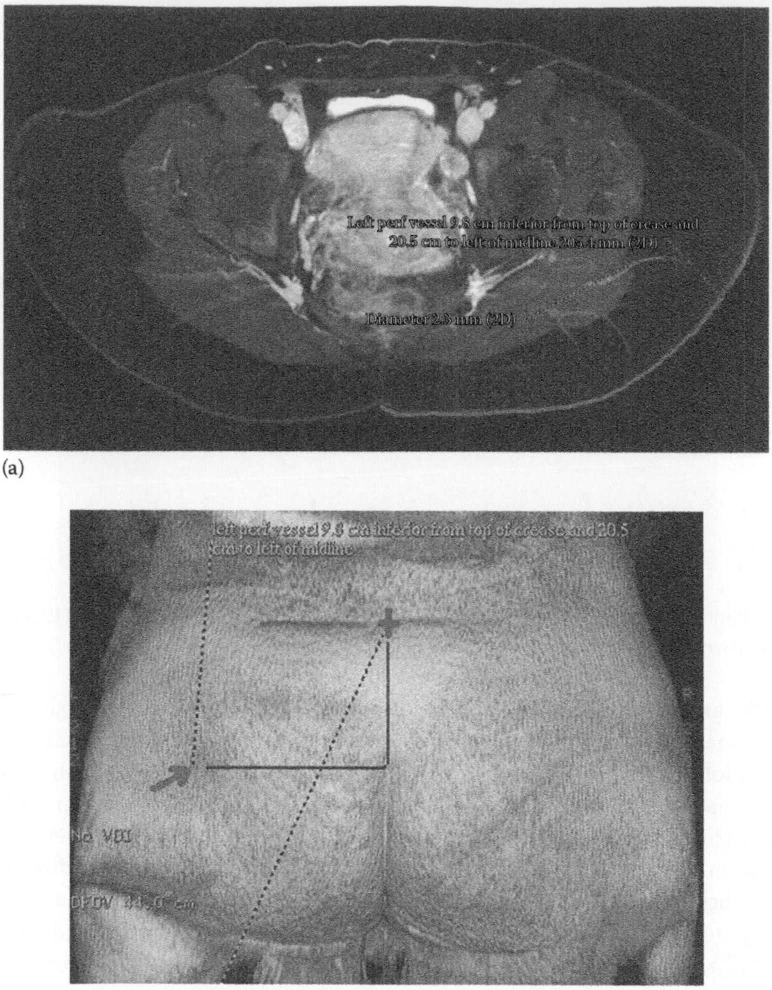

(a)

(b)

FIGURE 32.2 (a) Axial MRA. Arrow points to a gluteal perforator. Line along the curved skin surface illustrates how measurement is made. (b) Surface-rendered 3D reconstruction MRA. Same perforator located in reference to marker at top of gluteal crease. (Printed from Vasile, J.V. et al., *J. Reconstr. Microsurg.*, 26(1), 45, 2010. With permission.)

arborisation pattern within the subcutaneous fat. In this regard, a larger vessel diameter, pedicle of sufficient length for insetting, central location of the vessel on the flap, or a pattern of arborisation that suggests perfusion of the tissue to be transferred are all considered favourable. Vessels located laterally on the buttock produce longer pedicles, but if a vessel is located too laterally, it will be at the edge of the designed flap. An ideal vessel for insetting is one that will produce a pedicle length of between 8 and 10 cm. Special consideration in the selection of vessels is taken with bilateral gluteal flap procedures. To create symmetrical scars on the buttock, we try to select vessels that are located at a similar position on each buttock.

The course of a vessel is a secondary factor that influences vessel selection. If two vessels appear to be of similar size and both have equivalent vascular arborisation patterns within the subcutaneous fat of the planned flap, then the vessel that can be dissected more easily or with the least trauma to the muscle is selected. Provided there is adequate length for insetting, a perforator with a more direct intramuscular course is favoured because the dissection is usually technically easier, proceeds more quickly, and reduces trauma to the gluteal muscle. A septocutaneous branch of the superior gluteal artery, which travels around the gluteus muscles or between the gluteus maximus and medius muscles, may also be advantageous. However, sometimes the dissection can be tedious with gluteal septocutaneous vessels that are enveloped by thick fascia where they emerge laterally from the muscle, as in the case with deep femoral artery perforators.[12] IGAPs tend to have a more oblique course, yielding a longer pedicle than SGAPs. An IGAP flap typically yields a longer pedicle of 8–11 cm, compared with 6–8 cm in an SGAP flap. The longer perforator length may result in a longer dissection required to reach an arterial diameter of adequate length but may also be beneficial during microsurgical anastomosis and insetting of the flap.

32.5 FLAP DESIGN

In the office, on the day prior to the planned surgery, the patient is placed in the prone position for marking. The locations of the optimal vessels selected on MRA are marked with indelible ink on the gluteal skin using measurements calculated from the MRA. A handheld Doppler is also used to confirm location of the perforators. Ample time can be taken in the office to design the flap skin pattern. An elliptical skin pattern is drawn to incorporate the selected vessels. The width of the ellipse varies based on the location of the selected vessels that are to be incorporated, the amount of skin required to reconstruct the breast, and the laxity of a patient's buttock skin. Typical flap widths used to be 8–10 cm. With the increased certainty of an adequate vessel, MRA enables us to design flaps with smaller skin patterns. For immediate reconstruction when extra skin is not needed, the skin paddle width can be 6–8 cm. Flap lengths can vary from 20 to 26 cm. The planned pattern of bevelling of subcutaneous fat is outlined around the elliptical skin pattern based on tissue volume requirements to reconstruct the breast.

In contrast to an abdominal flap, the design of a buttock flap is not just influenced but determined by optimal perforator location. Only a small portion of the buttock is used in breast reconstruction, and precise flap design is important. The goal is to design a flap that incorporates the optimal perforator and a backup option while minimising the vertical skin width harvested. Because there are usually many large calibre perforators in the buttock, vessel location is an important determining factor in selecting the optimal vessel. Laterally positioned perforators will result in more lateral flaps that may spare the central aesthetic unit in superior buttock flaps or the medial cushioning fat in lower buttock flaps. An attempt is made to design flaps that will result in a scar that can be hidden. For inferior gluteal flaps, an inferiorly positioned perforator allows for design of an *in-the-crease* gluteal flap to enable most of the scar to be hidden in the inferior gluteal crease. In bilateral flaps, an attempt is made to design flaps that will result in symmetrical scars. Examples of MRA images of perforators with corresponding superior and inferior gluteal flap designed are shown in Figures 32.3 through 32.6.

Preoperative imaging gives us the opportunity to plan and contemplate the details of a GAP flap in a less stressful office environment. MRA is the preoperative imaging modality of choice because it provides accurate, high-resolution, anatomic images without radiation exposure or iodinated contrast agents to the patient and allows for serial image acquisitions to visualise multiple donor sites in one study. Advanced anatomic knowledge of the best perforators improves our ability to confidently select donor sites and to design flaps and our efficiency in the execution of the procedure.

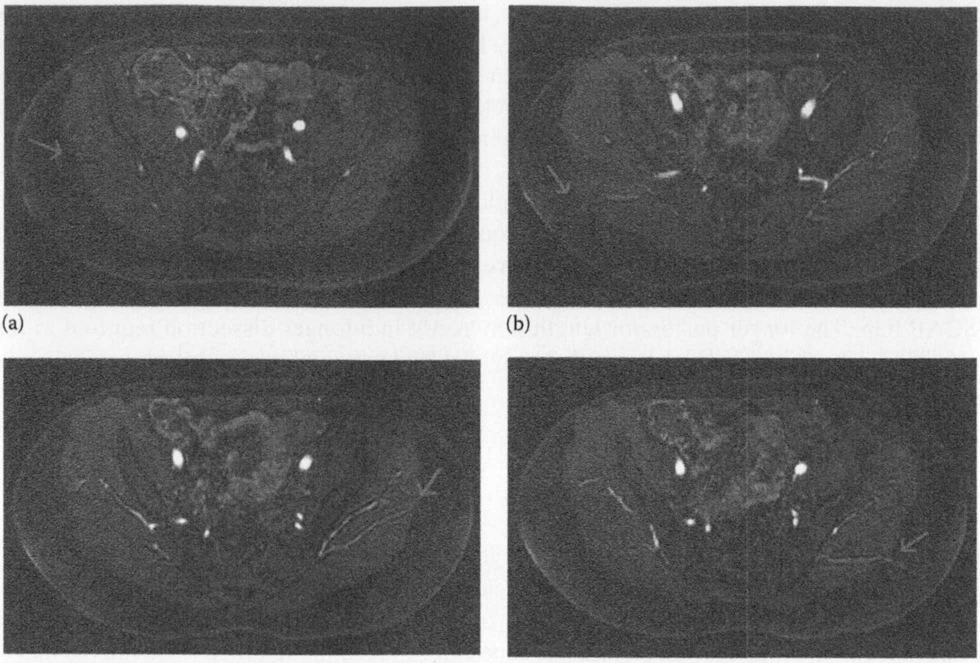

(a) (b) (c) (d)

FIGURE 32.3 (a) Axial MRA. Arrow points to a right laterally located septocutaneous SGAP that courses between the gluteus maximus and gluteus medius muscles. (b) Axial MRA. Arrow points to a right laterally located intramuscular SGAP. (c) Axial MRA. Arrow points to a left septocutaneous SGAP with similar location on the contralateral buttock. (d) Axial MRA. Arrow points to a left intramuscular IGAP with similar location on the contralateral buttock. (Printed from Vasile, J.V. et al., *J. Reconstr. Microsurg.*, 26(1), 45, 2010. With permission.)

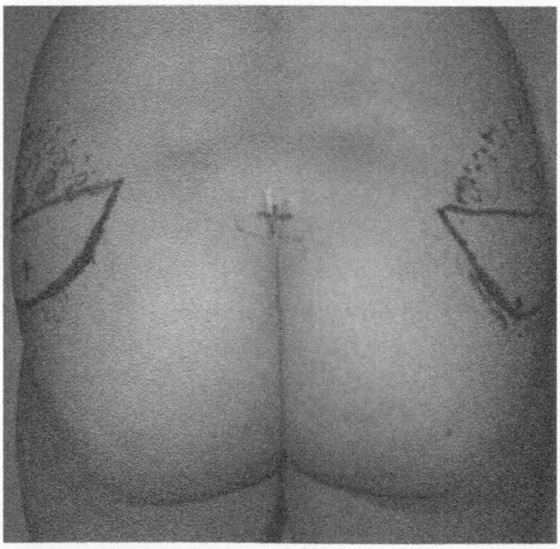

(a)

FIGURE 32.4 (a) Photograph of buttock (posterior view) of flap design for bilateral superior gluteal flaps. Two large perforators are located lateral on the buttock to preserve the upper central gluteal tissue on each buttock. SC marks the location of the septocutaneous perforator on each flap, and the other dot locates the intramuscular perforator. The width of the skin island of each flap is narrow, but designed to incorporate a large perforator and back up perforator, and results in two symmetrical scars. Planned bevelling of subcutaneous fat is marked.

(Continued)

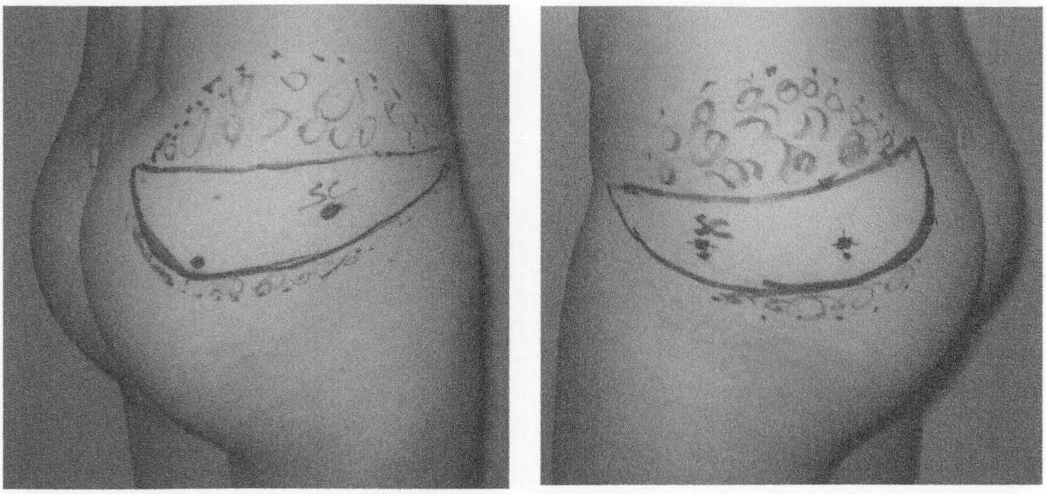

(b) (c)

FIGURE 32.4 (*Continued*) (b, c) Photograph of buttock (lateral views). (Printed from Vasile, J.V. et al., *J. Reconstr. Microsurg.*, 26(1), 45, 2010. With permission.)

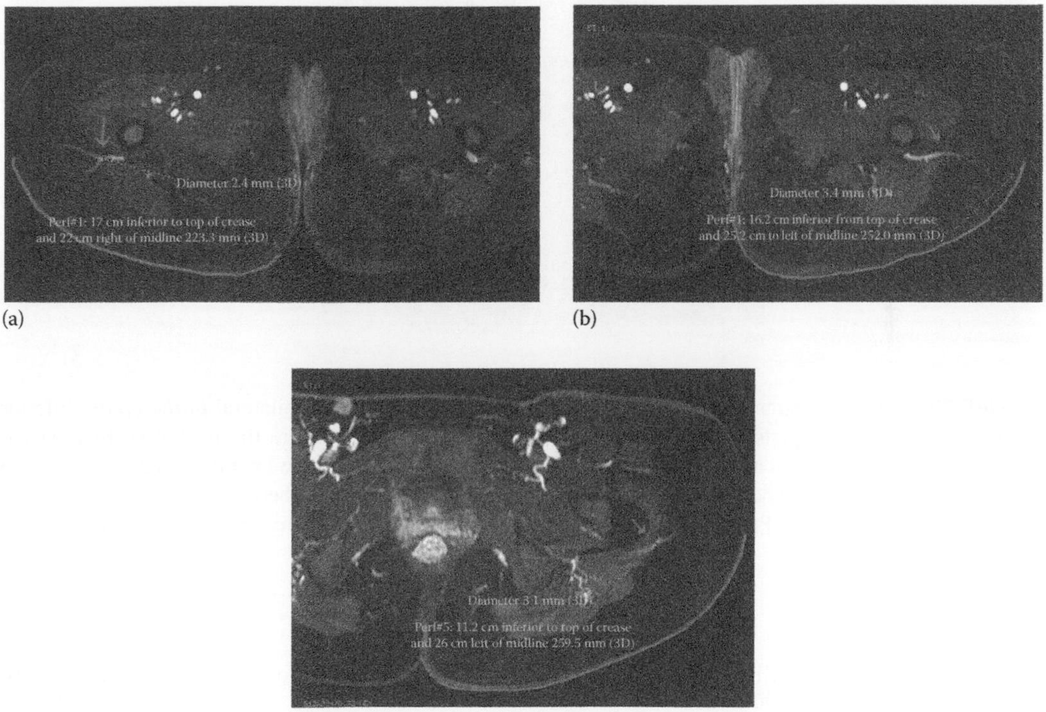

(c)

FIGURE 32.5 (a) Axial MRA. Arrow points to a right lateral and inferiorly located septocutaneous deep femoral artery perforator. (b) Axial MRA. Arrow points to a left septocutaneous deep femoral artery perforator, with similar location on the contralateral buttock. (c) Axial MRA. Arrow points to a left intramuscular IGAP coursing through the gluteus maximus muscle, with similar location on the contralateral buttock. (Printed from Vasile, J.V. et al., *J. Reconstr. Microsurg.*, 26(1), 45, 2010. With permission.)

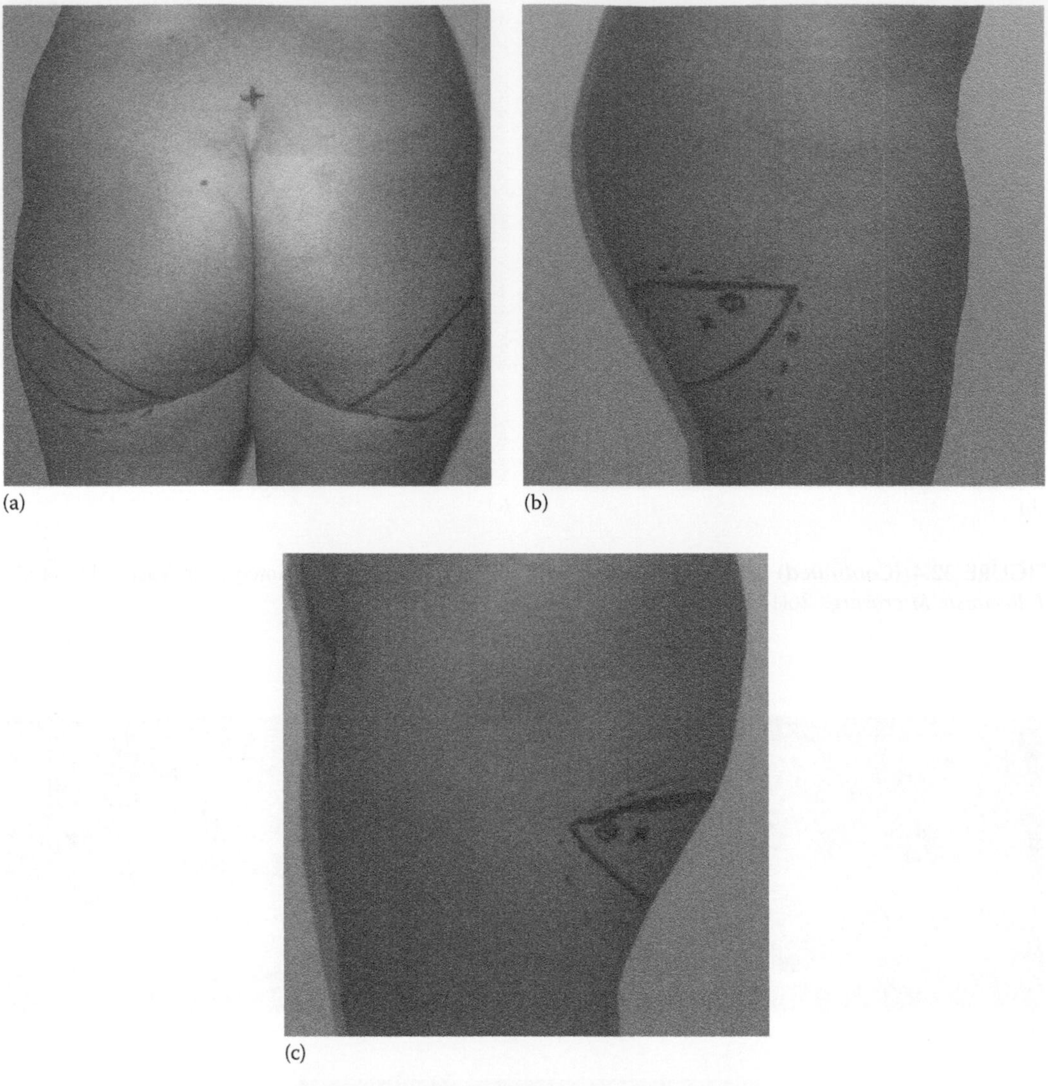

FIGURE 32.6 (a) Photograph of buttock (posterior view) of flap design for bilateral *in-the-crease* inferior gluteal flaps. Two large perforators are located lateral on the buttock to spare the medial cushioning fat. The width of the skin island of each flap is narrow and designed to harvest the lateral fat and results in two symmetrical scars. Planned bevelling of subcutaneous fat is marked with a dashed line. (b and c) Photograph of buttock (lateral views). (Printed from Vasile, J.V. et al., *J. Reconstr. Microsurg.*, 26(1), 45, 2010. With permission.)

REFERENCES

1. Allen RJ, Tucker C Jr. 1995. Superior gluteal artery perforator free flap for breast reconstruction. *Plast Reconstr Surg* 95(7):1207–1212.
2. Guerra AB, Metzinger SE, Bidros RS et al. 2004. Breast reconstruction with gluteal artery perforator (GAP) flaps: A critical analysis of 142 cases. *Ann Plast Surg* 52:118–125.
3. Allen RJ, Levine JL, Granzow JW. 2006. The in-the-crease inferior gluteal artery perforator flap for breast reconstruction. *Plast Reconstr Surg* 118(2):333–339.
4. Levine JL, Miller Q, Vasile J et al. 2009. Simultaneous bilateral breast reconstruction with in-the-crease inferior gluteal artery perforator flaps. *Ann Plast Surg* 63(3):249–254.

5. Ahmadzadeh R, Bergeron L, Tang M et al. 2007. The superior and inferior gluteal artery perforator flaps. *Plast Reconstr Surg* 120(6):1551–1556.
6. Heitmann C, Levine JL, Allen RJ. 2007. Gluteal artery perforator flaps. *Clin Plast Surg* 34(1):123–130.
7. Vasile JV, Newman T, Rusch DG et al. 2010. Anatomic imaging of gluteal perforator flaps without ionizing radiation: Seeing is believing with magnetic resonance angiography. *J Reconstr Microsurg* 26(1):45–58.
8. Greenspun D, Vasile J, Levine JL et al. 2010. Anatomic imaging of abdominal perforator flaps without ionizing radiation: Seeing is believing with magnetic resonance imaging angiography. *J Reconstr Microsurg* 26(1):37–44.
9. Vasile JV, Newman TM, Prince MR et al. 2011. Contrast-enhanced magnetic resonance angiography. *Clin Plast Surg* 38(2):263–275.
10. Newman TM, Vasile J, Levine JL et al. 2010. Perforator flap magnetic resonance angiography: A review of 25 deep inferior epigastric and gluteal perforator artery flap patients. *J Magn Reson Imaging* 31(5):1176–1184.
11. Zou Z, Lee HK, Cerilles M et al. 2012. Gadofosveset trisodium enhanced abdominal perforator MRA. *J Magn Reson Imaging* 35(3):711–716.
12. Schneider LF, Vasile JV, Levine JL et al. 2011. Deep femoral artery perforator flap: A new flap for breast reconstruction. *J Reconstr Microsurg* 27(9):531–536.

33 Imaging and Surgical Principles of Anterolateral Thigh Perforator Flap

Diego Ribuffo, Emanuele Cigna, Luca Saba, Francesco Serratore, and Arianna Milia

CONTENTS

33.1 HISTORY

The anterolateral thigh flap (ALTF) was originally described by Song in 1984 as a septocutaneous flap based on the descending branch of the lateral circumflex femoral artery (LCFA) [1]. Conversely to its first report, it was later determined that the flap was supplied only by musculocutaneous perforators in the majority of cases and that septocutaneous supply only occurred in a small percentage of cases [2–5].

In the past, the variable anatomy and the necessity for intramuscular dissection of perforators has given this flap the reputation of requiring a relatively difficult dissection. In recent years, advances in perforator flap dissection and in imaging techniques have provided familiarity of the technique required for safe harvest, and this has popularised the use of this flap for a wide variety of indications.

In 1991, Zhou et al. evaluated their results of utilising this flap for the reconstruction of defects in various regions of the body, with interesting preliminary results.

Koshima et al. [6,7] and Kimata et al. [8] have outlined the utility of this flap in head and neck reconstruction since it may be adapted to cover most defects of the face, neck, or intraoral regions [9–14].

After 20 years from its first clinical report, this flap has been extensively used and is becoming a workhorse flap for reconstruction of small or large defects, both simple and complex, in any part of the body with excellent results and minimal donor site morbidity.

This flap can provide muscle, fascia, skin, or any of these in combination, and the vascular pattern also allows the use of a more versatile design with double skin paddles based on multiple perforators.

It has a reliable blood supply despite some anatomic variability; it is pliable and can be thinned to a significant degree without compromising its blood supply and can provide a long pedicle with large-diameter vessels.

It can be used as a flow-through flap and, because of its unique position, allows a two-team approach to the reconstruction of most defects in the body.

As a sensate flap, using the lateral cutaneous femoral nerve, the superior perforator nerve, and the median perforator nerve [15], it has been proposed especially for hand [16], intraoral [17], and foot reconstruction [18–20].

As a functioning muscle flap, it can be used in combination with vastus lateralis muscle or combined with adjacent flaps according to the chimeric flap principle to reconstruct large or complex 3D defects. The ALTF can be harvested with fascia lata to provide a vascularised fascial sling when the facial nerve has been damaged or removed [21].

The ALTF is relatively easy to harvest once the technique of perforator flap dissection has been absorbed.

It has disadvantages such as a colour mismatch when reconstructing facial defects and the presence of hair in some patients. When large defects have to be reconstructed, skin grafts are required at the donor site.

33.2 FLAP ANATOMY

The ALTF is supplied by the descending branch of the LCFA, which is the largest branch of the profunda femoris system.

The pedicle lies in the groove between the rectus femoris and vastus lateralis muscles along with the motor nerve to the vastus lateralis.

The pedicle length ranges between 8 and 16 cm with a vessel diameter usually larger than 2 mm. The pedicle supplies perforating branches to the surrounding rectus femoris and vastus lateralis muscles and septocutaneous vessels to the (anterolateral thigh) ALT skin. In some instances, the predominant vascular supply to the flap may originate from the transverse branch of the LCFA or even directly from the profunda femoris system.

The descending branch usually courses inferiorly along the medial edge of the vastus lateralis muscle or, rarely, over the vastus intermedius muscle.

It exits in the majority of cases within a circle of 3 cm radius located at the midpoint of a line drawn between the anterior superior iliac spine (ASIS) and the superior lateral border of the patella as either a septocutaneous vessel or a musculocutaneous perforator, or both. Septocutaneous vessels run between the rectus femoris and vastus lateralis and traverse the fascia to supply the skin of the ALT. At the exit point, musculocutaneous perforators traverse through the vastus lateralis muscle, giving off numerous intramuscular branches before piercing through the fascia and supplying the skin.

In 30% of patients, the descending branch further divides into a medial and lateral branch at the midpoint of a line extending from the ASIS to the lateral aspect of the patella.

The medial branch courses medially under the rectus femoris muscle to supply both the rectus femoris and the skin overlying the anteromedial thigh. The lateral branch travels inferiorly along the intermuscular septum between the vastus lateralis and rectus femoris, giving rise to musculocutaneous perforators through the vastus lateralis or septocutaneous branches, or both, that supply the skin of the ALT.

In 2% of cases, there may be an absence of any skin vessels, or the perforator may be too small in diameter.

Two venae comitantes accompany the arterial pedicle of the ALTF. In rare instances, there may be no existing veins with the perforator pedicle.

The anterior branch of the lateral cutaneous nerve of the thigh, the superior perforator nerve, and the median perforator nerve can be included to create a sensory flap. The sensory nerve branches pierce the muscle fascia 10 cm below the inguinal ligament medial to the tensor fascia lata muscle.

The ALTF may also be harvested as a myocutaneous flap with the vastus lateralis muscle, thus including motor function.

33.3 IMAGING

The most critical factor to predict viability for any perforator flap is an adequate circulation.

Locating the cutaneous perforators is an important first step in ALTF design. Muscular and septal perforators may be present in different numbers and locations. Inaccurate localisation of these perforators may place the flap design outside the perforator location or limit the perfusion territory.

Precise preoperative mapping of the vascular system makes it possible to minimise the complications related to an untypical vessel distribution [22–24].

There are different imaging methods to investigate these perforators.

Doppler device is sufficient for vessel evaluation. It is a rapid and low-cost test which allows to obtain the information if a vessel with blood flowing through it is present in the examined area [25–28].

More advanced imaging techniques which include colour Doppler, computed tomographic angiography (angio-CT) scan, angio–magnetic resonance angiography (MRI), and angiography must be used for more precise evaluation of perforators.

33.4 DOPPLER DEVICES

The use of a handheld Doppler device to locate the cutaneous perforators of the ALTF is the most commonly used way, due to the device's simplicity and convenience [25–30]. Studies of the accuracy of these devices in locating cutaneous perforators of ALTFs have been reported in literature [29]. The cutaneous perforators can be examined in the clinic the day before surgery, and the Doppler examination can be repeated in the operating room. A handheld Doppler is a low-cost device and it is easy to use and allows identifying and locating the perforators. In contrast, the use of this device does not allow getting information on the course by subcutaneous or muscular vessel and does not identify precisely what the origin of the perforator vessel is. For Doppler examination, the patient has to be placed in the supine position with the leg straight in a neutral position. A line is then drawn connecting the ASIS and the superolateral corner of the patella (hereafter referred to as the A-P line) (Figure 33.1).

The majority of skin perforators are located within a circle of 3 cm radius centred at this midpoint. Xu et al. [2] located at least one perforator in the inferolateral quadrant of this circle in 80% of cases.

The long axis of the flap is designed parallel to that of the thigh.

Overall, the Doppler device is sensitive, and finding a signal with this device is very easy [31].

But during this examination, it is possible to find a vessel which is indeed located nearby and has a good flow but does not supply the skin in the supposed area. This is the consequence of a significant drawback of this procedure; in fact, the low accuracy of this method does not permit to identify the origin of the perforator vessel and its course. Thus, the sensitivity is 100%, the specificity is low (between 55% and 0%), and the positive predictive value is 89% [29]. Also, the probabilities of correct detection of cutaneous perforators with the Doppler device decrease while increasing body mass index. In fact, this device has low accuracy in patients with a higher body mass index. Some authors evaluate the accuracy of ALTF perforator mapping with the use of blind Doppler as 40% in relation to the intraoperative image. Nevertheless, with the current state of technology, Doppler sonography remains a more rapid, convenient, and simple method for perforator localisation.

33.5 COLOUR DUPLEX IMAGING

It is more strategic during preoperative planning having the characteristics of the cutaneous perforator. Colour duplex ultrasonography fulfils this requirement and permits the identification of additional characteristics, including calibre, course, and flow velocity of essential perforators and any source vessel [26]. This method, described for the first time by Hallock, allows also to

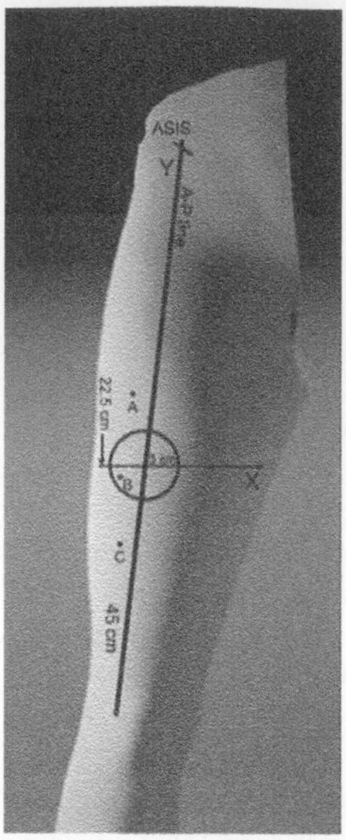

FIGURE 33.1 Graphical representation of cutaneous perforator locations in the x- (transverse) and y- (longitudinal) axes. The distance on the x-axis was that between the Doppler signal (or perforator) and the line connecting the ASIS and the superolateral corner of the patella (A-P line). The distance on the y-axis was that between the Doppler signal (or perforator) and the ASIS. (Graphic Design created by Massimiliano Scuderi.)

precisely measure the length of the vascular pedicle of the planned flap, to map the sites where the perforators pierce the fascia, and to determine the number and space orientation of the perforators [31]. It is a relatively accurate, cost-effective, and non-invasive examination using the ultrasound principle combined with flow evaluation based on the phenomenon described by Doppler.

The accuracy of this method in relation to the intraoperative image is rated highly, around 95%.

This is of particular importance when planning large flaps and flaps with independent skin islets used for the reconstruction of multilayer structures. It is also possible to trace the whole vascular pedicle of the planned flap. In older patients, if it is necessary to use a free flap for the reconstruction, this examination makes it possible to evaluate the condition of the vessel itself, the potential presence of wall thickening, or atherosclerotic plaques and thus enables the prediction of potential technical difficulties during the performance of the microvascular anastomosis.

Colour duplex ultrasonography will likely provide more accurate and detailed information regarding cutaneous perforators, but this modality is not readily available or easily accessible in many hospitals, thus is being rarely used.

33.6 COMPUTED TOMOGRAPHIC ANGIOGRAPHY

Computed tomography constitutes a modern useful tool in preoperative evaluation of an ALTF.

It allows to obtain 3D reconstructions of vessel course (size, location, and origin), which may help plan and significantly shorten the surgical time [32] (Figure 33.2).

Three-dimensional volume and maximum intensity projection renderings are created. The literature describes that the overall accuracy of angio-CT in predicting whether a perforator is septocutaneous or intramuscular is approximately 77.5% [33,34]. The accuracy of predicting perforator course decreases from proximal to distal. Factors such as the patient's age or sex or diseases do not favourably or unfavourably affect the detection of the perforators through angio-CT.

There is a trend toward perforators being more detectable in patients with a higher body mass index.

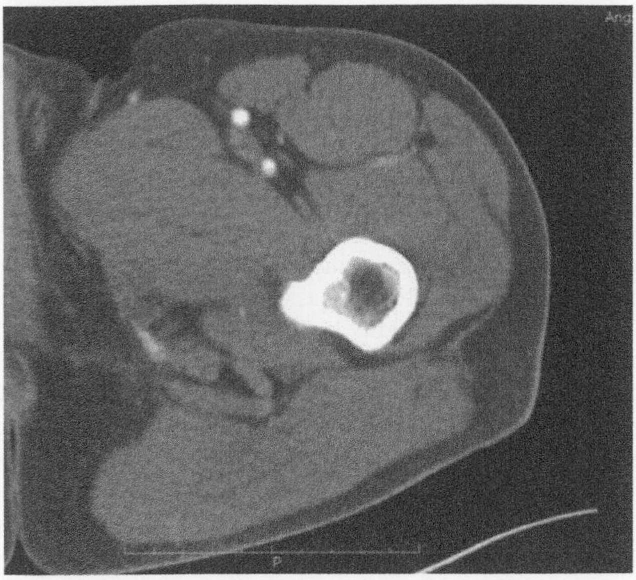

FIGURE 33.2 Axial computed tomographic angiographic image of a left lower extremity. The perforator that originated from the descending LCFA is easily identified as it pierces the fascia into the subcutaneous fat.

Perforators appear to be better visualised when surrounded by subcutaneous fat (as was the case in higher-body-mass-index patients or proximal perforators) than when surrounded by more radiopaque muscle, skin, or fascia [22]. The limitation of currently available computed tomographic scanners in imaging is that it does not show small perforators (less than 0.5 mm) for ALTF design.

This method is more expensive and requires contrast agent administration and patient's exposure to a dose of ionising radiation [35]. A 2007 study by Brenner and Hall raised concerns regarding the potential carcinogenic effects of repeated computed tomographic scans [32]. No large-scale epidemiologic studies of the cancer risks specifically associated with computed tomographic scans have been reported. Additional prospective studies of computed tomography are also needed with longer follow-up to better define potential risks.

Also, not every radiological laboratory has technical equipment and experience to allow the evaluation of small blood vessels.

33.7 NEAR-INFRARED LASER-ASSISTED INDOCYANINE GREEN IMAGING

Near-infrared laser angiography using indocyanine green (ICG), a water-soluble tri-carbocyanine dye, provides a useful adjunctive tool to more predictably assess the direct perforator perfusion zones [36]. It also allows for a dynamic, real-time evaluation of flap perfusion. ICG contains less than 5% sodium iodine and is contraindicated in patients with iodides or iodinated contrast allergies. ICG absorbs light in the near-infrared spectrum. It binds to plasma proteins with a peak absorption at 800–810 nm. The half-life of ICG is 3–5 min and it is metabolised hepatically and excreted renally. With the use of multiple injections, the dose should not exceed 1 mg/kg. The SPY system (Novadaq Technologies, Inc, Concord, Ontario, Canada) was originally developed to evaluate patency of coronary artery bypass grafts, with the approval of the Food and Drug Administration expanded to plastic surgical procedures in 2007. For breast reconstruction, the SPY system has been proposed to aid in perforator identification, evaluation of tissue perfusion, and predicting potential regions of tissue necrosis. SPY-Q analysis program can quantify relative and absolute tissue perfusion parameters based on the absorption patterns of light emitted from ICG, which is directly bound to intravascular proteins within the near-infrared spectrum.

Laser-assisted ICG angiography can not only reduce the incidence of poorly designed fasciocutaneous flaps by maximising flap perfusion zones but also preclude the need for other preoperative adjuncts that may be more costly and less efficient.

For this examination, a line is drawn from the ASIS to the lateral border of the patella, and the laser is centred over the midpoint. An X-Y system of 1 cm hatch marks, centred on the midpoint, is drawn onto the leg. ICG is injected intravenously and live fluorescence patterns are recorded using near-infrared laser angiography.

Optimal perforator perfusion zones are chosen using real-time imaging and SPY-Q analysis software. A template of the residual defect is made. Using the template, the skin paddle is centred over optimal perforator perfusion zones. Laser-assisted angiography can aid in optimising flap design while decreasing donor site morbidity by incorporating maximal flap perfusion patterns in a real-time setting. However, this method does not identify if a multipaddle ALT can be raised because the perforators are not directly visualised; but this can be utilised after flap elevation to assess viability of multiple paddles prior to separation. The intraoperative angiographic analysis can provide valuable information about the viability of a prospective flap. Thus, if the perforators are not visible on one thigh, the operation can be aborted and the contralateral thigh may be used. This could potentially avoid unnecessary flap dissection. A large experience using this imaging system could revolutionise and simplify the intraoperative design of perforator flaps.

33.8 MAGNETIC RESONANCE ANGIOGRAPHY

MRI is currently in the phase of clinical trials. It is one of the most advanced methods of obtaining 3D reconstruction of flap vessel images (Figure 33.3). Until recently, it has been an unreliable method in the evaluation of vessels with a diameter below 2 mm [37]. Presently, the most advanced devices allow to perform a technically perfect examination with 3D reconstruction. It is a non-invasive and accurate examination, for the time being used mainly for the evaluation of DIEP flap perforators. In the future, it will probably constitute the basis for preoperative evaluation of blood vessels in reconstructive surgery. Currently, the low availability and the high cost

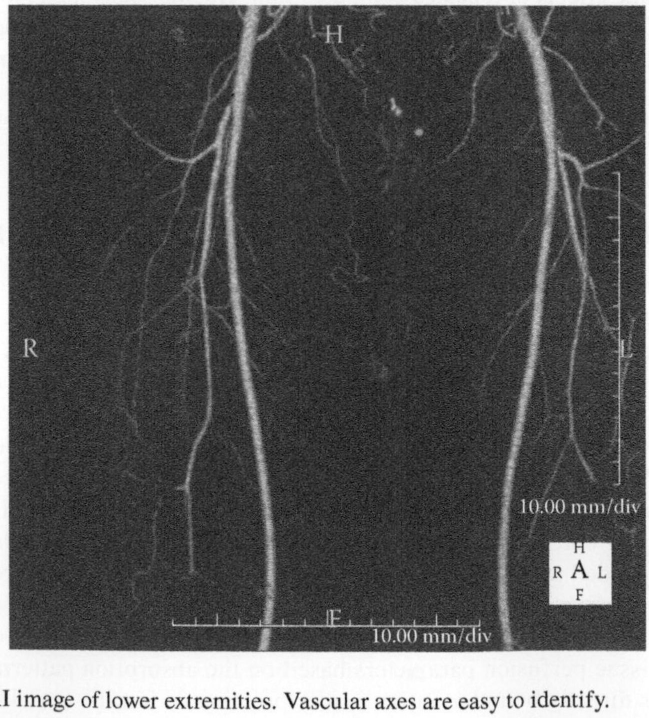

FIGURE 33.3 MRI image of lower extremities. Vascular axes are easy to identify.

of the procedure eliminate this method from the everyday clinical practice, but future studies are needed to determine the suitability of MRI for ALT perforator mapping and thus potentially avoid radiations.

33.9 FLAP DISSECTION

With the patient in a supine position, a line is drawn from the ASIS to the superolateral border of the patella, indicating the muscular septum between rectus femoris and vastus lateralis muscles.

Cutaneous perforators are mapped (in preoperative or intraoperative time) using a Doppler probe centred over the midpoint of this line [22,26–29]. Perforators are searched by slowly moving the device head along the traced line. The sites where the perforator pierced the deep fascia are marked with a colourful dot. Other imaging techniques may have been used to search the perforator vessels (i.e. angio-CT, MRI).

Preoperative angio-CT allows to obtain 3D reconstructions of vessel course. This imaging technique permits to predict whether a perforator is septocutaneous or intramuscular with 77.5% of accuracy.

The majority of skin perforators are located within a circle of 3 cm radius centred at this midpoint. Flap dimensions are marked based on the size of the recipient defect. Commonly, a flap of 8 or 9 cm by 22 cm is harvested based on one perforator.

Although experience with the ALTF has proven the reliability of a large skin paddle (up to 35 cm in length and 25 cm in width) based on one dominant perforator, when a large skin flap is to be harvested, the preference is to include more than one perforator for large flaps.

If a longer pedicle is required, the flap can be designed with the skin vessel in an eccentric position. The final design of the flap can be modified only after visualising and assessing the size and quality of the skin vessels intraoperatively.

The ALTF can be harvested in either a subfascial or suprafascial plane.

For thin flaps and when preservation of sensory innervation to parts of the thigh is required, a suprafascial dissection is preferred. Otherwise, a subfascial dissection is usually performed.

Loupe magnification during dissection is recommended as it aids in locating the skin vessels, avoids unnecessary injury to the pedicle, and helps to clearly visualise branches of the vessels.

In suprafascial dissection, the medial margin of the flap incision is first made through the skin and subcutaneous tissue, down to the level of the fascia of the thigh. Dissection usually begins at the medial border and proceeds above the fascia in a lateral direction using tenotomy scissors until the previously Dopplered skin vessels are reached.

After identifying a suitable skin vessel and confirming its course, piercing through the fascia and entering the subcutaneous tissue, the lateral skin flap incision is made down to the same suprafascial plane, and dissection proceeds in a medial direction until the same skin vessel is visualised. Dissection then proceeds in a retrograde fashion with all small branches carefully ligated or cauterised. Minimal and gentle manipulation of the skin vessel avoids vessel spasm.

In subfascial dissection, the medial incision is made down to and through the thigh fascia, exposing the rectus femoris muscle. Dissection usually begins at the medial border of the flap over the rectus femoris muscle.

The entire septum is exposed by retracting the rectus femoris medially. At this stage, the descending branch of the LCFA is identified in the groove between the rectus femoris and vastus lateralis.

In the largest series to date, septocutaneous vessels were encountered in only 12.9% of cases [5]. Therefore, in the majority of cases, flap harvest requires a careful dissection of a suitable intramuscular perforator.

For septocutaneous vessels, the dissection is performed in a retrograde fashion and the vessel is dissected away from the surrounding tissues. If the skin vessel is a musculocutaneous perforator, then intramuscular dissection is performed and the course of the perforator can easily be traced by dividing the muscle over the perforator and ligating or cauterising the small branches to the muscle.

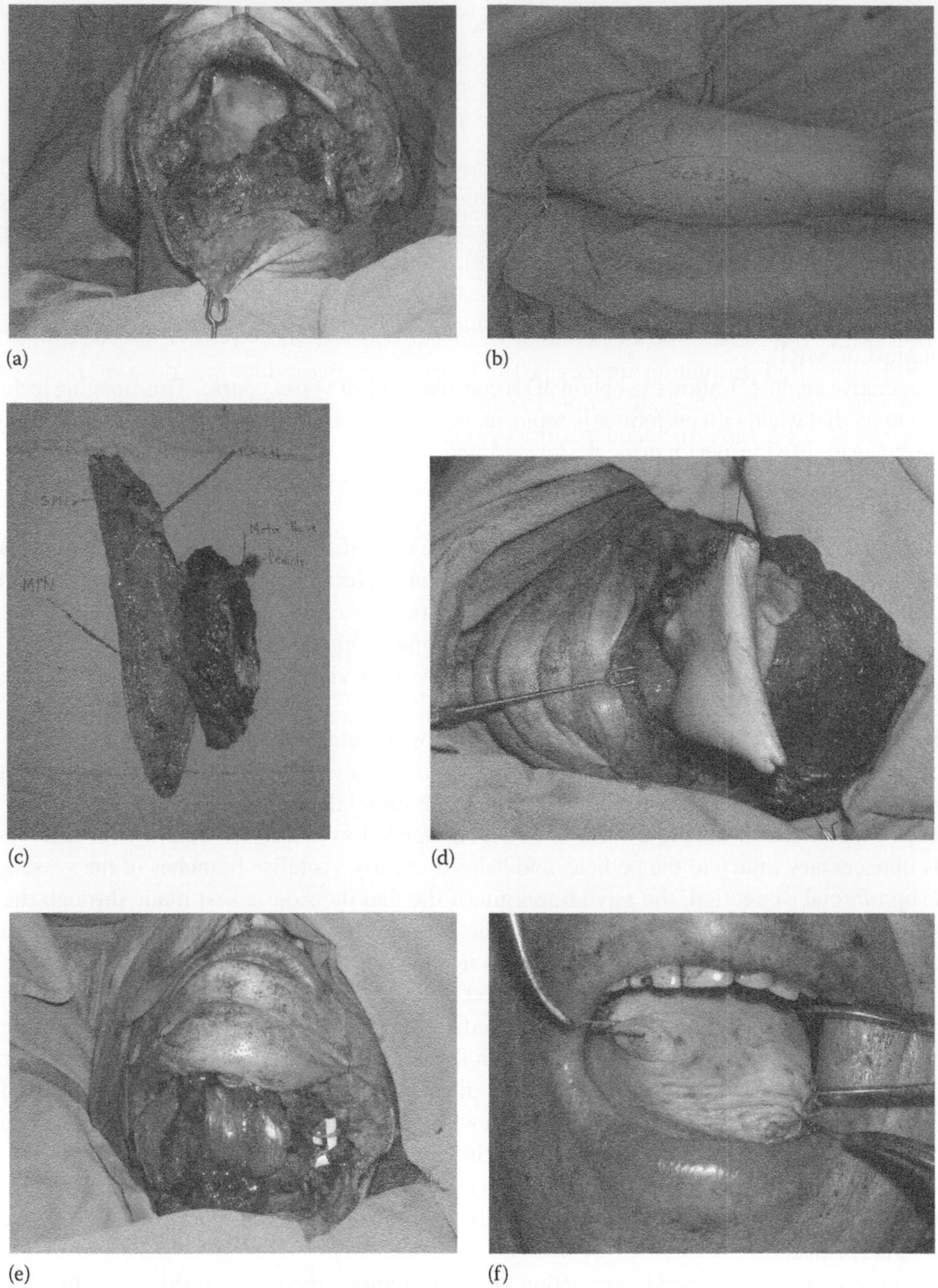

FIGURE 33.4 Case 1: (a) A 61-year-old man with tongue cancer. Intraoperative view of the defect after wide tumour's resection (glossectomy with selective neck dissection was performed). (b) An 8 cm × 23 cm right ALTF was designed with anterior branch of the lateral femoral cutaneous nerve of the thigh, the superior perforator nerve, and the median perforator nerve, to create a sensory flap. (c) The harvesting of the ALTF as a myocutaneous flap with the vastus lateralis muscle and its motor nerve pedicle. (d and e) The skin paddle was placed in order to reconstruct the tongue, and the vastus lateralis muscle was placed in order to cover the mouth floor. The pedicle was anastomosed to the recipient vessels. (f) Intraoperative final result.

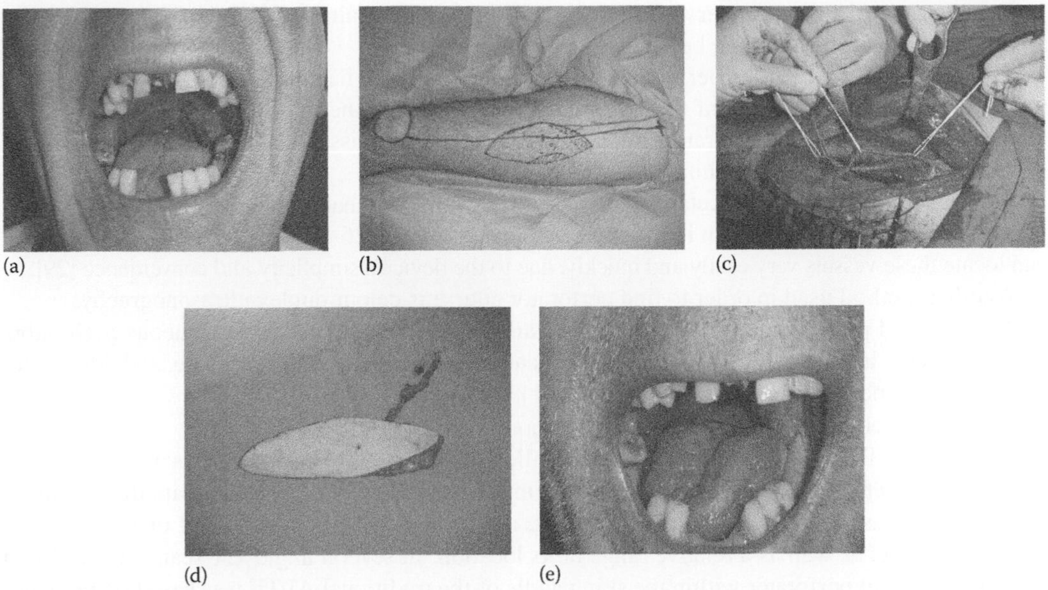

FIGURE 33.5 Case 2: (a) A 69-year-old man with retromolar trigone cancer. (b) An ALTF was designed on left lower limb. (c) An intraoperative view of the ALTF harvesting with perfect visualisation of the pedicle. (d) The skin paddle after the harvesting ready to be anastomosed to the receiving vessels. (e) Final result after 3 months of follow-up.

It is prudent to determine the course of the perforator to the source vessel by de-roofing the muscle fibres over the chosen perforator as the perforator may have a variable and tortuous intra-muscular course.

This manoeuvre avoids inadvertent injury to the perforator during incision of the muscle and also establishes that the perforator supplies the skin paddle of the musculocutaneous flap. Determining the course of the perforator to the source vessel is important because in 10% of cases, the perforator may arise from the transverse branch of the lateral circumflex artery, entering the muscle superiorly with a vertical course, and is liable to damage during muscle incision at the upper border of the flap [38].

The perforator is traced back to the main descending branch of the LCFA, which is divided according to pedicle length requirements (Figures 33.4a through f and Figures 33.5a through e).

33.10 CONCLUSION

The ALTF can be planned as a skin flap or skin-fascial one, may include a muscle fragment, may have sensory innervation, or may be used as a flow-through flap.

This flap has found universal applications for general-purpose reconstructive microsurgery [39–42].

The pedicled ALTF variant is used for the reconstruction of lower abdomen tissues and soft tissues of the pelvic girdle. An ALTF with sensory innervation and a muscle fragment is suitable for reconstructions within the lower extremity, including the load-bearing parts of the foot.

If separate vascular pedicles are used, the flap may have independent skin islets that can be used for the reconstruction of multilayer structures.

The use of an ALTF for the reconstruction of complex 3D structures requires careful planning and a meticulous study of its vascularisation [37].

The greatest difficulty in harvesting the ALTF is the uncertainty of the cutaneous perforator anatomy. These perforators can be found in consistent locations.

The correct location of the perforators allows planning of the flap appropriate architecture, and the determination of the type of these vessels allows planning the duration of the reconstructive surgery. In fact, muscular perforators take longer intramuscular dissection. It is also very important to select a better thigh with optimal distribution of perforators.

In patients with very thin subcutaneous tissue, the Doppler examination is usually more accurate and flap elevation is much easier than in patients with thicker tissues [26–31]. A handheld Doppler device can locate these vessels very easily and quickly, due to the device's simplicity and convenience [29].

Another method used in order to find perforator course is colour duplex ultrasonography.

This method provides more accurate and detailed information regarding cutaneous perforators and permits the identification of additional characteristics, including calibre, course, and flow velocity of essential perforators and any source vessel [31].

It is a relatively accurate, cost-effective, and non-invasive method.

The angio-CT is a more modern method that allows to obtain 3D reconstructions of vessel course (size, location, and origin). The use of this imaging technique permits to investigate the variables' range of the vessels' anatomic course. In effect, a potential concern is the point of origin of the perforator vessel as well as a relative range of its location. In several angio-CT scans, it was found that the dominant perforator within the skin paddle of the traditional ALTF was based on branches of the superficial (4.0%) or common femoral (1.1%) arteries [22]. This finding is a cause for concern, and recognition of this important variant is critical to avoid a potential complication in the distal extremity, in which case harvest of the flap may lead to devastating limb loss, a rare but possibly underreported complication. On these grounds, angio-CT is undoubtedly considered as the gold standard preoperative assessment tool in the study of variability of vascular anatomy, but it is more expensive and requires contrast agent administration and patient's exposure to a dose of ionising radiation [32–34].

However, the risk of radiation exposure from angio-TC must be weighed against the precise anatomical information gained by performing a high-resolution scan. Furthermore, a precise scan allows the choice of the side of the ALT to be harvested according to pedicle length requirements and septocutaneous or musculocutaneous perforator choice that may vary on the same patient's limbs. Although the use of MRI to study ALTF perforators is currently in the phase of clinical trials, this technology may provide the necessary anatomical and perforator information without unnecessary radiation exposure [37]. In the future, it will probably constitute the basis for preoperative evaluation of blood vessels in reconstructive surgery.

Laser-assisted angiography with SPY-Q analysis gives live localisation of the flap's dominant perforator perfusion zones while quantifying the relative tissue perfusion for immediate skin paddle design [36]. This method provides robust, intraoperative, objective data to optimise ALT skin paddle design while potentially minimising patient morbidity. But currently, the low availability and the very high cost eliminate this method from everyday clinical practice.

REFERENCES

1. Song YG, Chen GZ, Song YL. The free thigh flap: A new free flap concept based on the septocutaneous artery. *Br J Plast Surg* 1984;37:149–159.
2. Xu DC, Zhong SZ, Kong JM et al. Applied anatomy of the anterolateral femoral flap. *Plast Reconstr Surg* 1988;82:305–310.
3. Kimata Y, Uchiyama K, Ebihara S, Nakatsuka T, Harii K. Anatomic variations and technical problems of the anterolateral thigh flap: A report of 74 cases. *Plast Reconstr Surg* 1998;102:1517–1523.
4. Ao M, Uno K, Maeta M, Nakagawa F, Saito R, Nagase Y. De-epithelialised anterior (anterolateral and anteromedial) thigh flaps for dead space filling and contour correction in head and neck reconstruction. *Br J Plast Surg* 1999;52:261–267.

5. Wei FC, Jain V, Celik N, Chen HC, Chuang DC, Lin CH. Have we found an ideal soft-tissue flap? An experience with 672 anterolateral thigh flaps. *Plast Reconstr Surg* 2002;109:2219–2226; discussion 2227–2230.
6. Koshima I, Hosoda S, Inagawa K et al. Free combined anterolateral thigh flap and vascularized fibula for wide, through-and-through oromandibular defects. *J Reconstr Microsurg* 1998;14(8):529–534.
7. Koshima I. Free anterolateral thigh flap for reconstruction of head and neck defects following cancer ablation. *Plast Reconstr Surg* 2000;105(7):2358–2360.
8. Kimata Y, Uchiyama K, Ebihara S et al. Versatility of the free anterolateral thigh flap for reconstruction of head and neck defects. *Arch Otolaryngol Head Neck Surg* 1997;123(12):1325–1331.
9. Liu HW, Li ZD, Dong HL et al. Application of free anterolateral thigh flap in head and neck surgery. *Zhonghua Er Bi Yan Hou Tou Jing Wai Ke Za Zhi* 2011;46(5):378–381.
10. Demirkan F, Chen HC, Wei FC et al. The versatile anterolateral thigh flap: A musculocutaneous flap in disguise in head and neck reconstruction. *Br J Plast Surg* 2000;53(1):30–36.
11. Shieh SJ, Chiu HY, Yu JC et al. Free anterolateral thigh flap for reconstruction of head and neck defects following cancer ablation. *Plast Reconstr Surg* 2000;105(7):2349–2357; discussion 2358–2360.
12. Nakayama B, Hyodo I, Hasegawa Y et al. Role of the anterolateral thigh flap in head and neck reconstruction: Advantages of moderate skin and subcutaneous thickness. *J Reconstr Microsurg* 2002;18(3):141–146.
13. Cipriani R, Contedini F, Caliceti U, Cavina C. Three-dimensional reconstruction of the oral cavity using the free anterolateral thigh flap. *Plast Reconstr Surg* 2002;109:53–57.
14. Hu W, Zhang B. Anterolateral thigh flap for reconstruction of periorbital defect. *J Craniofac Surg* 2012;23(5):e437–e438.
15. Ribuffo D, Cigna E, Gargano F, Spalvieri C, Scuderi N. The innervated anterolateral thigh flap: Anatomical study and clinical implications. *Plast Reconstr Surg* 2005;115:464.
16. Luo S, Raffoul W, Luo J et al. Anterolateral thigh flap: A review of 168 cases. *Microsurgery* 1999;19:232.
17. Kekatpure VD, Trivedi NP, Shetkar G et al. Single perforator based anterolateral thigh flap for reconstruction of large composite defects of oral cavity. *Oral Oncol* 2011;47(6):517–521.
18. Kuo YR, Jeng SF, Kuo MH et al. Free anterolateral thigh flap for extremity reconstruction: Clinical experience and functional assessment of donor site. *Plast Reconstr Surg* 2001;107:1766.
19. Chang NJ, Waughlock N, Kao D et al. Efficient design of split anterolateral thigh flap in extremity reconstruction. *Plast Reconstr Surg* 2011;128(6):1242–1249.
20. Dayan JH, Lin CH, Wei FC. The versatility of the anterolateral thigh flap in lower extremity reconstruction. *Handchir Mikrochir Plast Chir* 2009;41(4):193–202.
21. Huang WC, Chen HC, Jain V et al. Reconstruction of through-and-through cheek defects involving the oral commissure, using chimeric flaps from the thigh lateral femoral circumflex system. *Plast Reconstr Surg* 2002;109:433–441; discussion 442–443.
22. Seth R, Manz RM, Dahan IJ et al. Comprehensive analysis of the anterolateral thigh flap vascular anatomy. *Arch Facial Plast Surg* 2011;13(5):347–354.
23. Lin SJ, Rabie A, Yu P. Designing the anterolateral thigh flap without preoperative Doppler or imaging. *J Reconstr Microsurg* 2010;26(1):67–72.
24. Knobloch K, Reuss E, Gohritz A et al. A survey of preoperative perforator mapping in perforator flap surgery. *Handchir Mikrochir Plast Chir* 2009;41(6):322–326.
25. Wei FC, Jain V, Celik N et al. Have we found an ideal soft-tissue flap? An experience with 672 anterolateral thigh flaps. *Plast Reconstr Surg* 2002;109(7):2219–2226.
26. Tsukino A, Kurachi K, Inamiya T, Tanigaki T. Preoperative color Doppler assessment in planning of anterolateral thigh flaps. *Plast Reconstr Surg* 2004;113(1):241–246.
27. Xu ZF, Duan WY, Shang DH et al. Preoperative Doppler evaluation of vascular perforators in the anterolateral thigh flap harvest. *Zhonghua Kou Qiang Yi Xue Za Zhi* 2011;46(5):290–292.
28. Ensat F, Babl M, Conz C et al. Doppler sonography and colour Doppler sonography in the preoperative assessment of anterolateral thigh flap perforators. *Handchir Mikrochir Plast Chir* 2011;43(2):71–75.
29. Yu P, Youssef A. Efficacy of the handheld Doppler in preoperative identification of the cutaneous perforators in the anterolateral thigh flap. *Plast Reconstr Surg* 2006;118:928–933.
30. Shaw RJ, Batstone MD, Blackburn TK et al. Preoperative Doppler assessment of perforator anatomy in the anterolateral thigh flap. *Br J Oral Maxillofac Surg* 2010;48(6):419–422.
31. Ulatowski Ł. Colour Doppler assessment of the perforators of anterolateral thigh flap and its usefulness in preoperative planning. *Pol Przegl Chir* 2012;84(3):119–125.
32. Garvey PB, Selber JC, Madewell JE et al. A prospective study of preoperative computed tomographic angiography for head and neck reconstruction with anterolateral thigh flaps. *Plast Reconstr Surg* 2011;127(4):1505–1514.

33. Ribuffo D, Atzeni M, Saba L et al. Angio computed tomography preoperative evaluation for anterolateral thigh flap harvesting. *Ann Plast Surg* 2009;62(4):368–371.
34. Chiu WK, Lin WC, Chen SY et al. Computed tomography angiography imaging for the chimeric anterolateral thigh flap in reconstruction of full thickness buccal defect. *ANZ J Surg* 2011;81(3):142–147.
35. Liu SC, Chiu WK, Chen SY et al. Comparison of surgical result of anterolateral thigh flap in reconstruction of through-and-through cheek defect with/without CT angiography guidance. *J Craniomaxillofac Surg* 2011;39(8):633–638.
36. Sacks JM, Nguyen AT, Broyles JM et al. Near-infrared laser assisted indocyanine green imaging for optimizing the design of the anterolateral thigh flap. *Eplasty* 2012;12:278–285.
37. Smit JM, Klein S, Werker PM. An overview of methods for vascular mapping in the planning of free flaps. *J Plast Reconstr Aesthet Surg* 2010;63(9):e674–e682.
38. Bayol JC, Sury F, Petraud A et al. The free anterolateral thigh flap for head and neck reconstruction: Technical particularities of the harvesting and results about six cases. *Ann Chir Plast Esthet* 2011;56(6):504–511.
39. Rashid M, Aslam A, Malik S et al. Clinical applications of the pedicled anterolateral thigh flap in penile reconstruction. *J Plast Reconstr Aesthet Surg* 2011;64(8):1075–1081.
40. Holzbach T, Giunta RE, Machens HG. Phalloplasty with pedicled anterolateral thigh flap. *Handchir Mikrochir Plast Chir* 2011;43(4):227–231.
41. Lannon DA, Ross GL, Addison PD et al. Versatility of the proximally pedicled anterolateral thigh flap and its use in complex abdominal and pelvic reconstruction. *Plast Reconstr Surg* 2011;127(2):677–688.
42. Zeng A, Qiao Q, Zhao R et al. Anterolateral thigh flap-based reconstruction for oncologic vulvar defects. *Plast Reconstr Surg* 2011;127(5):1939–1945.

34 Imaging and Surgical Principles of Anteromedial Thigh Perforator Flaps

Emanuele Cigna, Michele Maruccia, Alessandro Napoli, and Hung-Chi Chen

CONTENTS

34.1 INTRODUCTION

The distal anteromedial half of the thigh is a very adequate flap donor site for knee and upper leg soft tissue reconstruction. Different pedicle can be used to harvest skin flap as local or free flap. The perforator branches that supply this area originate from different principal vascular axis such as the saphenous artery [1–3], the musculoarticular or osteoarticular branch of the descending genicular artery [1,4], the superior medial genicular artery [5], the femoral artery [6], or the popliteal artery [1,5].

The anteromedial thigh flap (AMTF) is first described by Song et al. [7] but even though it has been reported more than 20 years ago there are only few descriptions concerning its clinical use, mostly case reports [8–10]. These described indications for AMTF use are generally related to chimeric flaps [8,10] or as an alternative procedure, in case of absence or intraoperative damage of perforators, during anterolateral thigh flap (ALTF) harvest [11]. Following these first descriptions, other studies were reported describing the origin of the pedicle of the AMTF [8–11]; however, just recently, detailed anatomical studies concerning the arterial anatomy of the thigh region have been reported [12–15], focusing on the number, position, calibre, and type of AMT perforators, nevertheless with a limited clinical impact.

One of the main problems in the harvesting of this flap is an inconstant anatomy of the pedicle, but with the development of imaging techniques and especially computed tomography angiogram (angio-CT) also with 3D reconstruction, this flap has become a viable alternative to ALTF [16] (Figures 34.1 and 34.2).

34.2 HISTORY

The restricted clinical use of the AMTF is simply due to the anatomical variations in the perforator of the flap. Its vascular anatomy is still a debated issue, concerning the point of origin of the pedicle, the perforator, and its nomenclature.

Initially, Song et al. [7] described an *innominate* branch of the lateral circumflex femoral artery (LCFA) which arises from the descending branch. Using this perforator, they transferred four AMTFs.

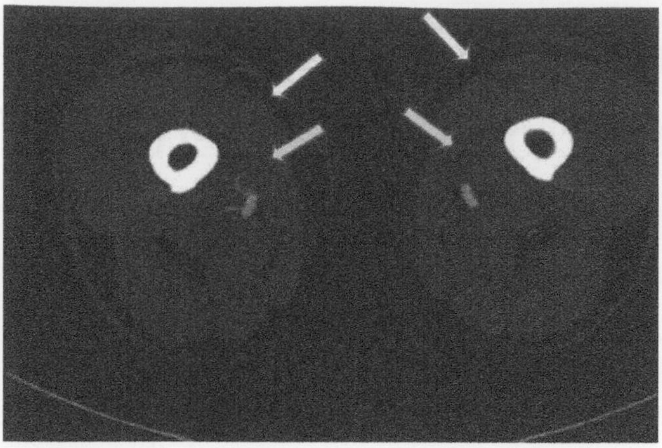

FIGURE 34.1 Preoperative angio-CT scan (axial view) of the left thigh demonstrating the bilateral course of a perforator of the AMTF with intramuscular course (inferior arrows) and subcutaneous course (superior arrows).

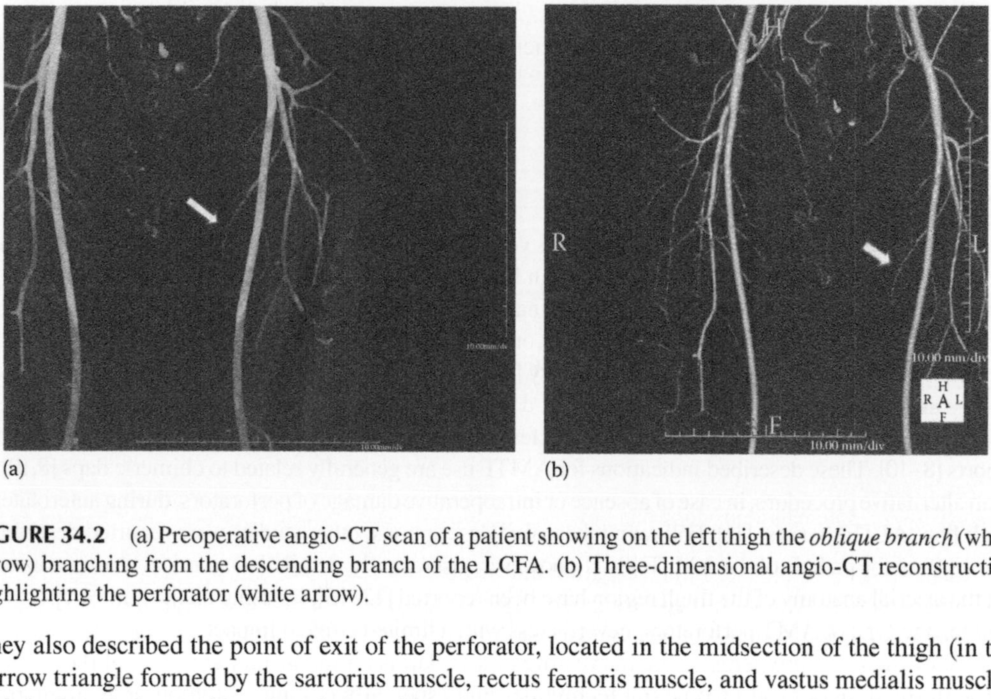

(a) (b)

FIGURE 34.2 (a) Preoperative angio-CT scan of a patient showing on the left thigh the *oblique branch* (white arrow) branching from the descending branch of the LCFA. (b) Three-dimensional angio-CT reconstruction highlighting the perforator (white arrow).

They also described the point of exit of the perforator, located in the midsection of the thigh (in the narrow triangle formed by the sartorius muscle, rectus femoris muscle, and vastus medialis muscle), and the length (up to 12 cm) and the calibre (more than 2 mm) of the artery. They stated that the venous network is double, one accompanies the artery and the second is superficial and tributary of the great saphenous vein; the nerves of the flap are anterior cutaneous branch of the femoral nerve.

Subsequently, Koshima et al. [17] reported three cases of free AMTF in which the origin of the perforator was from the LCFA and not from the descending branch, although there was correspondence with the previous report (and also the following) relating to the venous system and the sensory nerves of the flap.

In the last 10 years, several studies were carried out to define the anatomy of the ALTF. Among them, Shimizu in an anatomical study included the anteromedial region of the thigh and found the perforators of this flap in the 46% of the dissections only [18]. In their drawings, the authors represented a division of the descending branch in two branches of which the medial was considered the vessel that nourished the AMTF.

After 2 years, Ao et al. [19] reported a clinical series of four cases in which they used the AMTF and reviewed the anatomy of its pedicle. They defined a lateral and a medial descending branch of the LCFA and six more branching points where arises the cutaneous perforator for the AMTF. While the lateral branch supplies the ALT region through several perforators, the medial branch supplies the anteromedial skin of the thigh. This study introduced for the first time, regarding the anatomy of the AMTF, the term *medial* descending branch as part of the descending branch of the LCFA.

The division of the descending branch into lateral and medial branches was first reported by Xu and associates [20]. Based on a study on cadavers, to explain the anatomy of the ALTF, they stated that the descending branch divides into medial and lateral branches. While the medial branch continues downward until the geniculate network, the lateral one is the main nutrient vessel of the anterolateral skin of the thigh. They named lateral branch the perforator that supplies the skin and medial the one which is usually named descending branch, which runs distally until its connection with the lateral geniculate network. Between these two studies (Xu et al. [20] on ALTF and Ao et al. [19] on AMTF), the nomenclature is the same (medial and lateral descending branch of the LCFA) but the vessels clearly differ. Valdatta et al. [21], following the Ao and Xu nomenclature, described the vascular anatomy of the lateral circumflex femoral arterial system. In their work on cadavers, they found on 7/16 (43.75%) thighs a division of the descending branch of the LCFA in lateral and medial. In one case, the medial descending branch arose directly from the LCFA. As a result, the medial branch of the LCFA (which was considered the pedicle of the AMTF) was absent in the 50% of cases (54% following the previous anatomical study), thus suggesting to microsurgeons a low reliability of the anatomy of this flap.

Even though Schoeller and associates [8], as well as others [6–8], reported a 100% reliability of the pedicle of this flap and found that its branching point and the point of exit of the perforator correspond to the first description [7].

34.3 ANATOMY

The AMT skin is supplied by two sources of perforator: the rectus femoris branch from the descending branch of the lateral circumflex femoris artery and the superficial femoral artery itself. The perforators from the superficial femoral artery are more distally located and have a rather short and small pedicle vessel, making them less useful clinically. The perforators from the rectus femoris branch are clinically more useful because they can be traced back to the descending branch, obtaining a long and large vascular pedicle, and consequently can be used as an AMTF alone or as a chimeric ALT/AMTF. The main vascular pedicle of the AMTF, the rectus femoris branch, arises from the descending branch of the lateral circumflex femoris artery and travels underneath the rectus femoris muscle and enters the muscle on the deep medial edge. It then travels along the medial edge of the rectus femoris muscle and sends out cutaneous perforators to the AMT skin.

34.4 IMAGING EXAMINATION AND SURGICAL PRINCIPLES

There are many reports on anatomical variability of the perforator vessel of the upper third of the leg in particular in AMTF. Precise preoperative mapping of the vascular system makes it possible to minimise the complication related to an untypical vessel distribution and like in this flap where there is a high pedicle variability. A lot of methods for preoperative identification of the perforators have been described: handheld Doppler is mostly used but also colour Doppler, duplex ultrasound, arteriography, magnetic resonance angiography, and high-resolution CT. However, the handheld Doppler probe is adequate for the precise identification of perforators, while the colour Doppler can provide enough data regarding the internal diameter of the perforators [22–24].

Handheld Doppler is a non-invasive examination using the ultrasound principle combined with flow evaluation based on the phenomenon described by Doppler. It is possible to accurately

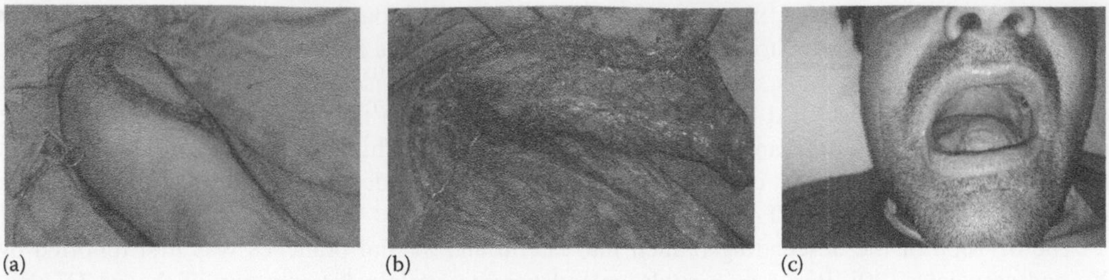

FIGURE 34.3 Patient with tongue cancer treated with hemiglossectomy and reconstruction with AMT perforator flaps. (a and b) Intraoperative view; (c) postoperative view (1 month).

determine the site where the perforator pierces the deep fascia. The number of perforators present can be determined and their diameters and blood flow can be evaluated. The accuracy of this method in the upper third of the leg in relation to the intraoperative image is rated highly – around 95% [25,26].

The perforators may be preoperatively identified with a Doppler probe and mapped on the skin. These are mainly distributed in the supero-medial quadrant of a circle of 3 cm in radius with its centre in the midpoint of a line connecting the anterior superior iliac spine and the adductor tubercle of the femur.

Angio-CT has a higher resolution than ultrasound, but if this examination is negative because the calibre of the vessel is less than 0.5 cm, in this case, it is advisable to evaluate the contralateral limb.

A 12–15 cm long incision is performed along the lateral border of the flap down to the underlying muscle. The deep fascia (fascia lata) is incised, and the rectus femoris muscle with its bi-pennate muscle fibres is exposed (a suprafascial elevation can also be performed). The fascia is sutured to the skin, and the undermining of the flap continues upward until the sartorius muscle overlying the rectus femoris muscle can be recognised and followed to reach the triangular intermuscular space, which it forms with the rectus femoris muscle and the vastus medialis muscle. The dissection proceeds carefully until the main perforator is identified and traced for few centimetres with the only intention to show if its pattern is septocutaneous or musculocutaneous. Musculocutaneous perforators are rare and their intramuscular course if present is minimal. The rectus femoris muscle is retracted laterally, and the perforators are dissected until the required length of the pedicle is achieved. The flap can now be isolated on its pedicle. Large superficial veins are clipped and spared. Sensory nerves can be harvested to provide a sensate flap (Figure 34.3).

The AMTF can be easily combined with the rectus femoris muscle or, as a chimeric flap, based on the lateral circumflex femoral system, with the vastus medialis muscle flap, the ALTF, the tensor fascia lata flap, and the iliac bone flap [27].

34.5 CONCLUSION

The AMTF has been described more than 20 years ago concurrently to the ALTF; however, there are numerous clinical reports concerning the use of the ALTF, while the AMTF vascular anatomy has not been clearly defined and only few reports describing this flap are available in the literature. The anatomy of the AMTF is reliable but the variability of diameter of its pedicle and of its origin may indicate the microsurgeon to perform an accurate preoperative evaluation.

In this flap, the preoperative mapping is extremely important to define the correct localisation of the pedicle, the calibre, and the perforator flap. At present, the clinical preoperative standard for mapping perforators is Doppler ultrasound and angio-CT.

REFERENCES

1. Acland RD, Schusterman M, Godina M et al. 1981. The saphenous neurovascular free flap. *Plast Reconstr Surg* 67:763–774.
2. Bertelli JA. 1992. The saphenous postero-medial island thigh flap and the saphenous supero-medial cutaneous island leg flap. *Surg Radiol Anat* 14:187–189.
3. Tsai CC, Lin SD, Lai CS et al. 1995. Reconstruction of the upper leg and knee with a reversed flow saphenous island flap based on the medial inferior genicular artery. *Ann Plast Surg* 35:480–484.
4. Ballmer FT, Masquelet AC. 1998. The reversed-flow medio-distal fasciocutaneous island thigh flap: Anatomic basis and clinical applications. *Surg Radiol Anat* 20:311–316.
5. Hayashi A, Maruyama Y. 1990. The medial genicular artery flap. *Ann Plast Surg* 25:174–180.
6. Koshima I, Hosoda M, Inagawa K et al. 1996. Free medial thigh perforator- based flaps: New definition of the pedicle vessels and versatile application. *Ann Plast Surg* 37:507–515.
7. Song YG, Chen GZ, Song YL. 1984. The free thigh flap: A new free flap concept based on the septocutaneous artery. *Br J Plast Surg* 37(2):149–159.
8. Schoeller T, Huemer GM, Shafighi M et al. 2004. Free anteromedial thigh flap: Clinical application and review of literature. *Microsurgery* 24(1):43–48.
9. Hayashi A, Maruyama Y. 1988. The use of the anteromedial thigh fasciocutaneous flap in the reconstruction of the lower abdomen and inguinal region; a report of two cases. *Br J Plast Surg* 41(6):633–638.
10. Koshima I, Hosoda M, Moriguchi T et al. 1993. A combined anterolateral thigh flap, anteromedial thigh flap, and vascularized iliac bone graft for a full-thickness defect of the mental region. *Ann Plast Surg* 31(2):175–180.
11. Koshima I, Fukuda H, Utunomiya R, Soeda S. 1989. The anterolateral thigh flap; variations in its vascular pedicle. *Br J Plast Surg* 42(3):260–262.
12. Pan WR, Taylor GI. 2009. The angiosomes of the thigh and buttock. *Plast Reconstr Surg* 123(1):236–249.
13. Hupkens P, Van Loon B, Lauret GJ et al. 2010. Anteromedial thigh flaps: An anatomical study to localize and classify anteromedial thigh perforators. *Microsurgery* 30(1):43–49.
14. Yu P, Selber J. 2011. Perforator patterns of the anteromedial thigh flap. *Plast Reconstr Surg* 128(3):151–157.
15. Cömert A, Altun S, Unlü RE et al. 2011. Perforating arteries of the anteromedial aspect of the thigh: An anatomical study regarding anteromedial thigh flap. *Surg Radiol Anat* 33(3):241–247.
16. Ribuffo D, Tenna S, Chiummariello S et al. 2003. Free anterolateral thigh flap for reconstruction of head and neck defects: Preliminary results and a comparison with the radial forearm flap. *Minerva Chir* 58(3):369–373.
17. Koshima I, Soeda S, Yamasaki M et al. 1988. The free or pedicled anteromedial thigh flap. *Ann Plast Surg* 21(5):480–485.
18. Shimizu T, Fisher DR, Carmichael SW, Bite U. 1997. An anatomic comparison of septocutaneous free flaps from the thigh region. *Ann Plast Surg* 38(6):604–610.
19. Ao M, Uno K, Maeta M et al. 1999. De-epithelialised anterior (anterolateral and anteromedial) thigh flaps for dead space filling and contour correction in head and neck reconstruction. *Br J Plast Surg* 52(4):261–267.
20. Xu DC, Zhong SZ, Kong JM et al. 1988. Applied anatomy of the anterolateral femoral flap. *Plast Reconstr Surg* 82(2):305–310.
21. Valdatta L, Tuinder S, Buoro M et al. 2002. Lateral circumflex femoral arterial system and perforators of the anterolateral thigh flap: An anatomic study. *Ann Plast Surg* 49(2):145–150.
22. Bhattacharya V, Deshpande SB, Watts RK et al. 2005. Measurement of perfusion pressure of perforators and its correlation with their internal diameter. *Br J Plast Surg* 58:759–764.
23. Panse NS, Bhatt YC, Tandale MS.2011. What is safe limit of the perforator flap in lower extremity reconstruction? Do we have answers yet? *Plast Surg Int* 2:349–357.
24. Saint-Cyr M, Schaverien MV, Rohrich RJ. 2009. Perforator flaps: History, controversies, physiology, anatomy, and use in reconstruction. *Plast Reconstr Surg* 123:132–145.
25. Taylor GI, Doyle M, McCarten G. 1990. The Doppler probe for planning flaps: Anatomical study and clinical applications. *Br J Plast Surg* 43:1–16.
26. Cheng MH, Chen HC, Santamaria E et al. 1997. Preoperative ultrasound Doppler study and clinical correlation of free posterior interosseous flap. *Changgeng Yi Xue Za Zhi* 20:258–264.
27. Cigna E, Chen HC, Ozkan O, Sorvillo V, Maruccia M, Ribuffo D. 2014. The anteromedial thigh free flap anatomy: a clinical, anatomical, and cadaveric study. *Plast Reconstr Surg*. Feb;133(2):420–429.

35 Imaging and Surgical Principles for Tensor Fascia Lata Flap

Ömer Özkan, Özlenen Özkan, Ahmet Duymaz, Kamil Karaali, and Can Çevikol

CONTENTS

35.1 INTRODUCTION

The tensor fascia lata (TFL) flap is one of the first described free flaps. It consists of the tensor muscle, the fascia lata, and the cutaneous coverage over the fascia. It is a type 1 muscle (Mathes & Nahai) with a single dominant pedicle known as the transverse branch of the lateral circumflex femoral artery and venae comitantes. The TFL is one of the most reliable and usually satisfactory flaps, due to its constant anatomy and the acceptable diameter and length of the vascular pedicle. The vascular pedicle gives three musculocutaneous perforators to nourish the overlying cutaneous region. Although the TFL muscle itself is too small, these perforators permit almost all the skin of the anterolateral thigh to be supplied, offering an extensive cutaneous territory, three times the size of the muscle. It may be used as a pedicled flap to adjacent defects involving the groin, vulva, perineum, sacrum, ischium, or trochanteric region or as a free flap for more distal reconstruction.

The TFL muscle was first used by Wangensteen in 1934 to reconstruct hernia defects as a pedicled flap without skin. It was used as a musculocutaneous flap by Baily in 1967 to cover acetabular defects. Surgeons such as Hill, Nahai, Bostwick, and McGregor and Buchan subsequently discovered a wide variety of applications in reconstructive surgery. Nowadays, it can also be used as a perforator flap, as described by Deiler in 2000 and Koshima in 2001.

35.2 REGIONAL ANATOMY

(Figure 35.1)

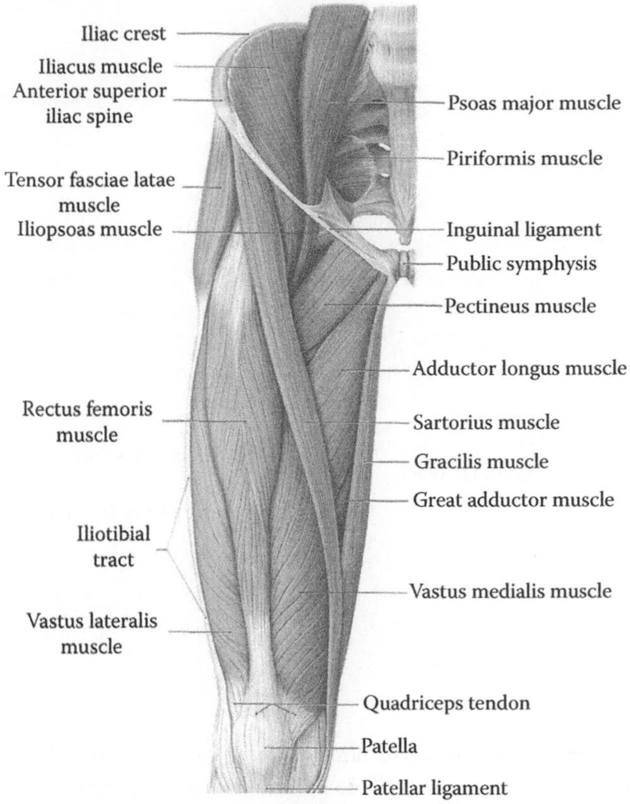

FIGURE 35.1 Regional anatomy and muscles of the thigh.

35.3 ARTERIAL ANATOMY OF THE THIGH

The femoral artery receives blood through the external iliac artery. This connection arises at the femoral triangle behind the inguinal ligament (Figure 35.2). After the femoral artery, known specifically as the common femoral artery, leaves the femoral triangle, it divides into superficial and deep (profunda) branches 2–4 cm inferior to the inguinal ligament. The adductor longus muscle serves as a separation between these branches. While the deep branches run posterolaterally to the adductor longus muscle, the superficial branch courses anterior to it. The deep femoral artery provides blood to the thigh, while the superficial femoral artery supplies blood to the arteries that nourish the knee and foot.

The deep femoral artery gives off the medial femoral circumflex artery and three perforating arteries when it runs posterior to the adductor longus muscle. The medial femoral circumflex artery gives off two branches, the ascending and descending branches, at the level of the upper border of the adductor brevis. The deep femoral artery generally has four perforating arteries, though this can range from 2 to 6. The lateral circumflex artery arises from the lateral side of the deep femoral artery 8–10 cm inferior to the anterior superior iliac spine (ASIS); runs transversally between the divisions of the femoral nerve, behind the sartorius and rectus femoris muscle; and then divides into ascending, transverse, and descending branches which supply the lateral and posterior thigh muscles. The ascending branch primarily supplies blood to the gluteus minimus muscle, and the transverse branch nourishes the TFL muscle, emerging through the anteromedial aspect of the muscle, while the descending branch supplies the vastus lateralis muscle.

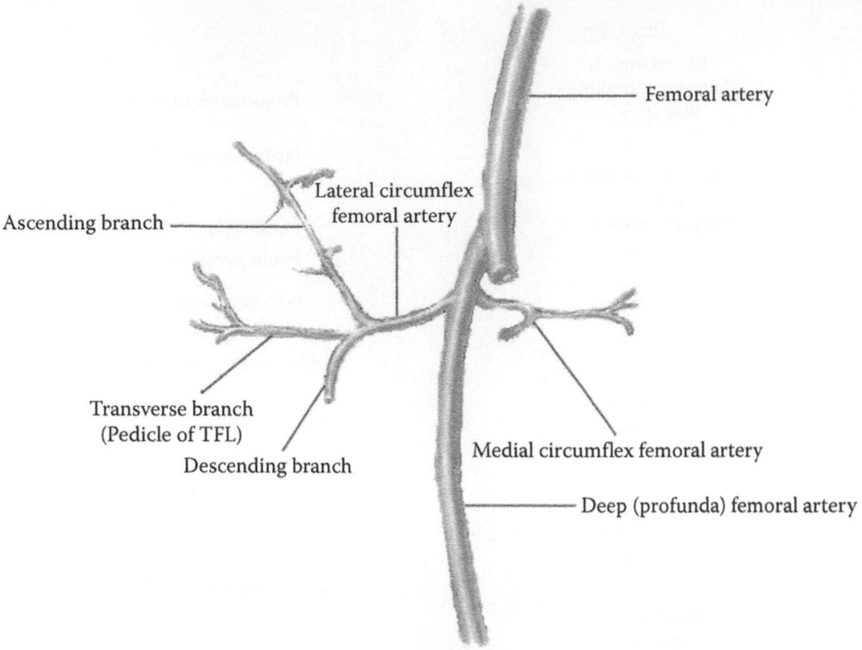

FIGURE 35.2 Arterial supply of the thigh.

The external diameter of the transverse branch of the lateral circumflex artery is 2–3 mm at its origin. Measured from its origin to the TFL muscle, the average length of the vascular pedicle is 4–6 cm in adults. It gives off three branches before emerging from the TFL muscle; superior, middle, and inferior. The superior branch supplies the proximal or upper one third of the muscle and neighbouring iliac bone at the origin of the muscle. The middle branch supplies the middle one third of the muscle, and the inferior branch supplies the lower third of the muscle and distal fascia.

Connections between the origin of the TFL muscle and outer lip of the anterior iliac crest permit transfer of the muscle with the bone as a vascularised bone flap based on the vascular pedicle of the muscle. The blood supply of the osseous segment is furnished by 2–3 small vessels emerging from the iliac bone through the muscle attachments.

Both the medial and lateral femoral circumflex arteries may rarely arise directly from the femoral artery.

The distal third of the thigh is also supplied by the perforating branches of the deep femoral artery.

35.4 VENOUS ANATOMY IN THE REGION

The venous system is usually through one or two venae comitantes which course with the arteries. The external diameter is approximately 2–4 mm at the level where the transverse branch connects to its main trunk. The lateral circumflex femoral vein then joins to the femoral vein (not the deep branch of the femoral vein or the profundus femoris vein), 2–4 cm inferior to the inguinal ligament.

35.5 NERVES IN THE REGION

The lateral femoral cutaneous nerve of the thigh is a nerve of the lumbar plexus which takes the form of the dorsal divisions of the second and third lumbar nerves (Figure 35.3). It enters from the lateral margin of the psoas major muscle at the level of its middle and runs in the pelvis beneath the iliac fascia, toward the ASIS. It then passes under the inguinal ligament 1–3 cm medial to the ASIS and over the sartorius muscle into the thigh, where it divides into an anterior and a posterior branch.

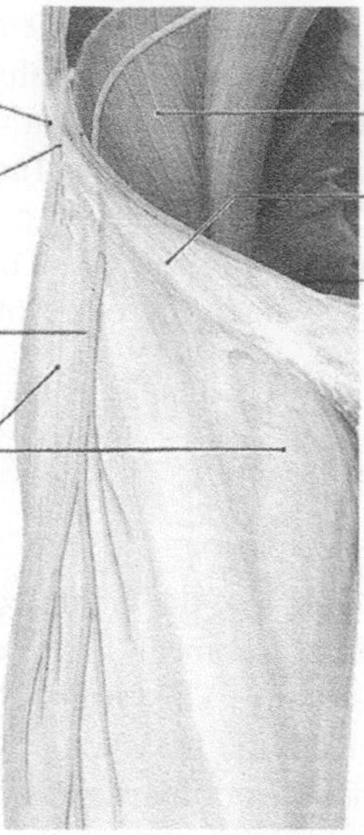

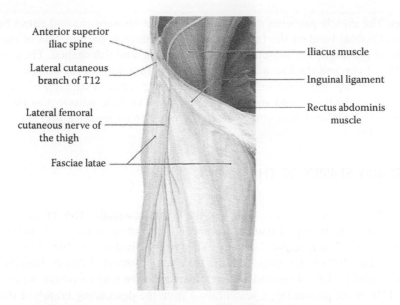

FIGURE 35.3 Sensorial territory of the overlying skin of the TFL muscle flap.

The anterior branch becomes superficial about 10 cm below the inguinal ligament and divides into branches which are distributed to the skin of the anterior and lateral parts of the thigh, as far as the knee. It measures 2–3 mm proximally and has 3–4 fascicles.

35.6 FLAP ANATOMY

The TFL muscle, located on the lateral side of the thigh, arises from the anterior part of the outer lip of the iliac crest between the gluteus medius and sartorius muscles (Figures 35.1 and 35.4). It extends 5 cm along the iliac crest toward the outer surface of the ASIS as a flat and

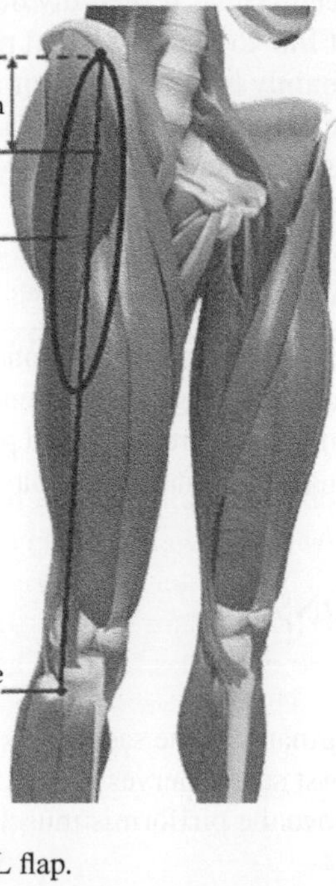

FIGURE 35.4 Anatomic landmarks for the TFL flap.

broad tendon. The muscle proceeds distally as a band-like aponeurosis and enters between two layers of the iliotibial band of the fascia lata approximately at the junction of the upper and middle thirds of the thigh. The muscle is small, broad, flat, and fish shaped. The average length is 13 cm, width 4 cm, and thickness 2 cm. The primary functions of the muscle are to provide stabilisation of the hip and lower extremity in standing posture; extension of the knee, as an accessory flexor of the thigh; and abduction of the hip. The TFL muscle may be sacrificed; it is not of primary functional importance since there are other muscles that can assume these functions.

35.7 ARTERIAL SUPPLY OF THE FLAP

(Figure 35.2)

The dominant artery is the transverse branch of the lateral circumflex femoral artery. There is no minor artery because of the type 1 muscle. The mean length of the pedicle is 5 cm (range 4–7 cm) and the diameter is 2.5 mm (range 2–3 mm). This artery divides into three branches, superior, middle, and inferior, before emerging from the muscle as mentioned earlier. However, while the ascending branch of the lateral circumflex femoral artery is the major vascular supply of the TFL flap in 10%–15% of the population, a vessel raised from the descending branch of the lateral circumflex femoral artery supplies the flap in 15%–20% of cases.

An average of 2–5 musculocutaneous perforators, measuring 0.8–1.0 mm in diameter, originate from the pedicle to supply the overlying anterolateral thigh skin. These perforators penetrate the muscle proximally and then run superficially to the fascia. More distally, fasciocutaneous perforators arise from either the descending branch of the lateral circumflex artery or the profunda femoris artery and also supply the distal skin of the thigh (within 4–6 cm of the knee). However, these fasciocutaneous perforators are not applicable to dissection based on the main vascular pedicle of the flap. Delay procedures and involving the fascia to the flap require elevating the flap in the caudal part of the thigh.

All three branches of the transverse branch of the lateral circumflex femoral artery send perforating branches into the skin. The perforator vessel runs in a posterolateral direction in adipose tissue after penetrating the deep fascia. It then divides into several branches in the middle of its course which run in a straight line to the subdermal plexus. The blood flow to the skin and lining of adipose tissue is supplied mainly by the perforator and partially by the capillary network in the adipose tissue. Aggressive thinning without leaving a large cuff of fat may sacrifice the blood circulation through this network, resulting in a less reliable area of skin.

35.8 VENOUS DRAINAGE OF THE FLAP

Generally, two venae comitantes of the transverse branch of the lateral circumflex artery provide the venous network of the flap. The mean length of the venae comitantes is 5 cm (range 4–7 cm) and the diameter 2.5 mm (range 2–3 mm). There are also small perforator vessels in the caudal thigh which join to the deep femoral vein. But this is not suitable as additional venous drainage for standard flap harvest.

35.9 FLAP INNERVATIONS

35.9.1 Motor

The superior gluteal nerve originates in the sacral plexus and arises from the ventral division of the fourth and fifth lumbar and first sacral nerves (L4–L5–S1). It exits the pelvis through the greater sciatic foramen and passes above the piriformis muscle. The nerve is accompanied by the superior gluteal artery and vein. It runs laterally between the gluteus medius and minimus muscles, innervating both. It then emerges from the middle third of the TFL muscle from the posterior surface, 4–5 cm below the iliac crest.

35.9.2 Sensory

(Figure 35.3)
The skin of the TFL flap is innervated by two different sensory nerves:

1. Lateral cutaneous branch of the 12th thoracic nerve
2. Lateral cutaneous of the thigh (L2–3)

35.9.2.1 Lateral Cutaneous Branch of the 12th Thoracic Nerve

The nerve perforates the oblique externus and internus muscle in the anterior axillary line and descends over the iliac crest approximately 6 cm posterior to the ASIS. It is distributed to the skin overlying the iliac crest, the front part of the gluteal portion, or the proximal region of the TFL. It measures 2–3 mm in diameter proximally and involves 2–3 fascicles.

35.9.2.2 Lateral Cutaneous of the Thigh (L2–3)

It enters 1–3 cm inferomedially to the ASIS as detailed earlier and courses over the sartorius, penetrating deep fascia, to innervate the distal two thirds of the anterolateral aspect of the thigh.

35.10 FLAP COMPONENTS

The flap can be elevated as a musculocutaneous, osteomusculocutaneous, musculo-osseous, musculofascial, or skin-only flap.

35.11 ADVANTAGES

1. This flap has a long vascular pedicle with a suitable external diameter for vascular anastomosis.
2. The TFL has an extensive and reliable skin vascular territory.
3. The vascular pedicle is located between the vastus lateralis and rectus femoris muscles, and variation is rare.
4. It does not require positional changing during surgery for most patients, since the flap can be harvested with the patient in the supine position.
5. The TFL can be elevated as fasciocutaneous, musculocutaneous, fascia or muscle-only, osteomusculocutaneous, or musculo-osseous flaps and harvested under spinal or epidural anaesthesia.
6. A sensate flap can be obtained by captation of the lateral cutaneous part of T12 and/or the lateral femoral cutaneous nerve of the thigh to the skin portion of the flap.
7. A functional muscle flap can also be achieved by including a branch of the superior gluteal nerve (motor nerve).
8. The flap can be harvested as a perforator flap and thinned to 5 mm by sectioning the TFL muscle between the medial and superior branches of the distal lateral femoral artery.
9. Primary closure of the donor site is possible if the width of the skin flap is less than 8–9 cm, and it does not cause major functional deficit in the lower extremity when harvesting the TFL muscle flap.

35.12 DISADVANTAGES

1. The donor site may be unacceptable and difficult to conceal, especially in patients who require skin grafting for closure.
2. Unless the flap is elevated as a perforator-based flap, it may be bulky.
3. In rare cases, loss of TFL muscle can cause minimal loss of knee stability. When the cutaneous flap can be harvested suprafascially, this risk can be minimised.

35.13 FLAP DIMENSION

35.13.1 Muscle Dimensions

The width of the TFL muscle is 4 cm (range 3–5 cm) with an average length of 13 cm (range 12–15 cm). It is 2 cm thick (range 1.5–3 cm).

35.13.2 Skin Island Dimensions

The width of the cutaneous paddle is 10 cm (range 7–20 cm); length and thickness are 20 cm (range 15–40 cm) and 10 mm (range 5–20 mm), respectively. The length of the cutaneous flap can be extended beyond 10 cm proximal to the knee if a delay procedure is performed. Otherwise, there is no possibility of the distal portion of the flap surviving.

35.13.3 Fascia Dimensions

The length of the flap is 10 cm (range 5–30 cm), width 10 cm (range 6–20 cm), and thickness 2 mm (range 1–2 mm).

35.13.4 Bone Dimensions

The average length of the bone segment is 5 cm (range 4–8 cm), width is 4 cm (range 2–5 cm), and thickness is 12 mm (range 10–17 mm). The bone segment that incorporates the origin of the TFL muscle flap is included in the flap (Figure). The vascular pedicle of the osseous segment is provided by two to three small vessels emerging from the iliac crest through the TFL muscle, which is supplied by an ascending branch of the main pedicle.

35.13.5 Preoperative Preparation

The side of the flap chosen is determined by the recipient site or the defect to be reconstructed. A Doppler probe can be used according the type of the flap to decide on the most reliable artery and its course, such as harvesting the perforator-based flap. The thigh is prepared and scrubbed. Shaving the hair is usually optional and depends on surgeon's choice, the nature and length of the hair, and the recipient site.

For most cases, the area of the thigh, hip, and entire leg is prepared down to the level of the knee to facilitate hip and knee flexion when required.

Computed tomography (CT) and magnetic resonance (MR) imaging can be performed to ensure extension of the wound and reliability of the pedicle and the flap in the case of decubitus ulcer defects before surgery.

35.13.6 Flap Markings

A line is drawn from the ASIS to the lateral condyle of the femur to expose the vascular pedicle (Figures 35.4 and 35.5). The flap is outlined on the lateral aspect of the thigh; the anterior border corresponds to this line. A point, demarcating the vascular pedicle, is marked 8 cm (range 6–10 cm)

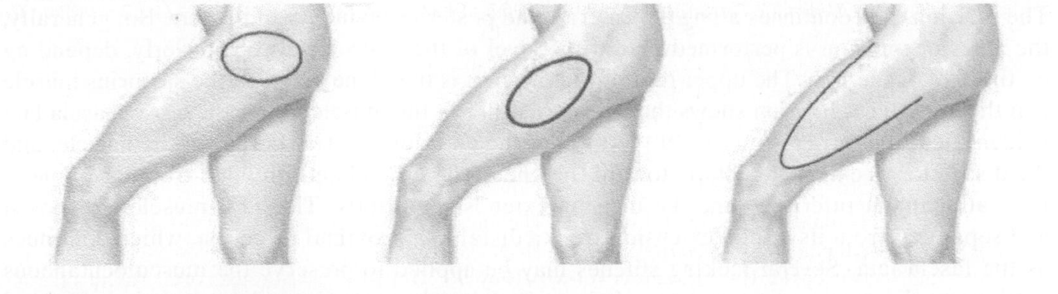

FIGURE 35.5 Flap markings.

caudal/inferior to the ASIS. This point also represents the central axis of the flap. The lateral femoral cutaneous nerve (also called the lateral cutaneous nerve of the thigh) emerges from the thigh below the inguinal ligament about 1–2 cm inferomedially to the ASIS and runs over the sartorius muscle into the thigh. A line 10 cm inferior to the ASIS at the anterior boundary of the flap represents the point for the lateral femoral cutaneous nerve of the thigh. The lateral cutaneous branch of the 12th thoracic nerve is located 6 cm posterior to the ASIS.

35.13.7 Patient Position

The patient is placed in the supine position to harvest the free flap and for the anterior arc of rotation or reconstruction of abdominal, inguinal, and trochanteric defects and in the prone position for the posterior arc of rotation or treatment of ischial and sacral defects. The lateral decubitus position can also be used for covering hip and ischial defects.

35.14 TECHNIQUE OF FLAP HARVEST

35.14.1 TFL Muscle Flap

(Figure 35.6)
An initial incision to elevate the flap can be made along the anterior, posterior, or distal border of the flap. If distal to proximal dissection is selected, the distal border of the flap is incised first.

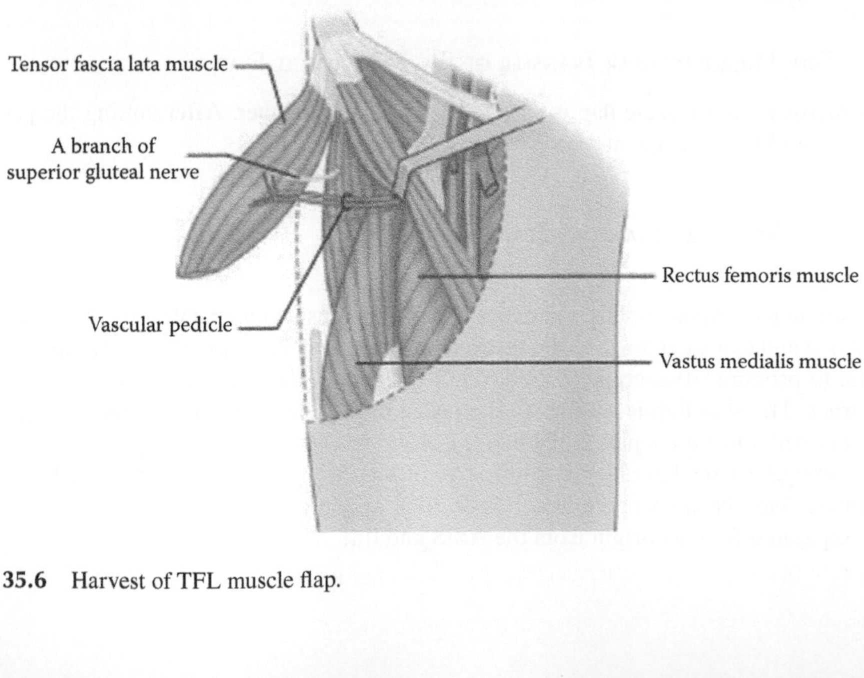

FIGURE 35.6 Harvest of TFL muscle flap.

The incision then continues along the anterior and posterior boundary of the flap. But generally, the anterior incision is performed first at the level of the ASIS or more anteriorly, depending on the size of the flap. The upper part of the incision is the plane between the sartorius muscle and the TFL. This incision shows the anterior border of the muscle. After the tensor fascia lata is identified, the fascia is incised at the level of the anterior–inferior border of the muscle, and the dissection is extended distally toward the knee. The fascia lata is divided from the aponeurotic attachment inferiorly, and the incision extends posteriorly. The TFL muscle is exposed and separated from its fascial extension from a distal to a proximal direction, which continues as the fascia lata. Several tacking stitches may be applied to preserve the musculocutaneous perforators. Dissection deep to the fascia lata overlying the vastus lateralis muscle is performed rapidly in a relatively bloodless field. The rectus muscle is exposed in the upper part of the incision and retracted medially to identify the neurovascular pedicle of the flap at the level of the middle third of the muscle between the rectus femoris and vastus lateralis muscles. When a pedicled flap is required, it is not necessary to pursue the dissection further proximally. If functional muscle transfer is planned, a branch of the superior gluteal nerve is identified between the gluteus medius and gluteus minimus muscles posterior to the vascular hilus. This should be carefully sought out at the posterior border of the muscle, 4–5 cm inferior to the iliac crest. Vascular branches of the gluteus minimus and vastus lateralis muscle are ligated, resulting in a pedicle length of 5–6 cm. Finally, the TFL muscle is completely freed from the vastus lateralis, rectus femoris, sartorius, and gluteal muscles. Dissection of the pedicle can be continued up to the profunda femoris artery to obtain more length when necessary. This can be achieved by further dissection to obtain a pedicle as long as 10 cm by ligating all branches, including the descending branch. During the dissection of the vascular pedicle, care should be taken deep to the rectus femoris muscle where the vessel is closely related to the muscular branch of the femoral nerve. For most purposes, it is not necessary to separate the origin of the muscle. However, to harvest a true island flap or to avoid a dog-ear deformity at the point of rotation, the origin of the muscle is divided from the iliac crest. The muscle flap is elevated based on its neurovascular pedicle.

To reduce flap bulk and donor site morbidity such as contour depression on the upper lateral region of the thigh, a small portion of the muscle can be elevated according to the defect requirement. This is achieved by preserving the superior, anterior, and posterior parts, including the muscle inferior to and around the vascular bundles.

35.14.2 Free Microvascular Transfer of the TFL Muscle Flap

The free microvascular muscle flap is elevated in the same manner. After cutting the pedicle, the flap is transferred to the recipient area.

35.14.3 TFL Musculocutaneous Flap

(Figure 35.7)

Markings are made similar to those mentioned earlier in muscle flap harvesting. All skin incisions are performed and extended down to the fascia lata. The flap is then elevated in the subfascial plane from distal to proximal dissection, at the level of the aponeurotic attachment of the muscle to the iliotibial tract. The skin flap is sutured to the fascia to prevent perforator damage. After the skin island is obtained, the muscle part of the flap is isolated based on its vascular pedicle. If a neurovascular flap is required, the lateral cutaneous nerve of the thigh is explored beforehand as described for the muscle flap, the appropriate length is decided on, and the nerve is sharply transected. The muscle is separated from its origin from the ASIS and iliac crest.

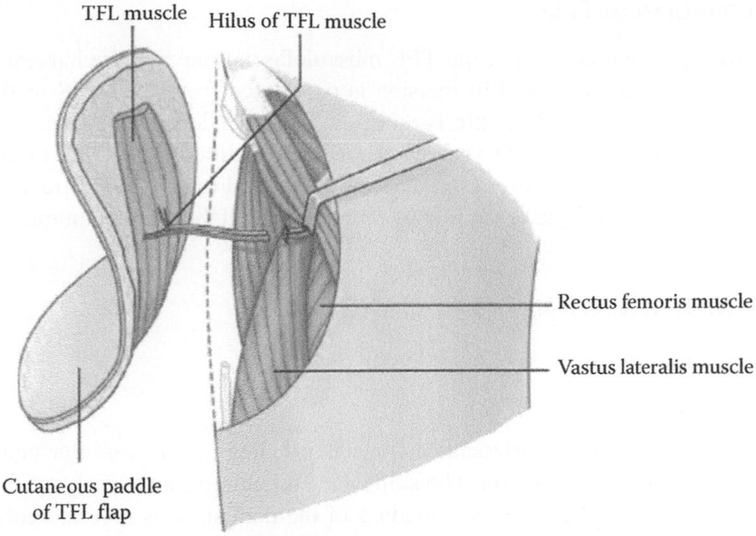

FIGURE 35.7 Harvest of TFL musculocutaneous flap.

35.14.4 TFL Osteomusculocutaneous Flap

(Figure 35.8)

An anterior segment of the iliac crest, connected to the origin of the TFL muscle and adjacent tissue, can be taken with the flap as a vascularised bone graft. The dissection is similar to those outlined earlier in the muscle or musculocutaneous flaps, with the exception that an upright incision proximal/superior to the ASIS might be involved to identify the osseous segment of the flap. Nourishment of the bony segment is from the periosteum at the muscle origin. After the vascular pedicle is isolated, ostomies are performed to elevate a segment of iliac bone without dividing the muscle origin from the iliac crest. Harvest of osseous segment is easier after ligation of the vascular pedicle.

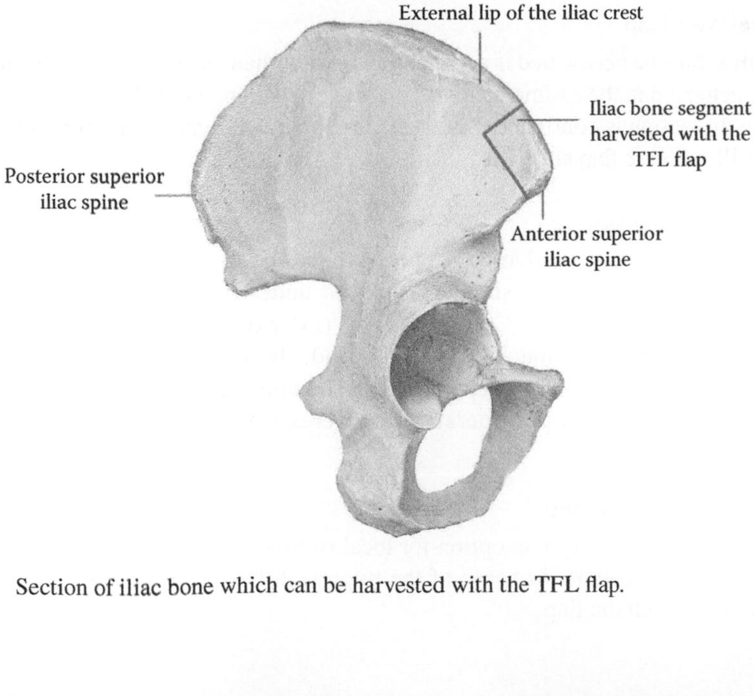

FIGURE 35.8 Section of iliac bone which can be harvested with the TFL flap.

35.14.5 Musculofascial Flap

If cutaneous coverage is not necessary, the TFL musculofascial flap may be harvested. The fascia lata is elevated with the muscle. A skin incision is performed from the ASIS to the knee along the midlateral point of the thigh. The skin is reflected on each side, and the fascia lata is exposed. The width and length of the fascia harvest are determined on the basis of the required flap size. The fascia lata is then incised and dissected as usual in a distal to proximal direction. However, a pure fascia flap without the muscle or cutaneous unit is not a reliable flap technique.

35.15 FLAP MODIFICATIONS/FLAP HANDLING

35.15.1 Transverse

35.15.1.1 Skin Island

An elliptical island marked in a horizontal manner is oriented on the vascular pedicle. This has been described for breast reconstruction. The skin island is centred transversely extending from the lateral thigh to the buttock. The superior boundary of the flap island is several centimetres below the iliac crest. The lower border is planned depending on the reconstructive needs. But this design is not to be preferred on account of unacceptable donor site appearance.

35.15.1.2 Osseomuscular or Osseomusculocutaneous Flap

An osseomusculocutaneous flap involving the outer side of the iliac bone at the origin of the muscle may be harvested in dimensions of 5 cm × 4 cm.

35.15.1.3 Extended Skin Island

This flap is much wider and longer than the standard flap. Planning of the cutaneous flap can be extended to 4 cm above the lateral femoral condyle, but the width of the flap should not be greater than 10 cm at the most distal level. The flap elevation is essentially the same as for the standard flap. Tissue expansion or flap delay is required for longer flap harvest. But the fascia lata must be involved with the skin flap at the distal level to prevent flap failure.

35.15.1.4 Delayed Flap

Delay procedures must be performed if a longer flap harvest than an extended skin island is required. This is usually achieved in the estimated distal margin of the flap. After the distal borders of the flap are incised, the dissection is continued subfascially, and finally, ligating small perforators from the main pedicle will increase flap survival.

35.15.1.5 Tissue Expansion

Tissue expansion makes it possible to increase the standard flap dimensions and functions as delay procedures. An expander should be placed under the fascia lata by a small incision anteriorly or posteriorly at least 2–3 cm away from (inferior to) the vascular pedicle. After the dissection is completed and homeostasis is achieved, the expander is located. Intraoperative expansion is performed minimally, depending on the volume of the expander. The expansion process is initiated 1–2 weeks postoperatively. Overexpansion is generally useful to achieve reasonable outcomes.

35.15.1.6 Neurosensorial Flap

The TFL is a good neurosensory flap option for local transfer or distant microvascular transplantation. The lateral femoral cutaneous nerve of the thigh (L2–L3) or the lateral cutaneous branch of T12 may be involved with the flap.

35.15.1.7 Functional Muscle Flap

The TFL muscle flap can be used as a dynamic functional flap. The branch of the superior gluteal nerve must be involved with the muscle flap for this purpose. It is preferred for upper extremity dynamic reconstructions, such as shoulder or elbow deficits. The maximum excursion of the muscle when properly sited is about 3 cm, and the muscle contractions can be shorted by an average fascicle length of 40%.

35.15.1.8 Chimeric Flap

Chimeric flaps can also be harvested based on the vascular pedicle of the TFL at the mid-part of the thigh and, more caudally, elevated based on the subcutaneous pedicle that is proximally supplied by the same pedicle. It permits mobilisation of the flap in many different planes. Each part of the flap may be transferred freely to cover more severe complex defects. This modification is reduced due to donor site morbidity, and more satisfactory aesthetic results can be achieved after flap inset due to pliability of the subcutaneous tissue. It may also be possible to harvest the vastus lateralis muscle pedicled on the descending branch of the lateral circumflex femoral artery with the chimeric TFL flap to obtain extensive volume and larger dimensions and also to give two units.

35.15.1.9 Perforator Flap

Perforators run in the posterolateral direction in fat tissue after penetrating the deep fascia. The diameters of these musculocutaneous perforators are 0.5–1 mm. Microdissection follows through the TFL muscle up to the transverse branch of the lateral circumflex femoral artery. After reaching the transverse branch of the artery, dissection proceeds up to the main trunk, the transverse branch is ligated, and finally, the perforator flap is elevated based on this vascular pedicle to use as a free or pedicled flap. The pedicle is longer than the musculocutaneous flap, with a mean length of 8 cm (range 7–10 cm). The adipose tissue of the skin flap is covered with deep fascia, which is trimmed sharply away from the perforator. This provides a thinned flap up to 5 mm. The disadvantage of this procedure is that it requires meticulous dissection and considerable experience. It is not always necessary to use Doppler USG to identify the perforator.

35.15.1.10 V–Y Advancement Flap

The V–Y advancement flap covers defects of the greater trochanter.

35.15.1.11 Special Instruments

Standard surgical instruments are adequate for the elevation of the pedicled musculocutaneous flap. However, microsurgical instruments, an operating microscope, and loupe magnification are required for the harvest of free or perforator flaps.

35.15.1.12 Donor Site Closure

Primary closure of the donor site is achieved when the width of the cutaneous flap is less than 6–8 cm. Otherwise, the donor site requires split-thickness skin graft closure. Before suction drains are placed, careful homeostasis to bleeding from the adjacent muscles is performed. Two-layer closures are then performed. Compression over the pedicle should be avoided when inserting the drains and applying the dressing. If even a small part of intact fascia is left in the donor site, this should be sutured back in an appropriate manner to preserve knee stability.

35.15.1.13 Precautions and Technical Tips

1. Donor site closure under tension should be avoided since this may lead to a compartment syndrome within the lower extremity.
2. Caution is advised, because the distal skin portion may be unreliable if extended too far. Flap delay or expander insertion is required.

3. The location of the vascular pedicle is not always constant; it may be found between 8 and 12 cm inferior to the ASIS. This should therefore be kept in mind during harvesting.
4. Elevating an osseous segment from the iliac bone may lead to contour deformity and possible herniation of the abdominal wall.
5. The superior gluteal nerve should be preserved during the flap dissection.
6. If a sensory flap is required, ultra-thinning of the flap should be avoided because of sensory nerve damage.
7. Injection of local anaesthesia over the proximal course of the lateral femoral cutaneous nerve is a very useful method in mapping the territory of the nerve if elevating a neurosensory flap.
8. The muscle attachment can be separated from the iliac crest to increase the arc of rotation of the flap and to avoid dog-ear formation.

35.16 FLAP USE

35.16.1 Pedicled

The TFL is used as a fascia–skin or the muscle–fascia–skin flap for reconstruction of defects in the

Groin
Ischium
Perineum
Lower abdomen
Sacrum
Trochanter

The pivot point of rotation of the flap is 10 cm below the ASIS that enters the vascular pedicle. Posterior and anterior arcs of rotation can cover the greater trochanter, ischium, perineum, and sacral area and the abdominal wall, groin, vulva, and perineum, respectively. Anterior rotation can extend to the xiphoid and the contralateral iliac bone. The TFL is an excellent choice for soft tissue closure of abdominal, trochanteric, ischial, perineal, and sacral defects. The fascia lata can provide additional fascial support for abdominal wall integrity. But in large abdominal defects or if there is an insufficient arc of rotation, a free TFL should be carried out. This flap is also used for penile reconstruction as a pedicled flap. The dimensions of the peninsular design as a rotation flap are 10–12 cm × 15–17 cm, but this can be up to 10–12 cm × 23–25 cm when the flap is designed as a free or island flap.

35.16.2 Microvascular Free Flap

The vascular territory of the TFL supplies a very large and reliable skin and muscle area. It is used as a free flap as described in the following:

Upper and lower extremity
Head and neck
Functional reconstruction
Upper abdominal wall reconstruction
Breast reconstruction

The standard TFL flap for closure of head and neck defects is not suitable where a thin flap is required involving intraoral mucosa defects and skin-only defects. But in composite or through-and-through defects, it may be an ideal option.

Osseomuscular or osseomusculocutaneous flaps are preferred for both bony and soft tissue repair, such as maxillofacial and long-bone reconstruction.

Functional muscle flap may be used for reconstruction of functional deficit in the extremities. The best options as an innervated flap are the restoration of knee extension, shoulder abduction, elbow flexion, and Achilles reconstruction. It can also be used for functional restoration of extensive tongue defects.

A neurosensory flap is also used as sole covering by including one or two sensory nerves to the flap.

The TFL perforator flap may be used either free or pedicled. As mentioned earlier, the TFL muscle is left intact in this modification to prevent excessive flap bulk and reduce donor site morbidity. The free TFL perforator flap is a good option for tendon coverage and reconstruction.

35.17 ATYPICAL INDICATIONS FOR THE USE OF THE FLAP

35.17.1 Pedicled

Penis reconstruction with an extended flap

35.17.2 Free

Maxillofacial and extremity bony reconstruction
Breast reconstruction with transverse skin island

35.17.3 Postoperative Care

Clinical observation is best for flap monitoring. This should be done hourly for the first 2 days after free TFL flap reconstruction. No medication for flap viability is given in our department. We use only antibiotics, pain medication, and fluid management. We recommend continuous heparin infusion in the postoperative period in heavy crush injuries and in patients undergoing flap re-exploration. Depending on the reconstructed site, in our clinic, the patient is usually kept in bed for 2–3 days and then mobilised. The supine position is preferred if the flap is placed on the ventral body surface or the extremities. The reconstructed extremity is slightly elevated. The prone or lateral decubitus position is recommended for dorsal flaps involving the ischial or sacral area for 12–15 days. The supine or lateral decubitus position is used for reconstruction of the trochanteric region.

The patient is discharged after 1 week postoperatively. However, this may be longer in cancer patients and patients with poor general condition.

35.17.4 MRI Appearance of the Tensor Fascia Lata Muscle

The tensor fascia lata muscle is clearly visible in routine MR images (Figure 35.9). It originates from the iliac crest, and its fibres run downward and slightly backward. Distally, the fibres are inserted into the iliotibial tract. The fibres appear isointense to the other muscles in the thigh, whereas the fascia lata is hypointense in all MR imaging sequences, since it is a dense fibrous tissue (Figure 35.10). Arteries and veins are usually seen as hypointense tubular structures in T2-weighted images. However, routine sequences are usually not sufficient for the visualisation of muscular perforators.

35.17.5 Demonstration of Vascular Pedicle and Perforators

CT or MR angiography techniques can be used for the demonstration of vascular pedicle and perforators.

CT angiography should be performed on multislice scanners, preferably at 64 or more slices. Iodine-based contrast materials are injected via antecubital veins, and bolus tracking techniques are necessary to achieve optimal enhancement and visualisation of the arteries.

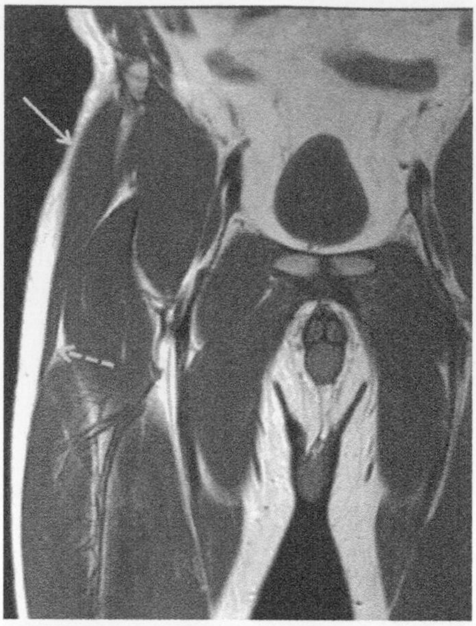

FIGURE 35.9 T1-weighted coronal MR image. The arrow shows the belly of the tensor fascia lata muscle. The dashed arrow shows the distal part of the muscle before insertion.

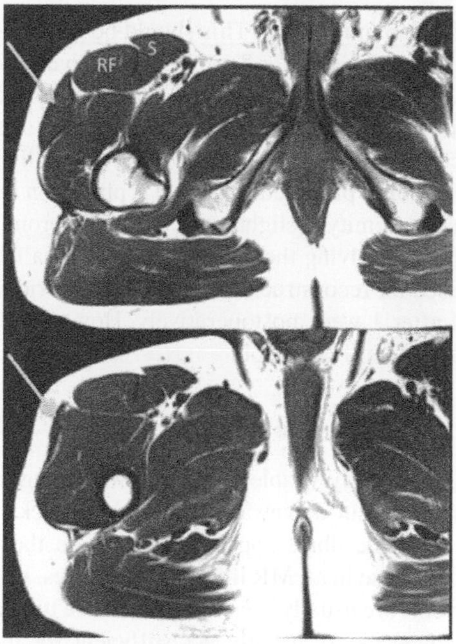

FIGURE 35.10 T1-weighted transverse MR images. The upper image is at the level of ischial tuberosity just below the iliac crest. The arrow shows tensor fascia lata muscle; RF, rectus femoris; S, sartorius muscle medial to the tensor fascia lata. Lower image, the arrow shows the distal part of the muscle before insertion to the fascia lata.

After obtaining the image data, reformatted images, such as multiplanar reformats and maximum and minimum intensity projections, are produced on workstations. At CT angiography, small perforators can be visualised better than with MR angiography (Figure 35.11). The soft tissue contrast is worse than with MRI. It also uses ionising radiation, which can be considered as another disadvantage.

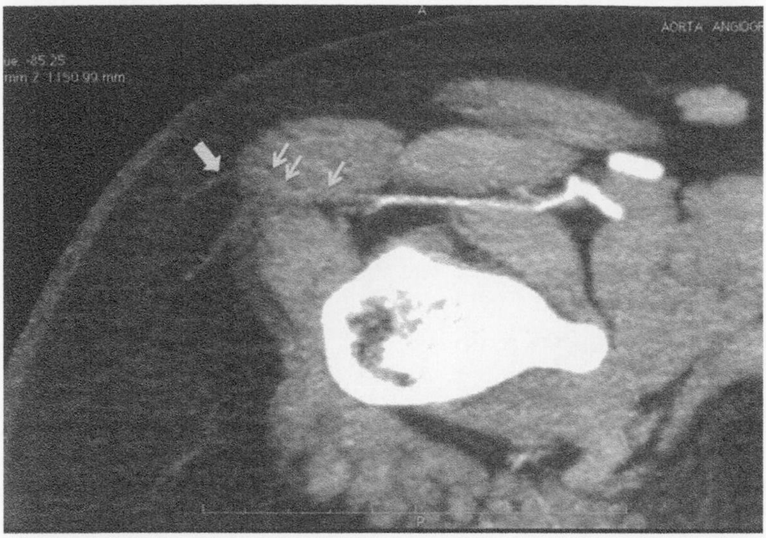

FIGURE 35.11 CT angiography, axial reformatted multi-planar reformatted (MPR) image showing the intramuscular (small arrows) and subcutaneous (large arrow) course of the perforator.

At MR angiography, breath-hold images are produced after obtaining localising scans. For the optimal enhancement of the arteries, accurate timing is necessary during the contrast injection. Fluorotriggering methods are used for this purpose. When optimal enhancement of the arteries within the area of interest is reached, the MR angiography sequence is started manually. After obtaining the image data, post-processing is performed on workstations, and 3D maximum intensity projection (MIP) images are produced. It is usually difficult to show small perforators at MR angiography. Perforator arteries may be visualised in routine MR sequences, such as T1- or T2-weighted spin echo/turbo spin echo. Additionally, 3D T2-weighted gradient echo sequences may be valuable for demonstrating small perforators (Figure 35.12). In this technique, contrast injection is not used, and vessels appear as bright linear intensities passing through muscles.

It is also possible to place external markers (such as fish oil capsules for MRI) to locate and mark perforators relative to the anterior superior iliac crest (Figure 35.13).

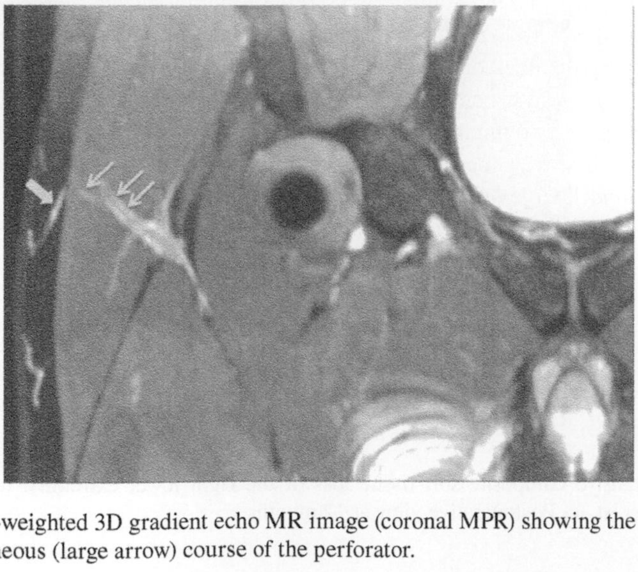

FIGURE 35.12 T2-weighted 3D gradient echo MR image (coronal MPR) showing the intramuscular (small arrows) and subcutaneous (large arrow) course of the perforator.

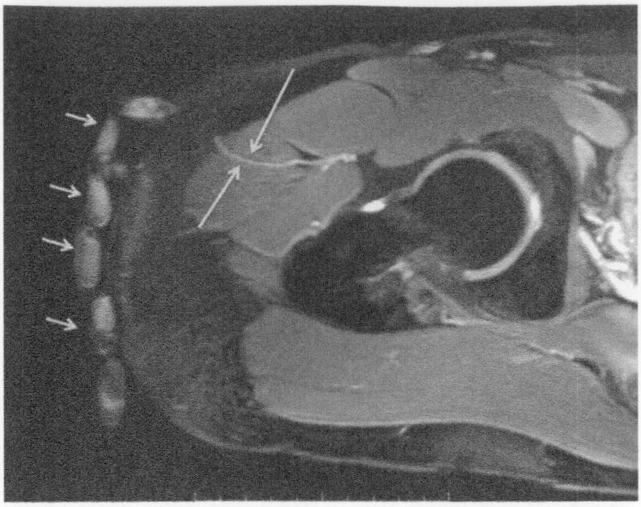

FIGURE 35.13 T2-weighted 3D gradient echo MR image (axial MPR) showing the intramuscular (long arrows) course of the perforator. Small arrows show fish oil capsules used for marking.

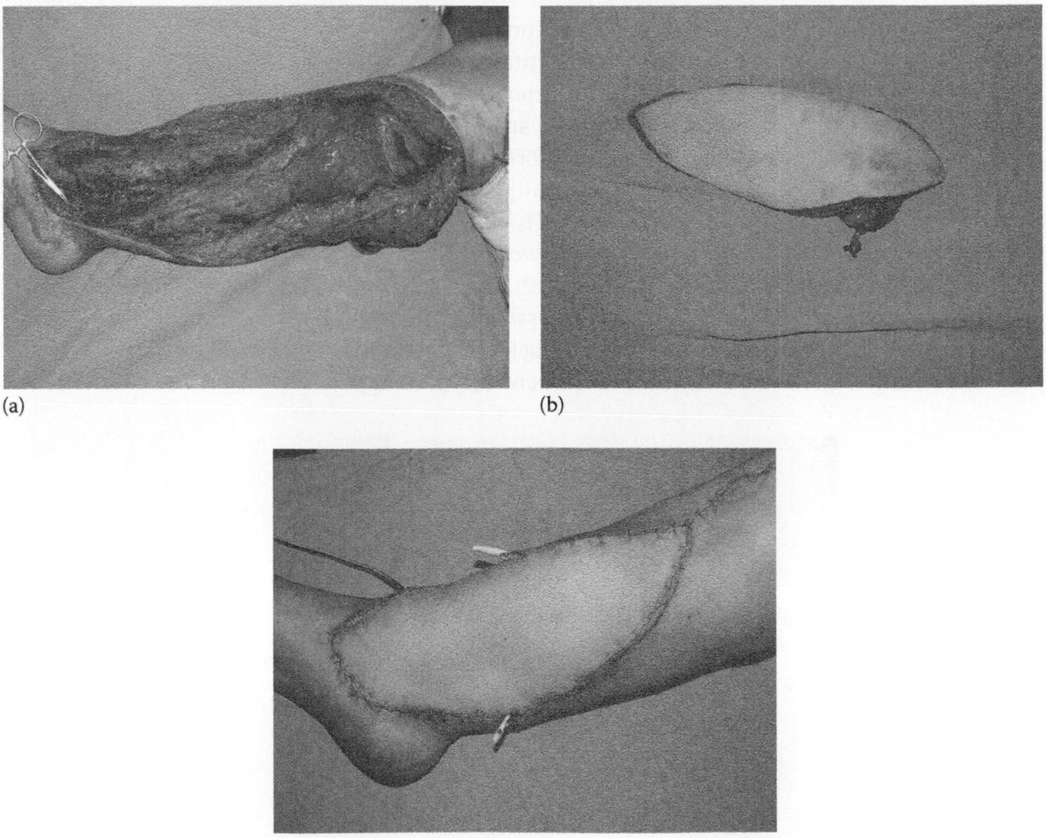

(a) (b) (c)

FIGURE 35.14 Extensive composite soft tissue loss of the right lower extremity. (a) Preoperative view. (b) TFL flap after harvest. (c) Postoperative view at 12 months.

35.17.6 Case Examples

Case 1: Extensive soft tissue reconstruction with exposed tibia of a lower extremity with a TFL myofasciocutaneous flap

A 44-year-old man suffered a traffic accident, which resulted in a composite tissue defect of the medial and distal anterior aspects of the lower extremity (Figure 35.14a). After sufficient debridement, a TFL flap (14 cm × 33 cm) was harvested (Figure 35.14b) and used to cover the defect (Figure 35.14c). The pedicle was anastomosed to the posterior tibial vessels. The donor area defect was closed using a split-skin graft. Postoperative recovery was uneventful.

Case 2: Subcutaneous pedicled TFL myocutaneous flap for reconstruction of a trochanteric decubitus ulcer

A 56-year-old paraplegic patient had a large trochanteric decubitus ulcer of 11 months duration (Figure 35.15a). A pedicled TFL flap (11 cm × 18 cm) was designed to close the defect (Figure 35.15b). The flap was rotated posteriorly, and the donor area was closed primarily (Figure 35.15c). Postoperative recovery was uneventful.

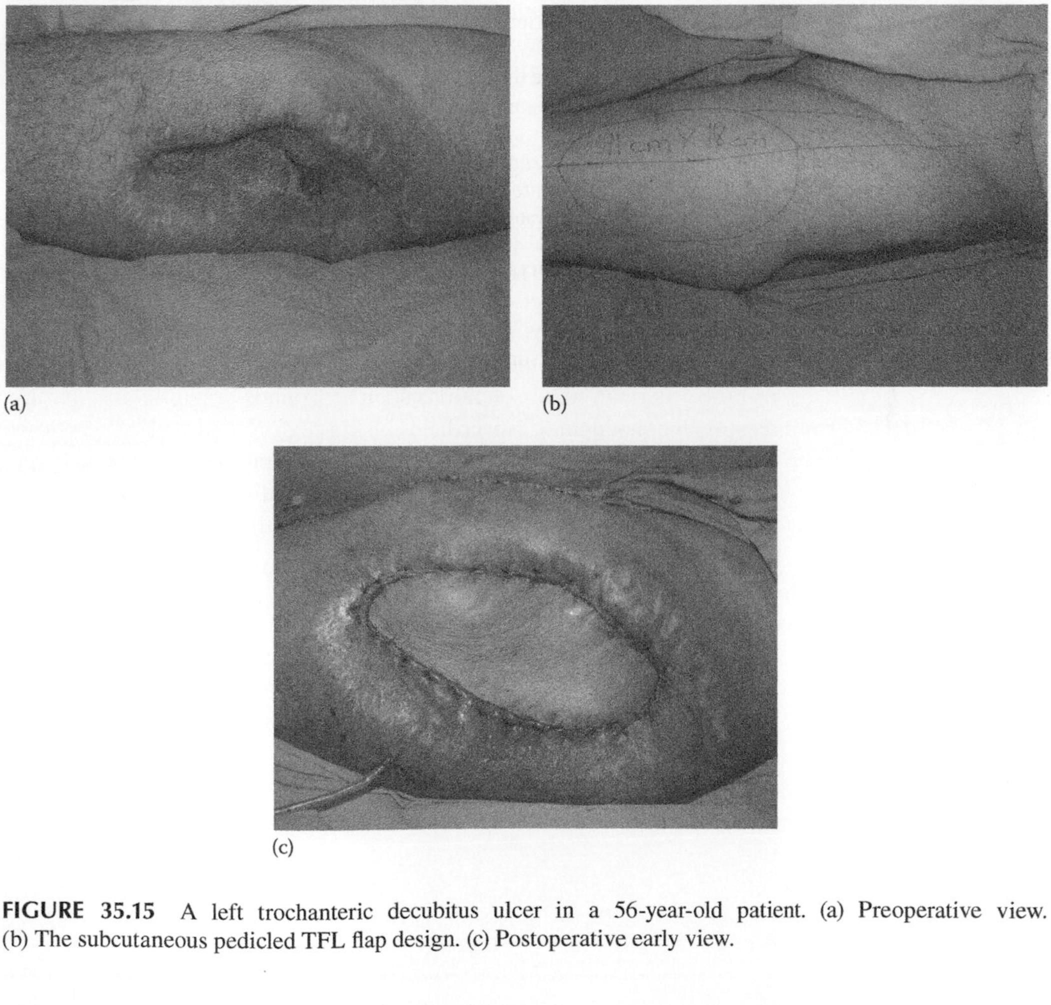

FIGURE 35.15 A left trochanteric decubitus ulcer in a 56-year-old patient. (a) Preoperative view. (b) The subcutaneous pedicled TFL flap design. (c) Postoperative early view.

FURTHER READING

Bostwick J, Hill NL, Nahai F. 1979. Repairs in the lower abdomen, groin, or perineum with myocutaneous or omental flaps. *Plast Reconstr Surg* 63:186–194.

Brand PW, Beach RB, Thompson DE. 1981. Relative tension and potential excursion of muscles in the forearm and hand. *J Hand Surg* 6A:209–219.

Caffee HH, Asokan R. 1981. Tensor fascia lata myocutaneous free flaps. *Plast Reconstr Surg* 68:195–200.

Cheng N, Shou B, Zheng M, Huang A. 1994. Microneurovascular transfer of the tensor fascia lata musculocutaneous flap for reconstruction of the tongue. *Ann Plast Surg* 33:136–141.

Coşkunfirat OK, Ozkan O. 2006. Free tensor fascia lata perforator flap as a backup procedure for head and neck reconstruction. *Ann Plast Surg* 57(2):159–163.

Hill HL, Nahai F, Vasconez LO. 1978. The tensor fascia lata myocutaneous free flap. *Plast Reconstr Surg* 61:517–522.

http://en.wikipedia.org. (Accessed on August 10, 2012).

Kimura NA. 2002. Microdissected thin tensor fasciae latae perforator flap. *Plast Reconstr Surg* 109:69–77.

Koshima I, Urushibara K, Inagawa K et al. 2001. Free tensor fasciae latae perforator flap for the reconstruction of defects in the extremities. *Plast Reconstr Surg* 107:1759–1765.

Manktelow RT, McKee NH. 1978. Free muscle transplantation to provide active finger flexion. *J Hand Surg* 3:416–426.

Masquelet AC. 2001. *An Atlas of Flaps of Musculoskeletal System*, Taylor & Francis Group, UK, pp. 141–142. Tensor fasciae latae myocutaneous flap.

Mathes SJ, Nahai F. 1997. *Reconstructive Surgery Principles, Anatomy and Technique Volume*, Tensor fascia lata TFL flap, eds. SJ Mathes and F Nahai, pp. 1271–1292. Churchill Livingstone, Inc. Printed in USA.

McGregor JC, Buchan AC. 1980. Our clinical experience with the tensor fasciae latae myocutaneous flap. *Br J Plast Surg* 33:270–276.

Nahai F, Hill L, Hester TR. 1979. Experiences with the tensor fascia lata flap. *Plast Reconstr Surg* 63:788–799.

Nahai F, Silverton JS, Hill HL et al. 1978. The tensor fascia lata musculocutaneous flap. *Ann Plast Surg* 1:372–379.

Ozkan O, Coskunfirat OK. 2009. *Flaps and Reconstructive Surgery*, Tensor fascia lata flap, ed. FC Wei and S Mardini, pp. 545–560. Elsevier, Inc., UK, Printed in China.

Ribuffo D, Cigna E, Gargano F et al. 2005. The innervated anterolateral thigh flap: Anatomical study and clinical implication. *Plast Reconstr Surg* 115(2):464–470.

Safak T, Klebuc MJ, Kecik A, Shenaq SM. 1996. The subcutaneous pedicle tensor fascia lata flap. *Plast Reconstr Surg* 97:765–774.

Strauch B et al. 1993. Atlas of microvascular surgery: The anatomy and operative techniques, pp. 174–179. Thieme Medical Publishers, New York, NY, tensor fascia lata flap.

36 Surgical Principles of Deep Circumflex Iliac Artery

Warren M. Rozen, Mark W. Ashton, Vachara Niumsawatt, Alberto Alonso-Burgos, Iain S. Whitaker, and Jeannette W. Ting

CONTENTS

36.1 INTRODUCTION

The deep circumflex iliac artery (DCIA) flap is a safe and versatile flap that has long been considered the gold standard flap for hemi-mandibular reconstructions.[1–4] The DCIA flap has a dependable vascular pedicle length, large diameter vessels, and wide arc of rotation for the flap.[5] The thick and sturdy iliac crest the DCIA supplies is associated with an inconspicuous donor scar and low donor site morbidity.[6,7] The iliac crest is rich in cortico-cancellous bone, the high osteogenicity and vascularity of which is particularly useful in the setting of previous infection.[8] Large volumes of vascularised bone and muscle can be used to close maxillectomy fistulas, create a contoured mandible, support the orbital contents, reconstruct the orbital rim, and provide sufficient bulk of bone for the placement of implants.[9] The DCIA flap has also been used for reconstruction of the maxilla, groin, lower limb, and upper limb.[8,10–18] Until recently, there was generally a poor understanding of the DCIA perforators (DCIA-Ps) of the skin overlying the iliac crest, leading to its reputation as having unreliable perforators. Recent computed tomography angiographic studies have dispelled this myth, and with appropriate imaging, the DCIA-P flap is a valuable tool in the reconstructive surgeons' repertoire.

36.2 HISTORY OF THE DCIA FLAP

The iliac crest flap has long been used for bony reconstruction of the mandible. Autologous cancellous bone from the ilium replaced prosthetic appliances in the 1890s as the reconstruction of choice for mandibular defects.[19] During World War I, non-vascularised iliac crest bone was used and held in place with external fixation. In World War II, internal fixation was used and antibiotics were introduced.[2] Although these techniques significantly impacted on wound healing, results remained poor, with a high rate of failure. From the 1960s, a combination of metallic plates and non-vascularised bone graft were used, but these were also complicated by infection, exposure, and fracture.[2,20] Regardless of whether the ilium, rib, or prosthetic material was used, it was finally recognised that non-vascularised bony grafts all tended to result in high rates of non-union, resorption, and infection.[5,21–23] In the 1970s, surgeons began to replace non-vascularised bone with their vascularised counterpart with significantly improved results.

Surgeons first used soft tissue free flaps (rectus abdominis, radial forearm) to cover mandibular reconstruction plates. However, erosion of the plate through the flap was common.[24] They then turned to vascularised bone and its associated muscle in myocutaneous flaps. These include pectoralis major and associated rib, sternocleidomastoid muscle with clavicle, trapezius with scapula, temporalis with parietal bone, and first dorsal metatarsal artery and the metatarsus.[20] With this new approach, the bone and soft tissue now began to survive, but results remained somewhat unsatisfactory as the bone quality of these flaps was often poor and function was sacrificed for form.[2,20,25,26]

Attention was turned back to the iliac crest. Surgeons attempted to raise the iliac crest as a free flap based on the superficial circumflex iliac artery (SCIA) as its vascular supply. This was met with less than ideal results.[1,27]

Reliable and successful elevation of a vascularised iliac crest flap was first described in 1979. Two landmark papers, one clinical and one experimental, by Taylor et al. described in detail the DCIA-P flap as an osteomusculocutaneous flap of the iliac crest, abdominal muscle, and overlying skin.[5]

Since then, various modifications of the flap have increased its repertoire of use. Smaller volumes of bone and muscle are also achievable with the DCIA flap cortex splitting technique first described by Taylor's group in 1982[28] and again described by Shenaq in 1994.[29] The muscle cuff-sparing variation has also been described by Safak in 1997 and Kimata in 2003 to allow harvesting of the overlying skin with less underlying muscle bulk.[6,12,30] The Rubens flap, a musculocutaneous flap based on the DCIA, was developed by Hartrampf as an extension of Taylor's work.[11] This was first described in 1994, and it utilises the DCIA's supply to the muscle and soft tissue of the iliac region for breast reconstruction. It was named the *Rubens* flap after Peter Paul Rubens' *The Three Graces* painting which clearly outlined the fat deposit in this area.[31] The Rubens flap is an option for breast reconstruction in a woman who has had previous abdominal lipectomy and therefore unable to have autologous breast reconstruction utilising the abdominal wall.

When perforator flaps became popular in the late 1980s, there was hesitancy by surgeons to use the DCIA for a perforator flap, believing that the DCIA had unreliable perforators. This is predominantly due to a poor understanding and lack of research into DCIA-Ps. Surgeons who use the DCIA flap tend to advocate including some overlying abdominal muscle to preserve the perforators. Interestingly enough, although several authors in the 1980s refer to these flaps as osteocutaneous flaps, they all include the cuff of muscle and therefore should be named osteomusculocutaneous flaps.[32]

Recent computer tomographic angiography studies have described the DCIA-P in detail and re-established the versatility of the DCIA flap.[33] Its successful use has been demonstrated in case series, and recent advancements in preoperative anatomical modelling have increased the repertoire of use.[34]

36.3 ANATOMY OF THE DCIA

The DCIA is the first lateral arterial branch of the external iliac artery as it passes under the inguinal ligament.[5] It ascends medial to the iliac bone towards the anterior superior iliac spine (ASIS) and branches into the main branch and the ascending branch.[35] The DCIA has been well described as a large vessel (routinely over 2 mm) arising from the lateral or posterolateral surface of the external iliac artery adjacent to the origin of the deep inferior epigastric artery[5,27] (Figure 36.1). Its territory of supply includes the iliac crest, and the vessel has been described into two parts: a straight (inguinal) part medial to the ASIS and a curved (iliac) part lateral to the ASIS.[27] It ends by piercing the transversus abdominis muscle at approximately the midpoint of the iliac crest[12] and anastomosing with the iliolumbar, superior gluteal, and intercostal arteries.[12,27,35] The main branch of the DCIA travels along the iliac crest also between transversus abdominis and internal oblique and then sends musculocutaneous perforators to the overlying skin.[35] It forms a rich anastomotic network with surrounding arteries including the superficial circumflex iliac, intercostal, lumbar, and iliolumbar arteries.[35] The iliac crest bone has been identified to be supplied by the DCIA in two ways: firstly, by the main branch on the medial side

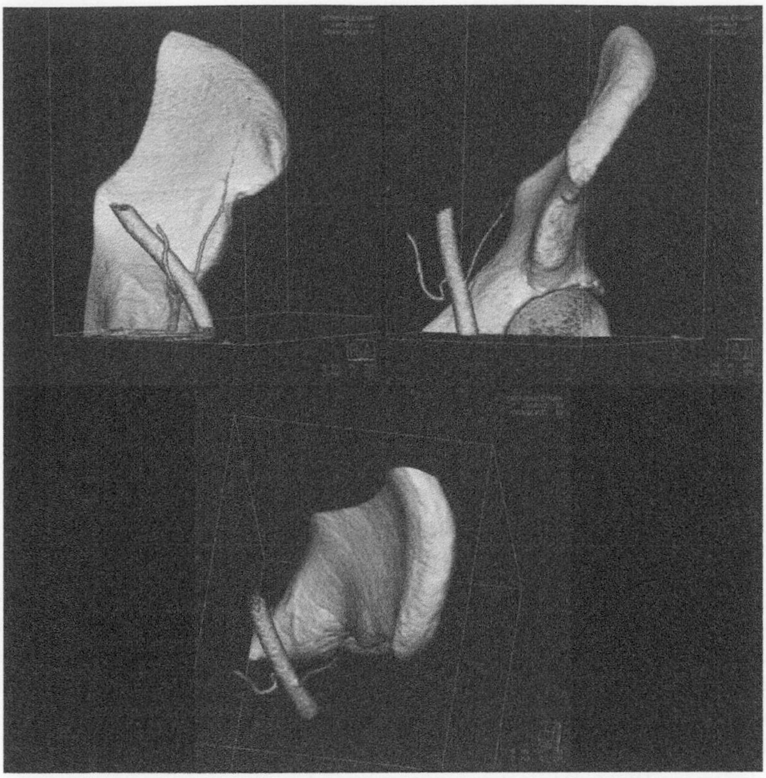

FIGURE 36.1 Preoperative VRT reconstruction of a CTA of the abdominal wall vasculature, demonstrating the left iliac bone in three dimensions and its mode of supply by the DCIA. (Reproduced from Ting, J.W.C. et al., *Microsurgery*, 30, 163, 2010. With permission.)

of the cortex and, secondly, to the periosteal vessels by branches to the iliacus muscle.[35] The DCIA supplies the whole iliac crest via multiple small branches which results in the ability to perform wedge osteotomy and reshaping of the iliac crest without compromising the blood supply to the iliac crest.[28]

Its most significant branch, the large ascending branch, is usually greater than 1 mm in diameter and arises 1 cm medial to the ASIS, to supply the internal oblique muscles, with almost no supply to the skin.[5,12,27,35,36] The ascending branch of the DCIA arises in 1 cm of the ASIS in 65% of cases, 2–4 cm medial to the ASIS in 15% of patients. In the remaining 20% of cases, the ascending branch exists as multiple branches rather than a single branch.[36]

36.4 IMAGING OF THE DCIA

Taylor et al.'s study found that the DCIA's supply to the iliac crest is extraordinarily robust[5] with perforators that are within centimetres of the ASIS.[35] The vascular pedicle of the source DCIA vessel for the perforator flap is of adequate length and calibre, comprising at least 2 mm diameter in calibre and 5–6 cm in length.

Computed tomographic angiogram (CTA) can be used to identify the bony supply by the DCIA to the iliac crest to guide the surgeon when harvesting small amount of iliac crest.[15] This may be particularly useful when the whole iliac crest is not required or in composite flaps, and morbidity to the patient may be reduced when only the required amount of bone is safely harvested.[15,34]

Researchers have attempted to achieve in improving the understanding of the perforators of the DCIA through studies such as whole body injection[37] and Doppler ultrasound.[10,29,35,37] Doppler ultrasound is known for its inter-individual variability, poor accuracy, and inability to accurately

TABLE 36.1
Summary Findings of the Anatomy of the DCIA-Ps in 44 Hemiabdominal Walls, Assessed with the Use of CTA

	Mean	Range
No. of perforators per hemiabdomen	1	0–4
Diameter	1.1 mm	0.8–1.8 mm
Distance from ASIS		
Vertical distance	5.1 cm	0.5–10.0 cm
Posterior distance	3.9 cm	0.5–6.7 cm

Source: Reproduced from Ting, J.W.C. et al., *Microsurgery*, 29, 326, 2009. With permission.

predict size differences between perforators. More so, aside from mere location, the Doppler probe is unable to identify the source artery or its intramuscular and extramuscular path. The region of supply is further confounded by the adjacent territory of supply by the SCIA.[5,27]

Computer tomographic angiographic study have now identified the size, number, and location of the perators.[33] A 2009 study was used, utilising a 64-slice multi-detector row CT scanner (Siemens Medical Solutions, Erlangen, Germany), with 100 ml of intravenous contrast (Omnipaque 350; Amersham Health, Princeton, NJ). CTA images were reformatted into maximum intensity projection (MIP) and 3D volume-rendered technique (VRT) images using commercially available software (Siemens InSpace; Version: nSpace2004A PRE 19, PA).

The summary findings of the number, size, and location of this largest computed angiographic tomographic studies on DCIA-P to date are shown in Table 36.1.
The use of CTA in this case enabled preoperative planning of the side of choice for flap harvest and to map the course of the DCIA throughout its path as a means to safe and rapid harvest.

In 60% of hemiabdominal walls, there are no identifiable perforators over 0.8 mm. Of these, over 50% have only one perforator of >0.8 mm diameter (32%), over ¼ hemiabdomens had two perforators, 15% had three perforators, and less than 4% had four perforators arising from the DCIA (Graph 36.1). The mean distances of the perforators are 5.1 cm cranial and 3.9 cm from the ASIS.

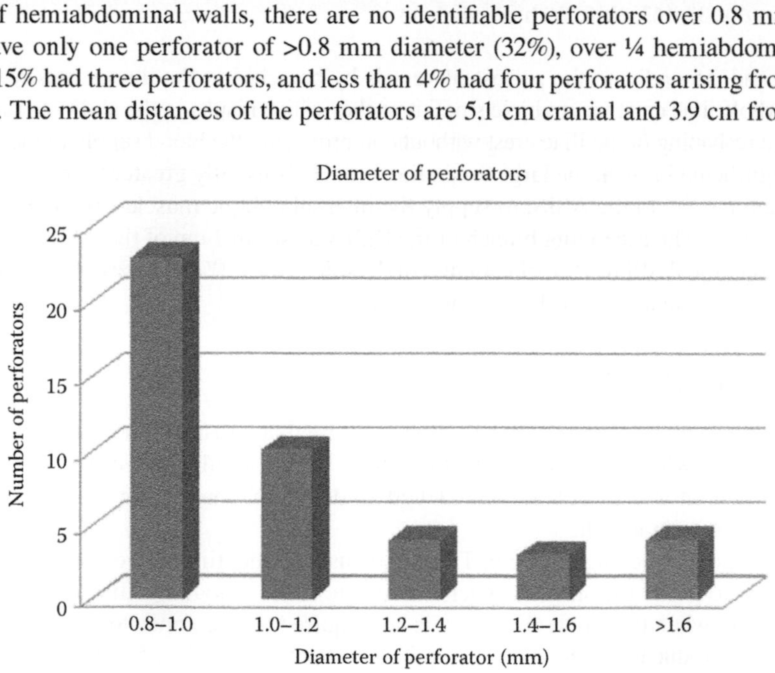

GRAPH 36.1 The diameter of DCIA-Ps over 0.8 mm. (Reproduced from Ting, J.W.C. et al., *Microsurgery*, 29, 326, 2009. With permission.)

In addition, the majority of perforators emerge from the muscle in a 4 cm × 4 cm area of skin 3 cm superior and 2 cm posterior to ASIS.[38] The location and number of perforators can be easily remembered by the 4, 3, 2, 1 rule – where within a square of 4 cm × 4 cm, 3 cm cranial, and 2 cm posterior to ASIS, one perforator may be found (Figures 36.2 through 36.4). Just over half of the perforators are between 0.8 and 1.0 mm in diameter with the majority of the remaining perforators being between 1.0 and 1.2 mm in diameter.

Most recent advancements of the use of CTA of the DCIA are its application to stereolithographic models. Stereolithographic biomodels have been described in the literature for a number

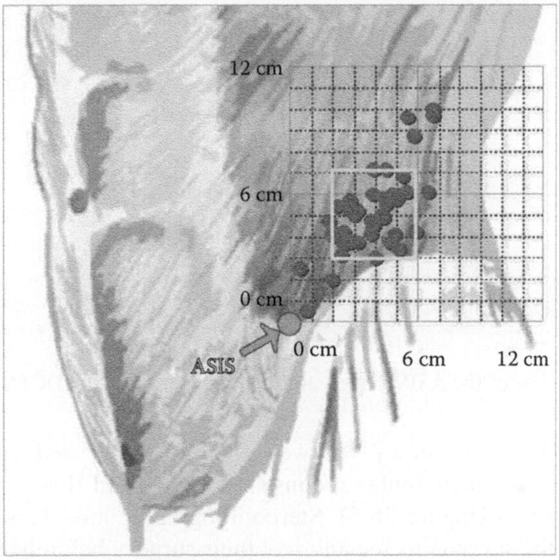

FIGURE 36.2 Schematic representation of the location of emergence of DCIA-Ps from the deep fascia, relative to the ASIS, for the 44 perforators identified. (Reproduced from Ting, J.W.C. et al., *Microsurgery*, 29, 326, 2009. With permission.)

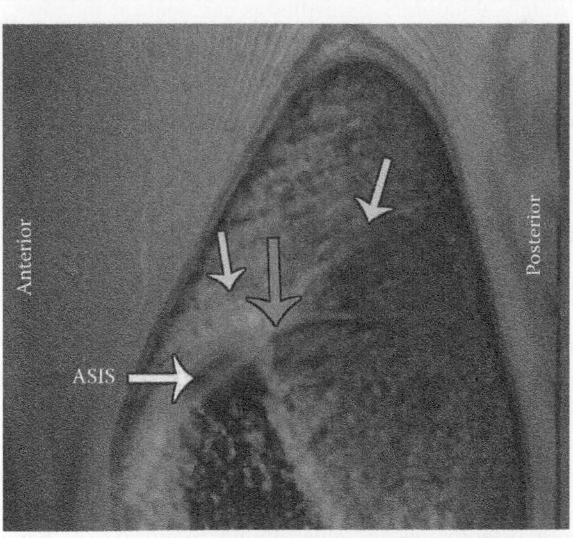

FIGURE 36.3 CTA with VRT reformat, performed for imaging of the vasculature of the torso. Multiple DCIA-Ps are demonstrated, two of which were 0.8 mm diameter (yellow arrows) and one 1.2 mm perforator (blue arrow). (Reproduced with permission from Ting, J.W.C. et al., *Microsurgery*, 29, 326, 2009. With permission.)

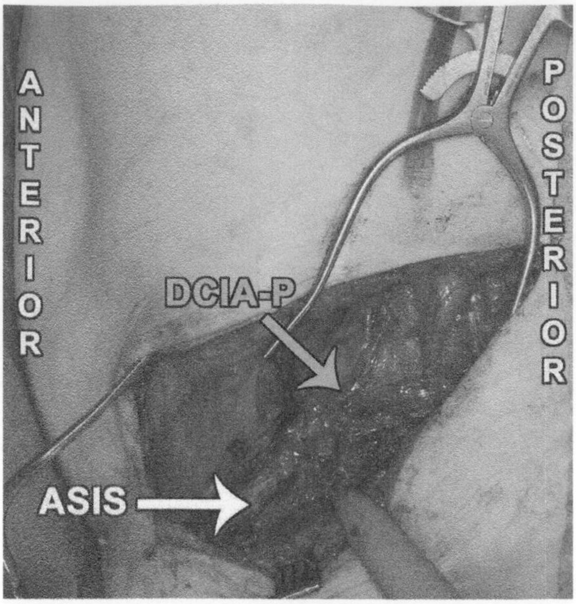

FIGURE 36.4 Surgical view of the ASIS demonstrating the location of the DCIA-P.

of years and with reproductive accuracy.[39] However, although it is used regularly in orthognathic surgery, their application to mandibular reconstruction[40–45] and iliac crest harvesting[46–50] has only recently been reported (Figure 36.5). Stereolithographic models add an extra element of tangibility that allows the surgeon to *see* and *feel* their surgery beforehand and, combined with imaging, can enable *virtual surgery* preoperatively. Surgeons can further use the models as guides during the surgery and modifications so the plan can be easily communicated between the surgical teams. The use of these biomodels can minimise bone harvest by selection of the most appropriately vascularised and best-fitting bone, spare donor site morbidity through more precise harvest, and improve bone-to-bone contact at the recipient site. Pre-moulding of plates and measurement of screws for mandibular reconstruction can reduce the time of operation and allow the resection and reconstruction teams to work simultaneously. Pedicle length of the DCIA and therefore arc of movement can also be measured preoperatively to determine if there is adequate length.

36.5 CLINICAL APPLICATION OF DCIA FLAP

As in the early landmark papers, the DCIA flap has predominantly been popularised for use in mandibular reconstruction. The DCIA flap has also been used for maxillary, upper limb, and lower limb reconstruction with various amounts of muscle used for bulk.[15,16,37,51–54] Although, traditionally, the ipsilateral pelvis is used for mandibular reconstruction, if only a short body of mandible is required, either iliac crest may be used.[28] DCIA-P flap, until recently, has been slow to gain popularity, but CTA studies of their perforators have changed this.

The associated bone, the iliac crest, is a strong bony construct allowing for harvesting of either cancellous or cortical bone depending on the requirements. The iliac crest shape is akin to that of the hemi-mandible; hence, osteotomies are generally not required to reshape the bone to the defect even for an extended hemi-mandible[28] (Figure 36.6). The bony stock and height also provides a solid base for osteointegrated dental implants and the ability to withstand the large amount of bite force and repetitive stress that the normal mandible is subjected to. The skin overlying the iliac crest is

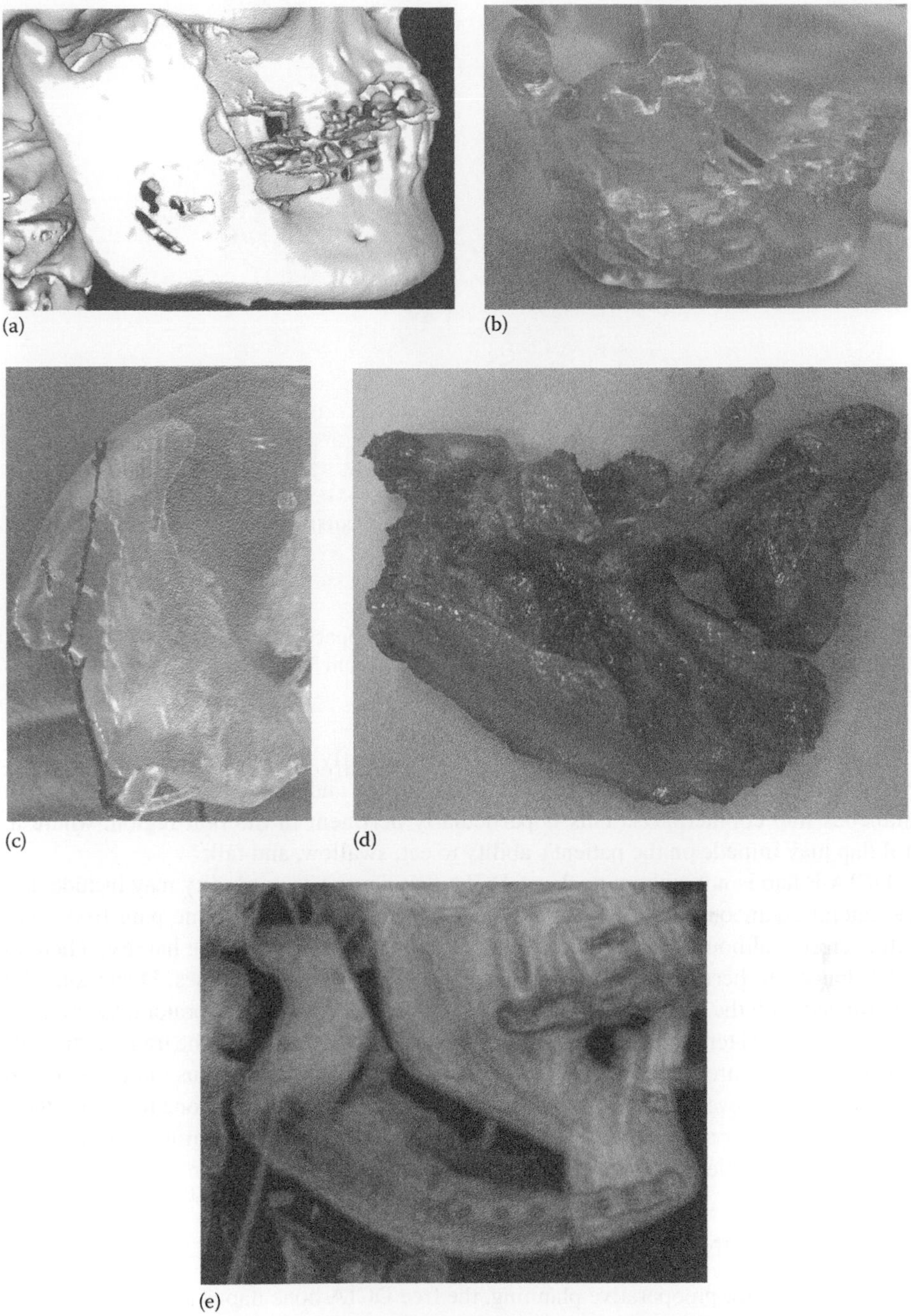

FIGURE 36.5 (a) 3D, multiplanar computed tomographic (CT) imaging of the mandible. (b) The stereolithographic BioModels made from the CT imagining. (c) BioModel constructed from CTA of the iliac crest and associated DCIA. (d) Intraoperative harvesting of the DCIA. Post-operative imagining of the DCIA flap based on the stereolithographic model. (e) Post-operative CT of DCIA reconstruction of the right hemi-mandible. (a and b: Reproduced from Rozen, W.M. et al., *Plast. Reconstr. Surg.*, 130, 227e, 2012. With permission; c: Reproduced from Rozen, W.M. et al., *Plast. Reconstr. Surg.*, 130, 380e, 2012. With permission.)

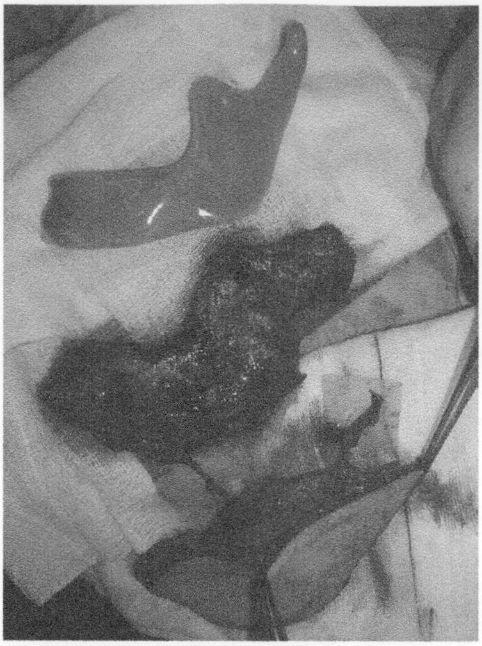

FIGURE 36.6 Intraoperative photographs demonstrating a comparison of the raised DCIA-P flap (below) to the preformed model of the mandible (above). (Reproduced from Ting, J.W. et al., *Microsurgery*, 31, 603, 2011. With permission.)

also, unlike the free fibula flap, hairless, which is particularly ideal for intraoral coverage. Unlike the myocutaneous flaps, perforator flaps contain no muscle and are generally less bulky than their myocutaneous flap counterparts. This is particularly pertinent in the oral region, where a bulky intraoral flap may impede on the patient's ability to eat, swallow, and talk.

The DCIA-P flap is not without its flaws. DCIA flap donor site morbidity may include numbness over the lateral cutaneous nerve distribution.[55] There is also reported bone pain from harvesting of the iliac crest,[55] although this is associated with any flap involving bone harvest. There are also reports of donor site hernia ranging from 0%–5%[27,38,56,57] to 33%[55] of cases. Donor site closure is easily facilitated with the preservation of all three muscle layers in the perforator dissection allowing suturing with minimal tension and mesh-free repair. From our experience, the transversus abdominis muscle needs to be sutured to the iliacus during closure, but often, the iliacus muscle is too feeble to hold the sutures. To prevent this, small holes may be drilled into the iliac bone to anchor the sutures in place. This allows for a solid closure of the iliacus and transversus abdominis muscle sandwiched around the iliac bone. Meticulous closure, therefore, is the key to prevention of hernia formation.

36.6 CONCLUSION

With the aid of CTA for preoperative planning, the free DCIA bone flap is a useful technique in the management of upper limb bony reconstruction. It is of particular usefulness in the setting of recent infection, since the iliac crest comprises cortico-cancellous bone, which has a high osteogenicity.

The role of CTA in modelling the iliac crest bone to be harvested and demonstrating its DCIA vascular anatomy cannot be understated. In addition to mapping the location and size of the DCIA-Ps, CTA can also demonstrate the cutaneous course of each perforator, allowing the safe design of a flap to capture an individual perforator territory.

REFERENCES

1. Daniel RK, Kerrigan CL. Mandibular reconstruction with free tissue transfers. *Ann Plast Surg* 1978;1:346.
2. Disa JJ, Cordeiro PG. Mandible reconstruction with microvascular surgery. *Semin Surg Oncol* 2000;19:226.
3. David DJ, Tan E, Katsaros J, Sheen R. Mandibular reconstruction with vascularized iliac crest: A 10-year experience. *Plast Reconstr Surg* 1988;82:792.
4. Jewer DD, Boyd JB, Manktelow R et al. Orofacial and mandibular reconstruction with the iliac crest free flap: A review of 60 cases and a new method of classification. *Plast Reconstr Surg* 1989;84:391.
5. Taylor GI, Townsend P, Corlett R. Superiority of the deep circumflex iliac vessels as the supply for free groin flaps: Experimental work. *Plast Reconstr Surg* 1979;64:595–604.
6. Safak T, Klebuc MJ, Mavili E, Shenaq SM. A new design of the iliac crest microsurgical free flap without including the 'Obligatory' muscle cuff. *Plast Reconstr Surg* 1997;100:1703–1709.
7. Bitter K, Schlesinger S, Westerman U. The iliac bone or osteocutaneous transplant pedicled to the deep circumflex iliac artery. *J Max Fac Surg* 1983;11:241–247.
8. Leung PC, Chan KT. Giant cell tumour of the distal end of the radius treated by the resection and free vascularized iliac crest graft. *Clin Orthop Relat Res* 1986;202:232–236.
9. Brown JS. Deep circumflex iliac artery free flap with internal oblique muscle as a new method of immediate reconstruction of maxillectomy defect. *Head Neck* 1996;18:412–421.
10. Brown JS. Reconstruction of the total maxillectomy defect using a pedicled coronoid flap and deep circumflex iliac artery free flap (letter to the editor). *Br J Oral Maxillofac Surg* 2008;26.
11. Akyurek M, Conejero A, Dunn R. Deep circumflex iliac artery perforator flap without iliac crest. *Plast Reconstr Surg* 2008;122:1790–1795.
12. Kimata Y. Deep circumflex iliac perforator flap. *Clin Plast Surg* 2003;30:433–438.
13. Akyurek M, Morse A, Safak T, Fudem G, Dunn R. Deep circumflex iliac artery perforator skin flap: Anatomic study and clinical application. American Society for Reconstructive Microsurgery (ASRM) (Abstracts). *J Reconstr Microsurg* 2006;22.
14. Blondeel PN, Van Landuyt K, Hamdi M, Monstrey SJ. Perforator flap terminology: Updated 2002. *Clin Plast Surg* 2003;30:343–346.
15. Ting JWC, Rozen WM, Leong J, Crock J. Free deep circumflex iliac artery vascularised bone flap for reconstruction of the distal radius: Planning with CT angiography. *Microsurgery* 2010;30:163–167.
16. Peek A, Giessle GA. Functional total and subtotal heel reconstruction with free composite osteofasciocutaneous groin flaps of the deep circumflex iliac vessels. *Ann Plast Surg* 2006;56:628–634.
17. Sanders R, Mayou BJ. New vascularized bone graft transferred by microvascular anastomosis as a free flap. *Br J Surg* 1979;66:787–788.
18. Gabl M, Reinhart C, Lutz M et al. Vascularized bone graft from the iliac crest for the treatment of nonunion of the proximal part of the scaphoid with an avascular fragment. *J Bone Joint Surg* 1999;81:1414–1428.
19. Bromberg BE, Walden RH, Rubin LR. Mandibular bone grafts – A technique in fixation. *Plast Reconstr Surg* 1963;32:589.
20. Genden EM. Reconstruction of the mandible and maxilla. The evolution of surgical technique. *Arch Facial Plast Surg* 2010;12:87–90.
21. Phillips CM. Primary and secondary reconstruction of the mandible after ablative surgery. *Am J Surg* 1967;114:601–604.
22. Kudo K, Fujioka Y. Review of bone grafting for reconstruction of the mandible after ablative surgery. *Am J Surg* 1978;114:601–604.
23. Rozen WM, Ashton MW, Ferris S et al. Developments in perforator imaging for the anterolateral thigh flap: CT angiography and CT-guided stereotaxy. *Microsurgery* 2008;28:227–232.
24. Cordeiro PG, Hidalgo DA. Soft tissue coverage of mandibular reconstruction plates. *Head Neck* 1994;16:112–115.
25. Snyder CC, Bateman JM, Davis CW, Warden GD. Mandibulo-facial restoration with live osteocutaneous flaps. *Plast Reconstr Surg* 1970;45:14–19.
26. Miyamoto Y, Tani T. Reconstruction of mandible with free osteocutaneous flap using deep circumflex iliac vessels as the stem. *Ann Plast Surg* 1981;6:354–361.
27. Taylor GI, Townsend P, Corlett R. Superiority of the deep circumflex iliac vessels as the supply for free groin flaps: Clinical work. *Plast Reconstr Surg* 1979;64:745–759.

28. Taylor GI. Reconstruction of the mandible with free composite iliac bone graft. *Ann Plast Surg* 1982;9:361–376.
29. Shenaq SM, Klebuc M. The iliac crest microsurgical free flap in mandibular reconstruction. *Clin Plast Surg* 1994;21:37–44.
30. Lee JS, Choyke LT, Locklin JK. Use of hydrodissection to prevent nerve and muscular damage during radiofrequency ablation of kidney tumors. *JVIR* 2006;17:1967–1969.
31. Hartrampf CR, Noel T, Drazan L et al. Ruben's fat pad for breast reconstruction: A peri-iliac soft tissue free flap. Case reports. *Plast Reconstr Surg* 1993;25:402–407.
32. Takada K, Yoshiga K, Amin HM, Miyamoto Y. Mandibular reconstruction with a microvascular free groin osteocutaneous graft based on the deep circumflex iliac vessels. *J Oral Maxillofac Surg* 1986;44:660–665.
33. Ting JWC, Rozen WM, Grinsell D, Stella DL, Ashton MW. The in vivo anatomy of the deep circumflex iliac artery perforators: Defining the role for the DCIA perforator flap. *Microsurgery* 2009;29:326–329.
34. Ting JW, Rozen WM, Chubb D et al. Improving the utility and reliability of the deep circumflex iliac artery perforator flap: The use of preoperative planning with CT angiography. *Microsurgery* 2011;31:603–609.
35. Bergeron L, Tang M, Morris S. The anatomical basis of the deep circumflex iliac artery perforator flap with iliac crest. *Plast Reconstr Surg* 2007;120:252–258.
36. Ramasastry SS, Granick MS, Futrell JW. Clinical anatomy of the internal oblique muscle. *J Reconstr Microsurg* 1986;2:117.
37. Shaw RJ, Brown JS. Osteomyocutaneous deep circumflex iliac artery perforator flap in the reconstruction of midface defect with facial skin loss: A case report. *Microsurgery* 2009;29:299–302.
38. Boyd JB, Rosen I, Rotstein L et al. The iliac crest and the radial forearm flap in vascularized oromandibular reconstruction. *Am J Surg* 1990;159:301–308.
39. Bouyssie JF, Bouyssie S, Sharrock P. Stereolithographic models derived from x-ray computed tomography: Reproduction accuracy. *Surg Radiol Anat* 1997;19:193–199.
40. Ro E, Ridge JA, Topham NS. Using stereolithographic models to plan mandibular reconstruction for advanced oral cavity cancer. *Laryngoscope* 2007;117:759–761.
41. Mavili ME, Canter HI, Salglam-Aydinatay B, Kamaci S, Kocadereli I. Use of three-dimensional medical modeling methods for precise planning of orthognathic surgery. *J Craniofac Surg* 2007;18:740–747.
42. Hallermann W, Olsen S, Bardyn T et al. A new method for computer-aided planning for extensive mandibular reconstruction. *Plast Reconstr Surg* 2006;117:2431–2437.
43. Liu XJ, Gui L, Mao C, Peng X, Yu GY. Applying computer techniques in maxillofacial reconstruction using a fibula flap: A messenger and an evaluation method. *J Craniofac Surg* 2009;20:372–377.
44. Vakharia K, Natoli N, Johnson T. Stereolithography-aided reconstruction of the mandible. *Plast Recons Surg* 2012;192:194e–195e.
45. Antony A, Wei FC, Kolokythas A, Weimer KA, Cohen MN. Use of virtual surgery and stereolithography-guided osteotomy for mandibular reconstruction with free fibula. *Plast Recons Surg* 2011;128:1080–1084.
46. Juergen P, Klug C, Krol Z et al. Navigation guided harvesting of autologous iliac crest graft for mandibular reconstruction. *J Oral Maxillofac Surg* 2011;69:2915–2923.
47. Modabber A, Gerressen M, Stiller MB et al. Computer-assisted mandibular reconstruction with vascularized iliac crest bone graft. *Aesth Plast Surg* 2012; Epub ahead of print.
48. Shen Y, Sun J, Li J et al. Using computer simulation and stereomodel for accurate mandibular reconstruction with vascularized iliac crest flap. *Oral Surg Oral Med Oral Pathol Oral Radiol Endod* 2012; Epub ahead of print.
49. Rozen WM, Ting JW, Leung M et al. Advancing image-guided surgery in microvascular mandibular reconstruction: Combining bony and vascular imaging with computed tomography-guided stereolithographic bone modeling. *Plast Reconstr Surg* 2012;130:227e–229e.
50. Rozen WM, Ting JW, Baillieu C, Leong J. Stereolithographic modelling of the deep circumflex iliac artery (DCIA) and its vascular branching: A further advance in CT guided flap planning. *Plast Reconstr Surg* 2012;130:380e–382e.
51. Nahai F, Hill HL, Hester H. Experiences with the tensor fascia lata flap. *Plast Reconstr Surg* 1979;63:788–799.
52. Cai J, Cao X, Liang J, Sun B. Heel reconstruction. *Plast Reconstr Surg* 1997;99:448–453.
53. Rieger UM, Haug M, Schwarzl F et al. Free microvascular iliac crest flap for extensive flap necrosis: Case report with a 16 year long-term follow-up. *Microsurgery* 2009;29:667–671.

54. Stevenson TR, Greene TI, Kling TF. Heel reconstruction with the deep circumflex iliac artery osteocutaneous flap. Case reports. *Plast Reconstr Surg* 1987;76:982.
55. Franklin JD, Shack RB, Stone JD, Madden JJ, Lymch JB. Single stage reconstruction of mandibular and soft tissue defects using a free osteocutaneous groin flap. *Am J Surg* 1980;140:492–497.
56. Iqbal M, Lloyd CJ, Paley MD, CN P. Repair of the deep circumflex iliac artery free flap donor site with Protack (titanium spiral tacks) and Prolene (polypropylene) mesh. *Br J Oral Maxfac Surg* 2007;45:596–597.
57. Kantelhardt T, Stock W, Stützle H, Deiler S. Results at the donor site after free microvascular iliac crest transplantation. *Eur J Plastic Surg* 1999;22:366–369.4

37 Imaging and Surgical Principles of the Propeller and Perforator Flaps of the Lower Limb

Emanuele Cigna, Michele Maruccia, Alessandro Napoli, Federico Lo Torto, Paola Parisi, and Diego Ribuffo

CONTENTS

37.1 INTRODUCTION

Preoperative imaging to assess the arterial anatomy of flaps has been of interest to reconstructive surgeons since the earliest days of reconstructive microsurgery. At that time, microsurgery was considered the *cutting edge*, and the imaging modality most often used was the handheld Doppler probe. Presently, it is fundamental to assess the perforator vasculature as part of the preoperative workup, due to the increasingly technically demanding flaps, designed on specific perforator vessels [1–4].

Free flap surgery has become progressively successful over the past 30 years; however, a failure rate of 2%–4% still remains. Flap failures and partial necrosis in technically successful operations may sometimes be attributed to anatomical variations in perforator topography. These could be congenital or acquired, secondary to previous trauma or surgery. In this setting, it is hypothesised that some form of preoperative perforator mapping would alert the surgeon to the anomalous anatomy and steer the choice of operation to a safer part of the body or facilitate planning. These variations, when detected intraoperatively, can lead to impromptu changes of plan that can further increase the operative times and surgeon fatigue and possibly contribute to aesthetically poorer outcomes [1,2].

To reduce the incidence of these complications, different imaging modalities have been adopted by plastic surgery units around the world, whereas many believe that no systematic imaging is required before surgery. These strategies appear to be ad hoc, and there is a general lack of consensus on whether imaging is required at all, required in all cases, or in select cases and if so, which imaging modality should be used. The ideal imaging modality would satisfy a number of key criteria. It would give accurate information about the course and calibre of perforating vessels down to the submillimetre level. It would be reproducible and have low inter-operator variability. The imaging technology would be fast, inexpensive, and readily available. There would be a low radiation dose allowing the test to be used in a routine screening capacity. If the scan provided information on incidental co-morbidities pertinent to the surgery or the patient's condition as a whole, this would be of additional value [1–3].

Regarding imaging of the lower limb, the literature is mixed. A number of studies have suggested that routine imaging of lower limbs before surgery is very low yield except in the context of abnormal pedal pulses or in severe trauma. These studies suggest that this low yield should be balanced against the potential harm of imaging, which traditionally was invasive catheter angiography. While it may be true that clinical examination is very sensitive for assessing the vasculature of the lower limb, arguments against low-yield imaging may be less relevant in the era of high-resolution non-invasive imaging such as computed tomography angiography (CTA) and magnetic resonance angiography (MRA) [1].

Regarding perforator mapping prior to reconstructive microsurgery, there is a large body of evidence to suggest that traditional methods such as the handheld Doppler and colour duplex have been superseded. Modern modalities such as CTA and MRA have been shown to be more accurate with less observer-dependent variations. Unlike other modalities, evidence exists showing improved outcomes when preoperative imaging with CTA and MRA are used. This is particularly true for CTA, in which a number of cohort studies have shown statistically significant reductions in the operative time and surgeons stress levels and improvements in flap outcomes. While this evidence has only been validated for the use of CTA in deep inferior epigastric perforator (DIEP) flap planning, the proof of concept may allow some extrapolation to other perforator flaps, and there are emerging series showing the use of these techniques in the planning of thigh and gluteal flaps as well as other more exotic perforator flaps. A recent review article on the subject of monitoring concluded that for flaps with *standard anatomy and superficial vasculature*, the handheld Doppler should remain the modality of choice [5]. While there were substantial methodological concerns with that study (limited search terms in that review resulted in some key studies demonstrating improved outcomes with CTA being omitted from consideration), preoperative imaging continues to enjoy widespread practice in a number of areas of reconstructive surgery. Even the *humble* handheld Doppler continues to be used in high profile units [6] and is enjoying a renaissance in the field of freestyle perforator flaps, no doubt thanks to its ubiquity and portability.

37.2 PERFORATOR AND PROPELLER FLAPS OF THE LOWER LEG: HISTORICAL EVOLUTION

Simple or complex defects in the lower leg continue to be a challenging task for reconstructive surgeons. The ideal reconstruction technique for both simple and complex defects of the lower limb should replace like-to-like tissue, minimise donor-site morbidity, preserve main vascular trunks, and reduce operating and hospitalisation time. A variety of flaps were used in the attempt to achieve excellence in form and function [7]. In the absence of specific knowledge of the pattern or reliability of the blood supply, the flaps were used initially as random pattern flaps constrained by length-to-width ratios to ensure viability [8]. These flaps are unreliable in the lower leg because of their small dimensions and restrictions in mobility [9]. Moreover, Almeida et al. [10] found a random pattern flap necrosis in 25% of cases. The axial pattern flap introduced by McGregor and Jackson [11] in 1972 and based on axial blood supply improved the quality of results, but with the sacrifice of a main artery [12–16]. Ger [17], in 1966, and Orticochea [18], in 1972, described the musculocutaneous flaps which became very popular in leg reconstruction because of their reliability [19], but with few indications as pedicle flaps in the distal third, because of inadequate pedicle length in this region [20–23]. In 1981, Ponten [24] demonstrated that by including the deep fascia in a cutaneous flap, it can be raised without respecting the length-to-width ratio, but only later other works [25–27] established the anatomical basis of his assumption. Despite their big advent, the fasciocutaneous flaps proved not to be a very safe procedure for defects in the lower third of the lower leg, as demonstrated by the experience of Chatre and Quaba with a necrosis rate of 25% [23]. The reappraisal of the works of Manchot [28] and Salmon et al. [29] by Taylor and Palmer [30], which defined the static vascular territories of source arteries as angiosomes, opened new perspectives in flap design. They defined an angiosome as a 3D vascular territory supplied by a source artery and vein through branches for all tissue layers between the skin and the bone and showed that between neighbouring angiosomes, there are choked and true anastomotic arteries [30]. Regarding the lower leg, Taylor and Pan [31] found that the branches of the cutaneous vessels radiate after piercing the deep fascia in all directions and interconnect to form a continuous vascular network within the integument.

37.2.1 Era of Perforator Flaps

As a result of this evolution, and following the works published by Koshima and Soeda [32] and Kroll and Rosenfield [33], in 1989, the era of perforator flaps began.

In fact, Koshima and Soeda [32] used the terminology *perforator flaps* for the first time in a clinical setting. In two cases, they had used a paraumbilical skin and fat island based on a muscular perforator to reconstruct the groin and the tongue. Koshima introduced the concept of perforator flaps to differentiate them from fasciocutaneous flaps, as he was convinced that the fascial vascular plexus was not fundamental for flap vascularisation. Since the first applications and the popularisation of the use of perforator-based lower abdominal wall skin flaps in breast reconstruction [1,5], the principle of perforator flaps has become more and more popular over the last decade. Its growing popularity is mainly related to the important decrease in donor-site morbidity as a consequence of the preservation of muscle functionality and vascularisation. In addition, it has been observed that patients in general have less postoperative pain and a quicker recovery.

The advantages of harvesting relatively large and thin skin flaps include the absence of postoperative muscle atrophy as seen in myocutaneous flaps, the presence of long vascular pedicles based on well-known source vessels, and the possibility of harvesting sensory nerves with the flap, thus providing a tool to perform more accurate and precise reconstructions. Given that an ideal reconstruction should replace *like with like*, and the knowledge that about 80% of free flaps are used for resurfacing purposes and only a minority of patients need a free flap to fill up dead space or deep defects, free flaps consisting of skin and subcutaneous fat tissue are predominantly needed in a daily practice.

In the pioneer phase, the principles of a perforator flap were defined as a flap consisting of skin and subcutaneous fat only, based on a perforator vessel (more frequently transmuscular) that was dissected by splitting the muscle and not harvesting it. Both vascularisation and innervation of that muscle were left intact. A perforator flap was seen as an ultimate upgrade of a myocutaneous flap because it preserves almost all the intrinsic advantages of its myocutaneous analogue.

In the last few years, the plastic surgery journals have been filled with reports of new perforator flaps. Slowly, perforator flaps have become a common denominator for any type of skin flap that is dissected on a single vascular pedicle consisting of one artery and one vein. The origin and the route the perforators followed have become less relevant and confusion has increased. The exact definition of a perforator flap is not clear, and the terminology and the classification of the different perforator flaps have not yet been identified. A perforating vessel, or, in short, a perforator, is a vessel that has its origin in one of the axial vessels of the body and that passes through certain structural elements of the body, besides interstitial connective tissue and fat, before reaching the subcutaneous fat layer and then the skin. Hallock [21] defines a perforator as any vessel that enters the superficial plane through a defined fenestration in the deep fascia, regardless of origin. Hallock discerns direct and indirect perforators according to the distinct origin of their vascular supply and the structures they traverse before piercing the deep fascia. Perforators that pierce the deep fascia without traversing any other structural tissue are called direct perforators. All other perforators that first run through deeper tissues, mainly muscle, septum, or epimysium, are called indirect perforators.

According to the Gent consensus [34], perforator flaps are constituted by areas of cutaneous and subcutaneous tissue nourished by perforator branches originating from deep vascular axis with an intramuscular (musculocutaneous perforator flap [MCPF]) or intraseptal (septocutaneous perforator flap [SCPF]) course [35–37].

Free perforator flaps such as anterolateral thigh (ALT) perforator flap [21,38], tensor fasciae latae muscle perforator flap [21,39], inferior epigastric artery perforator flap [40], thoracodorsal artery perforator flap [41–43], and medial sural artery perforator flap [21,44] are mostly used in the lower leg and foot. The revisiting vascular anatomy and the extensive clinical experience have confirmed that also local and regional perforator flaps are safe and reliable in achieving the goals of lower leg reconstruction. As shown by Geddes et al. [45], the lower extremity appears to have the greatest potential for harvesting new or modified perforator flaps. The work of Saint-Cyr and his co-workers, which defined the vascular territories of perforators as perforasomes, helped to better understand the dynamic potential of these perforasomes and their importance in harvesting pedicled perforator flaps in the lower leg [46–49]. As the adjacent angiosomes are connected through choke and true anastomotic arteries, between neighbouring perforasomes, there are direct and indirect linking vessels [46].

The big popularity gained by the local perforator flaps was due to their main advantages: (1) sparing of the source artery and underlying muscle and fascia; (2) combining the very good blood supply of a musculocutaneous flap with the reduced donor-site morbidity of a skin flap; (3) replacing like with like; (4) limiting the donor site to the same area; (5) possibility of completely or partially primary closure [50,51]; (6) technically less demanding, because they are microsurgical procedures, without the need of microvascular sutures; and (7) shorter operating time [16,20,23,51–54].

37.2.2 Propeller Flaps

The concept of propeller flap belongs to Hyakusoku et al. [55], which described in 1991 an adipocutaneous flap designed as a propeller, with blood supplied through a random subcutaneous pedicle and rotated 90°. The term was used for the first time to define a perforator flap based on a skeletonised perforator vessel and rotated 180° by Hallock [56] in 2006. The ultimate definition and terminology of propeller perforator flaps was reached by an Advisory Panel of the First Tokyo Meeting on Perforator and Propeller Flaps in 2009 [57]. According to this consensus, a propeller perforator flap is designed as a skin island with two paddles which can be of the same dimensions or with a larger and a smaller one, the demarcation limit between them being the perforator vessel. To be a propeller flap, it has to rotate around the perforator vessel for at least 90°–180°. A very detailed description of the surgical technique in harvesting propeller perforator flaps in the lower leg was presented by Teo [58] in 2006.

Starting from previous works [13–15,27–31,59–63], in the last 10 years, a large number of surgeons became interested in evaluating the perforator arteries and in performing pedicled perforator flaps in the lower leg [9,16,20–23]. Despite the aforementioned advantages, they were also confronted with some possible drawbacks. The general complication rate with propeller perforator flaps is similar to that observed with free flaps and consists mainly incomplete or partial flap loss mainly due to venous problems [20,23,49].

In the attempt to reduce the risk of these complications, a lot of artifices in flap design and harvesting technique were imagined. The venous supercharging by including in the flap and suturing a subcutaneous vein can avoid the venous congestion and related complications. Teo [58] considers that in designing the flap, to the distance between the perforator and the distal edge of the defect, 1 cm must be added, and half a centimetre to the width, also that the vascular pedicle has to be cleared of all muscular side branches for at least 2 cm, that the fascial strands must be divided especially around the venae comitantes, and that the flap should be left in its original position for 10–15 min after the tourniquet was released. To reduce the risk of vascular complications due to torsion and buckling of the pedicle, Wong et al. [64] suggested that a perforator of 1 mm diameter should be dissected for a length of at least 3 cm. Probably the main way to reduce the complication rate is the ability to establish the safe vascular limits of a pedicled perforator flap, in other words, the real potential dimensions of the flap. While 15 years ago the safe length of a perforator flap was considered to be the distance between two perforators [65–67], nowadays, according with the perforasome concept of Saint-Cyr et al. [46], in a perforator flap raised on a single perforator, this one will be hyperperfused resulting in its increased filling pressure with the possibility of recruitment of adjacent perforasome territories. It is easy to understand that as large the vessels' diameter is, as high is the pressure, with bigger potential to open the linking vessels. Based on haemodynamic studies, it was demonstrated that for a perforator in normal anatomic conditions, the flow through it is much smaller than in the source artery, while for the same perforator used as pedicle of a flap, the flow through it is still smaller than in the source artery, but much greater than in the former situation [68,69]. In each specific region, the greater is the number of perforators, the lesser will be the size of the potential territory of each perforator. This statement is obvious in the lower leg, in which the perforators from the posterior tibial artery are small in number, but of larger diameter than the perforators of the anterior tibial (AT) and peroneal arteries, which are more numerous, but with a smaller diameter [30]. The problem is if it's possible to establish before or during surgery the size of the perforators and their anatomic and potential territories, to be able to precisely approximate the safer dimensions of the flap. For this reason, the correct preoperative planning is very important. Panse et al. [69] performed a study in the attempt to find a relationship between the necrosis rate of the flap and the rate between the length of the lower leg and the length of the flap. They found a six times more chance of necrosis for a length of the flap more than one-third of the limbs' length.

37.2.3 Free-Style Free Flaps

Finally, the concept of free-style free flaps can be applied also for pedicled perforator flaps, meaning that those flaps can be designed in free-style fashion based on any major cutaneous perforator [70] and offering a large spectrum of local flap options [20]. The term *free-style free flap* was introduced in 1983 by Asko-Seljavaara [71] in a personal communication, to describe a flap harvested in the upper limb after dissection and visualisation of a main vessel and identification of its branches, the flap being supplied with blood by those vessels. In 1990, in the hand, and then in 2006, in the lower leg, Quaba et al. [20,72] developed the concept of ad hoc perforator flap which is analogous with the freestyle concept, but which considers as irrelevant the knowledge of source vessel and their anatomical variations. The difference consists in the fact that Quaba and Quaba [20] design the flap in a potential donor territory close to the defect, based on a perforator detected by handheld Doppler signal. Mardini et al. in 2003 [73] and Wei and Mardini in 2004 [74] brought some modifications to the original concept of free-style free flaps, very similar with the theory of Quaba and Quaba [20], consisting in incision of only one flap's edge at the beginning, with no need to visualise the source vessel of the perforator (the identification of the perforator should be done by Doppler preoperative examination), the dissection of the perforator starting from the skin level. Authors from the same collective elaborated in 2009 the main principles in harvesting such a flap and enlarged their application also as local perforator flaps [75]. Some other surgeons published also their experience with freestyle perforator flaps in various anatomical regions [76–78]. Georgescu et al. [79] and Matei et al. [80] published their experience in harvesting perforator flaps in the forearm without performing a preoperative exploration of the perforators, considering that because of the superficial location of the main axial source vessels, there can be a lot of false-positive or false-negative results. They conclude that the initial incision of only one edge of the future flap, followed by microsurgical dissection, identification, and isolation of the required perforator, represents more important considerations than preoperatively detecting the perforators for a successful flap in this region. This concept, which corresponds in part with the freestyle flap described by Asko-Seljavaara [71] except the identification first of the source vessels and its branches and the free-style flap described by other authors [81–84], can be extrapolated also for propeller perforator flaps harvested in the distal lower leg, where two main source arteries (anterior and posterior tibial arteries) have a relatively superficial location (Figure 37.1).

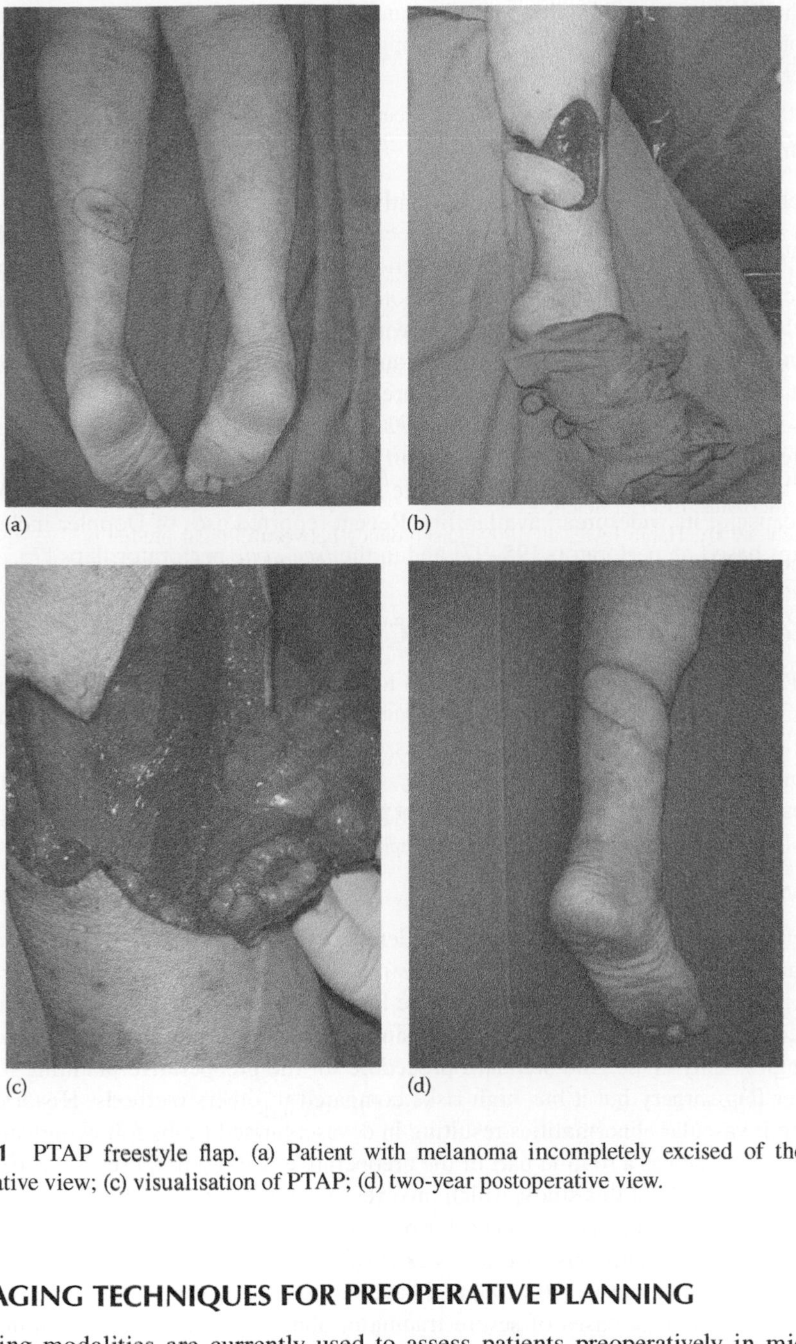

FIGURE 37.1 PTAP freestyle flap. (a) Patient with melanoma incompletely excised of the lower leg; (b) intraoperative view; (c) visualisation of PTAP; (d) two-year postoperative view.

37.3 IMAGING TECHNIQUES FOR PREOPERATIVE PLANNING

Many imaging modalities are currently used to assess patients preoperatively in microvascular reconstructive surgery. Until recently, their use has been ad hoc with some surgeons using preoperative imaging routinely, others in specific cases, and others not at all. In all cases where imaging is used, it is intuitively felt to reduce the risk associated with surgery such as the risk of partial and total flap loss due to anomalous perforator anatomy or risk due to the distal limb when raising a fibular free flap [1].

A lot of methods for preoperative identification of the perforators have been described: handheld Doppler is the mostly used, but also colour Doppler, Duplex ultrasound, arteriography, MRA, and high-resolution computed tomography (CT), but these examinations do not provide informations regarding the flap viability [54]. However, the handheld Doppler probe is adequate for the precise identification of perforators, while the colour Doppler can provide enough data regarding the internal diameter of the perforators [68–71,85].

37.3.1 Doppler Ultrasound

The handheld Doppler ultrasound probe is a relatively inexpensive, portable unit, which is readily available in most hospitals. This device was advocated for use in planning microvascular free flaps as early as 1975 [86,87] and was a common practice by 1990 [88]. The handheld Doppler has been mainly described for assisting in identifying donor vessels before perforator and propeller flap surgery of the lower leg. Many studies have shown the Doppler probe to have reasonable accuracy in identifying perforators in preparation for various free flap operations [88–91], although some of them report worrying inaccuracies when compared with operative findings, especially in smaller, deeper vessels (like intramuscular perforator) [92,93], and a number of comparative studies have found the technique to be less accurate and suffer higher inter-user variation when compared with newer modalities such as CTA [94]. Despite its drawbacks, Doppler continues to be popular, possibly because of its widespread availability. Recent reported uses of Doppler include planning pedicled flaps based on perforators [95–97] and in the *free-style* perforator flaps [73,74,98].

37.3.2 Colour Duplex Ultrasound (Eco-Colour Doppler)

In the lower leg, this technology has been shown to be useful in identifying the position of perforators preoperatively in the setting of gluteal flaps, and ALT flaps, and indeed to be more accurate than Doppler ultrasound in this setting [99]. Nonetheless, comparisons with more modern technologies such as CTA showed colour duplex to be less accurate; it provides less information on the intramuscular course of vessels, is a slow procedure, and does not provide information on other nearby vessels [100].

37.3.3 Angiography

Classic arterial catheter angiography and its modern day extension-digital subtraction angiography have been advocated for preoperative imaging since the early days of microvascular reconstructive surgery. This has predominantly been in the limbs, particularly the lower limb in the context of either reconstruction after trauma or in assessing the limb for suitability as a free fibular donor. Actually, angiography is the gold standard procedure for the preoperative planning for perforator and propeller flap surgery but it has high risks compared to others methods. Historically, due to concerns about vascular abnormalities resulting in devascularised limbs following vessel division, imaging was advocated as a routine part of the preoperative workup in these cases [101]. However, given the invasive nature of this study, which involves arterial puncture and the concomitant risk of pseudoaneurysm and thrombosis, the need for routine imaging of limbs has been frequently challenged in the literature. Numerous case series exist showing a very low rate of imaging abnormalities in limbs with normal pulses [102,103] and have suggested that routine imaging is not required and should be reserved for cases of severe trauma or abnormal pedal pulse examination. These arguments may be less compelling in the era of modern imaging techniques such as CTA and MRA, which have been proven to be equal to angiography for resolving detail and are non-invasive [104].

37.3.4 Computed Tomographic Angiography

CTA uses computer-analysed x-ray images in combination with a bolus of venous contrast medium to produce high-resolution reconstructions of vascular structures. Ongoing advances in CT technology such as increased number of detector rows now allow for faster, more detailed images to be produced, often with a lower radiation dose. Although CTA allows for the production of fine images of the vasculature down to the submillimetre level without the use of intra-arterial contrast, concerns regarding cost and radiation exposure have been raised. CTA has a number of distinct advantages over traditional imaging modalities. It is non-invasive, produces more accurate images than Doppler or colour Doppler [100], provides detailed information regarding the intramuscular course of perforating vessels, provides information about other vessels in the scan field, and may give valuable incidental findings. CT has been used in preoperative assessment of a number of areas of the body. Its initial application was to assess the vessels in settings where catheter angiography had previously been advocated, in particular, the assessment of the recipient vessels in lower limb trauma, avoiding the potential risks of pseudoaneurysm and embolism associated with classic catheter angiography [105,106]. Over time, this was expanded to include preoperative assessment of the donor limb in planning fibular free flaps [107,108] and in recent years to assess the perforators of donor flaps all over the body.

In addition to an extremely accurate spatial map, CTA provides information about the intramuscular course of the vessel. Numerous series have demonstrated the effectiveness of CTA in accurately predicting the location and calibre of the perforating vessels, particularly in ALT flaps [109]. However, recently, several studies have demonstrated concrete benefits associated with preoperative CTA using case-control models. These benefits include significantly shortened dissection times and operating times, reduced cost, reduced complications including flap complications and herniae, and reduced operator stress levels.

While CTA is criticised for its radiation exposure, some authors present low-dose protocols which still offer high-resolution images [110]. These protocols reduce the dose by reducing the scanning field of the study to include only the area of the abdomen in question. Recent applications of preoperative CTA have included perforator flaps such as superior and inferior gluteal artery perforator flaps [111], superficial inferior epigastric artery flaps [112], posterior interosseous artery flaps [113], internal mammary perforator flaps [114], thoracodorsal perforator flaps [115], and even mapping of bone perfusion in deep circumflex iliac artery bone flaps [116].

37.3.5 MRI/MRA

MRI was developed in the 1970s as an alternative to conventional x-rays for forming medical images. Since that time, it has become the imaging modality of choice for many applications, particularly imaging of the soft tissues. Despite this, MRI remains an expensive technology, and until recently, scanners were not available in all hospitals. In addition, scans are generally slow and many contraindications exist including ferrous medical implants and claustrophobia.

Visualisation of the vessels is possible using MRI alone. This technique called flow-related enhancement forms images of the vessels by selectively imaging blood which has moved into the receptor plane at the time of capture. Images produced using this technique were initially lower-resolution images, and studies investigating the potential of MRI for mapping the perforators of abdominal free flaps were promising, although of limited resolution. Advances in the field of flow-related enhancement have led to protocol changes and increasingly high-resolution images. MRI is now able to resolve detail to a sufficient level to produce acceptable perforator maps [117]. Supplementing the MR scan with non-ionising paramagnetic contrast material such as gadolinium can help to produce even sharper images of arteries [118]. Commonly referred to as MRA, this technique has rapidly found many applications in the preoperative imaging in reconstructive surgery and in particular in the lower limb reconstruction.

MRA has been investigated in the preoperative assessment of legs for free fibular harvest. Its accuracy has been compared with angiography and found to be comparable in this context [119]. Numerous series have demonstrated the utility of this modality for imaging the peroneal vessels [120], and recently, the technology has been shown to be even more useful in planning free fibular transfers as it is able to resolve detail about the septocutaneous perforators of the peroneal system, thus allowing planning of safe skin paddles [121]. MRA has also been used recently in the setting of perforator mapping (Figures 37.2 through 37.5).

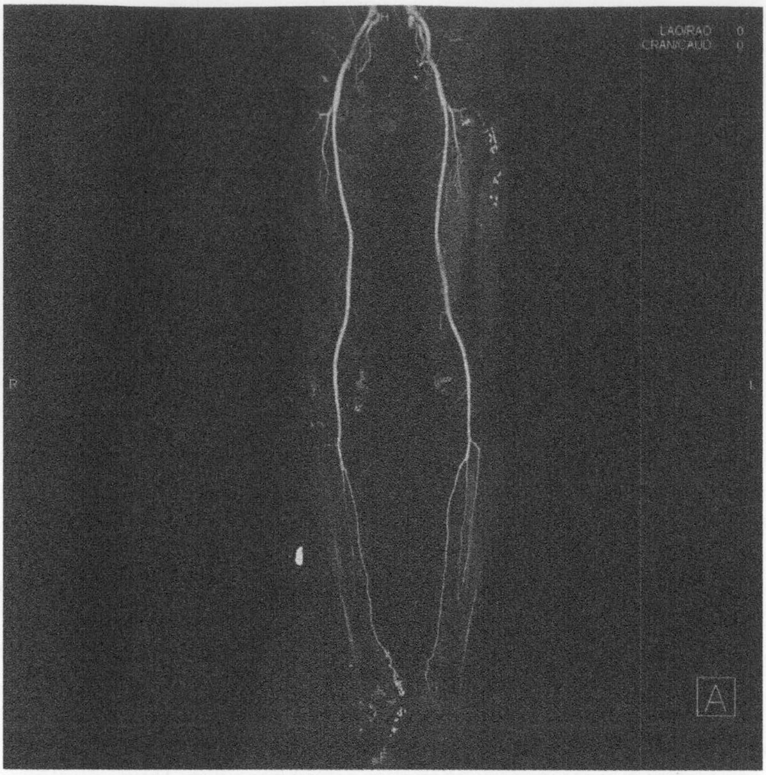

FIGURE 37.2 MRA of the lower limbs, showing a normal branching pattern of the vessel.

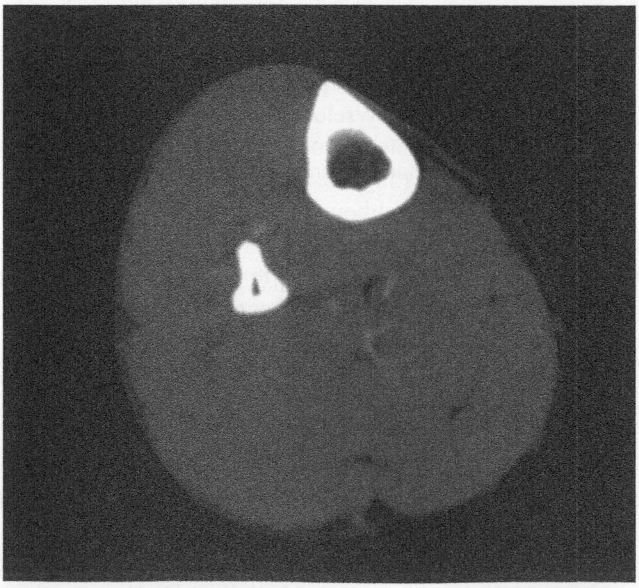

FIGURE 37.3 MRA in the axial plane of the lower leg, showing a perforator and its course through the muscle.

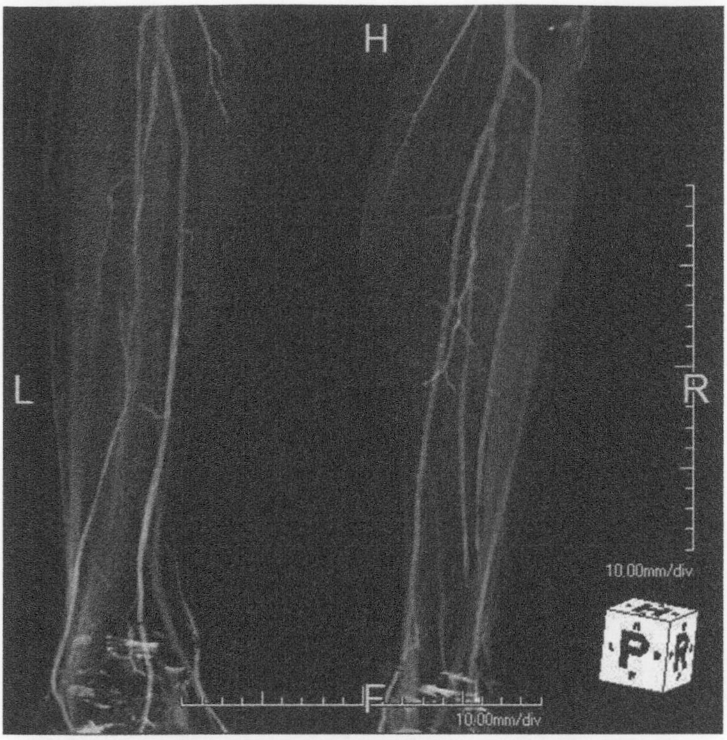

FIGURE 37.4 MRA in the longitudinal plan of the lower leg.

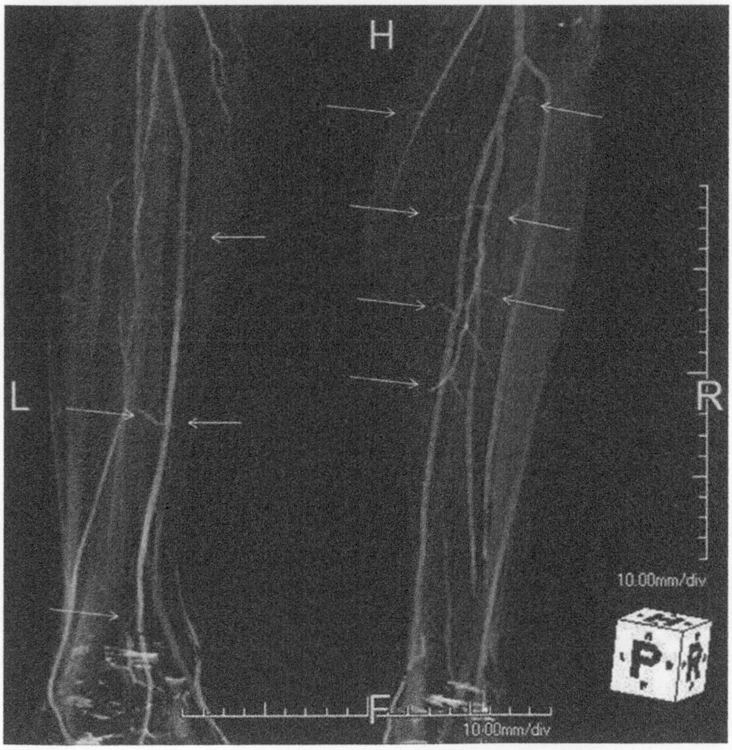

FIGURE 37.5 MRA of the lower leg, showing the perforator vessels (arrows).

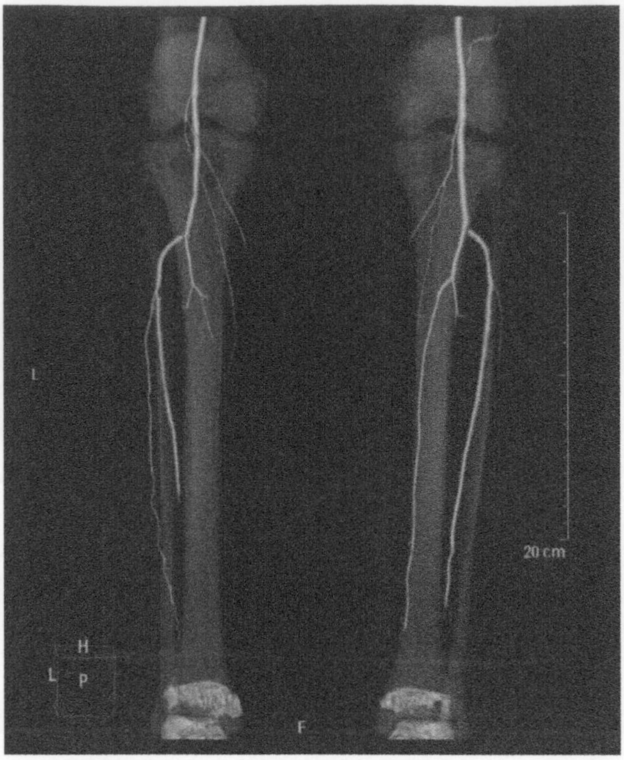

FIGURE 37.6 Three-dimensional magnetic resonance angiography (3D-MRA) of the lower leg.

MRA has begun to be used in perforator mapping in other anatomic regions including gluteal flaps [122] and in lower limb trauma to replace traditional angiography and CTA.

MRA is one of the most advanced methods of obtaining 3D reconstruction of flap vessel images. Until recently, it has been an unreliable method in the evaluation of vessels with a diameter below 2 mm. Currently, the most advanced devices and state-of-the-art software allow to perform a technically perfect examination with 3D reconstruction. It is a non-invasive and accurate examination (Figures 37.6 through 37.8).

In the future, it will probably constitute the basis for preoperative evaluation of blood vessels in reconstructive surgery. Currently, the low availability and the very high cost eliminate this method from everyday clinical practice.

37.3.6 Image-Guided Stereotactic Navigation

Stereotactic guidance systems have been used for spatial localisation in various surgical specialties for some time. They allow the surgeon to accurately define the location of structures and their own instruments relative to preoperatively captured CT or MR scans in real time. This is achieved by placing markers on anatomic landmarks which are then registered by an optical sensor on a computer system. The system can then relate the anatomy of the patient and of surgeons' tools to a precaptured CT scan in real time. Although relatively little published data exist regarding the use of these systems in plastic and reconstructive surgery, much data exist to support their use in other specialties [123], demonstrating improved operative safety and lower

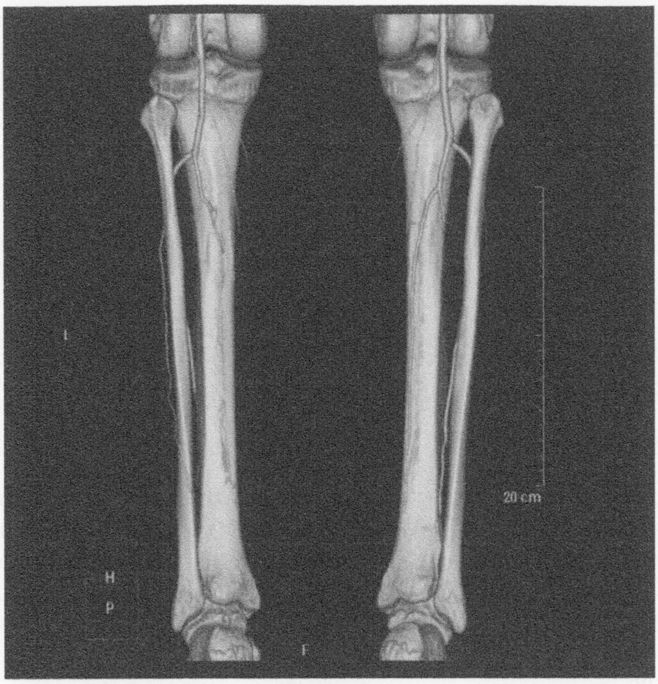

FIGURE 37.7 3D-MRA of the lower leg. With the bone.

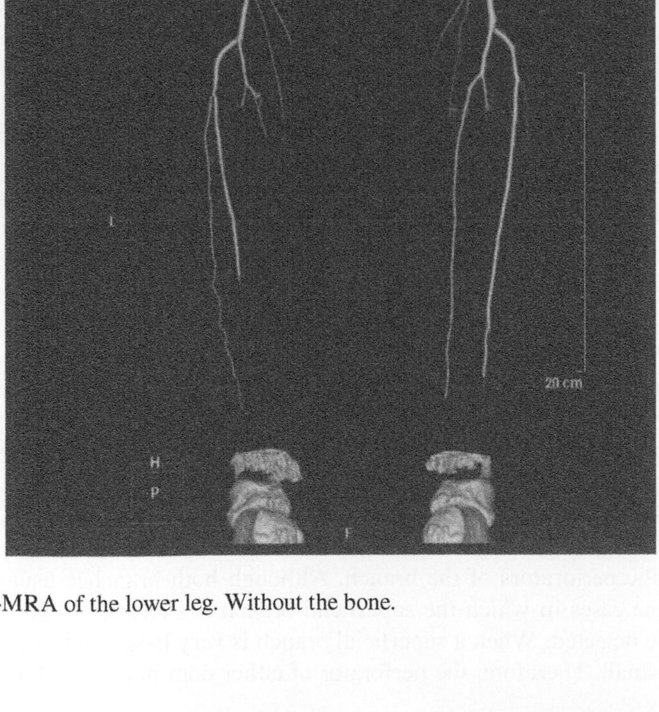

FIGURE 37.8 3D-MRA of the lower leg. Without the bone.

morbidity. This technology has now been used to map out the exact position of perforators in the preoperative assessment of patients undergoing DIEP flap breast reconstruction [124]. In this small series, use of stereotactic navigation software in conjunction with CTA was shown to be feasible and at least as accurate as CTA alone. In addition, this technology has been shown to be feasible in other flaps such as the ALT despite previous concerns regarding the suitability of fiducial marker fixation on non-bony landmarks. One study has examined other methods of computer registration such as registration with surface matching laser; however, it was found that the registration of soft tissue was not achievable with this technique and only fiducially was found to be effective [125].

37.4 PERFORATOR AND PROPELLER FLAPS OF THE LOWER LEG: ANATOMY, IMAGING, AND SURGERY TECHNIQUE

37.4.1 Superficial Circumflex Iliac Artery Perforator Flap

The groin flap, nourished by the superficial circumflex iliac artery, was the first successful free flap [126]. Nowadays, it is rarely used because flap elevation is generally difficult and presents anatomical variation in the course and size of the pedicle vessel. The superficial circumflex iliac artery perforator (SCIP) flaps are a pedicle flap based on only a perforator with a small segment of the superficial circumflex iliac vessel.

37.4.1.1 Anatomy

The superficial circumflex iliac artery and concomitant vein have superficial and deep branches. The superficial branch of the superficial circumflex iliac artery divides from the femoral artery and runs superolaterally to approach the anterior superior iliac spine. This branch locates proximally over the deep fascia of the sartorius muscle and distally in the fatty tissue. It gives off a few perforators (0.3–0.5 in diameter) at the middle portion of the anteromedial groin region. The deep branch of the superficial circumflex iliac artery system also derives from the femoral artery and vein and runs in a superolateral direction beneath the deep fascia of the sartorius muscle through the inguinal ligament. After penetrating the deep fascia at the lateral border of the sartorius muscle, the deep branch enters the suprafascial layer to give off several perforators (0.5–0.8 mm in diameter) in the anterolateral portion of the groin region. When a superficial branch is long and large, the deep branch is usually short and small. Sometimes, in cases in which the superficial branch is absent, only the long and large deep branch can be detected. The distal terminals of the superficial and deep branch sometimes connect to the perforators from the deep circumflex iliac system, deep inferior epigastric system, and lateral circumflex femoral system. Regarding the venous system, the superficial circumflex iliac artery accompanies the concomitant vein and also often accompanies a cutaneous vein, which also runs parallel to the superficial circumflex iliac artery system in the superficial layer of fatty tissue.

37.4.1.2 Principle of Surgical Technique

Preoperative Doppler examination is useful to confirm the course of the superficial circumflex iliac artery and localisation of perforators. The dominant perforator of the superficial and deep branches of the superficial circumflex iliac artery system is usually located at the cross-point, 3 cm medial from the anterosuperior iliac spine and through the course of the superficial circumflex iliac artery. The flap is outlined to include this point and a portion on the iliac spine. The first incision is made through the superior or inferior border of the outline to detect the deep or superficial branch and the perforators of the branch. Although both branches usually have dominant perforators, in some cases in which the superficial branch is short or absent, the long and large deep branch can be detected. When a superficial branch is very long and large, the deep branch is usually short and small. Therefore, the perforator of either dominant branch can be selected as a pedicle of the SCIP flap. During suprafascial flap elevation from the distal side, several perforators of the superficial circumflex iliac artery system can be easily identified under lower magnification with a loupe. The dominant perforator is dissected deeply to the level of the superficial or deep branch of the superficial circumflex iliac artery system. The cutaneous vein in the adiposal layer is included as a venous drainage system for the flap, because the concomitant vein of the superficial circumflex iliac artery is sometimes too small (0.5 mm in diameter) to anastomose. After dissection of the perforator and superficial circumflex iliac artery system, the other border of the flap is incised to elevate it as an island flap. If necessary, thinning, except around the perforator in the flap, is possible with removal of fatty tissue with scissors. The key point for this operation is bloodless flap elevation to detect and preserve the perforators and both superficial circumflex iliac artery branches. Finally, the superficial circumflex iliac artery, concomitant vein (usually one, sometimes two), and superficial circumflex iliac cutaneous vein are ligated. The proximal and distal portions of the perforator division of the superficial circumflex iliac artery system are transected, and a free groin perforator flap with a perforator and small segment of superficial circumflex iliac artery and concomitant vein (0.8–1 mm in diameter at the proximal transected end) and the cutaneous vein (1.5 mm) is transferred. As the vascular dissection for the proximal side of the superficial circumflex iliac artery system is not necessary, the flap can be elevated within a short time, about 30 min. Usually, the donor defect can be closed directly, but sometimes, a split-thickness skin graft is required [127].

37.4.2 Medial Circumflex Femoral Gracilis Perforator Flap

Orticochea [18] and McCraw et al. [128] were the first authors that reported the transfer of large skin flaps from the medial thigh, including the gracilis muscle to form a musculocutaneous flap. Hallock CG was the first who described the transfer of superior medial thigh skin as a free *muscle perforator flap* based on the gracilis musculocutaneous perforators alone [129,130].

37.4.2.1 Anatomy

Although the medial circumflex femoral artery has historically been considered the dominant source pedicle to the gracilis muscle, sometimes, the latter arises via the adductor branch of the profunda femoral artery [131,132]. This enters the muscle at a point usually within 6–10 cm below the pubic tubercle, with the exit of the pertinent musculocutaneous perforators restricted to a 6 cm wide area centred over this location [128,133,134]. Occasionally, septocutaneous perforators arise directly from the source pedicle medial to the adductor longus muscle, but these are always in addition to the musculocutaneous perforators [133,134]. Because multiple intramuscular branches pass proximally and distally within the muscle in primarily a longitudinal direction, this has been the basis for safely splitting the muscle without devascularisation [135,136]. The musculocutaneous perforators typically traverse the muscle anterior to these muscle branches so that they can be dissected independently. This permits creation of a combined conjoint flap [137] if desired. Of final importance, the corresponding venae comitantes follow the cutaneous perforators through the muscle [138] but are often minute so it is always advisable to also include branches of the greater saphenous vein as a secondary means for venous outflow [139].

37.4.2.2 Principle of Surgical Technique

At a point about 10 cm below the pubic tubercle, an audible Doppler probe is used to identify any gracilis perforators. A medial thigh incision is then made posterior to the course of the gracilis muscle to allow its elevation in the usual fashion, except for preservation of any large musculocutaneous perforators intact with the overlying skin [140,141]. The boundaries of the perforator flap were then centred around the largest perforator, with the posterior margin dictated by the original incision. An intramuscular dissection of the perforator back to the source vessels was completed by dividing muscle fibres and coagulating muscle side branches as necessary while protecting purely muscle branches by periodically inspecting the dominant pedicle on the lateral side of the muscle during this dissection. Any branches of the greater saphenous vein found passing within the flap boundaries were kept, with their separate dissection back to the saphenous bulb if necessary. After division of the muscle insertion, both flaps were passed through a subcutaneous tunnel into the groin. The muscle was independently inset over the exposed femoral vessels and the perforator flap used for closure of the groin skin wounds. The donor site was closed directly as in a medial thigh plastic.

37.4.2.3 Imaging

There are many reports on anatomical variability of the perforator vessel of the upper third of the leg. Precise preoperative mapping of the vascular system makes it possible to minimise the complication related to an untypical vessel distribution. More advanced imaging techniques, which include colour Doppler, must be used for more precise evaluation of perforators in this region of the leg [89,89]. This is a non-invasive examination using the ultrasound principle combined with flow evaluation based on the phenomenon described by Doppler. It is possible to accurately determine the site where the perforator pierces the deep fascia. The number of perforators present can be determined and their diameters and blood flow can be evaluated. The accuracy of this method in the upper third of the leg in relation to the intraoperative image is rated highly – around 95% [88,91]. This is of particular importance when planning large flaps and flaps with independent skin islets used for the reconstruction of multilayer structures. It is also possible to trace the whole vascular pedicle of the planned flap. Its length and diameter can be measured. If it is necessary to use a long pedicle, the most distal perforator should be used.

In older patients, if it is necessary to use a free flap for the reconstruction and is possible to evaluate the condition of the vessel itself, the potential presence of wall thickening or atherosclerotic plaques thus enables the prediction of potential technical difficulties during the performance of the microvascular anastomosis. In these cases, evaluation of blood flow rate seems to be invaluable, and it is impossible with any other of the methods discussed. The flap skin islet may be supplied by septal and muscular perforators. Isolation of septal perforators is incomparably quicker, easier, and less time consuming.

Mapping is easier for the obese patients since the vessel is demonstrated more prominently in the fatty tissue than in the muscle. On the other hand, it may be difficult to trace the perforator to the very end of the perforating point in very lean patients with little fat in the intermuscular septum and poorly developed subcutaneous fatty layer. This may explain the cases in which a perforator was actually present which was not identified preoperatively in CT angiography, or the vessel actually has a short intramuscular course before reaching the septum which was mistaken as a septocutaneous perforator preoperatively. It may be more problematic in relatively small perforators with weak signal intensities. Doppler mapping is still useful in the standpoint of sensitivity and also in very lean patients.

There is a more recent method of CT but it is more expensive and requires contrast agent administration and patient's exposure to a dose of ionising radiation.

MRA is currently in the phase of clinical trials.

37.5 FLAPS OF THE MIDDLE THIRD OF THE LEG

37.5.1 Soleus Perforator Flap

The proximal lateral leg flap transfer using the major nutrient vessel to the soleus muscle was first described in 1994 [142]. The most significant feature of this flap is that there is no need to sacrifice any main arteries in the lower leg.

37.5.1.1 Anatomy

This flap is based on the musculocutaneous perforator vessels that arise from one of the three main arteries in the proximal lower leg and pierce the soleus muscle bellies, giving off muscular branches before reaching the skin. This perforator vessel originated from the peroneal artery in only 40%, the posterior tibial artery in 21%, the tibio-peroneal trunk in 28%, and the trifurcation of the posterior tibial and peroneal arteries in 11% [143].

37.5.1.2 Principle of Surgical Technique

The location of perforator vessels was plotted preoperatively by using a Doppler flow metre. There were usually one or two points near the distal portion of the proximal third of the lower leg along the posterior margin of the fibula. The flap was designed to include these points according to the size of the defect. The first incision was made along the posterior border of the flap. The dissection was carried out carefully until the perforator vessels that penetrated the fascia of the soleus could be seen. After confirming the perforator vessels, the flap was elevated from anterior to posterior without the fascia of the soleus. The perforator vessels were then dissected deeply through the soleus muscles, with ligation of the muscular branches. Then, the soleus muscle was detached from the fibula, and the bifurcation of the perforator vessels from a main artery was easily located. The free soleus perforator flap was elevated to ligate the perforator vessels at their bifurcation. The arterial diameter of the perforator vessels was approximately 1.8 mm. The donor site could be closed primarily less than 6 cm in width; otherwise, it was closed with a skin graft.

37.5.2 Medial Sural Perforator Flap

The use of the gastrocnemius muscle flap for the reconstruction of complex lower extremity defects was described about 20 years ago [144,145]. Taylor and Daniel [146] and later Montegut et al. [147] showed the basis for a fasciocutaneous flap (the medial sural artery perforator flap) based on perforating branches of medial sural artery, avoiding the need for gastrocnemius muscle sacrifice, thus reducing the morbidity of the donor site. Other clinical studies [148] based on vascular anatomy investigations [149] showed that the medial sural artery perforator flap is an ideal thin cutaneous flap [150].

37.5.2.1 Anatomy

The vascular anatomy of the posterior calf region is based on the superficial sural artery and musculocutaneous perforators from medial and lateral sural arteries. The medial sural artery supplies the medial gastrocnemius muscle and sends perforating branches to the skin. Many studies evidenced that [148,151] almost all limbs had at least one large musculocutaneous perforator to the overlying calf skin that exited via the medial head of the gastrocnemius muscle, so that a true muscle perforator flap could be raised from that territory. The majority of these perforators were localised in the distal half of the muscle and emanated near the raphe separating the two heads of the gastrocnemius [148,151].

37.5.2.2 Principle of Surgical Technique

An incision near the midline is made to confirm the identification of two large musculocutaneous perforators over the medial gastrocnemius muscle. A medial sural flap slightly larger than the defect to cover is circumscribed. Intramuscular dissection of the perforators is stopped when tension-free transfer of the flap through a subcutaneous tunnel is possible. The donor site could be closed primarily. The island version of the medial sural perforator flap permits transfer as a local flap unconstrained except for the vascular pedicle itself. The flap can be tunnelled under adjacent skin to the defect, but venous compression causing flap congestion should always be a concern. Inclusion of a branch of the posterior femoral cutaneous nerve, which provides sensation to the skin overlying the medial gastrocnemius muscle, would require a dissection separate to that of the medial sural vessels and could compromise flap reach [152].

37.5.2.3 Imaging

A systematic and precise knowledge of the dominant perforating vessels in sural and medial soleus perforator flaps is not feasible due to high variability of the vascular plexus. For these reasons, the precise determination by instrumental exam of the dominant perforator regarding its position, course, and calibre for every patient would be extremely useful.

The most commonly used technique for preoperative localisation of perforating vessels in this flap is the Doppler ultrasound examination due to its simplicity and low costs. It gives a good correlation between the audible volume of signal and vessel diameter, but the results are imprecise [153] and the number of false-positive results can be high [154]. Besides, it cannot permit the distinction of the perforator from the main axial vessel. Colour Doppler imaging provides more information and higher results, such as good evaluation of the calibre and haemodynamic properties of both arterial and venous part of the perforator as well as main vascular trunk and its branches. It is an excellent tool in planning of other perforator flaps due to its high sensitivity and 100% predictive value [154]. Duplex Doppler does not expose patients to unnecessary high doses of radiation and its risks as the CTA. This property is very important in patients who require free flap reconstructions for non-cancer-related defects, such as trauma, congenital deformities, or burns sequelae. The comparative study by Damir Kosutic et al. [155] on Duplex-Doppler ultrasound showed high correlation between exact location of the dominant lateral and medial sural artery perforators and their most frequent position in the examined and dissected cadaver lower legs. According to the authors, "Duplex-Doppler imaging enables the surgeon not only to preoperatively choose the dominant perforator on the basis of its calibre but also to determine its precise location. This is important for dissection and makes the entire procedure safer and faster to perform with fewer intra and postoperative complications" [155].

37.5.3 Anterior Tibialis Perforator/Propeller Flap

The tibialis anterior perforator-based fasciocutaneous flap is an alternative for satisfactory coverage of proximal third tibial defects and patellar defects.

37.5.3.1 Anatomy

The blood supply of the lower leg derives from the popliteal artery, which ramifies into three main vessels: the AT artery, the posterior tibial artery, and the peroneal artery. The AT artery begins at the inferior border of the popliteus muscle, branching from the bifurcation of the popliteal artery, and passes between the two heads of the tibialis posterior and through the interosseous membrane, to the deep part of the anterior leg. It then descends on the anterior surface of the interosseous membrane, moving closer to the tibia, and becomes the dorsalis pedis artery at the level of the ankle joint [156] (Figure 37.9).

The AT artery is the origin of multiple septocutaneous or musculocutaneous perforators. The most proximal large perforator branches of the AT artery are Dopplered approximately 10–12 cm distal to the femoral condyle. The perforators then appear at approximately 5 cm intervals along a line longitudinally through the anterior intermuscular septum that is between the extensor digitorum longus and the peroneus muscles. These penetrate the deep fascia of the proximal one-third of the lower leg. The perforators course downward through the intermuscular space between the AT muscle and the extensor digitorum longus muscle to penetrate the deep fascial junction of the upper and middle third of the lower leg. This is measured out at approximately 17 cm distal to the tibial condyle and runs caudally beneath the extensor digitorum longus muscle. The vessel courses anteriorly through the lateral intermuscular septum between the extensor digitorum and peroneus muscles or through the medial anterior intermuscular septum between the anterior musculature and tibia. The perforators pierce the deep fascia to enter the skin of the middle third of the lower leg [157].

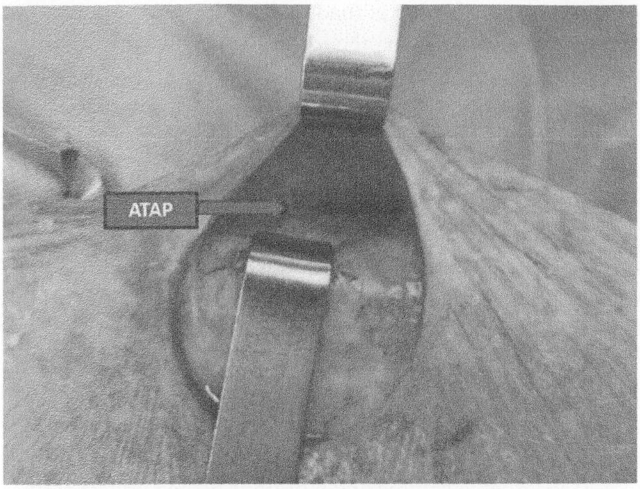

FIGURE 37.9 Anterior tibial artery perforator (ATAP). Intraoperative view.

37.5.3.2 Imaging

Accurate information on septocutaneous vessels that arise from the AT artery is needed in order to design safe and reliable flaps. Previous anatomical studies reported controversial results about the location and distribution of septocutaneous perforators of the AT artery.

The anatomic study of K. Panagiotopoulos et al. [158] reported that a series of septocutaneous perforators originates from the AT artery, courses along three intermuscular septa (I, II, and III), and penetrates the deep fascia to form an interconnecting network supplying the skin of the antero-lateral leg region. According to Haertsch [159] and Dong et al. [160], septocutaneous perforators of the AT artery course along the intermuscular septa I and III, while Rocha et al. [161] and Satoh et al. [162] reported only septum III, Morrison et al. [163] reported septa II and III, Stadler et al. [164] reported septa I and II, and, finally, Wee [165] and Whetzel et al. [166] reported septa I, II, and III. Other authors suggested that in the distal segment of the lower leg, there is a relative lack of large septocutaneous perforators (diameter ≥ 1 mm) of the AT artery, while Stadler et al. [164] found an adequate number of perforators in the distal segment.

As a result of individual anatomic variations, it is not possible to predict that a perforator actually exists at a particular site. The preoperative identification of septocutaneous perforators (especially those with a diameter ≥ 1 mm) is possible with colour Doppler assessment, which is non-invasive, causes no radiation exposure, and can be easily repeated if needed [167]. By mapping a particular perforator with preoperative colour Doppler, individual flaps may be designed to lie exactly over the perforator, ensuring blood supply to the flap.

37.5.3.3 Principle of Surgical Technique

Before the operation, perforator vessels are mapped using a handheld Doppler ultrasound probe. Flap design and orientations are marked on the skin around the sited perforators. An incision is made along only on the anterior edge of the marked flap. It is important to leave two or more skin bridges intact, preferably the proximal and distal margins, should the decision to delay the flap become necessary during periodic evaluation of flap perfusion. The proximal margin of the flap should also be left intact until the final choice of perforator to use has been made (a more proximal perforator will require a longer flap). The dissection extends to include the deep fascia, elevating the flap from the underlying muscle in the subfascial plane. Using loupe magnification, local fascial feeders and perforators are identified and protected. The remainder of the subfascial dissection is completed around the preserved perforating vessel(s), to all margins of the flap. When more than one perforator is identified, the choice of ideal perforator is made based on vessel calibre and the position which allows ease of flap transposition to resurface the wound under minimal tension. Assessment of flap perfusion and venous drainage based on the chosen feeder can be made with temporary atraumatic occlusion of deselected perforators with single Acland clamps. If flap colour and capillary refill suggest adequate perfusion and drainage over time, deselected perforators are ligated and divided. The flap is then completely islandised on the single perforator. Inadequate flap perfusion will warrant inclusion of a nearby perforator(s); this however precludes maximal rotation of the flap and thus the principal utility of rotation flaps. To maximise the arc of rotation of the flap, dissection of the perforator continues toward the tibialis anterior artery and its venae comitantes to minimise kinking by spreading out the twisting of the pedicle over a greater length. The option to delay the flap is only available if inadequate perfusion of the flap is observed before complete division of all skin attachments or final deselection of all extra perforators. During flap inset, undue tension on or twisting of the vessels will compromise circulation and therefore flap survival. Retrograde intramuscular dissection of the principal perforator maximises pedicle length. This distributes the 180° rotation over a greater pedicle length and minimises tension and twist on the pedicle. The flap is secured in place loosely with 3–0 and 4–0 absorbable sutures and a drain is placed underneath.

37.5.4 Posterior Tibialis Propeller/Perforator Flap

The posterior tibial artery perforators (PTAPs) are consistently the largest and easiest to dissect [168–171] (Figure 37.10), and the flap may be transposed or islanded and rotated through up to 180° about the perforator and may be proximally or distally based, enabling reconstruction of a variety of lower limb defects [172–175]. Flap harvest is relatively quick, and the recipient site has similar texture, thickness, pliability, and pigmentation to that which has been lost. V–Y or propeller flap designs may enable primary closure. These flaps are particularly suitable for complicated defects of the lower third of the leg, foot, heel, and ankle, where local flap options have previously not been available.

37.5.4.1 Anatomy

The posterior tibial artery, which is the dominant source of blood supply to the foot, is preserved, and the need for microvascular anastomoses is obviated [176,177].

The PTAPs are each accompanied by two venae comitantes and are predominantly septocutaneous, arising from within the intermuscular septum between the soleus and the flexor hallucis longus [168–171]. A large flap territory can be raised on a single perforator from the posterior tibial artery

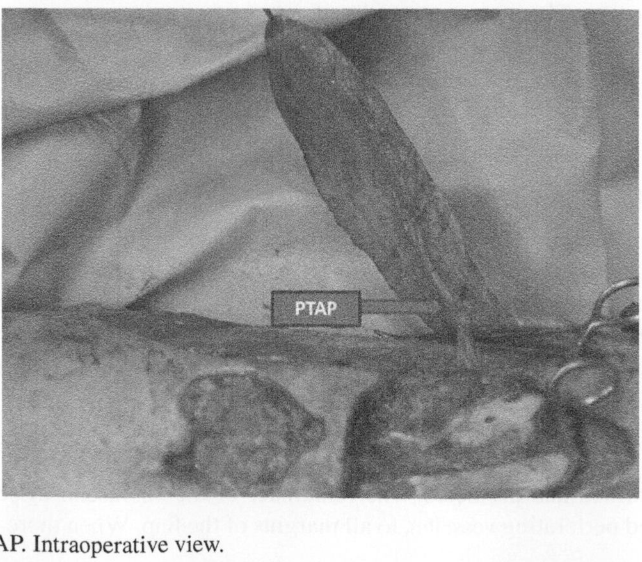

FIGURE 37.10 PTAP. Intraoperative view.

because of axial vessels communicating between the PTAPs within the flap [178]. Not including the long saphenous vein may lead to an increased rate of flap tip necrosis. Flap harvest does not necessitate exposure of the posterior tibial artery or skeletonisation of the perforator, reducing the risk of damage to the perforator and delicate venae comitantes.

37.5.4.2 Principle of Surgical Technique

Preoperatively, the PTAPs are identified and marked on the skin using handheld Doppler ultrasonography. The flap is designed with respect to the defect and a limited anterior incision as for a fasciotomy is made through which the perforators are identified by direct visualisation. The most reliable perforators are found at 6–8 cm and 10–12 cm from the tip of the medial malleolus, and the flap can be reliably harvested within 10 cm of the popliteal skin crease. If the perforator is of sufficient calibre, the anterior and posterior flap incisions are completed and the flap is raised from proximal to distal in the subfascial plane, identifying and preserving all of the perforators encountered, leaving the flap bridges proximally and distally. The largest suitable distal perforator is selected and single microclamps are placed on all other perforators. A soft non-crushing clamp is placed across the base of the flap and perfusion within the flap is evaluated. If flap perfusion is reliable, the other perforators are ligated and the proximal incision is made. The flap is only islanded if bleeding at the tip can be demonstrated. Care is taken to preserve the saphenous vein and saphenous nerve. If flap perfusion is compromised following application of the soft non-crushing clamp, the flap is transposed rather than islanded, with ligation of perforators as necessary to allow flap transposition, or abandoned. After islanding, the septum around the perforator is gently released to allow rotation of the flap up to 180° without occluding the pedicle. The donor site may be closed directly but often requires application of a split-thickness skin graft [179].

37.5.5 Peroneal Artery Perforator–Based Propeller Flap

The perforator-based propeller flap technique mitigates the use of either the posterior tibial or the peroneal arteries proper, as these major vessels themselves are not dissected or divided. Whichever main vessel is giving primary flow to the perforator will remain intact.

37.5.5.1 Anatomy

The peroneal artery branches off the tibio-peroneal trunk and courses along the medial aspect of the fibula in the deep compartment to supply the posterolateral lower leg, ankle, and heel. Perforating vessels branch from the peroneal artery at 3–5 cm intervals and course through or in close proximity to the posterolateral intermuscular septum before reaching the subdermal plexus of the posterolateral skin. They may be purely septal or course through the flexor hallucis muscle, the soleus muscle, or both [180]. Distally, the peroneal artery anastomoses with the posterior tibial artery via one to three transverse communicating branches deep to the Achilles tendon [181]. These branches are located about between 0 and 6 cm above the level of the ankle joint or just above the calcaneal insertion of the Achilles.

37.5.5.2 Imaging

Due to the anatomic characteristic of this vascular plexus, it is impossible by Doppler ultrasound to know whether the flow through the distal posterior tibial artery originates from the proximal posterior tibial artery or indirectly from the distal peroneal artery via the communicating branches. Conversely, it is also not possible to determine whether the flow through the peroneal artery originates from the peroneal artery proper or from the posterior tibial artery [182]. This fact becomes important in assessing the relative contribution of each major vessel to foot perfusion, particularly in the setting of peripheral vascular disease, and therefore the appropriateness of flaps based on these arterial systems. The perforating vessels may be identified with handheld unidirectional Doppler [183,184], colour duplex imaging [185], MRA [186], or similar to DIEP flap perforators [187,188], 3D CT scan angiography.

37.5.5.3 Principle of Surgical Technique

Flap design and orientations are marked on the skin around the sited perforators, ensuring adequate flap length proximally should the most proximal perforator be selected. This ensures that the perforator vessels remain fully dilated that aids in their identification. A longitudinal incision is made along the anterior edge of the flap. Using loupe magnification, the dissection continues posteriorly in either a suprafascial or subfascial plane and local perforators are identified and protected. During this dissection, the proximal margin of the flap should be left intact until the final choice of perforator to use has been made (a more proximal perforator will require a longer flap). The ideal perforator is selected based on vessel calibre and the most distal position possible. The posterior incision is then made and the flap completely undermined while protecting the isolated perforators. Assessment of flap perfusion and venous drainage based on the chosen vessel can be made with temporary atraumatic occlusion of deselected perforators with Acland clamps after the tourniquet is released. If flap colour and capillary refill suggest adequate perfusion and venous drainage over time, secondary perforators are deselected, ligated, and divided. Inadequate flap circulation or venous congestion warrants inclusion of nearby perforator(s) or flap delay. Thus, it is critical to leave one or more skin bridges intact (preferably the proximal and distal margins); so, the decision to delay the flap should become necessary during periodic evaluation of flap perfusion. If commitment to a single perforator is appropriate, the proximal and distal skin bridges are divided last. Retrograde intramuscular or intraseptal dissection of the principal perforator toward the peroneal artery maximises pedicle (perforator) length. This distributes the 180° rotation over a greater pedicle length to minimise tension and twist on the pedicle (perforator) and allows greater reach. During flap inset, undue tension on or twisting of the vessels is avoided, and the flap is secured with 3–0 and 4–0 absorbable sutures. A drain is placed subcutaneously and is removed after 24–48 h. A posterior foot-drop plaster splint is applied and strict elevation of the flap is enforced for 1–2 weeks postoperatively [189] (Figure 37.11).

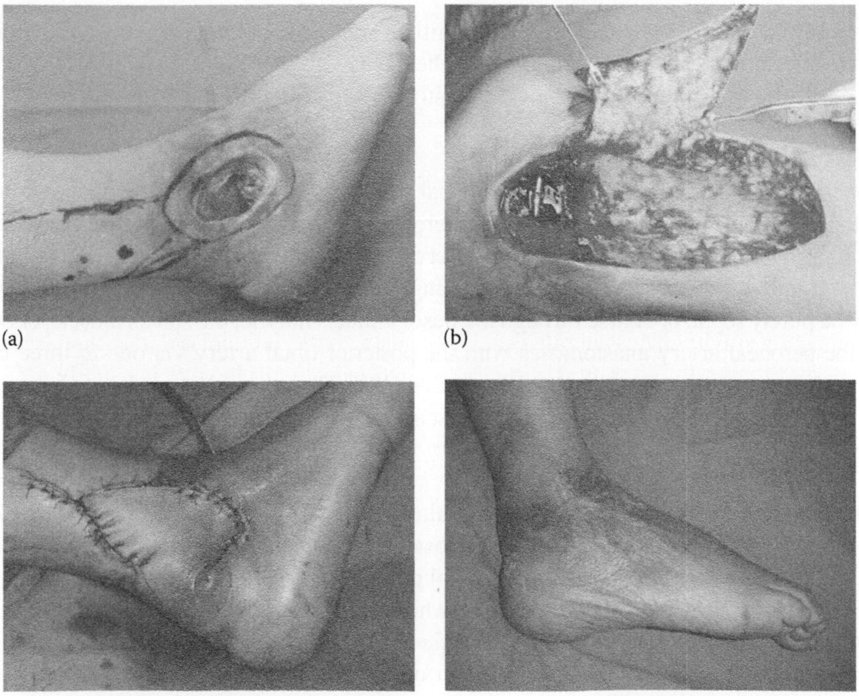

FIGURE 37.11 (a) Patient with lateral malleolar vascular ulcer; (b) hatchet flap based on the peroneal artery perforator; (c) positioning and suturing of the flap; (d) 2-year postoperative view.

37.5.6 Saphenous Perforator Flap

In 1986, Amarante et al. [190] forwarded the concept of the saphenous perforator flap based on cadaver studies. Later, Cavadas [191,192] reported clinical experiences with this type of neurocutaneous flap; this flap was termed neurocutaneous flap, because the perineural arterial network is important for flap survival.

37.5.6.1 Anatomy

The perforators of the posterior tibial artery emerge in the septum between the soleus and the flexor digitorum longus muscle and feed the axial suprafascial net of blood vessels accompanying the saphenous nerve and the greater saphenous vein. Magnifying loops (fourfold) are strongly recommended to localise the perforator at the estimated pivot point.

37.5.6.2 Principle of Surgical Technique

Without tourniquet, an 8–10 cm exploratory incision is made at the dorsal edge of the stripe of skin, and skin with 2 mm subcutaneous tissue is elevated in the direction of the Achilles tendon. The subcutaneous tissue and fascia are then incised for 8 cm along the ventral rim of the Achilles tendon and the fascia elevated dorsal to ventral from the soleus muscle up to the septum to identify perforator arteries. If no perforator is visualised at the dorsal aspect of the septum between soleus and flexor digitorum longus muscle, a second exploratory incision is made at the anterior edge of the skin stripe, elevating the skin with 2 mm subcutaneous tissue toward the tibia taking care to preserve the saphenous nerve. The subcutaneous fat and fascia are split along the dorsal rim of the tibia for about 8 cm and the fascia over the flexor digitorum longus muscle elevated from ventral to the intermuscular septum. In most cases, a perforator is visualised about 10 cm proximal to the tip of the malleolus. If no perforator is identified at this level, it may be located between the two layers of the septum. In that case, the pivot point is set at 10 cm. If, however, a strong perforator should be identified either proximal or distal to the 10 cm level, the flap design has to be adjusted to the new pivot level. At this stage of surgery, the definite proximal skin incision is outlined including the size and shape of the skin island. The skin over the subcutaneous pedicle is incised in the proximal direction with a seam of 1.5 cm fat and fascia around the skin island. Both from the ventral and the dorsal side, the fascia is elevated to the septum between soleus and flexor digitorum longus muscle, and the septum is severed from proximal to distal. During the dissection, the location and calibre of perforator arteries proximal to the pivot point should be registered. If more than one strong perforator has to be divided proximal to the pivot point and no perforator was found between the layers of the septum at the 10 cm level, the vascularisation of the flap may be at stake and staged surgery with delayed flap transfer should be considered. The flap is transposed to the site of insertion by a separate incision and not by subcutaneous tunnelling. Inserting the flap, the rims of the defect are elevated for 2 cm and the adipofascial seam of the skin island buried beneath the wound edges. The donor defect is preliminary covered by artificial skin grafts or by split-skin grafting. Through a window in the dressing, the flap condition is evaluated 2 h after surgery and later every 6 h for 48 h. Any haematoma is immediately evacuated. Skin sutures are removed in case of oedema formation. Minor flap necrosis (<1⁄4) is managed by early redebridement, split-skin grafts, and vacuum-assisted closure. Signs of flap infection indicate surgical revision.

37.6 FLAPS OF THE FOOT

37.6.1 Medial Plantar Artery Perforator Flap

This flap has been popularised for the repair of defects in the foot, palm, and fingers in 1954 when Mir y Mir introduced cross-leg medial plantar flap [193]. A pedicled instep flap based on the medial plantar artery and nerve was described by Shanahan and McCarthy [194] in 1979; Reiffel [195] also reported the calcaneal flap, medial plantar flap, and lateral plantar flap. An instep island flap was reported in 1981 by Harrison and Morgan [196]. In 1983, a free sensory instep flap with medial plantar artery for heel defects was developed by Morrison et al. [197]. Inoue et al. [198] and Lee et al. [199] reported free medial plantar flaps with short segmental vascular pedicle for finger reconstructions. Masquelet and Romana in 1990 [200] and Ishikura et al. [201] in 1995 reported the successful use of a new flap, the medialis pedis flap in the same donor area, for reconstruction of soft-tissue defects of the foot. In 2001, Koshima et al. described the free medial plantar artery perforator flap based on only the medial plantar artery perforator. This flap can be an island flap for coverage of the heel and forefoot plantar weight-bearing defects without transecting the medial plantar or posterior tibial systems [202,203].

The advantages of this flap are minimal donor-site morbidity, minimal damage to both the posterior tibial and medial plantar systems, no need for deep dissection, the ability to thin the flap by primary removal of excess fatty tissue, the use of a large cutaneous vein as a venous drainage system, a good colour and texture match for finger pulp repair, short time for flap elevation, possible application as a flow-through flap, and a concealed donor scar [202–204].

37.6.1.1 Anatomy

This perforator flap is nourished only by perforators of the medial plantar vessel and a cutaneous vein or with a small segment of the medial plantar vessel. It has no fascial component. There is a possibility of anatomic variation in the superficial branch of the medial plantar system. Based on the cadaver and clinical experiences of Koshima et al., superficial branches deriving from the proximal level of the medial plantar artery (pedicle artery of medialis pedis flap) showed irregular anatomy. But, perforators of the medial plantar artery always existed and were constant [202,203].

37.6.1.2 Imaging and Surgical Technique

Preoperative Doppler examinations are useful to confirm the localisation of the perforators of the medial plantar perforator flap. Using an air tourniquet and magnifying glass, before outlining the flap, the first incision is made parallel to the abductor hallucis muscle at the dorsal border of the flap. When the flap is elevated suprafascially above the flexor hallucis muscle, several perforators of the medial plantar vessel can be easily identified through the intermuscular septum between the abductor hallucis muscle and the flexor digitorum muscle. Perforator is usually composed of a 0.3 mm calibre artery and smaller concomitant vein. An important point is that a small amount of intermuscular septum and adiposal tissue should be included around the perforator, not to skeletonise a perforator in cases with island flap transfer. Because flap transfer usually requires 180° rotation of the pedicle perforator, it creates strong traction through short and bare perforators and results in poor flap circulation. With the use of retractors, the medial plantar vessel is exposed through the intermuscular space. Taking care to include the perforators, the plantar border of the perforator flap is outlined, and an additional skin incision is made through the inferior border of the flap. Preserving the medial plantar nerve, the perforator is deeply dissected to the division of the medial plantar vessel. The donor defect can usually be closed directly but sometimes requires a split-thickness skin graft or free flap in cases with large and deep defect [203,204].

37.6.2 Lateral Plantar Perforator Flap

Reconstruction of the forefoot plantar defect was made possible after the description of the reverse-flow medial and lateral plantar flaps [205–207]. These flaps have the advantage of moving healthy tissues from the non-weight-bearing area to the defect [208]. However, this flap has the drawbacks of venous congestion and an increased donor-site morbidity by transecting a major vessel of the foot. In some cases, this approach requires a skin graft thus adding a donor-site morbidity area [208]. Since then, different flaps and technique have been described [208–215].

37.6.2.1 Anatomy

This flap is based on the perforators arising from the lateral plantar artery [216]. It can be used to harvest a flap for the reconstruction of a plantar defect. Using this flap, there is no compromise of the dominant inflow source to the foot: the posterior tibial, the medial, and lateral plantar arteries and the dorsalis pedis artery and nerve are left intact. The dissection length of the perforators can be adjusted according to surgical requirements; there is no exposure of plantar sensory nerves and vessels; the flap elevation can be completed within a short operating time [217].

37.6.2.2 Imaging and Surgical Technique

Preoperative imaging techniques, such as Doppler examinations and/or angio-CT scans, are useful to confirm the localisation of the perforators of the lateral plantar, arising from the artery. A full-thickness incision of the lateral edge flap, up to the lateral edge of the abductor digiti minimi muscle, is performed. Once the muscle is reached, the flap is carefully undermined, laterally to medially, just above the abductor digiti minimi fascia, until reaching the medial edge of the muscle. Then, the lateral plantar artery perforators are found coming off between the abductor digiti minimi muscle and the flexor digitorum brevis muscle. The incision is then completed and the flap is advanced forward and sutured in a V–Y fashion (Figure 37.12).

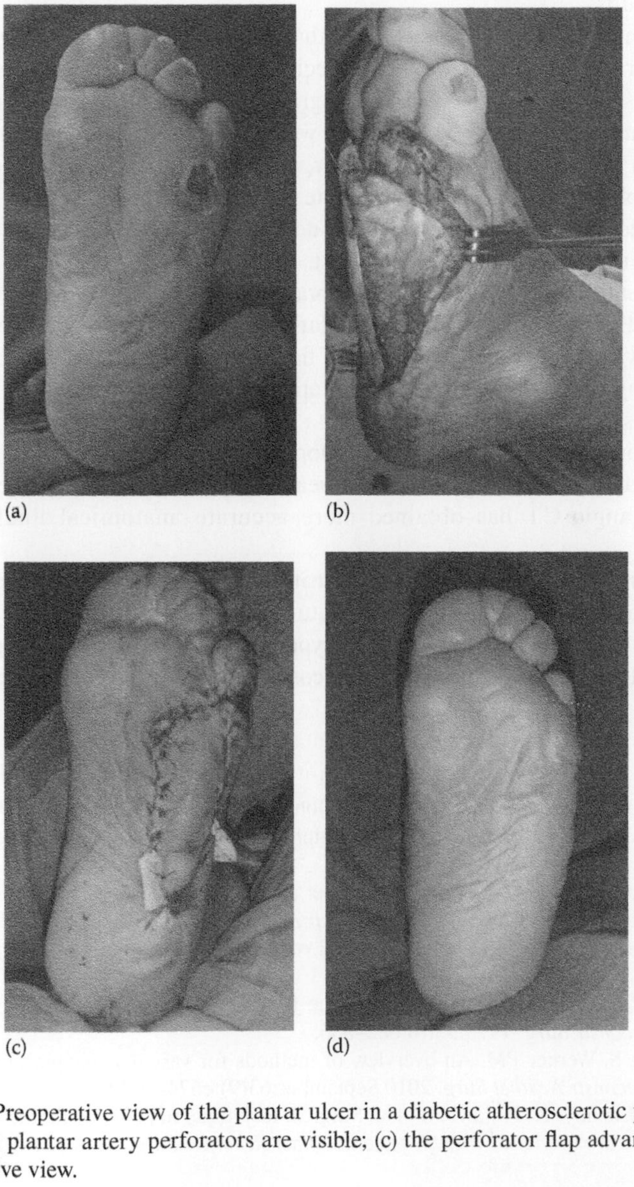

FIGURE 37.12 (a) Preoperative view of the plantar ulcer in a diabetic atherosclerotic patient; (b) the flap is raised and the lateral plantar artery perforators are visible; (c) the perforator flap advanced in V–Y fashion; (d) 2-year postoperative view.

37.7 CONCLUSION

The advent of perforator and propeller flaps represented a significant step forward in the treatment of lower limb defects in many cases, which previously could only be solved by free tissue transfers. Perforator flaps also obtain lower morbidity and better cosmetic results than pedicled fasciocutaneous, muscular, or myocutaneous flaps, which create excessive volume and achieve poor aesthetic results. Due to their great versatility, pedicled perforator flaps have become the first surgical choice for the reconstruction of lower extremities.

The disadvantage of perforator flaps is the technical difficulty of their insertion. There is a long learning curve and operative time is increased. However, the difficulty of the surgery can be reduced by prior knowledge of the vascular anatomy.

Many reports have described the anatomy of the perforator vessels of the lower extremities, but perforators and their vascular territory are highly complex and variable. At present, the clinical preoperative standard for mapping perforators is Doppler ultrasound, but the method does not produce entirely reliable results.

Angio-CT is a minimally invasive technique that provides a 3D image of the vascular anatomy and surrounding structures and gives a more precise anatomical description of the location, size, condition, and course of the vessel. The CT angiogram requires the IV administration of low-osmolar, nonionic iodinated contrast media, like other well-known radiologic examinations (i.e. chest or abdominal CT scan and urography). Low-osmolar, nonionic contrast media are considered safe and without effects on blood vessels. The reported rate of fatal reactions in man is 1/80,000. There are several recent articles in plastic surgery journals devoted to the use of CT angiogram, which demonstrate the lack of risks due to iodinated contrast.

Being able to identify a priori the largest perforator with the most favourable course reduces the time of dissection. Prior knowledge of the vascular anatomy helps us to customise the flap according to requirements and to decide which type of flap is the best option for a particular perforator. Angio-CT can change a surgical indication if no appropriate perforator branch is found, especially in traumatic and vascular disease.

Angio-CT is not intended to replace the Doppler sonography or surgical exploration, but it facilitates the work of the surgeon and increases the reliability of these other techniques. In many studies, angio-CT has obtained more accurate anatomical findings than Doppler sonography.

Three-dimensional images of microvascular anatomical vessels can provide a better understanding of how skin is perfused and may aid in the future design of new flaps. Nowadays, there are not any publications in which it is demonstrated beyond all doubt that CT angiogram could replace Doppler. Hence, CT angiogram and Doppler are complementary to one another.

REFERENCES

1. Pratt GF, Rozen WM, Chubb D, Ashton MW, Alonso-Burgos A, Whitaker IS. Preoperative imaging for perforator flaps in reconstructive surgery: A systematic review of the evidence for current techniques. *Ann Plast Surg*. 2012 July;69(1):3–9.
2. Rozen WM, Garcia-Tutor E, Alonso-Burgos A et al. Planning and optimizing DIEP flaps with virtual surgery: The Navarra experience. *J Plast Reconstr Aesthet Surg*. 2010 February;63(2):289–297.
3. Aoyagi F, Fujino T, Ohshiro T. Detection of small vessels for microsurgery by a Doppler flowmeter. *Plast Reconstr Surg*. 1975;55(3):372–373.
4. Karkowski J, Buncke HJ. A simplified technique for free transfer of groin flaps, by use of a Doppler Probe. *Plast Reconstr Surg*. 1975;55(6):682–686.
5. Smit JM, Klein S, Werker PM. An overview of methods for vascular mapping in the planning of free flaps. *J Plast Reconstr Aesthet Surg*. 2010 September;63(9):e674–e682.
6. Hamdi M, Van Landuyt K, Hijjawi JB et al. Surgical technique in pedicled thoracodorsal artery perforator flaps: A clinical experience with 99 patients. *Plast Reconstr Surg*. 2008;121(5):1632–1641.

7. Georgescu AV. Propeller perforator flaps in distal lower leg: Evolution and clinical applications. *Arch Plast Surg*. 2012 March;39(2):94–105.
8. McGregor IA, Morgan G. Axial and random pattern flaps. *Br J Plast Surg*. 1973;26:202–213.
9. Rad AN, Singh NK, Rosson GD. Peroneal artery perforator-based propeller flap reconstruction of the lateral distal lower extremity after tumor extirpation: Case report and literature review. *Microsurgery* 2008;28:663–670.
10. Almeida MF, da Costa PR, Okawa RY. Reverse-flow island sural flap. *Plast Reconstr Surg*. 2002;109:583–591.
11. McGregor IA, Jackson IT. The groin flap. *Br J Plast Surg*. 1972;25:3–16.
12. McCraw JB, Furlow LT Jr. The dorsalis pedis arterialized flap. A clinical study. *Plast Reconstr Surg*. 1975;55:177–185.
13. Torii S, Namiki Y, Hayashi Y et al. Reverse-flow peroneal island flap for the reconstruction of leg and foot. *Eur J Plast Surg*. 1988;11:26–31.
14. Liu K, Li Z, Lin Y et al. The reverse-flow posterior tibial artery island flap: Anatomic study and 72 clinical cases. *Plast Reconstr Surg* 1990;86:312–316.
15. Innocenti M, Menichini G, Baldrighi C, Delcroix L, Vignini L, Tos P. Are There Risk Factors for Complications of Perforator-based Propeller Flaps for Lower-extremity Reconstruction? *Clin Orthop Relat Res*. 2014 Apr 5.
16. Koshima I, Itoh S, Nanba Y et al. Medial and lateral malleolar perforator flaps for repair of defects around the ankle. *Ann Plast Surg*. 2003;51:579–583.
17. Ger R. The operative treatment of the advanced stasis ulcer. A preliminary communication. *Am J Surg*. 1966;111:659–663.
18. Orticochea M. The musculocutaneous flap method: An immediate and heroic substitute for the method of delay. *Br J Plast Surg*. 1972;25:106–110.
19. Ger R. The technique of muscle transposition in the operative treatment of traumatic and ulcerative lesions of the leg. *J Trauma*. 1971;11:502–510.
20. Quaba O, Quaba AA. Pedicled perforator flaps for the lower limb. *Semin Plast Surg*. 2006;20:103–111.
21. Hallock GG. Lower extremity muscle perforator flaps for lower extremity reconstruction. *Plast Reconstr Surg*. 2004;114:1123–1130.
22. Kamath BJ, Joshua TV, Pramod S. Perforator based flap coverage from the anterior and lateral compartment of the leg for medium sized traumatic pretibial soft tissue defects: A simple solution for a complex problem. *J Plast Reconstr Aesthet Surg*. 2006;59:515–520.
23. Jakubietz RG, Jakubietz MG, Gruenert JG et al. The 180-degree perforator-based propeller flap for soft tissue coverage of the distal, lower extremity: A new method to achieve reliable coverage of the distal lower extremity with a local, fasciocutaneous perforator flap. *Ann Plast Surg*. 2007;59:667–671.
24. Ponten B. The fasciocutaneous flap: Its use in soft tissue defects of the lower leg. *Br J Plast Surg*. 1981;34:215–220.
25. Haertsch P. The surgical plane in the leg. *Br J Plast Surg*. 1981;34:464–469.
26. Barclay TL, Cardoso E, Sharpe DT et al. Repair of lower leg injuries with fascio-cutaneous flaps. *Br J Plast Surg*. 1982;35:127–132.
27. Cormack GC, Lamberty BG. Fasciocutaneous vessels. Their distribution on the trunk and limbs, and their clinical application in tissue transfer. *Anat Clin*. 1984;6:121–131.
28. Manchot C. *The Cutaneous Arteries of the Human Body*. New York: Springer-Verlag; 1983.
29. Salmon M, Taylor GI, Tempest M. *Arteries of the Skin*. London, U.K.: Churchill Livingstone; 1988.
30. Taylor GI, Palmer JH. The vascular territories (angiosomes) of the body: Experimental study and clinical applications. *Br J Plast Surg*. 1987;40:113–141.
31. Taylor GI, Pan WR. Angiosomes of the leg: Anatomic study and clinical implications. *Plast Reconstr Surg*. 1998;102:599–616.
32. Koshima I, Soeda S. Inferior epigastric artery skin flaps without rectus abdominis muscle. *Br J Plast Surg*. 1989;42:645–648.
33. Kroll SS, Rosenfield L. Perforator-based flaps for low posterior midline defects. *Plast Reconstr Surg*. 1988;81:561–566.
34. Blondeel PN, Van Landuyt KH, Monstrey SJ, Hamdi M, Matton GE, Allen RJ, Dupin C, Feller AM, Koshima I, Kostakoglu N, Wei FC. The "Gent" consensus on perforator flap terminology: Preliminary definitions. *Plast Reconstr Surg*. 2003 October;112(5):1378–1383.
35. Allen RJ, Treece P. Deep inferior epigastric perforator flap for breast reconstruction. *Ann Plast Surg*. 1994;32:32.

36. Blondeel PN, Boeckx WD. Refinements in free flap breast reconstruction: The free bilateral deep inferior epigastric perforator flap anastomosed to the internal mammary artery. *Br J Plast Surg*. 1994;47:495.
37. Blondeel PN. One hundred free DIEP flap breast reconstructions: A personal experience. *Br J Plast Surg*. 1999;52:104.
38. Koshima I, Kawada S, Etoh H et al. Flow-through anterior thigh flaps for one-stage reconstruction of soft-tissue defects and revascularization of ischemic extremities. *Plast Reconstr Surg*. 1995;95:252–260.
39. Koshima I, Urushibara K, Inagawa K et al. Free tensor fasciae latae perforator flap for the reconstruction of defects in the extremities. *Plast Reconstr Surg*. 2001;107:1759–1765.
40. Koshima I, Nanba Y, Tsutsui T et al. Perforator flaps in lower extremity reconstruction. *Handchir Mikrochir Plast Chir.* 2002;34:251–256.
41. Angrigiani C, Grilli D, Siebert J. Latissimus dorsi musculocutaneous flap without muscle. *Plast Reconstr Surg*. 1995;96:1608–1614.
42. Koshima I, Saisho H, Kawada S et al. Flow-through thin latissimus dorsi perforator flap for repair of soft-tissue defects in the legs. *Plast Reconstr Surg*. 1999;103:1483–1490.
43. Kim JT, Koo BS, Kim SK. The thin latissimus dorsi perforator-based free flap for resurfacing. *Plast Reconstr Surg*. 2001;107:374–382.
44. Hallock GG, Sano K. The medial sural MEDIAL GASTROCNEMIUS perforator free flap: An 'ideal' prone position skin flap. *Ann Plast Surg*. 2004;52:184–187.
45. Geddes CR, Tang M, Yang D et al. Anatomy of the integument of the lower extremity. In: Blondeel PN, Morris SF, Hallock GG et al., editors. *Perforator Flaps: Anatomy, Technique & Clinical Applications*. St. Louis, MO: Quality Medical Publishing, Inc.; 2006; pp. 541–578.
46. Saint-Cyr M, Schaverien M, Arbique G et al. Three- and four-dimensional computed tomographic angiography and venography for the investigation of the vascular anatomy and perfusion of perforator flaps. *Plast Reconstr Surg*. 2008;121:772–780.
47. Schaverien M, Saint-Cyr M. Perforators of the lower leg: Analysis of perforator locations and clinical application for pedicled perforator flaps. *Plast Reconstr Surg*. 2008;122:161–170.
48. Saint-Cyr M, Wong C, Schaverien M et al. The perforasome theory: Vascular anatomy and clinical implications. *Plast Reconstr Surg*. 2009;124:1529–1544.
49. Lecours C, Saint-Cyr M, Wong C et al. Freestyle pedicle perforator flaps: Clinical results and vascular anatomy. *Plast Reconstr Surg*. 2010;126:1589–1603.
50. Cinpolat A, Bektas G, Ozkan O, Rizvanovic Z, Seyhan T, Coskunfirat OK, Ozkan O. Metatarsal artery perforator-based propeller flap. *Microsurgery*. 2014 May;34(4):287–291.
51. Georgescu AV, Matei I, Ardelean F et al. Microsurgical nonmicrovascular flaps in forearm and hand reconstruction. *Microsurgery* 2007;27:384–394.
52. Parrett BM, Talbot SG, Pribaz JJ et al. A review of local and regional flaps for distal leg reconstruction. *J Reconstr Microsurg*. 2009;25:445–455.
53. El-Sabbagh AH. Skin perforator flaps: An algorithm for leg reconstruction. *J Reconstr Microsurg* 2011;27:511–523.
54. Lee BT, Lin SJ, Bar-Meir ED et al. Pedicled perforator flaps: A new principle in reconstructive surgery. *Plast Reconstr Surg*. 2010;125:201–208.
55. Hyakusoku H, Yamamoto T, Fumiiri M. The propeller flap method. *Br J Plast Surg*. 1991;44:53–54.
56. Hallock GG. The propeller flap version of the adductor muscle perforator flap for coverage of ischial or trochanteric pressure scores. *Ann Plast Surg*. 2006;56:540–542.
57. Pignatti M, Ogawa R, Hallock GG et al. The "Tokyo" consensus on propeller flaps. *Plast Reconstr Surg*. 2011;127:716–722.
58. Teo TC. Perforator local flaps in lower limb reconstruction. *Cir Plast Iberlatinamer.* 2006;32:15–16.
59. Lineaweaver W, Zhang F. Cross-leg flaps and reconstructive surgery in the 21st century. *Ann Plast Surg*. 2014 May;72(5):491–492.
60. Carriquiry C, Aparecida Costa M, Vasconez LO. An anatomic study of the septocutaneous vessels of the leg. *Plast Reconstr Surg*. 1985;76:354–363.
61. Yoshimura M, Shimada T, Hosokawa M. The vasculature of the peroneal tissue transfer. *Plast Reconstr Surg*. 1990;85: 917–921.
62. Hwang WY, Chen SZ, Han LY et al. Medial leg skin flap: Vascular anatomy and clinical applications. *Ann Plast Surg*. 1985;15:489–491.
63. Koshima I, Moriguchi T, Ohta S et al. The vasculature and clinical application of the posterior tibial perforator-based flap. *Plast Reconstr Surg*. 1992;90:643–649.
64. Wong CH, Cui F, Tan BK et al. Nonlinear finite element simulations to elucidate the determinants of perforator patency in propeller flaps. *Ann Plast Surg*. 2007;59:672–678.

65. Taylor GI, Doyle M, McCarten G. The Doppler probe for planning flaps: Anatomical study and clinical applications. *Br J Plast Surg*. 1990;43:1–16.
66. Morris SF, Taylor GI. Predicting the survival of experimental skin flaps with a knowledge of the vascular architecture. *Plast Reconstr Surg*. 1993;92:1352–1361.
67. Dhar SC, Taylor GI. The delay phenomenon: The story unfolds. *Plast Reconstr Surg*. 1999;104:2079–2091.
68. Bhattacharya V, Deshpande SB, Watts RK et al. Measurement of perfusion pressure of perforators and its correlation with their internal diameter. *Br J Plast Surg*. 2005;58:759–764.
69. Panse NS, Bhatt YC, Tandale MS. What is safe limit of the perforator flap in lower extremity reconstruction? Do we have answers yet? *Plast Surg Int*. 2011;2011:349–357.
70. Saint-Cyr M, Schaverien MV, Rohrich RJ. Perforator flaps: History, controversies, physiology, anatomy, and use in reconstruction. *Plast Reconstr Surg*. 2009;123:132e–145e.
71. Asko-Seljavaara S. Free style free flaps. *Seventh Congress of the International Society of Reconstructive Microsurgery*; 1983 June 19–30; New York.
72. Quaba AA, Davison PM. The distally-based dorsal hand flap. *Br J Plast Surg*. 1990;43:28–39.
73. Mardini S, Tsai FC, Wei FC. The thigh as a model for free style free flaps. *Clin Plast Surg*. 2003;30:473–480.
74. Wei FC, Mardini S. Free-style free flaps. *Plast Reconstr Surg*. 2004;114:910–916.
75. Wallace CG, Kao HK, Jeng SF et al. Free-style flaps: A further step forward for perforator flap surgery. *Plast Reconstr Surg*. 2009;124:e419–e426.
76. Yildirim S, Taylan G, Akoz T. Freestyle perforator-based V-Y advancement flap for reconstruction of soft tissue defects at various anatomic regions. *Ann Plast Surg*. 2007;58:501–506.
77. D'Arpa S, Cordova A, Pirrello R et al. Free style facial artery perforator flap for one stage reconstruction of the nasal ala. *J Plast Reconstr Aesthet Surg*. 2009;62:36–42.
78. D'Arpa S, Cordova A, Pignatti M et al. Freestyle pedicled perforator flaps: Safety, prevention of complications, and management based on 85 consecutive cases. *Plast Reconstr Surg*. 2011;128:892–906.
79. Georgescu AV, Capota I, Matei I et al. The place of local/regional perforator flaps in complex traumas of the forearm. *J Hand Microsurg India* 2009;1:25–31.
80. Matei I, Georgescu A, Chiroiu B et al. Harvesting of forearm perforator flaps based on intraoperative vascular exploration: Clinical experiences and literature review. *Microsurgery* 2008;28:321–330.
81. Lee GK. Invited discussion: Harvesting of forearm perforator flaps based on intraoperative vascular exploration: Clinical experiences and literature review. *Microsurgery* 2008;28: 331–332.
82. Tang M, Mao Y, Almutairi K et al. Three-dimensional analysis of perforators of the posterior leg. *Plast Reconstr Surg*. 2009;123:1729–1738.
83. Zhang X, Wang X, Wen S et al. Posterior tibial artery-based multilobar combined flap free transfer for repair of complex soft tissue defects. *Microsurgery* 2008;28:643–649.
84. Wu WC, Chang YP, So YC et al. The anatomic basis and clinical applications of flaps based on the posterior tibial vessels. *Br J Plast Surg*. 1993;46:470–479.
85. Saba L, Atzeni M, Rozen WM, Alonso-Burgos A, Bura R, Piga M, Ribuffo D. Non-invasive vascular imaging in perforator flap surgery. *Acta Radiol*. 2013 February 1;54(1):89–98.
86. Wax MK. The role of the implantable Doppler probe in free flap surgery. *Laryngoscope*. 2014 Mar;124 Suppl 1:S1-12. doi: 10.1002/lary.24569.
87. Anderl H. Free vascularized groin fat flap in hypoplasia and hemiatrophy of the face (a three years observation). *J Maxillofac Surg*. 1979 Nov;7(4):327–332.
88. Sheena Y, Jennison T, Hardwicke JT, Titley OG. Detection of perforators using thermal imaging. *Plast Reconstr Surg*. 2013 Dec;132(6):1603–1610.
89. Giunta RE, Geisweid A, Feller AM. The value of preoperative Doppler sonography for planning free perforator flaps. *Plast Reconstr Surg*. 2000;105:2381–2386.
90. Shaw RJ, Batstone MD, Blackburn TK et al. Preoperative Doppler assessment of perforator anatomy in the anterolateral thigh flap. *Br J Oral Maxillofac Surg*. 2010;48:419–422.
91. Cheng MH, Chen HC, Santamaria E et al. Preoperative ultrasound Doppler study and clinical correlation of free posterior interosseous flap. *Changgeng Yi Xue Za Zhi*. 1997;20:258–264.
92. Yu P, Youssef A. Efficacy of the handheld Doppler in preoperative identification of the cutaneous perforators in the anterolateral thigh flap. *Plast Reconstr Surg*. 2006;118:928–933.
93. Khan UD, Miller JG. Reliability of handheld Doppler in planning local perforator-based flaps for extremities. *Aesthet Plast Surg*. 2007;31:521–525.
94. Rozen WM, Phillips TJ, Ashton MW et al. Preoperative imaging for DIEA perforator flaps: A comparative study of computed tomographic angiography and Doppler ultrasound. *Plast Reconstr Surg*. 2008;121:9–16.
95. Demirtas Y, Ozturk N, Kelahmetoglu O et al. Pedicled perforator flaps. *Ann Plast Surg*. 2009;63:179–183.

96. Cheng HT, Lin FY, Chang SC. Diagnostic efficacy of color Doppler ultrasonography in preoperative assessment of anterolateral thigh flap cutaneous perforators: an evidence-based review. *Plast Reconstr Surg*. 2013 Mar;131(3):471–473.
97. Bravo FG, Schwarze HP. Free-style local perforator flaps: Concept and classification system. *J Plast Reconstr Aesthet Surg*. 2009;62:602–608.
98. Vico PG, Cartilier LH. A new approach to the study of skin vascularization. *Plast Reconstr Surg*. 1993 Sep;92(3):463–468.
99. Tsukino A, Kurachi K, Inamiya T et al. Preoperative color Doppler assessment in planning of anterolateral thigh flaps. *Plast Reconstr Surg*. 2004;113:241–246.
100. Scott JR, Liu D, Said H et al. Computed tomographic angiography in planning abdomen-based microsurgical breast reconstruction: A comparison with color duplex ultrasound. *Plast Reconstr Surg*. 2010;125:446–453.
101. Dublin BA, Karp NS, Kasabian AK et al. Selective use of preoperative lower extremity arteriography in free flap reconstruction. *Ann Plast Surg*. 1997;38:404–407.
102. Lutz BS, Ng SH, Cabailo R et al. Value of routine angiography before traumatic lower-limb reconstruction with microvascular free tissue transplantation. *J Trauma*. 1998;44:682–686.
103. Lutz BS, Wei FC, Machens HG et al. Indications and limitations of angiography before free-flap transplantation to the distal lower leg after trauma: Prospective study in 36 patients. *J Reconstr Microsurg*. 2000;16:187–191.
104. Saba L, Atzeni M, Ribuffo D, Mallarini G, Suri JS. Analysis of deep inferior epigastric perforator (DIEP) arteries by using MDCTA: Comparison between 2 post-processing techniques. *Eur J Radiol*. 2012 August;81(8):1828–1833.
105. Klein MB, Karanas YL, Chow LC et al. Early experience with computed tomographic angiography in microsurgical reconstruction. *Plast Reconstr Surg*. 2003;112:498–503.
106. Bogdan MA, Klein MB, Rubin GD et al. CT angiography in complex upper extremity reconstruction. *J Hand Surg Br*. 2004;29:465–469.
107. Rozen WM, Ribuffo D, Atzeni M, Stella DL, Saba L, Guerra M, Grinsell D, Ashton MW. Current state of the art in perforator flap imaging with computed tomographic angiography. *Surg Radiol Anat*. 2009 October;31(8):631–639.
108. Ribuffo D, Atzeni M, Saba L, Guerra M, Mallarini G, Proto EB, Grinsell D, Ashton MW, Rozen WM. Clinical study of peroneal artery perforators with computed tomographic angiography: Implications for fibular flap harvest. *Surg Radiol Anat*. 2010 April;32(4):329–334.
109. Ribuffo D, Atzeni M, Saba L, Milia A, Guerra M, Mallarini G. Angio computed tomography preoperative evaluation for anterolateral thigh flap harvesting. *Ann Plast Surg*. 2009 April;62(4):368–371.
110. Phillips TJ, Stella DL, Rozen WM et al. Abdominal wall CT angiography: A detailed account of a newly established preoperative imaging technique. *Radiology* 2008;249:32–44.
111. Rad AN, Flores JI, Prucz RB et al. Clinical experience with the lateral septocutaneous superior gluteal artery perforator flap for autologous breast reconstruction. *Microsurgery* 2010;30:339–347.
112. Fukaya E, Kuwatsuru R, Iimura H et al. Imaging of the superficial inferior epigastric vascular anatomy and preoperative planning for the SIEA flap using MDCTA. *J Plast Reconstr Aesthet Surg*. 2010;64:63–68.
113. Rozen WM, Hong MK, Ashton MW et al. Imaging the posterior interosseous artery with computed tomographic angiography: Report of a rare anomaly and implications for hand reconstruction. *Ann Plast Surg*. 2010;65:300–301.
114. Wong C, Saint-Cyr M, Rasko Y et al. Three- and four-dimensional arterial and venous perforasomes of the internal mammary artery perforator flap. *Plast Reconstr Surg*. 2009;124:1759–1769.
115. Schaverien M, Wong C, Bailey S et al. Thoracodorsal artery perforator flap and Latissimus dorsi myocutaneous flap – Anatomical study of the constant skin paddle perforator locations. *J Plast Reconstr Aesthet Surg*. 2010;63:2123–2127.
116. Ting JW, Rozen WM, Grinsell D et al. The in vivo anatomy of the deep circumflex iliac artery perforators: Defining the role for the DCIA perforator flap. *Microsurgery* 2009;29:326–329.
117. Masia J, Kosutic D, Cervelli D et al. In search of the ideal method in perforator mapping: Noncontrast magnetic resonance imaging. *J Reconstr Microsurg*. 2010;26:29–35.
118. Haider CR, Glockner JF, Stanson AW et al. Peripheral vasculature: High temporal-and high-spatial-resolution three-dimensional contrast-enhanced MR angiography. *Radiology* 2009;253:831–843.
119. Mast BA. Comparison of magnetic resonance angiography and digital subtraction angiography for visualization of lower extremity arteries. *Ann Plast Surg*. 2001;46:261–264.
120. Lohan DG, Tomasian A, Krishnam M et al. MR angiography of lower extremities at 3 T: Presurgical planning of fibular free flap transfer for facial reconstruction. *Am J Roentgenol*. 2008;190:770–776.

121. Fukaya E, Grossman RF, Saloner D et al. Magnetic resonance angiography for free fibula flap transfer. *J Reconstr Microsurg*. 2007;23:205–211.
122. Newman TM, Vasile J, Levine JL et al. Perforator flap magnetic resonance angiography for reconstructive breast surgery: A review of 25 deep inferior epigastric and gluteal perforator artery flap patients. *J Magn Reson Imaging*. 2010;31:1176–1184.
123. Blomstedt P, Olivecrona M, Sailer A et al. Dittmar and the history of stereotaxy; or rats, rabbits, and references. *Neurosurgery* 2007;60:198–201.
124. Rozen WM, AshtonMW, Stella DL et al. Stereotactic image-guided navigation in the preoperative imaging of perforators for DIEP flap breast reconstruction. *Microsurgery* 2008;28:417–423.
125. Rozen WM, Buckland A, Ashton MW et al. Image-guided, stereotactic perforator flap surgery: A prospective comparison of current techniques and review of the literature. *Surg Radiol Anat*. 2009;31:401–408.
126. Daniel RK, Taylor GI. Distant transfer of an island flap by microvascular anastomoses. *Plast Reconstr Surg*. 1973;52:111.
127. Koshima I, Nanba Y, Tsutsui T, Takahashi Y, Urushibara K, Inagawa K, Hamasaki T, Moriguchi T. Superficial circumflex iliac artery perforator flap for reconstruction of limb defects. *Plast Reconstr Surg*. 2004 January;113(1):233–240.
128. McCraw JB, Massey FM, Shanklin KD et al. Vaginal reconstruction with gracilis myocutaneous flaps. *Plast Reconstr Surg*. 1976;58:176–183.
129. Hallock GG. The gracilis (medial circumflex femoral) perforator flap: A medial groin free flap? *Ann Plast Surg*. 2003 December;51(6):623–626.
130. Hallock GG. The conjoint medial circumflex femoral perforator and gracilis muscle free flap. *Plast Reconstr Surg*. 2004 January;113(1):339–346.
131. Holle J, Worseg A, Kuzbari R, Wuringer E, Alt A. The extended gracilis muscle flap for reconstruction of the lower leg. *Br J Plast Surg*. 1995;48:353–359.
132. Morris SF, Yang D. Gracilis muscle: Arterial and neural basis for subdivision. *Annal Plast Surg*. 1999;42:630–633.
133. Persichetti P, Simone P, Berloco M et al. Vulvo-perineal reconstruction: Medial thigh septo-fasciocutaneous island flap. *Annals Plast Surg*. 2003;50:85–89.
134. Giordano PA, Abbes M, Pequignot JP. Gracilis blood supply: Anatomical and clinical re-evaluation. *Br J Plast Surg*. 1990;43:266–272.
135. Manktelow RT, Zuker RM. Muscle transplantation by fascicular territory. *Plast Reconstr Surg*. 1984;73:751–755.
136. Wellisz T, Rechnic M, Dougherty W et al. Coverage of bilateral lower extremity calcaneal fractures with osteomyelitis using a single split free gracilis muscle transfer. *Plast Reconstr Surg*. 1990;85:457–460.
137. Hallock GG. Simplified nomenclature for compound flaps. *Plast Reconstr Surg*. 2000;105:1465–1470.
138. Watterson PA, Taylor GI, Crock JG. The venous territories of muscles: Anatomical study and clinical implications. *Br J Plast Surg*. 1988;41:569–585.
139. Wang TS, Whetzel T, Mathes SJ et al. A fasciocutaneous flap for vaginal and perineal reconstruction. *Plast Reconstr Surg*. 1987;80:95–102.
140. Hallock GG. Minimally invasive harvest of the gracilis muscle. *Plast Reconstr Surg*. 1999;104:801–805.
141. Hattori Y, Doi K, Abe Y et al. Surgical approach to the vascular pedicle of the gracilis muscle flap. *J Hand Surg*. 2002;27:534–536.
142. Yajima H, Ishida H, Tamai S. Proximal lateral leg flap transfer utilizing major nutrient vessels to the soleus muscle. *Plast Reconstr Surg*. 1994;93:1442.
143. Kawamura K, Yajima H, Kobata Y, Shigematsu K, Takakura Y. *Plast Reconstr Surg*. 2005 January;115(1):114–119. Clinical applications of free soleus and peroneal perforator flaps.
144. Feldman JJ, Cohen BE, May Jr JW. The medial gastrocnemius myocutaneous flap. *Plast Reconstr Surg*. 1978;61:531–539.
145. Dibbell DB, Edstrom LL. The gastrocnemius myocutaneous flap. *Clin Plast Surg*. 1980;7:45–50.
146. Taylor GI, Daniel RK. The anatomy of several free-flap donor sites. *Plast Reconstr Surg* 1975;56:243–253.
147. Montegut WJ, Allen RJ. Sural artery perforator flap as an alternative for the gastrocnemius myocutaneous flap. In *Proceedings of the 90th Annual Scientific Assembly of the Southern Medical Association*, Baltimore, MD, November 1996.
148. Cavadas PC, Sanz-Gimenez-Rico JR, Gutierrez-de la Camara A et al. The medial sural artery perforator free-flap. *Plast Reconstr Surg*. 2001;108:1609–1615.
149. Hallock GG. Anatomic basis of the gastrocnemius perforator based flap. *Ann Plast Surg*. 2001;47:517–522.
150. Hallock GG. Medial sural artery perforator free flap: legitimate use as a solution for the ipsilateral distal lower extremity defect. *J Reconstr Microsurg*. 2014 Mar;30(3):187–192.

151. Hallock GG. Invited discussion. A modified technique for harvesting the reverse sural artery flap from the upper part of the leg: Inclusion of a gastrocnemius muscle "cuff" around the sural pedicle. *Ann Plast Surg*. 2001;47:274–278.
152. Hallock GG. The medial sural (MEDIAL GASTROCNEMIUS) perforator local flap. *Ann Plast Surg*. 2004 November;53(5):501–505.
153. Jakubietz RG, Jakubietz MG, Grünert JG, Zahn RK, Meffert RH, Schmidt K. Propeller flaps: the reliability of preoperative, unidirectional Doppler sonography. *Handchir Mikrochir Plast Chir*. 2011 Apr;43(2):76–80.
154. Blondeel PN, Beyens G, Verghaege R et al. Doppler flowmetry in the planning of perforator flaps. *Br J Plast Surg*. 1998;51:202.
155. Kosutic D, Pejkovic B, Anderhuber F, Vadnjal-Donlagic S, Zic R, Gulic R, Krajnc I, Solman L, Kocbek L. Complete mapping of lateral and medial sural artery perforators: Anatomical study with Duplex-Doppler ultrasound correlation. *J Plast Reconstr Aesthet Surg*. 2012 November;65(11):1530–1536.
156. Gray H. *The Anterior Tibial Artery. Anatomy of the Human Body*, 20th edn. Philadelphia, PA: Lea and Febiger; 1918. Available at www.bartleby.com/107/. Accessed January 19, 2009.
157. Attinger CE, Evans KK, Bulan E et al. Angiosomes of the foot and ankle and clinical implications for limb salvage: Reconstruction, incisions, and revascularization. *Plast Reconstr Surg*. 2006;117(Suppl 7):261S–293S.
158. Panagiotopoulos K, Soucacos PN, Korres DS, Petrocheilou G, Kalogeropoulos A, Panagiotopoulos E, Zoubos AB. Anatomical study and colour Doppler assessment of the skin perforators of the anterior tibial artery and possible clinical applications. *J Plast Reconstr Aesthet Surg*. 2009 November;62(11):1524–1529.
159. Haertsch PA. The blood supply of the skin of the leg: A post mortem investigation. *Br J Plast Surg*. 1981;34:470.
160. Dong JS, Peng YP, Zhang YX et al. Reverse anterior tibial artery flap for reconstruction of foot donor site. *Plast Reconstr Surg*. 2003;112:1604.
161. Recalde Roccha JF, Gilbert A, Masquelet A et al. The anterior tibial artery flap: Anatomic study and clinical application. *Plast Reconstr Surg*. 1987;79:396.
162. Satoh K, Yoshikawa A, Hayashi M. Reverse-flow anterior tibial flap type III. *Br J Plast Surg*. 1988;41:624.
163. Morrison WA, Shen TY. Anterior tibial artery flap: Anatomy and case report. *Br J Plast Surg*. 1987;40:230.
164. Stadler F, Brenner E, Todorrof B et al. Anatomical study of the perforating vessels of the lower leg. *Anat Rec*. 1999;255:374.
165. Wee JTK. Reconstruction of the lower leg and foot with the reverse pedicled anterior tibial flap: Preliminary report of a new fasciocutaneous flap. *Br J Plast Surg*. 1986;39:327.
166. Whetzel TP, Barnard MA, Stokesl RB. Arterial fasciocutaneous vascular territories of the lower leg. *Plast Reconstr Surg*. 1997;100:1172.
167. Hallock GG. Evaluation of fasciocutaneous perforators using colour duplex imaging. *Plast Reconstr Surg*. 1994;94:644.
168. Lee JT, Chen PR, Hsu H, Wu MS, Cheng LF, Huang CC, Chien SH. The proximal lateral lower leg perforator flap revisited: Anatomical study and clinical applications. *Microsurgery* 2014 Apr 23. doi: 10.1002/micr.22264.
169. Eburdery H, Chaput B, Andre A, Grolleau JL, Chavoin JP, Lauwers F. Can we consider standard microsurgical anastomosis on the posterior tibial perforator network? An anatomical study. *Surg Radiol Anat*. 2014 Jan 31.
170. Georgescu AV, Matei IR, Capota IM. The use of propeller perforator flaps for diabetic limb salvage: a retrospective review of 25 cases. *Diabet Foot Ankle* 2012;3.
171. Heymans O, Verhelle N, Peters S. The medial adiposofascial flap of the leg: Anatomical basis and clinical applications. *Plast Reconstr Surg*. 2005;115:793–801.
172. Ozdemir R, Kocer U, Sahin B, Oruc M, Kilinc H, Takdemir I. Examination of the skin perforators of the posterior tibial artery on the leg and the ankle region and their clinical use. *Plast Reconstr Surg*. 2006;117:1619–1630.
173. Herlin C, Lievain L, Qassemyar Q, Michel G, Assaf N, Sinna R. Freestyle free perforator flaps for heel reconstruction. *Ann Chir Plast Esthet*. 2013 Aug;58(4):283–289.
174. Shalaby HA. The blood supply of the posterior tibial perforator-based flap. *Plast Reconstr Surg*. 1994;93:440.
175. Dong KX, Xu YQ, Fan XY, Xu LJ, Su XX, Long H, Xu LQ, He XQ. Perforator pedicled propeller flaps for soft tissue coverage of lower leg and foot defects. *Orthop Surg*. 2014 Feb;6(1):42–46.
176. John JR, Sharma RK. Local perforator island flaps in post-traumatic reconstruction of middle third of the leg. *Strategies Trauma Limb Reconstr*. 2014 Apr;9(1):59–61.
177. Satoh K, Sakai M, Hiromatsu N, Ohsumi N. Heel and foot reconstruction using reverse-flow posterior tibial flap. *Ann Plast Surg*. 1990;24:318–327.

178. Boucher F, Ho Quoc C, Pinatel B, Thiney PO, Mojallal A. Transtibial amputation salvage with a cutaneous flap based on posterior tibial perforators. *Ann Chir Plast Esthet.* 2013 Aug;58(4):342–346.
179. Schaverien MV, Hamilton SA, Fairburn N, Rao P, Quaba AA. Lower limb reconstruction using the islanded posterior tibial artery perforator flap. *Plast Reconstr Surg.* 2010 June;125(6):1735–1743.
180. Wolff K-D. Peroneal artery perforator flap. In: Blondeel PN, Morris SF, Hallock GG, Neligan PC, editors. *Perforator Flaps: Anatomy, Technique, & Clinical Applications*, Vol. 2. St. Louis: QMP Publishing; 2006. pp. 707–717.
181. Karki D, Narayan RP. The versatility of perforator-based propeller flap for reconstruction of distal leg and ankle defects. *Plast Surg Int.* 2012;2012:303247.
182. Attinger C, Cooper P, Blume P, Bulan E. The safest surgical incisions and amputations applying the angiosome principles and using the Doppler to assess the arterial-arterial connections of the foot and ankle. *Foot Ankle Clin.* 2001;6:745–799.
183. Purushothaman R, Balakrishnan TM, Alalasundaram KV. Anatomical study of terminal peroneal artery perforators and their clinical applications. *Indian J Plast Surg.* 2013 Jan;46(1):69–74.
184. Hallock GG, Wei F-C, Mardini S, Kimura N. Reconstruction of the lower extremity. In: Blondeel PN, Morris SF, Hallock GG, Neligan PC, editors. *Perforator Flaps: Anatomy, Technique, & Clinical Applications*, Vol. 2. St. Louis, MO: QMP Publishing; 2006. pp. 915–933.
185. Hallock GG. Color duplex imaging for identifying perforators prior to pretransfer expansion of fasciocutaneous free flaps. *Ann Plast Surg.* 1994 Jun;32(6):595–601.
186. Klein S, Van Lienden KP, Van't Veer M, Smit JM, Werker PM. Evaluation of the lower limb vasculature before free fibula flap transfer. A prospective blinded comparison between magnetic resonance angiography and digital subtraction angiography. *Microsurgery* 2013 Aug 27.
187. Masia J, Clavero JA, Larranaga JR, Alomar X, Pons G, Serret P. Multidetector-row computed tomography in the planning of abdominal perforator flaps. *J Plast Reconstr Aesthet Surg.* 2006;59: 594–599.
188. Rosson GD, Williams CG, Fishman EK, Singh NK. 3D CT angiography of abdominal wall vascular perforators to plan DIEAP flaps. *Microsurgery* 2008;28(8):663–670.
189. Rad AN, Singh NK, Rosson GD. Peroneal artery perforator-based propeller flap reconstruction of the lateral distal lower extremity after tumor extirpation: Case report and literature review. *Microsurgery* 2007;27:641–646.
190. Amarante J, Costa H, Reis J, Soares R. A new distally based fasciocutaneous flap of the leg. *Br J Plast Surg.* 1986;39:338–340.
191. Cavadas PC. Reversed saphenous neurocutaneous island flap: Clinical experience. *Plast Reconstr Surg.* 1997;99:1940–1946.
192. Cavadas PC. Reversed saphenous neurocutaneous island flap: Clinical experience and evolution to the posterior tibial perforator-saphenous subcutaneous flap. *Plast Reconstr Surg.* 2003;111:837–839.
193. Mir y Mir L. Functional graft of the heel. *Br J Plast Surg.* 1954;14:444–450.
194. Shanahan RS, McCarthy JG. Medial plantar sensory flap for coverage of heel defects. 1979;64:295–298.
195. Reiffel RS. Coverage of heel and sole defects: A new subfascial arterialized flap. 1980;66:250–260.
196. Harrison DH, Morgan BDG. The instep island flap to resurface plantar defects. 1981;34:315–318.
197. Morrison WA, Grabb DM, O'Brien BM et al. The instep of the foot as a fasciocutaneous island and as a free flap for heel defects. *Plast Reconstr Surg.* 1983;72:56–64.
198. Inoue T, Kobayash M, Harashina T. Finger pulp reconstruction with a free sensory medial plantar flap. *Br J Plast Surg.* 1988;41:657–659.
199. Lee HB, Tark KC, Rah DK et al. Pulp reconstruction of fingers with very small sensate medial plantar free flap. *Plast Reconstr Surg.* 1998;101:999–1005.
200. Masquelet AC, Romana MC. The medialis pedis flap: A new fasciocutaneous flap. *Plast Reconstr Surg.* 1990;85:765–772.
201. Ishikura N, Heshiki T, Tsukada S. The use of a free medialis pedis flap for resurfacing skin defects of the hand and digits: Results in five cases. *Plast Reconstr Surg.* 1995;95:100–107.
202. Koshima I, Urushibara K, Inagawa K et al. Free medial plantar perforator flaps for the resurfacing of finger and foot defects. *Plast Reconstr Surg.* 2001;107:1753–1758.
203. Koshima I, Nanba Y, Tsutsui T et al. Medial plantar perforator flaps with supermicrosurgery. *Clin Plast Surg.* 2003;30:447–455.
204. Koshima I, Narushima M, Mihara M, Nakai I, Akazawa S, Fukuda N, Watanabe Y, Nakagawa M. Island medial plantar artery perforator flap for reconstruction of plantar defects. *Ann Plast Surg.* 2007 November;59(5):558–562.
205. Amarante J, Martins A, Reis J. A distally based median plantar flap. *Ann Plast Surg.* 1988;20:468–470.
206. Butler CE, Chevray P. Retrograde-flow medial plantar island flap reconstruction of distal forefoot, toe, and webspace defects. *Ann Plast Surg.* 2002;49: 196–201.

207. Oberlin C, Vasconcellos ZA, Touam C. Medial plantar flap based distally on the lateral plantar artery to cover a forefoot skin defect. *Plast Reconstr Surg*. 2000;106:874–877.
208. Bhandari MS, Sobti C. Reverse flow instep island flap. *Plast Reconstr Surg*. 1999;103:1986.
209. Martin D, Legaillard P, Bakhach J, Hu W, Baudet J. L'allongement pediculaire en VY a flux retrograde: Un moyen pour doubler l'arc de rotation d'un lambeau sous certaines conditions. *Ann Chir Plast Esthet.* 1994;39:403.
210. Martin D, Gorowitz B, Peres JM, Baudet J. Le lambeau plantaire interne sur pedicule plantaire externe: Un moyen de couverture utilisable sur toute la surface du pied. *Ann Chir Plast Esthet.* 1991;36:544.
211. Oberlin C, Bastian D, Greant P. *Les Lambeaux Pedicules de Couverture des Membres*. Paris, France: Expansion Scientifique Francaise; 1994. pp. 117–121.
212. Rudig LL, Gercek E, Hessmann MH, Müller LP. The distally based sural neurocutaneous island flap for coverage of soft-tissue defects on the distal lower leg, ankle and heel. *Oper Orthop Traumatol*. 2008 Sep;20(3):252–261.
213. Wei JW, Ni JD, Dong ZG, Liu LH, Luo ZB, Zheng L. Distally Based Perforator-Plus Sural Fasciocutaneous Flap for Soft-Tissue Reconstruction of the Distal Lower Leg, Ankle, and Foot: Comparison between Pediatric and Adult Patients. *J Reconstr Microsurg*. 2014 May;30(4):249–254.
214. Zhu YL, Wang Y, He XQ, Zhu M, Li FB, Xu YQ. Foot and ankle reconstruction: An experience on the use of 14 different flaps in 226 cases. *Microsurgery* 2013 Sep 3. doi:10.1002/micr.22177.
215. Gu JH, Jeong SH. Radical resection of a venous malformation in middle finger and immediate reconstruction using medial plantar artery perforator flap: a case report. *Microsurgery*. 2012 Feb;32(2):148–152.
216. Koshima I, Urushibara K, Inagawa K, Hamasaki T, Moriguchi T. Free medial plantar perforator flaps for the resurfacing of finger and foot defects. *Plast Reconstr Surg*. 2001;107:1753–1758.
217. Cigna E, Fioramonti P, Fino P, Scuderi N. Island lateral plantar artery perforator flap for reconstruction of weight-bearing plantar areas. *Foot Ankle Surg*. 2011 March;17(1):e13–e16.

38 Lymphoscintigraphy for Extremities' Oedemas and for Sentinel Lymph Node Mapping in Cutaneous Melanomas of the Torso

Giuliano Mariani, Paola A. Erba, Gianpiero Manca, Luisa Locantore, Federica Orsini, Sara Mazzarri, Valerio Duce, Manuel Tredici, and Elisa Tardelli

CONTENTS

38.1 BACKGROUND

The earliest applications of lymphoscintigraphy date back to over 60 years ago, with an initial report on accumulation in regional draining lymph nodes of radioactive colloidal gold injected interstitially (Walker 1950), then with successful imaging of lymph flow and of regional draining lymph nodes (Sherman and Ter-Pogossian 1953). These seminal works opened new avenues to the investigation of the lymphatic system for diagnostic purposes, including both characterisation of peripheral oedemas (to distinguish lymph flow obstruction from venous obstruction as the cause of oedema) and lymph node mapping in patients with various malignancies. In the latter regard, the underlying rationale was quite different from the current application of sentinel lymph node (SLN) mapping, although based on the same event, that is, physiologic phagocytosis of radiocolloids by the macrophages that line the sinusal spaces of lymph nodes. In particular, the idea of imaging lymph nodes with radionuclides was initially considered simply as the nuclear medicine counterpart mimicking the more invasive x-ray lymphography (based on cannulation of lymphatic vessels and injection of an iodinated contrast medium), which at that time constituted the accepted modality of screening patients for lymph node metastases, especially in areas of the body with complex anatomy such as the pelvis, the head and neck, and the torso (Hultborn et al. 1955; Voutilainen and Wiljasalo 1965; Rossi and Ferri 1966; Santi and Zecchin 1968).

The common concept shared by x-ray lymphography and by lymphoscintigraphy was that lymph nodes invaded by metastasis would lose (at least in part) their physiologic function of accumulating either the contrast medium or the radiocolloid, respectively, and would therefore not be visualised (or poorly visualised) where they were expected to be present. This concept, initially conceived with the only radiocolloid that was available until the mid-1960s, colloidal ^{198}Au, expanded then at a tremendous pace in the 1970s and 1980s after the more favourable radiocolloids labelled with ^{99m}Tc (Stern et al. 1966; Hawkins and McAlister 1969; Kort 1969; Scheffel et al. 1972; Schneider et al. 1973) were introduced into clinical practice.

It is interesting to note that one of the most frequent clinical applications of lymph node mapping with the rationale outlined earlier (i.e. search for possible sites of lymph node metastasis pinpointed by absent/poor lymph node visualisation at lymphoscintigraphy) was in patients with breast cancer (perhaps the most frequent current application of lymphatic mapping for radioguided sentinel node biopsy) and more specifically exploration of the internal mammary chain (Rossi et al. 1966; Schenk et al. 1966; Matsuo 1974; Ege 1976; Turoglu et al. 1992). This is still today a major matter of ongoing debate when performing lymphoscintigraphy for sentinel node mapping and radioguided sentinel node biopsy in patients with breast cancer, with particular regard to the optimal route of interstitial radiocolloid injection, that is, superficial versus deep injection (Manca et al. 2013; *see also Chapter 39 of this book*). Clearly, the whole concept of lymphatic mapping has changed in 1992–1993 (Morton et al. 1992; Krag et al. 1993), when radioguidance for sentinel node biopsy based on radiocolloid uptake linked to the same physiologic function of lymph nodes as in the earlier investigations was originally described for patients with cutaneous melanoma or breast cancer, respectively. In the case of sentinel node biopsy, however, failed visualisation of lymph nodes due to massive substitution of the normal lymph node components with metastatic tumour cells (i.e. the abnormal scintigraphic finding leading to identify possible lymph node metastasis based on the earlier rationale) is an important cause of failure (therefore of false-negative findings) of the entire radioguided sentinel node procedure.

In parallel with the applications of lymphoscintigraphy for lymphatic mapping in patients with cancer, clinical applications of this imaging modality have also grown for identifying the cause of oedema of the extremities or of intracavitary effusions of lymph-like fluid, as in the peritoneal cavity, pleural space, and others (Pecking et al. 1980; Petronis et al. 1985; see most recent review by Erba et al. 2013). This particular application, specifically the use of lymphoscintigraphy for identifying the cause of oedema of the extremities, constitutes the first section of this chapter, while the second section concerns sentinel node mapping in patients with cutaneous melanoma located in the torso.

38.2 LYMPHOSCINTIGRAPHIC IMAGING OF THE EXTREMITIES

38.2.1 Lymphatic System

Lymphatic circulation is a one-way transport system operating in conjunction with the circulatory system. It should therefore be considered as part of the peripheral cardiovascular system, interlinking closely with blood circulation at its origins (the interstitial space) and at its drainage point (the thoracic duct). Lymph, the lymphatic vessels, and lymph nodes are part of the system; lymph nodes constitute stations along the drainage route where fluid and cellular exchange between blood and lymph occurs. Lymphocytes represent the cellular connection point between the peripheral lymphatic system, blood circulation, and the reticuloendothelial system (distributed in the bone marrow, spleen, and liver).

The primary function of the lymphatic system is to transport excess interstitial fluid, as well as excessive proteins and waste (including cell debris), from the interstitial space back to the blood circulation, via the thoracic duct. Moreover, the lymphatic system is an integral part of the immune system and plays an important role in the dissemination of cancer through the lymphatic route.

Colloids, several kinds of cells (extravasated red cells, macrophages, lymphocytes, tumour cells, etc.), bacteria, and other microorganisms are channelled through the lymphatics, presumably as a protective mechanism to prevent noxious agent from directly entering the bloodstream (this is the reason why cellulitis and erysipelas can be a recurrent problem in patients with lymphoedema). Similarly, inorganic particulate matters such as carbon and silica are removed by lymphatics.

Formation of lymph starts as the interstitial fluid enters the small, blind-ended lymphatic capillaries that are highly permeable to interstitial fluid and macromolecules because they are composed of a single layer of endothelial cells, without a continuous basement membrane and pericytes (contractile cells that surround the outer surface of blood capillaries).

Lymph is pumped against a pressure gradient towards the jugular vein by the rhythmic contractions of lymphangions and by external motion of skeletal muscles, arteries, and veins (a process called *lymph propulsion*). Additional factors that regulate lymph propulsion include streamwise pressure gradients, transmural pressure, nerves, and hormones.

Adequate lymphatic circulation requires three interconnected steps:

1. Transport of prelymph across the interstitial space into the initial lymphatics
2. Movement of lymph through the network of non-contractile initial lymphatics
3. Active pumping of lymph through a series of contractile collecting trunks, a process facilitated by the presence of unidirectional valves in lymphatic vessels

38.2.2 Pathophysiology of Lymph Drainage Failure

Lymphoedema is caused by a functional overload in which the lymph volume exceeds the transport capabilities of the lymphatic system. The ensuing accumulation of interstitial macromolecules leads to increased oncotic pressure in the tissues, thus producing more oedema. Persistent swelling and the build-up of stagnant protein eventually lead to fibrosis and provide an excellent medium for repeated bouts of cellulitis and lymphangitis. As the lymphatic vessels dilate, their valves become incompetent, thus causing further stasis (although this pattern is not obvious for lymphatic vessels draining skeletal muscles, below the deep fascia).

Failure of lymph drainage can be caused by various factors: reduced lymph-conducting pathways (aplasia–hypoplasia of whole vessel, acquired obliteration of lymphatic lumen), pump contractility failure, lymph pathway obstruction (scar post-lymphadenectomy, radiation, or infection), and incompetent lymphatic system (reflux, megalymphatics, lymphatic hyperplasia).

Primary lymphoedema is caused by intrinsic abnormalities of the lymph-conducting pathways, and it can be either sporadic (the most frequent form) or familial/genetic. The most common cause is distal hypoplasia of the leg lymphatics. The paradigms of familial forms are Milroy's disease and Meige's syndrome. The genetic forms can be associated with Turner's and Noonan's syndromes or with the congenital vascular syndrome Klippel–Trenaunay. The currently ascertained mutations of genes involved in lymphatic development associated with primary lymphoedema involve genes GJC2, FOXC2, CCBE1, VEGFR3, PTPN14, GATA2, and SOX18 (Kari 2011; Sutkowska et al. 2012).

Some primary forms present relatively late in life (*lymphoedema tarda*), thus suggesting that the real cause of oedema is a failure of growth or regeneration following damage, not an abnormal development of lymphatic vessels since birth.

Secondary lymphoedema is more common than primary lymphoedema. It is caused by a wide variety of damage to lymphatic vessels originating outside the lymphatic systems, such as chronic venous insufficiency and post-thrombotic syndrome, surgical or radiation therapy, trauma, and parasitic infections.

The incidence of upper-limb and trunk lymphoedema after axillary lymph node dissection for breast cancer and/or radiation therapy ranges from 6% to 70% (Pavlista and Eliska 2012) although it can be a common under-reported morbidity. In these patients, lymphoedema is generally localised at the arm on the side of breast surgery, and patients with a high peripheral blood vascular filtration rate seem to be predisposed to this complication (Stanton et al. 2009; McLaughlin 2012). The relationship between the number of lymph nodes removed and the risk of lymphoedema is not clearly established, but clinical trials are focusing on the reduction of the rate of axillary dissection even in the presence of positive SLN biopsy (Wjcinski et al. 2012). Cutaneous melanoma, sarcoma, and pelvic tumours (including cervical, endometrial, and prostate cancers) are the most common cancers in which treatment (surgery and/or radiation therapy) can cause lower-limb lymphoedema; moreover, pelvic cancers and infiltrating sarcomas can present with lymphoedema as the first clinical manifestation.

Because of the relatively great plasticity of the lymphatic system, any injury has to be extensive in order to induce lymphoedema. Secondary lymphoedema due to cancer treatment is probably due to the failure of lymphatic vessels to regenerate and reanastomose satisfactorily through scarred or irradiated tissue.

Parasitic lymphoedema is the most common cause of secondary lymphoedema worldwide (Campisi 1999); it is caused by the microfilariae of *Wuchereria bancrofti* and *Brugia malayi*, which can be transmitted to humans by different mosquito species. Elephantiasis is the end result of repeated infections over many years.

38.2.3 Clinical Features

Patients with lower-extremity lymphoedema present initially unilateral painless swelling that starts on the dorsal aspect of the foot, with eventual proximal involvement over time. The oedema is initially pitting, but over time, the subcutaneous tissue becomes fibrotic resulting in nonpitting brawny oedema. Oedema can then spread circumferentially and involve the skin, which becomes hyperkeratotic, hyperpigmented, and papillomatous or verrucous, with increased skin turgor. Ultimately, the skin is at risk for rupture and subsequent infection. The swelling associated with lymphoedema results in heaviness, discomfort, and impaired mobility of the limb. Angiosarcoma may develop in chronic lymphoedematous limbs (Stewart–Treves syndrome), but it is most commonly seen in the upper extremity following mastectomy with axillary lymph node dissection (Durr et al. 2000). This is often referred to as lymphangiosarcoma – a misnomer, since the tumour does not derive from lymphatic vessels but rather derives from vascular endothelial cells within chronic lymphoedema.

The *International Society of Lymphology* (ISL) has developed a staging system for defining the progression/severity of limbs' disease, based on the extent of swelling and condition of the skin and tissues at each stage. The current version consists of four levels numbered from 0 to 3 (Consensus Document of ISL 2009).

Stage 0 lymphoedema (or Ia): latent or *preclinical stage.* The patient is at risk of developing lymphoedema, but no swelling or other visible evidence of impaired lymph transport is present. Further stages of lymphoedema can be prevented if specialised treatment is started immediately.

Stage I lymphoedema: early accumulation of fluid. There is visible swelling with protein-rich lymph; the swollen tissues are soft and pitting oedema is present. Prompt treatment of this stage can often control the condition and may prevent it from becoming more severe.

Stage II lymphoedema: a further increase in the swelling and a change in the tissues, which become increasingly firm due to fibrosis. Tissue changes at this stage increase the risks of even greater swelling, fibrosis, infections, and skin problems. Stage II lymphoedema can usually improve with intense treatment.

Stage III lymphoedema or lymphostatic elephantiasis: the skin tissues become extremely swollen and thickened due to a blockage in the flow of lymph and a build-up of fluid in tissues. The tissues become increasingly fibrotic. Normal elasticity is lost, the skin hangs in folds, and it may change colour. *Papillomas* and *hyperkeratosis* can develop. Changes in the texture of the skin are disfiguring and mobility can be difficult. Infections become more common because of increased risks of ruptures in the skin. These infections include fungal infections and open wounds that form within the folds of skin. Only intense therapy can improve this stage.

38.2.4 Diagnosis of Lymphoedema

Treatment of lymphoedema is based on correct diagnosis, but lymphoedema can be surprisingly difficult to diagnose, especially in its early stages. Without a proper diagnosis, therapy is often delayed, allowing secondary fibrosis and lipid deposition to take place. Instead, early treatment can result in rapid clinical improvement and prevents progression to the chronic phase of the disease.

Many conditions that cause swelling (oedema) are not lymphoedema. Lymphoedema can also coexist with other medical conditions associated with non-lymphoedema swelling. Diagnostic evaluation for lymphoedema includes the following (Position Statement of National Lymphedema Network 2011):

- History and physical examination
- Measures of volume
- Changes in electrical conductance
- Changes in biomechanical properties
- Genetic testing
- Soft tissue imaging
- Lymph vessel and lymph node imaging

38.2.4.1 History and Physical Examination

History and physical examination are important for all patients with chronic swelling. It is important to note age of onset, location(s) of swelling, pain and other symptoms, medications that can cause swelling, the course of progression of the swelling, and factors associated with swelling onset such as cancer, injury, or infection. Family history is important for the diagnosis of inherited forms of lymphoedema (Bellini et al. 2009).

Physical examination includes an assessment of the vascular system (lymphatics, veins, and arteries), skin and soft tissues in the swollen body part(s), palpation of lymph nodes, and looking for changes in body systems associated with various forms of inherited lymphoedemas.

The results of diagnostic tests and imaging must be matched with the information from history and physical examination. For trunk, breast, genital, head, and neck lymphoedema, history combined with physical examination is the currently accepted diagnostic approach (Murphy and Ridner 2010).

38.2.4.2 Measures of Volume

Measures of limb (arm and leg) volume have proven diagnostic accuracy when properly done (Cheville et al. 2003; Hayes et al. 2005). Enlargement of the limb (increase in volume) is the end result of fluid building up in the tissues. Therefore, volume measurements are used to quantify the presence and severity of lymphoedema and to monitor response to treatment. Volume is measured by three main methods: tape measurements, perometry, and water displacement (Unno et al. 2008). Measures of volume cannot differentiate lymphoedema from other types of oedema and do not determine when temporary post-operative arm oedema becomes chronic lymphoedema. Therefore, they are best suited for assessing the effects of treatment rather than for diagnosing lymphoedema.

38.2.4.3 Changes in Electrical Conductance

Bioimpedance spectroscopy (BIS) is utilised for measuring water content in tissues and has been shown to provide reliable data for the diagnosis of breast cancer-related lymphoedema (Mayrovitz 2009). BIS, which can detect early changes associated with lymphoedema (Kramer 2004), is performed by passing a small, painless, electrical current through the limb and measuring the resistance to the current (impedance). The higher the water content in the interstitial tissue, the lower the resistance (impedance) (Mayrovitz 2009). BIS shows promise for detecting smaller areas of localised lymphoedema, although this application has not yet been sufficiently validated (Stout Gergich et al. 2008). On the other hand, BIS is not as accurate in advanced, fibrotic oedema and cannot distinguish lymphoedema from other types of oedema.

38.2.4.4 Changes in Biomechanical Properties of Tissues

Lymphoedema causes the affected skin and subcutaneous tissues to become inflamed and fibrotic (Lolzewski et al. 2009). Lymphoedema is graded clinically, not just by increased size or volume but also by the progressive change in the skin texture as it becomes denser and harder (Gniadecka 1996). Currently, these skin changes are evaluated by physical examination of tissue texture, pitting, enlarged skin folds, and other dermatologic conditions such as wounds or papillomas (benign growths on the skin in areas of lymphoedema). Nevertheless, skin texture and resistance can be measured quantitatively by tissue dielectric constant (Mayrovitz 2009) and tonometry (Mirnajafi et al. 2004), although technical difficulties and a number of environmental factors (including a certain operator dependency) represent drawbacks to a general utilisation of these techniques.

38.2.4.5 Genetic Testing

Genetic counselling and genetic testing are mandatory for patients with primary lymphoedema (Ferrel et al. 2008; Connell et al. 2009). All young children diagnosed with primary lymphoedema should have a karyotype test performed. In case of late-onset primary lymphoedema, genetic testing is of limited benefit, although genetic counselling may be offered on a case-by-case basis.

38.2.4.6 Vascular Imaging

For children and for some adults diagnosed with primary lymphoedema, it is important to assess for other vascular abnormalities. Conditions such as congestive heart failure, vein clots known as deep venous thrombosis (DVT), damaged vein valves known as venous insufficiency, and some arterial conditions can lead to swelling or exist concurrent with lymphoedema (Boon et al. 2011). In case of secondary lymphoedema from cancer, obstruction of a vein can contribute to worsen the severity of oedema (Szuba et al. 2002). Imaging of the heart, veins, or arteries may be needed to obtain a complete and accurate diagnosis of the cause(s), in order to select proper treatment for oedema. The most common cardiovascular tests utilised for the evaluation of complex oedemas are echocardiogram, venous ultrasound (US), and arterial US with ankle brachial index (ABI). While venous clots can be detected with the patient in supine position, in order to accurately assess venous insufficiency (incompetent valves), the US examination must be performed with the patient standing or on a tilt table that can be tipped into a standing position (for patients who cannot stand for the test). If abnormalities of blood vessels in the chest, abdomen or pelvis are suspected, more advanced imaging, such as computed tomography (CT) venograms or arteriograms, is recommended (Position Statement of the National Lymphedema Network 2011).

38.2.4.7 Other Diagnostic Tests

There is no specific blood test for lymphoedema. Other medical conditions such as hypothyroidism (myxoedema) or hypoproteinaemia can cause oedema and therefore need to be assessed for complete evaluation of swelling. If filariasis is suspected, a blood smear (collected at night) looking for the presence of microfilariae is helpful. Nevertheless, antigen testing by immunochromatographic card test (Binax) or enzyme-linked immunosorbent assay (TropBio) is more sensitive than microfilariae detection and can use blood collected during day or night (Weil and Ramzy 2007).

38.2.4.8 Soft Tissue Imaging

Magnetic resonance imaging (MRI), CT, and US are able to detect the presence of extra fluid in the tissues, showing the presence of increased interstitial fluid (Astrom et al. 2001).

CT and MRI are mostly used to identify the anatomic changes due to subcutaneous lipomatous hypertrophy. However, they cannot identify the cause and their results must be combined with history and physical examination and sometimes with other imaging tests. Other conditions, such as heart failure or hypoproteinaemia from liver disease or malnutrition, can cause fluid to build up in the tissues. MRI, US, and CT may be required to identify the cause of lymphoedema, especially when lymphoedema is suspected to constitute the sole manifestation of an unknown/untreated cancer.

CT scanning or MRI of the lower extremity can also detect a *honeycomb* pattern of the subcutaneous tissue that is characteristic of lymphoedema (Liu et al. 2009; Lohrmann et al. 2009; Notohamiprodjo et al. 2012), and MR lymphangiography (MRL), based on intracutaneous injection of an extracellular, paramagnetic contrast agent, identifies abnormal lymphatic pathways with high resolution and has proven to be of value in patients with primary and secondary lymphoedemas. This technique visualises lymphatic vessels in a limb with lymph flow disturbances, but not the lymphatic vessels of a healthy limb, most likely due to the faster speed of lymph flow in the healthy limb. Therefore, lymph circulation disorders should be suspected when contrast-enhanced lymphatics are visualised with this test. Drainage of the contrast agent to regional lymph nodes also allows real-time evaluation of the transport function of the lymphatic system and the lymph nodes within a reasonable length of time. Furthermore, absorption and drainage of the contrast agent by the lymphatic system permit to visualise detailed morphologic changes of lymphatic vessels and regional lymph nodes. Finally, quantitative assessment of abnormal lymph flow kinetics may be achieved by tracing the flow within the lymphatic vessels and comparing dynamic nodal enhancement and time–signal intensity curves between oedematous and contralateral limbs. However, MRL is still experimental since intracutaneous injection is an off-label use of the contrast agent.

Venous Doppler US examination is often needed to assess for DVT or venous disease, which can coincide with lymphoedema. Up to 20%–30% of patients with advanced chronic venous disease have associated lymphatic dysfunction, presumably due to secondary damage from overload or from recurrent cellulitis (Bull et al. 1993).

38.2.5 Lymphoscintigraphy

Interstitial injection of radiolabelled compounds with sequential gamma camera imaging has been used to investigate the lymphatic system since the 1950s, after the pioneer observation on accumulation of radioactive colloidal gold (^{198}Au) in regional lymph nodes reported by Walker (1950). The method has largely replaced the more invasive and technically difficult technique of lymphangiography (Weissleder and Thrall 1989).

Yet, even more than 60 years later, the protocol for lymphoscintigraphy, a minimally invasive procedure simply requiring intradermal or subcutaneous injection of a radiocolloid, is not standardised, and remarkable differences among centres still persist. The main differences include the type and site of injection, the use of dynamic and static acquisitions, and the acquisition times themselves.

38.2.5.1 Radiopharmaceuticals

The choice of the radiopharmaceutical for lymphoscintigraphy is crucial. Since a significant fraction of the activity remained at the injection site after subcutaneous administration of colloidal ^{198}Au (a radionuclide with a significant emission of beta particles), radiation burden at the injection site limited the administered activity. The search for agents with more favourable characteristics led to replace colloidal ^{198}Au with particulate materials labelled with ^{99m}Tc, the most widely employed radionuclide for routine diagnostic nuclear medicine. The agents explored include ^{99m}Tc-sulphur colloid, ^{99m}Tc-nano- and micro-aggregated albumin, and ^{99m}Tc-antimony sulphide (Moghimi et al. 1994; Phillips et al. 2006). In the United States, filtered ^{99m}Tc-sulphur colloid (to limit particle size to <100 nm) is one of the most commonly employed radiopharmaceuticals for lymphoscintigraphy, while ^{99m}Tc-nanocolloidal albumin is mostly used in Europe.

Factors influencing transport of molecules from the interstitium to the lymphatic vessels are weight, size, shape, and charge (Bourgeois 2007). Moreover, composition of the extracellular matrix and properties of the molecules have significant influence on their ability to move through the interstitium into the lymphatics (Swartz 2001).

The optimal colloidal size for lymphoscintigraphy is believed to be at least 80 nm and ideally around 200 nm in the case of lymphoscintigraphy for sentinel lymph node mapping (Chinol and Paganelli 1999); instead, smaller colloidal particles (but still larger than 5–10 nm in order to prevent prevailing clearance through the blood capillaries) allows for faster visualisation of lymph flow in the case of peripheral lymphoscintigraphy. ^{99m}Tc-labelled albumin nanocolloid (Nanocoll®) has a reproducible colloid size distribution (95% of the particles <80 nm) and ease of labelling. Its rapid clearance from the injection site makes it suitable for quantitative studies, and interstitial injections are virtually painless. Thus, ^{99m}Tc-nanocolloidal albumin may be more suitable for quantitative studies than ^{99m}Tc-sulphur colloid.

38.2.5.2 Injected Volume and Activity

Bourgeois (Bourgeois 2007) has investigated the effect of variable concentration (0.02 mg versus 0.2 mg) and volume (0.2 mL versus 1.0 mL) of ^{99m}Tc-nanocolloidal albumin injected subcutaneously in the foot on lymph-nodal uptake after 1 h and found that the activity retained in inguinal lymph nodes was highest using the highest quantity in the lowest volume.

38.2.5.3 Factors Affecting Radiopharmaceutical Uptake

Several factors can affect the degree of radiocolloid uptake in the regional draining lymph nodes, briefly summarised as follows: (1) mechanical massage over the colloid injection site and exercise

(Olszewski et al. 1977, 2011), (2) surface properties of the radiocolloid particles (Ikomi et al. 1999), (3) venous pressure (which decreases lymph colloid and lymph leukocyte concentration) (Ikomi et al. 1996), and (4) temperature and pH of lymph or interstitial fluid (O'Morchoe et al. 1984).

38.2.5.4 Methodological Aspects

Lymphoscintigraphy is based on the interstitial injection of a suitable radiopharmaceutical that enters from the extracellular space into the initial lymphatics through interendothelial openings and by vesicular transport through the endothelial cells. The selection of an interstitial route of radiopharmaceutical administration is due to the anatomy of the lymphatic circulation: lymphatic vessels originate in the connective interstitium near the blood vessels. Therefore, investigation of functional integrity of the lymphatic system begins with the demonstration of a normal transport from the extracellular fluid, followed by the evaluation of lymph flow along the collectors until the reticuloendothelial system. In fact, both subcutaneous and intradermal injections are utilised in routine studies of superficial lymphatics of the extremities, although with some difference of opinion about which injection technique is best. Subcutaneous injection is recommended by many investigators (Cambria et al. 1993; Mortimer 1995) because of negligible clearance of the radiocolloid through the blood vessels (Weissleder and Weissleder 1988). According to Mostbeck and Partsch (Partsch 1995; Mostbeck and Partsch 1999), who compared subdermal and intradermal injections of ^{99m}Tc-nanocolloidal albumin, subcutaneous injections produced more reliable results, since it allowed to distinguish patients with lymphoedema from healthy subjects, based on semiquantitative parameters. Nevertheless, the optimal injection route may vary with the tracer employed, subcutaneous injection being optimal for the colloidal agents (Partsch 1995; Mostbeck and Partsch 1999). Intradermal administration of non-colloidal agents (such as ^{99m}Tc-human serum albumin [^{99m}Tc-HSA]) is associated with very rapid lymphatic transport and therefore facilitates fast evaluation and better quantification of lymphatic flow. However, other authors prefer intradermal injection (McNeill et al. 1989; Suga et al. 1991). Comparison of intradermal and subdermal injections of ^{99m}Tc-HSA reveals better tracer kinetics after intradermal injection and slow or no transport after subcutaneous injections (Bräutigam et al. 1998).

Intramuscular (subfascial) radiopharmaceutical injection is utilised for investigations of the deep lymphatic system of the extremities. When both epifascial and subfascial injections are performed sequentially, the procedure is called *two-compartment lymphoscintigraphy*. This approach is preferable for distinguishing the various mechanisms of oedema of the extremities, since evaluating both the deep lymphatic circulation (DLC) and the superficial lymphatic circulation (SLC) increases the diagnostic accuracy, as it makes it possible to identify lymphatic abnormalities present at either the deep or the superficial circulation (Kataoka et al. 1991; Bräutigam et al. 1998).

In our centre, we follow an ad hoc protocol for peripheral lymphoscintigraphy, which is based on separate, sequential evaluation of the DLC and of SLC. Since lymphatic vessels of the superficial circulation have a more complex anatomy, we prefer to assess the DLC system first. For DLC, we inject about 10–20 MBq (0.3–0.5 mCi) ^{99m}Tc-nanocolloidal albumin divided into 2–4 aliquots under the aponeurotic fascia of the palms or soles; in particular, the intramuscular space is reached by injecting the radiocolloid in the intermetatarsal/carpal muscle below the deep fascia plantaris/palmaris (see Figure 38.1).

After radiocolloid injection, some exercise is recommended to enhance sensitivity, such as walking (Kataoka et al. 1991), standing (McNeill et al. 1989), limb massage (Rijke et al. 1990), standardised treadmill exercise (Mostbeck and Partsch 1999), bicycle exercise (Kataoka 1991), squeezing of a rubber ball, use of a handgrip exercise device (Kleinhans et al. 1985), or massage (Williams et al. 2000). Exercise can also be useful for the quantitation of lymphatic flow. Images should be recorded with a dual-head gamma camera, from feet to pelvis for lower limbs and from hands to axilla (including the thorax) for upper limbs, for about 3–5 min from the most distal to the most proximal portion of the limbs.

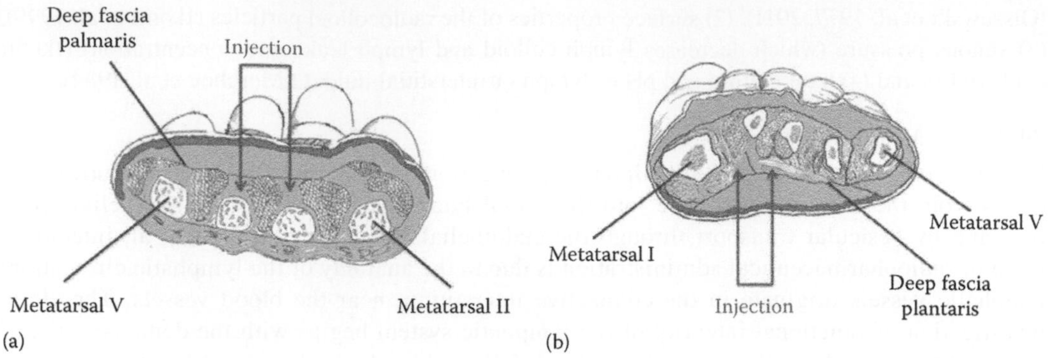

FIGURE 38.1 Schematic representation of the modality of radiocolloid injection for evaluating DLC of the extremities by the intramuscular route. A section of the hand (palm up) at the level of distal metacarpal bones II–V is shown in (a). Two aliquots of radiocolloid are injected under the deep *fascia palmaris* (inserting the needle about 10 mm deep), respectively, in the second and third intermetacarpal spaces, which are identified by palpating the palm immediately proximal to the distal head of the metacarpal bones. A similar section of the foot (sole down) at the level of distal metatarsal bones I–V is shown in (b). Two aliquots of radiocolloid are injected under the deep *fascia plantaris* (inserting the needle about 12–13 mm deep), respectively, in the first and second intermetatarsal spaces, which are identified by palpating the sole immediately proximal to the distal head of the metatarsal bones.

After evaluating the DLC, we evaluate the SLC by injecting a similar amount of the radiocolloid subdermally on the dorsum of each foot or hand in the II/III/IV metatarsal/metacarpal spaces (about 1–2 cm proximally to the interdigital web). We suggest not to inject directly into the interdigital web, since this may result in visualisation of either the SLC or the DLC. Images are then recorded in the same way as for DLC evaluation. Images of the abdomen should finally be acquired, to confirm passage of the radiocolloid to systemic blood circulation within a physiological time window until visualisation of the liver and spleen.

There is not yet a consensus on the criteria to visually interpret peripheral lymphoscintigraphy, and expertise plays a critical role in this setting, particularly for borderline situations (Jensen et al. 2010). Quantitative lymphoscintigraphy improves diagnostic accuracy of lymphoscintigraphy (Weissleder and Thrall 1989). Many procedures with semiquantitative indices have been proposed, among which the most relevant are transport index (TI, Damstra et al. 2008), transit time (TT), tracer appearance time (TAT, Tartaglione et al. 2010), transport capacity (TC, Carena et al. 1988, Cambria et al. 1993, Damstra et al. 2008), removal rate constant (RRC, Noer and Lassen 1979, Stanton et al. 2001), depot activity transported to inguinal lymph nodes after attenuation correction (Partsch 1995), uptake indices of the left inguinal (UIL) and right inguinal lymph nodes (UIR), washout rate constant (k) and depot half-life ($T_{1/2} = \ln 2/k$), and liver to nodal ratio (L/N ratio). However, all these parameters are affected by the injection technique (Brautigan et al. 1993, Modi et al. 2007). Weissleder and Thrall (1989) compared quantitative and qualitative lymphoscintigraphy and found that qualitative interpretation confirmed diagnosis of lymphoedema in 70% of extremities, while quantitative analysis detected abnormal lymphatic function in all the 308 examined limbs. The cases missed by qualitative interpretation are, in general, represented by patients with mild, grade I lymphoedema (Suga et al. 1991).

38.2.5.5 Image Interpretation

Qualitative lymphoscintigraphy is in many cases sufficient to establish a reliable diagnosis (Jensen et al. 2010). After intramuscular injection for DLC assessment, a normal lymphoscintigraphic pattern (see Figure 38.2) is represented by visualisation of both right and left limb lymphatic flow (usually only 1 main vessel for each side) within 5–10 min from the injection time.

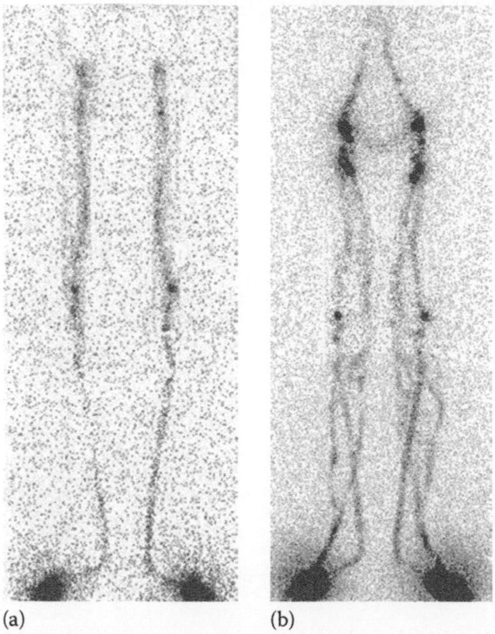

FIGURE 38.2 Normal lymphoscintigraphic pattern for the lower limbs following sequential intramuscular radiocolloid injection for visualising the DLC (a) and subdermal injection for visualising the SLC (b); since the two administration modalities are performed within about 1 h one after the other, the second scintigraphic acquisition (b) represents a combination lymphoscintigraphy in which the SLC pathways following intradermal injection are superimposed on the DLC pathways.

Deep lymphatic vessels course from the injection side along the medial part of leg/or arm until the knee/or elbow, in which it becomes lateral. When imaging the DLC, the popliteal, crural and inguinal lymph nodes are normally visualised. After intradermal injection for SLC assessment, the normal pattern similarly consists in visualisation of both right and left limb lymphatic flow within 5–10 min from the injection time. Superficial lymphatic flow courses in the opposite side with respect to DLC, from the injection side along the lateral part of leg/or arm until the knee/or elbow, in which it becomes medial. When imaging the SLC sequentially after evaluating DLC of the lower limbs, the normal visualisation pattern includes basically the same stations (crural and inguinal, to which both DLC and SLC contribute), but increasing in number and with increasing radiocolloid accumulation. For completion of lymphoscintigraphy, a whole-body image acquired in about 20 min will show the final appearance of the reticulo-endothelial system (spleen and liver) within physiological time.

38.2.5.6 Clinical Cases

Figure 38.3 shows an abnormal lymphoscintigraphic pattern due to congenital lower-limb lymphoedema secondary to angiodysplasia in a 1-year-old child. Abnormal findings include asymmetrical visualisation of lymphatic channels and collateral lymphatic channels, interrupted lymphatic vessels and lymph collection, asymmetrical or absent visualisation of regional lymph nodes, and the presence of *dermal flow* and/or of *dermal backflow*.

Figure 38.4 shows lymphoscintigraphic imaging in a case of primary monolateral lymphoedema affecting the right limb in a 12-year-old girl, with typical, isolated involvement of the affected side.

In case of cystic lymphangiomatosis (see Figure 38.5), a normal lymph flow can be observed bilaterally, but lymphoscintigraphy is recommended anyway for planning surgical correction, since it can guide this therapeutic option, in particular by identifying the component of lymphatic flow (deep or superficial) that supplies the lymph collection.

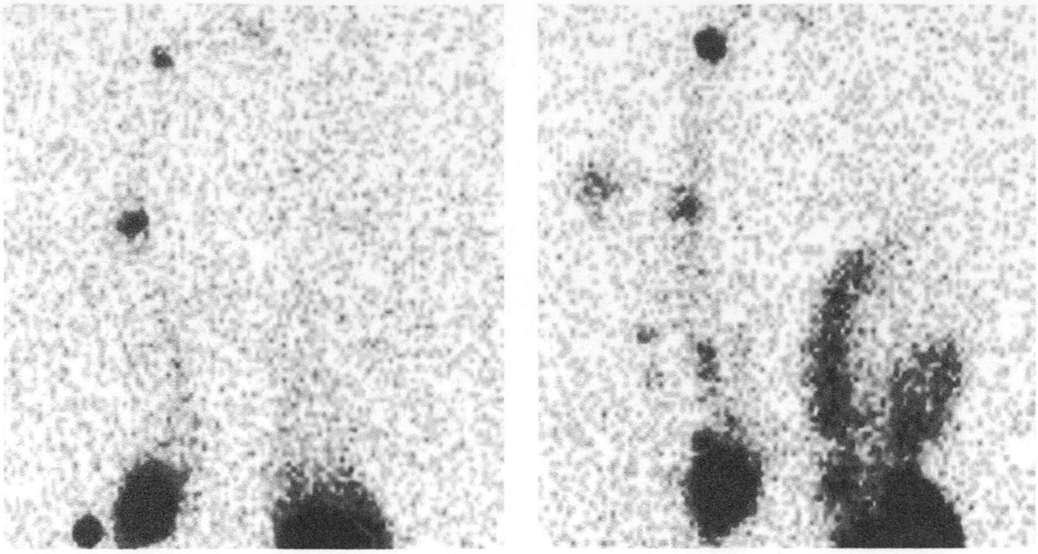

(a) (b)

FIGURE 38.3 Lymphoscintigraphy in a child with primary congenital lymphoedema. Pervious but delayed right DLC, with no visualisation of the left DLC (a). The SLC appears normal on the right side, while on the left side, there is only a partial and simultaneous visualisation of DLC and SLC, with dermal flow (b). Lymph node stations are normal on the right side, while they are absent on the left side.

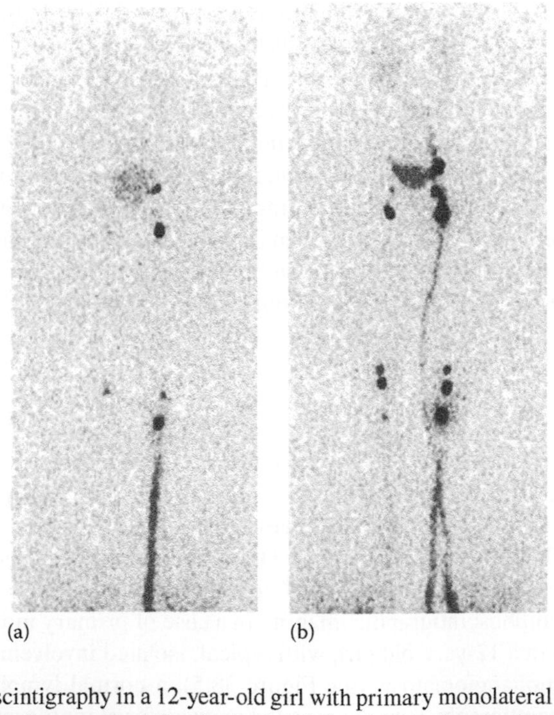

(a) (b)

FIGURE 38.4 Lymphoscintigraphy in a 12-year-old girl with primary monolateral lymphoedema at the right lower limb. Normal lymph flow on the left side, both DLC and SLC. Severe delay of right DLC (a), which appears only after injection for SLC visualisation, with absent SLC (b). Lymph nodes are present bilaterally, but fewer and/or less evident the right side.

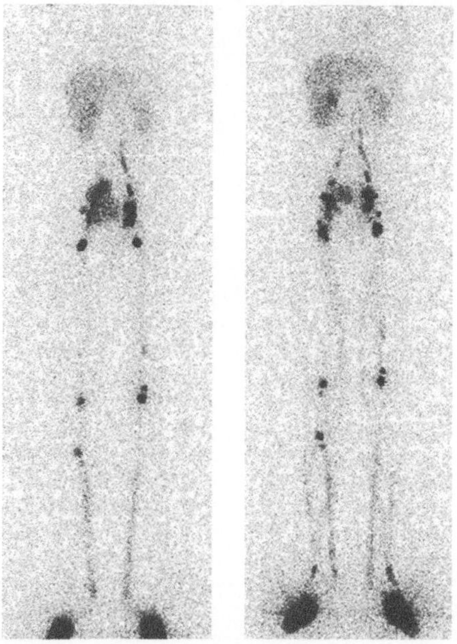

(a) (b)

FIGURE 38.5 Lymphoscintigraphy in a 33-year-old man with cystic lymphangiomatosis. Normal bilateral flow, in both the DLC (a) and the SLC images (b), with no lymph node abnormalities. The peculiarity of this lymphoscintigraphy is visualisation of two radiocolloid collections: one in the pelvis (supplied by the DLC) and the other at the upper pole of the right kidney (supplied by the SLC).

Lymphoscintigraphy can provide important diagnostic information also in patients with scrotal oedema, aiding in particular to choose the most suitable therapeutic options (see Figure 38.6). Sometimes, primary lower-limb lymphoedema can be associated with abdominal effusion (see Figure 38.7).

The typical cases of upper-limb lymphoedema encountered in the clinical practice include both primary forms of lymphoedema (see Figure 38.8) and acquired forms, due especially to surgery or therapy in patients undergoing treatment because of breast cancer (see Figure 38.9).

38.2.5.7 Lymphoscintigraphy in the Management of Lymphoedema

38.2.5.7.1 To Guide Therapeutic Options

Qualitative and semiquantitative lymphoscintigraphy has been widely used for guiding therapeutic options in patients with lymphoedema (Pecking 1999), treatment being constituted by either microsurgery (Gloviczky 1988; Ho et al. 1988; François et al. 1989; Gloviczky 1989; Brorson et al. 1998; Campisi et al. 2006), manual lymphatic massage (Leduc et al. 1988), pneumatic compression (Baulieu et al. 1987; Olszewski et al. 2011), hyperthermia (Liu and Olszewski 1993), hyperbaric oxygen therapy (Gothard 2004), or pharmacological interventions (Moore et al. 1996; Pecking et al. 1997). In unilateral lymphoedema, lymphoscintigraphic abnormalities may be also demonstrated at the contralateral limb in about 32% of the patients, thus suggesting either an early involvement of the contralateral side (Burnand et al. 2012) or an underlying (genetic?) condition predisposing to the development of lymphoedema following various types of injury.

38.2.5.7.2 During Follow-Up

Lymphoscintigraphy can be useful for monitoring lymphatic regeneration after both free-tissue transfer (Slavin et al. 1997) and lymphatic vessel transplantation (Weiss 2003); moreover, in patients with secondary lymphoedema, the lymphoscintigraphic patterns correlate well with the clinical stage and findings at intraoperative examination during lymphatico-venous anastomosis (Mikami 2011).

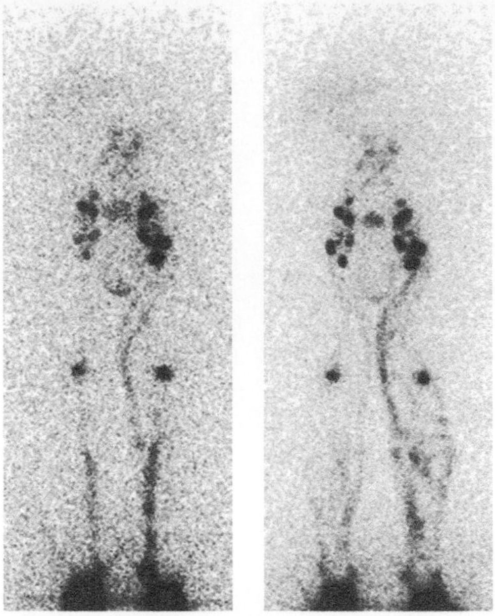

(a) (b)

FIGURE 38.6 Lymphoscintigraphy in a 73-year-old patient with scrotal oedema. Normal lymph flow on the right side. On the left side, there is a bypass of DLC to SLC (a), which is delayed with dermal backflow of the leg (b); this is a direct indication of an overloaded lymph flow (the radiocolloid cannot be drained by the lymphatics, so it takes the cutaneous route). Scrotal oedema is directly supplied by the left lymphatic flow.

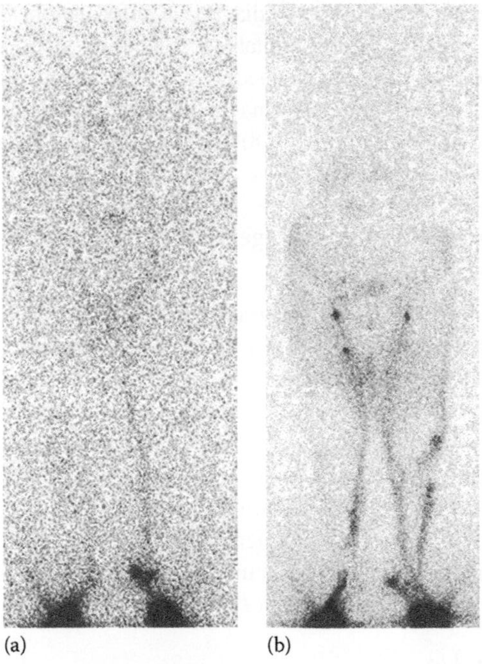

(a) (b)

FIGURE 38.7 Lymphoscintigraphy in a 62-year-old woman with bilateral lymphoedema localised at both thighs, associated with oedema of the lower abdominal wall. Severe impairment of the DLC, with absent visualisation bilaterally after radiocolloid injection of the radiocolloid (a). The SLC is delayed bilaterally with many collaterals, and there is dermal backflow at the thigh and abdomen (b).

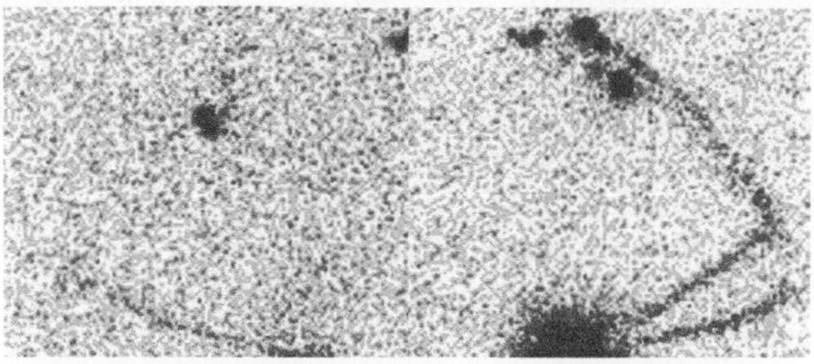

(a)

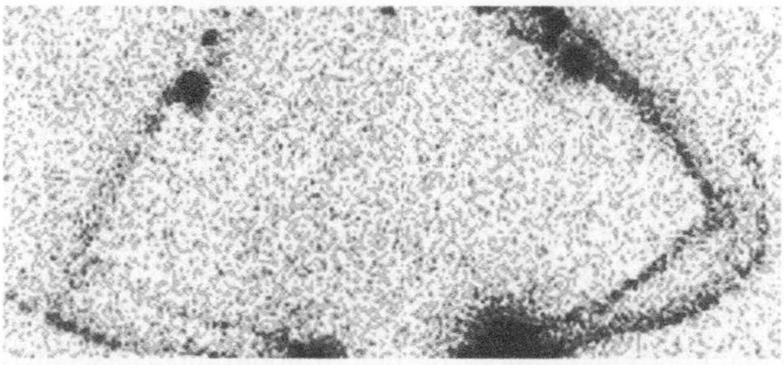

(b)

FIGURE 38.8 Lymphoscintigraphy in a patient with primary lymphoedema of the left upper limb (in each panel the injection sites at the hands are positioned in the bottom of the figure, while the axillae are depicted at the top of the figure). Normal lymph flow on the right side, both in the DLC and in the SLC images; bypass of left DLC on SLC, which appears normal (a). Epitrochlear lymph nodes are not visualised, with few axillary nodes (b).

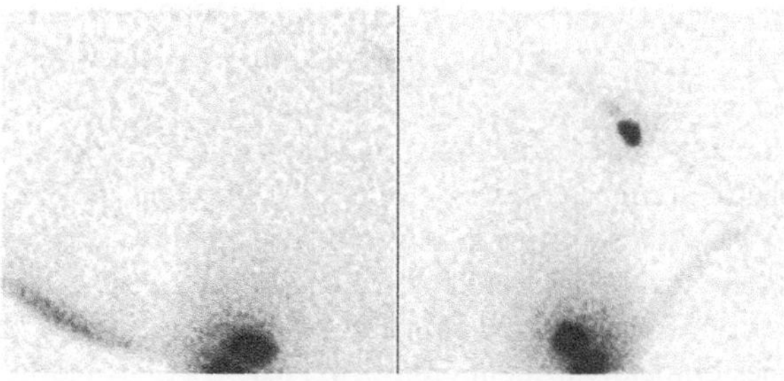

(a)

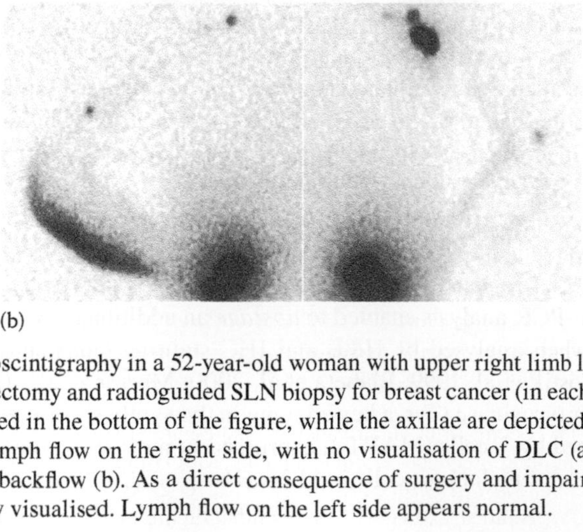

(b)

FIGURE 38.9 Lymphoscintigraphy in a 52-year-old woman with upper right limb lymphoedema secondary to homolateral quadrantectomy and radioguided SLN biopsy for breast cancer (in each panel the injection sites at the hands are positioned in the bottom of the figure, while the axillae are depicted at the top of the figure). Severe impairment of lymph flow on the right side, with no visualisation of DLC (a) and delayed SLC with dermal flow and dermal backflow (b). As a direct consequence of surgery and impaired lymph flow, the right axillary nodes are poorly visualised. Lymph flow on the left side appears normal.

38.2.5.7.3 *Lymphoscintigraphy for Prognostic Purposes*

Lymphoscintigraphy can predict the risk to develop lymphoedema in patients treated with surgery and/or radiotherapy for breast cancer (Pain et al. 2004), as disruption of the normal pattern of lymphatic drainage in postsurgical lymphoscintigraphy increases the risk of arm lymphoedema (Bourgeois et al. 1983; Pecking et al. 1988). Indications for lymphoscintigraphy performed with prognostic purposes include the following conditions: (1) women with postmastectomy lymphoedema, in whom the degree of lymphatic function impairment prior to treatment is well correlated with the outcome of manual lymphatic therapy (Szuba et al. 2000); (2) patients with clinical stage I unilateral lymphoedema, in whom visualisation of a main lymphatic vessel without collateral vessels is the best predictor for good response (Hwang et al. 2007) and also is continuing lymph node visualisation 4 h after radiocolloid administration (Gironet et al. 2004); and (3) patients with tibial fractures treated surgically in whom the lack of visualisation of inguinal lymph nodes predicts late post-operative leg oedema (Baulieu et al. 1985).

38.3 LYMPHATIC MAPPING AND RADIOGUIDED SENTINEL NODE BIOPSY IN CUTANEOUS MELANOMA

The number of metastatic nodes and tumour burden of nodal metastasis are the two major predictors of outcome in patients with melanoma of equivalent T classification (Balch et al. 2001, 2009). Therefore, accurate classification of the nodal status is of compelling prognostic value for patients with early-stage melanoma (Balch et al. 2009). The regional tumour-draining lymph node basin is the most frequent site of early melanoma metastases (Reintgen et al. 1994). As originally proposed, the SLN is defined as the first lymph node in the regional basin that receives a cutaneous afferent lymphatic vessel from the primary melanoma (Morton et al. 1992).

If the SLN is negative for metastases, then the probability for the remainder of the nodes in the basin to harbour melanoma cells is less than 1% (Morton et al. 1992). Therefore, full nodal classification can be obtained with lymphatic mapping and conservative SLN biopsy that is less invasive and less morbid and entails lower costs than elective lymph node dissection. Lymphadenectomy can thus be reserved for only those patients in whom a positive SLN has been detected (selective lymphadenectomy) (Essner et al. 1999). In fact, the disease-free survival rate is significantly greater when lymph node dissection is performed immediately after a positive SLN biopsy than when nodal metastasis becomes clinically evident (78.5% versus 73%, P = 0.009, at a median follow-up of 59.5 months) (Morton et al. 2006).

Another major advantage of lymphatic mapping is that only one or two SLNs per patient (instead of 10–40 lymph nodes deriving from complete lymphadenectomy) are processed for pathology. Since SLNs are the nodes most likely to contain metastatic disease, it is possible to analyse them more accurately, for instance, with serial sectioning (5 μm in thickness) and immunohistochemical (IHC) analysis with antibodies to S-100 or HMB (Walts et al. 1988; Cho et al. 1990). This procedure has 10%–30% higher sensitivity for identifying micrometastases compared with conventional haematoxylin and eosin (H&E) staining (Gibbs et al. 1999).

More recently, molecular techniques such as reverse transcriptase–polymerase chain reaction (RT–PCR) analysis (Wang et al. 1994; Reintgen et al. 1995; Goydos et al. 1998, 2003; Shivers et al. 1998; Ribuffo et al. 2003) are also being explored for their role in enhancing the detection of SLN metastases. In fact, RT–PCR analysis enabled to *upstage* an additional 13%–30% of patients whose SLNs were negative when analysed by H&E and IHC staining (conventional pathology, PATH) (Shivers et al. 1998; Bostik et al. 1999; Blaheta et al. 2000; Morton et al. 2003). Messenger RNAs (mRNAs) codifying for tyrosinase (Tyr, a key enzyme in the synthesis of melanin) and for the melanoma antigen recognised by T-cells (MART-1, expressed in most melanoma cell lines) are suitable markers for the presence of melanoma cells in SLNs (Hoon et al. 1995).

38.3.1 Lymphatic Drainage Relative to Cutaneous Melanoma

Lymphatic drainage from a melanoma lesion is usually predictable when the lesion is located in the extremities. Lower-extremity melanomas drain towards the homolateral groin, and upper-extremity lesions drain towards the homolateral axilla; if the melanoma is located in the hand/forearm or in the foot/leg, intercalated lymph nodes in epitrochlear or popliteal regions, respectively, can be imaged at lymphoscintigraphy. The pattern of lymphatic drainage from lesions of the head, neck, and trunk is instead much less predictable (Bennett and Lago 1983; Eberbach et al. 1987; Normal et al. 1991; Fisher et al. 1992; Uren et al. 1993; Berger et al. 1997; Roozendaal et al. 2000).

The first descriptions of the lymphatic drainage of the skin were based on the work of Sappey, a nineteenth-century anatomist who injected mercury into the lymphatic system of corpses to visualise the lymphatic channels (Sappey 1874). He reported drainage to the axilla and groin from the skin of the trunk and showed a vertical midline zone anteriorly and posteriorly where drainage to lymphatic basins in both sides of the body tended to overlap. A similar zone was identified horizontally around the waist, from the umbilicus to the region of the second lumbar vertebra. In these zones, called *Sappey's lines* by others, drainage was said to be possible to either side in the case of the vertical zone or to either the groin or the axilla in the case of the horizontal zone. On the other hand, outside these zones, lymphatic drainage always occurred to the ipsilateral groin or axilla, depending on whether the skin site of interest was above or below the horizontal band around the waist (Nieweg et al. 2004).

Nevertheless, lymphatic mapping with radiocolloids has revealed unsuspected routes of lymphatic drainage that contradict Sappey's anatomic drawings. The main advantage of lymphoscintigraphy over classic anatomic notions is that the lymphoscintigraphic pattern reflects the functional status of lymphatic drainage specifically in each patient and is more accurate than the typical distribution defined by the average anatomic appearance in a series of patients. Primary melanomas located in the trunk show a pattern of ambiguous drainage that is greatly expanded in comparison with the classic Sappey's watershed areas (Norman et al. 1991; Uren et al. 1993, 1998) (Figure 38.10).

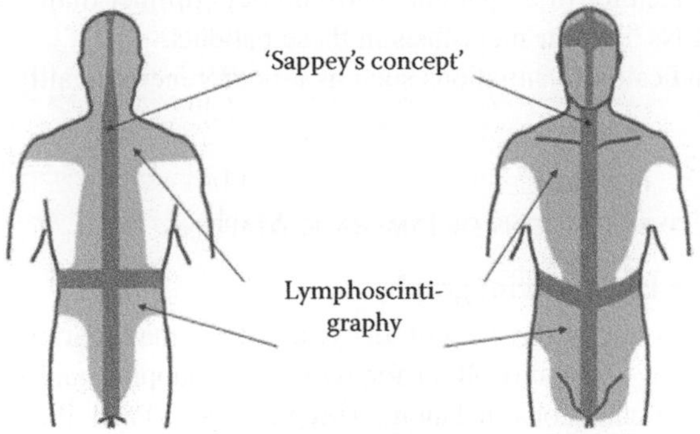

FIGURE 38.10 While the general pattern of lymphatic drainage from the extremities is quite predictable (from distal to proximal, i.e. towards the groin for lower limbs, towards the axilla for upper limbs), the direction of lymphatic drainage in other regions of the body can be ambiguous, especially for areas around midline of the body and around the waist. According to Sappey's notions (depicted in deep gray), ambiguous lymphatic drainage (i.e. possibility of draining towards either left-sided or right-sided lymph nodes for midline of the body or else cranially or caudally for the waist) corresponds to a restricted area extending only approximately 5 cm on each side. Experience with lymphoscintigraphy shows instead that ambiguous lymphatic drainage can extend to a much wider area (depicted in light gray): head, neck, and shoulders are virtually entirely included in this area, as is a relevant abdominal area around the waist.

These considerations explain why lymphoscintigraphy must be considered an essential part of radioguided SLN biopsy. In fact, the imaging phase performed on interstitial injection of the radiocolloid tracer should provide three pieces of information. The first is the identification of all lymph node basins at risk for metastatic disease, including those in unexpected locations (Uren et al. 1993; Leong et al. 1999; Roozendaal et al. 2000). If the primary site is a watershed area of lymphatic drainage to more than one nodal basin (McMasters 2000), preoperative lymphoscintigraphy provides the surgeon with a map of lymphatic flow from the primary site, so that all (and only) the nodal basins at risk for metastatic disease will be dissected. The second piece of information is the precise location of the SLN (or nodes), so that biopsy can be performed using a very limited skin incision and, whenever possible, local anaesthesia. The third is the identification of in-transit (or intercalated) nodes, defined as lymph nodes along the channel from the primary site to the regional basin, and marking of these for possible harvesting and histologic evaluation.

38.3.2 Clinical Indications and Contraindications for Sentinel Lymph Node Mapping in Cutaneous Melanoma

38.3.2.1 Indications

1. Intermediate-stage primary melanoma (1–4 mm Breslow).
2. Patients with high-risk lesions of 0.75–0.99 mm in thickness should be considered for SLN biopsy (SLNB) if their melanoma is Clark level IV or V, is ulcerated, shows a vertical growth phase, or has lymphatic invasion or a high mitotic rate.
3. Patients with tumours thicker than 4 mm may potentially benefit from SLNB.
4. No clinical evidence of lymph node involvement.
5. No clinical evidence of distant tumour spread (Balch et al. 2009).

38.3.2.2 Contraindications

1. Extensive previous surgery in the region of the primary tumour site or targeted lymph node circulation.
2. Patients with known distant metastases.
3. SLNB is not indicated for those patients with tumours thinner than 0.75 mm, because less than 2% of the SLNs harbour metastasis in these patients.
4. SLNB is contraindicated in situations such as a poor general health status or severe concurrent disease.

38.3.3 Technical Considerations of Lymphatic Mapping

38.3.3.1 Preoperative Lymphoscintigraphy

General consensus has developed over the last few years on the main parameters that define the optimal techniques of injecting the radiocolloid for lymphatic mapping and radioguided SLN biopsy in patients with malignant cutaneous melanoma (Moghimi and Patel 1989; Thompson et al. 1995; Alazraki et al. 1997; Borgstein and Meijer 1998; Krag et al. 1998; Borgstein 1999; Gennari et al. 1999, 2000; Keshtgar and Ell 1999; Keshtgar et al. 1999; Freeman and Blaufox 2000; Mariani et al. 2002).

Melanocytes, the cells that give rise to cutaneous melanomas, are located between the dermis and the epidermis. Transformed malignant melanocytes initially grow in this space, from which they spread elsewhere. Therefore, migration of tumour cells from cutaneous melanomas through the lymphatic route follows the general pattern of lymph flow in the skin.

Based on these considerations, the concept of intradermal/subdermal injection of radiocolloid for lymphatic mapping in patients with cutaneous melanoma is widely accepted and applied routinely. Preoperative lymphoscintigraphy is the first step in the lymphatic mapping procedure, as it constitutes a *road map* to guide the surgeon, especially useful for localising unpredictable

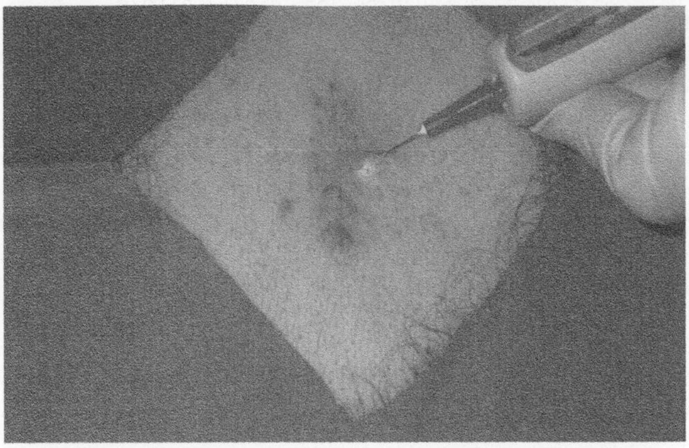

FIGURE 38.11 Intradermal–subdermal injection of radiocolloid for lymphatic mapping in a patient already submitted to excision of a cutaneous melanoma (with evident recent surgical scar).

lymphatic drainage patterns. Lymphoscintigraphy begins with a 2- to 8-point intradermal injection of ^{99m}Tc-labelled colloid using a 25- or 27-gauge needle (Figure 38.11).

Considering that sentinel node mapping is most frequently performed after removal of the melanoma (as histologic findings constitute part of the indications), the radiocolloid should be injected within 2–3 mm of the excision biopsy scar at the site of the original melanoma. Injections should not be given at the ends of a long excision biopsy scar, as this may cause drainage to lymph nodes that did not originally drain the melanoma site. Each injected aliquot is between 10 and 40 MBq, depending on whether same-day or next-day surgery is planned, respectively. Locally available radiocolloids generally include ^{99m}Tc-sulphur colloid in the United States, ^{99m}Tc-nanocolloidal albumin in Europe, ^{99m}Tc-stannous colloid in Japan, and ^{99m}Tc-antimony sulphide in Australia and Canada.

Following radiocolloid injection, dynamic images at 1 frame per minute are usually acquired over the injection site for 30 min (Figure 38.12), with further early imaging performed for 5–10 min

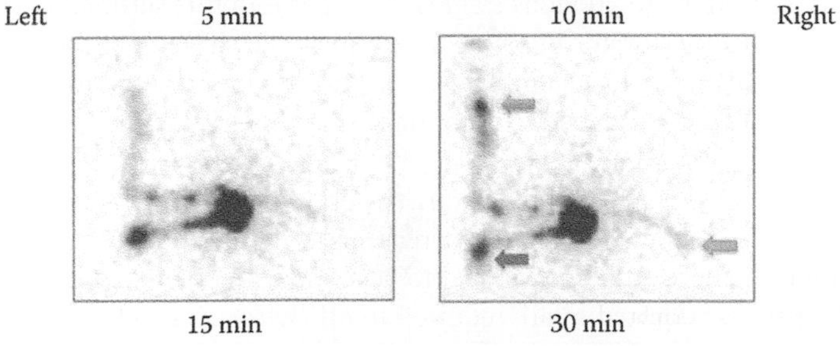

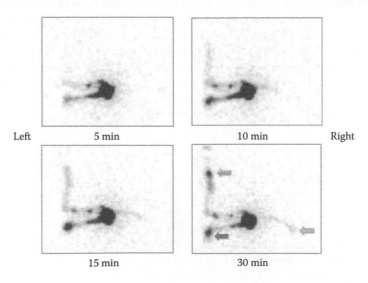

FIGURE 38.12 Representative sequential images extracted from a dynamic lymphoscintigraphic sequence recorded upon intradermal injection of ^{99m}Tc-nanocolloidal albumin in a patient with cutaneous malignant melanoma located on midline of the back. The radiocolloid follows initially lymphatic channels towards the left axilla (blue arrow), as well as towards the left groin (red arrow) and, at subsequent times, towards the right groin (green arrow).

over the draining node fields. Anterior (or posterior) and lateral views are obtained as necessary. Delayed imaging is performed 1–2 h later, again in the anterior/posterior and lateral projections to define the precise location of all SLNs. Examples of variable patterns of lymphatic drainage visualised by lymphoscintigraphy are shown in Figures 38.13 and 38.14.

Cutaneous projection of each SLN should be marked on the skin with an indelible marker, and a small point tattoo of carbon black is useful for later follow-up, especially if the sentinel nodes are not later removed. Skin marking should always be performed with the patient in the same position to be used at surgery.

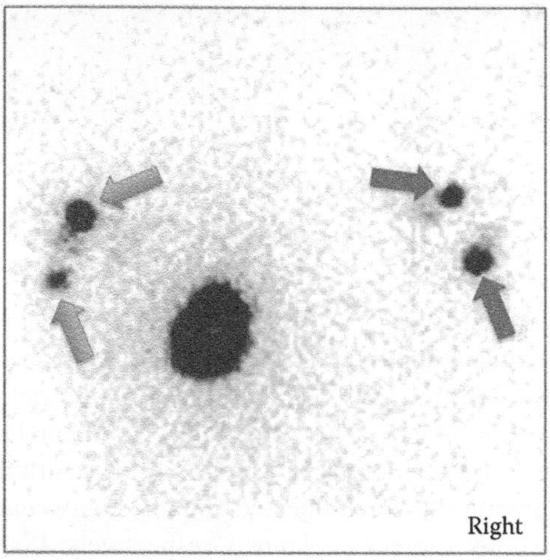

FIGURE 38.13 Lymphoscintigraphy (posterior view) in a male patient recently submitted to excisional biopsy of a cutaneous melanoma on his back (just about midline): lymph flows through several channels towards sentinel nodes in both axillae, with visualisation of two SLNs in right axilla (deep gray) and two SLNs in left axilla (light gray).

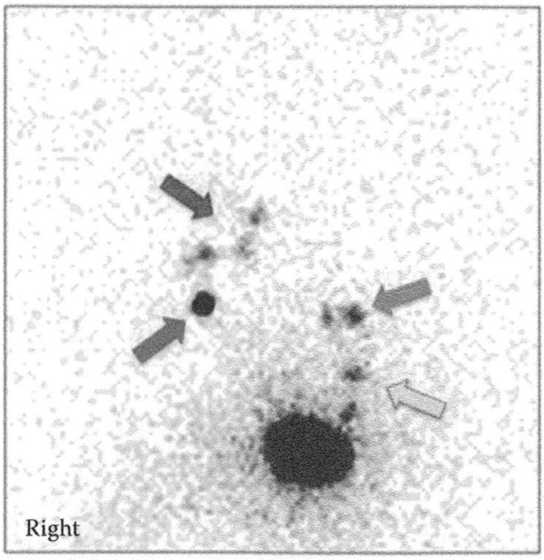

FIGURE 38.14 Lymphoscintigraphy (anterior view) in a male patient recently submitted to excisional biopsy of a cutaneous melanoma on his chest (just about right paramedian line): two separate lymphatic vessels lead, respectively, to an axillary SLN (red arrow) and to an internal mammary sentinel node on the right (yellow arrow). There is sequential visualisation of upper-tier nodes both in the axilla (blue arrow) and in the parasternal region (green arrow).

The last few years have seen the introduction of new technological possibilities for SLN detection. In particular, with the new generation of gamma cameras, the functional information from single-photon emission computed tomography (SPECT) can be combined with morphological information from CT (Statius et al. 2002; Even-Sapir et al. 2003; Ishihara et al. 2006; Valdés-Olmos et al. 2009).

In melanoma patients, SPECT/CT is especially helpful for localising the lymph nodes draining from primary tumours high on the trunk and in the head and neck area. This anatomic–functional imaging technique enables more accurate nodal staging and has the potential to reduce morbidity from primary melanomas of the trunk and the head and neck. The additional value of SPECT/CT is obvious for patients with non-visualisation on planar lymphoscintigraphy and for patients with SLNs close to the injection site. Another significant improvement added by the introduction of SPECT/CT in the clinical setting is the possibility of generating 3D images based on volume rendering software, to localise SLNs in relation to anatomical structures (Figure 38.15). The possibility of using different colours for different anatomical structures provides the surgeon with an excellent overview of SLNs, especially in areas such as the neck and upper part of the trunk. These images

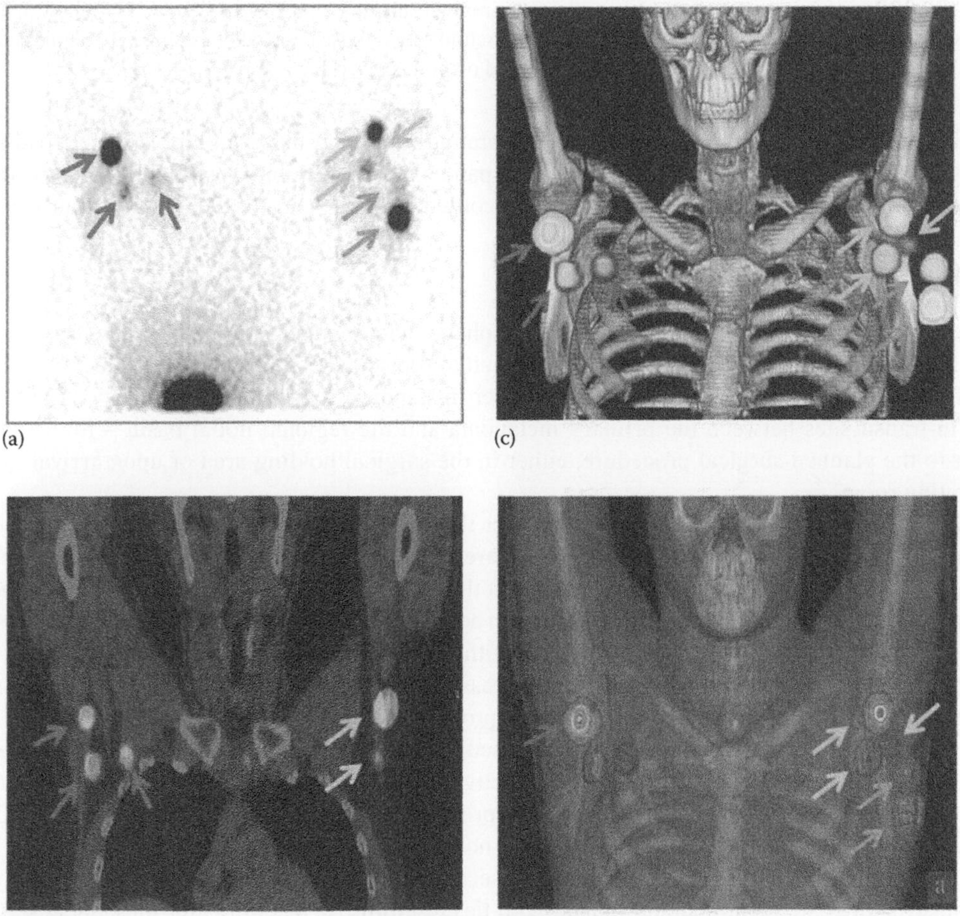
(a) (c) (b) (d)

FIGURE 38.15 Lymphoscintigraphy in a male patient recently submitted to excisional biopsy of a cutaneous melanoma on his back. Planar anterior view (a) shows some SLNs, seemingly located in the right axilla (red arrows) and in the left axilla (orange and blue arrows). Fused SPECT/CT images in coronal (b) and 3D volume rendering images with different levels of soft tissue visualisation (c and d) demonstrate that two out of the five left-sided lymph nodes (blue arrows) are actually located behind the shoulder blade and are related to subcutaneous (*in-transit*) SLNs.

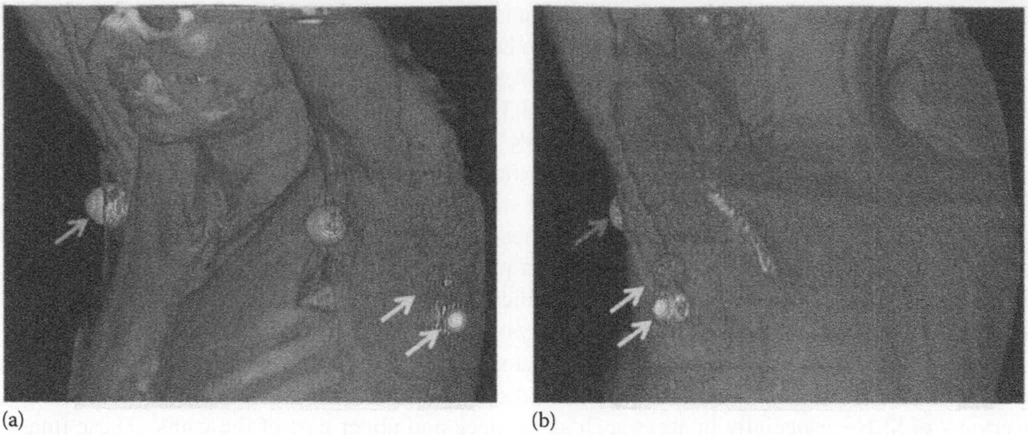

FIGURE 38.16 Same patient as in the previous figure: two subcutaneous (*in-transit*) SLNs (yellow arrows) located at the level of the lateral margin of the left latissimus dorsi muscle visualised using 3D volume rendering (a and b). In addition, an axillary SLN is displayed on both sides (blue and red arrows).

can be available on a separate screen in the operating room and thus facilitate a better road map for the surgeon. These images are very useful in patients with melanoma, especially in cases where the primary location is close to the site of radiocolloid injection and for depicting in-transit SLNs (Figure 38.16).

38.3.3.2 Intraoperative Procedure

As early as 1994, centres began performing lymphatic mapping and SLN biopsy using a handheld gamma probe. The handheld gamma probe is used to transcutaneously confirm the location of the SLN as marked at lymphoscintigraphy – whether in standard regional nodal basins or in ectopic and in-transit sites between the primary melanoma and the regional nodal basin – immediately prior to the planned surgical procedure, either in the surgical holding area or upon arrival in the operating room.

General anaesthesia is generally preferred for this procedure, since significant mobilisation of tissue is often required to achieve primary closure of the melanoma site following wide excision, and extensive dissection is occasionally needed at the SLN biopsy sites, especially in obese patients. In some cases, however, monitored sedation with adequate local anaesthesia may be sufficient.

Following external gamma-probe counting with the patient properly positioned for surgery and appropriately prepped and draped, areas of increased focal radioactivity accumulation in the first basin are confirmed with the handheld gamma probe. A small, usually approximately 3 cm, incision is then made overlying the area of increased focal uptake, identifying the sentinel node by blunt dissection towards the area of increasing activity detected by the intraoperative gamma probe. Subtle manipulation of the angle of the gamma probe helps to precisely locate the direction of the required dissection. Once identified the *hottest* node in the basin, it is secured with a suture and gently elevated. Surrounding fatty tissue is dissected with electrocautery, and vascular and lymphatic structures are identified and ligated with ties to minimise bleeding and subsequent seroma formation. In this fashion, the lymph node is harvested, and ex vivo radiotracer counts are obtained with the handheld gamma probe and recorded in the patient's chart, the operative record, and the pathology form. After removal of the SLN, the basin is rescanned using the gamma probe; if an area of increased focal activity is again identified, the preceding gamma-probe-guided searching procedure is repeated. In our experience, any lymph node whose counting rate is at least 20% of the counting rate of the hottest node in the basin should be considered an additional sentinel node (Manca et al. 2008).

The SLNs so harvested are numbered sequentially within a nodal basin and submitted for permanent section pathological analysis. Copious irrigation and verification of haemostasis of the sentinel node biopsy cavity is subsequently performed. In general, these incisions are closed in two layers using absorbable interrupted dermal sutures followed by a running subcutaneous stitch. Drains are rarely required for sentinel node biopsy sites, since in most cases, use of the handheld gamma probe permits limited dissection of the nodal basin (and therefore little disruption of the lymphatics).

38.3.4 Learning Curve for Radioguided Sentinel Lymph Node Biopsy in Cutaneous Melanoma

The learning curve for SLN biopsy reflects the time required to form a team of specialists in nuclear medicine, surgery, and pathology to work together (Mariani et al. 2001). Although some controversy exists on the number of procedures to be performed by a team to qualify for routinely performing lymphatic mapping in patients with cutaneous melanoma, we agree with Morton's suggestion of 30–50 procedures (Reintgen et al. 1997). Multidisciplinary teams for SLN biopsy in melanoma patients must achieve two important performance requirements for completing their learning phase: The SLN must be successfully identified in at least 97% of patients, and metastasis must be found in the sentinel node of between 12% and 20% of patients whose melanoma is >1 mm thick (Mariani et al. 2004).

38.3.5 Conclusions on Sentinel Node Biopsy in Cutaneous Melanoma

Despite some differences in the way radioguided SLN biopsy is being performed around the world, the excellent results reported univocally point to this procedure as the most safe, efficient, and cost-effective modality for lymphatic mapping in patients with primary cutaneous melanoma (Reintgen et al. 1997; Brobeil et al. 1999; Balch et al. 2000) due to the capability of the procedure to actually change surgical management of melanoma patients, by sparing them unnecessarily extensive surgery (Reintgen 1996; Balch and Ross 1999).

Although the reliability of SLN biopsy in patients with malignant melanoma is widely recognised both for staging purposes and for prognostic stratification, some issues are still open for discussion. In particular, the actual long-term impact of sentinel node biopsy (with the ensuing elective lymph node dissection of a metastatic basin) on the clinical outcome of patients has yet to be unequivocally defined. Critical meta-analysis of all the long-term follow-up and survival studies published so far helps to assess the actual benefit of the procedure for patients with cutaneous melanoma (Morton et al. 2006; Matias et al. 2011).

REFERENCES

Alazraki NP, Eshima D, Eshima LA et al. 1997. Lymphoscintigraphy, the sentinel node concept, and the intraoperative gamma probe in melanoma, breast cancer, and other potential cancers. *Semin Nucl Med* 27: 55–67.

Aström K, Abdsaleh S, Brenning C, Ahlström, K. 2001. MR imaging of primary, secondary, and mixed forms of lymphedema. *Acta Radiol* 42: 409–416.

Balch CM, Buzaid AC, Atkins MB et al. 2000. A new American Joint Committee on Cancer Staging system for cutaneous melanoma. *Cancer* 88: 1484–1491.

Balch CM, Gershenwald JE, Soong SJ et al. 2009. Final version of 2009 AJCC melanoma staging and classification. *J Clin Oncol* 36: 6199–6206.

Balch CM, Ross MI. 1999. Sentinel lymphadenectomy for melanoma – Is it a substitute for elective lymphadenectomy? *Ann Surg Oncol* 6: 416–417.

Balch CM, Soong SJ, Gershenwald JE et al. 2001. Prognostic factors analysis of 17,600 melanoma patients: Validation of the American Joint Committee on Cancer melanoma staging system. *J Clin Oncol* 19: 3622–3634.

Baulieu F, Baulieu JL, Mesny J et al. 1987. Visualization of the thoracic duct by lymphoscintigraphy. *Eur J Nucl Med* 13: 264–265.

Baulieu F, Itti R, Taieb W, Richard G, Martinat H, Barsotti J. 1985. Lymphoscintigraphy: A predictive test of post-traumatic lymphedema of the lower limbs. *Rev Chir Orthop Reparatrice Appar Mot* 71: 327–332.

Bellini C, Witte MH, Campisi C, Bonioli E, Boccardo F. 2009. Congenital lymphatic dysplasias: Genetics review and resources for the lymphologist. *Lymphology* 42: 36–41.

Bennett LR, Lago G. 1983. Cutaneous lymphoscintigraphy in malignant melanoma. *Semin Nucl Med* 13: 61–69.

Berger DH, Feig BW, Podoloff D et al. 1997. Lymphoscintigraphy as a predictor of lymphatic drainage from cutaneous melanoma. *Ann Surg Oncol* 4: 247–251.

Blaheta HJ, Ellwanger U, Schittek B et al. 2000. Examination of regional lymph nodes by sentinel node biopsy and molecular analysis provides new staging facilities in primary cutaneous melanoma. *J Invest Dermatol* 114: 637–642.

Boon LM, Ballieux F, Vikkula M. 2011. Pathogenesis of vascular anomalies. *Clin Plast Surg* 38: 7–19.

Borgstein P, Meijer S. 1998. Historical perspective of lymphatic tumour spread and the emergence of the sentinel node concept. *Eur J Surg Oncol* 24: 85–89.

Borgstein PJ. 1999. The sentinel node concept. Consequences of lymphatic tumour spread in melanoma and breast cancer, PhD thesis. University Hospital, Vrije Universiteit, Amsterdam, The Netherlands.

Bostick PJ, Morton DL, Turner RR et al. 1999. Prognostic significance of occult metastases detected by sentinel lymphadenectomy and reverse transcriptase-polymerase chain reaction in early-stage melanoma patients. *J Clin Oncol* 17: 3238–3244.

Bourgeois P. 2007. Scintigraphic investigations of the lymphatic system: The influence of injected volume and quantity of labeled colloidal Tracer. *J Nucl Med* 48: 693–695.

Bourgeois P, Frühling J, Henry J. 1983. Postoperative axillary lymphoscintigraphy in the management of breast cancer. *Int J Radiat Oncol Biol Phys* 9: 29–32.

Bräutigam P, Földi E, Schaiper I, Krause T, Vanscheidt W, Moser E. 1998. Analysis of lymphatic drainage in various forms of leg edema using two compartment lymphoscintigraphy. *Lymphology* 31: 43–55.

Bräutigam P, Vanscheidt W, Földi E, Krause T, Moser E. 1993. The importance of the subfascial lymphatics in the diagnosis of lower limb edema: Investigations with semiquantitative lymphoscintigraphy. *Angiology* 44: 464–470.

Brobeil A, Cruse CW, Messina JL. 1999. Cost analysis of sentinel lymph node biopsy as an alternative to elective lymph node dissection in patients with malignant melanoma. *Surg Oncol Clin N Am* 8: 435–445.

Brorson H, Svensson H, Norrgren K, Thorsson O. 1998. Liposuction reduces arm lymphedema without significantly altering the already impaired lymph transport. *Lymphology* 31: 156–172.

Bull RH, Gane JN, Evans JE, Joseph AE, Mortimer PS. 1993. Abnormal lymph drainage in patients with chronic venous leg ulcers. *J Am Acad Dermatol* 28: 585–590.

Burnand KM, Glass DM, Mortimer PS, Peters AM. 2012. Lymphatic dysfunction in the apparently clinically normal contralateral limbs of patients with unilateral lower limb swelling. *Clin Nucl Med* 37: 9–13.

Cambria RA, Gloviczki P, Naessens JM, Wahner HW. 1993. Noninvasive evaluation of the lymphatic system with lymphoscintigraphy: A prospective, semiquantitative analysis in 386 extremities. *J Vasc Surg* 18: 773–782.

Campisi C. 1999. Global incidence of tropical and non-tropical lymphoedemas. *Int Angiol* 18: 3–5.

Campisi C, Davini D, Bellini D et al. 2006. Lymphatic microsurgery for the treatment of lymphedema. *Microsurgery* 26: 65–69.

Carena M, Campini R, Zelaschi G, Rossi G, Aprile C, Paroni G. 1988. Quantitative lymphoscintigraphy. *Eur J Nucl Med* 14: 88–92.

Cheville AL, McGarvey CL, Petrek JA, Russo SA, Thiadens SR, Taylor ME. 2003. The grading of lymphedema in oncology clinical trials. *Semin Radiat Oncol* 13: 214–225.

Chinol M, Paganelli G. 1999. Current status of commercial colloidal preparations for sentinel lymph node detection. *Eur J Nucl Med* 26: 560.

Cho KH, Hashimoto K, Taniguchi Y et al. 1990. Immunohistochemical study of melanocytic nevus and malignant melanoma with monoclonal antibodies against S-100 subunits. *Cancer* 66: 765–771.

Connell FC, Ostergaard P, Carver C et al. 2009. Lymphoedema consortium analysis of the coding regions of VEGFR3 and VEGFC in Milroy disease and other primary lymphoedemas. *Hum Genet* 124: 625–631.

Consensus Document of the International Society of Lymphology. 2009. The diagnosis and treatment of peripheral lymphedema. *Lymphology* 42: 53–54.

Damstra RJ, vanSteensel MA, Boomsma JH, Nelemans P, Veraart JC. 2008. Erysipelas as a sign of subclinical primary lymphoedema: A prospective quantitative scintigraphic study of 40 patients with unilateral erysipelas of the leg. *Br J Dermatol* 158: 1210–1215.

Durr HR, Pellengahr C, Nerlich A et al. 2000. Angiosarcoma associated with chronic lymphedema (Stewart–Treves syndrome) of the leg: MR imaging. *Skeletal Radiol* 29: 413–416.
Eberbach MA, Whal RL, Argenta LC et al. 1987. Utility of lymphoscintigraphy in directing surgical therapy for melanomas of the head, neck and upper thorax. *Surgery* 102: 433–442.
Ege GN. 1976. Internal mammary lymphoscintigraphy. *Radiology* 118: 101–107.
Erba PA, Sollini M, Boni R. 2013. Lymphoscintigraphy for the differential diagnosis of peripheral edema and intracavitary lymph effusion. In *Atlas of Lymphoscintigraphy and Sentinel Node Mapping – A Pictorial Case-Based Approach*, eds. Mariani G, Manca G, Orsini F, Vidal-Sicart S, Valdés Olmos RA, pp. 39–86. Milan, Italy: Springer-Verlag Italy.
Essner R, Conforti A, Kelley MC et al. 1999. Efficacy of lymphatic mapping, sentinel lymphadenectomy, and selective complete lymph node dissection as a therapeutic procedure for early-stage melanoma. *Ann Surg Oncol* 6: 442–449.
Even-Sapir E, Lerman H, Lievshitz G et al. 2003. Lymphoscintigraphy for sentinel node mapping using a hybrid SPECT/CT system. *J Nucl Med* 44: 1413–1420.
Ferrell RE, Kimak MA, Lawrence EC, Finegold DN. 2008. Candidate gene analysis in primary lymphedema. *Lymphat Res Biol* 6: 69–76.
Fisher EB, Lewis VL Jr, Griffith BH, Spies W. 1992. The role of cutaneous lymphoscintigraphy in determining regional lymph node drainage of truncal melanomas. *Ann Plast Surg* 28: 506–510.
François A, Richaud C, Bouchet JY, Franco A, Comet M. 1989. Does medical treatment of lymphedema act by increasing lymph flow? *Vasa* 18: 281–286.
Freeman LM, Blaufox D. 2000. *Seminars in Nuclear Medicine*, Vol 30. Philadelphia, PA: WB Saunders.
Gennari R, Bartolomei M, Testori A et al. 2000. Sentinel node localization in primary melanoma: Preoperative dynamic lymphoscintigraphy, intraoperative gamma probe, and vital dye guidance. *Surgery* 127: 19–25.
Gennari R, Stoldt HS, Bartolomei M et al. 1999. Sentinel node localisation: A new prospective in the treatment of nodal melanoma metastases. *Int J Oncol* 15: 25–32.
Gibbs JF, Huang PP, Zhang PJ et al. 1999. Accuracy of pathologic techniques for the diagnosis of metastatic melanoma in sentinel lymph nodes. *Ann Surg Oncol* 6: 699–704.
Gironet N, Baulieu F, Giraudeau B, Machet L, Toledano C, Tiguemounine J, Lorette G, Vaillant L. 2004. Lymphedema of the limb: Predictors of efficacy of combined physical therapy. *Ann Dermatol Venereol* 131: 775–779.
Gloviczki P. 1989. Principles of surgical treatment of chronic lymphedema. *Int Angiol* 18: 42–46.
Gloviczki P, Fisher J, Hollier LH, Pairolero PC, Schirger A, Wahner HW. 1988. Microsurgical lymphovenous anastomosis for treatment of lymphedema: A critical review. *J Vasc Surg* 7: 647–652.
Gniadecka M. 1996. Localization of dermal edema in lipodermatosclerosis, lymphedema, cardiac insufficiency. High-frequency ultrasound examination of intradermal echogenicity. *J Am Acad Dermatol* 35: 37–41.
Gothard L, Stanton A, MacLaren J et al. 2004. Non-randomised phase II trial of hyperbaric oxygen therapy in patients with chronic arm lymphoedema and tissue fibrosis after radiotherapy for early breast cancer. *Radiother Oncol* 70: 217–224.
Goydos JS, Patel KN, Shih WJ et al. 2003. Patterns of recurrence in patients with melanoma and histologically negative but RT-PCR-positive sentinel lymph nodes. *J Am Coll Surg* 196: 196–204.
Goydos JS, Ravikumar TS, Germino FJ et al. 1998. Minimally invasive staging of patients with melanoma: Sentinel lymphadenectomy and detection of the melanoma specific proteins MART-1 and tyrosinase by reverse transcriptase polymerase chain reaction. *J Am Coll Surg* 187: 182–188.
Hawkins LA, McAlister J. 1969. The use of 99Tcm antimony sulphide colloid for liver scanning – Its preparation and some clinical and experimental observations. *Br J Radiol* 42: 234–235.
Hayes S, Cornish B, Newman B. 2005. Comparison of methods to diagnose lymphoedema among breast cancer survivors: 6-month follow-up. *Breast Cancer Res Treat* 89: 221–226.
Ho LY, Lay ME, Kenedy J. 1988. Micro-lymphatic bypass in the treatment of obstructive lymphoedema of the art: Case report of a new technique. *Br J Plast Surg* 36: 360–366.
Hoon DS, Wang Y, Dale PS et al. 1995. Detection of occult melanoma cells in blood with a multiple-marker polymerase chain reaction assay. *J Clin Oncol* 13: 2109–2116.
Hultborn RA, Larsson LG, Ragnhult I. 1955. The lymph drainage from the breast to the axillary and parasternal lymph nodes studied with the aid of colloidal ^{198}Au. *Acta Radiol* 43: 52–64.
Hwang JH, Choi JH, Lee JY et al. 2007. Lymphoscintigraphy predicts response to complex physical therapy in patients with early stage extremity lymphedema. *Lymphology* 40: 172–176.
Ikomi F, Hanna GK, Schmid-Schönbein GW. 1999. Size- and surface-dependent uptake of colloid particles into the lymphatic system. *Lymphology* 32: 90–102.

Ikomi F, Hunt J, Hanna G, Schmid-Schönbein GW. 1996. Interstitial fluid, plasma protein, colloid, and leukocyte uptake into initial lymphatics. *J Appl Physiol* 81: 2060–2067.

Ishihara T, Kaguchi A, Matsushita S et al. 2006. Management of sentinel lymph nodes in malignant skin tumors using dynamic lymphoscintigraphy and the single-photon-emission computed tomography/computed tomography combined system. *Int J Clin Oncol* 11: 214–220.

Jensen MR, Simonsen L, Karlsmark T, Bülow J. 2010. Lymphoedema of the lower extremities – Background, pathophysiology and diagnostic considerations. *Clin Physiol Funct Imaging* 30: 389–398.

Kari A. 2011. The lymphatic vasculature in disease. *Nat Med* 17: 1371–1380.

Kataoka M, Kawamura M, Hamada K, Itoh H, Nishiyama Y, Hamamoto K. 1991. Quantitative lymphoscintigraphy using ^{99}Tcm human serum albumin in patients with previously treated uterine cancer. *Br J Radiol* 64: 1119–1121.

Keshtgar MRS, Ell PJ. 1999. Sentinel lymph node detection and imaging. *Eur J Nucl Med* 26: 57–67.

Keshtgar MRS, Waddington WA, Lakhani SR et al. 1999. *The Sentinel Node in Surgical Oncology*. Berlin, Germany: Springer Verlag.

Kleinhans E, Baumeister RG, Hahn D, Siuda S, Büll U, Moser E. 1985. Evaluation of transport kinetics in lymphoscintigraphy: Follow-up study in patients with transplanted lymphatic vessels. *Eur J Nucl Med* 10: 349–352.

Kort W. 1969. 99mTc human serum albumin colloid for liver cirrhosis. *Strahlentherapie* 137: 420–423.

Krag D, Harlow S, Weaver D et al. 1998. Technique of sentinel node resection in melanoma and breast cancer: Probe-guided surgery and lymphatic mapping. *Eur J Surg Oncol* 24: 89–93.

Krag DN, Weaver DL, Alex JC, Fairbank JT. 1993. Surgical resection and radiolocalization of the sentinel lymph node in breast cancer using a gamma probe. *Surg Oncol* 2: 335–339.

Kramer EL. 2004. Lymphoscintigraphy: Defining a clinical role. *Lymph Res Biol* 2: 32–37.

Leduc O, Bourgeois P, Leduc A. 1988. Manual lymphatic drainage: Scintigraphic demonstration of its efficacy on colloidal protein reabsorption. In *Progress in Lymphology*, ed. Partsch H, pp. 551–554. Amsterdam, The Netherlands: Elsevier Science.

Leong SP, Achtem TA, Habib FA et al. 1999. Discordancy between clinical predictions versus lymphoscintigraphic and intraoperative mapping of sentinel lymph node drainage of primary melanoma. *Arch Dermatol* 135: 1472–1476.

Liu NF, Lu Q, Jiang ZH, Wang CG, Zhou JG. 2009. Anatomic and functional evaluation of the lymphatics and lymph nodes in diagnosis of lymphatic circulation disorders with contrast magnetic resonance lymphangiography. *J Vasc Surg* 49: 980–987.

Liu NF, Olszewski W. 1993. The influence of local hyperthermia on lymphedema and lymphedematous skin of the human leg. *Lymphology* 26: 28–37.

Lohrmann C, Foeldi E, Langer M. 2009. MR imaging of the lymphatic system in patients with lipedema and lipo-lymphedema. *Microvasc Res* 77: 335–339.

Lolszewski W, Jain P, Govinda A, Marzanna Z, Cakala M. 2009. Anatomical distribution of tissue fluid and lymph in soft tissues of lower limbs in obstructive lymphedema – Hints for physiotherapy. *Phlebolymphology* 64: 283–289.

Manca G, Romanini A, Pellegrino D et al. 2008. Optimal detection of sentinel lymph node metastases by intraoperative radioactive threshold and molecular analysis in patients with melanoma. *J Nucl Med* 49: 1769–1775.

Manca G, Tredici M, Duce V et al. 2013. Preoperative and intraoperative lymphatic mapping for radioguided sentinel node biopsy in breast cancer. In *Atlas of Lymphoscintigraphy and Sentinel Node Mapping – A Pictorial Case-Based Approach*, eds. Mariani G, Manca G, Orsini F, Vidal-Sicart S, Valdés Olmos RA, pp. 121–168. Milan, Italy: Springer-Verlag Italy.

Mariani G, Erba P, Manca G et al. 2004. Radioguided sentinel lymph node biopsy in patients with malignant cutaneous melanoma: The nuclear medicine contribution. *J Surg Oncol* 85: 141–151.

Mariani G, Gipponi M, Moresco L et al. 2002. Radioguided sentinel lymph node biopsy in malignant cutaneous melanoma. *J Nucl Med* 43: 811–827.

Mariani G, Moresco L, Viale G et al. 2001. Radioguided sentinel lymph node biopsy in breast cancer surgery. *J Nucl Med* 42: 1198–1215.

Matias E, Valsecchi DS, Silbermins D et al. 2011. Lymphatic mapping and sentinel lymph node biopsy in patients with melanoma: A meta-analysis. *J Clin Oncol* 29: 1479–1487.

Matsuo S. 1974. Studies of the metastasis of breast cancer to lymph nodes – II: Diagnosis of metastasis to internal mammary nodes using radiocolloid. *Acta Med Okayama* 28: 361–371.

Mayrovitz HN. 2009. Assessing lymphedema by tissue indentation force and local tissue water. *Lymphology* 42: 88–98.

Mayrovitz HN, Davey S, Shapiro E. 2009. Suitability of single tissue dielectric constant measurements to assess local tissue water in normal and lymphedematous skin. *Clin Physiol Funct Imaging* 29: 123–127.

McLaughlin SA. 2012. Lymphedema: Separating fact from fiction. *Oncology (Williston Park)* 26: 242–249.

McMasters KM. 2000. Multiple nodal basin drainage in truncal melanomas. *Ann Surg Oncol* 7: 249–250.

McNeill GC, Witte MH, Witte CL et al. 1989. Whole-body lymphangioscintigraphy: Preferred method for initial assessment of the peripheral lymphatic system. *Radiology* 172: 495–502.

Mikami T, Hosono M, Yabuki Y et al. 2011. Classification of lymphoscintigraphy and relevance to surgical indication for lymphaticovenous anastomosis in upper limb lymphedema. *Lymphology* 44:155–167.

Mirnajafi A, Moseley A, Piller N. 2004. A new technique for measuring skin changes of patients with chronic postmastectomy lymphedema. *Lymphat Res Biol* 2: 82–85.

Modi S, Stanton AWB, Svensson WE, Peters AM, Mortimer PS, Levick JR. 2007. Human lymphatic pumping measured in healthy and lymphoedematous arms by lymphatic congestion lymphoscintigraphy. *J Physiol* 583: 271–285.

Moghimi SM, Hawley AE, Christy NM, Grayb T, Illum L, Davisa SS. 1994. Surface engineered nanospheres with enhanced drainage into lymphatics and uptake by macrophages of the regional lymph nodes. *FEBS Lett* 344: 25–30.

Moghimi SM, Patel HM. 1989. Differential properties of organ-specific serum opsonins for liver and spleen macrophages. *Biochim Biophys Acta* 984: 379–383.

Moore TA, Reynolds JC, Kenney RT, Johnston W, Nutman TB. 1996. Diethyl-carbamazine-induced reversal of early lymphatic dysfunction in a patient with bancroftian filariasis: Assessment with use of lymphoscintigraphy. *Clin Infect Dis* 23: 1007–1011.

Mortimer PS. 1995. Evaluation of lymphatic function: Abnormal lymph drainage in venous disease. *Int Angiol* 14: 32–35.

Morton DL, Hoon DS, Cochran AJ et al. 2003. Lymphatic mapping and sentinel lymphadenectomy for early-stage melanoma: Therapeutic utility and implications of nodal microanatomy and molecular staging for improving the accuracy of detection of nodal micrometastases. *Ann Surg* 238: 538–549.

Morton DL, Thompson JF, Cochran AJ et al. 2006. Sentinel-node biopsy or nodal observation in melanoma. *N Engl J Med* 355: 1307–1317.

Morton DL, Wen DR, Wong JH et al. 1992. Technical details of intraoperative lymphatic mapping for early stage melanoma. *Arch Surg* 127: 392–399.

Mostbeck A, Partsch H. 1999. Isotope lymphography – Possibilities and limits in evaluation of lymph transport. *Wien Med Wochenschr* 149: 87–91.

Murphy B, Ridner H. 2010. Late-effect laryngeal oedema/lymphoedema. *J Lymphedema* 5: 92–93.

Nieweg OE, Estourgie S, Valdés Olmos RA. 2004. Lymphatic mapping and sentinel node biopsy. In *Nuclear Medicine in Clinical Diagnosis and Treatment*, 3rd edn., eds. Ell PJ and Gambhir SS, pp. 229–260. Edinburgh, U.K.: Churchill Livingstone.

NLN Medical Advisory Committee. 2011. The diagnosis and treatment of lymphedema, position statement of the national lymphedema network 2011: 1–2. http://www.lymphnet.org/pdfDocs/nlntreatment.pdf (last accessed: December 12, 2012).

Noer I, Lassen NA. 1979. Evidence of active transport (filtration?) of plasma proteins across the capillary walls in muscle and subcutis. *Acta Physiol Scand Suppl* 463: 105–110.

Norman J, Cruse CW, Espinosa C et al. 1991. Redefinition of cutaneous lymphatic drainage with the use of lymphoscintigraphy for malignant melanoma. *Am J Surg* 162: 432–437.

Notohamiprodjo M, Weiss M, Baumeister RG et al. 2012. Lymphangiography at 3.0 T: Correlation with lymphoscintigraphy. *Radiology* 264: 78–87.

O'Morchoe CC, Jones WR, Jarosz HM, O'Morchoe PJ, Fox LM. 1984. Temperature dependence of protein transport across lymphatic endothelium in vitro. *J Cell Biol* 98: 629–640.

Olszewski WL, Cwikla J, Zaleska M, Domaszewska-Szostek A, Gradalski T, Szopinska S. 2011. Pathways of lymph and tissue fluid flow during intermittent pneumatic massage of lower limbs with obstructive lymphedema. *Lymphology* 44: 54–64.

Olszewski WL, Engeset A, Sokolowski J. 1977. Lymph flow and protein in the normal male leg during lying, getting up, and walking. *Lymphology* 10: 178–183.

Pain SJ, Purushotham AD, Barber RW et al. 2004. Variation in lymphatic function may predispose to development of breast cancer-related lymphoedema. *Eur J Surg Oncol* 30: 508–514.

Partsch H. 1995. Assessment of abnormal lymph drainage for the diagnosis of lymphedema by isotopic lymphangiography and by indirect lymphography. *Clin Dermatol* 13: 445–450.

Pavlista D, Eliska O. 2012. Relationship between the lymphatic drainage of the breast and the upper extremity: A postmortem study. *Ann Surg Oncol* 19: 3410–3415.

Pecking A, Firmin F, Rain JD et al. 1980. Lymphoedema of the upper limb following surgery or radiotherapy. Investigation by indirect radioactive lymphography. *Nouv Presse Med* 9: 3349–3351.

Pecking AP. 1999. Possibilities and restriction of isotopic lymphography for the assessment of therapeutic effects in lymphedema. *Wien Med Wochenschr* 149: 105–106.

Pecking AP, Fevrier B, Wargon C, Pillion G. 1997. Efficacy of Daflon 500 mg in the treatment of lymphoedema (secondary to conventional therapy of breast cancer). *Angiology* 48: 93–98.

Pecking AP, Lasry S, Floiras J, Rambert P, Guérin P. 1988. Post surgical physiotherapeutic treatment: Interest in secondary upper limb lymphedemas prevention. In *Progress in Lymphology*, ed. Partsch H, pp. 561–564. Amsterdam, The Netherlands: Elsevier Science.

Petronis JD, LaFrance ND, Kaelin W. 1985. Lymphoscintigraphy. *Eur J Nucl Med* 10: 560–562.

Phillips WT, Goins BA, Medina LA. 2006. Targeting of liposomes to lymph nodes. Liposome technology, vol. III, chap. 3, pp. 231–252 in *Interactions of Liposomes with the Biological Milieu*, III edition, ed. Gregoriadis G. New York: Informa Healthcare.

Reintgen D. 1996. More rational and conservative surgical strategies for malignant melanoma using lymphatic mapping and sentinel node biopsy techniques. *Curr Opin Oncol* 8: 152–158.

Reintgen D, Albertini J, Berman C et al. 1995. Accurate nodal staging of malignant melanoma. *Cancer Control* 2: 405–414.

Reintgen D, Balch CM, Kirkwood J et al. 1997. Recent advances in the care of the patient with malignant melanoma. *Ann Surg* 1: 1–14.

Reintgen D, Cruse CW, Wells K et al. 1994. The orderly progression of melanoma nodal metastases. *Ann Surg* 220: 759–767.

Reintgen DS, Albertini J, Millotes G. 1997. Investment in new technology research can save future health care dollars. *J Fla Med Assoc* 84: 175–181.

Ribuffo D, Gradilone A, Vonella M et al. 2003. Prognostic significance of reverse transcriptase-polymerase chain reaction-negative sentinel nodes in malignant melanoma. *Ann Surg Oncol* 10: 396–402.

Rijke AM, Croft BY, Johnson RA, de Jongste AB, Camps JA. 1990. Lymphoscintigraphy and lymphedema of the lower extremities. *J Nucl Med* 31: 990–998.

Roozendaal GK, De Vries JDH, Van Poll D et al. 2000. Sentinel nodes outside lymph node basins in melanoma patients. *Br J Surg* 88: 305–308.

Rossi R, Ferri O. 1966. The visualization of the internal mammary chain with Au-198. Presentation of a new method of lymphoscintigraphy. *Minerva Med* 57: 1151–1155.

Rossi R, Ferri O, Trivellini G. 1966. Etude de la chained lymphatique mammaire interne par ^{198}Au colloidal. *J Chir* 95: 79–96.

Santi G, Zecchin R. 1968. Lymphoscintigraphy with Au-198 of the oropharynx and neck in normal and pathological conditions. *Minerva Otorinolairngol* 18: 167–175.

Sappey MPC. 1874. *Anatomie, Physiologie, Pathologie des Vaisseaux Lymphatiques Considerez Chez L'homme et les Vertebrés*. Paris, France: DeLahaye and Lecrosnier.

Scheffel U, Rhodes BA, Natarajan TK, Wagner HN Jr. 1972. Albumin microspheres for study of the reticuloendothelial system. *J Nucl Med* 13: 498–503.

Schenk P, Zum Winkel K, Becker J. 1966. Die Szintigraphie des Parasternalen Lymphsystems. *Nucl Med* 5: 388–396.

Schneider J, Glaubitt D, Gerhartz H. 1973. Bone marrow scintigraphy using 99m Technetium-sulfur-rhenium colloid in plasmacytoma patients. *Verh Dtsch Ges Inn Med* 79: 513–516.

Sherman AI, Ter-Pogossian M. 1953. Lymph-node concentration of radioactive colloidal gold following interstitial injection. *Cancer* 6: 1238–1240.

Shivers SC, Wang X, Li W et al. 1998. Molecular staging of malignant melanoma: Correlation with clinical outcome. *JAMA* 280: 1410–1415.

Slavin SA, Upton J, Kaplan WD, Van den Abbeele AD. 1997. An investigation of lymphatic function following free-tissue transfer. *Plast Reconstr Surg* 99: 730–743.

Stanton AW, Modi S, Mellor RH, Levick JR, Mortimer PS. 2009. Recent advances in breast cancer related lymphedema of the arm: Lymphatic pump failure and predisposing factors. *Lymphat Res Biol* 7: 29–45.

Stanton AW, Svensson WE, Mellor RH, Peters AM, Levick JR, Mortimer PS. 2001. Differences in lymph drainage between swollen and non-swollen regions in arms with breast-cancer-related lymphoedema. *Clin Sci (Lond)* 101: 131–140.

Statius Muller MG, Hennipman FA, van Leeuwen PA et al. 2002. Unpredictability of lymphatic drainage patterns in melanoma patients. *Eur J Nucl Med Mol Imaging* 29: 255–261.

Stern HS, McAfee JG, Subramanian G. 1966. Preparation, distribution and utilization of technetium-99m-sulfur colloid. *J Nucl Med* 7: 665–675.

StoutGergich NL, Pfalzer LA, McGarvey C, Springer B, Gerber LH, Soballe P. 2008. Preoperative assessment enables the early diagnosis and successful treatment of lymphedema. *Cancer* 112: 2809–2819.

Suga K, Uchisako H, Nakanishi T, Utsumi H, Yamada N, Oohara M, Esato K. 1991. Lymphoscintigraphic assessment of leg oedema following arterial reconstruction using a load produced by standing. *Nucl Med Commun* 12: 907–917.

Sutkowska E, Gil J, Stembalska A, Hill-Bator A, Szuba A. 2012. Novel mutation in the FOXC2 gene in three generations of a family with lymphoedema-distichiasis syndrome. *Gene* 498: 96–99.

Swartz MA. 2001. The physiology of the lymphatic system. *Adv Drug Deliv Rev* 50: 3–20.

Szuba A, Achalu R, Rockson SG. 2002. Decongestive lymphatic therapy for patients with breast carcinoma-associated lymphedema. A randomized, prospective study of a role for adjunctive intermittent pneumatic compression. *Cancer* 95: 2260–2267.

Szuba A, Cooke JP, Yousuf S, Rockson SG. 2000. Decongestive lymphatic therapy for patients with cancer-related or primary lymphedema. *Am J Med* 109: 296–300.

Tartaglione G, Pagan M, Morese R et al. 2010. Intradermal lymphoscintigraphy at rest and after exercise: A new technique for the functional assessment of the lymphatic system in patients with lymphoedema. *Nucl Med Commun* 31: 547–551.

Thompson JF, McCarthy WH, Bosch CM et al. 1995. Sentinel lymph node status as an indicator of the presence of metastatic melanoma in regional lymph nodes. *Melanoma Res* 5: 255–260.

Turoglu HT, Janjan NA, Thorsen MK et al. 1992. Imaging of regional spread of breast cancer by internal mammary lymphoscintigraphy, CT and MRI. *Clin Nucl Med* 17: 482–484.

Unno N, Nishiyama M, Suzuki M et al. 2008. Quantitative lymph imaging for assessment of lymph function using indocyanine green fluorescence lymphography. *Eur J Vasc Endovasc Surg* 36: 230–236.

Uren RF, Howman-Giles RB, Shaw HM et al. 1993. Lymphoscintigraphy in high-risk melanoma of the trunk: Predicting draining node groups, defining lymphatic channels and locating the sentinel node. *J Nucl Med* 34: 1435–1440.

Uren RF, Howman-Giles RB, Thompson JF, Roberts J, Bernard E. 1998. Variability of cutaneous lymphatic flow rates in melanoma patients. *Melanoma Res* 8: 279–282.

Valdés Olmos R, Vidal-Sicart S, Nieweg O. 2009. SPECT-CT and real-time intraoperative imaging: New tools for sentinel node localization and radioguided surgery? *Eur J Nucl Med Mol Imaging* 36: 1–5.

Voutilainen A, Wiljasalo M. 1965. On the correlation of lymphography and lymphoscintigraphy in metastases of tumours of the pelvic region. *Ann Chir Gynaecol Fenn* 54: 268–277.

Walker LA. 1950. Localization of radioactive colloids in lymph nodes. *J Lab Clin Med* 36: 440–449.

Walts AE, Said JW, Shintaku IP. 1988. Cytodiagnosis of malignant melanoma. Immunoperoxidase staining with HMB-45 antibody as an aid to diagnosis. *Am J Clin Pathol* 90: 77–80.

Wang X, Heller R, VanVoorhis N et al. 1994. Detection of submicroscopic lymph node metastases with polymerase chain reaction in patients with malignant melanoma. *Ann Surg* 220: 768–774.

Weil GJ, Ramzy RM. 2007. Diagnostic tools for filariasis elimination programs. *Trends Parasitol* 23: 78–82.

Weiss M, Baumeister RG, Hahn K. 2003. Planning and monitoring of autologous lymph vessel transplantation by means of nuclear medicine lymphoscintigraphy. *Handchir Mikrochir Plast Chir* 35: 210–215.

Weissleder H, Weissleder R. 1988. Lymphedema: Evaluation of qualitative and quantitative lymphoscintigraphy in 238 patients. *Radiology* 167: 729–735.

Weissleder R, Thrall J. 1989. The lymphatic system: Diagnostic imaging studies. *Radiology* 172: 315–317.

Williams WH, Witte CL, Witte MH, McNeill GC. 2000. Radionuclide lymphangioscintigraphy in the evaluation of peripheral lymphedema. *Clin Nucl Med* 25: 451–464.

Wjcinski S, Nuengsri S, Hillemanns P et al. 2012. Axillary dissection in primary breast cancer: Variations of the surgical technique and influence on morbidity. *Cancer Manag Res* 4: 121–127.

39 Nuclear Medicine as an Aid to Minimally Invasive Surgery, with Emphasis on Hybrid SPECT/CT Imaging

Federica Orsini, Alessandra Serra, Mario Piga, and Giuliano Mariani

CONTENTS

The increase in detection of occult lesions has led to the development of new methods to identify foci or tissues that have been preoperatively labelled with a radioactive tracer. The identification of occult lesions for radioguided surgery can be carried out in two ways. The first approach consists of systemic administration of a specific radiopharmaceutical that exhibits tropism for a tumour or tissue, such as ^{99m}Tc-sestamibi for the identification of parathyroid adenomas or hyperplasia (Mariani et al. 2003) or ^{111}In-DTPA-octreotide for the identification of neuroendocrine tumours (Gulec and Baum 2007). In the second approach, the tissue to be excised is labelled by intratumoural injection of ^{99m}Tc-albumin macro-aggregate or ^{99m}Tc-colloid guided by ultrasound (US), CT, or another imaging methods. This technique, known as radioguided occult lesion localisation (ROLL), was first described in 1998 for the preoperative localisation of occult lesions of the breast (Paganelli et al. 1997). Both techniques require preoperative imaging of radioactivity accumulation in the target tissue. Preoperative imaging may be performed by planar or SPECT/CT images depending of complexity of the anatomical site of lesion (head and neck, abdomen). Often, presurgical imaging should be preferably carried out with SPECT/CT, which enables simultaneous detection of the distribution of the radiopharmaceutical and its precise anatomical location for an accurate planning of the surgical approach. Intraoperative detection of the *hot targets* is performed using a gamma probe, which leads to smaller and less traumatic excisions. The ROLL technique has mainly been used for the preoperative labelling of occult breast lesions, although this technique has been described in other oncological pathologies such as recurrence of thyroid cancer in non-palpable cervical lymph nodes (Tükenmez et al. 2007; Borsò et al. 2013), non-palpable colonic lesions (Rezzo et al. 2002), and localisation of pulmonary nodules during thoracoscopy (Sortini et al. 2006).

At present, the main clinical application of radioguided surgery in oncology is to identify the sentinel lymph node (SLN) and occult lesions or to find lesions that are difficult to locate intraoperatively. A recent review (Povoski et al. 2009) reports the concept that radioguided surgery is modifying the surgical management of many malignancies. This technique does not have any side effects, involves minimal dose radiation, and enables less invasive procedures with accurate information regarding the location and extent of disease as well as regarding the assessment of surgical resection margins. Furthermore, the approach reduces surgery time and shortens the patient's hospital stay, while still maintaining maximum benefit to the patient.

39.1 SENTINEL LYMPH NODE MAPPING IN EARLY BREAST CANCER

Over the last three decades, surgical treatment of breast cancer has become increasingly conservative, in particular by adopting limited tumour resections, such as lumpectomy or quadrantectomy, in place of the mutilating mastectomy (which is now reserved to few advanced, selected cases). Sentinel lymph node biopsy (SLNB) has further revolutionised the approach to early-stage breast cancer, by allowing minimally invasive staging of the axilla based on resection of few lymph nodes rather than the more aggressive complete lymph node dissection. In this regard, tumour status of axillary lymph nodes is the most significant prognostic factor for patients with early-stage breast cancer. Predictors of lymph node metastases include tumour size, lymph vascular invasion, tumour grade, and patient's age. Accurate assessment of the lymph node status (parameter N of the TNM staging system) is important not only for staging and prognosis but also for guiding treatment selection (Carter et al. 1989; Carlson et al. 2009).

The lymphatic system of the breast is classically made up of four intercommunicating lymphatic plexi: two superficial and two deep. The superficial plexi are located in the dermis (cutaneous plexus) and in the superficial subcutaneous region (subcutaneous plexus). One of the deep plexi is located in the mammary gland, including lobes and ducts (glandular plexus). This plexus, through lymphatic vessels that accompany the lactiferous ducts, communicates with a region of the subcutaneous plexus located immediately below the areola, known as the Sappey's sub-areolar plexus (Turner-Warwick 1959). The superficial plexi drain directly to the axillary lymph nodes. The deep plexi also drain to the axillae but may initially drain into intramammary and interpectoral lymph nodes. Breast lymphatic drainage may occur also into parasternal lymph nodes (*internal mammary* lymph nodes), although this drainage pattern is almost exclusive to the deep lymphatic plexi. Most of the lymph drains to the axillary lymph nodes, and consequently, in the case of breast cancer, they are the main location for metastasis.

Axillary lymph node dissection (ALND) has long remained a standard treatment for breast cancer, because it was thought to be the most accurate method for assessing spread of disease to the axillary lymph nodes. However, anatomical disruption caused by ALND may result in complications, such as lymphedema, nerve injury, and shoulder dysfunction, that may impair the quality of life.

The SLN is defined as the first node that receives lymphatic flow from a primary tumour site; therefore, the SLN should be the first node to be involved in metastasis. This concept assumes that lymphatic metastasis proceeds through an orderly pattern of lymphatic drainage from the primary site to each regional lymph node basin. In principle, a tumour-free SLN excludes metastatic involvement of other nodes. As a consequence, accurate identification of the SLN and its biopsy (with extensive histologic analysis) can reduce the number of ALNDs in SLN-negative patients, so that only patients who have clinically palpable axillary lymph nodes or positive nodes confirmed by ultrasound-guided fine-needle aspiration would undergo ALND de novo; on the other hand, a positive SLNB justifies ALND.

Thus, the fundamental issue concerning radioguided SLNB as the *standard of care* in breast cancer is its reliability as a prognostic factor of the true axillary lymph node status. Different approaches have been employed to assess how reliable is this technique, in order to ensure with certainty that if SLNB is negative and ALND is not performed, other axillary lymph nodes do not contain metastasis. In the initial studies, patients underwent SLNB and completion ALND in the same surgical session, regardless of the result of SLN analysis. SLN(s) and the remaining axillary lymph nodes were then analysed separately. As reviewed by Mariani et al., the results of these studies consistently showed that false-negative rates (the detection of metastasis in axillary lymph nodes when the SLN was tumour-free) only occurred in about 3%–7% of the cases (Mariani et al. 2001). False-negative SLNBs are very rare in patients with early breast cancer (Veronesi et al. 1999), probably because of the low rate of nodal involvement combined with accuracy of the procedure. Long-term follow-up of patients whose SLNB is negative and who do not undergo ALND can also prove the efficacy of the technique. Results of a recent meta-analysis based on 48 studies involving almost 15,000 patients with a median follow-up of 34 months show that only 0.3% of the patients develop axillary metastasis when ALND had not been performed after a negative SLNB (van der Ploeg et al. 2008). These results support the routine use of SLNB in the clinical management of patients with early breast cancer.

The American Society of Clinical Oncology in 2005 (Lyman et al. 2005) and more recently the British Association of Surgical Oncology (Association of Breast Surgery 2009) recommended SLNB as the method of staging early breast cancer in clinically node-negative patients. The European Association of Nuclear Medicine recommends SLNB in women who have a biopsy-proven carcinoma of the breast in whom definitive surgery and axillary node clearance is planned and in whom there are no palpable axillary lymph nodes (Buscombe et al. 2007).

From the histopathologic point of view, the resected SLN(s) can be further stratified as to contain macrometastases (>2 mm in size), micrometastases (between 0.2 and 2 mm), and submicrometastases (<0.2 mm), as specified in the latest edition of the Cancer Staging Manual of the American Joint Committee on Cancer (Edge et al. 2010). Such detailed classification is possible because attention of the pathologist can now focus on much fewer lymph nodes than those normally retrieved during conventional axillary dissection, so that a more detailed histopathologic examination of the SLN(s) can be carried out, for instance, obtaining more histologic sections (to encompass virtually the entire lymph node) and employing more sensitive techniques (immunohistochemistry in addition to haematoxylin and eosin and even molecular analysis).

Radiopharmaceuticals commonly employed for SLN mapping (SLNM) consist of colloidal particles labelled with ^{99m}Tc. A uniform number of small (<100 nm in diameter) colloid particles are essential to clear the radiocolloid from the interstitial space to the lymphatic channels and on to regional lymph nodes. ^{99m}Tc-nanocolloidal human serum albumin (in which about 80% of the particles have size between 40 and 50 nm, an overall 95% have size <80 nm, 4% have size between 80 and 100 nm, and only 1% >100 nm) is the radiopharmaceutical most commonly used in Europe for lymphoscintigraphy, while ^{99m}Tc-sulfur colloid (which is composed of larger particles and has a wider range of particle size distribution) is utilised in the United States. In most nuclear medicine centres around the world, for mapping of lymphatic drainage to the axilla, radiocolloids are injected either intradermally (at the skin projection just above the primary breast tumour site) or through the sub-areolar or peri-areolar route, with a mean radioactivity amount of 20 MBq in a volume of 0.2–0.4 mL (Mariani et al. 2001; Manca et al. 2013; Orsini et al. 2013). The injection site can be gently massaged after radiocolloid administration. After interstitial injection, particles constituting the radiocolloids are cleared by lymphatic drainage with a speed inversely proportional to their size.

Nevertheless, the optimal site of the radioactive tracer injection is still controversial, in particular whether it should be *superficial* (sub-areolar, peri-areolar, intradermal) or *deep* (peritumoural, intratumoural) (Pelosi et al. 2004; Orsini et al. 2013). The superficial injection is based on the concept that there is a common lymphatic drainage pathway from the whole breast to the axilla, thus implying that the site of injection is irrelevant for SLN identification. The superficial injection techniques have several advantages; they are easier to perform in all patients, including those with non-palpable lesions, and axillary lymph nodes are rapidly and intensely visualised.

A sub-dermal injection of radiotracer just above the primary breast tumour site is sufficient for all but the deepest tumours. A peritumoural injection of 0.5 mL (at different spots equatorially around the tumour) is recommended in all deep tumours or using a peri-areolar or sub-areolar injection in particular in upper quadrant tumours to avoid possible crosstalk due to short distance between peritumoural depots and the axillary sentinel node (Pelosi et al. 2004; Chakera et al. 2005). Nearly all breast lymphatic drainage passes through the sub-areolar plexus of Sappey and then into the axillary nodal basin; hence, sub-areolar injections are potential approaches for the injection of mapping agents, also in patients with non-palpable or multifocal/multicentric tumours. A potential disadvantage of the sub-areolar injection route is that approximately 10% of breast cancers may demonstrate non-axillary lymphatic drainage, the SLNs being located in the internal mammary or supraclavicular nodal basins; hence, not all breast tumours will have the same drainage patterns as the overlying skin and nipple areas. On the other hand, the issue of whether or not to perform biopsy of SLNs located in the internal mammary chain is still highly debated from the purely oncologic surgery point of view.

Lymphoscintigraphy is performed in most nuclear medicine centres as an integral, mandatory step for radioguided SLNB. It is generally performed in the afternoon of the day preceding surgery if the operation is scheduled in the early morning or on the same day 4–6 h prior to surgery, depending on logistics of the institution. For lymphoscintigraphy, the patient lies supine on the gamma-camera imaging table, with her arm in the same position as during surgery (extended laterally at 90°). Planar anterior and 45° anterior oblique and lateral images are generally acquired (see Figures 39.1 and 39.2). Images should be recorded within 10 min after radiocolloid injection, but, if required, later images can be acquired 2–3 h or up to 16–18 h afterwards (see Figure 39.3). The first hotspots identified along the pathways of lymphatic drainage visualised by the radiocolloid are defined as SLNs. The anatomical site of any suspected SLN can be localised in the skin using a ^{57}Co source and marked with a small spot of indelible ink (Mariani et al. 2001). Lymphoscintigraphy is normally performed with conventional gamma cameras. When the gamma camera is combined with a CT component to constitute a hybrid SPECT/CT, the fused images so obtained are highly useful, especially in case of complex anatomical regions and/or in case of unusual lymphatic drainage patterns. In fact, they provide to the surgeon a morphologic and functional roadmap (CT component and SPECT component, respectively) for planning the procedure with minimal surgical access and operating time (see Figure 39.4).

Intraoperative SLN detection is performed with a handheld gamma probe. Intraoperative probes are capable of detecting a very low flow of gamma photons. The gamma probe is generally a cylindrical tube 1–2 cm in diameter and about 15 cm long, at the tip of which there is a sensitive part represented either by a gamma-ray detector crystal [such as NaI(Tl) and CsI(Tl)] or by a semiconductor-type detector (such as CdTe and CdZnTe). To ensure sterility, the gamma probe is placed into a disposable, sterile flexible sleeve. The gamma probe is connected, by cable or wireless by Bluetooth technology, with an electronic unit which analyses the signal, displays the count rate, and emits a sound (beeps) whose tone/pitch is modulated according the level of radioactivity detected. The intraoperative detection probes currently available have a very high sensitivity to gamma photons emitted by technetium-99m. Moreover, handheld gamma probes are nowadays smaller and more manoeuvrable, with better shielding for directional detection of gamma rays, thus making the method even more applicable. Moreover, the recently developed portable gamma

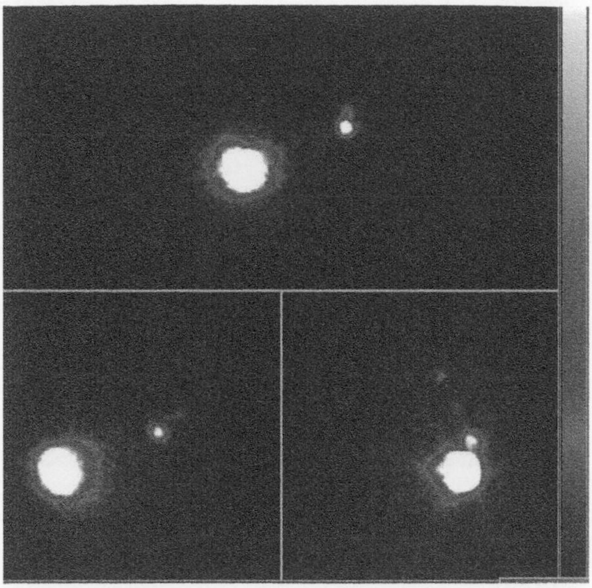

FIGURE 39.1 Planar lymphoscintigraphy in the oblique anterior view (upper panel), lateral view (lower left panel), and anterior view (lower right panel) obtained in a patient with left breast cancer following sub-dermal radiocolloid injection on the cutaneous projection of the tumour, showing one left axillary SLN and visualisation of a further radioactive second-echelon lymph node.

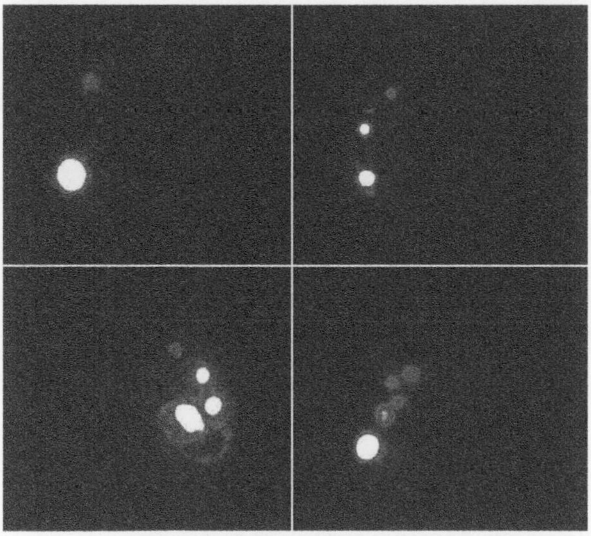

FIGURE 39.2 Planar lymphoscintigraphic imaging obtained in the anterior view in four different patients with breast cancer. Upper left panel: visualisation of one single SLN in the right axilla after intradermal injection. Upper right panel: one right axillary SLN and visualisation of further radioactive axillary second-echelon lymph nodes. Left lower panel: two lymphatic pathways leading to two left axillary SLNs with visualisation of a second-echelon radioactive axillary lymph node. Lower right panel: four right axillary SLNs after intradermal injection on the cutaneous projection of a cancer in the external-lower quadrant of the breast.

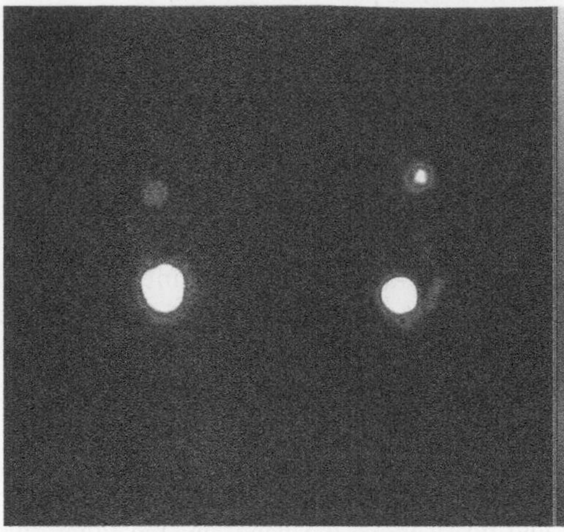

FIGURE 39.3 Planar lymphoscintigraphy in the anterior view obtained in a patient with bilateral breast cancers, showing one SLN for each axilla.

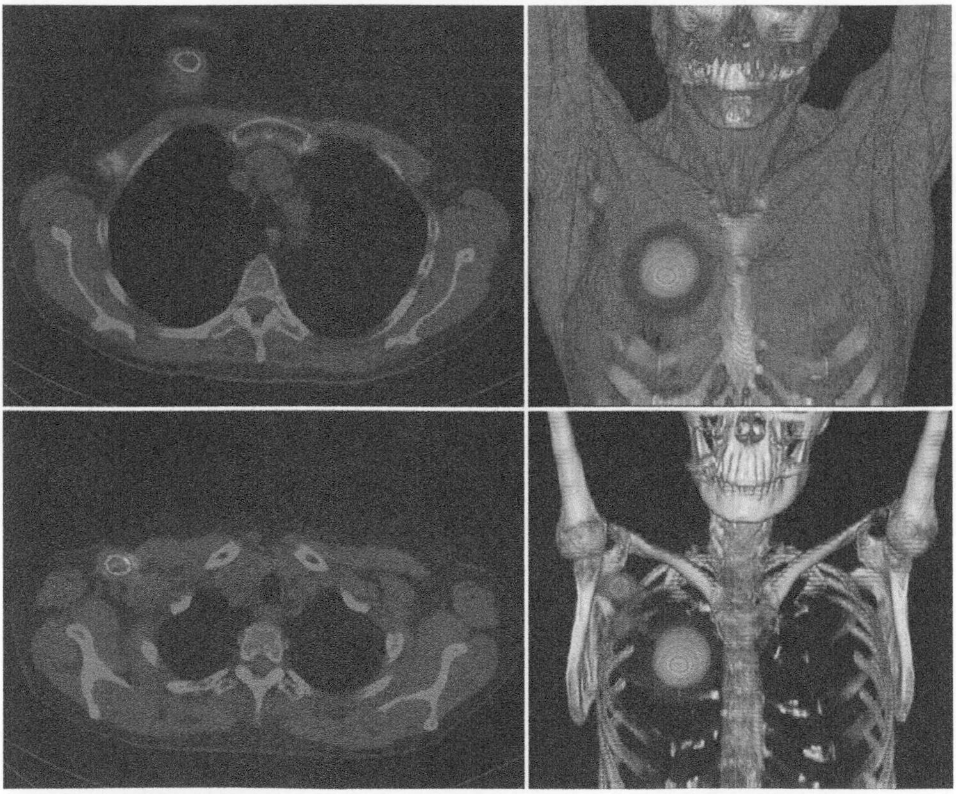

FIGURE 39.4 Fused transaxial SPECT/CT sections showing two SLNs following intradermal injection (upper and lower left panels) in a patient with right breast cancer. Three-dimensional SPECT/CT volume rendering images obtained by selecting the soft tissue window (upper right panel) and the bone window (lower right panel), demonstrating better anatomo-topographic localisation of the two SLNs.

cameras enable real-time scintigraphic imaging of the surgical field, for checking the surgical bed for any residual radioactive spot after SLN resection. This interaction between technologies and medical disciplines permits to continuously refine the methodology and to improve the outcomes of radioguided surgery.

Under general or local anaesthesia according to the findings of preoperative SLNM, the surgeon uses the probe to guide dissection to the hot node(s) and places the probe in the surgical bed after node excision to confirm removal of the hot node(s). Counts are recorded with the probe in the operative field, over the node before excision (in vivo), and after excision (ex vivo). Comparative studies suggest that SLNs are identified more frequently with radiocolloid than with blue dye and that the combination of both agents is associated with a higher sensitivity in the detection of SLNs with metastatic disease (Tsugawa et al. 2000; Takei et al. 2006).

To ensure and maintain the high accuracy and low false-negative rate of the radioguided SLN procedure, several selection criteria and relative contraindications for the procedure have been reported (Filippakis and Zografos 2007). The absolute contraindications for SLNB include patients with palpable axillary nodes or other evidence of axillary node metastatic disease, patients with large breast cancer above stage T2 (>5 cm), patients with multifocal or multicentric cancer (although the prevailing trend in these patients is now to adopt the sub-areolar or peri-areolar route of radiocolloid injection) and inflammatory breast cancer, and patients who previously underwent any surgical procedures in the axilla that may have altered the regional pattern of lymphatic drainage. Some additional contraindications to SLNB in patients with breast cancer are still debated, for instance, patients previously treated with wide excisional biopsy or patients undergoing neoadjuvant chemotherapy for locally advanced cancer. In these patients, the potential benefit of SLNB should be considered on a case-by-case basis (Buscombe et al. 2007; Orsini et al. 2013).

Since radioguided SLNB requires close integration among different specialists (nuclear physician, oncologic surgeon, medical oncologist, pathologist, medical physicist), an initial learning phase is recommended to harmonise and optimise interaction between such different components involved, in order to merge into a real multidisciplinary *team work*. It is often considered that 20–40 procedures with completion ALND are sufficient in order to implement radioguided SLNB into the routine clinical practice of a given hospital. These numbers, however, are highly variable and SLNB should only be introduced to clinical practice where the team demonstrates high identification rate and accuracy (Lyman et al. 2005).

39.2 RADIOGUIDED OCCULT LESION LOCALISATION

Breast cancer is the most frequent malignant tumour in women, and its treatment is constantly evolving towards more conservative techniques. In fact, screening mammography allows detection of an increasing number of locally invasive, occult, or even in situ carcinomas (Franceschi et al. 1990; Goedde et al. 1992). In 1997, Paganelli and coworkers proposed a radionuclide method to localise non-palpable lesions called ROLL, which is based on intratumoural injection of a suitable radiopharmaceutical (usually ^{99m}Tc-macroaggregated albumin, ^{99m}Tc-MAA, whose large particle does not appreciably migrate from the site of interstitial administration), preoperative scintigraphy to display the injection site, and surgical excision of the lesion localised with the aid of an intraoperative gamma detector probe (Paganelli et al. 1997). This procedure allows fast and accurate surgical removal of occult lesions and has several advantages in comparison with traditional procedures (De Cicco et al. 2004; van der Ploeg et al. 2008a). The goal of ROLL is to ensure precise preoperative localisation of the lesion, its complete removal and sufficient margin of healthy tissue, and accurate intraoperative histological examination to identify any early invasive component, particularly for intraductal carcinomas. Efficient multidisciplinary cooperation is crucial to attain this goal. Following the mammographic or ultrasound detection of a suspicious breast lesion (typically as a cluster of microcalcifications, opaque spot or parenchymal distortion), the use of ROLL facilitates lesion localisation by intratumoural injection of the radioactive particles under stereotactic or ultrasound guidance. The ROLL procedure is not applicable in women with diffuse microcalcifications and multifocal or multicentre lesions.

39.2.1 ROLL Technique

A single amount of 7–12 MBq ^{99m}Tc-MAA (particle size 10–150 μm) is injected into the breast lesion. After interstitial injection, such MAA particles remain almost stationary, with minimal local diffusion. Particle degradation, slow lymphatic absorption, and phagocytosis constitute the principal mechanisms for ^{99m}Tc-MAA clearance from the injection site. When the primary lesion has no definite mass but consists only of microcalcifications, the entire radioactive bolus is injected among these calcifications. Using the same needle, a radiographic contrast medium can be injected immediately after tracer injection, in order to confirm by mammography satisfactory positioning of the radioactive marker. Then, a few minutes after radiopharmaceutical injection, scintigraphy is performed in anterior and lateral views to obtain information on its localisation. The patient is positioned supine with the arm ipsilateral to the lesion in maximum abduction in order to achieve the same position as on the surgical bed. At the end of the examination, both the anterior and the lateral cutaneous projections of the lesion are marked on the overlying skin. The surgeon localises the lesion using the gamma probe placed on the previously marked breast skin. Surgical excision of the occult lesion is then carried out, and correct lesion resection is confirmed by high level of radioactivity in the resected tissue and no residual radioactivity in post-excision biopsy cavity evaluated by gamma probe. The excised specimen is marked for correct orientation (for subsequent histologic analysis), and the ex vivo tissue specimen is imaged by scintigraphy and mammography to verify the presence of the lesion within the specimen itself (De Cicco et al. 2002). ROLL enables to reduce the volume of healthy breast tissue to be excised, associated with good lesion centring and satisfactory cosmetic results. Different studies have addressed the feasibility of ROLL in connection with lymphoscintigraphy and SLNB. To this purpose, the same radiopharmaceutical (^{99m}Tc-nanocolloidal albumin) can be used both for ROLL (injecting half the radioactivity amount intratumourally) and for SLNB (injecting the remaining half superficially to facilitate its drainage to the regional lymph nodes) (Feggi et al. 2001).

39.3 OTHER APPLICATIONS OF SENTINEL NODE MAPPING UNDER CLINICAL VALIDATION

As described earlier, radioguided SLNM procedures in patients with breast cancer or cutaneous melanoma have already achieved the status of standard of care for N-staging purposes, so that further management of cancer patients after primary surgery can adequately be planned. Nevertheless, potential benefits of this approach can be envisaged for other solid cancers of plastic surgery interest, with the rationale of accurately mapping the status of loco-regional lymph nodes, therefore of avoiding aggressive procedures based on extensive lymph node dissection.

The general term *radioguided surgery* includes a set of pre-, intra-, and post-operative techniques and procedures that are designed to optimise oncologic surgery. The feature that most obviously characterises radioguided surgery is the intraoperative use of a handheld radioactivity counting probe (most often the so-called gamma probe) that facilitates the task of the surgeon, that is, identification and removal of the target tissue, either a lymph node or the tumour itself, by virtue of preferential radioactivity accumulation in the target tissue. Intraoperative exploration of the surgical field with the gamma probe (which has recently evolved so as to allow intraoperative imaging as well) is made possible by a set of preoperative techniques employed by the nuclear medicine physician to achieve accumulation of the radiopharmaceutical in the specific target lesion.

Several clinical trials have explored the feasibility and accuracy of SLNM in oncologic conditions, regarding in particular squamous cellular carcinomas; these include, among others, penile cancer, vulvar cancer, and anal tumours, as well as tumours of the oral cavity. In squamous cell carcinomas, the pattern of tumour dissemination is predominantly lymphogenic, although the hematogenous route is also possible. In all these clinical settings, SLNM procedures should still be considered within well-designed experimental clinical trials, as further investigations are required for defining the long-term clinical impact of such procedures. Technological advances in nuclear medicine equipment (including especially SPECT/CT) and the use of dedicated intraoperative gamma cameras may improve SLNB outcomes in all these tumours, where SLNM does not yet represent the standard of care. Investigations are also ongoing regarding the development of new radiotracers for lymphatic mapping.

The whole procedure of SLNM for SLNB was first originally proposed for *penile cancer* (Cabanas 1997), in order to identify the exact side of possible tumour metastasis in the loco-regional lymph nodes. In fact, in penile cancer, the injection of a radiotracer and/or blue dye is easy to perform, due to the easily accessible superficial localisation of the tumour. Furthermore, penile cancer is a typical case of possible ambiguous lymphatic drainage for its anatomical structure in midline position; in this condition, the application of SLNM procedures is expected to aid in identifying the occurrence of ipsi- or bilateral drainage.

The feasibility of radioguided SLNB for penile cancer is currently being increasingly explored because of the high incidence of morbidity (such as wound infection and lymphedema) after standard surgery with full lymph node dissection. Moreover, the introduction of microinvasive surgical techniques implies the possibility to achieve proper evaluation of the lymph node status, even with a small surgical incision. This goal can be reached by analysing SLNs with serial sectioning and extensive histopathologic analysis, including immunohistochemical staining.

SLNM in penile cancer is very promising in patients with clinically negative lymph nodes, in order to select patients who can benefit from lymph node dissection (Horenblas et al. 2008). In fact, there is no consensus on the management of patients with clinically node-negative penile carcinoma, in whom radical inguinal lymph node dissection is routinely performed, although it turns out to be unnecessary in approximately 75%–80% of patients (Wespes 2007). In the earlier phases of development of SLNM for penile cancer, there were reservations about the accuracy/reliability of SLNB for penile cancer, because of the supposedly long learning curve associated with the procedure and because of possible false-negative cases (reported in up to 21% of the procedures) (Kroon et al. 2004). At present, radioguided SLNB has evolved into a reliable minimally invasive staging technique with an associated high sensitivity (90%–95%) and low morbidity in experienced centres (Leijte et al. 2007); as a consequence, this procedure has been recently included in the European Association of Urology guidelines on penile cancer, with level of evidence 2b (Pizzocaro et al. 2010).

Patients with >T1G2 penile tumours and negative groins (as defined by ultrasound-guided fine-needle cytology) are the best candidates for SLNB. In fact, it has been suggested that extensive metastatic involvement of a SLN can lead to blocked inflow and rerouting of lymph fluid to a *neo-sentinel node* that may not yet contain tumour cells, thus spuriously causing a false-negative result (Leijte et al. 2009).

The highest sensitivity/detection rate is achieved using both radiocolloid and blue dye for SLNM (Sadeghi et al. 2012). Administration of the radiopharmaceutical/blue dye is usually performed by intradermal peritumoural injection of the radiocolloid, with the recommendation of injecting within a 1 cm radius from the primary tumour (or from the surgical scar in case of prior excision of the primary tumour). Immediately after injection, dynamic lymphoscintigraphy is generally performed in order to identify lymphatic ducts and the first directly draining lymph nodes. The early planar images visualise the first draining lymph nodes in about 85% of the cases. Nevertheless, delayed static planar imaging (after 20–30 min and/or 2 h, depending on protocols) is generally acquired in order to identify slow drainage.

Generally, the lymph nodes draining directly from the injection site are classified as SLNs. In the case of multiple visible nodes without visible afferent vessels, the first node appearing in a basin is considered to be the SLN. The most frequently visualised lymphatic drainage pattern is bilateral drainage to both groins (80%). This pattern is, however, asynchronous in two-thirds of the cases, and visualisation of the contralateral lymph nodes is often only possible on delayed imaging (Valdés Olmos et al. 2001). Drainage from the injection site mostly occurs through one or two visualised afferent lymphatic ducts leading to one or two SLNs in each groin. In some cases, a cluster of inguinal lymph nodes is observed. During the intraoperative phase, the surgeon removes the SLN(s) with the help of gamma probe, for histopathologic analysis. If the SLN is tumour positive, completion ipsilateral lymphadenectomy is performed. Groins with tumour-free SLNs are managed with close surveillance, thereby avoiding the morbidity associated with de novo lymphadenectomy.

However, there are still important differences in the clinical protocols employed worldwide; harmonisation of the different phases of the SLNB procedure in patients with penile cancer (including how to implement the learning curve) is therefore highly needed (Sadeghi et al. 2012). SPECT/CT imaging contributes to better anatomical localisation of the SLNs, especially in order to discriminate inguinal (superficial) from iliac (deep) lymph nodes (see Figures 39.5 and 39.6) (Leijte et al. 2008). Moreover, the introduction of a hybrid fluorescent-radioactive imaging agent (indocyanine green-^{99m}Tc-nanocolloid) has recently been tested in penile cancer patients, and the conclusion was reached that fluorescence guidance can be considered as an added value for the intraoperative SLN search (Brouwer et al. 2012).

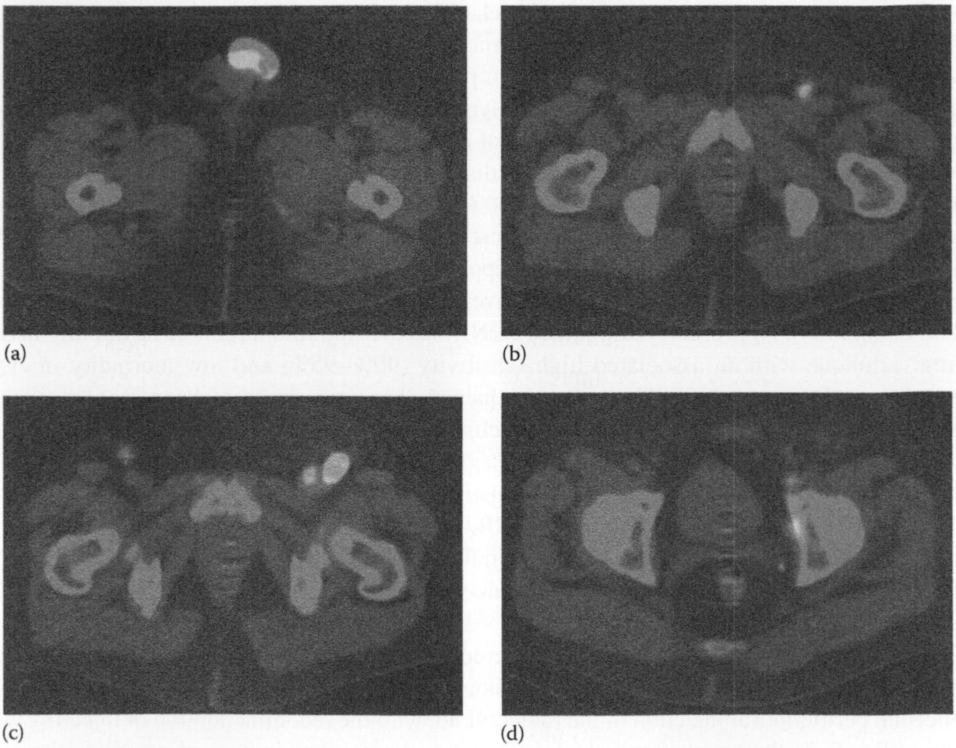

(a) (b) (c) (d)

FIGURE 39.5 Fused transaxial SPECT/CT sections obtained at various levels during lymphoscintigraphy in a patient with penile squamous cell carcinoma. After administration of ^{99m}Tc-nanocolloidal albumin (injection site in panel (a), there is visualisation of two left and one right superficial inguinal SLNs (b and c); in addition, lymphatic drainage visualises radiocolloid accumulation also in deep SLNs, corresponding to the external iliac area (d).

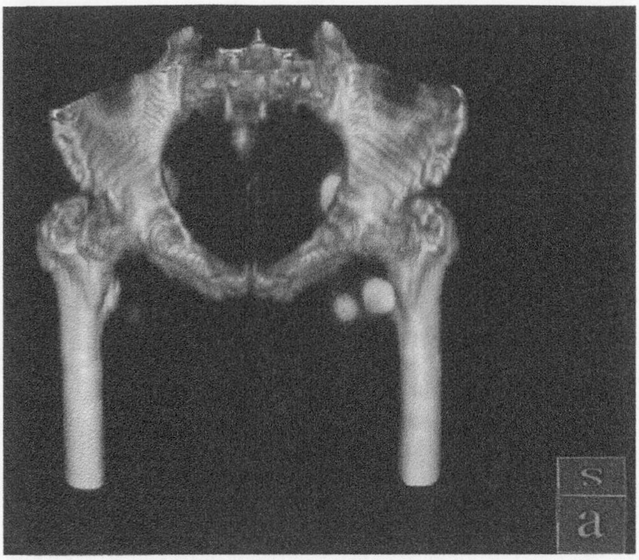

FIGURE 39.6 Three-dimensional SPECT/CT volume rendering of SLNM in the same patient as in Figure 39.1 (penile cancer), obtained through selecting the window for bone. Clear anatomo-topographic localisation of the SLNs shown in Figure 39.1.

As for the majority of other solid tumours, also in patients with early malignant tumours of the vulva, cervix, and uterus, the most important prognostic factor for optimising the therapeutic strategy is tumour status of loco-regional lymph nodes. *Vulvar cancer* usually metastasises to inguinal lymph node(s) that can easily be explored clinically but are often enlarged due simply to inflammatory processes. Moreover, lymphatic drainage from the vulva frequently crosses the midline. Based on this consideration, lymphoscintigraphy and radioguided SLNB holds potential for staging purposes, although this procedure is still in an experimental phase of clinical validation. In particular, the technique of radiocolloid injection has not yet been standardised, and there is no consensus on choice of the optimal radiocolloid, site of injection, protocols for scintigraphic acquisition, etc.

Nevertheless, despite the aforementioned limitations, the SLNM/SLNB application that is more close to achieving a recognised status of standard of care among all gynaecologic malignancies is probably radioguided SLNB in patients with vulvar cancer. Vulvar cancer is an excellent target for the SLN concept because the tumour is easy to inject with blue dye and/or radiocolloid and because lymph drainage is predictable to one or both of the groins. Standard treatment consists of wide radical excision of the primary tumour and inguino-femoral lymphadenectomy. With the use of such current surgical technique, half the women who undergo treatment for vulvar cancer suffer from post-surgical complication, such as wound disruption and acute infections, lymphedema, and cellulitis (Gaarenstroom et al. 2003). Concerning the prognostic value of regional lymph node status in vulvar cancer, the 5-year survival rate decreases from 94.7% when the nodes are negative to 62% when they are positive (Burger et al. 1995). When first diagnosed, 30% of cases show nodal invasion, 10%–20% of these tumour-positive lymph nodes being in the pelvic area. When the tumour is confined to one side of the vulva, more than 80% of nodal metastases are ipsilateral.

Similarly as for other applications in solid epithelial cancers, the aim of SLNM/SLNB in patients with vulvar cancer is to provide opportunity for early intervention in women with SLN metastases and to spare the morbidity of unnecessary regional lymphadenectomy to SLN-negative women.

The superficial location of vulvar tumours makes tracer injection easier than in patients with other gynaecological tumours, which explains the greater experience reported in the literature for this application (van der Zee et al. 2008). Inguino-femoral lymphadenectomy is performed only when metastasis in SLN(s) has been confirmed. The results reported so far show a decrease in

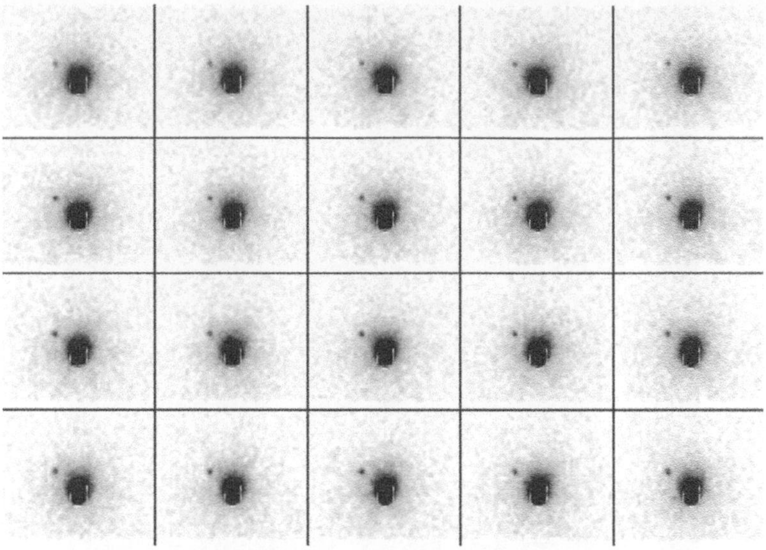

FIGURE 39.7 Dynamic lymphoscintigraphy recorded in the anterior view at the frame rate of 1/min (64 × 64 matrix), starting about 2–3 min after peritumoural injection of ^{99m}Tc-nanocolloidal albumin in a patient with vulvar cancer. Radiocolloid migration is very fast, so that a right inguinal SLN is already visible in the first frame of dynamic recording. Intensity of uptake continues to rise throughout the 20 min recording period.

morbidity both in the short term (wound breakdown, cellulitis) and in the long term (lymphoedema) in patients who underwent SLN biopsy versus patients submitted to de novo lymphadenectomy.

Early studies in vulvar cancer were performed with blue dye as the sole imaging agent, with a detection rate approaching 90% (86%–88%) (Levenback et al. 2001); the introduction of radiocolloid and radioguidance has improved the detection rate to 95%–100% (Hampl et al. 2008; Johann et al. 2008). Currently, the accepted SLNM technique includes injection of both tracers (radiocolloid and blue dye) after the application of an anaesthetic cream or spray such as lidocaine or ethyl chloride. Lymphoscintigraphy starts with a dynamic acquisition and planar images (see Figure 39.7). SPECT/CT is generally performed in the delayed phase, in order to include also lymph nodes with slow draiange and delayed viualisation.

Indications to SLNM in patients with vulvar cancer are well established: SLNM/SLNB is accepted as standard of care in squamous cell carcinoma in stages Ib–II less than 4 cm in size, without presurgical detection of nodal metastases. Although there is more scarce reported experience, SLNB in vulvar melanoma is also accepted with the same indications as cutaneous melanoma (Trifirò et al. 2010).

Despite the fact that the vulva is a central, midline organ, the rate of unilateral drainage is quite high (Vidal-Sicart et al. 2007). In this regard, several groups avoid bilateral lymphadenectomy when the tumour and its lymphatic drainage are unilateral, while other groups prefer to perform complete contralateral lymphadenectomy to ensure against a possible lymphatic blockage due to massive nodal metastatic invasion. The advantages of SLNB over de novo, standard lymphadenectomy include reduced morbidity, possible upstaging, and, according to some authors, reduced surgical time (Hefler et al. 2008).

Tomographic acquisitions (SPECT/CT) help in the 3D location of the SLN, but not in the surgical management or the final number of depicted nodes. There are only three published studies, all performed in vulvo-vaginal melanoma, showing a higher detection rate due to the increase in the number of SLN locations identified by SPECT/CT versus planar imaging (Beneder et al. 2008; Kobayashi et al. 2009; Trifirò et al. 2010).

Regarding the use of novel imaging agents, the use of a multispectral fluorescence camera and of indocyanine green has been reported in 10 patients with vulvar cancer (Crane et al. 2010).

During surgery, the fluorescence camera allows the visualisation of the fluorescent tracer, precisely locating the SLN. The detection rate using a handheld gamma probe was compared with the fluorescence camera and blue dye, and better results were found with the new tracer (89% versus 72%).

SLNB in squamous cellular *carcinoma of the anal canal* as standard of care is a further challenge for radioguided surgery. This procedure has been demonstrated to be technically feasible, with SLN visualisation rates generally reported in 75%–100% of the patients (Mistrangelo et al. 2009). At diagnosis, synchronous inguinal metastasis occurs in 10%–25% of patients and constitutes an independent prognostic factor for local failure and overall mortality (Gerard et al. 2001). Most inguinal lymph nodes site of metastasis (40%–50%) are smaller than 5 mm in size (Wade et al. 1989).

At present, the standard treatment is radiochemotherapy, which achieves similar clinical outcomes as surgery, without however requiring a permanent stoma (Nigro et al. 1974). This squamous cell carcinoma has a low tendency to spread by a hematogenous route, although it may also spread to loco-regional lymph nodes. Depending on its location, it may drain to the perirectal, iliac, or inguinal nodes. Inguinal lymph node metastases cannot be accurately predicted by either clinical examination or imaging techniques. According to current guidelines, selection of patients with anal cancer for irradiation including the groin is based on tumour size, palpation, ultrasound, and fine-needle cytology (Benson et al. 2012). Thus, current staging of anal cancer may result in under-treatment for patients with small tumours and, conversely, in overtreatment for patients with large tumours.

SLNB can be considered as a minimally invasive, safe, and effective method for adequate pretreatment lymph node staging in patients with squamous cell carcinoma of the anal canal (De Nardi et al. 2011) and has proven to be more reliable for inguinal lymph node staging than the currently available imaging techniques (Mistrangelo et al. 2009). In this particular application, SLNB allows to identify those patients for whom inguinal radiotherapy is not necessary, thereby sparing the unwanted side effects of such treatment. Recent investigations performed in patients with anal cancer have shown the feasibility and accuracy of radioguided SLNB, with better performance even if compared to [^{18}F]FDG-positron emission tomography (PET)/CT (which has sensitivity close to 100%, but specificity lower than that of SLNB) (Mistrangelo et al. 2010).

Similarly as accepted in the case of other tumours, SLN biopsy should not be performed in patients presenting with clinically positive lymph nodes (Krontiras and Bland 2003). Clinically obvious nodal involvement and lymphatic invasion have been related with obstruction of the normal drainage pathways. In this setting, lymphatic drainage will occur via alternative routes to secondary non-SLNs, making SLNM/SLNB unreliable and possibly associated with high false-negative rates. Thus, suspicious palpable lymphadenopathy should be considered a formal contraindication to SLNM/SLNB.

The anal canal is relatively easy to assess. Thus, during digital examination, it is possible to define size and location of the tumour, therefore identifying exactly where the radiocolloid or the blue dye should be injected. SLNM/SLNB generally consists of combined injection of patent blue dye and of radiocolloid, followed by intraoperative localisation of lymph nodes that concentrate these markers. Preoperative lymphoscintigraphy (see Figures 39.8 and 39.9) and gamma-probe mapping are routinely employed to localise the SLN(s) and to search for bilateral inguinal SLNs. Such bilateral exploration seems to be particularly important for those tumours involving the midline of the anal canal, in which diffusion to both inguinal lymphatic basins is expected. Radioguidance makes the detection of SLNs technically easier and less time-consuming than inguinal exploration based solely on visualisation of the blue dye (Damin et al. 2006).

At present, there are no publications regarding the advantages of SPECT/CT imaging, intraoperative imaging, and new combined imaging agents in patients with tumours of the anal cancer, even if such novel combined approaches have been applied with excellent results to colorectal cancer SLNM (Kusano et al. 2008).

It should be noted that because of the reported occurrence of inguinal lymph node metastasis after a tumour-negative SLNB, special caution must be adopted for considering this procedure as the standard of care in all patients with anal carcinoma, in order to avoid under-treatment of patients

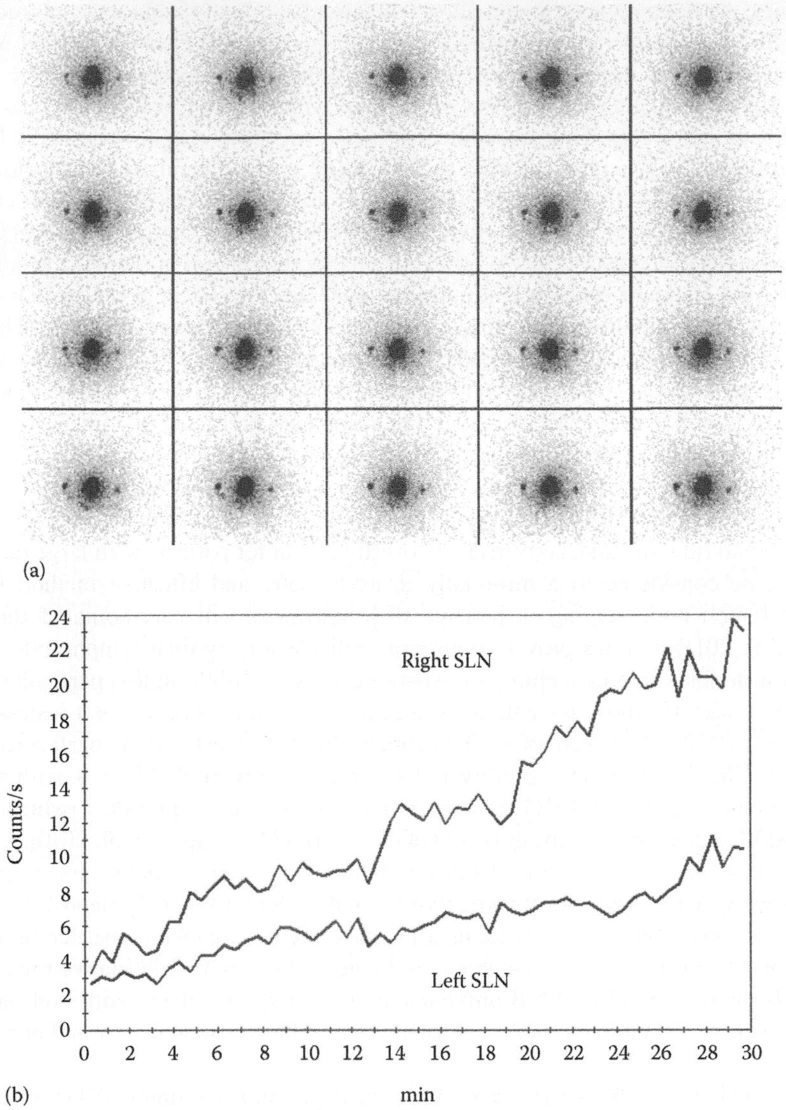

FIGURE 39.8 Dynamic lymphoscintigraphy recorded in the anterior view at the frame rate of 1/min (64 × 64 matrix), starting about 2–3 min after peritumoural injection of ^{99m}Tc-nanocolloidal albumin in a patient with cancer of the anal canal. (a) Individual frames, showing very fast radiocolloid migration, so that inguinal SLNs are already visible in the first frame of dynamic recording, both on the right side (earlier and more intense) and on the left side (apparently a single SLN). Intensity of uptake continues to rise throughout the 20 min recording period, as shown in (b).

who would otherwise benefit from inguinal radiotherapy. In this regard, because of the low incidence of this tumour, multi-institutional studies should be implemented to assess the effect of this technique on clinical outcomes before it can be systematically implemented into clinical practice. Furthermore, patients should be referred to specialised centres to allow enrollment on to the appropriate trials (De Jong et al. 2010).

Finally, applications of radioguided surgery, and especially of SLNB, are growing also in patients with squamous cell *carcinoma of the head and neck* region. The most important applications of SLNM/SLNB for tumours of this region concern cancers of the oral cavity (Calabrese et al. 2008). Similarly as in the case of cutaneous melanoma located in the head and neck region,

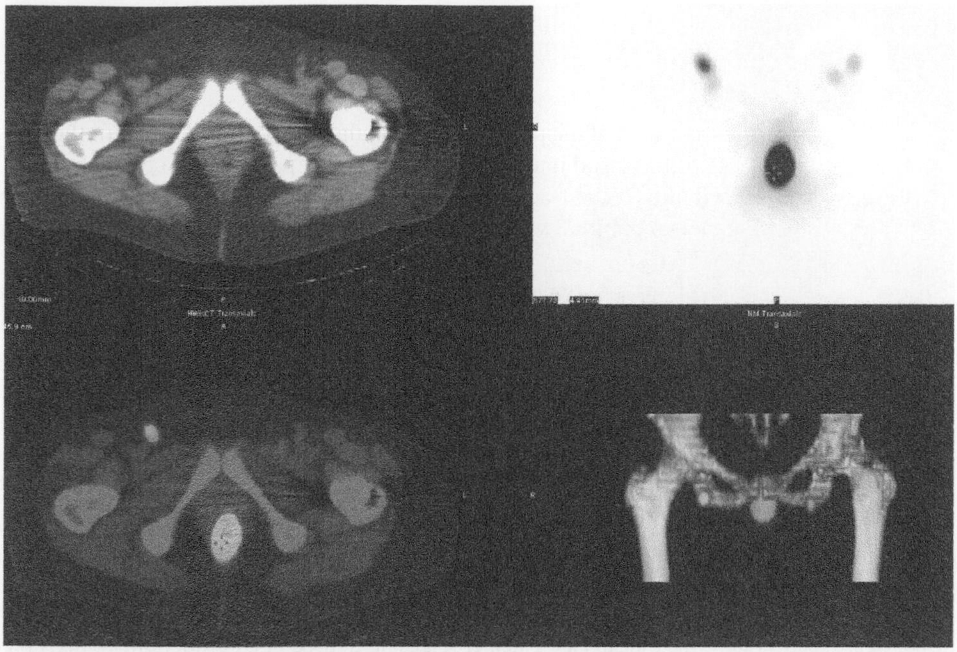

FIGURE 39.9 SPECT/CT imaging obtained during SLNM in the same patient as in Figure 39.4 (cancer of the anal canal). Transaxial CT section (upper left panel), SPECT section (upper right panel), fused SPECT/CT (lower left panel), and 3D SPECT/CT volume rendering obtained through selecting the window for bone (lower right panel). Clearer anatomo-topographic localisation of the SLNs shown in Figure 39.4, demonstrating that on the left side there are actually two SLNs (while planar imaging only showed one SLN).

tumour status of loco-regional lymph nodes is an important prognostic factor in patients with head and neck cancers, in whom cervical node dissection has a potential curative role. In these patients, radioguided SLNB is emerging as a highly promising modality to stage the clinical and radiological N0 neck, considering the poor sensitivity of other commonly used radiologic and nuclear medicine staging modalities. A positive SLN is considered as an unfavourable prognostic factor (Kovács et al. 2009).

At present, the management of clinically node-negative patients with head and neck cancer remains controversial, because the probability of micrometastasis is about 20% in these patients and their management is still debated, especially for what concerns prophylactic neck node dissection versus a wait-and-see approach. SLNB has the potential of enabling accurate selection of patients for elective lymph node dissection. The anatomy of lymph nodes in the head and neck region is very complex, and the patterns of lymph drainage from the oral cavity, oropharynx, larynx, and hypopharynx exhibit numerous inter-individual variations even from the same primary tumour site. Moreover, lymph drainage from a primary tumour located in a given side may cross the midline, or for primary tumours located in/around the midline, it may be directed to either side. While lymphoscintigraphic mapping offers definite advantages over the blue-dye technique as a guide to SLNB, the procedure is still experimental and is therefore to be employed only within controlled clinical trials before its feasibility and accuracy for routine clinical application become clearly established.

SLNM/SLNB has been used to stage T1 or T2 lesions (Paleri et al. 2005; Civantos et al. 2008), although for T2 tumours several authors find selective neck dissection more appropriate in view of the high risk of nodal metastasis. In general, patients with trans-orally resectable T1–T2 tumours and with negative lymph node assessment on clinical and radiological examination (including FNAC) are considered for SLNB.

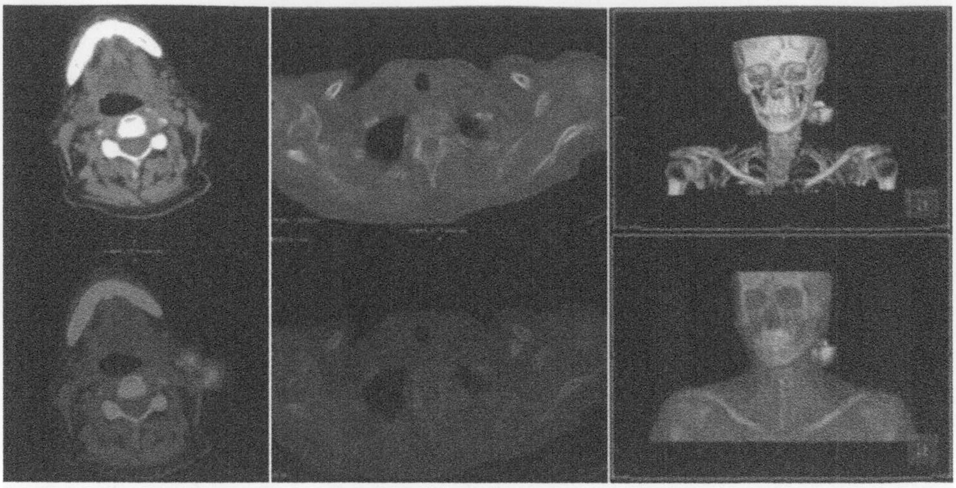

FIGURE 39.10 SLNM in a patient with melanoma located in the left sub-auricular region. Left panels show the transaxial CT (upper image) and fused SPECT/CT (lower image) sections obtained at the level of the post-surgical scar (where ^{99m}Tc-nanocolloidal albumin was injected; injection corresponds to the more external radioactivity accumulation, while one area of radiocolloid uptake) very close to the injection site is also visualised. Centre panels show the transaxial CT (upper image) and fused SPECT/CT (lower image) sections obtained at the level of supraclavicular SLN. Right panels show 3D SPECT/CT volume rendering obtained through selecting the window for muscle (lower image) and for bone (upper image), respectively; the images show clear anatomo-topographic localisation of the left supraclavicular SLN, while intense radioactivity accumulation at the injection site masks the SLN better depicted in the left panels.

Early results regarding accuracy of SLNB in patients with oral cavity malignancies, in whom both SLNB and completion selective neck dissection were performed, showed quite accurate staging of regional lymph nodes, with a 96% negative predictive value (Civantos et al. 2010).

Lymphoscintigraphy for SLNM is generally performed in the afternoon or some hours before the scheduled time for surgery. After peritumoural or intratumoural radiocolloid injection, both planar lymphoscintigraphy and SPECT/CT imaging are generally acquired (see Figure 39.10). Intraoperatively, the search for the radioactive SLNs is generally performed with a conventional handheld gamma probe. However, the advent of new techniques such as the use of a portable gamma camera for intraoperative SLN detection or the concomitant injection of radiolabelled and fluorescent colloidal agents may improve accuracy of SLNB in head and neck cancers, especially when the injection site is close to the SLN basin; such combined imaging may in fact help the surgeon to localise the SLNs in relation to the anatomic level in the neck (Vermeeren et al. 2010).

SPECT/CT imaging allows SLN visualisation in relation to anatomical structures, and 3D reconstructions help the surgeon to better plan the optimal surgical approach. In fact, in the head and neck area, it is important to identify the relation of SLNs to several vital vascular and neural structures, as well as other anatomical structures (such as the mandible, parotid gland, jugular vein, and sternocleidomastoid muscle), in order to be able to safely remove these lymph nodes. Moreover, it has been demonstrated that SPECT/CT imaging increases the number of recorded SLNs up to 100% of the surgically demonstrated radioactive lymph nodes, compared with 76% for planar imaging, with visualisation of one or more additional SLNs in more than half of the patients (Wagner et al. 2004; Bilde et al. 2006; Khafif et al. 2006). These additionally found SLNs on SPECT/CT imaging might be tumour positive. Especially lymph nodes adjacent to the injection area are better detected by SPECT/CT, while they are easily missed on planar imaging. Furthermore, areas of radioactivity accumulation that had been classified as SLNs on the basis of planar imaging can correctly be interpreted as non-nodal areas of accumulation (radiocolloid leakage or contamination) on the basis of SPECT/CT imaging.

Recently, the use of combined preoperative SLN identification and intraoperative radio and fluorescence guidance was proven feasible using ICG-^{99m}Tc-nanocolloid during SLNB for oral cavity cancer. The addition of fluorescence imaging was of particular value when SLNs were located in close proximity to the primary tumour (van den Berg et al. 2012). Moreover, the use of intraoperative imaging provides the possibility of assessing completeness of excision, thus also leading to detection of additional SLNs that had not been identified during preoperative imaging. In this regard, a recent study has demonstrated identification and excision of an additional SLN in 24% of patients with head and neck malignancies (including one tumour-positive node) (Vermeeren et al. 2010).

39.4 SPECT/CT IN ONCOLOGY

SPECT/CT imaging offers many clinical applications in oncology, some of which are well established and some still in the stage of potential perspectives. In the same way as PET benefited from the addition of CT, functional SPECT and anatomical CT data, obtained as a single imaging session, have ensued improvements in diagnostic sensitivity (better disease localisation) and specificity (exclusion of false-positive findings due to physiological tracer uptake/excretion). Furthermore, the anatomical imaging better localises the functional data, which can be critical in surgical and radiotherapy planning. Integrated SPECT/CT has a wide range of clinical applications in the assessment of oncologic patients, particularly those with endocrine malignancies, as well as in some in benign conditions such as infection.

39.4.1 Hybrid SPECT/CT Imaging in Endocrine and Neuroendocrine Tumours

39.4.1.1 Differentiated Thyroid Carcinoma

Differentiated follicular or papillary thyroid carcinoma (DTC) is one of the commonest endocrine tumours and generally has an excellent prognosis (Schlumberger 1998). Diagnostic localisation and therapy of these tumours are generally based upon their capacity to concentrate radioiodide (^{131}I) via specific uptake through the sodium-iodide symporter, with consequent retention within the tumour. The initial treatment of patients with DTC is based on a combination of surgery followed by administration of high-activity ^{131}I-iodide, at least in high-risk patients (Cooper et al. 2006; British Thyroid Association 2007). The goal of radioiodine ablation is to destroy post-surgical normal thyroid remnants and any residual loco-regional disease (mostly represented by lymph node metastasis) or distant metastases (mainly lung and bone lesions). Post-therapy scintigraphy is then generally performed about 7 days after administration of ^{131}I-iodide, in order to localise the radioiodide uptake foci and identify possible lymph node or distant metastasis (see Figure 39.11). Lifelong follow-up is required for high-risk patients, since potentially curable local recurrences and distant metastases may occur even decades after primary treatment (Vorburger et al. 2009). Routine surveillance is conducted using serial measurements of serum thyroglobulin (Tg), neck ultrasound, and whole-body radioiodide scintigraphy (although the role of the latter has recently been downscaled and put in a different perspective, with particular reference to therapy of iodide-concentrating tumour recurrences).

Diagnostic total body scintigraphy is usually performed 72 h after administration of ^{131}I-iodide (or 24–48 h with ^{123}I-iodide) and 5–10 days after administration of ^{131}I-iodide for therapy; post-therapy scintigraphy is more sensitive than diagnostic scintigraphy, due to the much higher activity administered. Radioiodine scintigraphy usually includes a whole-body scan (WBS) associated with spot acquisitions on the neck and mediastinum (Luster et al. 2008). Some factors can limit the performance of this procedure. In particular, the low resolution of gamma camera due to the unfavourable physical properties of ^{131}I associated with a relatively low count density in the target lesions and with non-negligible background activity of radioiodide can yield false-negative results for small lesions. Additionally, the presence of areas of physiological uptake that cannot always easily be distinguished from tumour recurrence due to the lack of anatomical landmarks can result in false-positive findings (Sutter et al. 1995; Mitchell et al. 2000; Shapiro et al. 2000). Sensitivity around 45%–75% and specificity around 90%–100% have been reported for diagnostic planar ^{131}I-iodide whole-body imaging in detecting recurrences or metastases from DTC (Simpson et al. 1998; Lind and Kohlfürst 2006).

SPECT/CT imaging increases both the sensitivity and the specificity of radioiodide scintigraphy. In fact, the hybrid system provides a definite added value over WBS and stand-alone SPECT for characterising equivocal foci of tracer uptake, as well as for precise localisation of malignant lesions in the neck, chest, and skeleton (Wong et al. 2008). ^{131}I-iodide SPECT/CT is also able to differentiate normal residual thyroid tissue from cervical lymph node metastases (Wong et al. 2008; Spanu et al. 2009). The use of this procedure in post-surgical diagnostic ^{131}I-iodide imaging allows more accurate risk stratification of patients with DTC before administration of ^{131}I-iodide for ablation of post-surgical remnants, with the consequent advantage to deliver high doses of ^{131}I-iodide to high-risk patients and lower doses for thyroid remnant ablation in low-risk patients (Wong et al. 2008, 2010b). In patients with non-iodine-avid tumours (negative ^{131}I-iodide scan associated with elevated serum Tg levels indicating persistent or recurrent disease), [^{18}F]FDG-PET/CT is used to identify areas with enhanced glucose metabolism and source of thyroglobulin production.

(a)

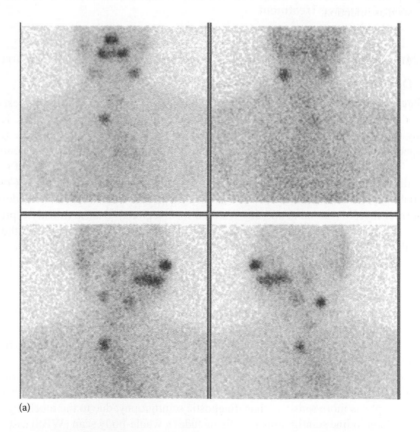

FIGURE 39.11 (a) Planar images of the neck region obtained 7 days after ^{131}I-iodide therapy for ablation of post-surgical remnants in a patient with DTC. The upper panels (anterior and posterior views) show focal uptake in the right paratracheal region and two areas in left and right submandibular regions. Lower panels (right and left lateral views) show the three areas of focal uptake from different point of views. *(Continued)*

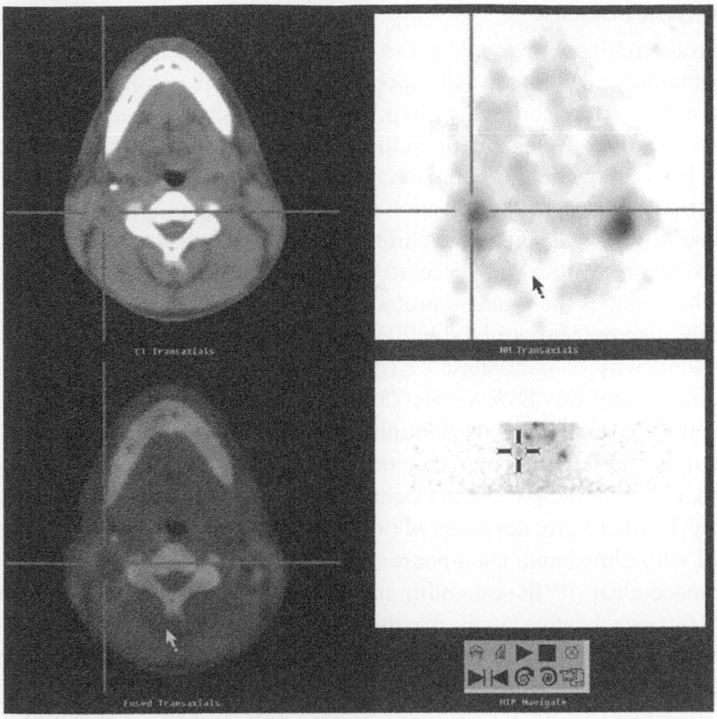

(b)

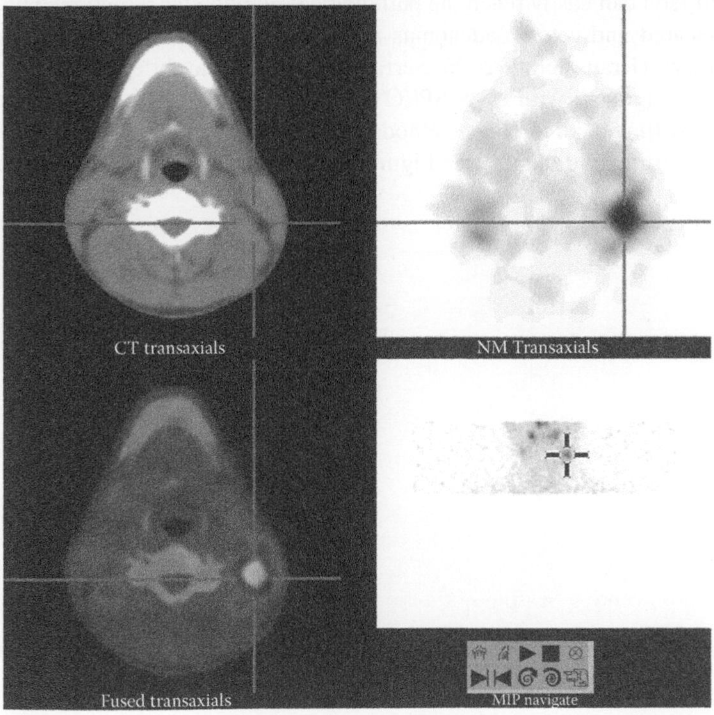

(c)

FIGURE 39.11 (*Continued*) (b and c) SPECT/CT images at different neck levels clearly show that the two areas of focal uptake in the submandibular regions actually correspond to two metastatic cervical lymph nodes.

39.4.1.2 Parathyroid Disease

Primary hyperparathyroidism is caused by a single parathyroid adenoma in up to 80% of the clinical cases. The remaining cases are usually secondary to hyperplasia and, less commonly, to parathyroid carcinoma. Secondary and tertiary hyperparathyroidism are usually linked to chronic renal failure and are frequently associated with multigland disease. Surgical resection of the hyperfunctioning adenoma is the only curative approach for this disease, and the main clinical indication for parathyroid imaging is presurgical localisation of pathological gland(s). Over the past decade, with the increasing use of minimally invasive parathyroidectomy, presurgical localisation of parathyroid adenoma has become critical for successful surgery. Parathyroid ^{99m}Tc-sestamibi scintigraphy combined with ultrasound is the standard protocol employed for preoperative localisation of pathological parathyroid glands (Mariani et al. 2003; Rubello et al. 2007). One meta-analysis reported that the overall sensitivity of dual-phase ^{99m}Tc-sestamibi scintigraphy in comparison with high-resolution ultrasonography was 88% versus 78% for single adenomas, 30% versus 16% for double adenomas, and 44% versus 35% for multiple gland hyperplasia (Ruda et al. 2005). Ultrasound allows anatomical detection of an enlarged parathyroid gland and accurate localisation relative to the thyroid gland, although the presence of coexisting nodular thyroid disease reduces its sensitivity and specificity. Furthermore, deep-seated or ectopic adenomas in the neck or mediastinum are poorly visualised with ultrasound. Dual-phase scintigraphy with early and delayed images using a single radiopharmaceutical (^{99m}Tc-sestamibi) or dual-isotope subtraction scintigraphy using ^{99m}Tc-sestamibi and ^{99m}Tc-pertechnetate are the two most commonly performed procedures. SPECT imaging had already demonstrated higher sensitivity than planar imaging scintigraphy, often translating into increased lesion detection particularly of ectopic adenomas, which are mainly located in the mediastinum (Schachter et al. 2004; Slater and Gleeson 2005; Rubello et al. 2006). The introduction of hybrid SPECT/CT imaging has allowed even more accurate lesion localisation; consequently, the endocrine surgeon can easily reach the pathological gland(s) for resection. This is of particular benefit in deep-seated and ectopic adenomas and in patients with altered neck anatomy following previous surgery (Krausz et al. 2006; Serra et al. 2006). Lavely et al. recommend dual-phase ^{99m}Tc-sestamibi scintigraphy with early SPECT/CT combined with delayed images as a superior imaging protocol with respect to other methods, because of improved preoperative localisation of hyperfunctioning parathyroid glands (see Figure 39.12); whenever available, this imaging protocol

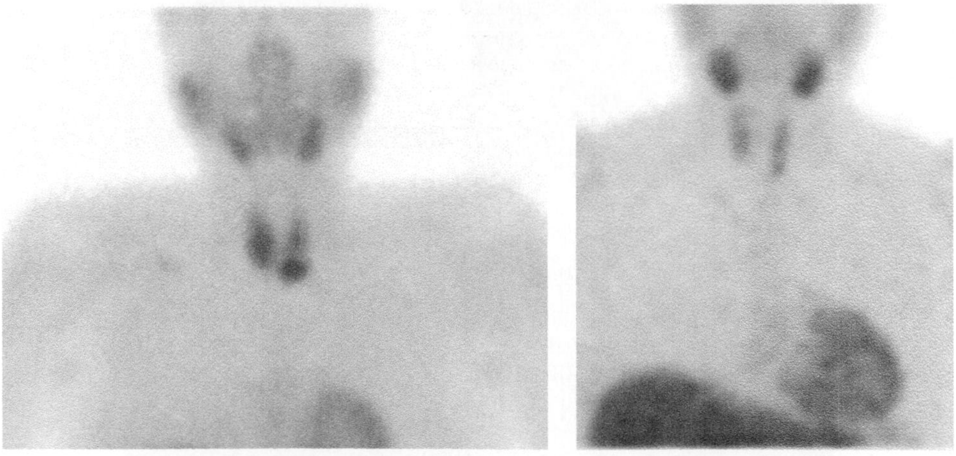

(a) (b)

FIGURE 39.12 (a) Early planar images and (b) early maximum intensity projection (MIP) obtained after administration of ^{99m}Tc-Sestamibi, showing an area of focal uptake below the lower pole of the left thyroid lobe, interpreted as a hyperfunctioning parathyroid adenoma. *(Continued)*

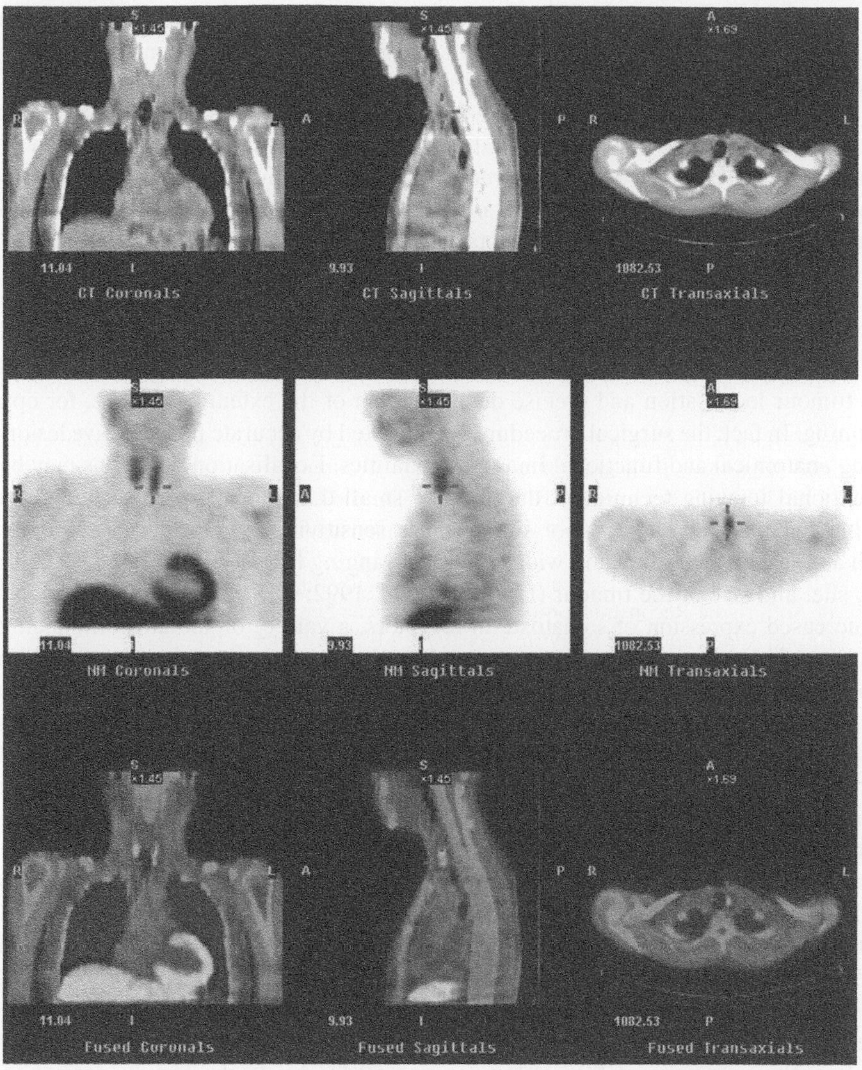

(c)

FIGURE 39.12 (*Continued*) (c) SPECT/CT images (CT component in upper row, SPECT component in middle row, fused SPECT/CT in lower row) confirm exact location of the parathyroid adenoma.

should therefore be part of the routine preoperative evaluation of patients with primary hyperparathyroidism for planning minimally invasive parathyroidectomy (Lavely et al. 2007). Image fusion as obtained by hybrid SPECT/CT with ^{99m}Tc-sestamibi has a significant impact on surgical planning in both primary and secondary hyperthyroidism, although accurate detection of multigland disease remains still problematic (Serra et al. 2006; Harris et al. 2008).

39.4.1.3 Adrenocortical Tumours

Adrenocortical scintigraphy with ^{131}I-labelled 6-β-iodomethyl-19-norcholesterol provides information about functional and tumour characterisation of adrenocortical masses in patients with biochemically proven disorder and/or with incidentaloma (Barzon et al. 2001). Reports on the impact of hybrid SPECT/CT imaging on the performance of functional imaging with ^{131}I-iodocholesterol imaging remain limited. In a recent study comparing SPECT/CT with planar imaging, hybrid imaging significantly improved the diagnostic accuracy in patients who had inconclusive adrenal venous sampling and equivocal CT results, allowing the identification of small adrenal lesions and discriminating hyperfunctioning adenomas from idiopathic adrenal hyperplasia (Yen et al. 2009). Thus, SPECT/CT is redefining the role of functional imaging in clinical practice by integration of morphological information which can assist interpretation of scintigraphy by localising focal uptake to the adrenal glands, allowing direct assessment of function within adrenal nodules, and distinguishing physiological bowel activity from adrenal uptake (Yen et al. 2009; Wong et al. 2010a).

39.4.2 Neuroendocrine Tumours

The clinical outcome of patients with neuroendocrine tumours (NETs) is significantly affected by accurate tumour localisation and precise determination of the extent of disease, for optimal surgery planning. In fact, the surgical procedure is facilitated by accurate preoperative lesion localisation, using anatomical and functional imaging modalities. Localisation of lesions may be difficult by conventional imaging techniques, due to their small diameter or because they are obscured by structural changes related to prior surgery. The sensitivity of conventional imaging modalities, such as CT and US, is low and widely variable ranging between 13% and 85% depending on the type, site, and size of the tumour (Lamberts et al. 1992; Kaltsas et al. 2004). As many NETs exhibit increased expression of somatostatin receptors, a variety of somatostatin analogues with high binding affinity to somatostatin receptors have been synthesised for diagnostic imaging or for targeted therapy. In particular, somatostatin receptor scintigraphy (SRS) is a functional imaging modality based on the use of somatostatin analogues that preferentially bind to somatostatin subtypes 2 and 5. At present, SRS with ^{111}In-pentetreotide (Octreoscan®) is predominantly used for the detection of primary tumours (gastro-enteropancreatic tumours) or of their liver and/or mesenteric metastases.

SRS has been used for diagnosis, staging, and follow-up of NET, as well as for facilitating the detection of microscopic foci during radioguided surgery. In addition, SRS is being increasingly used to define the receptor status of NET metastases for potential treatment with *cold* (unlabelled) somatostatin analogues or for targeted peptide radio-receptor therapy (PRRT) using somatostatin analogues labelled with either ^{90}Y or ^{177}Lu. SRS imaging has a reported sensitivity of 82%–95% and can detect sites of disease undetected by conventional imaging techniques in 30%–50% of the patients, depending on the different NETs considered (Krenning et al. 1994; Shi et al. 1998). Nevertheless, the specificity of SRS is low (around 50%), due to the lack of precise anatomical localisation and to physiological tracer accumulation/excretion; furthermore, these tracers accumulate also in benign conditions, which may potentially be misinterpreted as pathological foci.

NETs are often localised in the abdomen and, without anatomic correlations, it can be difficult to precisely identify whether a suspicious focus is located in the pancreas, small bowel, or liver. Because of these limitations, SRS may benefit from co-registration with CT images. Indeed, SPECT/CT improves the localisation of scintigraphic findings especially for lesions located in the abdominal area, by distinguishing physiological uptake/accumulation or activity due to benign lesion from pathological foci (see Figures 39.13 and 39.14). A recent study with Octreoscan® SPECT/CT showed 95% accuracy for identifying and localising NETs, significantly higher than 46% for standalone SPECT, especially for lesions located in the abdominal area (Perri et al. 2008). Another study has evaluated the impact of SRS SPECT/CT on the diagnostic accuracy in 72 patients with various NETs, including 45 carcinoid tumours, medullary thyroid carcinoma, or islet cell tumours (Krausz et al. 2003). Additional information beyond that provided by planar imaging or by standalone SPECT was obtained in 24 patients, whereas SPECT/CT improved the localisation of the planar/SPECT findings in 23 patients (32%) and changed clinical management in 10 patients (14%). In particular, SPECT/CT improved localisation of the SPECT-detected lesions in 23 of the 44 positive studies. It defined the extent of disease in 17 patients, showed unsuspected bone involvement

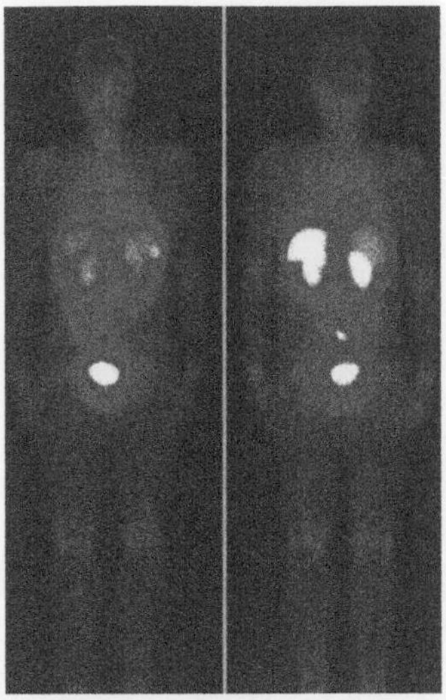

(a)

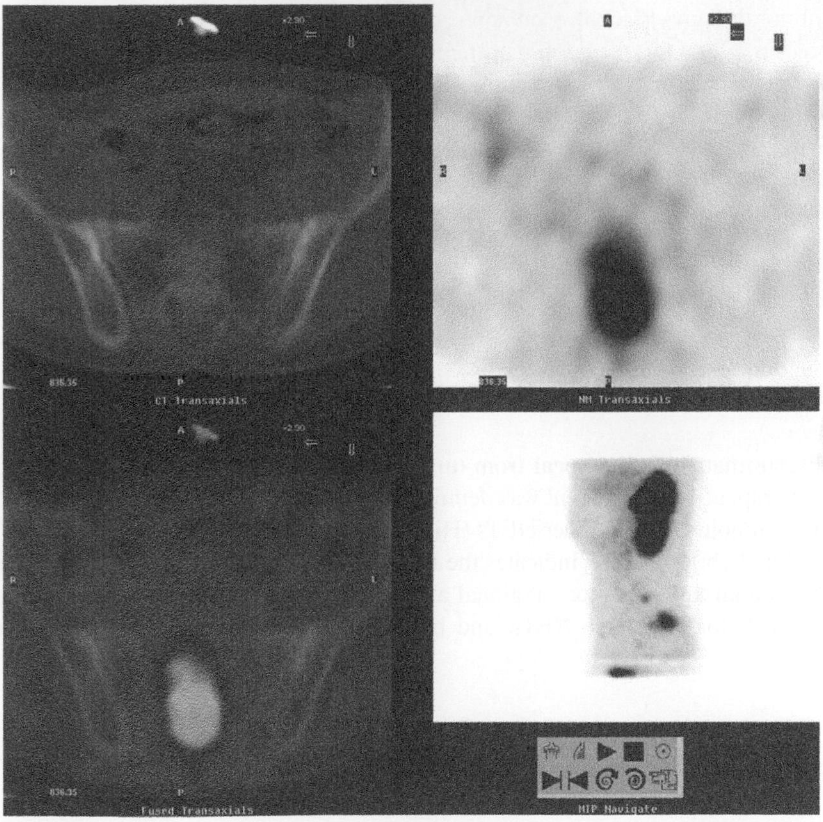

(b)

FIGURE 39.13 (a) Planar images in anterior and posterior whole-body views (left and right panel, respectively) obtained 4 h after administration of ^{111}In-pentetreotide in a patient with lung carcinoid, showing two focal uptake areas in the chest (corresponding to enlarged lymph nodes according to the CT scan) and an additional area of uptake in the abdomen/pelvis. SPECT/CT images of the abdomen clearly (b) localise the latter focal uptake area to a sacral lesion and (c) show a further small lytic bone lesion in the L4 body. *(Continued)*

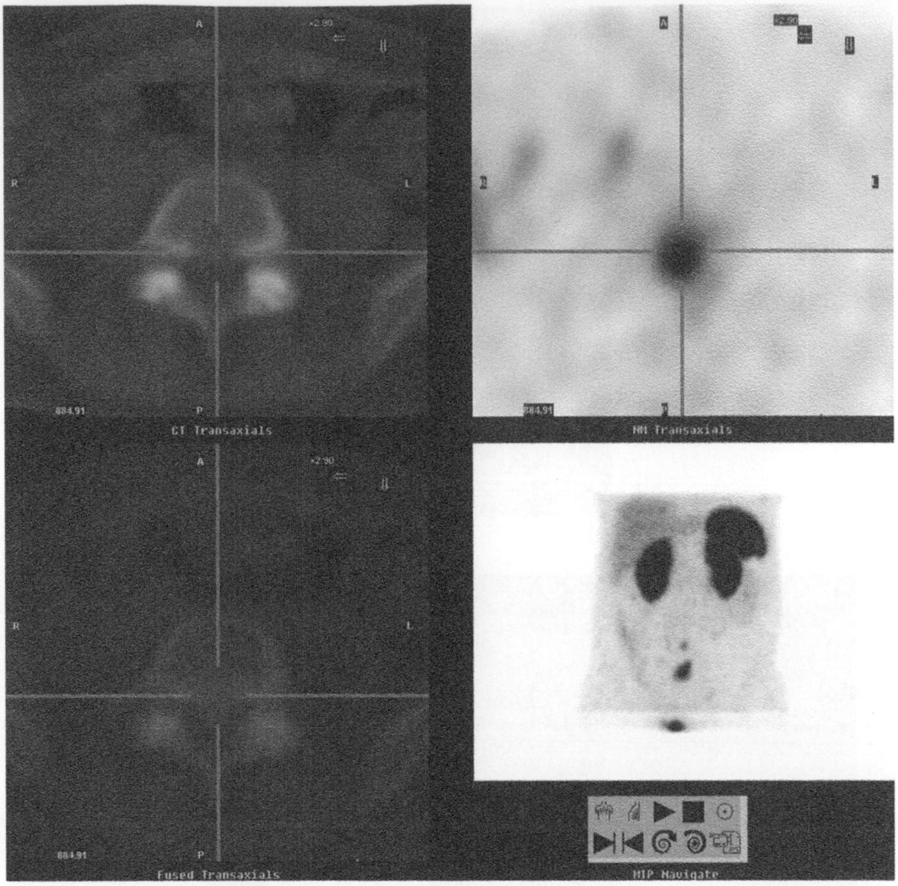

(c)

FIGURE 39.13 (*Continued*) (c) show a further small lytic bone lesion in the L4 body.

in 3, and discriminated physiological from tumour uptake in 3. Significant impact of SPECT/CT imaging on therapeutic management was demonstrated also by Hillel and coworkers in 29 patients with carcinoid tumours or with other NETs (Hillel et al. 2006).

In conclusion, hybrid imaging indicates the functional status of the disease, defines exact localisation of the tumour and of its loco-regional and/or distant metastases, optimises planning of the surgical approach for resectable NETs, and helps to choose the optimal treatment strategy for advanced disease.

39.4.2.1 Sympathetic Nervous System Tumours

This group includes benign and malignant tumours that are generally classified as NETs but that arise from the neural crest, such as phaeochromocytoma, paraganglioma, neuroblastoma, and medullary thyroid carcinoma. Since surgical resection remains the only curative treatment, accurate preoperative staging is critical for optimal surgery planning. Morphological imaging modalities, such as CT or MRI, offer high sensitivity for the detection of tumours of the sympathetic nervous system. Functional imaging is frequently required as a complementary imaging modality because its high specificity enables to better characterise the lesions. Some NETs, particularly those that produce catecholamines (i.e. phaeochromocytoma and paraganglioma) and neuroblastoma, can be successfully imaged with radiolabelled guanethidine analogues, such as ^{123}I- or ^{131}I-labelled

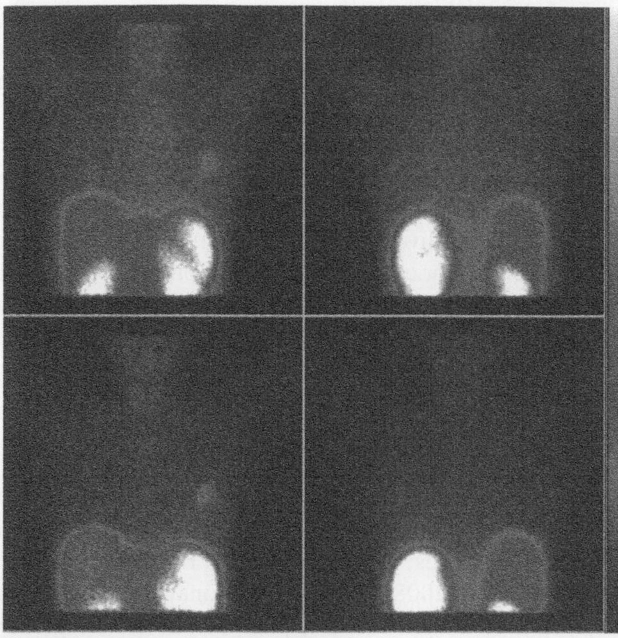

(a)

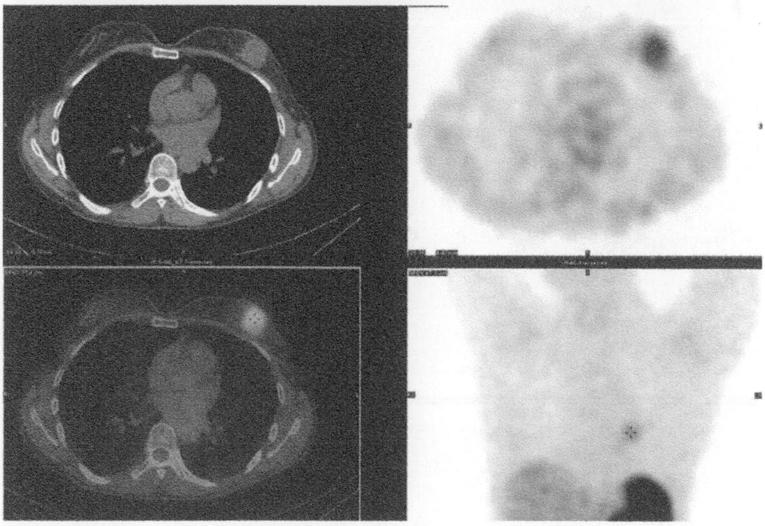

(b)

FIGURE 39.14 (a) Planar images in the anterior (left panels) and posterior (right panels) views in a patient with NET (which was not possible to classify further) of the left breast 4 h (upper panels) and 24 h (lower panels) after administration of ^{111}In-Pentetreotide, showing a focal uptake area in the left breast. (b) SPECT/CT images such as transaxial CT (left upper panel), SPECT (right upper panel), fused SPECT/CT (lower left panel) sections, and 4 h MIP images confirm expression of somatostatin receptors by the lesion in the left breast.

meta-iodobenzylguanidine (MIBG), which is taken up by tumour cells via an active pathway (Shapiro et al. 1995). Radionuclide imaging is also helpful for the detection of extra-adrenal tumour sites and is superior to anatomical imaging for distinguishing scar tissue from residual tumour after surgery (Avram et al. 2006; Gross et al. 2007). In addition, in advanced or recurrent disease, MIBG scintigraphy allows to select patients suitable for radiometabolic therapy with high doses of

^{131}I-MIBG (Avram et al. 2006; Gross et al. 2007) and for monitoring response to treatment (Rufini et al. 2006) (see Figure 39.15).

Sensitivity and specificity of ^{123}I-MIBG for the detection of neuroblastoma and phaeochromocytoma lesions are over 90% (Jacobson et al., 2010). Despite such high sensitivity in selected patients, it is reasonable to assume that further improvement in diagnostic accuracy can be achieved using SPECT/CT, considering that specificity of planar and stand-alone SPECT imaging can be limited because of the normal biodistribution of the radiotracer especially for lesions adjacent to high physiological activity organs, such as liver and myocardium. In 31 patients undergoing ^{123}I-MIBG scintigraphy because of biochemical or clinical suspicion of phaeochromocytoma, the incremental diagnostic value of fused SPECT/CT images in identifying physiological tracer uptake was demonstrated in 74% of the cases (Ozer et al. 2004). By correctly localising recurrent disease or metastases, hybrid imaging provided additional diagnostic information over planar imaging both for diagnostic ^{123}I-MIBG scintigraphy and for post-therapy high-dose ^{131}I-MIBG scintigraphy (Meyer-Rochow et al. 2010; Fukuoka et al 2011).

Pathologic findings on MIBG scintigraphy (planar and SPECT) and on diagnostic CT are sometimes difficult to correlate because of anatomical distortion caused by prior surgery or irradiation. Rozovsky et al. evaluated the impact of fused SPECT/CT images on correlation and image analysis of both techniques; overall, SPECT/CT provided additional information in 8/15 cases (53%) (Rozovsky et al. 2008). In four additional neuroblastoma patients in whom a residual mass was present on diagnostic CT, planar MIBG scintigraphy was negative; in

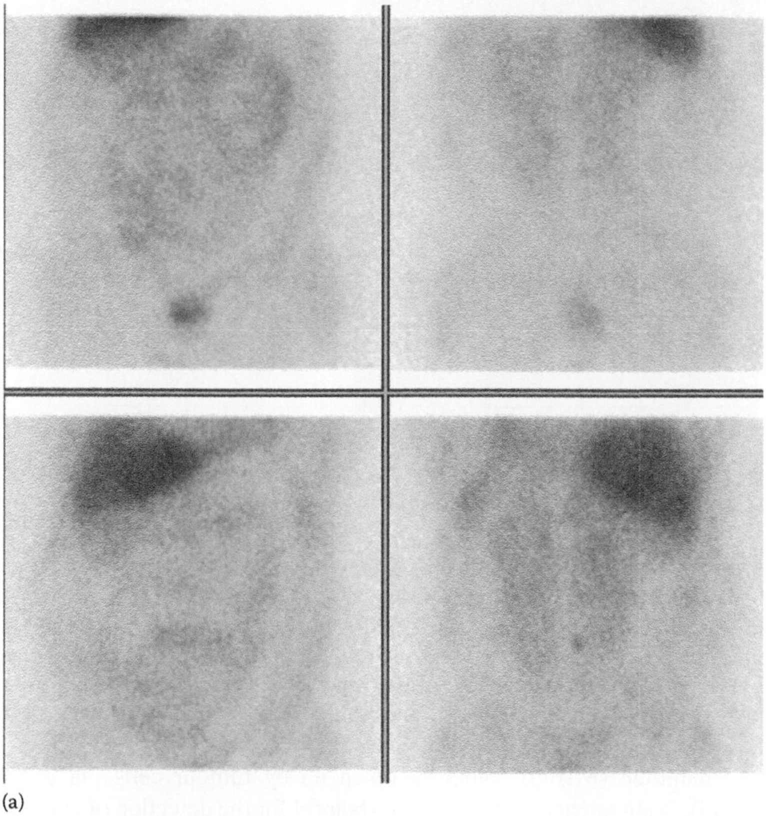

(a)

FIGURE 39.15 (a) Planar images of ^{123}I-MIBG scintigraphy in a patient with biochemical recurrence of malignant phaeochromocytoma, showing a small area with faint focal uptake in the abdomen, better visualised in the posterior view (left panels) of the late acquisitions (lower panels). *(Continued)*

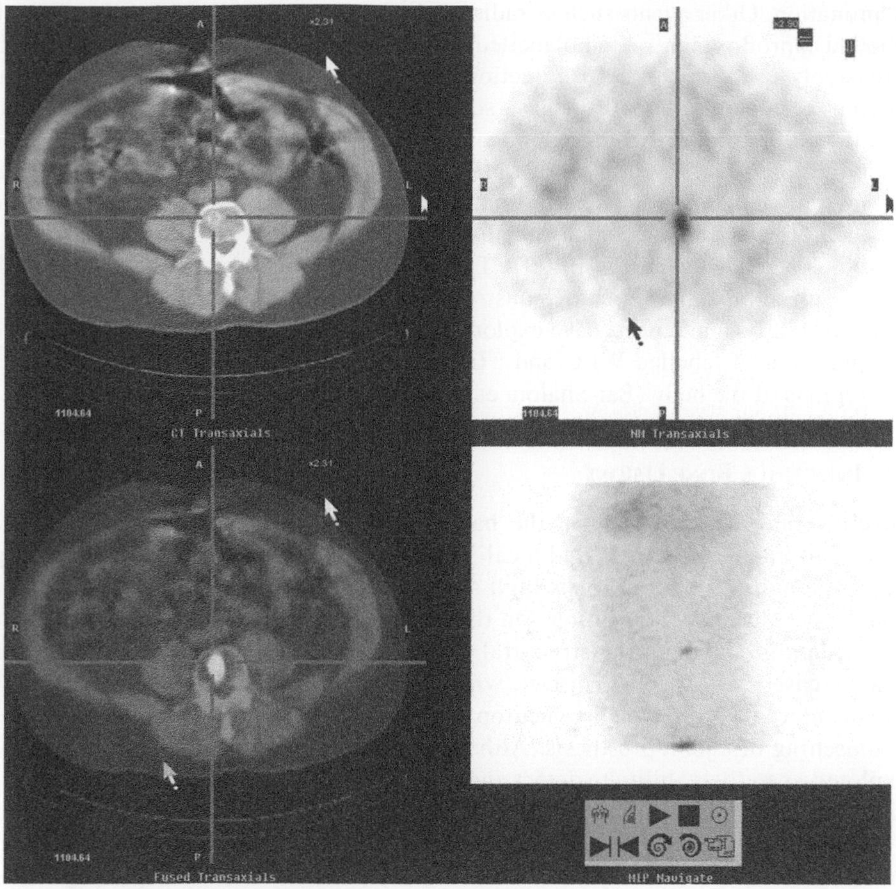

(b)

FIGURE 39.15 (*Continued*) (b) SPECT/CT images clearly localise the uptake area to the body of L4.

these cases, SPECT/CT imaging focused on the area of the diagnostic CT abnormality and showed no focal MIBG uptake, thus increasing the diagnostic certainty of disease remission. Anatomical–functional image fusion allows for improved localisation and characterisation of NETs with resultant modification of the treatment approach (Pfannenberg et al. 2003; Meyer-Rochow et al. 2010). Finally, in patients who are candidates for radiometabolic therapy with ^{131}I-MIBG, a CT-based measurement of the target volume of interest is useful to quantify the effective radiation dose.

39.5 HYBRID SPECT/CT IMAGING OF INFECTION

Infection and inflammation often represent a diagnostic challenge for physicians. Both morphological and functional imaging modalities have been extensively employed for diagnosing and monitoring these conditions. Although CT and MRI provide high-quality anatomical details, the structural abnormalities underlying the infectious process are, in some cases, nonspecific or appreciable only in a subacute or late phase of the disease. Nuclear medicine can play a crucial role in the evaluation of patients suspected of infection, because of its capability of demonstrating physiologic processes and metabolic changes before structural changes, by several days or weeks (Love and Palestro 2004; Auler et al. 2007). ^{67}Ga-citrate imaging and radiolabelled white blood cell (WBC) imaging have long been used to evaluate infection and inflammation. Other agents such as radiolabelled anti-granulocyte monoclonal antibodies, radiolabelled ciprofloxacin, or radiolabelled natural antimicrobial peptides are also becoming increasingly used for suspected infection (although radiolabeled ciprofloxacin is not longer avaialbel commercially). All of these scintigraphic approaches mainly reflect functional data, and the ability to define fine anatomical detail may be critical in discriminating between pathologic and physiologic sites/foci of radioactivity accumulation. SPECT/CT scanning has offered new opportunities for infection imaging, especially for facilitating precise localisation and accurate characterisation of infectious foci (Filippi and Schillaci 2006; O'Conno and Kemp 2006). The added value of SPECT/CT for diagnosing infections with labelled WBC and ^{67}Ga-citrate scintigraphy has been demonstrated by several authors (Bar-Shalom et al. 2006; Bajaj et al. 2008). Recent reports have explored the contribution of SPECT/CT to a more accurate interpretation of labelled WBC and ^{67}Ga-citrate scintigraphy for suspected infection in different regions of the body (Bar-Shalom et al. 2006).

39.5.1 Infectious Bone Lesions

Osteomyelitis may be suspected on the basis of a 3-phase bone scintigraphy with ^{99m}Tc-labelled diphosphonates, as increased localised accumulation/uptake during all three phases. However, although this approach has high sensitivity, it lacks specificity for discriminating infection versus sterile inflammation. On the other hand, CT and MRI provide high-quality anatomical details, although the structural abnormalities underlying the infectious process are, in some cases, non-specific. In fact, with morphological imaging alone, it is difficult to distinguish infection from fracture, neuropathic joint changes, post-operative changes, and aseptic loosening of a joint prosthesis. Although a variety of new radiopharmaceuticals have been explored as to their ability to detect and localise infectious and inflammatory processes, ^{67}Ga-citrate scintigraphy and scintigraphy with ^{111}In- or ^{99m}Tc-HMPAO-labelled autologous WBCs remain the functional imaging techniques of choice for diagnostic work-up of infection. Although PET with the metabolic tracer [^{18}F]FDG is gradually replacing ^{67}Ga-citrate scintigraphy in many clinical settings related to infection, ^{67}Ga-citrate scintigraphy is still employed to evaluate in particular osteomyelitis of the spine (Prandini et al. 2006). While ^{99m}Tc-HMPAO-WBC scintigraphy has been found to be the most accurate in detecting acute osteomyelitis affecting the peripheral bones, anti-granulocyte antibody radiopharmaceuticals have been used in patients with joint prosthesis (Filip Gemmel et al. 2012). In particular, major benefits of the radionuclide imaging modalities were achieved in the diagnosis of relapsing osteomyelitis in patients with structural bone abnormalities after trauma or orthopaedic implants. Suspected infection of orthopaedic prosthetic implants requires anatomical imaging that is usually restricted to conventional x-ray, since tomographic modalities such as CT or MRI are limited by artefacts, depending on the type of prosthesis. Scintigraphic imaging is less affected by artefacts but suffer from poor spatial resolution utilising only planar imaging; even stand-alone SPECT imaging can be problematic for distinguishing soft tissue from bone infection. These difficulties have been overcome with the use of SPECT/CT. The contribution of SPECT/CT to ^{99m}Tc-HMPAO-WBC or ^{67}Ga-citrate scintigraphy has been evaluated, demonstrating its definite added value in distinguishing physiological uptake from infectious processes and in defining the precise anatomical location of infection (Horger et al. 2004; Bar-Shalom et al. 2006; Bunyaviroch et al. 2006; Filippi and Schillaci 2006). In this regard, Filippi and Schillaci have recently evaluated the usefulness of SPECT/CT imaging for interpreting ^{99m}Tc-HMPAO-WBC scintigraphy in 15 patients with suspected osteomyelitis and in 13 patients with suspected infection of orthopaedic prosthesis. Hybrid SPECT/CT provided more accurate data on the anatomical localisation and extent of disease, with accurate information about bone infection complicating orthopaedic joint prosthesis and hardware, which better guides clinical management (see Figures 39.16 and 39.17).

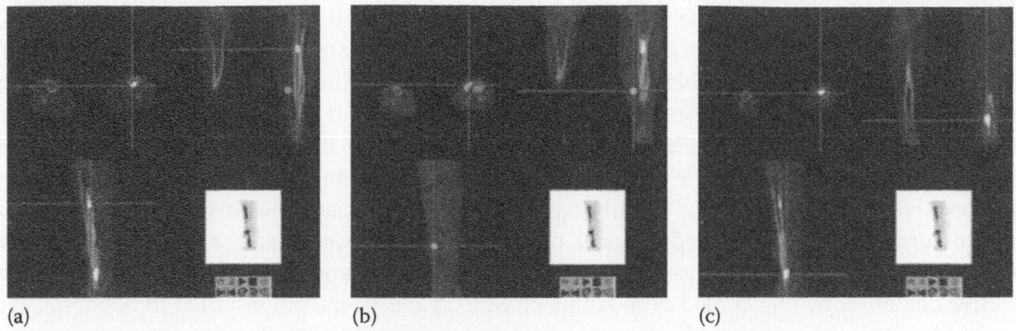

FIGURE 39.16 ^{99m}Tc-HMPAO-WBC scan obtained in a 37-year-old man with osteomyelitis of the left tibia. The patient underwent the examination because of suspected exacerbation of prior infection at the diaphysis of the left tibia. (a–c) depict the SPECT/CT images at different levels, showing sites of infection (a) at the primary, already known site, but also (b) in the soft tissue in the medial portion of the calf, and (c) in an additional focus of osteomyelitis at the distal tibia. Each panel shows the fused SPECT/CT images in the transaxial (upper left), coronal (upper right), and sagittal (lower left) sections; MIP shown in lower right image. (Courtesy of Dr. Elena Lazzeri and Roberto Boni, Regional Center of Nuclear Medicine, University of Pisa, Pisa, Italy.)

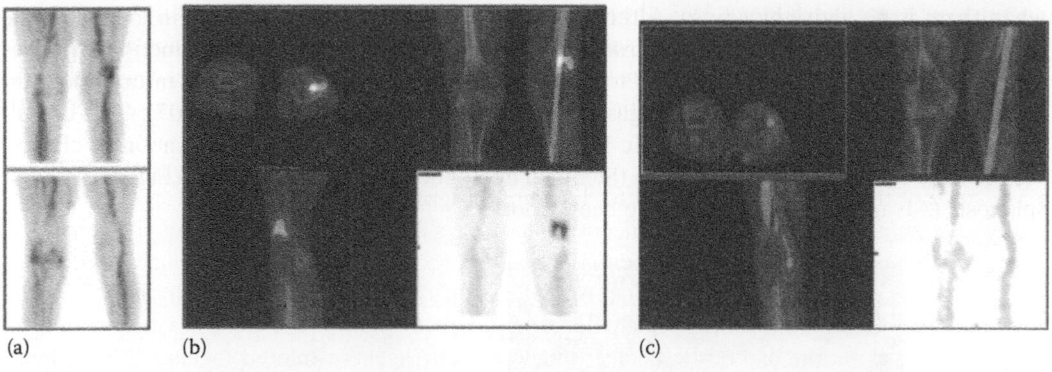

FIGURE 39.17 ^{99m}Tc-HMPAO-WBC scans obtained in two different occasions in a 46-year-old woman with rheumatoid arthritis who had been submitted 2 years earlier to immobilisation of the left knee with surgical implant of a left femoral endomedullary nail. (a) Planar scans recorded 4 h after reinfusion of radiolabelled leukocytes, respectively, during clinical signs of infection at the left knee (upper panel) and at follow-up after antibiotic therapy and clinical recovery (lower panel): the first scan shows an area of accumulation at the left knee, which was not detected in the second scan, after successful therapy. (b and c) show the corresponding SPECT/CT acquisitions, respectively, during infection and after therapy. Each panel shows the fused SPECT/CT images in the transaxial (upper left), coronal (upper right), and sagittal (lower left) sections; MIP shown in lower right image. Infection is clearly shown in (b), involving both the bone around the endomedullary nail and the adjacent soft tissues. (Courtesy of Dr. Elena Lazzeri and Roberto Boni, Regional Center of Nuclear Medicine, University of Pisa, Pisa, Italy.)

39.6 HYBRID SPECT/CT IMAGING IN OTHER NON-ONCOLOGIC DISORDERS

Fusion SPECT/CT imaging has been widely employed in various non-oncologic diseases localised in the abdomen (Schillaci et al. 2007). Evaluation of gastrointestinal bleeding depends on the suspected source of the bleeding. The diagnostic tool of choice for all cases of upper gastrointestinal bleeding is esophagogastroduodenoscopy; for acute lower gastrointestinal bleeding, it is colonoscopy or arteriography. Both techniques can directly localise the bleeding source, and in some cases, local therapy in the same session can be performed. If no upper gastrointestinal or large bowel source of bleeding is identified, small bowel or intermittent bleeding can be investigated using ^{99m}Tc-labelled red blood cell (RBC) scintigraphy. This radionuclide procedure is the best suited for identifying slow-bleeding sources, with rates of 0.1–0.4 mL per minute (Zuccaro 1998), but it is not as accurate as arteriography in identifying the exact location of a bleeding site. A retrospective study of ^{99m}Tc-RBC scintigraphy showed that an early positive scan had a high positive predictive value for identifying patients with associated positive active bleeding that requires urgent angiography and surgical treatment. On the other hand, a negative or delayed positive ^{99m}Tc RBC scan predicts a negative angiogram, a finding that indicates observation and elective colonoscopy (Ng et al. 1997). Although SPECT has been demonstrated to be more accurate in identifying the sites of bleeding than planar imaging, SPECT/CT offers even more precise localisation of the bleeding site, by providing anatomical landmarks (see Figure 39.18) (Kimura et al. 2006; Schillaci et al. 2009).

The Meckel diverticulum represents in the adult life a remnant of the omphalomesenteric or vitelline duct; heterotopic tissue, including gastric mucosa and pancreatic tissue, is present in 50% of the subjects. Symptoms resulting from the presence of ectopic gastric mucosa in the Meckel diverticulum (recurring postprandial pain, sometimes accompanied by bleeding) are usually due to erosion of the adjacent ileal mucosa by acid secretion produced by the ectopic gastric tissue. The most sensitive technique for confirming the presence of ectopic gastric mucosa in a Meckel diverticulum is ^{99m}Tc-pertechnetate scintigraphy (which should be performed when there is no active bleeding). Although ultrasonography and CT can help in localising the Meckel diverticulum, the fusion of structural images (provided by CT) with functional images (provided by SPECT) of the same tomographic sections provides helpful information for an exact localisation of heterotopic gastric mucosa (Papathanassiou et al. 2007). The usefulness of SPECT/CT imaging with ^{99m}Tc-RBCs in patients with equivocal localisation or clinical significance of hepatic haemangiomas (Schillaci et al. 2004; Zheng et al. 2005) (Figure 39.19) or splenosis (Alvarez et al. 2007) has also been reported.

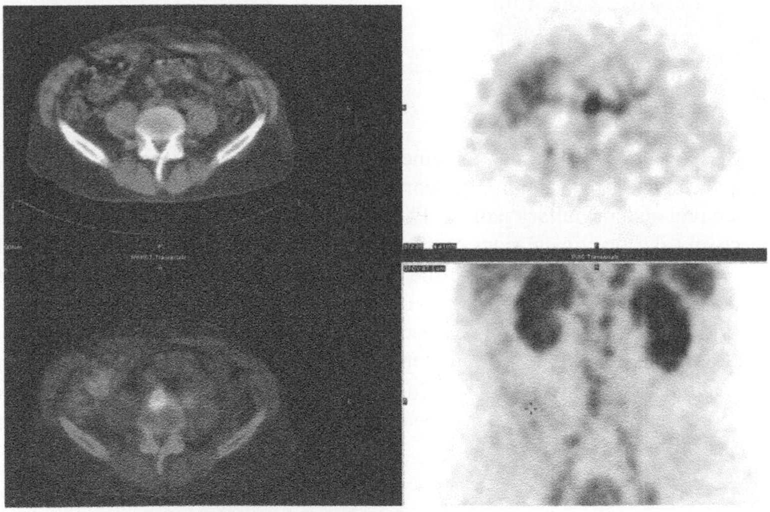

FIGURE 39.18 SPECT/CT images obtained during ^{99m}Tc-labelled RBC in a patient with suspected gastrointestinal bleeding (transaxial CT in left upper panel, transaxial SPECT in right upper panel, fused SPECT/CT in lower left panel, MIP image in lower right panel); sections at the level of the pelvis. The site of bleeding (indicated by the cross-reference lines) can be localised in the terminal ileum and/or lumen of the cecum.

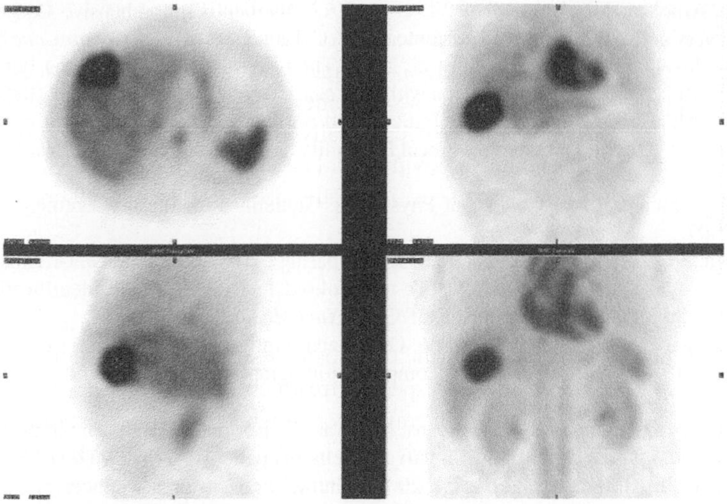

FIGURE 39.19 SPECT images obtained during ^{99m}Tc-labelled RBC scintigraphy in a patient with suspected haemangioma of the liver (segment VIII). Transaxial section is shown in left upper panel, coronal section in right upper panel, sagittal section in lower left panel, and MIP image (in lower right panel). Intense accumulation of the labelled RBCs confirms that the lesion detected at ultrasound is hepatic haemangioma.

39.7 CONCLUSION

A combined imaging technique such as SPECT/CT provides morpho-functional information that constitutes an important tool in diagnostic imaging for a wide spectrum of disease. In surgery, these procedures should be performed with the purpose of planning the surgical approach most suited to the individual patient avoiding, whenever possible, the use of invasive procedures, or prior to adopting miniinvasive approaches.

Advances in SPECT instrumentation, CT technology, and radiopharmaceutical development have the potential to advance SPECT/CT beyond its current level of performance with high-quality imaging that will provide useful diagnostic information for better clinical management and patients' care.

REFERENCES

Association of Breast Surgery at Baso 2009. Surgical guidelines for the management of breast cancer. *Eur J Surg Oncol.* 2009;35 Suppl 1:1–22.

Alvarez, R., Diehl, K.M., Avram, A., Brown, R., Piert, M. 2007. Localization of splenosis using ^{99m}Tc-damaged red blood cell SPECT/CT and intraoperative gamma probe measurements. *Eur J Nucl Med Mol Imaging* 34:969.

Auler, M.A., Bagg, S., Gordon, L. 2007. The role of nuclear medicine in imaging infection. *Semin Roentgenol* 42;117–121.

Avram, A.M., Fig, L.M., Gross, M.D. 2006. Adrenal gland scintigraphy. *Semin Nucl Med* 36:212–227.

Bajaj, S.K., Seitz, J.P., Qing, F. 2008. Diagnosis of acute bacterial prostatitis by Ga-67 scintigraphy and SPECT-CT. *Clin Nucl Med* 33:813–815.

Bar-Shalom, R., Yefremov, N., Guralnik, L. et al. 2006. SPECT/CT using ^{67}Ga and ^{111}In-labeled leukocyte scintigraphy for diagnosis of infection. *J Nucl Med* 47:587–594.

Barzon, L., Zucchetta, P., Boscaro, M., Marzola, M.C., Bui, F., Fallo, F. 2001. Scintigraphic patterns of adrenocortical carcinoma: Morpho-functional correlates. *Eur J Endocrinol* 145:743–748.

Beneder, C., Fuechsel, F.G., Krause, T., Kuhn, A., Mueller, M.D. 2008. The role of 3D fusion imaging in sentinel lymphadenectomy for vulvar cancer. *Gynecol Oncol* 109:76–80.

Benson, A.B. 3rd, Arnoletti, J.P., Bekaii-Saab, T. et al. 2012. National Comprehensive Cancer Network. Anal Carcinoma, Version 2.2012: Featured updates to the NCCN guidelines. *J Natl Compr Canc Netw* 10:449–454.

Bilde, A., Von Buchwald, C., Mortensen, J. et al. 2006. The role of SPECT-CT in the lymphoscintigraphic identification of sentinel nodes in patients with oral cancer. *Acta Otolaryngol* 126:1096–1103.

Borsò, E., Grosso, M., Boni, G. et al. 2013. Radioguided occult lesion localization of cervical recurrences from differentiated thyroid cancer: Technical feasibility and clinical results. *Q J Nucl Med Mol Imaging* 57:401–411.

British Thyroid Association, Royal College of Physicians. Guidelines for the management of thyroid cancer, 2nd edn., 2007.

Brouwer, O.R., Buckle, T., Vermeeren, L. et al. 2012. Comparing the hybrid fluorescent-radioactive tracer indocyanine green-^{99m}Tc-nanocolloid with ^{99m}Tc-nanocolloid for sentinel node identification: A validation study using lymphoscintigraphy and SPECT/CT. *J Nucl Med* 53:1034–1040.

Bunyaviroch, T., Aggarwal, A., Oates, M.E. 2006. Optimized scintigraphic evaluation of infection and inflammation: Role of single-photon emission computed tomography/computed tomography fusion imaging. *Semin Nucl Med* 36:295–311.

Burger, M.P., Hollema, H., Emanuels, A.G., Krans, M., Pras, E., Bouma, J. 1995. The importance of the groin node status for the survival of T1 and T2 vulval carcinoma patients. *Gynecol Oncol* 57:327–334.

Buscombe, J., Paganelli, G., Burak, Z.E. et al. 2007. Sentinel node in breast cancer procedural guidelines. *Eur J Nucl Med Mol Imaging* 34:2154–2159.

Cabanas, R.M. 1977. An approach for the treatment of penile carcinoma. *Cancer* 39:456–466.

Calabrese, L., Soutar, D., Werner, J., Bruschini, R., De Cicco, C., Chiesa, F. 2008. Sentinel lymph node biopsy in cancer of the head and neck. In *Radioguided Surgery: A Comprehensive Team Approach*. G. Mariani, A.E. Giuliano, W.H. Strauss (eds), pp. 120–129. New York, NY: Springer Science.

Carlson, R.W., Allred, D.C., Anderson, B.O. et al. 2009. Breast cancer: Clinical practice guidelines in oncology. *J Natl Compr Canc Netw* 7:122–192.

Carter, C.L., Allen, C., Henson, D.E. 1989. Relation of tumor size, lymph node status, and survival in 24,740 breast cancer cases. *Cancer* 63:181–187.

Chakera, A.H., Friis, E., Hesse, U., Al-Suliman, N., Zerahn, B., Hesse, B. 2005. Factors of importance for scintigraphic non-visualization of sentinel nodes in breast cancer. *Eur J Nucl Med Mol Imaging* 32:286–293.

Civantos, F. Jr, Zitsch, R., Bared, A., Amin, A. 2008. Sentinel node biopsy for squamous cell carcinoma of the head and neck. *J Surg Oncol* 97:683–690.

Civantos, F. Jr, Zitsch, R.P., Schuller, D.E. et al. 2010. Sentinel lymph node biopsy accurately stages the regional lymph nodes for T1-T2 oral squamous cell carcinomas: Results of a prospective multi-institutional trial. *J Clin Oncol* 28:1395–1400.

Cooper, D.S., Doherty, G.M., Haugen, B.R. et al. 2006. Management guidelines for patients with thyroid nodules and differentiated thyroid cancer. *Thyroid* 16:109–142.

Crane, L.M., Themelis, G., Buddingh, K. et al. 2010. Multispectral real-time fluorescence imaging for intraoperative detection of the sentinel lymph node in gynecologic oncology. *J Vis Exp* 44:22–25.

Damin, D.C., Rosito, M.A., Schwartsmann, G. 2006. Sentinel lymph node in carcinoma of the anal canal: A review. *Eur J Surg Oncol* 32:247–252.

De Cicco, C., Pizzamiglio, M., Trifirò, G. et al. 2002. Radioguided occult lesion localisation (ROLL) and surgical biopsy in breast cancer. Technical aspects. *Q J Nucl Med* 46:145–151.

De Cicco C1, Trifirò G, Intra M, Marotta G, Ciprian A, Frasson A, Prisco G, Luini A, Viale G, Paganelli G. 2004. Optimised nuclear medicine method for tumour marking and sentinel node detection in occult primary breast lesions. *Eur J Nucl Med Mol Imaging*. 31:349–54.

De Jong, J.S., Beukema, J.C., van Dam, G.M., Slart, R., Lemstra, C., Wiggers, T. 2010. Limited value of staging squamous cell carcinoma of the anal margin and canal using the sentinel lymph node procedure: A prospective study with long-term follow-up. *Ann Surg Oncol* 17:2656–2662.

De Nardi, P., Carvello, M., Canevari, C., Passoni, P., Staudacher, C. 2011. Sentinel node biopsy in squamous-cell carcinoma of the anal Canal. *Ann Surg Oncol* 18:365–370.

Edge, S.B., Byrd, D.R., Compton, C.C., Fritz, A.G., Greene, F.L., Trotti, A. (eds). 2010. Breast cancer. In *AJCC Cancer Staging Manual*, 3rd 7th edn. pp. 241–249. New York, NY: Springer.

Feggi, L., Basaglia, E., Corcione, S. et al. 2001. An original approach in the diagnosis of early breast cancer: Use of the same radiopharmaceutical for both non-palpable lesions and sentinel node localisation. *Eur J Nucl Med* 28:1589–1596.

Filippakis, G.M., Zografos, G. 2007. Contraindications of sentinel lymph node biopsy: Are there any really? *World J Surg Oncol* 5:10.

Filippi, L., Schillaci, O. 2006a. SPECT/CT with a hybrid camera: A new imaging modality for the functional anatomical mapping of infections. *Expert Rev Med Devices* 3:699–703.

Filippi, L., Schillaci, O. 2006b. Usefulness of hybrid SPECT/CT in ^{99m}Tc-HMPAO labeled leukocyte scintigraphy for bone and joint infections. *J Nucl Med* 47:1908–1913.

Franceschi, D., Crowe, J., Zollinger, R. et al. 1990. Biopsy of the breast for mammographically detected lesions. *Surg Gynecol Obstet* 171:449–455.

Fukuoka, M., Taki, J., Mochizuki, T., Kinuya, S. 2011. Comparison of diagnostic value of I-123 MIBG and high-dose I-131 MIBG scintigraphy including incremental value of SPECT/CT over planar image in patients with malignant pheochromocytoma/paraganglioma and neuroblastoma. *Clin Nucl Med* 36:1–7.

Gaarenstroom, K.N., Kenter, G.G., Trimbos, J.B. et al. 2003. Postoperative complications after vulvectomy and inguinofemoral lymphadenectomy using separate groin incisions. *Int J Gynecol Cancer* 13:522–527.

Gemmel, F., Van den Wyngaert, H., Love, C., Welling, M.M., Gemmel, P., Palestro, C.J. 2012. Prosthetic joint infections: Radionuclide state-of-the-art imaging. *Eur J Nucl Med Mol Imaging* 39:892–909.

Gerard, J.P., Chapet, O., Samiei, F. et al. 2001. Management of inguinal lymph node metastases in patients with carcinoma of the anal canal: Experience in a series of 270 patients treated in Lyon and review of the literature. *Cancer* 92:77–84.

Goedde, T.A., Frykberg, E.R., Crump, J.M., Lay, S.F., Turetsky, D.B., Linden, S.S. 1992. The impact of mammography on breast biopsy. *Am Surg* 58:661–666.

Gross, M.D., Avram, A., Fig, L.M., Rubello, D. 2007. Contemporary adrenal scintigraphy. *Eur J Nucl Med Mol Imaging* 34:547–557.

Gulec, S.A., Baum, R. 2007. Radio-guided surgery in neuroendocrine tumors. *J Surg Oncol* 96:309–315.

Hampl, M., Hantschmann, P., Michels, W., Hillemanns, P., German Multicenter Study Group. 2008. German multicenter study group. Validation of the accuracy of the sentinel lymph node procedure in patients with vulvar cancer: Results of a multicenter study in Germany. *Gynecol Oncol* 111:282–288.

Harris, L., Yoo, J., Driedger, A. et al. 2008. Accuracy of technetium-99m SPECT-CT hybrid images in predicting the precise intraoperative anatomical location of parathyroid adenomas. *Head Neck* 30:509–517.

Hefler, L.A., Grimm, C., Six, L. et al. 2008. Inguinal sentinel lymph node dissection vs. complete inguinal lymph node dissection in patients with vulvar cancer. *Anticancer Res* 28:515–517.

Hillel, P.G., van Beek, E.J., Taylor, C. et al. 2006. The clinical impact of a combined gamma camera/CT imaging system on somatostatin receptor imaging of neuroendocrine tumours. *Clin Radiol* 61:579–587.

Horenblas, S., Kroon, B.K., Valdes Olmos, R.A., Nieweg, O.E. 2008. Dynamic sentinel lymph node biopsy in penile carcinoma. In: *Radioguided Surgery: A Comprehensive Team Approach*, G. Mariani, A.E. Giuliano, H.W. Strauss (eds). pp. 117–125. New York: Springer.

Horger, M., Eschmann, S.M., Pfannenberg, C. et al. 2004. Evaluation of combined transmission and emission tomography for classification of skeletal lesions. *AJR Am J Roentgenol* 183:655–661.

Jacobson, A.F., Deng, H., Lombard, J., Lessig, H.J., Black, R.R. 2010. ^{123}I-*Meta*-Iodobenzylguanidine scintigraphy for the detection of neuroblastoma and pheochromocytoma: Results of a meta-analysis. *J Clin Endocrinol Metab* 95:2596–2606.

Johann, S., Klaeser, B., Krause, T., Mueller, M.D. 2008. Comparison of outcome and recurrence-free survival after sentinel lymph node biopsy and lymphadenectomy in vulvar cancer. *Gynecol Oncol* 110:324–328.

Kaltsas, G.A., Besser, G.M., Grossman, A.B. 2004. The diagnosis and medical management of advanced neuroendocrine tumors. *Endocr Rev* 25:458–511.

Khafif, A., Schneebaum, S., Fliss, D.M. et al. 2006. Lymphoscintigraphy for sentinel node mapping using a hybrid single photon emission CT (SPECT)/CT system in oral cavity squamous cell carcinoma. *Head Neck* 28:874–879.

Kimura, Y., Yama, N., Isobe, M. et al. 2006. A novel method for the detection and the localization of intestinal bleeding using a fusion image of Tc-99m-labeled RBC SPECT and X-ray CT. *J Abdom Emerg Med* 26:387–389.

Kobayashi, K., Ramirez, P.T., Kim, E.E. et al. 2009. Sentinel node mapping in vulvovaginal melanoma using SPECT/CT lymphoscintigraphy. *Clin Nucl Med* 34:859–861.

Kovács, A.F., Stefenelli, U., Seitz, O. et al. 2009. Positive sentinel lymph nodes are a negative prognostic factor for survival in T1–2 oral/oropharyngeal cancer-a long-term study on 103 patients. *Ann Surg Oncol* 16:233–239.

Krausz, Y., Bettman, L., Guralnik, L. et al. 2006. Technetium-99m-MIBI SPECT/CT in primary hyperparathyroidism. *World J Surg* 30:76–83.

Krausz, Y., Keidar, Z., Kogan, I. et al. 2003. SPECT/CT hybrid imaging with ^{111}In-pentetreotide in assessment of neuroendocrine tumours. *Clin Endocrinol* (Oxf). 59:565–573.

Krenning, E.P., Kwekkeboom, D.J., Oei, H.Y. et al. 1994. Somatostatin-receptor scintigraphy in gastroenteropancreatic tumors: An overview of European results. *Ann NY Acad Sci* 733:416–424.

Krontiras, H., Bland, K.I. 2003. When is sentinel node biopsy for breast cancer contraindicated? *Surg Oncol* 12:207–210.

Kroon, B.K., Horenblas, S., Estourgie, S.H., Lont, A.P., Valdés Olmos, R.A., Nieweg, O.E. 2004. How to avoid false-negative dynamic sentinel node procedures in penile carcinoma. *J Urol* 171:2191–2194.

Kusano, M., Tajima, Y., Yamazaki, K., Kato, M., Watanabe, M., Miwa, M. 2008. Sentinel node mapping guided by indocyanine green fluorescence imaging: A new method for sentinel node navigation surgery in gastrointestinal cancer. *Dig Surg* 25:103–108.

Lamberts, S.W., Chayvialle, J.A., Krenning, E.P. 1992. The visualization of gastroenteropancreatic endocrine tumors. *Metabolism* 41:111–115.

Lavely, W.C., Goetze, S., Friedman, K.P. et al. 2007. Comparison of SPECT/CT, SPECT, and planar imaging with single- and dual-phase ^{99m}Tc-sestamibi parathyroid scintigraphy. *J Nucl Med* 48:1084–1089.

Leijte, J.A., Kroon, B.K., Valdés Olmos, R.A., Nieweg, O.E, Horenblas, S. 2007. Reliability and safety of current dynamic sentinel node biopsy for penile carcinoma. *Eur Urol* 52:170–177.

Leijte, J.A., Valdés Olmos, R.A., Nieweg, O.E., Horenblas, S. 2008. Anatomical mapping of lymphatic drainage in penile carcinoma with SPECT-CT: Implications for the extent of inguinal lymph node dissection. *Eur Urol* 54:885–890.

Leijte, J.A., van der Ploeg, I.M., Valdés Olmos, R.A., Nieweg, O.E., Horenblas S. 2009. Visualization of tumor blockage and rerouting of lymphatic drainage in penile cancer patients by use of SPECT/CT. *J Nucl Med* 50:364–367.

Levenback, C., Coleman, R.L., Burke, T.W., Bodurka-Bevers, D., Wolf, J.K., Gershenson, D.M. 2001. Intraoperative lymphatic mapping and sentinel node identification with blue dye in patients with vulvar cancer. *Gynecol Oncol* 83:276–281.

Lind, P., Kohlfürst, S. 2006. Respective roles of thyroglobulin, radioiodine imaging, and positron emission tomography in the assessment of thyroid cancer. *Semin Nucl Med* 36:194–205.

Love, C., Palestro, C.J. 2004. Radionuclide imaging of infection. *J Nucl Med Technol* 32:47–57.

Luster, M., Clarke, S.E., Dietlein, M. et al. 2008. Guidelines for radioiodine therapy of differentiated thyroid cancer. *Eur J Nucl Med Mol Imaging* 35:1941–1959.

Lyman, G.H., Giuliano, A.E., Somerfield, M.R. et al. 2005. American Society of Clinical Oncology. American Society of Clinical Oncology guideline recommendations for sentinel lymph node biopsy in early-stage breast cancer. *J Clin Oncol* 23:7703–7720.

Manca, G., Tredici, M., Duce, V. et al. 2013. Preoperative and intraoperative lymphatic mapping for radioguided sentinel node biopsy in breast cancer. In *Atlas of Lymphoscintigraphy and Sentinel Node Mapping*, G. Mariani, G. Manca, F. Orsini, S. Vidal-Sicart, R.A. Valdés Olmos (eds). pp. 121–168. Milan: Springer.

Mariani, G., Gulec, S.A, Rubello, D. et al. 2003. Preoperative localization and radioguided parathyroid surgery. *J Nucl Med* 44:1443–1458.

Mariani, G., Moresco, L., Viale, G. et al. 2001. Radioguided sentinel lymph node biopsy in breast cancer surgery. *J Nucl Med* 42:1198–1215.

Meyer-Rochow, G.Y., Schembri, G.P., Benn, D.E. et al. 2010. The utility of metaiodobenzylguanidine single photon emission computed tomography/computed tomography (MIBG SPECT/CT) for the diagnosis of pheochromocytoma. *Ann Surg Oncol* 17:392–400.

Mistrangelo, M., Bellò, M., Mobiglia, A. et al. 2009. Feasibility of the sentinel node biopsy in anal cancer. *Q J Nucl Med Mol Imaging* 53:3–8.

Mistrangelo, M., Pelosi, E., Bellò, M. et al. 2010. Comparison of positron emission tomography scanning and sentinel node biopsy in the detection of inguinal node metastases in patients with anal cancer. *Int J Rad Oncol Biol Phys* 77:73–78.

Mitchell, G., Pratt, B.E., Vini, L., McCready, V.R., Harmer, C.L. 2000. False positive ^{131}I whole body scans in thyroid cancer. *Br J Radiol 73*:627–635.

Ng, D.A., Opelka, F.G., Beck, D.E. et al. 1997. Predictive value of technetium Tc99m-labeled red blood cell scintigraphy for positive angiogram in massive lower gastrointestinal hemorrhage. *Dis Colon Rectum* 40:471–477.

Nigro, N.D., Vaitkevicious, V.K., Considine, B. 1974. Combined therapy for cancer of the anal canal: A preliminary report. *Dis Colon Rectum* 17:354–356.

O'Conno, M.K., Kemp, B.J. 2006. Single-photon emission computed tomography/computed tomography: Basic instrumentation and innovations. *Semin Nucl Med* 36:258–266.

Orsini, F., Rubello, D., Giuliano, A.E., Mariani, G. 2013. Radioguided surgery. In *Nuclear Oncology – Pathophysiology and Clinical Applications*, H.W. Strauss, G. Mariani, D. Volterrani, S.M. Larson (eds), pp. 731–762. New York: Springer.

Ozer, S., Dobrozemsky, G., Kienast, O. et al. 2004. Value of combined XCT/SPECT technology for avoiding false positive planar ^{123}I-MIBG scintigraphy. *Nuklearmedizin* 43:164–170.

Paganelli, G., De Cicco, C., Luini, A. et al. 1997. Radioguided surgery in non-palpable breast lesions. *Eur J Nucl Med* 24:893.

Paleri, V., Rees, G., Arullendran, P., Shoaib, T., Krishman, S. 2005. Sentinel node biopsy in squamous cell cancer of the oral cavity and oral pharynx: A diagnostic meta-analysis. *Head Neck* 27:739–747.

Papathanassiou, D., Liehn, J.C., Meneroux, B. et al. 2007. SPECT-CT of Meckel's diverticulum. *Clin Nucl Med* 32:218–220.

Pelosi, E., Bellò, M., Giors, M. et al. 2004. Sentinel lymph node detection in patients with early-stage breast cancer: Comparison of periareolar and subdermal/peritumoral injection techniques. *J Nucl Med* 45:220–225.

Perri, M., Erba, P., Volterrani, D. et al. 2008. Octreo-SPECT/CT imaging for accurate detection and localization of suspected neuroendocrine tumors. *Q J Nucl Med Mol Imaging* 52:323–333.

Pfannenberg, A.C., Eschmann, S.M., Horger, M. et al. 2003. Benefit of anatomical-functional image fusion in the diagnostic work-up of neuroendocrine neoplasms. *Eur J Nucl Med Mol Imaging* 30:835–843.

Pizzocaro, G., Algaba, F., Horenblas, S. et al. 2010. European Association of Urology (EAU) Guidelines Group on Penile Cancer. EAU penile cancer guidelines 2009. *Eur Urol* 57:1002.

Povoski, S.P., Neff, R.L., Mojzisik, C.M. et al. 2009. A comprehensive overview of radioguided surgery using gamma detection probe technology. *World J Surg Oncol* 7:11.

Prandini, N., Lazzeri, E., Rossi, B., Erba, P., Parisella, M.G., Signore, A. 2006. Nuclear medicine imaging of bone infections. *Nucl Med Commun* 27:633–644.

Rezzo, R., Scopinaro, G., Gambaro, M., Michetti, P., Anfossi, G. 2002. Radioguided occult colonic lesion identification (ROCLI) during open and laparoscopic surgery. *Tumori* 88:S19–22.

Rozovsky, K., Koplewitz, B.Z., Krausz, Y. et al. 2008. Added value of SPECT/CT for correlation of MIBG scintigraphy and diagnostic CT in neuroblastoma and pheochromocytoma. *Am J Roentgenol* 190:1085–1090.

Rubello, D., Gross, M.D., Mariani, G., AL-Nahhas A. 2007. Scintigraphic techniques in primary hyperparathyroidism: From pre-operative localisation to intra-operative imaging. *Eur J Nucl Med Mol Imaging* 34:926–933.

Rubello, D., Massaro, A., Cittadin, S. et al. 2006. Role of ^{99m}Tc-sestamibi SPECT in accurate selection of primary hyperparathyroid patients for minimally invasive radio-guided surgery. *Eur J Nucl Med Mol Imaging* 33:1091–1094.

Ruda, J.M., Hollenbeak, C., Stack, B.C. Jr. 2005. A systematic review of the diagnosis and treatment of primary hyperparathyroidism from 1995 to 2003. *Otolaryngol Head Neck Surg* 132:359–372.

Rufini, V., Calcagni, M.L., Baum, R.P. 2006. Imaging of neuroendocrine tumors. *Semin Nucl Med* 36:228–247.

Sadeghi, R., Gholami, H., Zakavi, S.R., Kakhki, V.R., Tabasi, K.T., Horenblas, S. 2012. Accuracy of sentinel lymph node biopsy for inguinal lymph node staging of penile squamous cell carcinoma: Systematic review and meta-analysis of the literature. *J Urol* 187:25–31.

Schachter, P.P., Issa, N., Shimonov, M., Czerniak, A., Lorberboym, M. 2004. Early, postinjection MIBI-SPECT as the only preoperative localizing study for minimally invasive parathyroidectomy. *Arch Surg* 139:433–437.

Schillaci, O., Danieli, R., Manni, C., Capoccetti, F., Simonetti, G. 2004. Technetium-99m-labelled red blood cell imaging in the diagnosis of hepatic haemangiomas: The role of SPECT/CT with a hybrid camera. *Eur J Nucl Med Mol Imaging* 31:1011–1015.

Schillaci, O., Filippi, L., Danieli, R., Simonetti, G. 2007. Single-photon emission computed tomography/computed tomography in abdominal diseases. *Semin Nucl Med* 37:48–61.

Schillaci, O., Spanu, A., Tagliabue, L. et al. 2009. SPECT/CT with a hybrid imaging system in the study of lower gastrointestinal bleeding with technetium-99m red blood cells. *Q J Nucl Med Mol Imaging* 53:281–289.

Schlumberger, M.J. 1998. Papillary and follicular thyroid carcinoma. *N Engl J Med* 338:297–306.

Serra, A., Bolasco, P., Satta, L., Nicolosi, A., Uccheddu, A., Piga, M. 2006. Role of SPECT/CT in the preoperative assessment of hyperparathyroid patients. *Radiol Med* 111:999–1008.

Shapiro, B., Rufini, V., Jarwan, A. et al. 2000. Artifacts, anatomical and physiological variants, and unrelated diseases that may cause false-positive whole-body 131-I scans in patients with thyroid cancer. *Semin Nucl Med* 30:115–132.

Shapiro, B., Sisson, J.C., Shulkin, B.L. 1995. The current status of meta-iodobenzylguanidine and related agents for the diagnosis of neuroendocrine tumors. *Q J Nucl Med* 39:3–8.

Shi, W., Johnston, C.F., Buchanan, K.D. et al. 1998. Localization of neuroendocrine tumors with [^{111}In] DTPA-octreotide scintigraphy (Octreoscan): A comparative study with CT and MR imaging. *QJM* 91:295–301.

Simpson, W.J., Panzarella, T., Carruthers, J.S., Gospodarowicz, M.K., Sutcliffe, S.B. 1998. Papillary and follicular thyroid cancer: Impact of treatment in 1578 patients. *Int J Radiat Oncol Biol Phys* 14:1063–1075.

Slater, A., Gleeson, F.V. 2005. Increased sensitivity and confidence of SPECT over planar imaging in dual-phase sestamibi for parathyroid adenoma detection. *Clin Nucl Med* 30:1–3.

Sortini, D., Feo, C., Maravegias, K. et al. 2006. Intrathoracoscopic localization techniques. Review of literature. *Surg Endosc* 20:1341–1347.

Spanu, A., Solinas, M.E., Chessa, F., Sanna, D., Nuvoli, S., Madeddu, G. 2009. ^{131}I SPECT/CT in the follow-up of differentiated thyroid carcinoma: Incremental value versus planar imaging. *J Nucl Med* 50:184–190.

Sutter, C.W., Masilungan, B.G., Stadalnik, R.C. 1995. False-positive results of I-131 whole-body scans in patients with thyroid cancer. *Semin Nucl Med* 25:279–282.

Takei, H., Suemasu, K., Kurosumi, M. et al. 2006. Added value of the presence of blue nodes or hot nodes in sentinel lymph node biopsy with breast cancer. *Breast Cancer* 13:179–185.

Trifirò, G., Travaini, L.L., Sanvito, F. et al. 2010. Sentinel node detection by lymphoscintigraphy and sentinel lymph node biopsy in vulvar melanoma. *Eur J Nucl Med Mol Imaging* 37:736–741.

Tsugawa, K., Noguchi, M., Miwa, K. et al. 2000. Dye- and gamma probe-guided sentinel lymph node biopsy in breast cancer patients: Using patent blue dye and technetium-99m-labeled human serum albumin. *Breast Cancer* 7:87–94.

Tükenmez, M., Erbil, Y., Barbaros, U. et al. 2007. Radio-guided non palpable metastatic lymph node localization in patients with recurrent thyroid cancer. *J Surg Oncol* 96:534–538.

Turner-Warwick, RT. 1959. The lymphatics of the breast. *Br J Surg* 46:574–582.

Valdés Olmos, R.A., Tanis, P.J., Hoefnagel, C.A. et al. 2001. Penile lymphoscintigraphy for sentinel node identification. *Eur J Nucl Med* 28:581–585.

van den Berg, N.S., Brouwer, O.R., Klop, W.M. et al. 2012. Concomitant radio- and fluorescence-guided sentinel lymph node biopsy in squamous cell carcinoma of the oral cavity using ICG-99mTc-nanocolloid. *Eur J Nucl Med Mol Imaging* 39:1128–1136.

van der Ploeg, I.M., Hobbelink, M., van den Bosch, M.A., Mali, W.P., Borel Rinkes, I.H., van Hillegersberg, R. 2008a. Radioguided occult lesion localisation (ROLL) for non-palpable breast lesions: A review of the relevant literature. *Eur J Surg Oncol* 34:1–5.

van der Ploeg, I.M., Nieweg, O.E., van Rijk, M.C., Valdés Olmos, R.A., Kroon, B.B. 2008b. Axillary recurrence after a tumour-negative sLNB in breast cancer patients: A systematic review and meta-analysis of the literature. *Eur J Surg Oncol* 34:1277–1284.

van der Zee, A.G., Oonk, M.H., De Hullu, J.A. et al. 2008. Sentinel node dissection is safe in the treatment of early-stage vulvar cancer. *J Clin Oncol* 26:884–889.

Vermeeren, L., Valdés Olmos, R.A., Klop, W.M., Balm A.J., van den Brekel M.W. 2010. A portable gamma-camera for intraoperative detection of sentinel nodes in the head and neck region. *J Nucl Med* 51:700–703.

Veronesi, U., Paganelli, G., Viale, G. et al. 1999. Sentinel lymph node biopsy and axillary dissection in breast cancer: Results in a large series. *J Natl Cancer Inst* 91:368–373.

Vidal-Sicart, S., Puig-Tintoré, L.M., Lejárcegui, J.A. et al. 2007. Validation and application of the sentinel lymph node concept in malignant vulvar tumours. *Eur J Nucl Med Mol Imaging* 34:384–391.

Vorburger, S.A., Ubersax, L., Schmid, S.W., Balli, M., Candinas, D., Seiler, C.A. 2009. Long-term follow-up after complete resection of well-differentiated cancer confined to the thyroid gland. *Ann Surg Oncol* 16:2862–2874.

Wade, D.S., Herrera, L., Castillo, N.B., Petrelli, N.J. 1989. Metastases to the lymph nodes in epidermoid carcinoma of the anal canal studied by a clearing technique. *Surg Gynecol Obstet* 169:238–242.

Wagner, A., Schicho, K., Glaser, C. et al. 2004. SPECT-CT for topographic mapping of sentinel lymph nodes prior to gamma probe-guided biopsy in head and neck squamous cell carcinoma. *J Craniomaxillofac Surg* 32:343–349.

Wespes, E. 2007. The management of regional lymph nodes in patients with penile carcinoma and reliability of sentinel node biopsy. *Eur Urol* 52:5–6.

Wong, K., Zarzhevsky, N., Cahill, J.M., Frey, K.A., Avram, A.M. 2008. The value of diagnostic 131-I SPECT-CT fusion imaging in the evaluation of differentiated thyroid carcinoma. *Am J Roentgenol* 191:1785–1794.

Wong, K.K., Komissarova, M., Avram, A.M., Fig, L.M., Gross, M.D. 2010a. Adrenal cortical imaging with I-131 NP-59 SPECT-CT. *Clin Nucl Med* 35:865–869.

Wong, K.K., Sisson, J.C., Koral, K.F., Frey, K.A., Avram, A.M. 2010b. Staging of differentiated thyroid carcinoma using diagnostic ^{131}I SPECT/CT. *Am J Roentgenol* 195:730–736.

Yen, R.F., Wu, V.C., Liu, K.L. et al. 2009. ^{131}I-6β-Iodomethyl-19-norcholesterol SPECT/CT for primary aldosteronism patients with inconclusive adrenal venous sampling and CT results. *J Nucl Med* 50:1631–1637.

Zheng, J.G., Yao, Z.M., Shu, C.Y., Zhang, Y., Zhang, X. 2005. Role of SPECT/CT in diagnosis of hepatic hemangiomas. *World J Gastroenterol* 11: 5336–5341.

Zuccaro, G. Jr. 1998. Management of the adult patient with acute lower gastrointestinal bleeding. American College of Gastroenterology. Practice Parameters Committee. *Am J Gastroenterol* 93:1202–1208.

40 Preoperative Imaging for Reconstruction of the Lower Extremities

Hidehiko Yoshimatsu and Takumi Yamamoto

CONTENTS

Whether the lower extremity is serving as a donor site, a recipient site for a vascularised tissue flap, or the subject for lymphatic surgery, a safe, accurate, and cost-effective imaging strategy is necessary to prevent potential complications of foot ischemia and to find aberrant anatomy that might change the surgical procedure. In this chapter, multiple imaging modalities are described.

40.1 MULTI-DETECTOR ROW CT

In many institutions, multi-detector row CT has taken over conventional angiography as the primary modality for preoperative evaluation for vascularised free-flap reconstruction of the lower extremity. When compared with angiography, it is less invasive and more cost-effective and is not associated with substantial complications potentially seen with angiography, including access site haematoma, pseudoaneurysm, dissection, and arterial occlusion.

One of the most important factors that can influence the strategy of reconstructive surgery is the arterial occlusion and arterial anomaly. This includes identification of occult vascular injury, in which arterial injury is found during operation in the presence of a normal preoperative physical examination. The occurrence of occult vascular injury can be as high as 28% in the setting of long bone injury.[1] In addition, special attention should be paid to venous thrombosis and pre-existing atherosclerotic disease demonstrated by intramural calcification. CT angiography also provides information regarding surrounding tissues and bone fractures. Using 3D volume-rendering technique, 3D image of the vessels can be obtained, which easily indicates the site of occlusion and variant anatomy. However, these sites should be confirmed with axial imaging (Figures 40.1 through 40.3).

Duymaz and colleagues confirmed the reliability of the preoperative CT angiography within a trauma setting, demonstrating preoperative arterial occlusion as a significant predictor of limb loss.[2]

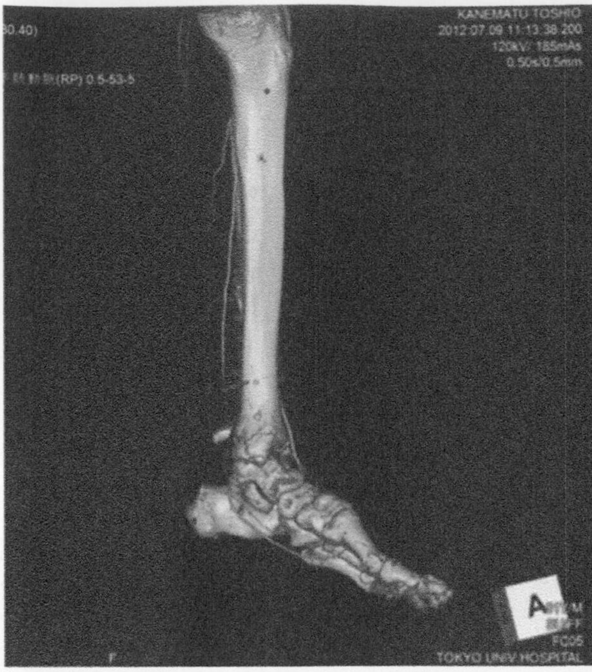

FIGURE 40.1 Three-dimensional reformatting CT angiography of the left leg of a 51-year-old man with fracture of the distal left tibia. The occlusion of the posterior tibial artery is identified, as indicated by the arrow. Reformatted images should be confirmed with axial imaging.

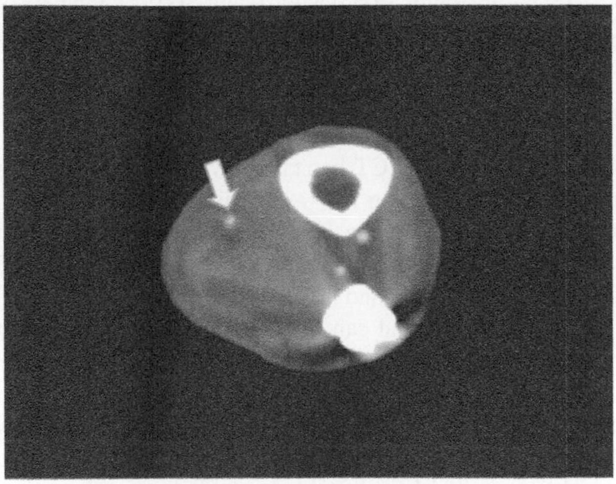

FIGURE 40.2 Image showing a patent posterior tibial artery proximal to the site of the injury.

40.1.1 When CT Angiography Can Be Misleading

One of the disadvantages of CT angiography is that it can produce false-positive readings caused by vasospasm, in which a vessel appears to be occluded. However, the rate of false-positive readings has been reported to be 1.3%, with a sensitivity of 95.1% and a specificity of 98.7%.[3]

CT angiography can visualise vessels as small as 1 mm. However, when dealing with reconstruction necessitating supermicrosurgery, where the diameter of the vessels can be as small as 0.3 mm, preoperative detection of the vessels can be challenging.

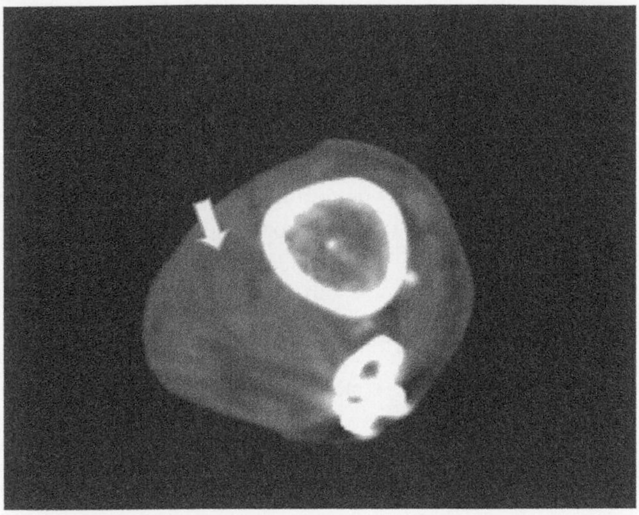

FIGURE 40.3 Image showing the occluded part of the posterior tibial artery distal to the site of the injury, as indicated by the absence of contrast.

40.2 ICG LYMPHOGRAPHY

Secondary lymphedema of the lower extremity can be a considerable burden to patients following cancer treatment, restricting their daily activities. Most cases of lymphedema progress over time despite conservative therapies.[4–6] Conservative therapies are mainstay method of lymphedema treatment and are required to continue for a life-long period.[7] Lymphaticovenular anastomosis (LVA) has become one of the treatment options for extremity lymphedema, and several studies have reported the efficacy of the treatment.[8–11] A significant problem lies as to when treatments for lymphedema should be commenced to achieve prevention of overtreatment and treatment delay. It is imperative to distinguish cases at high risk of developing lymphedema at an early stage and to establish indications for treatments.

Yamamoto and colleagues have reported indocyanine green (ICG) lymphography for evaluation of lower extremity lymphedema (LEL) and demonstrated its clinical utility for severity scaling and early diagnosis.[12] ICG lymphography is a non-invasive test which allows real-time evaluation. Unlike lymphoscintigraphy, it has no risk of radiation exposure, making it the modality of choice for routine evaluation of lymphedema.[13–16]

40.2.1 Procedures

For the lower extremities, lymphatic channel imaging is performed as follows: 0.2 mL of ICG (Diagnogreen 2.5 mg/mL; Daiichi Pharmaceutical, Tokyo, Japan) is subcutaneously injected into the bilateral lower extremities at the first web space of the foot and the lateral border of the Achilles tendon. After injection, circumferential fluorescent images of lymphatic drainage channels are obtained using an infrared camera system (Photodynamic Eye; Hamamatsu Photonics K.K., Hamamatsu, Japan) (Figure 40.2). Fluorescent images are observed immediately and at 12–24 h after ICG injection, because in lymphedema cases, it takes several hours for the ICG to spread to the whole leg, which is necessary for accurate evaluation of the ICG findings.

ICG lymphography can detect lymphatic channels located up to 2 cm deep from the skin surface if there is no fascia, muscle, or bone above the channels. Normal ICG lymphography shows superficial lymphatic channels as a white line on the screen. ICG lymphography can show lymphatic channels, lymphatic valves, and lymphatic flow immediately after injection of ICG (Figure 40.4).

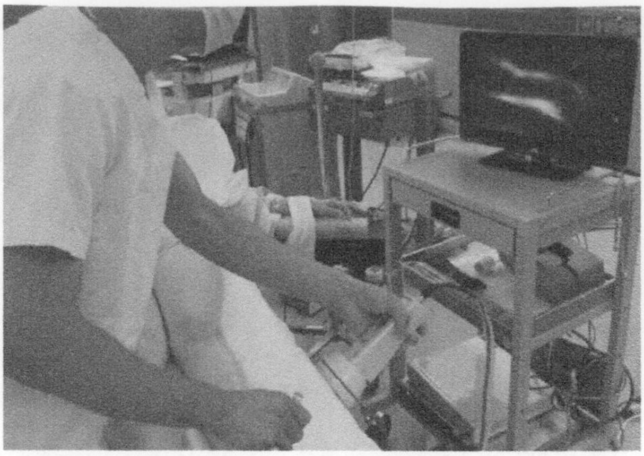

FIGURE 40.4 Marking the lymphatic channels using ICG lymphography.

40.2.2 ICG Lymphography Findings and Progression of Lymphedema

ICG lymphography pattern changes from normal linear pattern to abnormal DB patterns in obstructive peripheral lymphedema; with progression of lymphedema, DB patterns change from splash pattern, to stardust pattern, and finally to diffuse pattern (Figure 40.5). Lymph flow obstruction leads to lymphatic hypertension, lymphangiectasis, lymphatic valve insufficiency, lymphosclerosis, and lymph backflow. ICG lymphography visualises lymph backflow as DB patterns. Splash pattern on ICG lymphography represents dilated superficial lymphatics such as lymphatic precollectors and capillaries.

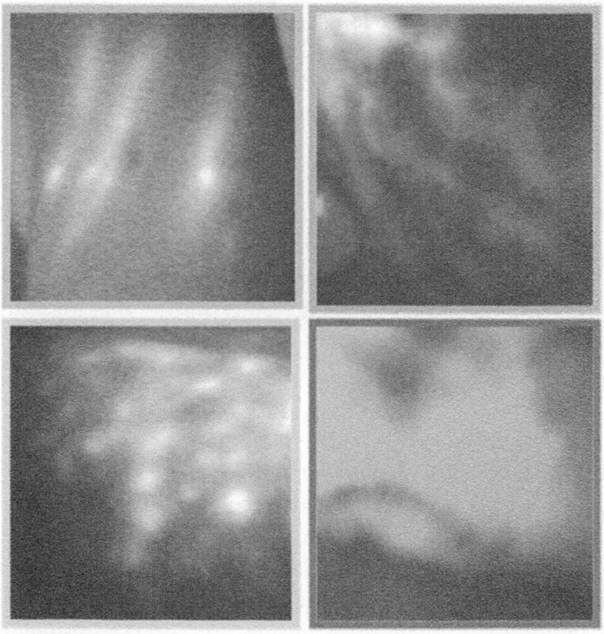

FIGURE 40.5 The linear pattern and three types of dermal backflow pattern observed in ICG lymphography. (Above, left) Linear pattern showing normal lymphatic channel. (Above, right) Splash pattern consisting of scattered dye twinkling in tortuous lymphatic channels. (Below, left) Stardust pattern demonstrating dimly luminous, spotted fluorescent signals. (Below, right) In diffuse pattern, dye is widely distributed without twinkling spots. with progression of lymphedema, the dermal backflow patterns change from splash, to stardust, and eventually to diffuse pattern.

Extravasation of lymph fluid occurs with progression of lymphedema, which is represented as spots on ICG lymphography – stardust pattern. Finally, the number of spots visualised on ICG lymphography increases the point where spots merge and cannot be distinguished from each other – diffuse pattern.

40.2.3 Leg DB Stage

In leg DB (LDB) stage 0, no DB pattern is seen on ICG lymphography (Figure 40.6). In LDB stage I, a splash pattern is seen around the groin (Figure 40.7). In LDB stage II through V, a stardust pattern is detected. In LDB stage II, the stardust pattern is limited proximally to the superior border of the patella (Figure 40.8). In LDB stage III, the stardust pattern exceeds the superior border of the patella

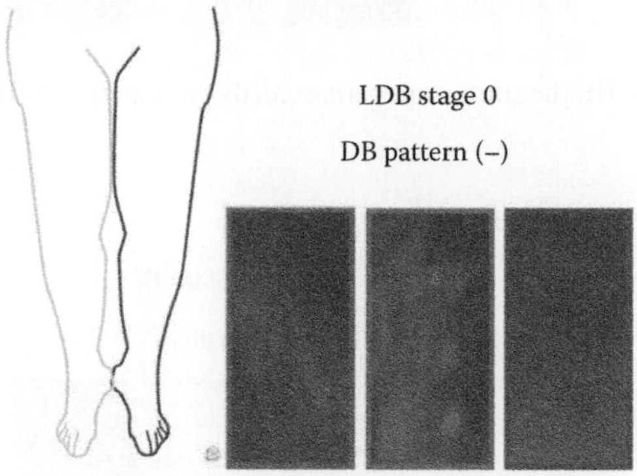

FIGURE 40.6 In LDB stage 0, no DB pattern is seen on ICG lymphography.

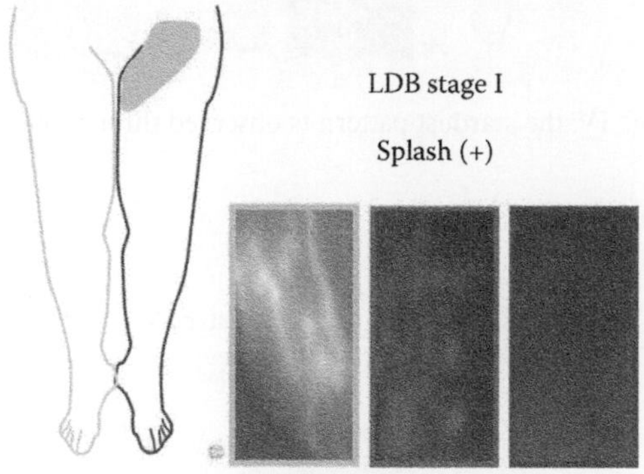

FIGURE 40.7 In LDB stage I, a splash pattern is seen around the groin.

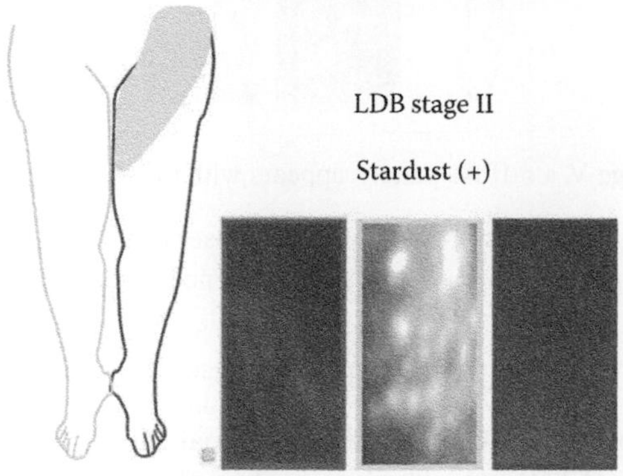

FIGURE 40.8 In LDB stage II, the stardust pattern is limited proximally to the superior border of the patella.

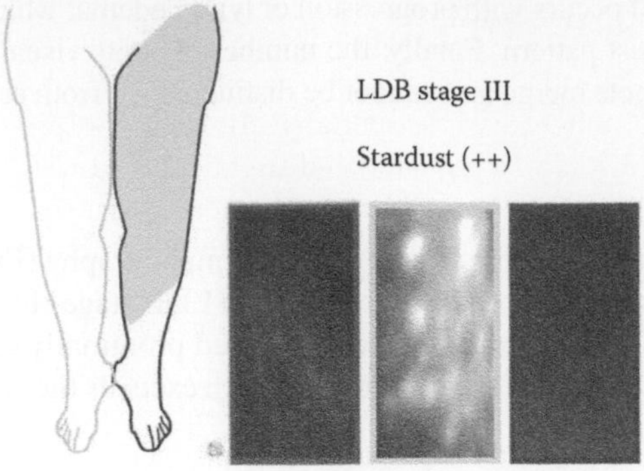

FIGURE 40.9 In LDB stage III, the stardust pattern exceeds the superior border of the patella.

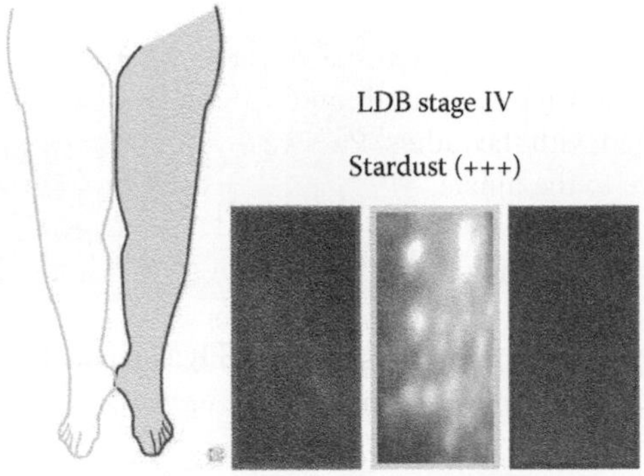

FIGURE 40.10 In LDB stage IV, the stardust pattern is observed throughout the limb.

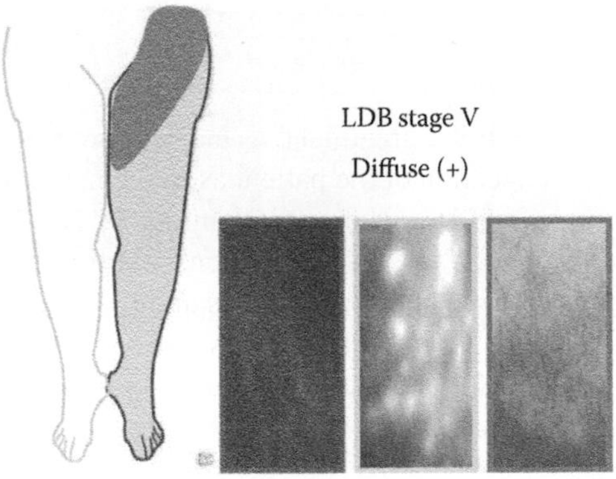

FIGURE 40.11 In LDB stage V, a diffuse pattern appears with the presence of the stardust pattern.

(Figure 40.9). In LDB stage IV, the stardust pattern is observed throughout the limb (Figure 40.10). In LDB stage V, a diffuse pattern appears with the presence of the stardust pattern (Figure 40.11).

40.3 NON-ENHANCED ANGIOGRAPHY

Non-enhanced angiography (NEA; Genial Viewer; Genial Light, Shizuoka, Japan) emits infrared light with the wavelength of 850 nm, which is exclusively absorbed by haemoglobin. The light penetrates the bones and other soft tissues, effectively visualising vessels containing blood, and

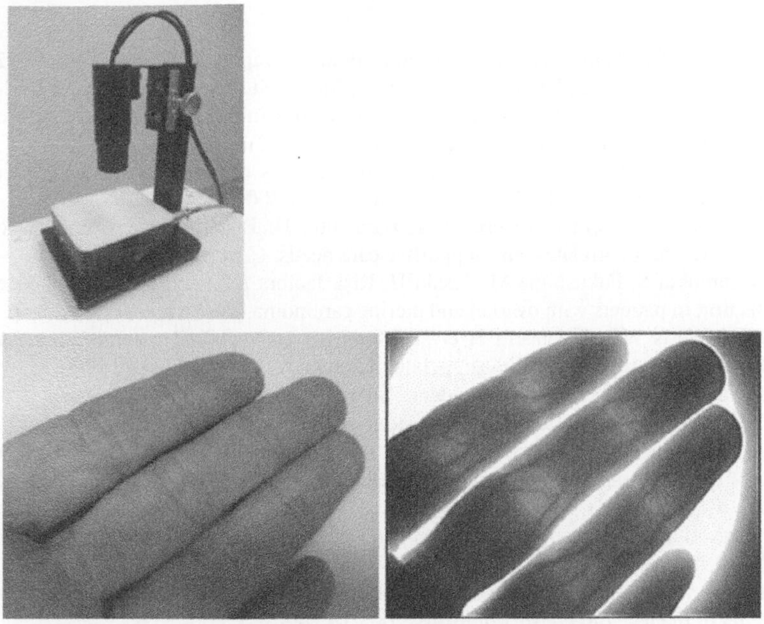

FIGURE 40.12 NEA.

the image is shown in real time on the screen of a laptop computer (Figure 40.12). NEA does not require contrast or will not expose patients to radiation, which makes it safe to use even on children and infants.[17]

NEA can be helpful in finding adequate vessels in replantation of amputated fingers. However, its application in toe transfer maximises the advantage of this device. In toe transfer, identification and procurement of the veins in the donor toe is the most challenging procedure. Using NEA preoperatively can significantly facilitate this step, allowing safer operation (Figure 40.13).

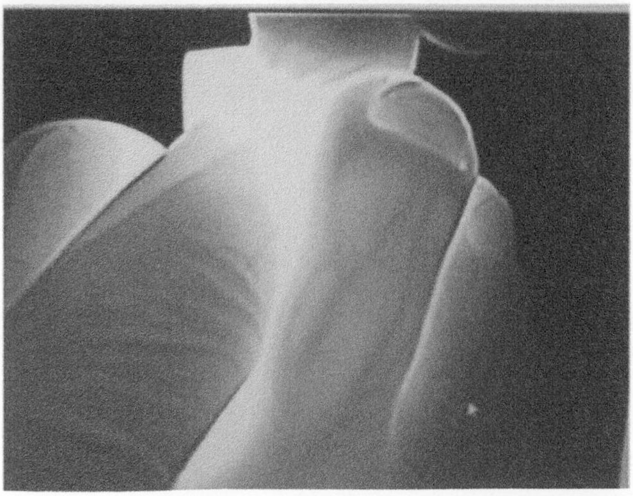

FIGURE 40.13 Visualisation of the dorsal veins of the second toe.

REFERENCES

1. Hessel SJ, Adams DF, Abrams HL. Complications of angiography. *Radiology* 1981;138:273–281.
2. Duymaz A, Karabekmez FE, Vrtiska TJ, Mardini S, Moran SL. Free tissue transfer for lower extremity reconstruction: A study of the role of computed angiography in the planning of free tissue transfer in the posttraumatic setting. *Plast Reconstr Surg* 2009 August;124(2):523–529.
3. Soto JA, Munera F, Morales C et al. Focal arterial injuries of the proximal extremities: Helical CT arteriography as the initial method of diagnosis. *Radiology* 2001;218:188–194.
4. Beesley V, Janda M, Eakin E, Obermair A, Battistutta D. Lymphedema after gynecological cancer treatment: Prevalence, correlates, and supportive care needs. *Cancer* 2007;109(12):2607–2614.
5. Tada H, Teramukai S, Fukushima M, Sasaki H. Risk factors for lower limb lymphedema after lymph node dissection in patients with ovarian and uterine carcinoma. *BMC Cancer* 2009;5:47.
6. Fiorica JV, Roberts WS, Greenberg H et al. Morbidity and survival patterns in patients after radial hysterectomy and postoperative adjuvant pelvic radiotherapy. *Gynecol Oncol* 1990;36(3):343–347.
7. Cohen SR, Payne DK, Tunkel RS. Lymphedema: Strategies for management. *Cancer* 2001;92(4):980–987.
8. Yamada Y. Studies on lymphatico-venous anastomoses in lymphedema. *Nagoya J Med* 1969;32:1–21.
9. Koshima I, Inagawa K, Urushibara K et al. Supermicrosurgical lymphaticovenular anastomosis for the treatment of lymphedema in the upper extremities. *J Reconstr Microsurg* 2000;16:432–437.
10. Yamamoto T, Narushima M, Kikuchi K et al. Lambda-shaped anastomosis with intravascular stenting method for safe and effective lymphaticovenular anastomosis. *Plast Reconstr Surg* 2011 May;127(5):1987–1992.
11. Koshima I, Nanba Y, Tsutsui T et al. Long-term follow-up after lymphaticovenular anastomosis for lymphedema in the leg. *J Reconstr Microsurg* 2003;19:209–215.
12. Yamamoto T, Narushima M, Doi K et al. Characteristic indocyanine green lymphography findings in lower extremity lymphedema: The generation of a novel lymphedema severity staging system using dermal backflow patterns. *Plast Reconstr Surg* 2011 May;127(5):1979–1986.
13. Henze E, Schelbert HR, Collins JD, Najafi A, Barrio JR, Bennett LR. Lymphoscintigraphy with Tc-99m-labeled dextran. *J Nucl Med* 1982;23(10):923–929.
14. Szuba A, Shin WS, Strauss HW, Rockson S. The third circulation: Radionuclide lymphoscintigraphy in the evaluation of lymphedema. *J Nucl Med* 2003;44(1):43–57.
15. Tomczak H, Nyka W, Lass P. Lymphoedema: Lymphoscintigraphy versus other diagnostic techniques – A clinician's point of view. *Nucl Med Rev Cent East Eur* 2005;8(1):37–43.
16. Modi S, Stanton AW, Mortimer PS, Levick JR. Clinical assessment of human lymph flow using removal rate constants of interstitial macromolecules: A critical review of lymphoscintigraphy. *Lymphat Res Biol* 2007;5(3):183–202.
17. Yoshimatsu H, Yamamoto T, Seki Y, Narushima M, Iida T, Koshima I. A new device expanding operability of fingertip replantation: Subzone 1 fingertip replantation assisted by non-enhanced angiography in a 2-year-old boy. *J Plast Reconstr Aesthet Surg* 2012 November;65(11):1592–1594. doi: 10.1016/j.bjps.2012.03.039. Epub 2012 April 17.

41 Imaging and Surgical Principles in Hand Surgery

Giorgio Pajardi and Andrea Ghezzi

CONTENTS

Standard and new imaging techniques are available and are necessary for the diagnosis and treatment of hand and wrist pathology. Despite the increasing use and availability of newer imaging modalities, radiographs remain an important technique for evaluating the patient with hand and wrist pathology. Plain x-rays are still the imaging technique of first choice for the assessment of abnormalities of wrist and hand. Magnetic resonance imaging (MRI) and computed tomography (CT) may be indicated depending on the clinical findings. If a bone injury is suspected, CT is the better choice. For soft tissue disorders, MRI is indicated, except for intrinsic ligaments and cartilage, for which arthrogram followed by CT (arthro-CT) is the most sensitive tool.

41.1 STANDARD RADIOGRAPHS

Radiographic evaluation of the hand and wrist should be performed, following a thorough history and physical exam. The standard studies that should be ordered include a posteroanterior (PA) and lateral view of the hand and wrist. Additional studies that may be indicated, depending upon the clinical findings, include the oblique view, the scaphoid view or ulnar-deviated PA view, the PA 45° pronated oblique view, the carpal tunnel view and the anteroposterior (AP) 30° supinated view and the stress-test view. Adequate radiographic evaluation of the hand and wrist is predicated upon standard positioning of the patient.

41.2 TECHNIQUE

Careful positioning of the upper limb is mandatory to obtain reproducible and comparable views. It is mandatory to perform comparative x-rays for children and sometimes also for adults.

Numerous techniques and measurements have been published in the literature, but the authors discuss those routinely used by radiologists and surgeons.

41.2.1 Hand

Posteroanterior (Figure 41.1) and lateral views of hand or digit are easy to perform. The 30° oblique views may be necessary to avoid superimposition of distal or proximal ends of metacarpals.

Carpometacarpal joints are also difficult to visualise when injured. Stress views are necessary when a subluxation or a ligament sprain has occurred (Figure 41.2). Trapeziometacarpal joint, scaphotrapezial and trapeziotrapezoid joints are seen on Kapandji views.

In the lateral view, the abducted thumb rests with its radial border against the cassette and the remaining fingers are elevated by a pad.

Measurement of maximum opening of the first cleft is obtained by a view with the hand in forced pronation and the cleft resting against the plate on its dorsal aspect.

Enlargements are useful in these circumstances, for a small bony fracture, particularly intraarticular, for the study of the bony texture, and in cases of bone infections.

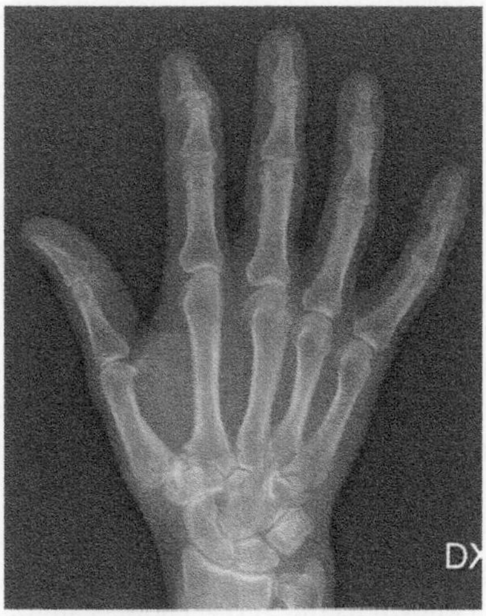

FIGURE 41.1 Posteroanterior view of the hand.

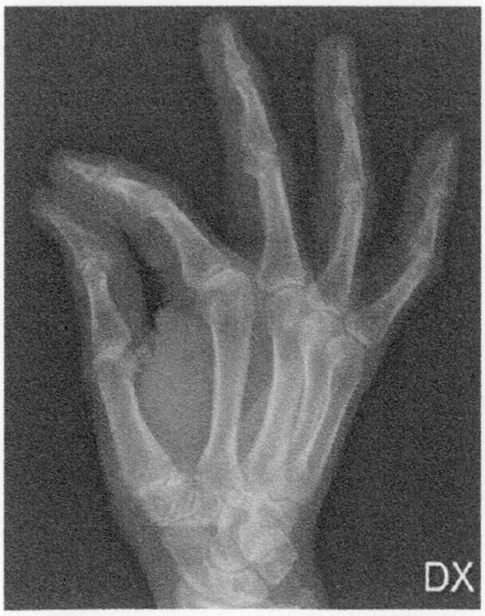

FIGURE 41.2 Stress view for CMC joint.

41.2.2 Wrist

Positioning of the wrist on the plate is mandatory. A malposition may induce an error of interpretation in radiological findings and calculation of indices. The usual incidence is PA and not AP, as often described. The standard way to obtain a reproducible PA view is an x-ray with the shoulder abducted 90°, the elbow flexed 90° and the hand flat on the plate with the fingers and thumb in stable position.

Some bones are difficult to visualise. The triquetrum in lateral view has been suggested to draw the bisector of this bone to calculate its position. It is also visible in films in 45° of pronation or supination. The pisiform and the pisotriquetral joints are visible when the hand lies with its ulnar border on the plate in 30° of supination. The hook of hamate may be seen in an oblique lateral view in 20° or 45° of supination plus maximal radial deviation and hyperextension. The scaphoid is the most investigated bone. Classic views have been described: Schreck's view, in which the hand is flat in forced ulnar deviation; Schreck's view, in which the hand rests on the plate in writing position; Stecher's view, in which the wrist is clenched and in ulnar deviation; and Bridgman's view, in which the hand is flat and the fingers elevated 20°.

In neutral position, the ulnar styloid is peripheral in PA and central in AP. This is a way to recognise the incidence. On PA view, the third metacarpal should be aligned with the radial axis.

From a PA view, clinical information available begins with evaluation of the joint surfaces. A perfect parallelism of the joint surfaces of the wrist is a normal condition, and this condition is evident on a correctly performed study and should be evident between the surfaces of the radius, scaphoid and lunate, the proximal and distal rows, and the distal carpus and the metacarpals. Overlapping of these normally parallel surfaces should alert to the possibility of subluxation or dislocation.

Gilula's arcs can be described on a normal PA view of the wrist. Arc 1 follows the main convex curvatures of the scaphoid, lunate and triquetrum proximal surface. Arc 2 corresponds to the distal borders of the same bones. Arc 3 is drawn close to the proximal borders of the capitate and hamate (Figure 41.3). These arcs in normal condition should be smooth, but if broken or not well delineated are suggestive of fracture, subluxation or dislocation or ligament lesions. The presence of a foreshortened scaphoid, or signet ring sign, on a PA view may signify a tear or attenuation of the scapholunate ligament, which is known as the Terry Thomas sign.

The slope of the distal radius is measured by calculating the angle between the perpendicular to its axis and the tangent to the distal end of this bone, which passes through the radial styloid and the distal-medial extremity of the radius, and it measures 25° (Figure 41.4). This slope falls into two

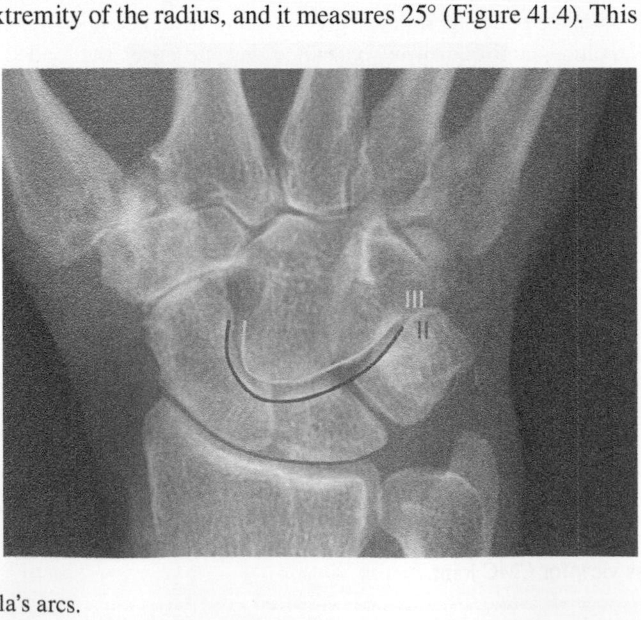

FIGURE 41.3 Gilula's arcs.

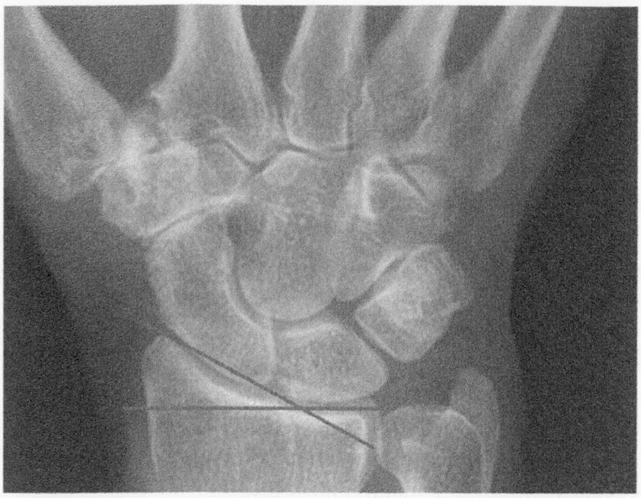

FIGURE 41.4 Radial slope.

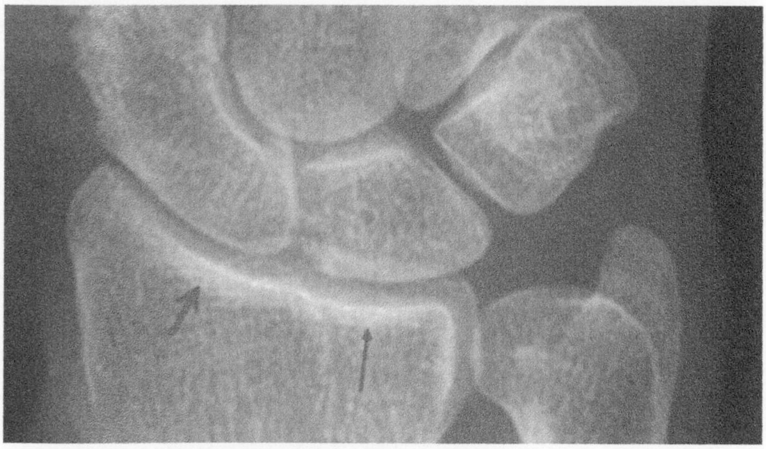

FIGURE 41.5 Two different slopes between scaphoid articular facet of the radius and lunate facet of the radius.

parts with different slopes: the scaphoid articular facet of the radius, which has the major slope, and the lunate facet, which is much more horizontal (Figure 41.5).

The distal ulna morphology is variable. The distal radioulnar joint (DRUJ) slope may be vertical or oblique distally or proximally. The ulnar styloid process is also variable in length and width.

41.2.3 PA View

How the PA radiograph is taken is important to assess the alignment of the carpal bones and to measure ulnar variance. To be in neutral position, the shoulder should be abducted 90°, the elbow flexed 90°, the hand and wrist flat on the plate, and the patient seated.

The ulnar styloid is peripheral in PA and central in AP. This is a way to recognise the incidence.

Ulnar variance has been shown to change with pronosupination. Supination will decrease the apparent length of the ulna, whereas pronation will increase the apparent length of the ulna as compared with the radius.

The convexity of the dorsal aspect of the hand makes AP positioning unreliable, but with the fingers in extension and the thumb in radial abduction, the PA position is stable and reproducible, remembering that, on PA view, the third metacarpal should be aligned with the radius axis.

At the DRUJ joint, there is no overlap of the articular surfaces, and the joint space is clearly outlined. Distally, all the carpometacarpal joint spaces are well outlined, and all the intermetacarpal joint spaces are of equal width.

The slope of the distal radius is measured calculating the angle between the perpendicular to its axis and the tangent to the distal end of this bone, passing through the radial styloid and the distal-medial extremity of the radius. It measures 25°. This slope divides into two parts with different slopes: the scaphoid articular facet of the radius (major slope) and the lunate facet (much more horizontal) (Figure 41.5).

In a normal radius, the anterior margin is virtually identical with this dense zone, whereas the posterior margin projects below it. The anterior margin is more prominent on the ulnar side, whereas the posterior has a minor slope corresponding to Lister's tubercle.

The distal ulna is variable. DRUJ slope may be vertical or oblique, distally or proximally. The ulnar styloid process is also variable in length and width.

41.2.4 Lateral View

The lateral view is best taken with the arm adducted against the chest, the elbow flexed to 90°, and the forearm and hand lying with their ulnar borders on the plate. To confirm the adequacy of a lateral view, the ulnar head and distal radius should be superimposed, the ulnar styloid should be in the centre of the ulnar head and the bases of the index, middle and ring finger metacarpals should overlap; the pisiform should overlap the midportion of the scaphoid.

For proper calculation of the angles specifying the intracarpal relationships, it is essential to insist on a perfect technique in performing the films.

Normally the lateral articular angle (the angle on an x-ray film between the axis of the radius and the articular cup the angle) is tilted towards the thumb (volar/ventral tilt) by 11° (Figure 41.6). A scaphopisocapitate alignment may define a true neutral lateral view of the wrist.

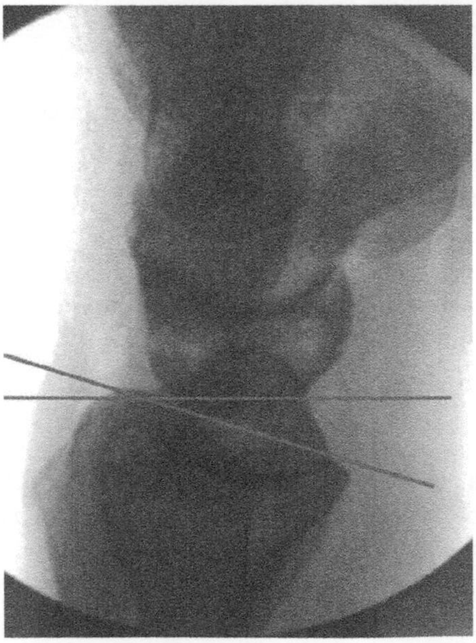

FIGURE 41.6 Angles in lateral view: volar tilt.

41.3 OTHER VIEWS

41.3.1 Carpal Tunnel View

In plain x-ray projections, the anterior surface of the forearm and wrist is held firmly against the cassette. It is obtained by maximally extending the wrist (the wrist is extended 60° and placed on a wedge-shaped foam block) using either the patient's opposite hand or a strap to hold the position. The central ray is directed along the longitudinal axis of the third metacarpal in ulnar deviation.

This view affords an excellent projection of the hook of the hamate, the pisiform and the volar aspect of the triquetrum.

41.3.2 Scaphoid View

The scaphoid view is also called the ulnar-deviated PA view.

The hand and wrist are placed on the IR with the palmar/volar aspects of the hand and wrist in contact with the IR. The wrist is ulnar deviated and the tube angled 20°–30° towards the patient's elbow. This aligns the long axis of this irregularly shaped bone perpendicular to the x-ray beam.

This is the commonly performed 'scaphoid view' that is an essential inclusion in any scaphoid series. This view provides an often elongated image of the scaphoid that can reveal a fracture that is not evident in any of the other views. The scaphoid fat pad is also demonstrated best with the wrist in ulnar deviation.

41.3.3 PA Clenched-Fist View

The patient makes a full fist with maximal force in the PA position. In this way, the capitate falls down into the fossa formed by the scaphoid and the lunate. If the scapholunate ligament is torn or attenuated, the scapholunate interval widens.

41.3.4 Oblique Views

With the ulnar border of the hand placed on the plate, a film could be taken in 30° of supination or in 45° of pronation.

1. AP 30° supinated oblique view: The ulnar side of the hand is placed against the film cassette at a 30° angle with the beam directed at the wrist. This is the best way to assess the pisotriquetral joint for fracture or osteoarthritic changes. The pisotriquetral joint is seen in profile without bony overlap.
2. PA 45° pronated oblique view: It is obtained by placing the ulnar border of the hand on the cassette and pronating the hand approximately 45°. This view demonstrates the dorsal aspect of the triquetrum, the body of the hamate, the radiovolar border of the scaphoid, as well as the best view of the scaphotrapezial joint and the trapeziotrapezoid joint.
3. PA 45° supinated oblique view: A film in 45° of supination shows part of the pisiform, the hamulus of the hamate and the triquetrum.
4. Carpal boss view: It is obtained by taking a lateral view and slightly supinating the hand. This is used for the identification of secondary ossicles or fracture of the base of the second or third metacarpal.
5. Reverse oblique view: An infrequent view of the wrist is obtained by taking a PA view with the ulnar border of the hand elevated above the cassette; it is useful to visualise an avulsion fracture from the dorsoradial border of the scaphoid.

41.3.5 Static Wrist Instability Series

Sometimes, a wrist instability series may be indicated. This can be done with plain films or by fluoroscope. The series consists of frontal films taken of both wrists in neutral, radial and ulnar deviation, as well as lateral views of the wrist in neutral, flexion and extension. These films allow visualising all the carpal bones to assess their movement during the different positions of the wrist and comparing with the opposite side, they are also important to differentiate pathological motion from natural anatomy and physiological biomechanics.

41.3.6 Dynamic Series

Wrist is in radial deviation: the scaphoid is in flexion, and the semicircle of the tuberosity is completed and becomes an entire circle delineating the ring sign. This is a normal aspect. The scaphoid is then squat and shortened.

Wrist is in ulnar deviation: the scaphoid is in extension. It has an elongated and regular appearance, and the outline of the tuberosity is no longer visible. The dynamics of the four medial carpal bones are less known. In radial deviation, the capitate is in contact with the triquetrum, and the lunate is well away from the hamate. In ulnar deviation, the tip of the hamate comes into contact with the lunate. Cineradiography may be useful to localise a midcarpal or SL clicking, especially for hypermobile persons.

In lateral views, flexion and extension of the wrist demonstrates motion of the lunate relative to the radius at the radiocarpal joint and the capitate relative to the lunate at the midcarpal joint; scaphoid motion is also assessed.

41.3.7 Stress Views

The most common is the fist view. A strong finger flexion is performed on the PA view. On the PA view, passive traction, compression and, in lateral view, the drawer sign, may display abnormal signs.

41.4 FLUOROSCOPY

The wrist instability series can be performed fluoroscopically; it is especially helpful in the patient with painful clicking or popping and for patients who have pain related to a specific motion. The wrist should be evaluated while watching the exact motion that causes pain, and in particular midcarpal instability can only be demonstrated by using dynamic motion studies.

41.4.1 Measurements, Angles, Indices and Ratios

41.4.1.1 Angles

1. The SL angle: It is the angle between the scaphoid axis and the axis of the lunate. This angle is considered as normal between 30° and 60° (Figure 41.7). It is calculated using the lateral view.
2. The radiolunate angle (Figure 41.8): The lunate is generally in 10° of flexion but may be considered normal between 15° of flexion and 20° of extension.
3. The radioscaphoid angle is between 35° and 65°: A dorsal intercalated segmental instability (DISI) angle of more than 60° and volar intercalated segmental instability (VISI) angle of less than 30° are then defined.
4. The lunocapitate angle: It is more or less equivalent to the radiolunate axis. It is abnormal if it exceeds 15°.

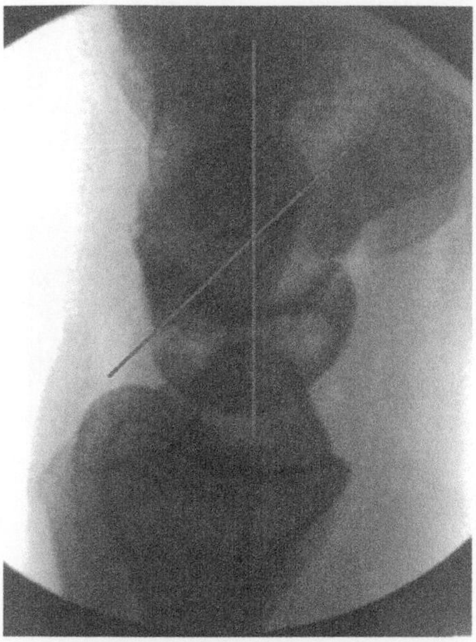

FIGURE 41.7 Scapholunate angle.

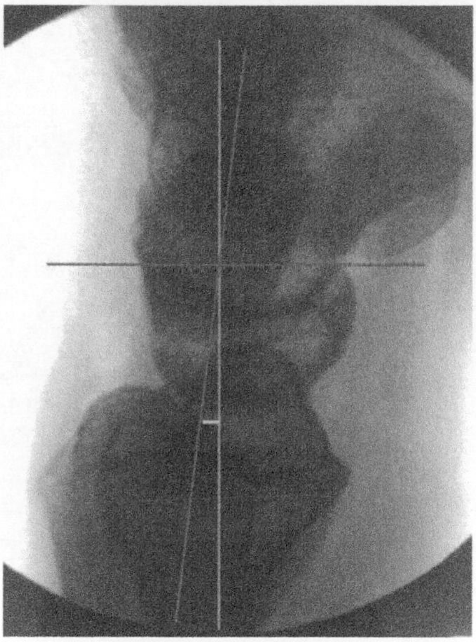

FIGURE 41.8 Radiolunate angle.

41.4.2 Carpal Height

Carpal height measurement of Youm and McMurtry: This is an indice used to measure carpal collapse in some different cases. It is calculated measuring the distance between the base of the third metacarpal and the subchondral region of the distal radius (Figure 41.9). The ratio of this distance to the length of the third metacarpal is equal to 0.54 ± 0.03. It remains constant in all movements of the wrist.

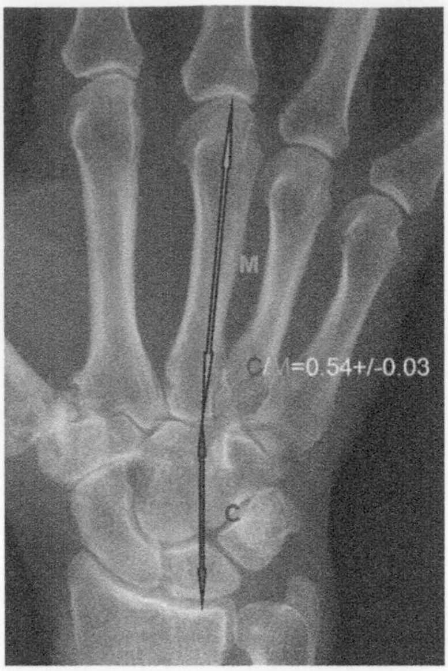

FIGURE 41.9 Carpal height measurement of Youm and McMurtry.

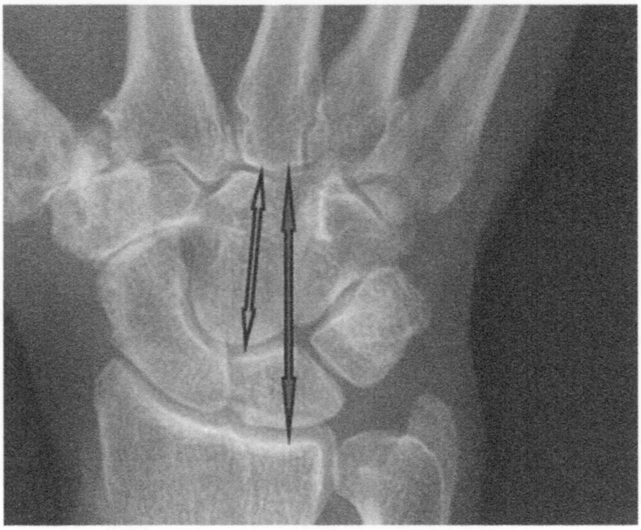

FIGURE 41.10 Carpal height measurement of Nattrass.

Carpal height measurement of Nattrass: This is an alternative method for measuring carpal height ratio. It is useful when wrist x-rays do not include the entire third metacarpal. It consists in carpal height along the third metacarpal axis and divided by the length of the capitate: 1.57 ± 0.05 (Figure 41.10).

41.4.3 Carpal Arcs

Three carpal arcs have been described on PA radiographs as mentioned previously. Arc 1: the main convex curvatures of the scaphoid, lunate and triquetrum proximal surface. Arc 2: the distal border of the same three bones. Arc 3: is close to the proximal curvatures of the capitate and hamate.

41.4.4 Index of Ulnar Variance

Three methods of measurement have been described and seem reliable:

1. The index is provided by the distance between a horizontal line perpendicular to the axis of the radius starting from the ulnar border of radius distal end and the ulnar distal rim.
2. The distance between the first circle passing as close as possible to the contour of the radius distal end and the distal cortex of the ulna.
3. The distance between perpendicular to the axis of the radius through the distal ulnar aspect of this bone and the ulnar distal cortical rim.

41.5 COMPUTED TOMOGRAPHY

CT is useful for hand and wrist pathologies because of its high resolution and multiplanar capabilities. It has limited use in the routine evaluation of the painful wrist. It is excellent in evaluating healing of scaphoid fractures, for demonstrating occult fractures, and is useful in the evaluation of the DRUJ with respect to subluxation. The asymptomatic wrist can be scanned for comparison.

There are two types of acquisition modes: direct and helical.

1. Direct acquisition: It provides a very high spatial resolution. And each plane is acquired separately in four different positionings: in coronal series, the patient lies prone with the elbow in flexion and wrist above the head and the ulnar surface lying against the table. In sagittal series, the wrist lies palm against the table, with mild ulnar deviation for radioscaphoid and radiolunate joint study and radial deviation for ulnar wrist compartment study. In axial view, the patient lies prone on the table with the arm extended above the head. In sagittal oblique series, the principal disadvantage is a long acquisition time.
2. Helical mode or spiral: CT is a whole-volume acquisition generally performed in an axial plane. It allows a large variety of reconstruction in two dimensions and three dimensions (Figure 41.11). It assures the advantage of a faster scan opposite to spatial resolution of reconstructed images that may be less acute than by direct acquisition.

It is useful for comparative and dynamic studies and also postoperatively (cast, surgical device). In all cases, high resolution is required.

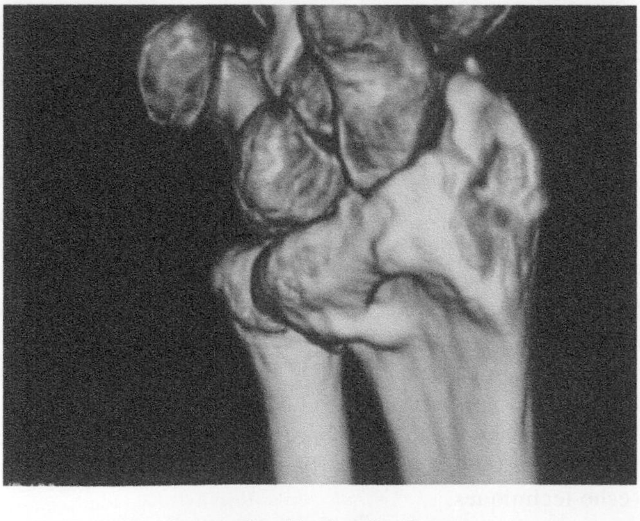

FIGURE 41.11 3-D reconstruction of a complex distal radius fractures.

41.6 BONE SCAN

Bone scintigraphy of the hands and wrists represents an important adjunct imaging technique that complements plain film radiographic examination. A bone scan may be useful for evaluating the patient who has normal radiographs but unexplained pain.

The use of the three-phase bone scan provides clinical information not only regarding osseous uptake but also the blood flow and extravascular distribution of the radiotracer as well and is used in the evaluation of hands and wrists both in acute and chronic conditions.

Its utility lies primarily in its specificity; however, a normal bone scan essentially rules out significant bone or joint pathology. A positive result is usually less diagnostic other than by confirming a pathological condition. Technically bone scans are generally performed by injecting an intravenous compound labelled with technetium-99m and three-phase imaging are identified. Phase 1 consists of multiple images taken in the first 1–2 min following injection, while the isotope is still intravascular. Phase 2 is the soft tissue pooling phase obtained 5–10 min after injection in which the isotope diffusing into the extracellular fluid. While delayed bone images correspond to the third phase whose are taken 2–3 h after injection when the isotope is bound to bone. In the event of an equivocal or negative plain film, the bone scan can identify occult fractures and also, of particular concern, is the identification of scaphoid fractures due to the higher incidence of osteonecrosis, work-related injuries represent a significant health issue, and can be a part of the algorithm for evaluating chronic pain syndromes including reflex sympathetic dystrophy. The complimentary roles of bone scanning and imaging with gallium-67 citrate or radiolabeled leukocytes have proven useful in the evaluation of acute or chronic osteomyelitis. In addition, the diphosphonates are useful in identifying solitary and multiple primary bone tumours. In the case of primary bone tumour, thallium-201 can be used to evaluate response to therapy. Finally, bone scintigraphy may be useful in identifying location and extent in a variety of conditions such as fibrous dysplasia, histiocytosis X and Paget's disease.

41.7 MAGNETIC RESONANCE IMAGING

MRI is widely used in the evaluation of internal derangement of joints. In the past, the use of hand and wrist MRI lagged behind imaging of larger joints, largely because of technical limitations of spatial resolution and signal-to-noise ratio (SNR) when imaging the small anatomic structures [1]. However, with recent technical advances, MRI has provided us with new insights into the difficult anatomy of the wrist by allowing improved visualisation of the relationship of the muscles, ligaments, tendons and bone (Figure 41.12).

There is great interest in using MRI for the diagnosis of hand and wrist pain due to its non-invasive nature and absence of ionising radiation.

To visualise the small structures of the hand and wrist, spatial resolution and image quality must be optimised. At 1.5 T, MRI quality is enhanced with the application of dedicated extremity coils, a small field of view (8–12 cm) and thin-slice thickness, on the order of 1–2 mm. Higher field strength magnets have the ability to produce images that are high in both SNR and contrast-to-noise ratios (CNR) and, thus, have the capability of generating images with higher spatial resolution, such as the 3.0 T MR or the super high-field magnets at 8 T that have been shown to have an in-plane resolution of 100–140 μm.

Standard MRI has the ability to demonstrate osteonecrosis, to give an accurate imaging of the triangular fibrocartilage complex (TFCC), but concern has been raised regarding the sensitivity and specificity of MRI for the extrinsic and intrinsic ligaments. Ideally, MRI of the wrist should be performed using dedicated wrist surface coils and by a radiologist skilled in interpreting the images.

Numerous pulse sequences are currently available: spin-echo, two- and three-dimensional Fourier transformation sequences, and fat-suppression techniques all have been used in the assessment of the wrist. More sophisticated software has introduced newer techniques, including thin-slice spin-echo techniques.

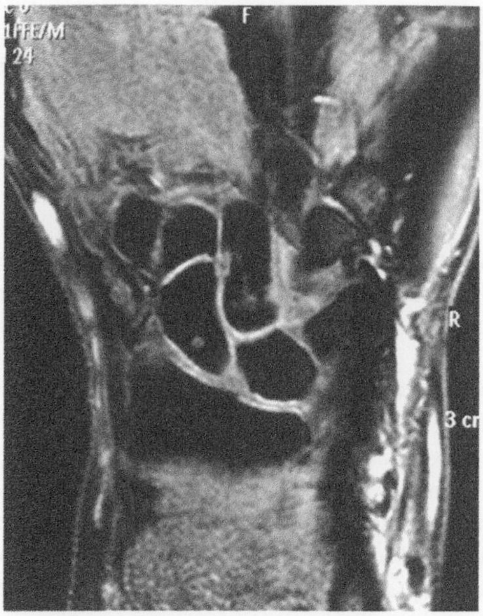

FIGURE 41.12 Wrist MRI image.

The use of volumetric gradient-recalled echo (GRE) sequences provides thin sections at a higher SNR than routine two-dimensional Fourier transform imaging.

T1-weighted sequences and short tau inversion recovery are useful for depiction of marrow pathology. The outstanding contrast afforded by these MRI techniques provides excellent depiction of the anatomy of the hand and wrist, including the intrinsic and extrinsic ligaments and components of the TFCC of the wrist, the components of the carpal tunnel and the tendons, ligaments and interstitial soft tissues of the hand and fingers.

Current research is focused upon enhancing the ability to differentiate between symptomatic and asymptomatic lesions. MRI is the gold standard for the diagnosis of osteonecrosis, such as in Kienböck's disease, which has an absent signal on both T1- and T2-weighted images while other pathophysiological processes, such as active bone healing, bone bruises and marrow oedema, have an absent or diminished signal on T1-weighted images but increased signal on T2-weighted images.

The TFCC will appear as a band of low-signal intensity on both T1- and T2-weighted images. Tears of the TFCC will appear as discontinuities or fragmentation of the TFCC, which is highlighted by interposed high-signal intensity, and the vast majority of these tears will be found along the ulnar insertion. The major current limitation of identifying TFCC pathology with MRI is the inability to differentiate between lesions causing pain and those associated with the normal aging process. Most degenerative tears will be located centrally, where the substance of the complex is thinner.

The extrinsic ligaments can be seen on both sagittal and coronal sections as low-signal bands on both T1- and T2-weighted images where the discontinuity of these ligaments is easily seen.

While evaluation of the intrinsic ligaments of the wrist, and in particular the scapholunate and lunotriquetral, is somewhat more difficult due to their small size and curved shape. Normally, these ligaments should be seen as a continuous, low-signal band on at least two images when using 3 mm cuts, and so discontinuity, elongation, absence or high-signal intensity on T2-weighted images is associated with a significant tear.

41.8 WRIST ARTHROGRAPHY

Wrist arthrography is a standard technique for the evaluation of wrist pain or instability when injuries to the triangular fibrocartilage, carpal ligaments or capsule are suspected. Single-, double- and triple-compartment injection protocols have been described [2–4]. The technique involves injecting radiopaque contrast dye into the compartments of the wrist. Dye leakage between the compartments suggests the location of causative wrist pathology when correlated with a physical exam.

Arthrography of the wrist and hand is easy to perform, but accurate diagnosis requires meticulous technique and thorough knowledge of anatomy, pathology and imaging principles. A complete examination usually requires injection of the RC, midcarpal and distal radioulnar joints.

Abnormalities that can be detected include interosseous ligament tears, capsular tears, triangular fibrocartilage perforations and separations, cartilaginous defects, loose bodies and synovial abnormalities including adhesive capsulitis.

Arthrography can also be useful in the evaluation of masses and scaphoid non-union. Finger arthrography can demonstrate capsular injury, ligament tears, tendon derangement, volar plate disruption, cartilage abnormalities, fibrous ankylosis, synovial abnormalities and ganglia. Tenography is seldom performed; this technique can delineate synovial abnormalities and can be used to evaluate tendon subluxation.

While the compartments are initially separate, it has been noted that communication between compartments due to attritional changes may be seen in asymptomatic wrists as early as the third decade of life, and that 50% of patients aged 50 years may have attritional tears.

It is important to remember that results of an arthrogram may not correlate with traumatic injury to the intercarpal ligaments or the TFCC due to the incidence of intercompartmental communication in asymptomatic wrists. Moreover, it has also been shown that a negative arthrogram does not preclude a ligament tear.

Arthrography remains a useful technique, especially in the diagnosis of intercarpal ligament tears. It may ultimately be replaced by the MRI as a diagnostic intervention in evaluating the painful wrist as that imaging technique is refined and becomes more cost-effective.

41.9 ULTRASOUND

The quality of ultrasound imaging to examine anatomical structures in the wrist and hand has improved highly over the last years due to high-frequency technology improving ultrasound. This technique offers the advantage of a quick, non-invasive, easily accessible and inexpensive examination. Comparative and dynamic studies are easily performed.

Ultrasound is useful in superficial plane pathology, and well described are tears of the collateral ligaments of the thumb with the typical Stener lesion, tendon ruptures and sheath lesions, annular pulley lesions in 'climber's finger' and the detection of foreign bodies in the soft tissue.

Combined with Doppler or pulsed Doppler, it helps in characterisation of a vascular mass. Ultrasound may help in early diagnosis of infection.

Ultrasound is a powerful modality for evaluation of pathological conditions in the hand and wrist and helps in some locoregional anaesthesiologic procedure (Figure 41.13). It provides a cost-effective and expedient alternative and/or adjunct to MRI. It is best used when there is a specific clinical question regarding a well-localised abnormality.

However, ultrasound has several disadvantages. Bone causes acoustic shadows; images are operator-dependent and not reproducible; specificity is lower than MRI; and ultrasound is limited when the finger is flexed.

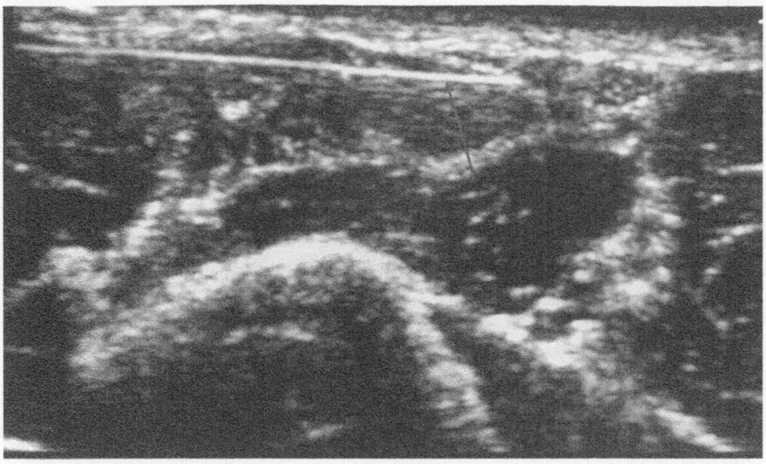

FIGURE 41.13 Locoregional anaesthesiologic procedure under ultrasound guide.

41.10 SPECIFIC LESIONS

A number of different studies may be helpful in establishing the proper diagnosis in a patient with hand or wrist pain. The choice of technique should be based on a careful history such as patient's hand dominance, age, gender and occupation, as well as any hobbies that require hand dexterity or strength. Other important aspects that must be considered are the time of onset of symptoms, the date and mechanism of injury and whether the injury occurred. Also, a complete physical examination should be investigated for a best evaluation of the nature pain, whether night symptoms are present and whether the pain is worse or whether the symptoms include numbness or tingling, specific motor difficulties and are unilateral or bilateral. A careful history will suggest the correct diagnosis in approximately 90% of patients with hand problems.

41.11 FRACTURES AND DISLOCATIONS OF THE HAND

41.11.1 Fractures and Dislocations of the Phalanges and Metacarpals

41.11.1.1 Fractures of the Phalanges and Metacarpals

41.11.1.1.1 Introduction

Fractures of the phalanges and metacarpals account for approximately 10% of all fractures. More than half of all hand fractures are work-related cause of the body position of the hand and wrist. The most common fractures in the hand are located at the border digits, thumb and little finger, and the most commonly fractured bone is the distal phalanx (about 45%–50% of all hand fractures).

Because metacarpal or phalangeal rotational malalignment is difficult to evaluate from a radiograph, physical examination is essential. However, a lot of radiological investigations should be performed in helping diagnosis and choosing conservative or surgical treatments, such as CT scan in case of intraarticular fractures, non-union and malunion, MRI in case of a soft tissue complication around a non-union or malunion, while arthrography or arthro-CT may provide information on cartilage finger joints.

41.11.1.1.2 Physical Examination

Examination of the hand is essential to identify the area of maximal tenderness and to visualise the location, type and severity of any deformities, the function of tendons and the neurovascular status.

Angular, rotational and shortening deformities should be catalogued clinically, assessing nail rotation, finger direction and overlapping of the fingers, and then radiographically.

41.11.1.1.3 Imaging Studies

Standard x-rays are usually the basic in evaluation of phalangeal shaft fractures and should include AP and lateral views. A true lateral view is especially important in accessing angulation in the sagittal plane, and an additional oblique view helps in defining fracture type. Description of a phalangeal or metacarpal fracture should include notation of the bone involved, the location within the bone (base, shaft or neck), open or closed fractures, configuration, displacement, deformity, fragment relationships and intraarticular component.

41.11.1.1.4 Treatment

Treatment of metacarpal and phalangeal fractures requires accurate fracture diagnosis, reduction, sufficient immobilisation to maintain the fracture reduction and early motion of the uninvolved fingers to prevent stiffness.

Fracture management should be principle-driven. These principles include anatomic position of reduction and an adequate stability to allow fracture healing and early active motion, minimising additional soft tissue damage when fracture fixation is required. Immobilisation after surgery or in case of conservative treatment (exception in specific cases) should place the hand in an intrinsic plus or a safe position to avoid secondary joint stiffness contractures.

In case of conservative treatment, immobilisation for phalangeal fractures should rarely exceed 3 weeks and for metacarpal fractures 4 weeks.

When external immobilisation is impossible or is unlikely to maintain fracture reduction, internal fixation is required and the type of fixation is directly dependent upon the fracture characteristics and surgical technique performed should minimise additional soft tissue damage when fracture fixation is required.

Internal fixation techniques include Kirschner wire fixation (is versatile but lacks the rigidity of other techniques), interosseous wiring, tension band wiring, interfragmentary screw fixation that is the ideal fixation for long oblique fractures (Figure 41.14), in which the obliquity of the fracture is

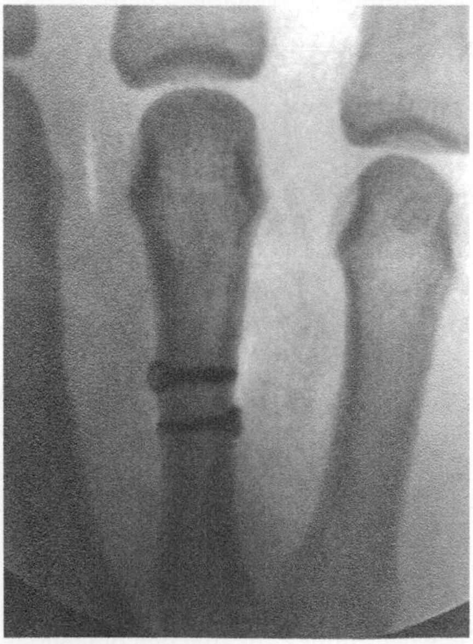

FIGURE 41.14 Screw fixation for an oblique metacarpal fracture (post-op).

more than two times the diameter of the fractured bone, or fixation with plates and screws that are particularly helpful in open metacarpal fractures with bone loss.

Stable fractures may be treated by either buddy taping the affected finger to an adjacent finger and allowing early motion or with a short period of splint immobilisation. Initially displaced unstable fractures that require closed reduction to achieve proper alignment will require external immobilisation with a cast or splint.

41.11.1.1.5 Follow-up

Repeat radiographs at 7–10 days to document maintenance of fracture reduction. A second radiographic look is indicated 4–5 weeks after the beginning of treatment to ensure the proceeding with bone healing.

41.11.1.2 Physeal Fractures

Approximately one-third of all fractures of the immature skeleton involve the epiphysis. The paediatric hand is vulnerable to injury for several reasons. Usage pattern of the exposed hand and the child's curiosity about the surrounding world are prime factors. Youngsters often are unaware of dangers and place their hands in vulnerable situations [5–11]. Hand and wrist injuries account for up to 25% of paediatric fractures. Salter–Harris physeal fractures are divided into five types.

41.11.1.2.1 Radiographic Examination

Several paediatric imaging factors complicate interpretation of plain x-rays, including lack of bony detail and normal variations. The normal ossification pattern of the immature hand creates problems with the detection of fractures and also promotes false interpretation of ligamentous injuries. Uncertain interpretation requires comparison to the non-injured hand or consultation with a paediatric atlas of child development and normal radiographic variants [12,13].

AP, lateral and oblique views are needed for complete evaluation of the injured hand or digit. Mini-fluoroscopy units are useful and allow a real-time assessment of articular congruity and joint stability and have considerable advantages, such as the ability to obtain multiple views and stress views with low-radiation exposure for the patient and physician.

41.12 ARTICULAR FRACTURES

41.12.1 Distal Interphalangeal Joint

The most common intraarticular fracture of the distal interphalangeal joint is a bony mallet finger, in which a portion of the articular surface is avulsed by the extensor tendon. If the fracture is large, when articular surface loss is greater than 30% and subluxation of the joint is present (the joint may sublux volarly), treatment requires stabilisation with a percutaneous pin for 4–5 weeks, followed by external splintage. In this case, we used the Hishiguro technique that consist in a dorsal block-pinning K-wire to reduce the dorsal fragment and a second K-wire to reduce and stabilise the DIP joint.

Most bony mallet injuries can be treated with splinting in extension for 6 weeks but just in case of a perfect reduction after hyperextension splinting. Dislocation of the distal interphalangeal joint is uncommon without an associated fracture.

41.12.2 Condylar Fractures

41.12.2.1 Introduction

Condylar fractures may occur in either the proximal or middle phalanges. These fractures are most often athletic injuries.

Patients are usually in their early 1920s, and males predominate. Between half and four-fifths of these injuries are due to sport, usually a ball sport [14,15]. Weiss and Hastings suggested that the outstretched digits are suddenly forced apart, such as when a ball strikes the hand, causing an oblique fracture of one condyle. Coronal shear fractures occur in hyperflexion or extension. The sudden impact with rapid loading of the digit may predispose to a fracture rather than a ligamentous injury.

41.12.2.2 Physical Examination

The patient usually presents swelling and pain in the region of the proximal interphalangeal joint, and its movement is restricted both by pain and swelling. Bruising may be seen. A haemarthrosis in the joint can occur, sideways angulation of the digit should suggest a condylar fracture and palpating the finger on its dorsal surface identifies spot tenderness over one or the other condyle.

41.12.2.3 Imaging Studies

AP, lateral and oblique radiographs are necessary to identify the fracture fragments. If the injury is inadequately appreciated, angulation of the finger and joint incongruity may lead to degenerative arthritis.

The radiographs should be viewed to determine whether the fracture is split by more than 1 mm or whether it is depressed by any extent. In addition, the inclination of the middle phalanx to the axis of the proximal phalanx should be noted in the PA projection. Clinical examination and plain radiographs are usually sufficient to establish the diagnosis. Clinically, a note should also be made of any compound or complicated injury. The presence of the injury, its displacement and any associated injury help decide management and prognosis.

41.12.2.4 Treatment

Displaced fracture should be openly reduced and internally fixed if the condylar fracture is displaced by more than 2 mm. If both condyles are fractured, they must be precisely secured together and then secured to the phalangeal shaft. The collateral ligament insertion to the condyle must be preserved as it is the only blood supply to the fragment. Permanent loss of motion may be anticipated in complex condylar fractures.

41.13 DISLOCATIONS OF THE PHALANGES AND METACARPALS

41.13.1 Introduction

Fracture dislocation of the proximal interphalangeal joint is a common injury of the proximal interphalangeal joint, and stability is the principal concern in management. These lesions are frequently associated with an injury to the volar plate, collateral ligament, extensor tendon (central slip) and joint articular surface.

The more common injuries occur secondary to a hyperextension force (dorsal subluxation or dislocation, volar plate rupture), longitudinal compression and hyperextension force (dorsal fracture dislocation), lateral deviation force (collateral ligament injuries) and combined rotatory and longitudinal compression force (rotatory dislocations).

41.13.2 Physical Examination

The patient is usually a young adult, and the majority of these injuries are acquired during sporting activity. Sometimes, the appearance of the digit can be normal when seen by the clinician. The degree of swelling of the digit and bruising depends on the severity of the injury. Often, apart from the general discomfort, point tenderness is difficult to elicit. Active range may be only restricted by swelling or be severely reduced if the joint is in a dislocated position. If there is comminution of the dorsal part of the articular surface in particular, it would remain in a dislocated position. Diffuse swelling can sometimes mask the displaced position of the digit.

41.13.3 Imaging Studies

Assess these structures and take true AP and lateral radiographs of the digit, particularly of the PIP joint. A careful positioning of the digit provides posterior, anterior and true lateral radiographs. The radiographs should then be viewed to document the position of the joint. There are many factors to investigate in an x-ray evaluation: in a reduced joint, the dorsal articular surface should be congruent with the dorsal surface of the condyles on a true lateral view. Any loss of congruence creates a divergence of the two articular surfaces. The second clue is in the alignment of the shaft of the middle phalanx to that of the proximal phalanx. The next factors to document are the size and separation of the volar fragment. If it is more than 40%, it is likely that all or most of the collateral ligament is attached to the volar fragment and that the injury is potentially unstable. The degree of separation of the fragments indicates the axial rent in the collateral ligament.

In some cases, stress views are important to assess collateral ligament injuries. Some authors demonstrate the usefulness of sonography in non-acute injuries, particularly using a stress test. MRI can detect the torn ligament and reveal displacement if present. One additional benefit of MRI in the assessment of these lesions is in the detection of associated clinically occult injuries involving bone or soft tissues.

41.14 PIP JOINT DISLOCATIONS

41.14.1 PIP Joint Dorsal Dislocations

Dorsal dislocations are more common than palmar or lateral dislocations. Dorsal dislocations can be classified into three types.

Type 1: Hyperextension injury avulses the volar plate from the base of the middle phalanx, whereas the collateral ligaments partially split from the middle phalanx and the joint surface is intact, usually with subluxation but not dislocation.

Type 2: Dorsal dislocations with a larger portion of the collateral ligament torned.

Type 3: Dorsal dislocation with proximal retraction of the middle phalanx, with a shear fracture of the volar base of the middle phalanx, producing a fracture dislocation.

41.14.2 Treatment

Treatment of proximal interphalangeal joint dislocations depends on the dislocation type.

Stable type 1 and 2 injuries should be treated by closed reduction and immobilisation in a dorsal splint in 30° of flexion for 1 week. The acute dorsal injury without fracture can be usually treated by closed reduction. A digital block is often unnecessary. The volar plate is ruptured, usually from the middle phalanx, but the collateral ligaments rarely are ruptured completely from their attachments [16,17].

After reduction and splinting, a radiograph should document the reduction. After first week of static splint, a cross-‘8’-shaped splint is dressed for other 3–4 weeks encouraging flexion and protecting maximal extension of the PIP joint. The finger may be buddy taped to an adjacent finger during sports for the next month.

Unstable fracture dislocations should be treated with closed reduction. Radiographs must document congruent joint reduction. When a reduction is possible, the splint is the first option. If closed reduction cannot be achieved, open reduction is required. When a single, large, palmarly displaced articular fragment is present, internal fixation may be attempted. If the fracture is comminuted, however, either volar plate arthroplasty or an axial traction technique that allows early controlled passive joint motion is necessary.

41.14.3 PIP Joint Lateral Dislocations

Lateral proximal interphalangeal dislocation is six times more common on the radial than on the ulnar side. Collateral ligament injuries are usually caused by an abduction or adduction force with the PIP joint in extension [18]. The radial collateral is more commonly injured than the ulnar one. These dislocations are associated with avulsion of the volar plate, extensor mechanism or a portion of the phalangeal base.

Clinically, tenderness occurs over the site of injury, and joint laxity to lateral stress may be present. In any case, an RX evaluation is necessary to assess the entity of trauma and the mutual location of the proximal and medial phalanx, particularly in AP view (Figure 41.15) and in a perfect lateral view. After the reduction of the PIP joint, some authors suggest to evaluate the integrity of the extensor bands and the collateral ligament by an ultrasound evaluation.

41.14.4 Treatment

Most PIP joint collateral ligament injuries are incomplete and need only to be protected by splinting and taping to a lateral digit for 3–6 weeks. However, lateral dislocations of the PIP joint can result in complete rupture of a collateral ligament and at least a portion of the volar plate. Angulation greater than 20°–30° by lateral stress testing indicates a complete collateral ligament injury.

Treatment of complete collateral ligament injuries is controversial.

After the joint is reduced, the residual joint stability should be assessed by observing the active range of motion and confirm joint congruency on radiographs. Stable fracture dislocations are immobilised at 5°–10° of flexion for 2–3 weeks, and then active range-of-motion activities are allowed and for the following 3–4 weeks dorsal splinting or an '8'-shaped PIP splint is worn, encouraging full active motion in flexion.

The surgical procedure to repair the collateral ligament has been described, but joint stiffness is a problem. The index radial collateral ligament is probably the only ligament that needs early surgery.

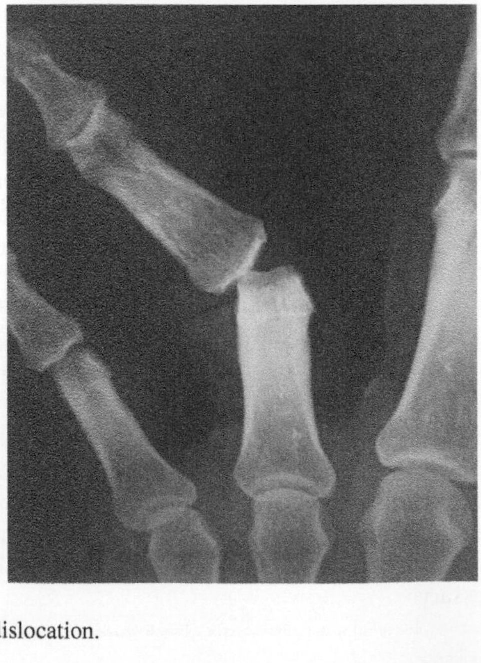

FIGURE 41.15 X-ray PIP dislocation.

41.14.5 Chronic Collateral Ligament Ruptures

Chronic collateral ligament injuries are rarely sufficiently symptomatic to require reconstruction. Often, there are degenerative changes in the joint, and ligament reconstruction cannot be expected to alleviate symptoms due to arthritis.

Pain, instability, loss of motion and arthrosis can occur from incomplete joint reduction, lateral translocation or uneven forces within the joint secondary to excessive scarring.

Once again, if reconstruction of a chronic PIP collateral ligament rupture is necessary, it is on the radial side of the index finger.

Reconstruction of the collateral ligament can be done by shortening or imbricating the remaining ligament or by augmenting the repair, usually with a slip of the superficialis or with a tendon grafting by transosseal holes.

41.14.6 PIP Joint Palmar Dislocations

Palmar proximal interphalangeal dislocations are unusual and are rare injuries.

The base of the middle phalanx may dislocate volarly without rotation (volar dislocation) or may rotate on one intact collateral ligament so that the opposite side subluxates in a volar direction (volar rotatory subluxation).

The condyle of the proximal phalanx may buttonhole between the central slip and the lateral bands.

Occasionally, when a volar dislocation occurs without a rotatory component, the central slip is ruptured. If the dislocation is irreducible, there is a high likelihood of an inter-posed structure such as the central slip, a collateral ligament or a fracture fragment.

41.14.7 Treatment

Closed reduction may be attempted by applying traction to the fingers after flexing both the metacarpophalangeal and the proximal interphalangeal joints. If closed reduction is successful, the digit should be splinted for 3–6 weeks to allow healing of the extensor rent. If closed reduction is unsuccessful, because of the interposition of the volar fibres of the lateral bands, open reduction will be necessary to free the condyle from the rent in the extensor mechanism.

Volar fracture dislocations are also rare. In particular, when these fractures include a large dorsal fragment, they may be treated with ORIF.

The management of chronic volar dislocations of the PIP joint is complex and requires the simultaneous surgical correction making a straight dorsal or slightly curvilinear incision, mobilising the lateral bands, reducing the joint and transfixing it in extension with smooth K-wire. After that, it is necessary to reattach the central slip to the base of the middle phalanx with non-absorbable sutures to remaining periosteum through bone holes or with suture anchors and finally repairing the interval between each lateral band and the central slip with non-absorbable sutures. Postreduction radiographs should confirm congruous reduction of the joint. Remove the pin after 6 weeks, having allowed active motion at the MP and DIP joints during that time.

There may be degeneration of the articular cartilage; if so, the prospect of restoring normal joint function is greatly diminished.

41.15 DIP JOINT DISLOCATIONS

The ligamentous anatomy of the distal articulation of the finger and the anatomic features are similar but less well defined in comparison with the same structure in the proximal interphalangeal joint. However, the enhanced stability of the DIP joint is provided by the adjacent insertions of the flexor and extensor tendons and so dislocations at this level are not as frequent.

Dislocations of the DIP joint are almost always dorsal and are rare [19,20].

Dislocations of the DIP joint are usually dorsal or lateral and often are associated with an open wound because of the snug skin fixation about the joint.

These injuries are usually produced by a longitudinal compression and hyperextension of the joint. Occasionally, a lateral, and even less commonly a palmar, dislocation can occur.

The most common injuries at this level are the jersey finger and the mallet finger in avulsion injuries.

41.15.1 Treatment

Treatment is similar to the treatment of the proximal interphalangeal joint. Avulsion of the extensor tendon insertion to the base of the distal interphalangeal joint is a particularly common injury and can be associated with a fracture. If the fracture is large, the joint may sublux volarly and require stabilisation with a percutaneous pin for 3 weeks, followed by external splintage using stack splint for a further 3 weeks or so.

In case of complete dislocations, treatment consists of closed reduction under digital anaesthesia. The reduction manoeuvre consists of longitudinal traction, direct pressure on the dorsum of the distal phalanx and manipulation of the distal phalanx into flexion. Then, place direct pressure on the dorsal base of the distal phalanx, displacing it distally and palmarly. Postreduction radiographs should confirm congruous reduction of the joint.

After joint reduction it is necessary to assess joint stability and flexor and extensor tendon function. If joint is stable after reduction, splint the joint for 2–3 weeks in a small DIP flexion splint in case of dorsal dislocations.

With a palmar dislocation avoid splinting the DIP joint in hyperextension. This prevents dorsal skin wound problems.

If the dislocation is open, the joint is contaminated by definition and treatment should include thorough irrigation and debridement in a controlled, sterile setting. Postreduction radiographs are mandatory to confirm congruous reduction.

Digital DIP dislocations are rarely irreducible, and when they occur, it is the result of proximal disruption of the volar plate, which then becomes interposed between the head of the digital middle or thumb proximal phalanx and the base of the distal phalanx, preventing reduction. Irreducible dislocations require surgical removal or manipulation of the offending anatomic structure to facilitate reduction.

41.16 MP JOINT DISLOCATIONS

Dislocations of the MCP joint are less common than proximal interphalangeal joint dislocations, and the border digits of the hand (index and small fingers) are most vulnerable to injury, in particular the index finger. The thumb is also more frequently injured than the small finger.

Most of these occur with the fingers in some extension when the collateral ligaments are more lax and the most common mechanism of injury is hyperextension or ulnar deviation of the joint.

Metacarpophalangeal joint injuries are frequently associated with an injury to the volar plate, collateral ligament and joint articular surface, which require adequate assessment and AP, lateral and oblique radiographs of the hand.

A Brewerton view or oblique view of the metacarpal heads may be helpful to identify small fractures.

Metacarpophalangeal joint injuries are classified according to dislocations or type of collateral ligament injuries. The dislocations are based on the direction of the dislocation (dorsal versus volar dislocation) and whether they are easily reducible (simple dislocation) or irreducible without surgical intervention (complex dislocation).

41.17 DORSAL MP DISLOCATIONS

Dorsal dislocations of the MP joints of the fingers (Figure 41.16) are relatively uncommon injuries, and the most frequently involved digit is the index followed by the small finger.

The mechanism of injury is usually forced hyperextension of the digit as might occur from falling on an outstretched hand.

The volar plate is avulsed from its attachment on the metacarpal in its membranous proximal portion and becomes interposed dorsally between the base of the proximal phalanx and the dorsal metacarpal head.

In a reducible dislocation, the proximal phalanx cartilage remains in contact with the dorsal articular cartilage of the metacarpal head and the volar plate is not interposed in the joint and the collateral ligament may be torn but it also may be intact.

If this was the only structure blocking reduction, it could be accomplished by using traction sufficient to draw the proximal edge of the volar plate over the metacarpal head. This is not possible, however, because of the taut medial and lateral structures drawn tightly around the narrow metacarpal neck, which become even more taut with traction.

Regarding irreducible dislocation, it occurs by the same mechanism as reducible dislocations, but in this case, the volar plate becomes interposed in the joint and in addition the metacarpal head can also become entrapped in the tendons and ligamentous structures as it displaces volarly.

Clinically, the joint is hyperextended with the phalanx appearing parallel to the metacarpal with a tendency for the digit to overlap one of the lateral digits while on the palmar surface, the skin is puckered or dimpled.

Radiographically, the joint space is widened, the joint surfaces are offset and the sesamoid appears to lie within the joint.

41.17.1 Treatment

41.17.1.1 Non-Operative Treatment

Sometimes, simple distraction of the joint as a reduction manoeuvre can convert a reducible dislocation to an irreducible dislocation because of its extremely complex pathomechanic. In fact, many MCP joint dislocations still require open reduction.

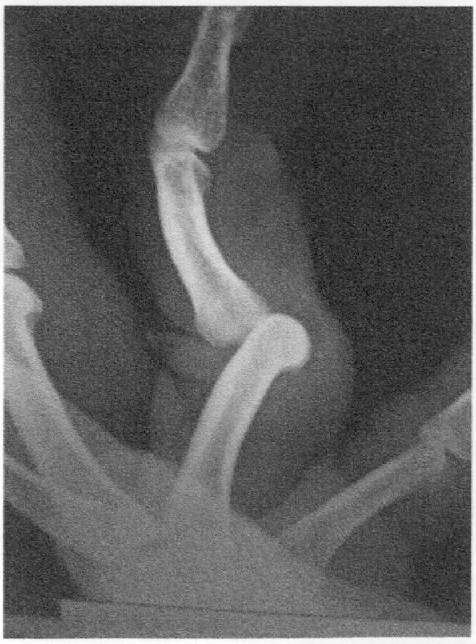

FIGURE 41.16 Dorsal MP dislocation.

An atraumatic reduction is the prior approach. Adequate anaesthesia is the key associated with the wrist and the proximal interphalangeal joint flexed to relax the flexor tendons. The MCP joint is then hyperextended to 90°, applying pressure dorsally and distally to the base of the proximal phalanx at the level of the MCP joint while attempting to slide the proximal phalanx over the metacarpal head. After this manoeuvre, confirm reduction clinically and radiographically, assess active and passive joint stability and splint the hand with the MP joints flexed for a few days and start early active motion with a dorsal extension-block splint.

If this fails, this means that either the volar plate is interposed in the joint or that the metacarpal head is buttonholed through the volar structure. In this case, performing an open reduction is recommended.

41.17.1.2 Surgical Treatment

Open reduction may be accomplished through either a palmar or a dorsal approach.

The dorsal approach consists of a straight or slightly curvilinear dorsal incision over the joint. Then, longitudinally release the extensor tendon or the sagittal band (usually on the ulnar side) and a dorsal midline capsulotomy is performed.

Identify and carefully incise longitudinally the volar plate in the midline avoiding damaging the metacarpal head articular surface. Flex the wrist to relax the flexor tendon and reduce the joint. After the joint is reduced, repair the capsule, the extensor tendon or sagittal band, and the skin. Intraoperative postreduction radiograph is mandatory to confirm congruous reduction of the joint. Splint the hand with the MP joints flexed for a few days and then begin active motion with an extension-block splint.

If the palmar approach is used, care should be taken to avoid injury to the radial digital nerve of the index finger or the ulnar digital nerve of the small finger. The A1 pulley is incised to release the tension of the flexor tendons on the volar plate. If the dorsal approach is used, the volar plate is longitudinally incised. Postoperatively, the metacarpophalangeal joint is immobilised in approximately 30° of flexion for 3–5 days. Splinting with active motion is then continued for 3 weeks.

Although lateral dislocations of the metacarpophalangeal joint are rare, isolated radial collateral ligament ruptures may occur. These injuries should also be immobilised in approximately 30° of flexion for 3 weeks. The fingers should be protected from ulnar stress for an additional 3 weeks. Unstable index and middle finger radial collateral ligament tears should be surgically repaired.

41.18 VOLAR MP DISLOCATIONS

Palmar MP joint dislocations are extremely rare. Avulsion of either the dorsal capsule from the metacarpal proximally or the volar plate from the proximal phalanx, or collateral ligament avulsion, can occur. In a border digit, a junctura tendinum may slip distal and volar to the metacarpal neck, also leading to an irreducible MP joint. Interposition of these structures between the metacarpal head and proximal phalanx can occur, and it produces a complex dislocation. If an attempt at a closed reduction under adequate anaesthesia is unsuccessful, an open reduction through a dorsal approach is necessary.

41.19 CARPOMETACARPAL JOINT DISLOCATIONS

Dislocations of the CMC joint are uncommon injuries and are present in less than 1% of hand injuries [21]. In isolated CMC dislocations, the most frequently injured CMC joint is the fifth. Although volar dislocations have been reported.

The fifth and fourth metacarpals may dislocate together. Often, an intraarticular fracture is associated with dislocation of the CMC joint and this type of lesion occurs when a longitudinal compressive force is applied to the dorsal aspect of the metacarpal head.

An high-energy trauma, from motor vehicle and motorcycle accidents and falls, or a direct blow to the dorsum or palm of the hand or a clenched fist against something or someone are generally the causes in these kind of lesions. In addition, extensive soft tissue damage and swelling can obscure subtle deformities. Tenderness and swelling at the CMC joints, prominence of the metacarpal head and/or base, deviation and malrotation of the involved digits should be present.

If the fracture fragment is small, the diagnosis may easily be missed in the PA radiograph.

Careful evaluation of AP, lateral and oblique radiographs helps in diagnosing the injury. In the lateral radiograph, displacement is obscured by superimposition of the central metacarpals. An additional 30° pronated lateral view (Figure 41.17), which places the fourth and fifth CMC joints in profile, will help in diagnosing dislocations or fracture dislocations of these joints because in this view the fifth CMC joint is projected in profile to demonstrate displacement. Tomography or CT scan can be used to further delineate the injury or help diagnose occult fractures (Figure 41.18).

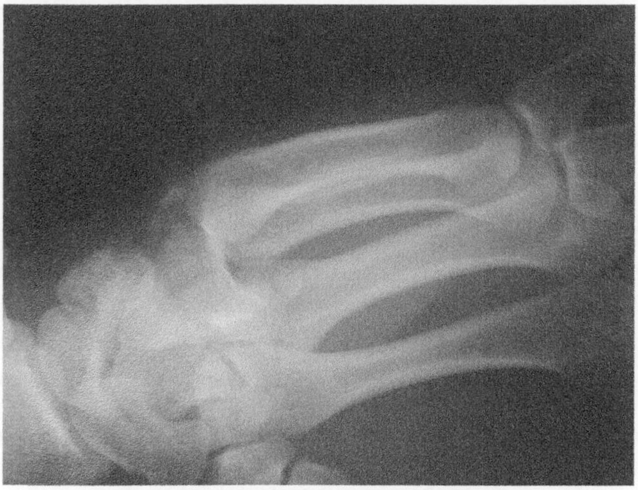

FIGURE 41.17 30° Pronated view for the evaluation in a 5th CMC joint dorsal dislocation.

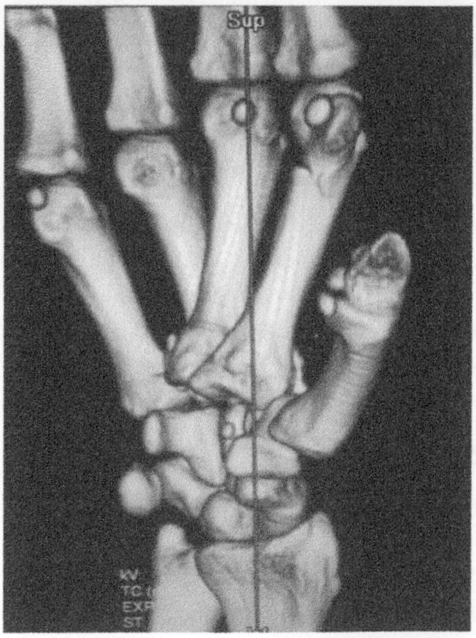

FIGURE 41.18 3-D CT reconstruction in a 2nd and 3rd CMC joint volar fracture dislocation.

41.19.1 Treatment

For dislocations without fracture, treatment options include a closed reduction, closed reduction and percutaneous K-wire fixation, and open reduction with internal fixation of the dislocation.

Closed reduction is usually possible by an adequate analgesia, applying a longitudinal traction to the involved digits, pressing over the dorsal base of the dislocated metacarpal in a distal and volar direction, and then extend the metacarpal to help reduce the dislocated joint. If the reduction is successful, immobilise the hand with the wrist extended, the MP joints flexed and the IP joints extended for 3–4 weeks.

In case of failure of conservative treatment, closed reduction will fail because of interposed soft tissues or chondral fragments open reduction is indicated.

Acute CMC dislocation makes a dorsal longitudinal or oblique incision over the affected joint. Than retract the extensor tendons and visualise the injured joint. Retract the ruptured ligaments, debride the joint, reduce it and also reduce any intraarticular fractures by K-wires. If no fracture is present, reduce the dislocation and fix it using smooth K-wire placed obliquely from the metacarpal across the joint into the appropriate carpal bone or to an adjacent stable metacarpal. Then repair the ligaments involved and capsular closure. Confirm reduction of the joint with radiographs. Splint the hand for 3–4 weeks, allowing full finger motion after the first few days. Remove the pins at 6 weeks.

41.19.2 Complications

If symptomatic post-traumatic arthrosis is present, a resection or resection on and interposition arthroplasty is useful, and an arthrodesis remains an option.

41.20 THUMB METACARPOPHALANGEAL JOINT DISLOCATIONS

The assessment and indications for treatment are similar to those of the MP joint of the fingers. Thumb MP joint injuries are frequently associated with collateral ligament and volar plate injuries, as well as an occasional intraarticular fracture.

The dislocations are based on the direction of dislocation of the phalanx (dorsal versus volar) and whether they are easily reducible (simple versus complex).

Dislocations of the MP joint usually are dorsal, resulting from hyperextension. The dislocation results in a complete tear of the volar plate proximally and usually of a portion of the collateral ligaments. Volar MP dislocations are quite rare.

Clinically and radiographically, hyperextension of the MP joint is noted. Widening of the joint space is suggestive of soft tissue interposition. Dislocations of the MP joint of the thumb usually can be treated conservatively.

Under adequate analgesia with the wrist and IP joint flexed to relax the flexor tendon, perform closed reduction of the dislocated joint, pushing the base of the proximal phalanx distally and palmarly. After that confirm congruous reduction of the joint on radiographs and test for active and passive joint stability.

In case of an irreducible dislocation, because of interposition of the volar plate or other structures, do an open reduction. Volar, dorsal or lateral approaches to the MP joint have been described.

41.21 THUMB UCL LESION

The most common injury to the metacarpophalangeal joint is sprain of the ulnar collateral ligament of the thumb known as gamekeeper's thumb or skier's thumb. This injury occurs when the ulnar collateral ligament is stressed by forcing the thumb into radial deviation. When the ulnar collateral ligament tears from its phalangeal insertion, the adductor aponeurosis should interpose between the retracted ligament, preventing healing of the ligament to the proximal phalanx with closed treatment (Stener's lesion).

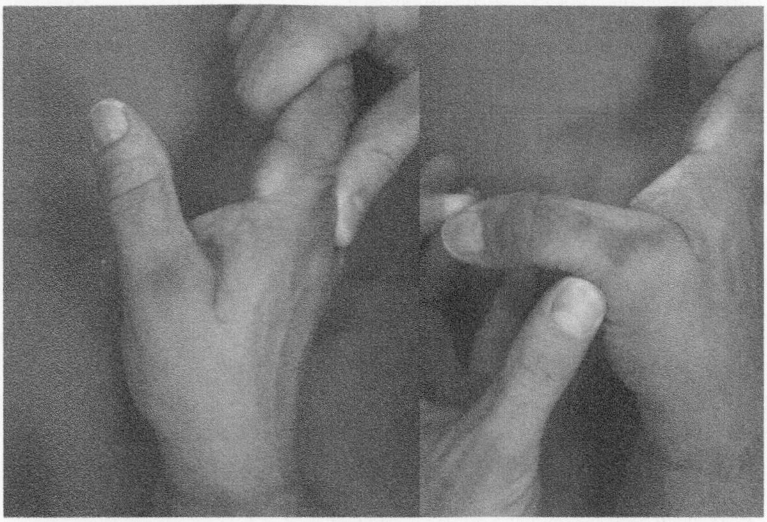

FIGURE 41.19 Stress test for the clinical evaluation in a complete injury of the UCL of the thumb.

41.21.1 Physical Examination

Evaluation of the integrity of the ligament may be made by radially stressing the flexed metacarpophalangeal joint under local anaesthesia. Radial deviation that is more than 30° from that of the opposite thumb is diagnostic of a totally disrupted (Figure 41.19), incompetent ligament, but pain, swelling, bruising and muscle spasm make the clinical assessment difficult in the acute phase.

41.21.2 Imaging Studies

Standard radiographs will exclude obvious fractures and dislocation or subluxation. The use and limitations of stress radiography, arthrography and MRI have been described. Ultrasound has been shown to be of some value in the diagnosis of acute UCL ruptures. There are many diagnostic tests useful to confirm the diagnosis, but the clinical examination with routine x-rays is still the most consistent.

41.21.3 Treatment

Three grades of the injury have been identified:

1. The ligament is intact but strained.
2. The ligament demonstrates mild laxity.
3. The ligament shows complete laxity.

Grade I and II injuries can be treated conservatively with a cast for 3–4 weeks. In grade III injuries, a Stener's lesion develops, and the ulnar collateral ligament is displaced above the adductor tendon aponeurosis. In this case, healing by casting is not possible because the ligament is no longer attached to the bone and it necessitates an operative procedure. For repairing a grade III ulnar collateral ligament injury, use a suture anchor for repair. The suture anchor is placed after abrading the surface where the collateral ligament usually originates on the proximal phalanx.

Avulsion of the ulnar collateral ligament may also be associated with a bony fragment. If the fragment is greater than 20% of the articular surface or if the avulsed fragment is displaced more than 4–5 mm, an open repair of the ligament is mandatory.

Chronic symptomatic ulnar collateral ligament injuries may be repaired if the residual ligament is of sufficient quality. Supplementation of the repair with either tendon transfer or tendon grafting may be useful. In patients who have developed traumatic arthritis or if ligament reconstruction is not deemed feasible, fusion of the metacarpophalangeal joint is preferred.

41.22 MALUNION AND NON-UNION OF THE PHALANGES AND METACARPALS

41.22.1 Malunion

Malunion is a common complication of phalangeal fractures owing to a lack of understanding regarding hand biomechanics.

Without appropriate treatment, injury to the phalanges and metacarpals of the fingers and thumb can produce shortening, angular and rotatory deformities of the digits.

Malunion has been subclassified into four types: malrotation, volar angulation, lateral angulation and shortening.

History and clinical examination and patients' daily working are mandatory to approach these lesions. This should elucidate pertinent details of the severity of the original injury and to the original treatment if a high-energy or open injury expands the traumatised zone far beyond the bone or joint in question, and if it is compromised, the soft tissues envelope. The patient's symptoms, the extent of rehabilitation and the patient's ability to comply with the prescribed treatments must be evaluated.

41.22.1.1 Physical Examination

Examination of the injured hand begins with a visual inspection. Palpation of the injured part helps distinguish non-union from malunion and reveals the function of the joints. Fixed angular deformities of the digits should be carefully measured and joint motion should be measured by a goniometer and always compared with the contralateral. Assess joint stability by stress tests.

41.22.1.2 Imaging Studies

Imaging of complicated hand injuries starts with plain radiographs. A standard PA, lateral and oblique view of all injured parts should be performed. The quality of the injured bone and the extent of bony union as well as the degree of angular malalignment can be gauged directly from the plain films. CT scans are useful adjuncts for any fracture involving a joint, allowing a more detailed evaluation of the number and potential viability of articular fragments. MRI in the evaluation of complicated injuries of the bones and joints of the hand is poorly indicated.

41.22.1.3 Treatment

According to malrotation, a small malrotation may be acceptable to many patients. However, significant malrotation results in functional impairment, pain and diminished grip strength. So in these cases, an osteotomy is recommended, preferably through the phalanx. Phalangeal osteotomy offers the advantage of correcting the malunion at its site of origin (Figure 41.20). Malrotation should be corrected by an osteotomy through the metacarpal shape. This technique is technically easier, but multiplanar correction is not possible.

The deformity in volar angulation is often aesthetically unacceptable and can result in a fixed PIP flexion contracture. The osteotomy is performed making an opening or closing wedge at the level of the malunion.

For lateral angulation, the correction is obtained by either opening or closing wedge osteotomy. Alternatively, corrective opening wedge osteotomy can be accomplished.

Shortening may occur after a comminuted fracture or after a long spiral fracture. However, a diaphyseal osteotomy with an appropriately fashioned intercalary graft may be indicated.

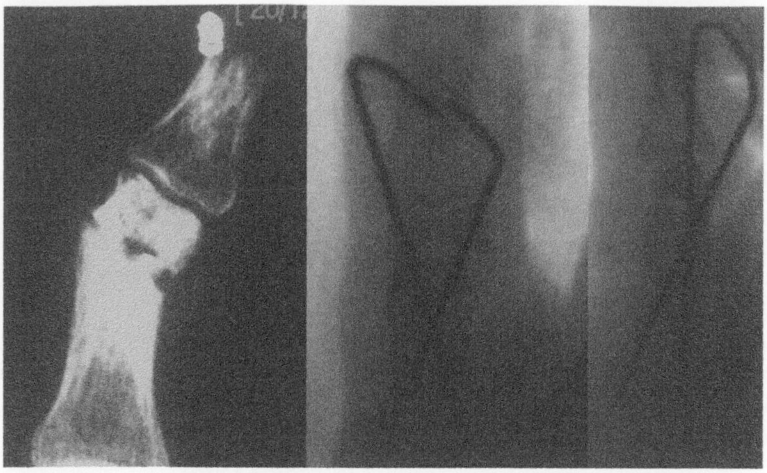

FIGURE 41.20 Osteotomy of the proximal phalanges and deformity correction with bone graft.

41.22.2 Non-Union

Non-union of the proximal and middle phalangeal shafts is a rare complication in hand fractures, with the exception of distal phalanx fractures, although delayed union is seen quite often.

41.22.2.1 Imaging Studies

Imaging starts with plain radiographs by a standard PA, lateral and oblique. The quality of the injured bone and the extent of bony non-union are investigated by CT scans, while MRI is useful in the evaluation of the quality of the bones and joints of allowing a more detailed evaluation.

41.22.2.2 Treatment

It is mandatory to remove fibrous tissue until there are fresh fracture ends. An intercalated cortico-cancellous bone grafting is indicated if bone loss is present. Plate fixation gives the advantage of being stable. Also, it gives the opportunity for a tenolysis and capsulotomy when indicated.

Avascular necrosis of the metacarpal head remains a concern in periarticular fractures, as an independent blood supply may be absent in 35% of cases.

41.23 DISTAL RADIUS FRACTURES

Fractures of the distal radius are the most common injuries. The majority are extraarticular fractures. Current diagnosis and treatment involve understanding the physiology and biomechanics of the fracture. The complexity of any kind of fracture, the age and patient activity give the indications of which kind of treatment is indicated. An accurate imaging study differentiates fractures features and determines the most appropriate form of treatment.

PA, lateral and oblique plain x-rays may demonstrate all the fracture features: extraarticular or intraarticular; number of fragments; dorsal comminution, volar comminution, or both; and volar or dorsal and medial or lateral displacement; an alteration of ulnar variance; and the direction of fracture displacement or shortening and DRUJ integrity.

41.24 INCIDENCE

Distal radius fractures represent approximately one-sixth of all fractures treated in emergency departments. Only 8% of fractures are caused by severe trauma. The remaining are a result from a fall at standing height or less.

41.25 DIAGNOSIS

41.25.1 Physical Examination

The majority of the external physical findings seen with this fracture may be related to the fact that the fractured radius has shortened relative to the intact strut of the ulna.

A comprehensive history should include the patient's activity level, age, handedness, medical conditions and occupation.

Regarding physical examination, the displaced fracture is quite noticeable, with deformity of the distal radius resulting in abnormal positioning of the hand dorsally or volarly. Usually swelling and ecchymosis are also noted. Sometimes an open injury is present.

When examining the patient, particular attention should be given to median nerve function and to any evidence of decreased sensory or motor function. Also, vascular status of the hand must be assessed, and flexor and extensor tendon function and distal ulna and DRUJ stability. Concomitant injuries may exist.

41.25.2 Imaging Studies

The PA view for extraarticular fractures assesses a radial shortening/comminution and ulnar styloid fracture location such as tip, waist or base (Figures 41.21 and 41.22). For intraarticular fractures, assess a depression of the lunate facet, a gap between scaphoid and lunate facet, a central impaction fragments and an interruption of the proximal carpal row.

The lateral view for extraarticular fractures is useful to assess the extent of metaphyseal comminution, palmar tilt, displacement of the volar or dorsal cortex, the scapholunate angle and the position of DRUJ.

In case of intraarticular fractures, lateral views give information about the lunate articular surface, depression of the central fragment (Figure 41.23) and the gap between palmar and dorsal fragments.

Oblique view for extraarticular fractures assesses radial comminution. For intraarticular fractures, assess the radial styloid for split or depression and depression of the dorsal lunate facet.

Additional views may be obtained as needed to assess for displacement or additional injuries.

The tilted lateral view is a lateral view with an inclination of the radius of about 20°. It eliminates the shadow of the radial styloid and provides a clear tangential view of the lunate facet and a possible hardware penetration into the articular surface.

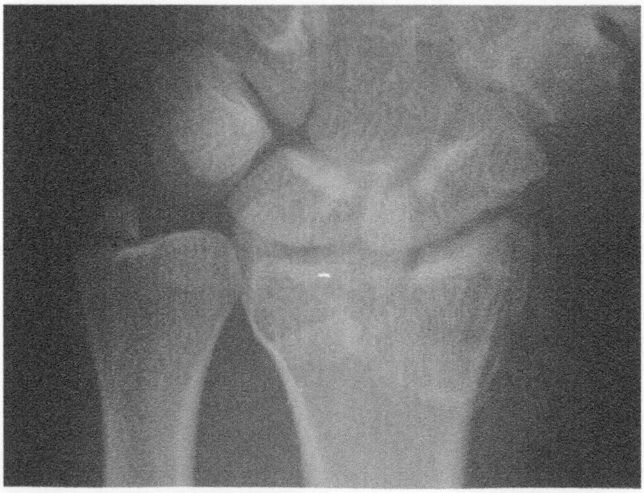

FIGURE 41.21 X-ray evaluation: posteroanterior view for extraarticular radius fracture.

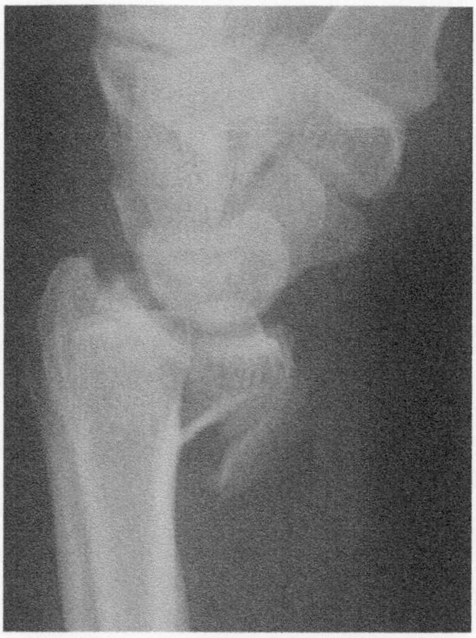

FIGURE 41.22 Lateral view of an intraarticular radius fracture.

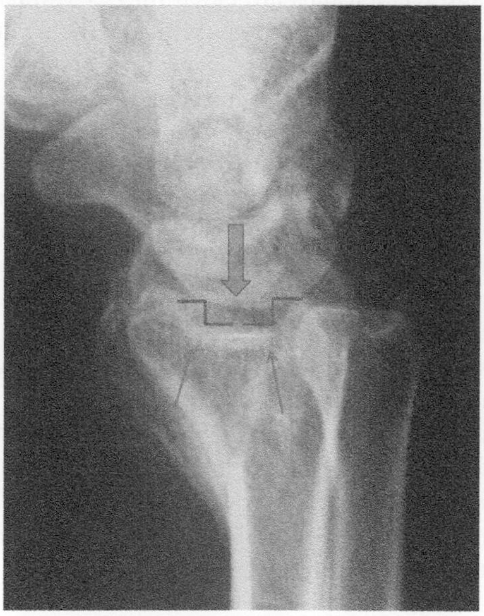

FIGURE 41.23 Step-off in an intraarticular radial fracture (radial depression in articular surface for the lunate bone).

AP and lateral traction views are taken with manual traction or finger traps applied after reduction helping during external fixation manoeuvres and the presence of incongruity consistent with interosseous ligament injury.

AP and lateral contralateral wrist x-rays may be useful during the diagnosis process before surgery to compare the patient's normal angles.

Relevant information of the articular injury can be obtained with oblique radiographs, taken with forearm partially pronated or partially supinated that shows the dorsomedial part of the distal radius.

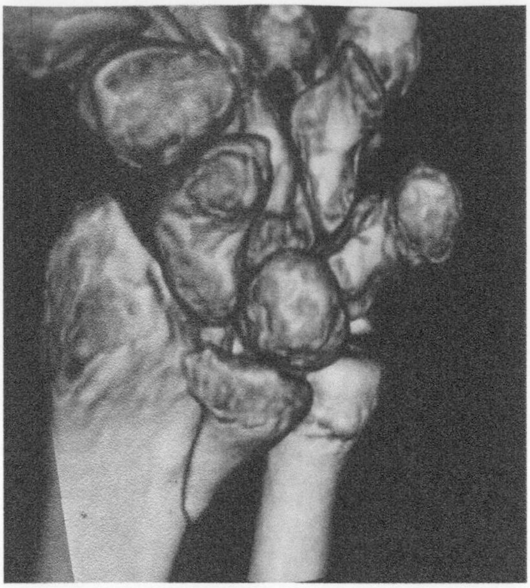

FIGURE 41.24 CT scan with 3-D elaboration for intraarticular radial fracture.

The important radiographic relationships are radial tilt (23°), volar tilt (11°), DRUJ reduction and radial height (12 mm), while radial width is useful for the evaluation of possible articular involvement.

In case of high-energy fractures, for the evaluation of multifragmented articular injuries, CT scan and CT scan with 3D elaboration is mandatory and is important in more accurately identifying these (Figure 41.24). It is also helpful in detecting intraarticular fractures with step-off during healing and early displacements. It provides a more accurate visualisation of the morphology of the fracture, the direction and extent of articular fragment displacement, and guides the surgeon in the determination of the optimal surgical approaches and methods of stable internal or external skeletal fixation.

CT with 3-D reconstruction or arthro-CT is useful to assess bone deformity, joint congruity, intraarticular fibrosis and DRUJ position.

Arthro-CT also assesses intraarticular malunion, distal radius cartilage condition, DRUJ and combined carpal cartilage and ligament tears.

In the assessment and management of intraarticular distal radius fractures for recognition of the potential association of intercarpal ligament injury with certain fractures, arthrography and arthroscopy has elevated the role of the wrist investigation.

MRI is useful in the acute setting unless concomitant wrist injuries are being evaluated, such as scaphoid fracture, scapholunate ligament injury or TFCC tears.

41.26 TREATMENT

For a successful outcome treatment, planning is basic. The rationale of treatment of these fractures is a wrist that provides sufficient pain-free motion and stability to permit activities reducing the risks to evolve in future degenerative changes.

41.26.1 Non-Operative Management

Closed reduction and cast immobilisation is the mainstay of treatment for these fractures. Cast immobilisation is indicated in stable fractures and in case of low-demand elderly patients in whom future functional impairment is a minimal concern for operative risks.

Conservative treatment for minimally to non-displaced fractures is a forearm cast for about 30–35 days to an evidence of radiographic healing. This is then followed by 2 weeks in a palmar wrist removable splint.

Displaced fractures are reduced in the emergency room if possible by longitudinal traction and gentle manipulation. Successful reduction requires adequate pain relief to overcome muscle spasm. Traction is used for reallineation/reduction of the bone surfaces; the thumb, index finger and long finger are placed in finger traps, and then direct pressure is applied on the displaced radial metaphyseal fragment.

Reduction may be confirmed using fluoroscopy or with plain x-rays after the manoeuvre.

The position of immobilisation of the radius is critical after reduction. The splint or cast should provide a dorsal supporting structure to prevent collapse, avoiding an excessive palmar flexion of the radius.

Follow-up consist in PA and lateral x-rays at 7–10 days after closed reduction or after cats immobilisation and a further x-ray evaluation after 30–35 days monitoring bone healing.

41.26.2 Surgical Management

Indications for surgery depend on fractures with loss of radial inclination, radial height, volar tilt, radial width and DRUJ injury that cannot be reliably maintained by non-operative means alone, also in those situation in which redisplacement occurs after reduction and cast immobilisation, comminuted displaced intraarticular fracture, open fractures, associated carpal fractures, associated neurovascular injury or tendon injury, bilateral fractures and impaired contralateral extremity.

Percutaneous pinning, external fixation and internal fixation (Figure 41.25) are the surgical options for treatment of distal radius fractures; these techniques may be used individually or in combination to maintain adequate reduction and to obtain optimal stability.

Many investigators have shown the importance of articular congruity in the outcome after distal radius fractures; there is concern regarding whether we can adequately visualise the articular surface intraoperatively.

Wrist arthroscopy has become an important adjunct in the reduction of these fractures [22–25]. The arthroscopic approach has the benefit of giving a perfect view of the fracture system, and

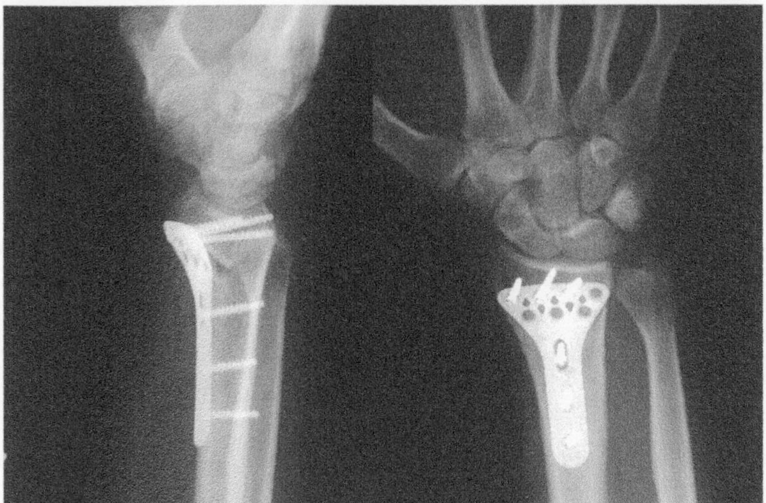

FIGURE 41.25 Internal fixation with plate for distal radial fracture.

the possibility to detect and treat osteochondral loose bodies and associated ligament injuries such as interosseous ligament injuries and avulsions of the triangular fibrocartilage.

After adequate surgical reduction and stable fixation, follow-up consist in PA and lateral x-rays at 7–10 days after closed reduction or after cats immobilisation and a further x-ray evaluation after 30–35 days monitoring bone healing.

In case of comminuted articular displaced fractures, after reduction and fixation, some authors suggest to perform a CT of the wrist checking the articular surface congruity.

41.27 COMPLICATIONS

41.27.1 Non-Union and Malunion

Non-union is an uncommon outcome in distal radius fractures, and is extremely rare, but does occur and is usually symptomatic. Excessive alcohol consumption, external fixator overdistraction, inadequate immobilisation, multiple medical problems, peripheral neuropathy and tobacco product use are the risk factors for this complication. Treatment for non-union of distal radius must be individualised and based on the patient's symptoms, functional deficit and bony substance and includes bone grafting and rigid internal fixation and, when possible, correction of the factor or factors that are compromising bone healing.

Symptomatic ulnar styloid non-unions are best treated with fragment excision, and when DRUJ instability is present, the TFC should be reattached by anchor screw to the fovea.

Malunion of the distal radius is a relatively common but complex problem that can occur and results in significant patient morbidity, in wrist pain (radiocarpal, radioulnar and/or ulnocarpal), decreased range of motion and/or midcarpal instability and limitation of function, and it continues to be a significant complication following non-operative management.

The effect of these changes can be significant with regard to both immediate functional impairment and the development of late degenerative changes.

The decision to do a simultaneous procedure at the DRUJ depends on the amount of radial shortening and the presence of osteoarthritic changes or instability of the joint.

Depending on extraarticular, intraarticular or complex malunion, post-traumatic wrist deformity can be corrected with extraarticular osteotomies, intraarticular osteotomies, or both.

41.27.1.1 Radiographic Evaluation

AP and lateral x-ray are the initial evaluation. An oblique x-ray may add additional information and is not mandatory, but an ulnar variance film is necessary whenever radial shortening is suspected and should be compared with the ulnar variance of the opposite wrist.

If a complex intraarticular malunion is suspected, computed tomography (CT) and reconstruction in the sagittal and coronal planes is mandatory and also 3-D CT scan reconstruction may be useful. All carpal angles and indices should be measured, and in particular the scapholunate, radiolunate, capitolunate angles and ulnar variance. Intraarticular malunions of the radial carpal joint and DRUJ should be noted, as well as the presence of associated arthritis. The CT scan is a good tool for the observation of congruent reduction of the DRUJ.

41.28 TREATMENT

41.28.1 Non-Operative Treatment

Non-operative treatment is used most commonly in the older, more debilitated patient, in older patient who is pain free or in a young person with a minimal extraarticular malunion. If the patient was referred late and if the fracture has healed, wait and see is the best indication; also if the malunion is extraarticular, a trial of non-operative treatment may be indicated.

41.28.2 Indication for Operative Treatment

Correcting the deformity at the level of the old fracture site to reorient the joint surface, to guarantee normal load distribution, to reestablish the mechanical balance of the midcarpal joint and to restore the anatomic relationships of the DRUJ, restoring the normal aspect and function of the wrist, is the aim of the distal radial osteotomy.

The absolute indications for osteotomy include intraarticular malunion, malunion that is associated with subluxation of the DRUJ or radial carpal or midcarpal joints, and malunion that is associated with progressive median neuropathy at the wrist.

41.29 CARPUS

It is not easy to differentiate clinically the presence of an injury of the wrist or to an injury of the carpus. The two most important views to diagnose an injury are the PA and lateral views taken in neutral position.

Special views are always necessary to diagnose a fracture and its displacement such as radial oblique (supinated PA) and ulnar oblique views.

These four standard views detect most of the carpal injuries. If there is the suspicion of carpal instability, additional views in maximal radial and ulnar deviation are recommended. Further views can be done in maximal flexion and extension.

41.30 SCAPHOID FRACTURE

Fractures of the scaphoid are common and affect predominantly young and productive individuals.

41.30.1 Physical Examination

The diagnosis of a scaphoid fracture is made from the clinical history with about 90% of patients recalling a hyperextension injury.

Sometimes, swelling, pain and ecchymosis are minimal, and not infrequently, serious injuries are dismissed as minor trauma. Tenderness in the anatomic snuffbox has been described as a classic physical finding for scaphoid fractures.

Range of motion is reduced, and there is usually pain at the extremes of motion.

41.30.2 Radiographic Evaluation

Because of the inaccuracy of clinical signs, the diagnosis of scaphoid fracture rests on high-quality radiographs. Initial radiographs include standard PA, lateral, oblique and ulnar deviation PA grip views (Figure 41.26) [26].

If standard views are non-diagnostic, several views have been described. They include a clenched-fist PA view and an ulnar deviation PA view in 20° of supination, a 45° pronated view, a 'carpal box' series of magnified and elongated radiographs.

Comparative views of the opposite uninjured wrist are often helpful.

If clinical findings are positive and there is presumptive evidence of an occult scaphoid fracture, and x-ray evaluation is negative, many authors suggest the use of palmar cast for 10 days and then repeating the scaphoid series.

In case of persistent tenderness and pain localised to the scaphoid waist, several diagnostic options are necessary.

Motion views of the wrist (flexion, extension and radial and ulnar deviation) may demonstrate fracture displacement, which indicates an unstable scaphoid fracture.

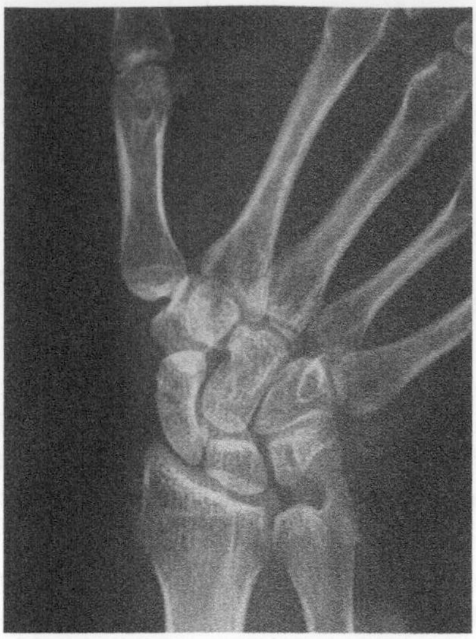

FIGURE 41.26 X-ray evaluation in ulnar deviation.

CT scans can produce high-resolution fine-cut images of the scaphoid in multiple planes and also three-dimensional reconstructions of these scans can be helpful for planning operative procedures of scaphoid reconstruction. It is indicated primarily for preoperative analysis of scaphoid non-union for planning of scaphoid reconstruction.

Technetium-99m bone scans also have a high sensitivity in diagnosing occult fractures of the carpus.

An MRI scan is a high accurate modality for early diagnosis of scaphoid fractures. It may be helpful in the differentiation between an acute scaphoid fracture and a scaphoid non-union. It has an excellent interobserver agreement. Most centres recommend a combination of sequences, including T1-weighted spin echo and short inversion time inversion-recovery imaging to maximise diagnostic yield (Figure 41.27).

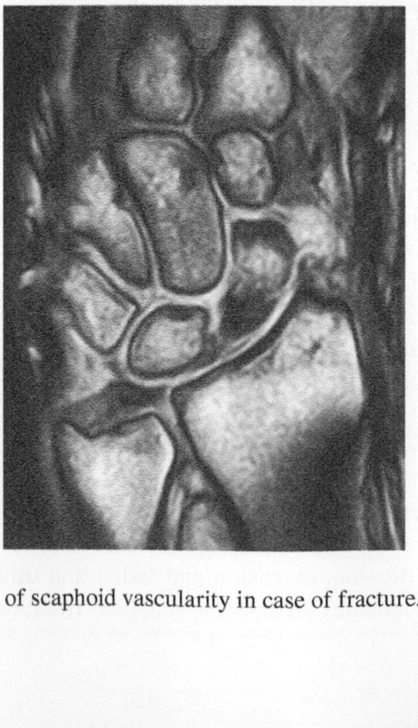

FIGURE 41.27 MRI evaluation of scaphoid vascularity in case of fracture.

With the additional advantage of its ability to identify bone marrow abnormalities, MRI imaging, over CT, is the best option in the detection of occult scaphoid fractures.

Additionally, MRI has the potential to diagnose other bony and soft tissue injuries simultaneously.

Ultrasound enjoyed some popularity as a diagnostic modality in the early 1980s, but subsequent reports refuted its reliability, showing a low sensitivity.

Scintigraphy and MRI are very efficient in the early detection of scaphoid fracture also demonstrated by a displacement of fat tissues surrounding this bone. CT may be used during the healing period to detect a displacement or a delayed healing. Arthro-CT may demonstrate combined ligament and cartilage injuries.

41.31 TREATMENT

41.31.1 Non-Operative Management

Non-operative management with cast immobilisation when applied during the acute injury period has a good healing rate. The indications for closed treatment of a scaphoid fracture include an isolated, acute, undisplaced fracture of the waist or distal pole.

Chest x-rays should be obtained at the time of cast removal. If there are still clinical and radiological signs of a scaphoid fracture, another cast is applied for two more weeks.

Therefore, careful clinical and radiographic follow-up examinations at the time of cast removal are essential. It is recommended that the patient be reviewed 6 weeks after cast removal for clinical and radiological examination and then every 3 months until the outcome is clear. Patients should be seen for a final checkup after 1 year.

If healing failed, a surgical approach is mandatory.

41.31.2 Operative Treatment in Acute Scaphoid Fractures

In all other patients with acute scaphoid fractures, the main choice is percutaneous screw fixation (Figure 41.28). This includes the majority of young high-demand patients. The method is relatively

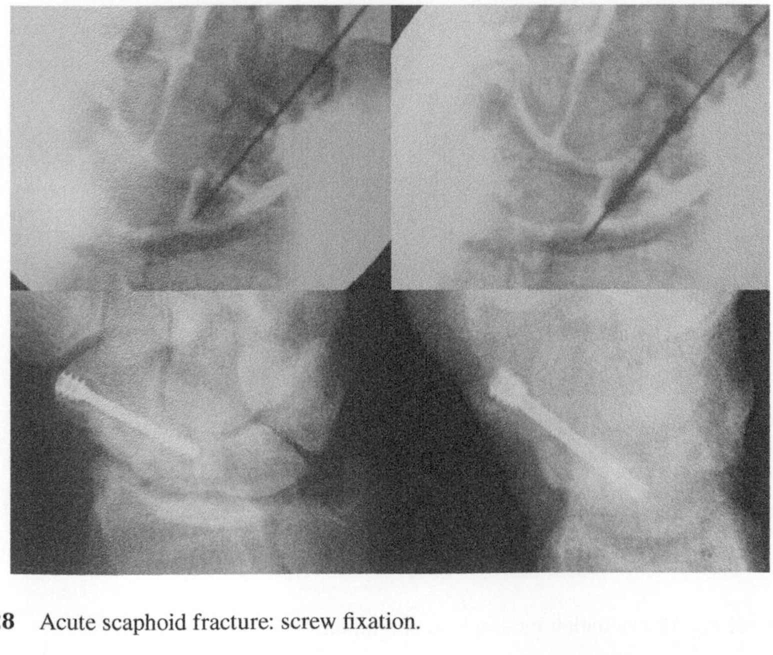

FIGURE 41.28 Acute scaphoid fracture: screw fixation.

easy and allows postoperative treatment early mobilisation, and the use of a removable cast for the immobilisation period. The advantage of this minimally invasive method is early return to sports and work in a young and active population.

41.32 SCAPHOID NON-UNION

Scaphoid fractures are the most common of carpal bone fractures, and it therefore follows that scaphoid non-union is the most common non-union of the wrist.

Clinically, the patient who presents with a scaphoid non-union has pain that is associated with activity and is relieved with rest, pain at the extremes of motion and diminished grip strength. Sometimes, pain is only with activity, and occasionally, there may be pain with rest; it varies with the extremes of motion, usually increasing with radial deviation and extension and decreasing with wrist flexion and ulnar deviation. Pain at rest is usually not present unless there is advanced post-traumatic arthritis.

41.32.1 Imaging Studies

Radiographic imaging is the hallmark in the diagnosis of scaphoid non-union and is an essential part of the decision-making process with respect to treatment.

A total of six views of the wrist is generally recommended in radiographic evaluation of the patient with suspected scaphoid non-union and wrist instability such as an AP (Figure 41.29), lateral and scaphoid views, as well as motion views, of the wrist.

An x-ray of the opposing wrist is occasionally recommended in the operative planning of scaphoid non-unions to compare with the normal scaphoid and normal carpal indices and angles.

CT is mandatory to establish the degree of scaphoid displacement and to determine the size of replacement bone grafting, and is recommended for three-dimensional reconstruction.

MRI is a useful procedure when one has concern regarding scaphoid non-union and avascular necrosis (AVN), and is mandatory to assess medullar bone vascularity (Figure 41.30) especially

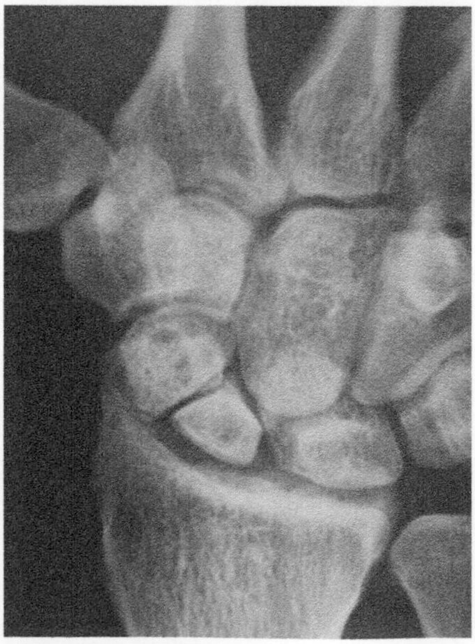

FIGURE 41.29 X-ray AP evaluation for scaphoid non-union.

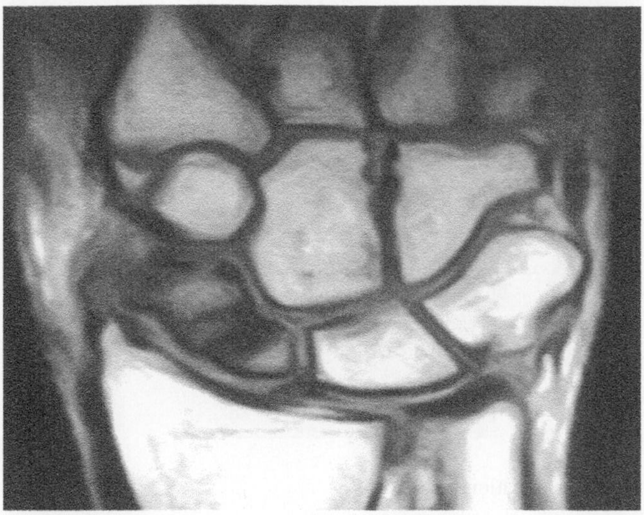

FIGURE 41.30 MRI scaphoid bone vascularity.

of the proximal pole. It is also useful to differentiate a delayed union from a non-union, depending on the junction aspect that is avascular with hypointense fibrous tissue or articular fluid, or the vascular junction with enhancement during gadolinium injection. It may also provide indication of fragment position and of approximate ligament status.

Arthroscopy is the final imaging technique that is used to assess scaphoid non-unions.

The stage of non-union indicates the types of investigations required. The presence of OA modifies the surgical indications.

41.33 SURGICAL MANAGEMENT

The operative procedure consists of an open procedure. The fracture is exposed and fibrous tissue removed. Cancellous bone is harvested from distal radius or from iliac crest. The two fragments of the scaphoid are fixed with a compression screw, which is inserted as previously described. Specific treatments, which are based on the location and vascularity of the non-union site, of a scaphoid non-union have also been described.

41.33.1 Other Carpal Bones

For other carpal bones, the decision-making procedure should be the same.

Some carpal fractures need special views already described or CT to be visualised: hook of hamate, trapezial ridge fracture, triquetrum chip fractures and fracture of the pisiform. MRI and sometimes CT may be used for occult fractures.

41.34 DISLOCATIONS AND LIGAMENT INJURIES OF THE WRIST

41.34.1 Carpal Dislocations

While several x-rays indicate the bone situation such as small fractures and scaphoid involvement for carpal trans-scapho-perilunate dislocations (Figures 41.31 and 41.32), CT is useful for a missed dislocation (Figure 41.33). MRI may assess vascularisation of the lunate or the scaphoid proximal pole and the extrinsic volar ligament plane.

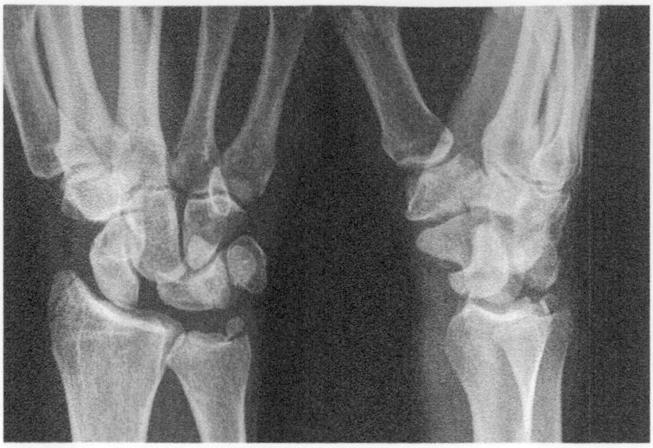

FIGURE 41.31 Perilunate dislocation.

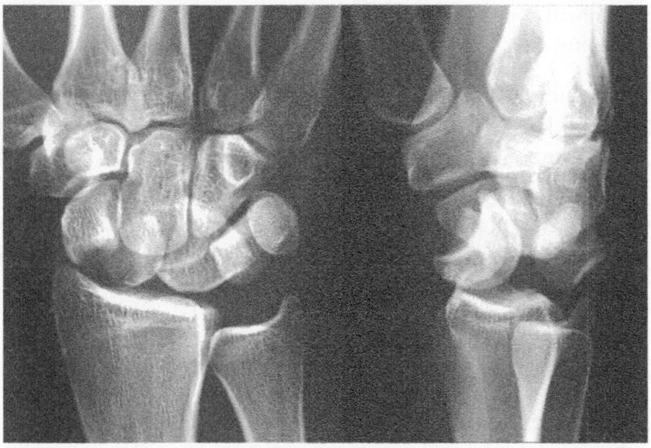

FIGURE 41.32 Transcapho-perilunate dislocation.

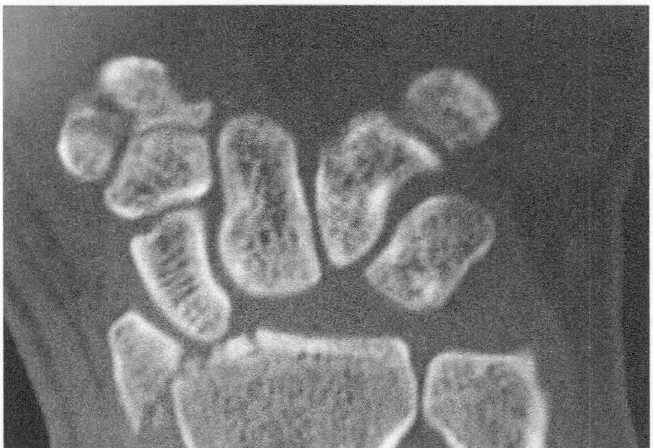

FIGURE 41.33 CT scan in a transtilo-transcapho-perilunate dislocation.

41.34.2 Carpal Instability

41.34.2.1 Scapholunate Instability

Scapholunate dissociation is the most frequent pattern of carpal instability occurring alone and in association with wrist fractures and without treatment evolves to progressive arthritis. The mechanism of injury usually consists in a dorsiflexion ulnar-deviation injury with an axial compression.

41.34.2.1.1 Physical Examination

The external appearance of SL instabilities may not be particularly dramatic. The wrist is often swollen and tender over the SL joint (the dorsum of the capsule distal to Lister's tubercle) and sometimes there is pain over the radial styloid and in particular tenderness in the anatomical snuffbox and over the palmar scaphoid tuberosity.

Acute carpal tunnel syndrome can occur with carpal fractures and dislocations. Most of these patients also have a reduction of range of motion in acute cases, whereas it may be normal in chronic cases. A positive Watson's manoeuvre may be present in this injury. This manoeuvre is the principal provocative test to assess scapholunate instability is the scaphoid shift test. This test evaluates motion of the scaphoid during radial deviation and wrist flexion while pressure is applied to the tubercle of the scaphoid in a volar to dorsal direction. Other tests are the resisted finger extension test and the scapholunate ballottement test.

41.34.2.1.2 Imaging Studies

Radiographs are essential in the evaluation of SL dissociation. Four views of the wrist are mandatory: PA view, lateral view, scaphoid and 45° semioblique views. The lateral radiograph must be a true lateral, with the wrist in neutral rotation.

In the PA view, the scaphoid is in flexion, and the semicircle at the distal end of the scaphoid is completed and becomes an entire circle delineating the ring sign. A gap between scaphoid and lunate may be present (Figure 41.34). This distance should be less than 3 mm even if this measurement varies for age of patient, weight, sex and height. A static instability identified by a significant gap between the scaphoid and lunate asserts an SL dissociation. Also, carpal height is decreased, and the capitate tends to move proximally between the lunate and the scaphoid.

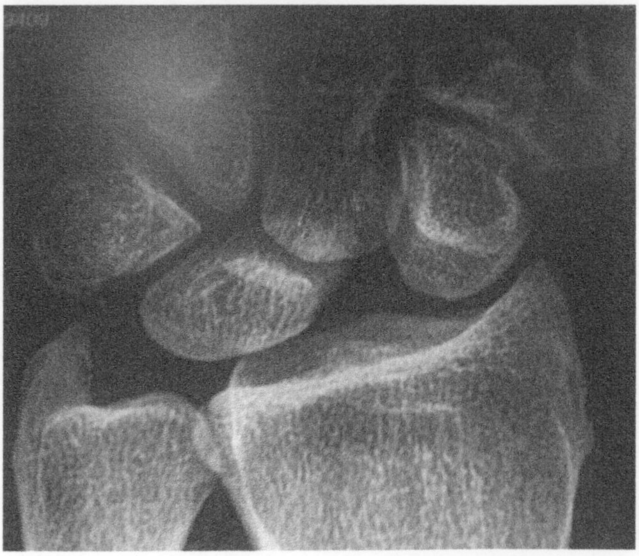

FIGURE 41.34 Scapholunate dissociation (Terry-Thomas sign).

In the PA view, three smooth radiographic arcs may be drawn to define normal carpal relationships. A step-off in the continuity of any of these arcs indicates an intracarpal instability. Any overlap between the carpal bones or any joint width exceeding 4 mm strongly suggests a carpal ligamentous injury.

The angle defined by a tangent to the two proximal and distal convexities of the palmar aspect of the scaphoid and a line through the central axis of the lunate determines the lunate angle. In the lateral view, normal values range between 30° and 60°, with an average of 47°; when the SL angle is increased to more than 60°, it should be considered a definite indication of scapholunate instability; in this case, the lunate is dorsally flexed in the so-called DISI deformity.

Dynamic series in ulnar deviation the SL gap increases and the scaphoid remains flexed, while on lateral x-rays the lunate remains in extension during wrist flexion (Figure 41.35). During a strength fist, SL gap increases and carpal height decreases (Figure 41.36).

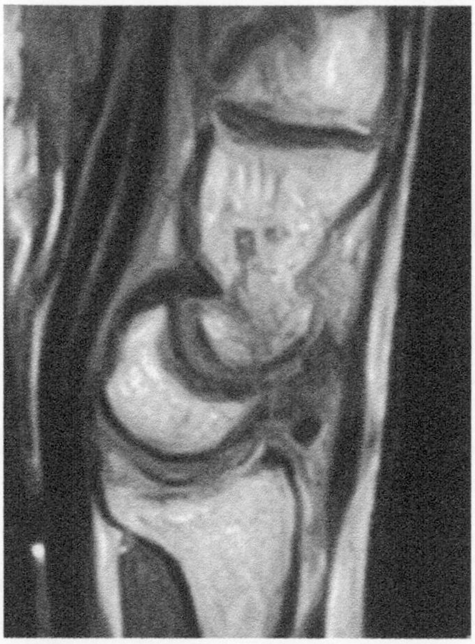

FIGURE 41.35 MRI: DISI view in SL injury.

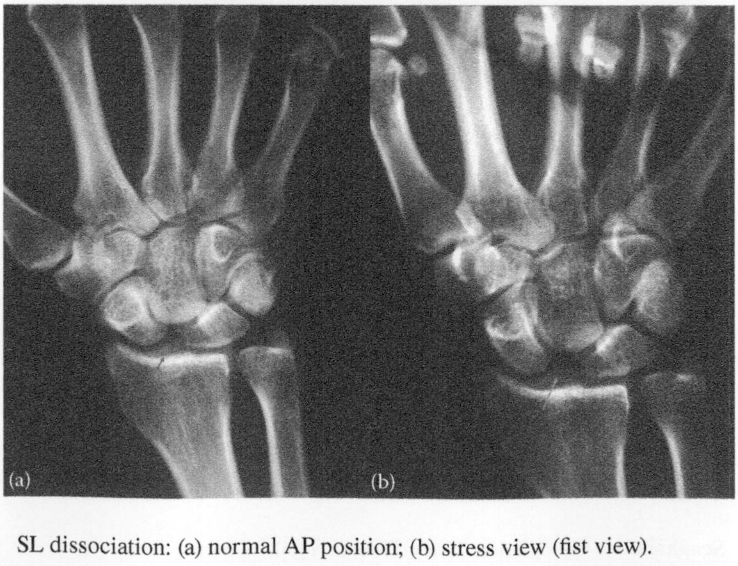

FIGURE 41.36 SL dissociation: (a) normal AP position; (b) stress view (fist view).

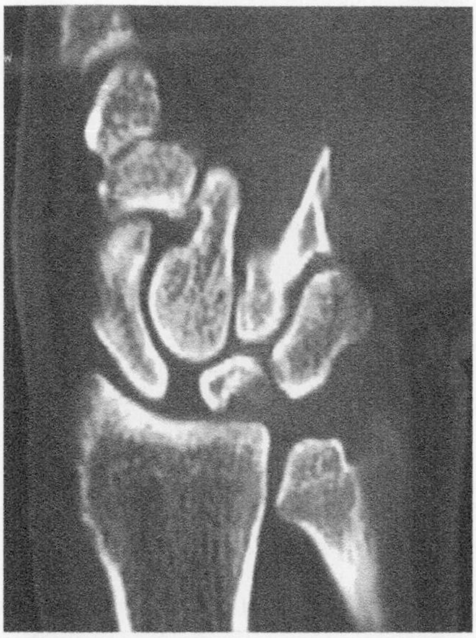

FIGURE 41.37 CT scan in SL dissociation.

Arthrography may be useful in defining partial tears of the SL ligaments even if some arthrograms confuse degenerative perforations of the central portion of the SL membrane with true ligament ruptures. In addition, a tear may be identified, but it is not possible to evaluate its extension and location and also poor information is provided on the status of the remaining ligament stump.

Because of these limitations, the use of arthrography has diminished substantially in favour of arthroscopy.

According to some authors, arthro-CT using millimetric slices is the most precise technique to assess ligament and cartilage status (Figure 41.37) because it is able to depict a thinned or stretched ligament and is helpful for diagnosis and treatment options.

MRI scans are more sensitive in detecting soft tissue injuries, including ruptures of the scapholunate ligament. Tears appear hyperintense on T2-weighted images. The diagnosis is certain when the signal is very intense in case of a large tear (Figure 41.38) while diagnosis of small tears is more difficult giving a frequent number of false-positive results even using arthro-MRI. MRI is less sensitive than arthro-CT.

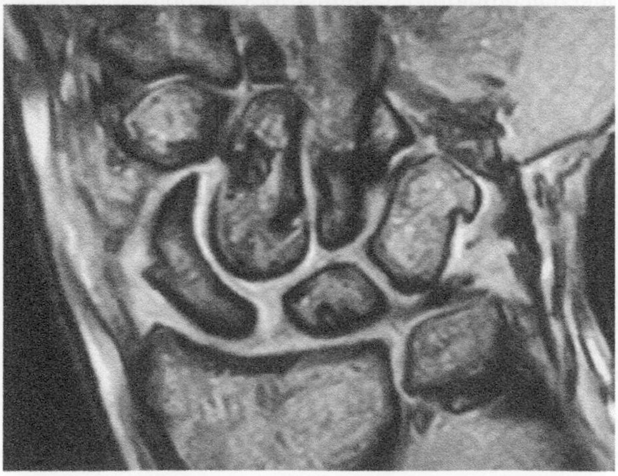

FIGURE 41.38 MRI in SL dissociation.

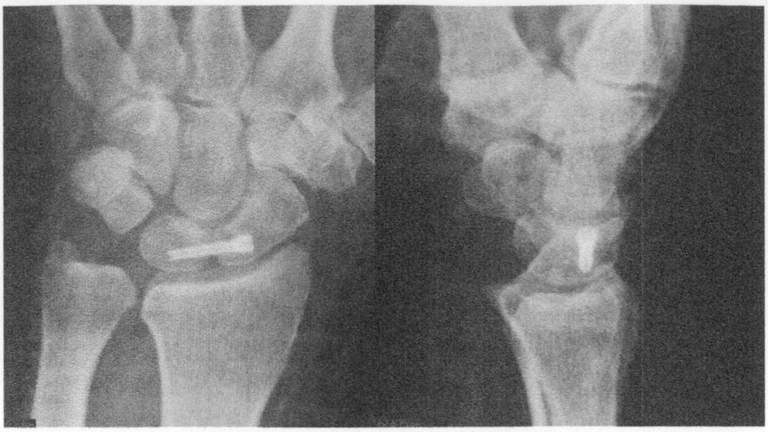

FIGURE 41.39 Capsulodesis with screw scapholunate fixation.

Arthroscopy has improved diagnostic capabilities and accuracy in wrist pathology. Some authors have reported that wrist arthroscopy is a more specific study than wrist arthrography [27,28]. Regarding most authors, arthroscopy is the gold standard technique in the diagnosis of intracarpal derangements.

41.34.2.1.3 Treatment

41.34.2.1.3.1 Acute Scapholunate Dissociation Patients with partial ligament tears without carpal instability may be treated conservatively with cast immobilisation and with re-education of wrist proprioception.

Surgical treatment depends on the SL dissociation degree.

In predynamic (occult) scapholunate dissociation, the main treatment described in literature are percutaneous Kirschner wire fixation of the SL Joint, arthroscopically guided Kirschner wire fixation of the SL Joint, arthroscopic debridement or electrothermal shrinkage.

In dynamic scapholunate dissociation, an open reduction and internal fixation, and repair of the dorsal SL ligament is the main choice (Figure 41.39). Alternatively, a dorsal radioscaphoid capsulodesis or soft tissue reconstruction of the dorsal SL ligament or bone ligament bone grafts are described.

In static reducible scapholunate dissociation, the main choice is based on tendon reconstruction techniques. Others are reduction association of the SL Joint (RASL procedure).

Postoperative care and rehabilitation are similar for both bony and soft tissue repair techniques. Support the wrist in the neutral position for 6–8 weeks or more and then remove K-wires. Initiate ROM exercises and in particular introduce forearm motion gradually if there is no associated ulnocarpal or forearm problem.

Begin wrist motion keeping the exercise limited, light and isokinetic and begin grip strengthening later than 4 months.

Follow-up consist in PA and lateral x-rays at 7–10 days after reduction and pin stabilisation and a further x-ray evaluation after 6 weeks and a final x-ray evaluation after 4–6 months.

41.34.2.1.3.2 Chronic Scapholunate Dissociation See Section 41.37.

41.35 CONCLUSION

A number of options are available for SL instability but no one treatment has proven to be the best choice because SL dissociation is complex. This injury leads to significant post-traumatic arthritis if left untreated and so a symptomatic or an instable lesion should be treated by the most reliable method of treatment.

41.35.1 Lunotriquetral Instability

Triquetrolunate dissociation may occur as an isolated injury or as part of the spectrum of perilunate dislocations Ulnar-sided wrist injuries can result from repetitive trauma or a single traumatic event, such as a twisting injury or a fall on an outstretched hand with a pronated forearm in which the wrist is extended and radially deviated. This injury is generally more stable than the scapholunate joint lesions. Often, these lesions are associated with other ulnar wrist problems such as ulnocarpal impingement, TFCC tears and DRUJ instabilities.

Injuries of the LT ligament should first be divided into degenerative stable and traumatic unstable conditions. Degenerative conditions are stable and largely involve disruption of only the proximal region of the LT ligament and are age-related degeneration. Traumatic conditions are a part of a spectrum of progressive ligament disruption that is associated with a lunate or perilunate dislocation. There are two directions in which the perilunate dislocation occurs: classic and reverse. Some authors describe several non-traumatic aetiologies that may contribute to an LT dissociation–like condition such as inflammatory and crystalline arthropathies, developmental extreme ulnar-plus variance of the ulna and generalised joint laxity.

41.35.1.1 Physical Examination

Patients complain of pain localised to the ulnar half of the wrist that is often accompanied by a sensation of weakness, worsened with activity, but the presentation is quite variable. Pain is sometimes intermittent or constant, such as a 'sprained wrist', with a loss of motion and may even experience ulnar nerve dysesthesias, a sense of 'clunk' in the wrist during radial-ulnar deviation.

Physical examination reveals tenderness specific to the lunotriquetral articulation and exacerbation of pain with ballottement of the unstable triquetrum.

A history of some specific injury is usually present.

Several provocative manoeuvres have been developed to increase the specificity of diagnosis for LT dissociation. Ballottement of the triquetrum, the shear test and compression of the LT joint can be accomplished by pressing laterally on the medial tubercle of the triquetrum.

41.35.1.2 Imaging Studies

Radiographs, as well as MRI or arthrography, often do not reveal the full extent of an injury. As in all conditions of the wrist, imaging studies should be considered largely as confirmatory tools rather than diagnostic ones. However, routine wrist radiographs, motion studies, tomography, arthrography, videofluoroscopy, scintigraphy and MRI could be used for the diagnosis of LT dissociation.

Plain radiographs of stable LT tears usually demonstrate normal intercarpal relationships; in fact, unless there is a significant static deformity (VISI pattern on lateral radiographs of the wrist) radiographic documentation of lunotriquetral dissociation may be difficult. However, they may demonstrate associated findings of ulnar-positive variance and cystic degeneration of the ulnar one-half of the proximal surface of the lunate.

In the PA view, a step-off may be present visualising a malalignment between the lunate and triquetrum so true LT dissociation may result in a disruption of Gilula's arc I and II, with proximal translation of the triquetrum or LT overlap, or both. The scaphoid is in extension. It has an elongated and regular appearance, and the outline of the tuberosity is no longer visible. In the lateral view, the SL angle may be normal or decrease under 30°, and there is a VISI.

However, such disruptions may be seen only in motion series views. On dynamic x-rays in radial deviation, the first Gilula's arc is interrupted; in particular, it has been noted preoperatively when the ligament tear is complete. Again, comparisons with the contralateral extremity should be made. If a VISI deformity is present with LT dissociation, the radiolunate and capitolunate angles are altered.

Arthro-CT remains the examination of choice. Arthrography and MRI can demonstrate a defect in the lunotriquetral membrane suggesting triquetrolunate dissociation. Technetium-99m bone scans can help identify the site of acute injury but are less specific than arthrography. MRI technology is not yet reliable for LT ligament imaging and is limited to the same constraints as arthrography. However, MRI as scintigraphy is useful to identify problems other than the LT ligament lesions.

Arthroscopy has become the most definitive diagnostic tool for *confirming* the presence and defining the stage of LT dissociation. The arthroscopic staging is applicable to scapholunate and LT injuries.

41.35.1.3 Treatment

Treatment options for LT ligament tears cover from conservative care to surgical procedures up to LT fusion. Treatment of triquetrolunate dissociation may not be necessary if symptoms are relieved after correction of the associated conditions. The final choice of treatments is based on the pathology that is present, patient factors and the experience of the surgeon.

Above all, the treating surgeon wants to be certain that matters are not worse after treatment, so more conservative steps are probably indicated more often than not, particularly early on in the care of a patient.

Conservative management is indicated for stable, degenerative conditions of the LT ligament, the patient who presents with an end-stage VISI deformity that is secondary to a long-standing LT dissociation. It includes the use of a supportive splint, particularly when sleeping, antiinflammatory medications (systemic or injected), and activity modifications. Also, conservative treatment with cast immobilisation is indicated in acute LT injury, with no radiographic changes, in static deformities.

Surgical management is useful to improve current symptoms and to stabilise the unstable joint to prevent recurrence of symptoms. It includes arthroscopy, percutaneous K-wire fixation or screw fixation (Figure 41.40), open repair with direct suture or ligament reconstruction up to LT fusion.

The application of individual surgical techniques is dependent on the skill and experience of the surgeon and the diagnosis.

41.35.2 Midcarpal Instability

The term *midcarpal instability* MCI does not refer to one specific pathology but to a number of conditions. MCI represents an entity with a loss of normal alignment or relationship between the bones in the proximal and distal carpal rows when they are placed under physiological loads or

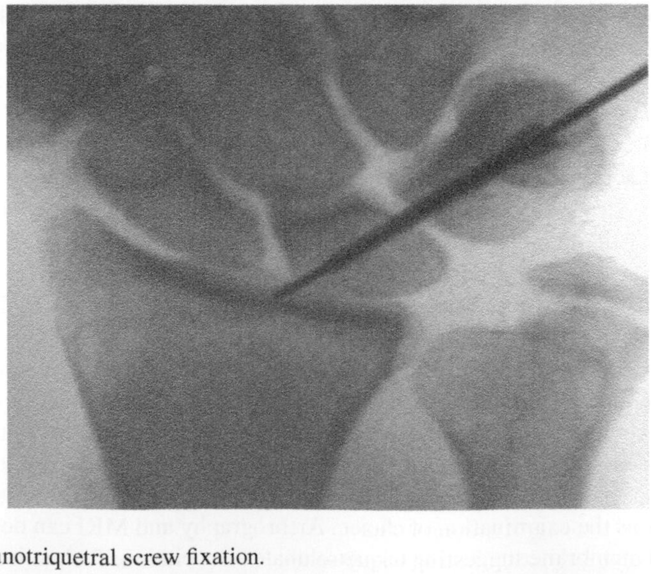

FIGURE 41.40 Lunotriquetral screw fixation.

pathological loads, due to ligamentous disruption or attenuation. Still, all these conditions present with a more or less similar alteration of the kinematics of the midcarpal joint.

41.35.2.1 Physical Examination

For many patients, especially those who are only occasionally symptomatic, understanding the problem and avoiding aggravating activities are sufficient. Some of these patients also experience hyperlaxity of other carpal joints, such as the radiocarpal joint, and MCI is only part of their problem. Patients often complain of disabling ulnar-sided wrist pain during all types of activities and in particular report a sudden painful clunk.

In midcarpal instability, diagnosis is essentially clinical. The provocative manoeuvre is performed by applying an axial load to a pronated and slightly flexed wrist, which is then brought into ulnar deviation (name catch-up clunk test). The contralateral wrist should be examined in a similar fashion because nearly 50% of patients with MCI have a non-symptomatic contralateral sign.

41.35.2.2 Imaging Studies

Because MCI is a dynamic condition, wrist arthrograms are commonly normal, not diagnostic, and of little use but may show evidence of incompetent ligaments that cross the midcarpal joint or even, occasionally, a leak in the capsule; at times they may show a mild VISI.

In the PA view, a slight palmar translation of the distal carpal row can be present with the entire first row in flexion and the ring sign present; however, the lunate is also in flexion, and its small pointed posterior horn appears at its lower border.

In the lateral projection, instead of the normal smooth translation of proximal row from flexion to extension stance a sudden snap of the proximal carpal row can be noted in ulnar deviation of the wrist. Also, the SL angle is always decreased, and VISI is present in even a severe VISI pattern. The second row is not aligned with the radius. Passive posterior drawer sign demonstrates a capitate subluxating dorsally relative to the lunate.

Abnormal alignment between the proximal and distal carpal rows can be defined by a capitolunate angle less than –30°, when the dorsal surfaces of the metacarpals and radius are parallel.

The definitive diagnosis of MCI is made by videofluoroscopy, which may demonstrate the sudden relocation of the second row under the first row correlating with the clinical clunk, and which shows a shift at the midcarpal joint during ulnar deviation of the pronated wrist, while axial compression is applied.

Arthrography is normal, or just the SL and lunotriquetral ligaments stretched. Arthro-CT shows the ligament in continuity. CT has no indication.

MRI has not yet proven useful in the evaluation of MCI.

41.35.2.3 Treatment

41.35.2.3.1 Non-Operative Treatment

Conservative therapy should be the initial treatment, as many patients respond well to non-operative management. This begins with education of the patient as to the nature of the problem, activity and job modification, and the use of non-steroidal antiinflammatory medications using also a steroid injection into the symptomatic joint. Wrist immobilisation by splinting may reduce symptoms.

By training and strengthening the hypothenar muscles and the extensor carpi ulnaris (as secondary dynamic stabilisers of the midcarpal joint), patients can learn to control their symptoms and to avoid the symptomatic clunking. If these active and passive measures fail, surgical treatment is recommended.

41.35.2.3.2 Operative Treatment

The surgical treatment of MCI is still evolving and aims to prevent the pathological motion at the midcarpal joint and to stabilise the proximal carpal row. This can be achieved by ligament reconstruction or capsular tightening, joint levelling procedures or limited midcarpal fusion.

41.35.2.3.4 DRUJ Pathology

The TFCC is one of many structures on the ulnar aspect of the wrist.

In addition to this complex, multiple structures contribute to the anatomy on the ulnar side of the wrist including the shape of the distal ulna and the carpal bones, the dorsal ligamentous complex of the wrist, the extensor carpi ulnaris and its subsheath and the ulnocarpal ligaments.

The DRUJ provides several key functions to the articulation between the forearm and hand-wrist unit and the goal in treating is to restore a pain-free, stable and a strength wrist.

TFC injury may be isolated or combined with other pathology. It should always be differentiated from degenerative changes. Acute injuries could occur by a compressive load on the ulnocarpus and forearm rotation or it could occur by repetitive-type activity, such as gripping associated with pronation and ulnar deviation and this could lead to TFC perforation and articular cartilage degeneration.

41.35.2.3.5 Physical Examination

Clinical evaluation should start with a detailed and accurate history to understand the mechanism of injury. A history of falling on the outstretched hand which causes hyperextension of the wrist or an onset of ulnar-sided wrist pain after lifting a heavy object gives a suspect of a traumatic lesion.

During the physical examination, measure the patient's wrist and forearm ranges of motion, both active and passive and compare with the opposite side. Increased AP translation of the ulna on the radius during passive manipulation is evidence of DRUJ instability. Decreased motion and crepitus during pronation/supination are signs of DRUJ arthritis, which may be accentuated by manually compressing the joint. Look for subluxation of the ECU during active supination and pronation of the forearm. Provocative manoeuvres and applied stresses can be helpful. Dynamic loading of the ulnocarpal joint by the patient can be done using the press test.

41.35.2.3.6 Imaging Studies

The most common study is plain radiographs. TFCC is composed of soft tissue and therefore cannot be seen on routine x-rays, but a variety of bony abnormalities can be evaluated, such as fractures or non-unions of the ulnar styloid and arthritic processes and evidence of carpal instability. The ulnar variance of the patient can be evaluated, and it is important to obtain a standard view.

Radiographic evaluation of the DRUJ should begin with standard PA and lateral views. A standard PA radiograph (neutral forearm rotation) is taken with the shoulder abducted 90°, the elbow flexed 90°, the forearm in neutral rotation and the wrist in neutral flexion-extension and neutral radial-ulnar deviation. This standard view allows comparison between patients and evaluation of the effects of various surgical procedures to unload the ulnocarpal articulation.

A standard lateral radiograph is taken with the shoulder at the patient's side, the elbow flexed 90° and the wrist in neutral position. An accurate view is marked by the pisiform palmar surface visualised.

Semi-supinated and semi-pronated views demonstrate the rims of the sigmoid notch and the dorsal and volar aspects of the ulnar head, and are also useful to evaluate for any fractures or arthritis.

Wrist arthrography once had an important role in assessing lesions of the TFCC but was subsequently criticised for poor clinical correlation a high incidence of perforations in asymptomatic wrists, low sensitivity compared with arthroscopy, even if some authors consider it as a useful tool for evaluating the DRUJ, especially TFCC tears, and in particular dynamic images of the arthrogram. These images can be stored on clip and studied in detail to detect subtle abnormalities and localise ligament and cartilage tears precisely.

Computed tomography (CT) scans can be useful for evaluating the DRUJ and in particular its deformity of the sigmoid notch and ulnar head related to the joint with pain and lost motion, for evaluating fractures, and degenerative arthritis.

Several measurement methods have been used to assess subtle DRUJ instability. These include the use of dorsal and palmar radioulnar lines described by Mino and associates [29], the epicentre and congruency methods proposed by Wechsler and colleagues [30] and, more recently, the radioulnar ratio described by Lo and coworkers [31].

For a complete evaluation, take three sets of scans, one each with the forearm in pronation, supination and neutral rotation and compare with the contralateral wrist to assess joint instability accurately. The scan with the forearm in pronation is most sensitive for detecting palmar subluxation, whereas the neutral image is best for detecting dorsal subluxation and DRUJ diastasis and the supination view is best for confirming the degree of reduction or subluxation of the DRUJ.

CT scans can be considered as an imaging tool for the wrist. It is an important test when evaluating the patient for DRUJ instability but its ability to image soft tissue structure is limited compared with MRI.

MRI is used to diagnose TFCC tears, but its sensitivity, specificity and accuracy vary widely among reports. There is no doubt that this structure can be visualised, but its accuracy is different, and according to some authors, MRI has a sensitivity of 100% and accuracy of 97% when evaluating the TFCC [32], while for others MRI has only 73% accuracy [33].

Similar to CT, MRI can be used to make anatomic measurements to assess instability.

MRI has seen an increase in use for the investigation of TFC pathology.

Degenerative defects are more common than traumatic defects. Either type of lesion may result in full-thickness defects of the TFCC, and these can be visualised on MRI exam or at MRI arthrography. Radial tears of the TFC appear as a linear band of increased signal intensity on short TR/TE and proton density-weighted spin echo (SE) or gradient echo (GRE) images. With complete tears the signal extends to proximal and distal articular surfaces. The signal will increase on long TR/TE images SE images, or T2-weighted GRE images or T2-weighted FSE sequences with fat suppression, consistent with synovial fluid trapped in the defect. There are no specific differentiating features on MRI exam separating a traumatically induced tear of the TFCC from one caused by degeneration.

Scintigraphy has a limited role in assessing the DRUJ but may be useful when the diagnosis is in question or other concurrent problems are suspected; a chronic inflammation in the bone and soft tissues show an increased uptake.

Arthroscopy allows a direct view of the anatomic elements of intraarticular structures and by palpation, using a probe, permit to detect the amount of tension on the TFCC; this is called 'trampolining effect'. In particular, gives some information regarding intraarticular soft tissues, chondral wear and synovitis, location and dimensions of ligamentous injuries, partial ligamentous injuries that at present cannot be shown even with the most sophisticated imaging equipment.

41.35.2.3.7 Treatment

Ulnar-sided tears should be differentiated from central ones because of the different therapeutic strategies. Peripheral tears have a good vascular supply and are thus repaired, whereas central lesions are avascular and are treated with debridement.

Treatment options chosen for individual patients should be based on an understanding of the underlying pathology and specific pathoanatomic disorders.

Recent advances have greatly expanded our knowledge of this portion of the wrist. Treatment options have also multiplied.

The advent of wrist arthroscopy has been an impetus in this direction. At present, debridement, surgical repair and a variety of mechanical unloading procedures have been devised to deal with this problem.

A trial of non-operative management is helpful and is warranted for patients with minor disorders of the DRUJ like strains of the radioulnar or other ulnar-sided wrist ligaments, tendonitis of the ECU, may respond to rest, ice after activity, oral antiinflammatory medications, splints or a steroid injection.

Surgical treatment of TFCC lesions is most commonly based on the classification of Palmer.

In type 1A lesions, TFCC should be treated by arthroscopic debridement, while in type 1B, 1C and 1D injuries it should be repaired either arthroscopically or by an open procedure with an anchor. In type 2, perforations represent a degenerative process, so these lesions should be treated conservatively. In type 2C, TFCC can be treated by a wafer procedure. In type 2D, TFCC lesions should be treated depending on the amount of lunotriquetral instability: a wafer procedure can be performed, if there is no instability of the carpal bones; an ulnar shortening is the main choice in a mild diastasis. In type 2E, distal ulnar resection and Sauve–Kapandji are two of the limited options available.

41.36 OSTEOARTHRITIS

41.36.1 Arthritis of the Hand and Wrist

41.36.1.1 Introduction

Osteoarthritis is a slowly progressive polyarticular disorder of unknown cause, predominantly affecting the hands. It is considered as a universal problem of humans, and women are more often affected than men of the same age. It is a condition that is characterised by articular cartilage deterioration. Involvement in the hand is seen most commonly at the thumb carpometacarpal joint and at the interphalangeal (IP) joints, and at the wrist joint as a post-traumatic condition.

41.36.1.2 Imaging Studies

Plain radiographs are generally all that is needed to confirm the diagnosis of an osteoarthritic joint. Dedicated, true, orthogonal PA, lateral and oblique views are required to accurately evaluate the joint line. For the evaluation of the hand joints, magnified views are helpful to identify subtle abnormalities.

Asymmetric joint space narrowing with articular cartilage space loss is evident on radiographic examination as the earliest radiographic finding, followed by marginal osteophyte formation (Figure 41.41). Focal erosions, subchondral sclerosis, cyst formation and peripheral joint osteophytes are the hallmark findings of advanced OA at the DIPJ and the PIPJ.

41.36.1.3 Physical Examination

Clinically, osteoarthritis is characterised by joint pain, limitation of motion, joint enlargement, swelling, stiffness, contracture and angular deformity, which interfere with function of the digit or hand, making pinch and grip activities difficult.

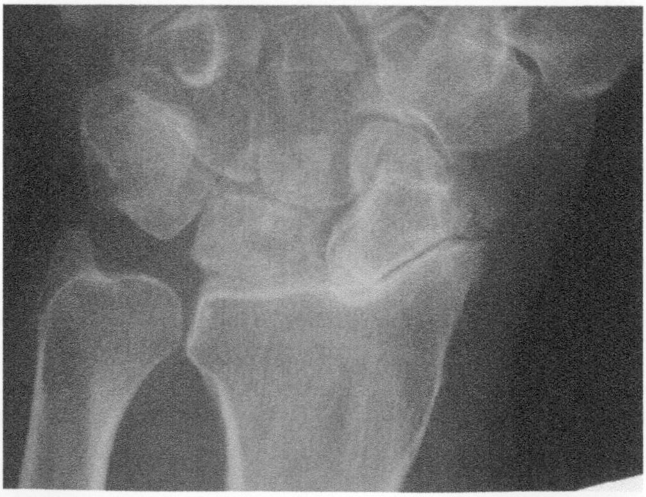

FIGURE 41.41 Radioscaphoid arthritis in SLAC wrist.

In some cases, however, cosmetic concerns may be the sole reason that a patient presents to the surgeon's office. Heberdens's nodes and Bouchard's nodes are noted at the DIPJ and the PIPJ, respectively. Angular deformity can range from minimal to quite dramatic. Large mucous cysts that are adjacent to the joint can cause longitudinal grooving of the nail plate. Similarly, the PIPJ usually shows some sign of enlargement. Palpation of the joint line at the PIPJ or DIPJ elicits tenderness and may demonstrate an effusion. Degrees of instability could be demonstrated during radial and ulnar deviation stress.

41.36.2 Treatment

41.36.2.1 Non-Operative Treatment

Because there is currently no medical therapy for the underlying disease process in OA, treatment is symptomatic only. Consequently, patient education is crucial.

Non-operative therapy is the cornerstone of treatment. The primary goal of non-operative treatment is pain relief. Symptomatic treatment includes controlling exposure to provocative activities that produce pain, swelling and stiffness. This includes modification of work and leisure activities, hand therapy to instruct patients on joint protection techniques, techniques for oedema control and the use of adaptive devices, splinting to immobilise a tender joint during a flare-up, to provide rest at night or after activities, or to provide support and protection during activities, medical treatment with analgesic or intraarticular steroid injections.

41.36.2.2 Operative Treatment

41.36.2.2.1 DIP, PIP, and MP Joint

The primary indication for surgery is pain unresponsive to oral medication and splinting. Distal interphalangeal joint arthrodesis relieves pain, corrects deformity, and resolves joint instability. Because the severely arthritic distal interphalangeal joint is often stiff, the additional loss of motion occasioned by arthrodesis is usually well tolerated. At the proximal interphalangeal joint, pain is the primary indication for surgery. Implant arthroplasty may be helpful in relieving pain and retaining motion in the ring and little fingers. The motion attained from implant arthroplasty is less in the proximal interphalangeal joints than in the metacarpophalangeal joints. Implant arthroplasty is usually avoided in the index finger or middle finger proximal interphalangeal joint because of residual instability to lateral or key pinch.

Fusion relieves pain at the proximal interphalangeal joint and provides pinch stability.

41.36.2.2.2 TM Joint

41.36.2.2.2.1 Imaging Studies Standard x-rays of the thumb CMC joint include PA 30° oblique stress view (Figure 41.42), pronated AP (Robert view), oblique and true lateral views. These show all four trapezial facets. The oblique and lateral x-rays show the severity of CMC disease and the palmar beak. Osteoarthritis may be confined to the TM joint or it may involve the pantrapezial joint complex. Indeed, the staging system originated by Eaton and Littler, who have proposed the pathological changes observed on x-ray, described four stages. In stage 1, x-rays show a normal joint with the exception of possible widening from synovitis; in stage 2, joint space is narrowing with debris and osteophytes less than 2 mm. Stage 3 has a joint space narrowing with debris and osteophytes greater than 2 mm in size. In stage 4, scaphotrapezial joint space involvement in addition to narrowing of the TM joint (Figure 41.43).

Although x-ray studies are helpful in staging the patient's disease, treatment of the patient is dependent on the patient's signs and symptoms.

Sometimes for a better visualisation of the space between the base of the first and second metacarpal bone, some authors suggest a CT scan; in fact, it helps to visualise some osteophytes placed in that space.

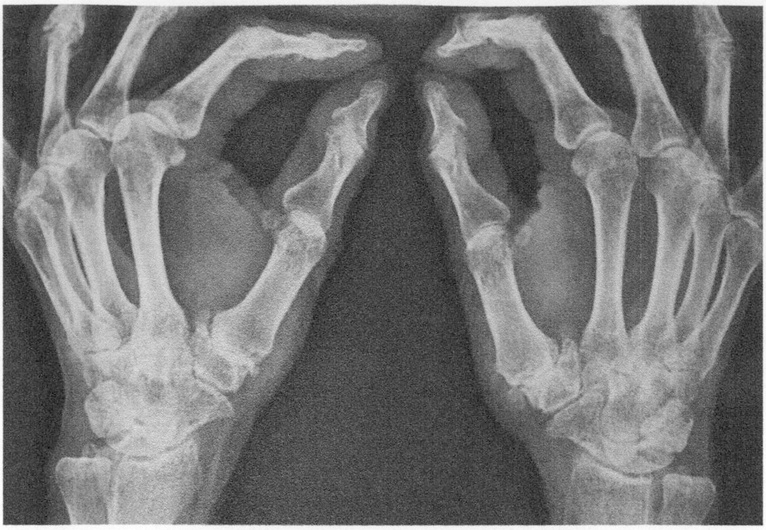

FIGURE 41.42 Comparative posteroanterior oblique stress view.

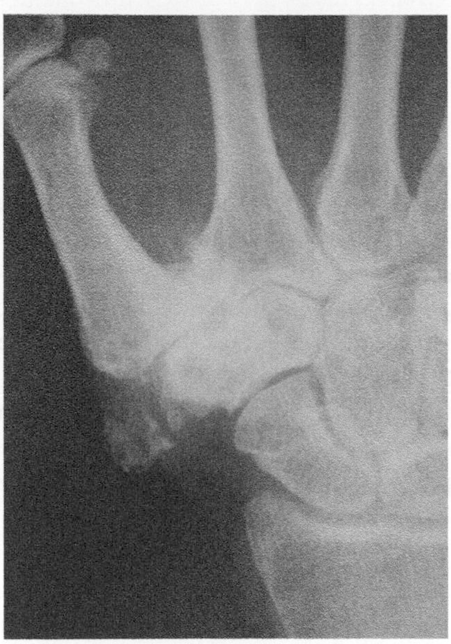

FIGURE 41.43 Stage 4th: thumb CMC joint arthritis.

41.36.2.2.2.2 Non-Operative Treatment At the trapeziometacarpal joint, conservative treatment includes a hand-based thumb splint with the interphalangeal joint left free, antiinflammatory medication, intraarticular corticosteroid injection and thenar muscle isometric conditioning.

All these measures may provide temporary pain relief.

41.36.2.2.2.3 Operative Treatment Indications for surgical intervention of basal joint disease of the thumb include pain, deformity, and/or weakness that interfere with daily function and are unresponsive to non-operative measures.

The primary indication for surgery is persistent pain.

According to Eaton x-ray classification, in stage 1 disease a hemi-trapeziectomy is the first choice. TM fusion, or implant arthroplasty, is indicated in stages 2 and 3 while in case of a pantrapezial arthritis (stage 4 disease) a trapezium complete excision with or without ligament reconstruction and with or without a tendon interposition using either the flexor carpi radialis or portion of the abductor pollicis longus placed in the articular surface of the thumb metacarpal surface.

Obviously, pantrapezial involvement contraindicates procedures such as TM arthrodesis or hemitrapeziectomy alone.

After surgery, the thumb is immobilised in a cast for 2 weeks followed by a removable thumb splint for 2–4 weeks. Arthrodesis of the thumb carpometacarpal joint is an alternative to trapeziectomy and suspension sling arthroplasty.

41.36.2.2.3 Wrist Joint

Osteoarthritis of the wrist is a common malady that is seen in multiple age groups. Rheumatoid arthritis of the wrist is far less common. In cases of severe arthritic damage to the radiocarpal or midcarpal joint where reconstructive procedures are excluded, salvage procedures are required. If the degenerative changes affected carpus and radiocarpal joint, the treatment choice is generally fusion of the entire wrist or total wrist arthroplasty.

In some patients, the osteoarthritis only affects a few of the intercarpal wrist joints or a portion of the radiocarpal joint, so in these cases, partial fusion of the wrist can provide a pain-free, stable wrist and preserve some motion. The principle of this treatment strategy consists of eliminating the destroyed articular surfaces by partial wrist fusion, in which are fused only the damaged or unstable articular surfaces while motion is maintained in the uninjured or stable regions of the joints. The benefit of limited wrist fusion is well documented.

41.36.2.2.4 Clinical Evaluation

It is always important to obtain a full history at the start of any evaluation. Patients with advanced wrist arthritis typically present with measurable limitation of motion and function. Local tenderness and specific abnormal motion are revealed by clinical examination. Pain is variable and is usually aggravated by loading activities. The passive and active ranges of motion should be recorded. Soft tissue swelling on the dorsoradial aspect of the wrist is not uncommon. Sometimes, extensor or flexor lags should be noted as possible signs of tendon rupture.

The DRUJ may also be affected; if symptomatic, and so clinical features are associated to other clinical signs and symptoms localised to other wrist regions.

41.36.2.2.5 Imaging Studies

Plain radiographs are necessary to confirm the diagnosis of wrist osteoarthritis (Figure 41.44). Imaging studies should be standardised within a clinic. A baseline study should consist of PA and lateral radiographs in the neutral position, and OA is diagnosed by joint narrowing, subchondral bone sclerosis, osteophytes, geodes and loose bodies. Additional views may occasionally add useful information.

Sclerosis and joint space narrowing are easily identified in advanced cases, but simple articular cartilage loss is better visualised by a CT scan.

Coronal and transverse CT, arthro-CT and MRI may be helpful to assess DRUJ and to evaluate the cartilage at the radioulnar joint or in case of ulna abutment syndrome. MRI shows the disease progression while CT depicts the magnitude of bone involvement.

41.36.2.3 Post-Traumatic Carpal Osteoarthritis

41.36.2.3.1 Scapholunate Advanced Collapse

Scapholunate advanced collapse (SLAC) refers to a specific pattern of osteoarthritis and subluxation which most commonly results from untreated chronic scapholunate dissociation (scapholunate

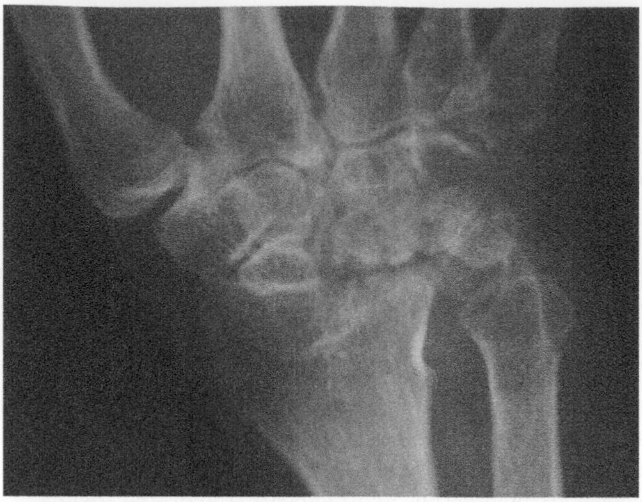

FIGURE 41.44 Wrist arthritis.

ligament injury). Degenerative changes occur most often in areas of abnormal loading usually at radial-scaphoid joint, followed by degeneration in the unstable lunocapitate joint, as capitate subluxates dorsally on lunate.

In plain x-rays, progression of OA is well demonstrated. The first joint which develops degenerative changes is the radioscaphoid joint. Capitolunate and STT joints follow in order degenerative changes and capitate migrates proximally into space created by scapholunate dissociation. Radiolunate joint is usually spared because of concentric articulation of lunate in lunate fossa. In the end stage, SLAC midcarpal joint collapses under compression and lunate assuming an extended or dorsiflexed position called DISI deformity.

PA view and arthro-CT demonstrate stages of collapse. Stage 1 shows a radiostyloid arthritis alone with modification of radial styloid. In stage 2, the radioscaphoid joint is completely narrowed with complete cartilage defect. Stage 3 shows involved degeneration of the lunocapitate joint.

The proximal migration of the capitate decreases the carpal height.

In the lateral view, it is possible to observe an increase in SL angle and capitolunate angles and DISI deformity is constant. CT does demonstrate only indirect signs.

41.36.2.3.2 Scaphoid Non-Union Advanced Collapse

In scaphoid non-union advanced collapse (SNAC), progression of OA is slightly different from SLAC and is assessed by plain x-rays and more precisely by arthro-CT.

Long-standing scaphoid non-union leads to a pattern of arthritis. It is described in a four-stage progression. Stage 1 shows arthritis and osteophyte formation at radial styloid (Figure 41.45). In stage 2, patients have arthritis at the radioscaphoid joint. In stage 3, patients have arthritis at the capitolunate and scaphocapitate joints. In stage 4, patients have arthritis involving all the radiolunate joints. This progression is described as SNAC wrist.

Diagnosis is evident on plain x-rays. It is characterised by radioscaphoid joint narrowing, sclerosis, osteophytes, cysts, scapholunate dislocation and carpal collapse. SLAC progression is faster than that of SNAC because lunate ulnar shift is more important in SLAC.

41.36.2.3.3 Conservative Treatment

Conservative treatment measures splintage of the wrist, antiinflammatory drugs, intraarticular cortisone injections or hyaluronic acid injections and modification of daily activity. Once advanced carpal degeneration is present, the wrist can be treated only by salvage procedures.

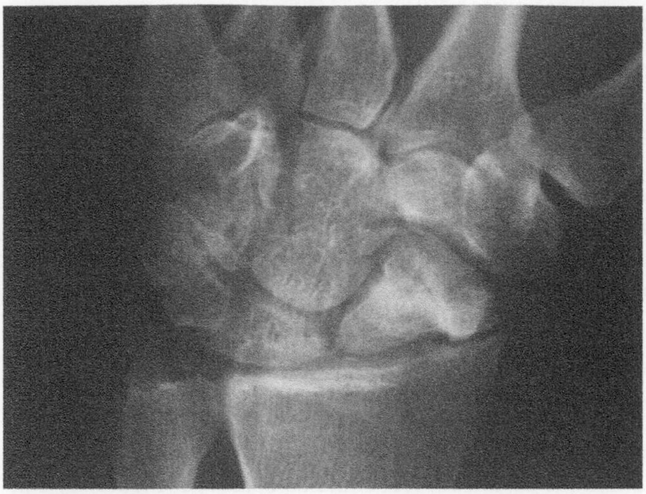

FIGURE 41.45 SNAC stage 1.

41.36.2.3.4 Operative Treatment

In case of radioscaphoid arthritis according to the amount of cartilage degeneration, different options could be chosen. From a styloid excision alone, or a radioscapholunate fusion, or scaphoid excision combined with four corner fusion, capitolunate fusion, proximal row carpectomy or midcarpal tenodesis. With the arthritis extended to the scaphocapitate joint, a scaphocapitate fusion or scaphoid excision and midcarpal fusion are necessary, or a proximal row carpectomy with a replacement capitates prosthesis or with a dorsal capsular flap interposition are described. The use of arthroscopy may help determine the best operative approach in these patients. With a radioscaphocapitate arthritis plus lunocapitate arthritis, a scaphoid excision and midcarpal fusion or a total wrist fusion is required to obtain a stable, painless wrist.

41.37 AVASCULAR NECROSIS AT THE CARPUS

Lunate and scaphoid are the two bones of the carpus mainly involved in avascular necrosis.

41.37.1 Kienböck's Disease

The aetiology of Kienböck's disease is still unknown. From multiple, repetitive microtrauma to a negative ulnar variance for developing a lunate fracture, it is likely that multiple factors contribute to the necrosis of the lunate. These factors are grouped into extrinsic and intrinsic factors.

Extrinsic factors includes an ulnar-minus variance that increases the load stresses acting on the lunate due to the differential hardness of the lunate fossa of the radius and the triangular fibrocartilage or the morphology of the distal radius in which the slope may be slightly more horizontal in Kienböck's patients than in the normal population [34,35] or traumas with an acute lunate fracture, and the subsequent development of Kienböck's disease in some cases is possible. Also, activities with use of vibrating tools may cause a direct vascular or trabecular fatigue fractures or a ligament instability.

Intrinsic factors include the shape of the lunate bone about the relationship between trabecular than cortical support, so the lunate is more at risk for microfractures of the trabeculae, arterial blood flow interruption such as in acute traumatic disruption at the time of ligament disruption and lunate fracture or in patients with inflammatory conditions or vasculopathy. Also, an association between Kienböck's disease and the use of oral steroids has also been reported.

41.37.2 History and Clinical Evaluation

Lunatomalacia is more common in men than in women and affecting mostly individuals in young adulthood at the level of dominant wrist. Bilateral occurrence has been reported in adolescents.

Symptoms developed first before imaging presentation sometimes with a history of trauma. Symptoms include limitation of motion in particular affecting extension more than flexion but usually in all directions, and a weakness, sometimes extensor tendon rupture, or symptoms of carpal tunnel syndrome or dorsal wrist pain, have also been reported. Patients may also note dorsal wrist swelling. Grip strength is diminished substantially in the involved wrist. Palpation demonstrates tenderness overlying the dorsal aspect of the lunate, and pain is accentuated by passive motion and by strength testing.

41.37.3 Imaging Studies

Radiographs may appear normal in the early stages of the disease, except for the ulnar-minus variant. Typical x-rays in the advance stages could be observed (Figure 41.46).

PA radiographs should be made with the shoulder abducted, elbow flexed 90°, forearm in neutral rotation and wrist in neutral flexion-extension. Lateral radiographs are made in the neutral position. In case of negative x-ray evaluation and persistent clinical features and suspect of lunatomalacia, other further evaluations are required such as MRI, CT scan or bone scan.

MRI is extremely well suited for detection of early phases of AVN. This investigation permits the diagnosis before collapse of the carpal bones and demonstrates a substantial decrease in the signal intensity on T1-weighted, T2-weighted and fat-suppressed images of the entire lunate (Figures 41.47 and 41.48). It may be used to demonstrate adequacy of treatment, either by demonstrable lack of improvement or with evidence of revascularisation. In addition to gadolinium enhancement, it allows a more accurate assessment of bone marrow vascularity, improving diagnostic accuracy and therapeutic responses. Care must be taken when interpreting MRI of the lunate; some subchondral inflammatory changes and oedema associated with ulnolunate impaction have similar signal changes to those seen in lunatomalacia, but in these cases the changes are limited to the ulnar side of the lunate.

Conventional tomography and CT are useful for structural changes including sclerosis, compression and fractures of the lunate, fracture patterns and displacement, and the amount of collapse in the lunate.

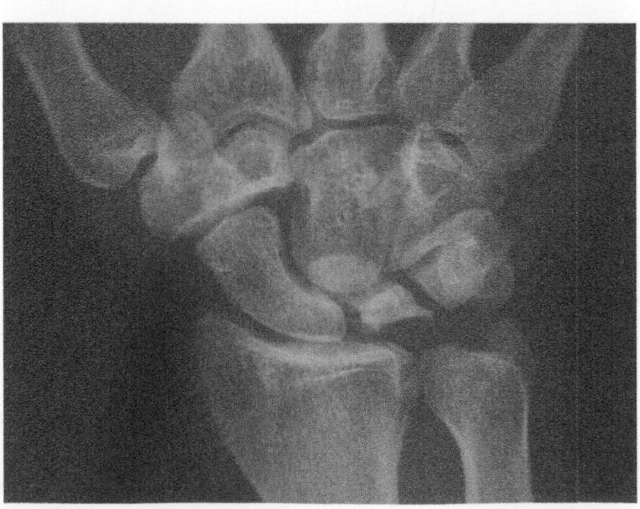

FIGURE 41.46 Kienböck's disease: x-ray evaluation.

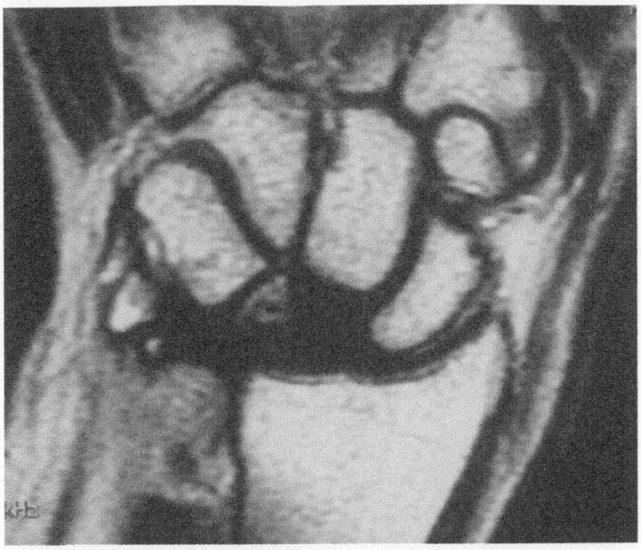

FIGURE 41.47 Kienböck's disease: MRI evaluation.

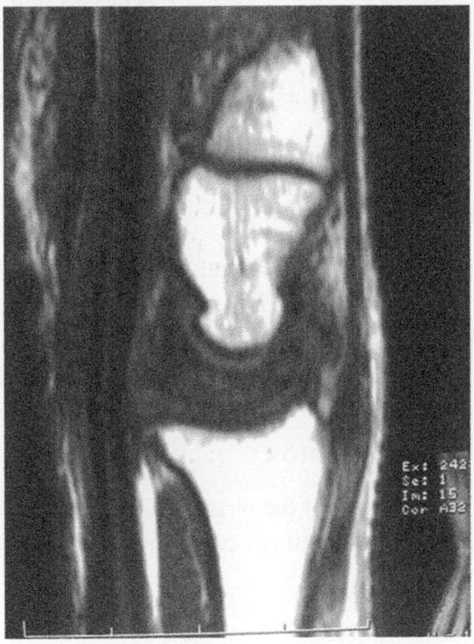

FIGURE 41.48 Kienböck's disease: MRI evaluation. Sagittal plane.

Bone scintigraphy may also show abnormally high uptake by the lunate in early Kienböck's disease. The use of a three-phase bone scan may provide some useful prognostic information about arterial and venous blood flow to the region of the lunate. Although scintigraphic findings may be non-specific or non-diagnostic of lunate AVN, because it is an important diagnostic tool with a high sensitivity but low specificity for carpal pathology.

Arthroscopic examination can provide very accurate information to radiocarpal and midcarpal joints, allowing an accurate assessment of the status of articular surfaces and the integrity of the scapholunate and lunotriquetral interosseous ligaments. Also, chondral fractures or defects may be identified before committing to a particular course of treatment. It is also a useful staging tool for Kienböck's disease and can be used to guide patient management.

41.37.4 Treatment

There are many treatment options for Kienböck's disease, from observation to complex surgical reconstruction, and it is based, at least in part, on radiographic staging, taking into account other clinical, radiographic, arthroscopic or surgical findings.

41.37.4.1 Conservative Treatment

Treatment of AVN with prolonged immobilisation by casting is the treatment of choice for Kienböck's disease. It is based on the principle of diminishing the forces responsible for the usual progression of lunatomalacia from ischaemia to collapse and arthrosis and to allow reconstitution of the lunate.

At present, immobilisation is the primarily choice in stage 1 disease, when spontaneous revascularisation may possible and allows the lunate to heal. Antiinflammatory drugs can be associated. If pain persists, efficient treatment must be based on surgical methods.

41.37.4.2 Surgical Treatment

Three different categories of surgical treatment can be identified: lunate unloading, lunate revascularisation and salvage options.

The unloading methods described include temporary use of external fixators or midcarpal distraction pinning, radial shortening, ulnar lengthening, angular or wedge osteotomies of the radius, capitate shortening and intercarpal arthrodesis such as scaphocapitate fusion or capitate-hamate fusion.

Revascularisation procedures consist in arteriovenous pedicle implantation or various vascularised bone grafts.

Salvage options include total wrist arthrodesis, proximal row carpectomy, proximal row fusion, total wrist arthroplasty and lunate arthroplasty. Also, a combination of these procedures is frequently used.

41.38 PREISER'S DISEASE

The Preiser's disease is a clear, progressive, clinical and radiographic sequence of osteosclerosis and subsequent fragmentation of the scaphoid. The pathogenesis of total scaphoid necrosis remains unclear. Unlike Kienböck's disease, there is no association with mechanical factors such as ulnar variance, although repetitive trauma has been suggested as a possible cause in some cases.

41.38.1 History and Clinical Evaluation

Clinical features include pain and stiffness of the wrist and swelling over the dorsoradial aspect of the wrist due to reactive synovitis. Diagnosis requires confirmation by x-ray and other imaging studies.

41.38.2 Imaging Studies

X-ray imaging of Preiser's disease demonstrates changes in the scaphoid. Initial mixed sclerotic and cystic changes are associated with collapse of the bone. The entire bone is involved in the process.

As in other bones with AVN, early diagnosis depends on MRI and bone scan.

AVN of the scaphoid are divided into four stages: in stage 1, x-rays are normal, but bone scan changes similar to Kienböck's disease are present; in stage 2, an increased density or generalised osteoporosis is present; in stage III, a fragmentation of the scaphoid is present; and in stage IV, a carpal collapse is evident.

41.38.3 Conservative Treatment

Rest, splintage or casting, and other conservative measures generally have no effect on the progressive collapse of the bone, and may be sufficient to reduce symptoms in some patients.

41.38.4 Operative Treatment

Early operation in an effort to salvage the scaphoid and reverse avascular changes has seldom been reported. The use of radial styloidectomy or arthroscopic debridement has also been reported to be successful in this condition.

Most authors have suggested salvage procedures including proximal row carpectomy, four-corner fusion with scaphoid resection or complete wrist arthrodesis and wrist denervation.

41.39 HAND TUMOURS

41.39.1 Soft Tissue Tumours

Usually all mass lesions in the hand or wrist are benign conditions. Foreign body granulomas, epidermoid inclusion cysts and neuromas are usually related to prior trauma. Ganglions and fibroxanthomas arise adjacent to joints or tendon sheaths.

41.39.1.1 Ganglion

Ganglions are the most common soft tissue mass of the hand and, as such, have inspired debate about their aetiology and treatment. Even within the hand, a ganglion can present in multiple sites, including the dorsal and volar wrist, the volar retinacular sheath, mucous cysts and intraosseous ganglions.

They are cystic structures filled with a mucinous fluid but without a synovial or epithelial lining. In most cases, a stalk can be identified communicating between the cyst and an adjacent joint or tendon sheath.

Ganglions are commonly located near joints and tendon sheaths and may be related to trauma.

Early theories of ganglion formation can be divided into neoplasms, myxoid degeneration or synovial herniations. Theories described ganglions as degenerated connective tissue with subsequent formation of cystic spaces or degenerative tissues that underwent liquefaction, or related to the joint capsule or distensions of bursae possibly related to trauma, or as a result of a one-way valve, with communication between the joint space and the main cyst, or more recent studies have focused on the relationship of the ganglions to the wrist ligaments.

41.39.1.2 Dorsal Wrist Ganglion

Dorsal wrist ganglions arise from the dorsal capsule of the scapholunate joint. Small dorsal ganglions may be barely palpable but highly symptomatic, whereas large ganglions are often soft and only mildly symptomatic.

Patients complain of pain with direct pressure or for impingement on the terminal branches of the posterior interosseus nerve, stiffness or weakness which may be attributed to interference with normal extensor tendon gliding. Also, ganglion size gets larger with activity and smaller with rest.

41.39.1.3 Imaging Studies

Plain radiographs of the involved region are often unremarkable, but sometimes can identify the presence of an intraosseous ganglion and any carpal pathology present at the wrist. Osteoarthritic changes are commonly seen with cysts at the DIP or carpometacarpal joints.

Arthrograms can demonstrate a communication between the wrist joint and the cyst.

MRI may confirm the cystic nature of the ganglion and to delineate the extent of the ganglion and any underlying ligamentous pathology. MR characteristics are those of most cysts, low-signal intensity at T1-weighted imaging and high-signal intensity at T2-weighted imaging. Peripheral enhancement following gadolinium administration is typical.

Ultrasound is maybe the prior examination to use in the study of a suspected ganglion cyst. It shows an anaecogen signal with a pedicle originating from the articular capsula. MRI and U/S are equally sensitive in the detection of wrist ganglions.

41.39.1.4 Differential Diagnosis

The differential diagnosis includes carpometacarpal boss, extensor tenosynovitis or lipoma. Also in a wrist pain with a non-evident ganglion cyst, differential diagnosis should be differentiated from carpal instability, carpal avascular necrosis, capsulitis and posterior interosseous nerve syndrome.

41.39.1.5 Treatment

Aspiration and steroid injection may provide transient symptomatic relief, but recurrence is frequent. Symptomatic lesions can be surgically excised taking care to preserve the ligament or a scapholunate dissociation may occur.

41.39.1.6 Palmar Wrist Ganglion

Second to dorsal wrist ganglions in frequency, volar wrist ganglions comprise 13%–20% of all ganglions. They may be located at radial-sided volarly at the level of the scaphoid tubercle or between the flexor carpi radialis and the radial artery. The most common sites of origin are the scaphotrapezoid or the radioscaphoid joints. Ulnarly ganglions arise from the pisotriquetral joint adjacent to the flexor carpi ulnaris tendon.

Patients complain of a cosmetic deformity, a wrist mass or pain and numbness. Palmar wrist ganglions present as swellings on the palmar radial aspect of the wrist.

An ultrasound may be helpful for diagnosis. An MRI can be obtained to define the nature and extent of the ganglion and also helps with preoperative planning if surgical excision is anticipated.

Differential diagnosis includes vascular lesions, venous or arterial aneurysms and other types of tumours, such as lipomas or a giant cell tumour of the tendon sheath.

41.39.1.7 Treatment

Aspiration and steroid injection may provide transient symptomatic relief, but recurrence is frequent. Symptomatic lesions can be surgically excised taking care to preserve the ligament or a scapholunate dissociation may occur.

41.39.1.8 Flexor Sheath Ganglion

Flexor sheath ganglions present as firm mass lesions over the palmar aspect of the flexor sheath and is sonographically anaecogen (Figure 41.49). Sometimes, MRI could be helpful for a better location and an adequate surgical approach. Treatment of symptomatic lesions is accomplished with aspiration or excision.

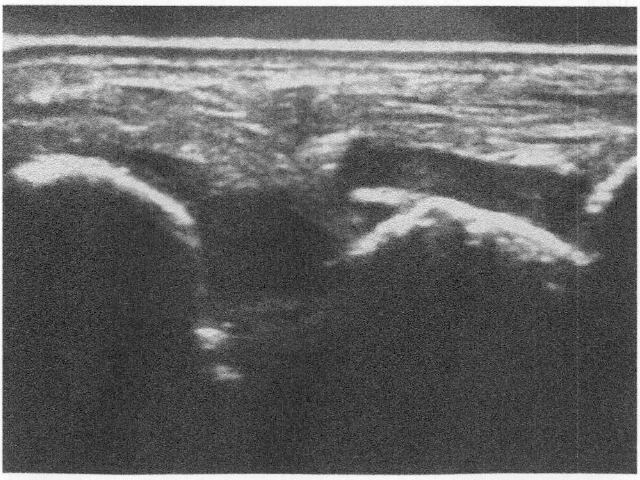

FIGURE 41.49 Sonography in flexor sheath ganglion.

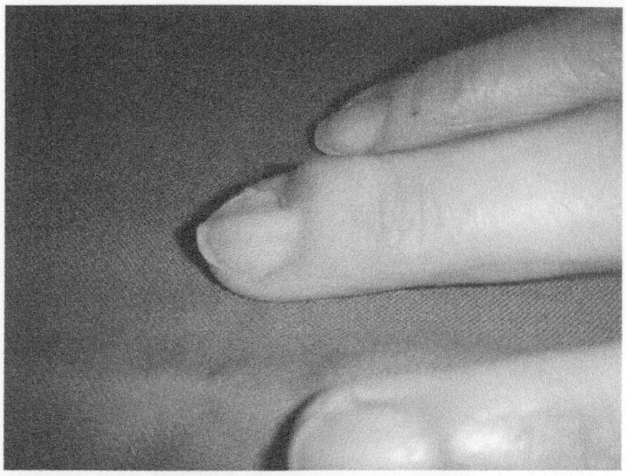

FIGURE 41.50 Clinical evidence of a mucous cyst.

41.39.1.9 Mucous Cyst

Mucous cysts are ganglions arising from the distal interphalangeal joint. The neck of the ganglion arises either radially or ulnarly to the extensor terminal tendon. Their precise aetiology is unclear and theories including synovial herniation, extensor retinacular metaplasia and myxomatous degeneration. They are cystic, smooth, translucent masses with viscous fluid (Figure 41.50).

Treatment options in the past have included aspiration, electrocautery, chemical cautery and various types of surgical excisions. Multiple incisions have been described, including H, T and U shapes or a transverse curving shape and an excision with debridement of the joint osteophyte is indicated. In the event of significant DIP joint arthritis and pain, a fusion can be performed. The patient should consent, if the skin is thinned, for a skin graft or a local flap coverage if the extensor tendon or joint is exposed.

Recent studies have shown the necessity of excision of not only the cyst but also the underlying DIP osteophyte.

41.39.1.10 Fibroxanthoma

Also known as giant cell tumours of tendon sheath or tendon sheath xanthomas, or localised nodular pigmented tenosynovitis, is the second most common soft tissue tumour of the hand and wrist. Most often involve the volar aspect of the digits, usually, the first, second and third fingers. Typically involved young patients or middle-aged adults. These lesions are usually painless, and the mass has a slowly growing and are usually fixed to deep tissues often on the palmar aspect of the hand or finger.

Conventional radiographs show the mass, which may uncommonly produce periosteal reaction, demonstrate calcification and erode adjacent bone.

A preoperatory ultrasound study or an MRI in case of a complex region (such as in the palm or in the first web space) is recommended.

MR shows a mass adjacent to a tendon. Signal characteristics reflect the degree of histiocytes, giant cells, fibrous stroma with hemosiderin and lipid-laden macrophages. Low-signal intensity is typical at T1-weighted imaging with low to mixed signal intensity at T2-weighted imaging. Hemosiderin is responsible for the low-signal intensity areas often seen on all pulse sequences.

Surgical resection requires delineation of adjacent nerves that may be displaced, compressed or encircled by a fibroxanthoma.

41.39.1.11 Foreign Bodies

Foreign bodies may act as a nidus, inciting the development of a surrounding granuloma. This may be associated with a local inflammatory reaction (Figure 41.51) or frank infection. Treatment consists of excision.

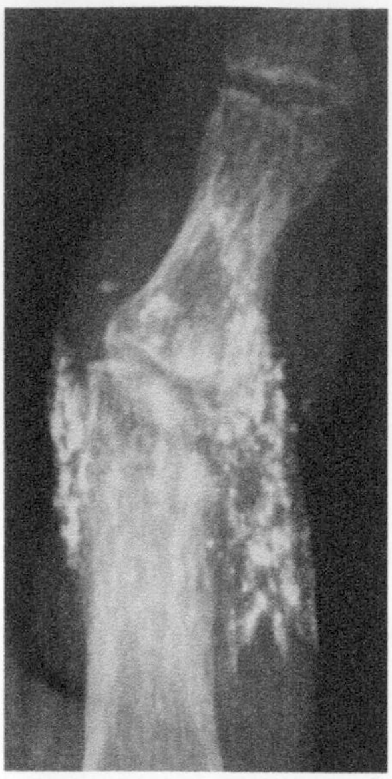

FIGURE 41.51 X-ray evidence of an infiltration of soft tissue by lead.

41.39.1.12 Glomus Tumour

Glomus tumours are benign hamartomas arising at the neuromyoarterial glomus and are concentrated at the tips of the digits. They are painful, tender and often sensitive to cold.

MRI has recently detected such lesions: they are isointense or slightly hyperintense to the dermal layer of the nail bed at T1-weighted imaging and strongly hyperintense at T2-weighted imaging (Figures 41.52 and 41.53). Most enhance following gadolinium administration, often heterogeneously. Bone erosion is common.

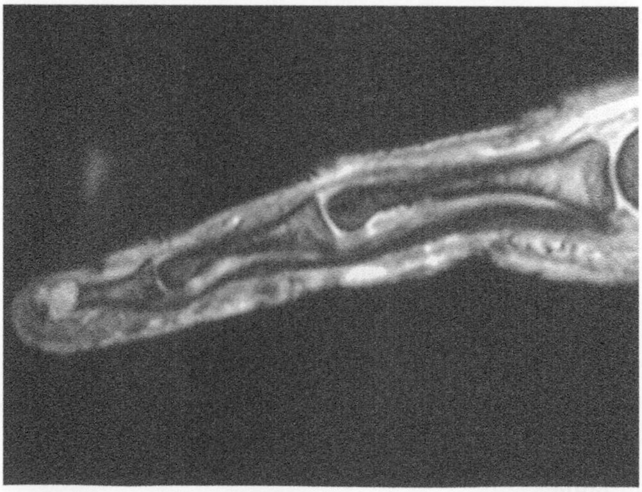

FIGURE 41.52 MRI evaluation of a glomus tumour.

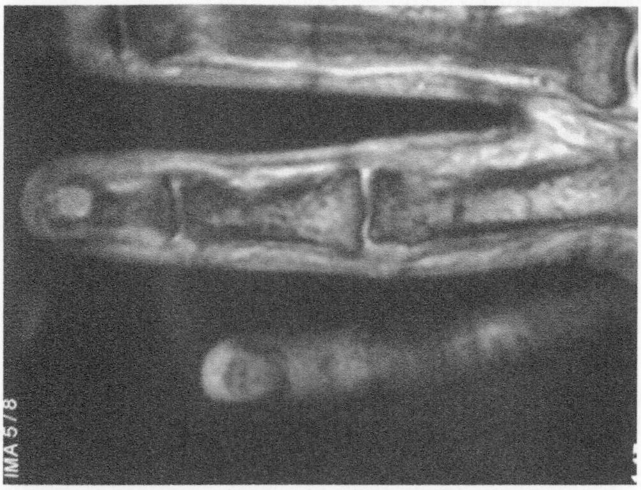

FIGURE 41.53 MRI evaluation of a glomus tumour.

41.40 SARCOMAS

41.40.1 Soft Tissue Sarcoma

Hand sarcomas are exceedingly rare, life-threatening diseases that must be managed according to oncologic principles; they encompass a wide range of tumour types. These originate from the mesenchyme and involve muscle, fat, nerve, vessels, synovium, joint capsule and tendons. Soft tissue sarcomas encompass diverse cell types, some of which have normal correlates. Examples include liposarcoma, which resembles fat, and rhabdomyosarcoma, which resembles muscle.

Approximately 75% of patients are treated with surgical resection and, in some cases, radiation therapy and chemotherapy, and 25% ultimately succumb to metastatic disease.

The main surgical principles are to not cause undue contamination at the time of biopsy or unplanned resection and to obtain a wide surgical margin at the time of definitive resection.

41.40.1.1 Imaging Studies

The role of MRI for detection of soft tissue sarcomas of the extremity has been well established. The ideal imaging modality for masses suspected to be sarcoma is MRI. MRI does a greater spatial resolution and superior contrast resolution versus CT scan, while CT scan remains a better method in assessing calcification and ossification.

MRI can define the local extent of the tumour and help in preoperative planning.

Gadolinium contrast can be helpful in postoperative studies in trying to distinguish scar from recurrent tumour.

Before excising a mass without a pathological diagnosis, a biopsy should be performed. Much depends on where the mass is anatomically located. For large masses, deep masses or clinically suspicious masses, MRI should be performed before excision or biopsy. MRI can be used to diagnose an intramuscular lipoma.

Small, subcutaneous, discrete lesions are homogeneous with low-signal intensity at T1-weighted imaging and high-signal intensity at T2-weighted imaging. Large, deep, infiltrative lesions may appear more heterogeneous.

41.41 BONE TUMOURS

Primary bone tumours are unusual, accounting for only a small portion of all neoplasms. The number of bone tumours and tumour-like lesions, unique to the upper extremity, are fewer in number than the soft tissue lesions described. Most bony lesions encountered at the upper extremity occur as frequently or perhaps more frequently at the lower extremity or axial skeleton.

Benign bone neoplasms are encountered with greater frequency.

41.41.1 Benign Bone Tumours

The majority of all primary bone tumours of the hand and wrist are benign.

41.41.1.1 Aneurysmal Bone Cysts

Aneurysmal bone cysts can arise alone or in association with another tumour, but are not considered to be of neoplastic origin. The aetiology is uncertain.

It is within the first two decades of life the incidence is equal with the male to female. The hand and wrist account for only 5% and the predominant location in the hand is at the level of metacarpals and the proximal phalanges. The patient presents with persisting pain and swelling and also pathological fracture has also been reported.

Radiographically the lesion shows expansion of the cortex of the involved bone with a sclerotic rim and periosteal new bone formation and no calcification is seen. Eccentric, lytic lesion, without internal mineralisation, with expansile remodelling, and extending to the end of the bone in the mature skeleton. CT scan has often demonstrated this finding.

MR is superior for evaluating the extent of the lesion in the medullary canal and the soft tissues. It appears well defined with a low-signal intensity margin representing osseous sclerosis or pseudocapsule. The solid component exhibits low to intermediate signal intensity at T1- and T2-weighted imaging.

Success in treatment has been reported with marginal curettage of the lesion and bone grafting. Curettage and cryosurgery as opposed to simple curettage and bone grafting is another choice of treatment.

41.41.1.2 Enchondroma

Enchondroma is the most common bone tumour in the hand and wrist. It is a benign cartilaginous lesion. It is diagnosed in all ages and has a relatively equal male to female distribution. The majority of lesions occur between the ages of 10 and 40 and the proximal phalanx is the most common site of involvement.

Largely asymptomatic, these benign tumours may present due to a pathological fracture or may be observed incidentally on routine hand radiographs obtained for other reasons. Clinically these lesions are asymptomatic and give manifestation of themselves only after pathological fractures or may be observed incidentally on routine hand radiographs obtained for other reasons.

The diagnosis of enchondroma in the overwhelming majority of cases can be made with plain radiographs without the need for axial images obtained with CT or MRI (Figures 41.54 and 41.55).

Radiographically they are medullary in origin, showing sharp, sclerotic margins, often are expansile lesions, with distortion of the cortex and punctate calcification of the matrix (Figure 41.56).

Small lesions are asymptomatic with a typical radiographic appearance.

The diagnosis of multiple enchondromas in the same extremity is known as the non-hereditary condition Ollier's disease.

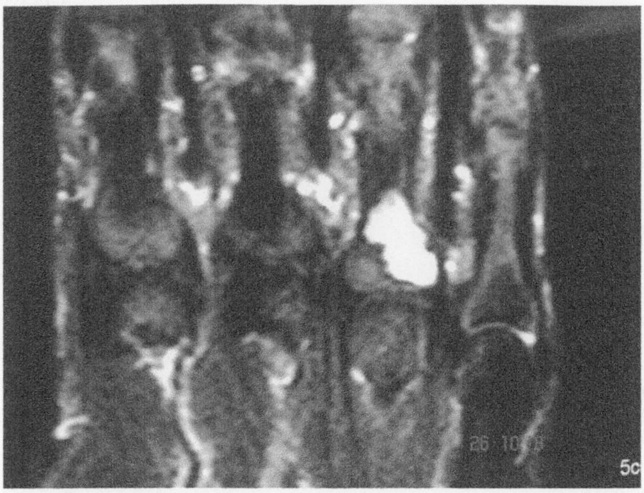

FIGURE 41.54 MRI evaluation of enchondroma.

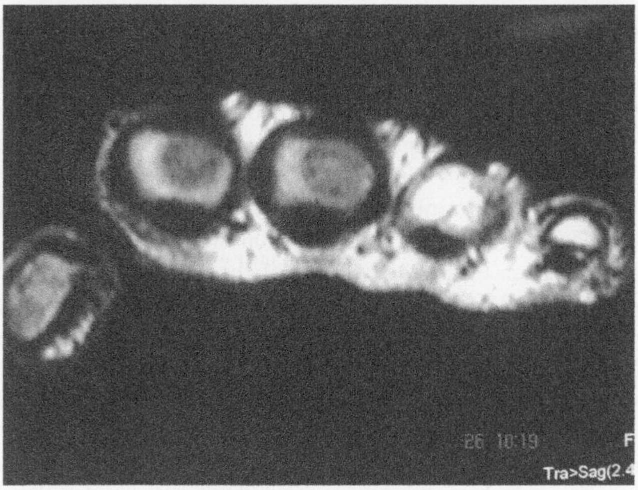

FIGURE 41.55 MRI evaluation of enchondroma. Coronal plane.

Maffucci's syndrome is an extremely rare non-hereditary condition composed of multiple enchondromas and associated hemangiomata. Radiographically, the enchondromas in Maffucci's syndrome appear identical to the solitary enchondromas.

Incidentally recognised, small, asymptomatic enchondromas require no specific treatment, while for those lesions compromising more than 50% of the bone's cortical integrity, impending pathological fracture must be considered and enchondroma excision must be planned. Pathological fractures may be treated acutely using whatever means necessary. The lesion discovered after a fracture may be treated acutely or after the pathological fracture has healed.

The digital enchondroma is generally approached dorsally, and the tumour removed by curettage and cancellous bone from the anterior iliac crest is harvested using separate instruments to prevent cross-contamination. Using the method of treatment, recurrence is approximately 4.5%. Alternatives to this method of removal include the use of allograft bone or simply curettage alone without bone grafting.

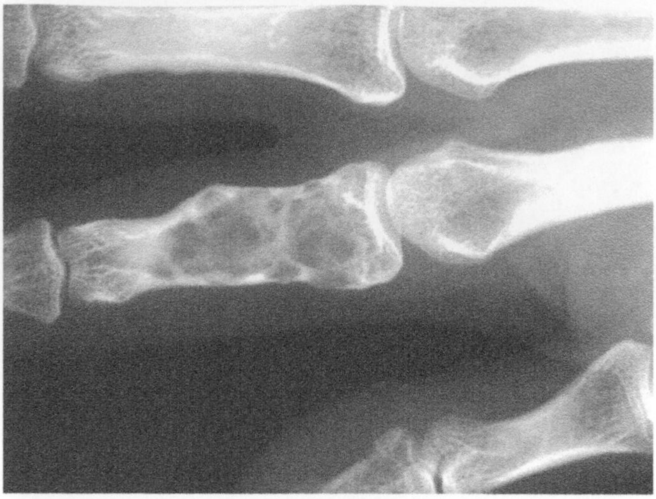

FIGURE 41.56 X-ray evaluation in enchondroma at proximal phalanx of a long finger.

41.42 EVALUATION OF VASCULAR SYSTEM IN UPPER EXTREMITIES

Vascular imaging is often necessary for preoperative planning of complex upper extremity reconstructions. In cases of trauma, indications include abnormal distal pulses, signs of haemorrhage, limb ischaemia, turbulent blood flow, injury of an adjacent structure or a penetrating injury close to a major vessel in particular in blast injuries and gunshot wounds or patients with non-traumatic vascular insufficiency with either diminished peripheral pulses or clinical signs of ischaemia. Also, these examinations are advocated in case of vascular malformations or tumours near to vessels.

Free tissue transfer has been established as one of the possible choices in the reconstructive option to cover large resection defects following traumatic events, tumour surgery or others problems that necessitate amputation surgery. Preoperatively, detailed information on the vascular status of both graft and host region has to be gained as one of the decisive factors for the success of these microvascular reconstructions is a sufficient perfusion of the graft that has to be provided by the host vessels.

To ensure the survival of the extremity after flap harvest, it is necessary to determine the adequate perfusion to the donor site because vascular variations and peripheral arterial occlusive disease can cause ischaemia in the extremities.

Many procedures have been described in order to identify these problems, the status of the host and graft vessels before the reconstruction procedure commences, such as the use of invasive procedures (conventional angiography) and non-invasive procedures like duplex ultrasonography, computed tomography angiography and magnetic resonance angiography (MRA).

According to any of these procedures, contrast angiography remains probably the gold standard for evaluating the anatomy of the upper extremity vasculature. This technique can also demonstrate the anatomy of the dominant circulation and collaterals, also identifying stenoses, occlusions, vascular malformations and eventually vasospasm. However, the test is expensive, time-consuming and carries potential risks of arterial puncture, radiation exposure and dye load to the patient. Although digital subtraction angiography has limitations including that it mainly evaluates the arterial system and gives little information regarding the venous anatomy or soft tissue anatomic relationships, and it is relatively expensive, it also has significant potential complications, including bleeding, haematoma, thrombosis, pseudoaneurysm, arteriovenous fistula and those related to the contrast medium. MRA is another imaging modality that has been used for preoperative evaluation prior to reconstructive surgery. It is an emerging technology that may hold great promise for investigations

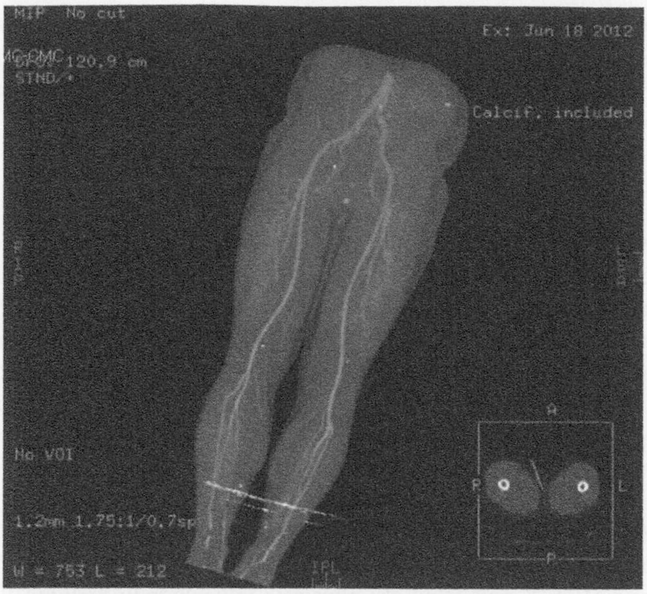

FIGURE 41.57 Angio-CT scan complete view of main vessels.

of upper extremity vasculature, there is no ionising radiation, there is no risk of allergic reaction to iodine contrast or potential toxicity to the kidney. It requires high-resolution equipment and specialised computer processing. One potential benefit of MRA is that it is less invasive than traditional angiography but is highly susceptible to movement artefact (due to long acquisition time) and it provides poor visualisation of intravascular calcifications and bony landmarks and cannot be performed if the patient has metallic implants in situ and patients with claustrophobia do not tolerate the procedure well.

CT angiography is a relatively new procedure that provides high-resolution vascular images and detailed images of the adjacent bone and soft tissue. It is relatively non-invasive and is base on injection of the contrast medium through a peripheral vein. The accuracy of arterial visualisation obtained is comparable to that of DSA. Additionally, three-dimensional reformatting allows for excellent appreciation of anatomic relationships between bones, soft tissues and the vascular system.

Application of CT angiography is becoming more widespread, both for major vessel and smaller vascular beds, and its potential utility in planning microsurgical reconstruction was recently described (Figure 41.57). Indications for upper extremity vascular imaging are varied.

41.43 SOFT TISSUES AND TENDON

41.43.1 Tendon Disorders: Trigger Finger and De Quervain's Disease

Inflammatory tendon pathologies at the wrist and hand are commonly found during clinical evaluation in hand surgery department. Such conditions are often defined as tenosynovitis due to inflammation of the tendon's synovial lining [36,37], and this is an associated reactive form with an increase in the tendon's volume or retinacular lining.

Other relatively common forms of tendon dysfunction are represented as proliferating tenovaginalitis, such as that which is found in cases of rheumatoid arthritis characterised by a diffuse and invasive synovial involvement, marked erosion throughout the tendinous sheath, the tendon itself and eventually leads to tendon weakening and possible rupture.

41.43.1.1 Trigger Finger

Trigger finger is the most common cause of finger and thumb pain and causes an alteration in hand function. This condition is characterised by a painful hand grasp or the presence of a trigger finger during finger flexion or extension movements.

It is due to a discrepancy between the flexor's circumference and that of its pulley system at the metacarpophalangeal level.

41.43.1.1.1 Physical Examination

The clinical story almost always refers to a slow onset of pain or trigger finger that occurs more frequently after exercise or repetitive heavy labour. Palpation at the level of metacarpophalangeal joint volarly evokes pain. Pain and tenderness in the palm at the proximal edge of the A1 pulley are the main symptoms. Patients frequently note catching or triggering of the affected finger or thumb after forceful flexion. The finger interesting by triggering may become locked in a flexed position. Triggering is often more pronounced in the morning than later in the day. In some cases, it is possible to feel crepitus at the tendon sheath.

41.43.1.1.2 Imaging Studies

There are various examinations that are required for the verification of the presence of this pathology: x-rays, ultrasound and MRI. X-rays allow the physician to exclude underlying skeletal pathologies. Ultrasound is useful to the physician for making an accurate diagnosis verifying tendon's movement and the anatomic level of tendon alteration, the presence of irritative liquid.

MRI is able to confirm more clearly the anomalies and tendon or tendon sheath alterations, but it still does not permit a dynamic evaluation.

41.43.1.1.3 Conservative Treatment

Most primary trigger digits in adults can be successfully treated non-surgically with the use of splinting eventually associated or not with a cortisone injection.

Most triggering digits may be successfully treated by long-acting steroid injection into the flexor sheath in fact cortisone infiltrations are usually an efficient treatment procedure with a small isolated nodule and a short time of onset even if flexor tendon rupture is a possible secondary complication that is caused by this procedure.

41.43.1.1.4 Surgical Treatment

Surgical release of the A1 pulley is recommended in digits refractory to steroid injection. Release is accomplished by directly exposing the pulley and longitudinally incising its transversely oriented fibbers. Percutaneous release of the A1 pulley may be done on the middle and ring fingers, especially if they actively lock.

41.43.1.2 De Quervain's Tenosynovitis

Stenosing tenovaginalitis in the wrist's first dorsal compartment is a frequent cause of wrist pain and subsequent hand function deficit. This pathology can be caused by activities that require frequent thumb abduction that is associated with wrist ulnar deviation or repetitive hand pronosupination. It is usually found in women after they give birth because they perform repetitive activities of hand and forearm pronosupination while they care for their newborn infants.

41.43.1.2.1 Physical Examination

The diagnosis is usually made without difficulty after eliciting a complaint of several weeks or months of pain localised to the radial side of the wrist and aggravated by movement of the thumb. A local tenderness and swelling 1–2 cm proximal to the radial styloid and knifelike pain when the thumb is clasped in the palm and the wrist forced into ulnar deviation are diagnostic of the disease. Symptoms are provoked by lifting activity in which the thumb is adducted and flexed while the

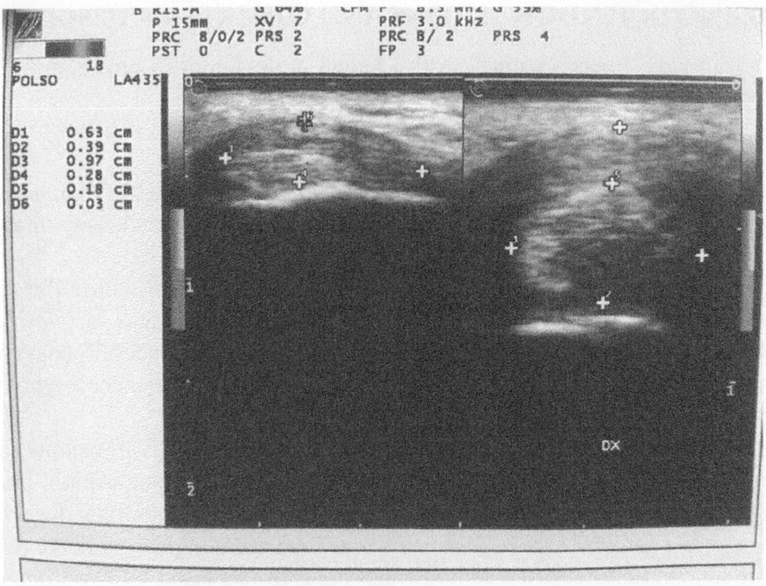

FIGURE 41.58 Ultrasound in De Quervain's disease.

hand is ulnarly deviated. Activities such as inflating a blood pressure cuff, picking up a new baby out of a crib or lifting a heavy frying pan off the stove may provoke pain along the radial aspect of the wrist.

The Finkelstein test and Brunelli test may be helpful in diagnosing this disorder.

41.43.1.2.2 Imaging Studies

De Quervain's disease should be differentiated by radiograph and physical examination from arthritis of the thumb carpometacarpal and/or STT joints arthritis or to exclude underlying skeletal pathologies, such as esostosis or poor consolidation from old radial fractures. Calcifications rarely occur.

An ultrasound examination (Figure 41.58) is important to do because it can verify that the tendon glides well or that there are anatomic alterations and also it is helpful to show any pulley cysts present at this level. MRI studies are not useful in these cases; however, a tenosynovitis manifests on MRI as fluid within the tendon sheath, with or without tendon sheath thickening. Low-signal intensity within the sheath indicates fibrosis, which has a poorer clinical prognosis and is usually seen in chronic tenosynovitis.

41.43.1.2.3 Conservative Treatment

Initial treatment includes immobilisation with a forearm-based thumb splint with the thumb placed in a hyperabduction position, which prevents both wrist deviation and thumb carpometacarpal and metacarpophalangeal joint motion while allowing interphalangeal joint motion. Steroid injection into the first extensor compartment may diminish swelling and pain but a corticosteroid infiltration is not always efficient for resolving symptoms and it is even less efficient in diabetic patients.

41.43.1.2.4 Surgical Treatment

If De Quervain's tenosynovitis is unresponsive to conservative care, surgical release of the overlying retinaculum may be elected. In some cases, the first extensor compartment is divided by a septum, creating two separate tendon sheaths so each one of the component sheaths must be opened.

41.44 IMAGING IN TENDON LESIONS AND OTHER SOFT TISSUE PATHOLOGY

Hand surgeons routinely evaluate patients with a defect in flexion or extension movement due to a prior tendon pathology.

There are several types of tendon pathology and can be grouped into five categories: tendinosis, peritendinitis/tenosynovitis, entrapment, rupture and instability.

MRI characteristics of tendinosis include fusiform shape or focal areas of increased tendon girth associated with increased intrasubstance signal on T1-weighted or proton density images; T2 hyperintensity is noted when severe degeneration is present.

In peritendinitis and tenosynovitis, MRI reveals fluid accumulation within the tendon sheath, synovial proliferation or scarring. In stenosing tenosynovitis, some areas of intermediate to low signal in the soft tissues around the tendon are seen on all MRI sequences. Tenosynovitis appears under ultrasound views as a tendon sheath distention from fluid and thickened synovium and flow on power Doppler sonography indicates synovial inflammation.

Tendon rupture can be acute or chronic and partial or complete. Ultrasound can effectively diagnose tendons that have ruptured by demonstrating tendon non-visualisation, blunt torn ends, refractive shadowing and adjacent fluid. Ultrasound can identify the retracted proximal tendon, facilitating appropriate surgical access. Moreover, real-time scanning can evaluate tendon gliding.

MRI in acute tendon ruptures often demonstrates areas of increased T2 hyperintensity owing to the presence of oedema and haemorrhage; in chronic tendon ruptures due to scar tissue formation, MRI shows areas of low-signal intensity on all pulse sequences. Tendon dislocation and subluxation are easily detected on MRI.

Ultrasonography may be a viable diagnostic tool in preoperatively evaluating flexor tendon injuries assessing the status of potentially injured flexor tendons and can help identify the location of the proximal tendon stump. Postoperatively, ultrasound can distinguish between the rupture of a repaired flexor tendon from limited motion that is secondary to the presence of intrasynovial adhesions.

The major advantage of ultrasonography lies in its ability to provide real-time dynamic images of a moving flexor tendon, unlike the static images provided by MRI and CT.

A2 or A4 pulley rupture can be inferred by the observation of bowstringing of the tendon away from the volar surface of the proximal or the middle phalanx respectively during digital flexion.

Carpal tunnel syndrome is a peripheral neuropathy frequently related to occupational causes. Compression of the median nerve may result in neuropathy with pain and paresthesias in a typical distribution. Sonographically, carpal tunnel syndrome appears as enlargement and hypoechogenicity of the median nerve. In general, the diagnosis of compression europathies at the wrist, particularly the carpal tunnel syndrome, is made by clinical exam and electrodiagnostic studies.

Recent technological advances have led to improved MR image quality resulting in high-resolution images. However, MRI imaging in the diagnosis of compressive neuropathy at the wrist should not be performed indiscriminately; it should be reserved, for instance, in which the clinical and electrodiagnostic findings are inconclusive. It is useful in severe form or in case of an infiltrative process or when a local tumour is suspected. This is particularly true for compressive neuropathy in Guyon's canal, where the prevalence of tumours or aberrant muscles is high.

Ultrasound also provides additional information regarding the aetiology of a neuropathy in cases such as masses and tenosynovitis.

41.45 RHEUMATOID ARTHRITIS

Rheumatoid arthritis is a very common disease that affects up to 1% of the world's population. The disease predominates in the elderly population but can occur at any age. Synovitis, which progresses to joint space destruction and long-term disability, is known to begin as early as 2 years after disease onset.

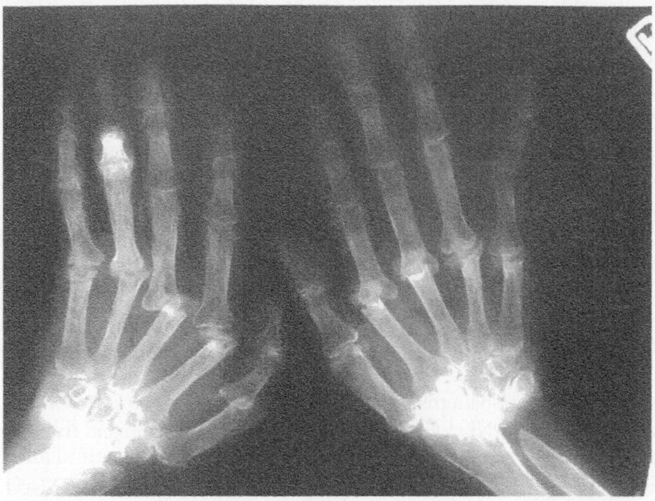

FIGURE 41.59 X-ray evaluation in rheumatoid arthritis.

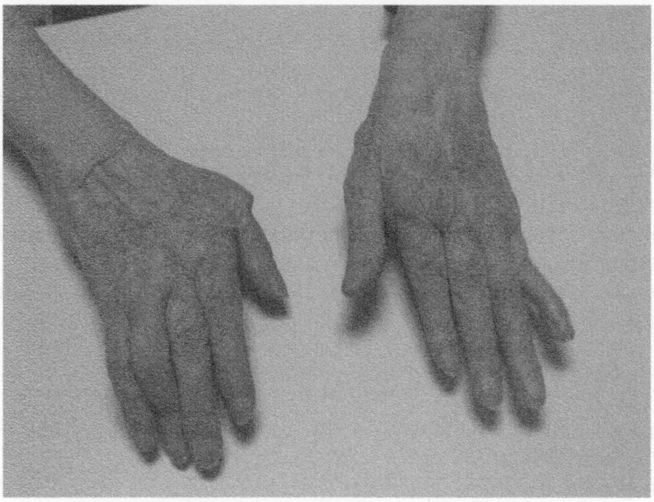

FIGURE 41.60 Clinical aspect in rheumatoid arthritis.

In the evaluation of inflammatory arthritis, ultrasound is one of the useful tools in the diagnostic process. Even if radiography remains the central diagnostic tool in these conditions (Figures 41.59 and 41.60), ultrasound can play a useful adjunctive role showing joint space widening, loss of cartilage definition, bone erosions and changes in tendons and tendon sheaths. Colour Doppler can quantify blood flow to inflamed tissues. Some studies suggest ultrasound detects more erosions than does radiography, especially early in the course of the disease, using MRI as the standard. MRI has emerged as the most sensitive means of identifying rheumatoid arthritis (RA) in its earliest stages. MRI permits to identify many findings and complications from RA. Tenosynovitis from inflammation of the extensor carpi ulnaris tendon sheath as it passes the ulnar styloid is a well-recognised cause of ulnar styloid erosion. In addition, synovial cyst formation is easily identified using MRI, with heterogeneous internal signal representing the synovial fronds. A variety of pathology directly related to inflammation of the tendons, tendon sheaths, bursae and soft tissues also can be evaluated with MRI.

REFERENCES

1. Mesgarzadeh M, Schneck CD, Bonakdarpour A. Carpal tunnel: MR imaging. I. Normal anatomy. *Radiology* 1989;171:743–748.
2. Linkous MD, Gilula LA. Wrist arthrography today. *Radiol Clin North Am* 1998;36:651–672.
3. Cerezal L, Abascal F, Garcia-Valtuille R, del Pinal F. Wrist MR arthrography: How, why, when. *Radiol Clin North Am* 2005;43:709–731.
4. Malfair D. Therapeutic and diagnostic joint injections. *Radiol Clin North Am* 2008;46:439–453.
5. Bhende MS, Dandrea LA, Davis HW. Hand injuries in children presenting to a pediatric emergency department. *Ann Emerg Med* 1993;22:1519–1523.
6. Hastings H 2nd, Simmons BP. Hand fractures in children. A statistical analysis. *Clin Orthop* 1984;34: 120–130.
7. Worlock PH, Stower MJ. The incidence and pattern of hand fractures in children. *J Hand Surg [Br]* 1986;11:198–200.
8. Worlock P, Stower M. Fracture patterns in Nottingham children. *J Pediatr Orthop* 1986;6:656–660.
9. Benson LS, Waters PM, Kamil NI et al. Camptodactyly: Classification and results of nonoperative treatment. *J Pediatr Orthop* 1994;14:814–819.
10. Wood VE. Fractures of the hand in children. *Orthop Clin North Am* 1976;7:527–542.
11. Grad JB. Children's skeletal injuries. *Orthop Clin North Am* 1986;17:437–449.
12. Stuart HC, Pyle SI, Cornoni J et al. Onsets, completions and spans of ossification in the 29 bonegrowth centers of the hand and wrist. *Pediatrics* 1962;29:237–249.
13. Greulich WW, Pyle SI. *Radiographic Atlas of Skeletal Development of the Hand and Wrist*, 2nd edn. Stanford, CA: Stanford University Press, 1959.
14. Weiss APC, Hastings H. Distal unicondylar fractures of the proximal phalanx. *J Hand Surg [Am]* 1993;18:594–599.
15. Ramos LE, Becker GA, Grossman JAI. A treatment approach for isolated unicondylar fractures of the proximal phalanx. *Ann Chir Main* 1997;16:305–308.
16. Benke GJ, Stableforth PG. Injuries of the proximal interphalangeal joint of the fingers. *Hand* 1979;3:263.
17. Bowers WH. The proximal interphalangeal joint volar plate. II: A clinical study of hyperextension injury. *J Hand Surg* 1981;6:77.
18. McCue FC, Honner R, Johnson MC, Gieck GH. Athletic injuries in the proximal interphalangeal joint requiring surgical treatment. *J Bone Joint Surg* 1970;52A:937.
19. Green DP, Butler TE. Fractures and dislocations in the hand. In: Rockwood CA, Green DP, Bucholz RW, Heckman JD, eds. *Fractures in Adults*, 4th edn. Philadelphia, PA: Lippincott-Raven, 1996:607.
20. Lenzo SR. Distal joint injuries of the thumb and fingers. *Hand Clin* 1992;8:769.
21. Mueller JJ. Carpometacarpal dislocations: Report of five cases and review of the literature. *J Hand Surg [Am]* 1986;11:184–188.
22. Adolfsson L, Jörgsholm P. Arthroscopically-assisted reduction of intra-articular fractures of the distal radius. *J Hand Surg Br* 1998;23:391–395.
23. Cooney WP, Berger RA. Treatment of complex fractures of the distal radius. Combined use of internal and external fixation and arthroscopic reduction. *Hand Clin* 1993;9:603–612.
24. Geissler WB. Arthroscopically assisted reduction of intra-articular fractures of the distal radius. *Hand Clin* 1995;11:19–29.
25. Geissler WB, Freeland AE. Arthroscopically assisted reduction of intraarticular distal radial fractures. *Clin Orthop* 1996:125–134.
26. Russe O. Fractures of the carpal navicular. *J Bone Joint Surg Am* 1960;42:759–768.
27. Cooney WP. Evaluation of chronic wrist pain by arthrography, arthroscopy, and arthrotomy. *J Hand Surg* 1993;18A:815–822.
28. Roth JH, Haddad RG. Radiocarpal arthroscopy and arthrography in the diagnosis of ulnar wrist pain. *Arthroscopy* 1986;2:234–243.
29. Mino DE, Palmer AK, Levinsohn EM. Radiography and computerized tomography in the diagnosis of incongruity of the distal radio-ulnar joint: A prospective study. *J Bone Joint Surg Am* 1985;67:247–252.
30. Wechsler RJ, Wehbe MA, Rifkin MD, Edeiken J, Branch HM. Computed tomography diagnosis of distal radioulnar subluxation. *Skeletal Radiol* 1987;16:1–5.
31. Lo IK, MacDermid JC, Bennett JD, Bogoch E, King GJ. The radioulnar ratio: A new method of quantifying distal radioulnar joint subluxation. *J Hand Surg [Am]* 2001;26:236–243.

32. Potter HG, Asnis-Ernberg L, Weiland AJ et al. The utility of high resolution magnetic resonance imaging in the evaluation of the triangular fibrocartilage complex of the wrist. *J Bone Joint Surg Am* 1997;79:1675–1684.
33. Shionoya K, Nakamura R, Imaeda T et al. Arthrography is superior to magnetic resonance imaging for diagnosing injuries of the triangular fibrocartilage. *J Hand Surg [Br]* 1998;23:402–405.
34. Tsuge S, Nakamura R. Anatomical risk factors for Kienböck's disease. *J Hand Surg [Br]* 1993;18(1):70–75.
35. Mirabello SC, Rosenthal DI, Smith RJ. Correlation of clinical and radiographic findings in Kienböck's disease. *J Hand Surg [Am]* 1987;12(6):1049–1054.
36. Thomas CL. *Taber's Encyclopedic Medical Dictionary*, 13th edn. Philadelphia, PA: FA Davis Co, 1977, pp. 1–17.
37. Wolfe SW. Tenosynovitis. In: Green DP, Hotchkiss RN, Pederson WC, eds. *Green's Operative Hand Surgery*, 4th edn. New York: Churchill Livingstone, 1999, pp. 2022–2044.

42 Imaging and Surgical Principles of Osteomyelitis and Pressure Ulcers

Bruno Carlesimo, Marco Ruggiero, Federico Lo Torto, and Marco Marcasciano

CONTENTS

Osteomyelitis is a pyogenic bone infection that may be acute, subacute, and chronic.

Infections may occur from haematogenous spread, spread from a contiguous source, direct implantation, or after trauma or surgery.

Aerobic Gram-positive cocci are the predominant microorganisms that colonise and acutely infect breaks in the skin. *Staphylococcus aureus* and the haemolytic streptococci (groups A, C, and G, but especially group B) are the most commonly isolated pathogens. Chronic wounds develop a more complex colonising flora, including enterococci, various Enterobacteriaceae, obligate anaerobes, *Pseudomonas aeruginosa*, and, sometimes, other nonfermentative Gram-negative rods. Hospitalisation, surgical procedures, and, especially, prolonged or broad-spectrum antibiotic therapy may predispose patients to colonisation and/or infection with antibiotic-resistant organisms (e.g. methicillin-resistant *S. aureus* [MRSA] or vancomycin-resistant enterococci [VRE]). Although MRSA strains have previously been isolated mainly from hospitalised patients, community-associated cases are now becoming common and are associated with worse outcomes in patients with diabetic foot infections. Acute infections in patients who have not recently received antimicrobials are often monomicrobial (almost always with an aerobic Gram-positive coccus), whereas chronic infections are often polymicrobial.[1]

TABLE 42.1
Imaging Steps for Osteomyelitis

Radiographic Features	Following Steps
Negative; low suspicion	Technetium scan
	Negative: stop
	Positive: MRI or combined radionuclide studies
Negative; high suspicion	Combined radionuclide studies and/or MRI
MRI	

Moreover, osteomyelitis is present in a substantial portion of patients with diabetes, and the risk of amputation is much higher than in patients without diabetes.[2] The most important underlying condition leading to diabetic foot problems is a neuropathy that involves sensory, motor, and autonomic nerves:

- Sensory neuropathy results in a loss of protective sensation and therefore foot trauma is not recognised and leads to ulcer formation. The ulcer often is the portal of entry for bacteria, leading to cellulitis and/or abscess formation.
- Motor neuropathy results in muscle atrophy, foot deformity, and altered biomechanics. This leads to areas of high pressure during standing or walking and repeated trauma that may go unrecognised because of sensory deficits.
- Autonomic neuropathy results in dry skin, leading to cracks and fissures, which serve as sites of entry for bacteria. Autonomic neuropathy also leads to an alteration of the neurogenic regulation of cutaneous blood supply that can contribute to ulcer formation and altered response to infection.[3]

Distinguishing osteomyelitis from aseptic neuropathic arthropathy is not easy, and all imaging studies must be interpreted in conjunction with the clinical findings (Table 42.1).[4]

The diagnostic modalities that have received the most attention in the published literature are

- Plain radiographs
- Radionuclide bone scans
- Radionuclide white blood cell scans (WBCS)
- Magnetic resonance imaging (MRI)

42.1 PLAIN RADIOGRAPHS

Conventional radiology is still the first-line modality in the study of the diabetic foot owing to its rapidity, ease of performance, and inexpensiveness, even though it is the least sensitive of all imaging modalities.

Radiographs can detect osteomyelitis, osteolysis, fractures, dislocations seen in neuropathic arthropathy, medial arterial calcification, soft-tissue gas, and foreign bodies as well as structural foot deformities, presence of arthritis, and biomechanical alterations.

Radiographic signs of osteoarthropathy and osteomyelitis are often interchangeable, particularly when the atrophic form of osteoarthropathy is present. These signs consist of demineralisation, periosteal reaction, and bony destruction; the same findings are also seen in fractures, joint deformities, and tumours.

Some 30%–50% of bone must be destroyed before osteomyelitis can be diagnosed radiographically, a process taking up to 2–3 weeks from the onset of infection. It is therefore important to maintain a high index of suspicion to make the proper diagnosis in the early stages of the disease process, because if the diagnosis is made early, 25% of patients may not develop deformity. The presence of soft-tissue swelling, periosteal reaction, permeative radiolucency, and focal erosion of cortical or medullary bone are diagnostic for osteomyelitis.

To date, plain radiographs have a sensitivity of 28%–93% and a specificity of 25%–92%.

42.2 RADIONUCLIDE BONE SCANS

The bone scan is more sensitive than plain radiography, but not specific for diagnosing osteomyelitis. The 3-phase bone scan is made up of an initial postinjection intravenous of radioactive technetium-99m methylene diphosphonate (MDP) angiogram (2–5 s), then a *blood-pool* image (10 min), followed by a delayed static image 2–3 h or 5–7 h later. The image produced by bone scan is affected by rate of bone turnover, capillary permeability, tissue perfusion, and regional blood flow. Conditions producing hyperaemia or ischemia will affect the bone scan. Although a positive bone scan is not necessarily indicative of osteomyelitis, a negative study excludes it with a higher degree of probability. The reported performance characteristics of various types of nuclear medicine scans varies, but the specificity of technetium bone scans is generally low. Sensitivity of radionuclide bone scan is reported to be between 50% and 83%, whereas specificity is not good (averaging ~50%), because almost any type of bone disorder (including neuroarthropathy and healing osteomyelitis) can cause increased isotope uptake on a bone scan. There are many causes of positive bone scans. In general, a positive delayed phase scan is seen when there is an underlying process that promotes bone remodelling (healing fracture, neuropathic osteoarthropathy, recent surgery). False negatives may occur when the radiotracer fails to reach the foot because of diminished vascular flow (patients with diabetes who have atherosclerotic disease).

42.3 RADIONUCLIDE WHITE BLOOD CELL SCANS

Other agents that are known to localise in areas of infection, such as labelled leukocytes, have been explored through dual tracer studies in an attempt to enhance specificity, and at the present time, labelled leukocyte imaging is the nuclear medicine procedure of choice for investigation of diabetic foot infections. The sensitivity of these tests can be limited in some situations as ischemic foot.[5] Furthermore, as infection resolves, the labelled leukocyte uptake decreases and then normalises, making it useful for assessing response to therapy.

WBC can be labelled with Tc-99 hexamethylpropyleneamine oxime (Tc-99-HMPAO), indium-111, or gallium-67 citrate.[6–10]

When using Indium-111, images are performed routinely the day after injection of labelled cells, which is more specific for acute infections than Tc-99 MDP scanning because indium-111 selectively labels polymorphonuclear leukocytes. On the other hand, chronic infections and inflammation are not well imaged with indium-111, because chronic inflammatory cells (i.e. lymphocytes) predominate and are not well labelled with indium.

Despite Indium-111, Tc-99-HMPAO images are performed 4 h after injection of labelled cells, using a smaller radiation dose. Moreover, it is less expensive and offers improved resolution compared with indium scanning. The sensitivity and specificity of both techniques are comparable.

The labelled autologous WBCS is relatively expensive, is technically demanding, and involves radiation exposure but can be helpful in demonstrating that an infection has resolved.

Image resolution is poor and it may not always be possible to separate soft tissue from bony infection. In our opinion, leukocyte scans are useful only when MRI scans are unavailable. Combining Tc-99 MDP and indium-111 increases the specificity of diagnosing osteomyelitis. This combined technique is useful, because the Tc-99 MDP scan localises the anatomic site of inflammation and the indium-111 labels the infected bone. The indium-111 scan is not typically positive in aseptic neuropathic arthropathy, although false-positive indium scans can occur.

A 100% sensitivity and 89% specificity have been reported with the combined technique in evaluating diabetic infections.

The precise mechanism by which ^{67}Ga citrate accumulates in normal and pathologic tissues is not completely understood. It is widely accepted that ^{67}Ga citrate, as an analog of iron, binds in ionic form to circulating transferrin, uses transferrin receptors to access cells, and then becomes highly stable within cells (except red blood cells). In acute inflammation, ^{67}Ga citrate is thought to leak through the vascular epithelium and bind to lactoferrin excreted in loco by leukocytes or to siderophores produced by the infecting microorganisms themselves. Approximately 25% is excreted through the urinary system in the first 24 h, and excretion is then through the colon. About 75% of the injected dose is retained in the liver, bone, bone marrow, and soft tissues at 48 h.

It is easy to prepare and has low toxicity and a low target-to-background ratio. ^{67}Ga citrate scanning has been described as outperforming most other techniques in detecting infection of both bacterial and nonbacterial origin, leading to its usefulness in immunosuppressed patients. Accumulation is normally present in liver, spleen, gastrointestinal tract, and kidneys but can vary significantly between individuals. With a physical half-life of 78 h and decay occurring through a broad range of gamma-ray emissions, ^{67}Ga has unfavourable physical characteristics for gamma-camera imaging. ^{67}Ga citrate imaging is an acceptable substitute when cell imaging is not possible, is an important infection localiser in its own right, and can be an important complement to leukocyte imaging. The use of 67Ga citrate is generally limited to the study of chronic osteomyelitis. To increase its low specificity, it is often used in combination with other radiopharmaceuticals.[11]

42.4 MAGNETIC RESONANCE IMAGING

There is general agreement that this is the most useful imaging study for diagnosing diabetic foot osteomyelitis (DFO), as well as for evaluating the extent of both bone and soft-tissue involvement and for planning surgery. MRI has replaced computed tomography (CT), as it is better able to identify bone marrow changes and evaluate septic involvement of the soft tissues, which allows surgery to be planned in such a way as to prevent recurrence of infection after amputation or abscess drainage.

Scintigraphy with technetium-labelled granulocytes is slightly less accurate than MRI in the diagnosis of osteomyelitis and is more time consuming and expensive. It is thus reserved for patients with contraindications to MRI or with doubtful MRI findings, or to assess response to antibiotic therapy during the follow-up. Recently, MRI has demonstrated good diagnostic accuracy in the evaluation of diabetic foot infections. Diagnostic sensitivity for osteomyelitis has generally been reported to be 90%–100%. Specificity is somewhat limited by difficulty in distinguishing osteomyelitis from other causes of marrow oedema, including acute neuropathic osteoarthropathy. Nevertheless, positive and negative predictive values as high as 93% and 100%, respectively, have been reported.

42.5 TREATMENT

All devitalised and fibrotic soft tissue are excised. Bone debridement is undertaken to remove all nonviable bones. The end point of bony debridement is marked by the appearance of bleeding in the cortical bone. The timing and type of coverage depend on the size of the bony and soft-tissue defects. With minimal bone debridement and bone stability, immediate soft-tissue coverage with local pedicle muscle flap or distant microvascular tissue transplantation is undertaken. With more extensive bone debridement, either cancellous bone grafting or microsurgical vascularised bone transfer is undertaken.

42.6 STERNAL OSTEOMYELITIS AND OTHER POSTSTERNOTOMY COMPLICATIONS

Plastic surgeons are often called to take part to the reconstruction of chest wall defects, after tumour resection or for chronic or complicated deep sternal osteomyelitis following open heart surgery (Figures 42.1 and 42.2).

Sternal osteomyelitis can be classified into primary (PSO) or secondary sternal osteomyelitis (SSO).

PSO is quite rare and represents the 0.3% of all causes of osteomyelitis described in literature. It is basically secondary to haematogenous spread of organism in the absence of a contiguous focus of infection. PSO may occur in patients with a history of intravenous drug abuse, acquired immunodeficiency syndrome, haemoglobinopathy, or other immune deficiency states.[12]

The most common organisms isolated in patients who abuse intravenous drugs are *S. aureus* and *P. aeruginosa*; Chen et al.[13] report other infectious causes, including *Salmonella* species (in patients with sickle cell disease), *Candida albicans*, *Aspergillus fumigatus*, and *Mycobacterium tuberculosis*.

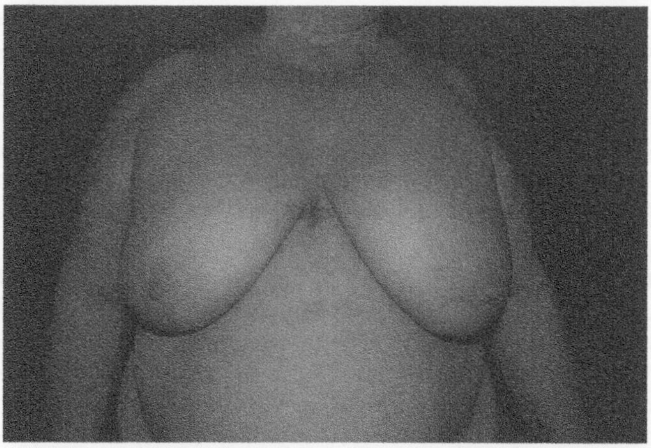

FIGURE 42.1 Clinical case: woman with sternal osteomyelitis (preoperative view).

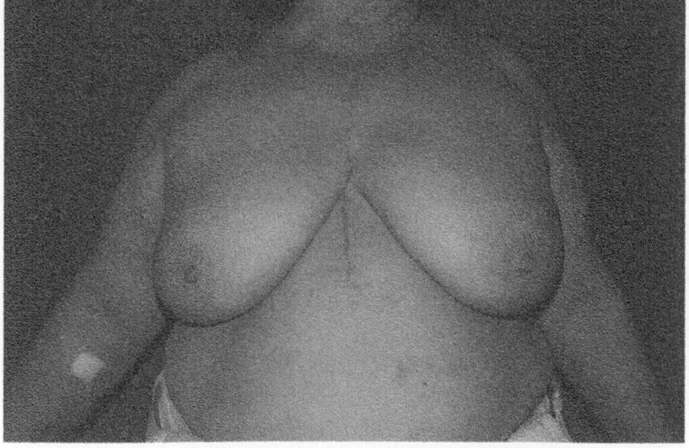

FIGURE 42.2 Clinical case: sternal osteomyelitis (postoperative view).

Changes are usually evident at radiography within 10–12 days and may include swelling of soft tissue and demineralisation, destruction, and sequestrum of bone. CT may depict soft-tissue swelling, irregular sternal contours, and inflammatory changes with small fluid collections at the level of the parasternal region. Earlier stage of infection can be evidenced by performing a skeletal scintigraphy that may show increased radiotracer uptake in the sternum and sternoclavicular regions. On the other hand, MRI findings with all pulse sequences include a lack of signal hypointensity in cortical bone and abnormal signal intensity (hypointense signal on T1-weighted images, hyperintense signal on T2-weighted images) in bone marrow. In fact, MRI imaging investigates the presence of abscess and evaluates the extension of the infectious process into adjacent joints and sinus tract formation. SSO has a higher incidence compared to the primary form (PSO), especially after sternotomy. However, it is not considered a frequent complication showing a reported incidence that ranges between 0.47%–8% and 0.22%–1.97% for deep sternal wound infections (SWIs) specifically. Mortality can vary from 1% with mortality rates reported from 0.5% to 9.1% for superficial SWIs and 1.0% to 36% for deep SWIs.[14]

Median sternotomy is the incision of choice for cardiac surgery and is also useful for accessing anterior mediastinal lesions and for bilateral pulmonary procedures. The operative approach begins with a vertical skin incision made from below the suprasternal notch to a point between the xiphoid process and umbilicus. Next, the sternum is divided with a power saw. A sternal spreader is then inserted and opened, exposing the anterior mediastinum. At the end of surgery, the sternum is closed with four to seven stainless steel parasternal sutures, the ends of which are securely twisted and buried in the sternal tissues. There several risk factors that are directly related to the development of wound complications. Obesity, diabetes, corticosteroid treatment, bilateral harvesting of the internal mammary artery, and prolonged procedural times are the most important[15] (Table 42.2).

Clinical diagnosis of SSO with sternal separation is usually based on local findings of sternal instability, erythema, fluid collection, wound dehiscence, and purulent discharge. Objective and subjective feelings of throbbing and looseness of the repair should be noticed. The clinical perception of a sternal click may be indicative of the presence of sternal instability. The evidence of systemic signs, such as pyrexia or leukocytosis at daily evaluation, and a high index of suspicion by the surgeon are essential to make the correct diagnosis. At this regard, mediastinitis should always be considered in cases of slow postoperative recovery since the depth of infection is difficult to be clinically determined and a purulent wound drainage can originate from a superficial infection in the presternal compartment or from the deep mediastinal tissues with mediastinitis.

Nevertheless, there are no single tests that can make or exclude the diagnosis. This complication must be differentiated from normal postsurgical changes that can persist for 3 weeks and include minimal soft-tissue infiltration with oedema and blood in the presternal and retrosternal compartments, focal air, and localised marginated fluid or hematoma. Focal dots of mediastinal air usually resolve in 7 days. On the other hand, normal postoperative events do not completely obliterate mediastinal fat planes, mostly or at least partially maintaining the mediastinal fat radiolucency.

TABLE 42.2
Risk Factors for SWI

Preoperative	Perioperative	Postoperative
Diabetes mellitus	Prolonged bypass time	Transfusions
Chronic obstructive airway disease	Use of internal thoracic arteries (ITA)	Surgical chest re-exploration
Smoking	Prolonged mechanical ventilation	Prolonged postoperative ventilation
Obesity		Longer stay in the ICU
Larger female breast size		

Defects of the sternum including gaps up to 4 mm wide, stepoffs (sternal tables at different levels), and impaction (overriding of the sternal halves) are usually present in these patients.

Callus formation begins after the 3rd postoperative month, and after 6 months, only 50% of surgical sternotomies heal completely and sternal union is definitely obtained within 1 year after the procedure.[16]

The diagnostic modalities that have received the most attention in the published literature are

- Chest radiographs
- CT
- MRI
- CT sinography
- Radionuclide WBCS

42.7 CHEST RADIOGRAPHS

Chest radiograph is a first step exam and is routinely performed during admission. In the past years, it was considered a primary diagnostic tool; nevertheless, this radiological exam (even if performed with different projections, including a sternum-specific oblique views) is nonspecific and offers only little contribution for the diagnosis and preoperative planning of surgical treatment of sternal infections. In particular, there are different conditions such as the presence of sinuses, costochondral retrosternal, or mediastinal infections that are virtually undetectable. Radiographic visualisation of the sternum in the frontal projection is often limited because of the thinness of the cortex and the low mineral mass, as well as the superimposition of the ribs, spine, and mediastinum.

The sternum is well depicted on lateral projections though abnormalities that do not involve its entire width may not be apparent and small or tricky findings might be especially difficult to appreciate. X-ray examination of the sternum can show broken metallic wires, sternal dehiscence, wire malposition, fracture, and pseudoarthrosis.[17]

Gross changes as well as small variations in the position of the wires on postoperative plain x-ray are indicative of sternal separation.

42.8 COMPUTED TOMOGRAPHY

CT is the modality of choice to evaluate anatomic details as well as pathologic conditions of the sternum, sternoclavicular joints, and adjacent soft tissues.[18] CT scan delineates changes in bone configuration and distinguishes insignificant infections from major infective processes, accurately depicting its extent and depth. Any persistent or recurrent fluid collection suggests localised sepsis, and CT-guided needle aspiration can help determine whether this collection is infected or needs a more invasive surgical treatment. Complications such as dehiscence, paramedian sternotomy, and osteomyelitis can be detected with CT scan.

A paramedian sternotomy is defined as an off-centre sternotomy incision and predisposes the patient to dehiscence as a consequence of the pressure exerted by the wires. In fact, they can break the delicate, thin side of the sternum when they are closed by the surgeon. CT findings of dehiscence include displaced sternal wires and progressive widening of the incisional gap. Early sternal osteomyelitis is often difficult to be recognised and it can be frequently mistaken for minor sternal irregularities caused by the bone saw and anatomic variants. Eventually, frank bone destruction, severe demineralisation, and dehiscence are seen. CT can show subtle erosions, periosteal reaction, sharply marginated sclerosis, and swelling in the adjacent soft tissues (Figures 42.3 and 42.4).

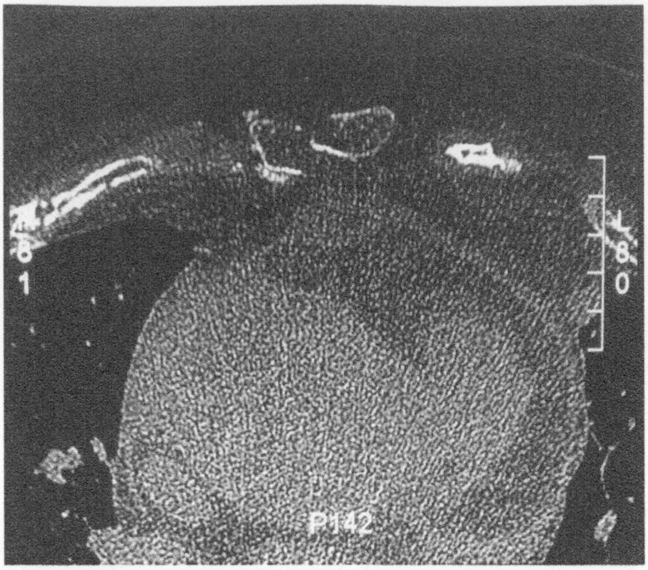

FIGURE 42.3 Sternal osteomyelitis. CT image.

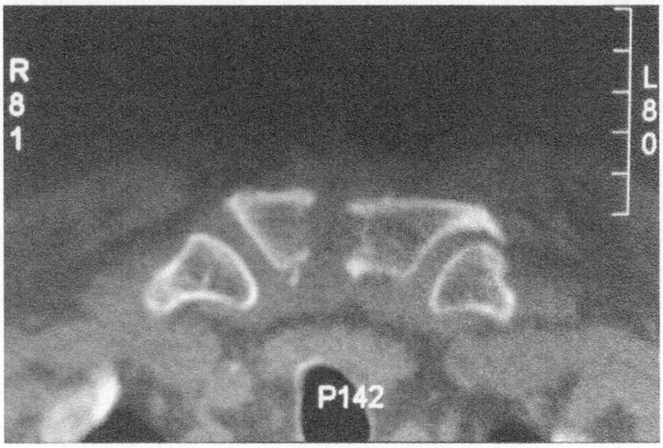

FIGURE 42.4 Sternal osteomyelitis. CT image showing sternal bone gap.

42.9 MAGNETIC RESONANCE IMAGING

MRI is of great value as a secondary modality. It can help clarify CT findings and can provide additional information about the bone marrow and soft tissues adjacent to the sternum. MRI is useful for determining the extent of the lesion. In particular, marrow involvement and soft-tissue spread are well determined and depicted, as well as abscess formation, destruction of articular cartilage, and sinus tract formation. These findings are not evident on a plain x-radiography until the process of bone destruction is advanced. Nevertheless, MRI has some limitations due to artefacts produced by the presence of sternal wires (Figures 42.5 through 42.8).[19]

At MRI, the sternal anatomy is best depicted with T1-weighted spin-echo pulse sequences. The coronal plane displays the articular surfaces, as well as the intra-articular disk; the sagittal

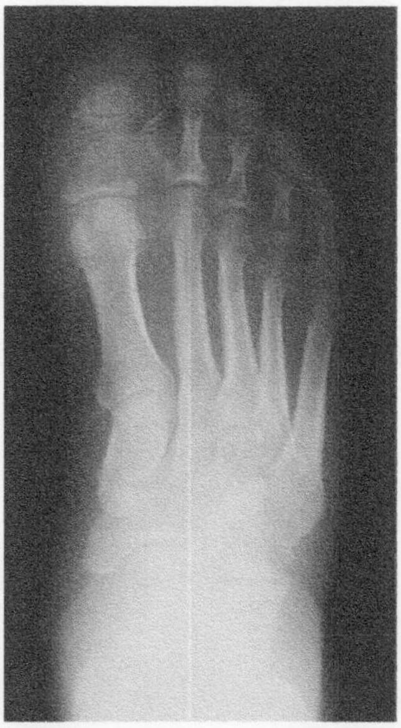

FIGURE 42.5 First toe osteomyelitis: plain radiograph image.

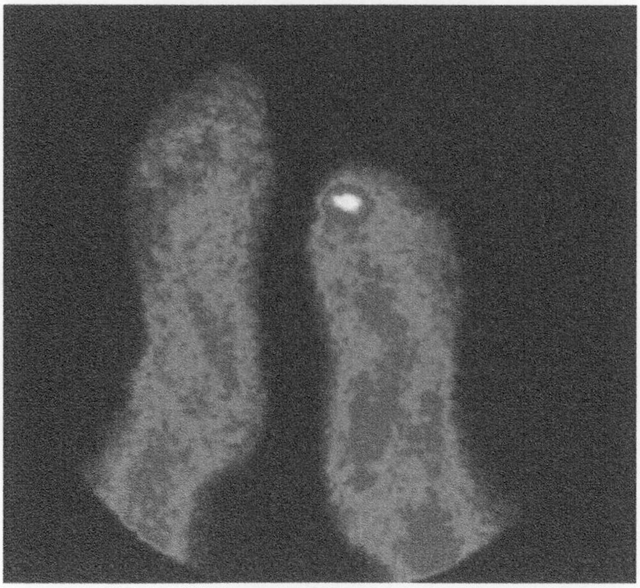

FIGURE 42.6 First toe osteomyelitis: radionuclide WBCS.

plane is useful for depicting the costoclavicular ligament; and the axial plane best delineates the anterior and posterior parts of the sternoclavicular joint capsule and the anterior and posterior sternoclavicular ligaments. Normal findings that should not be mistaken for disease including small amounts of joint collections, nonfatty bone marrow, and poorly defined cortical margins.

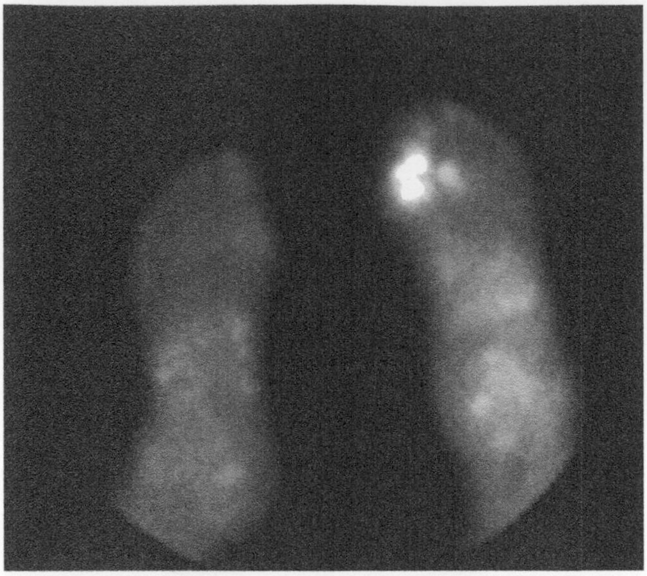

FIGURE 42.7 First toe osteomyelitis: bone scintigraphy.

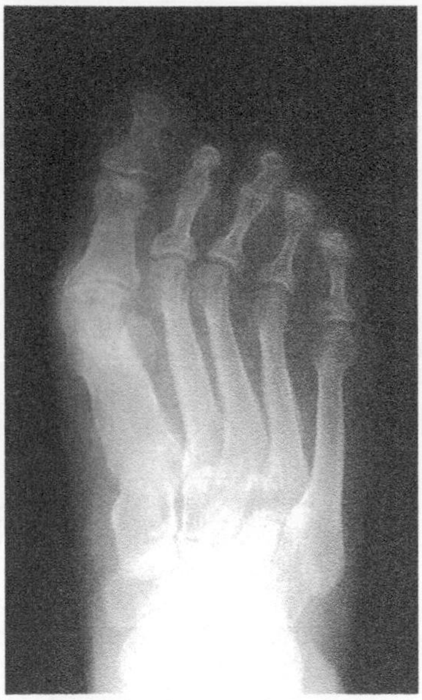

FIGURE 42.8 First metatarsal osteomyelitis in diabetic patient: plain radiograph.

42.10 CT SINOGRAPHY

CT sinography offers a simple and anatomical picture, which serves as a good guideline for the operator during surgery. Regular sinography is performed in frontal and lateral views that are mandatory to assess the extent of infection and penetration in both dimensions.

CT sinography can depict the depth of sinus tracts, reveal any mediastinal communication, and also demonstrate its relation to a retained foreign body. Sinus tracts that reach the outer plate of the sternum are suggestive of osteomyelitis.

42.11 NUCLEAR MEDICINE

Nuclear medicine procedures have been shown to be sensitive and are used as a functional adjunct to complement morphologic imaging techniques.

Common conventional nuclear medicine procedures include 3-phase bone scintigraphy, 67Ga citrate, and Indium-111 and *technetium-99m* HMPAO-labelled leukocytes (Figures 42.9 and 42.10).

The 3-phase bone scan has been shown to be sensitive for the diagnosis of PSO. The study consists of the flow phase (to examine perfusion), the blood-pool phase, and the delayed (2–4 h) bone phase.

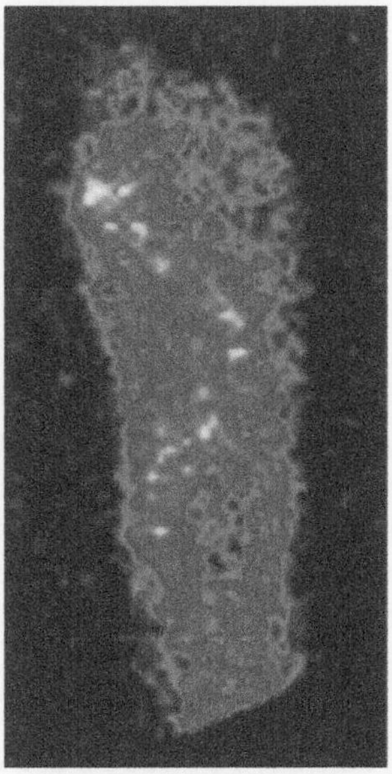

FIGURE 42.9 First metatarsal osteomyelitis in diabetic patient: single-photon emission CT (*technetium-99m* HMPAO).

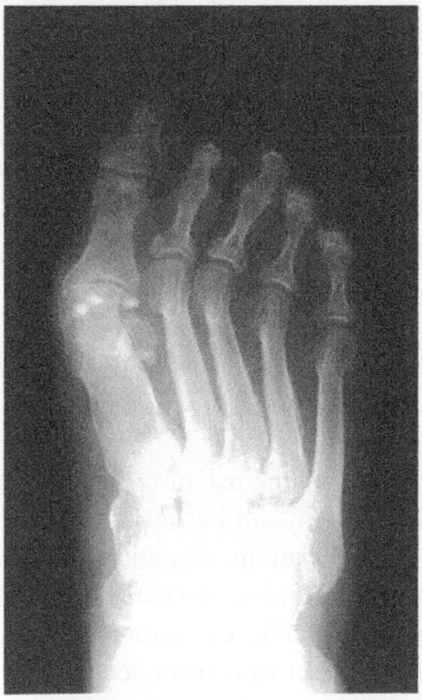

FIGURE 42.10 Osteomyelitis in diabetic patient: plain RX + SPECT 99 mTc-HMPAO.

Osteomyelitis demonstrates increased flow activity, blood-pool activity, and positive uptake on 3-h images in the area; when all these events occur, the bone scintigraphy is highly sensitive for osteomyelitis (73%–100%).[20,21]

In patients with previously violated bone and with pre-existing conditions such as fractures, median sternotomy, and orthopaedic hardware, bone turnover is constant and 3-phase bone scan is not reliable. Therefore, in these patients, this procedure is nonspecific, necessitating the performance of additional imaging studies. 67Ga imaging combined with bone scan was first suggested to increase specificity.

67Ga citrate has gained the greatest attention for its known capacity to localise in cases of active infection. Combined bone/gallium imaging provide complementary information about the disease process with overall specificities of 50%–100%.[22–25]

The need to perform two imaging procedures and delayed imaging (Ga-67 imaging requires at least 48 and sometimes 72 h postinjection to complete the study) is a major disadvantage.

Among the various conventional nuclear medicine procedures, the use of labelled leukocytes is one of the most specific imaging and almost replaced 67Ga citrate scintigraphy,[26] but often it must be performed in combination with bone marrow imaging to maximise accuracy.

WBCS has been reported to be a useful tool in the diagnosis of deep SWIs, independently of the radionuclide used for leukocyte labelling (111 In- and 99m Tc-HMPAO).

However, in our experience, we have found several false-positive cases presumably due to the fact that surgical toilette of the wound was not performed daily and it is possible that leukocytes will accumulate in soft tissues, giving rise to areas of increasing sternal uptake which can be misinterpreted as bone infection. We believe that the most benefit from this method results from its use when inflammation indexes (ESR, PRC, WBC count, etc.) are normalised and clinical features of infection have disappeared after performing the surgery and specific antibiotic therapy, in the assessment of the effective healing.

42.12 RADIONUCLIDE WHITE BLOOD CELL SCANS

WBCS has been reported to be a useful tool in the diagnosis of deep SWI, independently of the radionuclide used for leukocyte labelling.[27]

42.13 SURGICAL APPROACH

Superficial infections defined as presternal infections must be treated conservatively by simple incision, drainage, and open dressing changes.

Deep SWIs are harder to manage and many therapeutic options and combinations exist ranging from open wound treatment to early closure with irrigation and reconstruction with muscular and fasciocutaneous local and free flaps. Up to the 1960s, the main treatment for a mediastinal infection was an initial surgical debridement followed by frequent dressing changes, to promote granulation and facilitate secondary wound closure. This approach is incredibly slow since the time required for granulation tissue to cover the mediastinum is very long. Moreover, patients suffer significant physical and psychological stress, with high incidence of reoperation and mortality, which has been assessed around 22%.[28]

Schumacker and Mandelbaum reported the use of continuous mediastinal irrigation with iodine and local antibiotic[29] and later with the only antibiotic solution.[30]

Despite the disadvantages such as limitations on patient mobility, slow rehabilitation, toxicity of iodine used for lavage, fungal overgrowth, and fungal mediastinitis secondary to prolonged local antibiotic administration, continuous mediastinal lavage remains a valid nonsurgical therapeutic option.[31]

Among surgical procedures, the greater omentum seems an ideal and outmost viable solution for the repair of infected sternotomy wounds, thanks to its rich vascularisation and angiogenic and immunogenic features.[32]

This procedure, however, shows several disadvantages: It requires laparotomy, which can lead to additional complications especially in septic and critically ill patients, with high morbidity rate, and does not improve sternal stability and frequently necessitates skin transfer.[33–37]

Muscle flap transposition is also reported as an effective and feasible surgical option. Nowadays, many authors believe that this is the treatment of choice for most patients with sternal and mediastinal infection.

The first muscular option is usually offered by the harvesting of a pectoralis major flap (PMF) as turnover flap based on the perforating branches from the internal thoracic artery (ITA), advancement flap based on the blood supply from the thoracoacromial vessel, and bilateral flaps. Anyways, many different techniques of dissecting, mobilising, and transferring the pectoral muscle have been suggested. From 2004 to 2012 in the University of Rome *La Sapienza*, we treated 86 cases of SSO with PMF. The protocol was composed by surgical time associated with administration of specific and targeted antibiotics selected on the basis of intraoperative biopsies. During surgery, wound margins, soft tissues, bone, and cartilage are checked for signs of infections; metallic sternal sutures are removed, and toilette of the bone is needed in case of evidences of sequestrectomy. Then sternotomy and a partial costectomy are performed. Costal cartilage is frequently found to be necrotic especially after attempts of sternal refixation with Robicsek type of longitudinal wiring. Wound is irrigated by using hydrogen peroxide and physiologic solution. In all patients, a removable cardiac device (not attached to the pericardium) and/or metallic sternal sutures have to be removed so that the infection resolves without any relapse during the following months. Sometimes in several patients, fixed pacemaker with electrodes sutured to the pericardium cannot be completely extracted leading to higher incidences of relapse within 10 months. The coverage is performed by mobilising the left pectoral muscle from the chest wall and subcutaneous tissue to a distance of about 10 cm from the median line. The humeral attachment of the left pectoral muscle is never detached. After dissection of the muscle from the boundary to the rectus abdominis muscle, the flap could be mobilised to reach the right edge of the sternal defect and anchored to the contralateral muscle insertion fibres, previously arisen and disinserted. The contralateral muscle is then sutured to the previously anchored muscle, creating a multilayer covering of the sternal bone and avoiding the direct contact of the wound with the osteomyelitic site. Based on our experience, we suggest not to restore the bone continuity, avoiding the placement of metallic stitches and plaques. The suture of superficial and deeper tissues is always made by layers, with polyfilament absorbable wires and monofilament nonabsorbable wire for the skin.

42.14 PRESSURE ULCERS

Pressure sores are ischaemic damages to soft tissues resulting from unrelieved pressure, usually over a bony prominence.[38] They are commonly termed as bedsores, decubitus ulcers, or pressure sores, and sometimes as pressure necrosis or ischemic ulcers.[39]

The definition has been further refined by the European Pressure Ulcer Advisory Panel as 'areas of localized damage to the skin and underlying tissue caused by pressure, shear, friction and/or a combination of these'.[40] Pressure ulcer prevalence rate has been estimated as 0.4%–28% in the United States, 4.18% in Japan, and 18.1% in Europe.[41]

The complex aetiology of pressure sores requires a multidisciplinary approach to treatment and often the plastic surgeon is called to examine the patient for severity of the wound and to determine the best surgical approach, if necessary. Thus, before proceeding with a surgical treatment, plastic surgeons should coordinate and mobilise the many team members, clearly considering and understanding the physiology, classification, and cause of the pathology, in order to choose the correct strategies to prevent recurrence.[42] Sometimes, it can be very difficult to treat and evaluate chronic non-healing ulcers and their underlying complications such as osteomyelitis, heterotopic ossification, abscess, soft-tissue infection, sinus tract, fistula, septic arthritis, or squamous cell carcinoma.[43] All these conditions may lead to a failure or delay of normal healing process and postposition of the resolutive surgical treatment, resulting in prolonged hospitalisation. Nowadays more than ever, pressure sores have a substantial impact on the health-related quality of life of patients and in terms of the financial burden on the health service, patients and their families, and the society as a whole. From this perspective, a correct diagnosis, proper treatment, and prevention of such a disease became a priority in health-care structures, because management of a late-stage pressure ulcer may reach unsustainable costs.[44,45]

In this regard, different diagnostic exams and risk assessment tools and scales have been described with the primary aim of identifying those individuals at risk of developing pressure ulcers (older people and pregnant women; seriously ill patients; neurologically compromised individuals, e.g. those with spinal cord injuries [SCIs]; patients with impaired mobility or those who are immobile, including those wearing a prosthesis, body brace, or plaster cast, or who suffer from impaired nutrition, obesity, or poor posture, or who use equipment such as seating or beds which do not provide appropriate pressure relief) or find out related hidden complications, in order to treat it or prevent the onset.[46]

Pressure ulcer diagnosis and management approaches and techniques are continuously developing, but there remains no overall consensus about them, and accepted standard diagnostic guidelines still have not been developed for evaluating non-healing pressure ulcers, to assess the best clinical decisions in the perioperative period.[47]

In literature, there are different classifications that use external signs such as erythema, blistering, and outright skin breakdown to identify the lesions from least to most severe and determine the severity of necrosis.

Grade 1: Non-blanchable erythema of intact skin. Discolouration of the skin, warmth, oedema, induration, or hardness may also be used as indicators, particularly on individuals with darker skin.

Grade 2: Partial thickness skin loss involving epidermis, dermis, or both. The ulcer is superficial and presents clinically as an abrasion or blister.

Grade 3: Full-thickness skin loss involving damage to or necrosis of subcutaneous tissue that may extend down to, but not through, the underlying fascia.

Grade 4: Extensive destruction, tissue necrosis, or damage to muscle, bone, or supporting structures with or without full-thickness skin loss.

We reported a four-stage system guideline for pressure sores classification but it is important to keep in mind that the external appearance underestimates the extent of the injury.[48]

In fact, we believe that changes in subcutaneous deep tissues occurs much before the onset of visible external clinical signs of pressure damages. Several recent studies seem to confirm that inflammation or ischaemia caused by pressure has a greater effect on subcutaneous tissues and in particular on fat than cutaneous surface.[49,50]

The fat and the superficial fascia protect muscles and bone from the external forces, and their early damage represents the first step for a progressive ulceration process. This acquisition could lead to the formulation of a *reverse classification* of pressure sores on the basis of a progressive process for pressure ulcer development, which begins from deep subdermal to superficial dermal layers and only then shows up with epidermal layer ulceration. This would change completely the diagnosis protocols, medical approach, and surgical management of pressure sores.

In this regard, ultrasound (US) (10 MHz probe) can be used for visualising the dermis, the subcutaneous fatty tissue, and muscle up to 20–30 mm below the skin surface, in order to search for soft-tissue oedema and early damages and changes.[12] It can detect deep soft-tissue oedema and subperiosteal collections as well as the presence of fluid in a joint or extra-articular soft tissue. Moreover, US assessment can provide guidance for diagnostic or therapeutic aspiration, drainage, or biopsy, but the use of sonography in the diagnosis of pressure sores complications such as osteomyelitis is limited.[51] Current imaging modalities used in identifying the presence of complications in pressure ulcers include plain radiographs, sinograms, isotope bone scans, bone biopsy, CT, leukocyte scintigraphy, and MRI.[10,52–61]

These debilitated patients frequently have many co-morbidities with a high risk for developing pressure ulcer and its main related complications such as osteomyelitis. Authors report a pressure sores prevalence between 23% and 33% and a lifetime risk estimated between 25% and 85% for SCI patients.[62–64]

When a surgeon faces a chronic, non-healing wound, he or she must keep in mind that osteomyelitis may be present, and if possible, a bone biopsy is necessary to make the correct diagnosis. In fact, any non-healing wound in which the bone is either visible or can be easily palpated or any ulcer that does not heal after at least 6 weeks of appropriate care and off-loading is likely to be complicated by osteomyelitis.[65,66]

The reference standard for diagnosing osteomyelitis remains microbiologic analysis after bone biopsy. In fact, a diagnosis and moreover a long-term antibiotic therapy should not be set only on the basis of bone culture report. In literature, Darouiche et al. report on the accuracy of a simple clinical evaluation for osteomyelitis, showing that the sensitivity and specificity of the clinical examination resulted correct between 33% and 60%, respectively.[67] Nevertheless the surgical plan and the role of preoperative antibiotics without a definitive culture, are difficult to evaluate by physical examination alone, and may depend on an accurate preoperative radiological diagnosis of the bone infection.[68] Unfortunately, patients with pressure sores are very difficult to manage, and the radiological diagnosis of osteomyelitis can be very challenging. In this regard, imaging is used to confirm the presumed clinical diagnosis and to provide information regarding the exact site and extent of the infectious process, in order to help the clinician in medical planning or surgical treatment. White cell count and erythrocyte sedimentation rate are recommended in association to a plain x-ray as well as other imaging techniques. The combination of these exams leads to a higher rate of sensitivity and specificity in making the diagnosis of osteomyelitis. Nevertheless, laboratory findings, such as an elevated erythrocyte sedimentation rate and leukocytosis, are nonspecific for bone infection in its early stage and sometimes can even be normal. Serial blood cultures are positive in 32%–60% of cases[69] and cultures of blood and material aspirated by needle aspiration of the involved bone result positive in up to 87% of cases, while the outcome deriving from subperiosteal aspiration approaches 90%.[70]

Several authors stress on the importance of Jamshidi core needle bone biopsy in predicting or making early diagnosis of osteomyelitis in grade IV pressure ulcer patients.[71]

This technique shows a sensitivity and specificity of 73% and 96%, respectively, and can be incorporated to bone biopsy histopathology and bone cultures for a correct diagnosis and treatment of osteomyelitis. Radiographic imaging of the affected area includes conventional radiography and CT scans. Using a plain x-ray, there are several radiological findings that show the presence of bone infections. In fact, a positive score is obtained in the presence of signs of cortical destruction, osteopenia with appreciable loss of mineralisation, aggressive periosteal reaction, and intraosseous gas.[72] Moreover, it shows the details of the bony cortex and trabeculae, in the presence of ectopic bone or its deformation. Radiolucent areas associated with mild periostitis, endosteal scalloping, and intracortical tunnelling or subperiosteal gaps can be identified. When an abscess is present, it appears radiolucent and well defined by an inflammatory granulation tissue surrounded by spongy bone eburnation. In this case, a guided closed needle biopsy or aspiration can be performed to obtain a bacteriologic diagnosis. Nevertheless, the interpretation of such a pathological condition can be complicated by heterotopic ossification, demineralisation, and presence of air in the soft tissues. Negative scores with no diagnostic evidence of osteomyelitis are represented by the presence of a well-incorporated surface demineralisation and proliferation without signs of bony destruction.[73]

Wrobe et al.[74] report that plain films have a diagnostic sensitivity and specificity of 50% and 80% in identifying osteomyelitis in patients with diabetic foot, but recent studies by Larson et al. show that a plain x-ray has a sensitivity of 88%, when bone infection is demonstrated through a bone biopsy.[10] It is a first step radiological exam and, when positive, is helpful and useful to lead the suspect for pathologic conditions and to eventually exclude other pathologies. On the other hand, if negative, it does not exclude diagnosis of osteomyelitis. Most of the reduction of bone density may occur before it is detectable and it usually takes 10–21 days for an osseous change or lesion to become visible.[75]

In comparison to plain films, CT is a more expensive test but offers good resolution with the advantage of the possibility of manipulating the digital images. CT allows the operator to obtain information about the fibrous tissue surrounding the ulcer cavity, the position of ectopic bone (paraosteopathy), and the decreased volume of the fat planes or to evaluate the presence and thickness of a fibrotic wall when air is stored inside.[11] It may help to diagnose or better define deep, soft-tissue purulent collections and is usually needed to detect pathological findings or any signs of infectious reactivation in any skeletal location. A positive score is provided by evidences of intraosseous gas or abscess formation, direct contact with a soft-tissue abscess, cortical or medullary focal destruction, aggressive periosteal reaction, or exposed bone. All data can be elaborated with multi-planar or 3D reconstructions in order to obtain same anatomic images with better definition between muscle masses and a clear assessment of very small erosions of bone surfaces, located in areas that are not visible on conventional x-ray (anterior or posterior trochanter and ischial pubic branch). Local well-incorporated surface proliferation or sclerosis and simple demineralisation with no presence of trabecular or cortical destruction are not considered negative scores enough to make diagnosis of osteomyelitis. Even though it shows a lower sensitivity if compared to MRI, CT is considered superior for the detection of small necrotic bony fragments and abscesses, thanks to its excellent multi-planar reconstructions of the axial images.[76] It gives the operator the possibility to set the best surgical plan for a complete debridement of infected site, excision of soft-tissue fistulae, or guidance of interventional procedures (biopsies and aspirations).[77] In the same series cited before, Larson et al. report that the 50% of patients with biopsy-proven osteomyelitis could be identified by using a CT scan (88% for plain x-ray). On the other hand, if the percentage of patients with biopsy-proven osteomyelitis that were correctly identified as not having osteomyelitis by CT scan imaging was 85%, the results obtained with the conventional plain film did not exceed 32%.[10]

Plain radiography and CT scan may be useful in many cases, but MRI is more sensitive and specific, especially in differentiating between bone and soft-tissue infection. MRI relies on the mobile hydrogen concentration of blood and tissues to generate an image, and in particular, the difference in the concentration of water protons between the normal and abnormal bone marrow determines the ability of MRI to visualise areas of bone infection. It could be useful to help clarify CT findings providing additional information about the bone marrow and soft tissues. In fact, it can demonstrate marrow oedema and cortical erosion in addition to depicting adjacent soft-tissue changes, including deep collections and fistula formation.[78]

MRI is considered the modality of choice in cases of well-established osteomyelitis and in determining the extent of infection, since its sensitivity for a correct diagnosis ranges from 82% to 100%, with a specificity that varies between 75% and 96%.[79,80]

MRI is highly sensitive for detecting early-onset osteomyelitis (3–5 days),[81] though the interpretation of MRIs performed in SCI patients with pressure ulcers is frequently complicated by local conditions such as deformity of the pelvic skeleton, asymmetric muscle atrophy, subcutaneous oedema, myositis, and secondary bone modifications. For this reason, clinical correlation and risk factor considerations are very important to assist the MRI findings in achieving a correct diagnosis. Moreover, MRI plays a key role for identifying hidden, abnormal soft-tissue masses (squamous cell carcinoma) that sometimes develop at the level of the sinus tract in those patients with long history of non-healing wounds and concomitant bone infection.[82] According to Huang et al.,[58] who collected and compared the results deriving from MRI investigations, microbiological cultures, and histologic findings in SCI patients with pressure sores and suspect of osteomyelitis, MRI has an overall accuracy of 97%.

Different pulse sequences and imaging protocols can be used in the evaluation of this kind of patients and usually an MRI screening includes T1-weighted and T2-weighted spin-echo pulse sequences. Multi-plane images are produced and they represent useful tools in the hands of the surgeon to evaluate the extension of necrotic tissue, abscess, and infection to the adjacent areas and to determine the presence of heterotopic bone formation and the evidence of adjacent bone marrow oedema, in order to plan a correct surgical management of the lesions.[83]

Bone scintigraphy is one of the most frequently performed of all radionuclide procedures for the diagnosis of many different pathologic conditions, and it is the most sensitive and most specific imaging modality for the detection of osteomyelitis. Nevertheless, nuclear scintigraphy has a high false-positive rate and sometimes is not very helpful for the preoperative evaluation of pressure sores.[84,85] Three-phase bone scanning is the radionuclide procedure of choice for diagnosing osteomyelitis in a bone not affected by underlying conditions with a percentage of accuracy that approaches over 90%. It typically becomes positive within 24–48 h after the onset of symptoms and is fast, relatively inexpensive, widely available, and particularly sensitive in identifying bone multifocal involvement. The procedure is performed with technetium-99m-labelled diphosphonates that accumulate in bone by 2–6 h after injection, but complicating conditions such as grade IV pressure sores with overlying soft-tissue inflammation and reactive bone formation, recent trauma, surgery, placement of orthopaedic devices, or diabetes decrease the specificity, as the results are always positives.[86] In these kind of patients, when complicating conditions are superimposed, the WBCS was shown to be more specific compared with bone scans. It can be performed with indium111-labelled WBCs or *technetium-99m* HMPAO-labelled white cells.[87] Indium scanning involves the use of radiolabelled leukocytes that accumulate in sites of infection and inflammation and in the bone marrow. Approximately 50–60 mL of the patient's blood is previously taken and centrifuged to isolate WBCs that are subsequently exposed to indium. Images are taken in approximately 24 h after cells' reintroduction in patient's blood.

Melkun ET et al. reported on the efficacy of indium scanning in the chronic setting in patients with grade IV pressure ulcers to estimate the sensitivity, specificity, positive predictive value, and negative predictive value of this test.[88] They performed a bone biopsy and/or ostectomy specimen for tissue diagnosis in all patients who have undergone indium scanning and then compared their results with those of other diagnostic modalities used in these patients and the existing literature. The sensitivity and specificity obtained were 100% and 50%, respectively, with a positive predictive value of 63%.[54] High specificity and low sensitivity reflect the literature trend, and we believe that indium scanning has a limited role as a primary diagnostic test in patients with complicated pressure sores, since it is burdened by high costs and variable specificity limits and only allows to perform an exclusion diagnosis of osteomyelitis.[89]

42.15 TREATMENT

There is little agreement regarding the effective and appropriate surgical treatment of pressure ulcers.

In fact, even after surgery, complication rates vary from 16.6% to 46% and recurrence rates 12%–82%.[90] The management of pressure sores poses a significant reconstructive challenge for plastic surgeons and there is no overall consensus on whether musculocutaneous, fasciocutaneous, or perforator-based flaps provide superior results for treating pressure sores (Figures 42.11 through 42.13).[91]

Here we summarise the seven main points that are claimed to be the goals of treatment of pressure sores:

1. Total excisional debridement of the necrotic tissue, ulcer base, scar tissue, bursa, undermined skin (if not extensive), and heterotopic calcification
2. Excision of infected bone and bony prominence recontouring to eliminate isolated pressure points
3. Acquisition of haemostasis after debridement to healthy tissue and placement of low suction drainage(s), if appropriate
4. Obliteration of the anatomical dead space using muscle, myocutaneous, and/or de-epithelialised skin flaps to provide sufficient bulk to cushion bony prominences
5. Coverage of the wound with vascularised flaps placed to create a tension-free repair over the defect
6. Placement of the flap so as to position the stress point away from the suture line, a point of diminished blood flow
7. Restoration of the patient's activities of daily living before developing the pressure sore

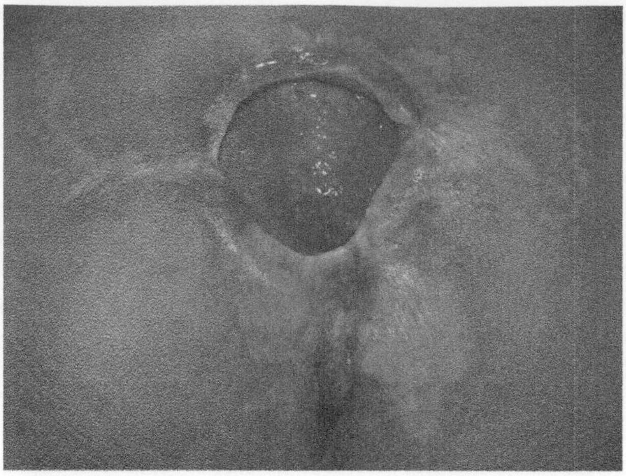

FIGURE 42.11 Clinical case: sacral pressure sore (preoperative view).

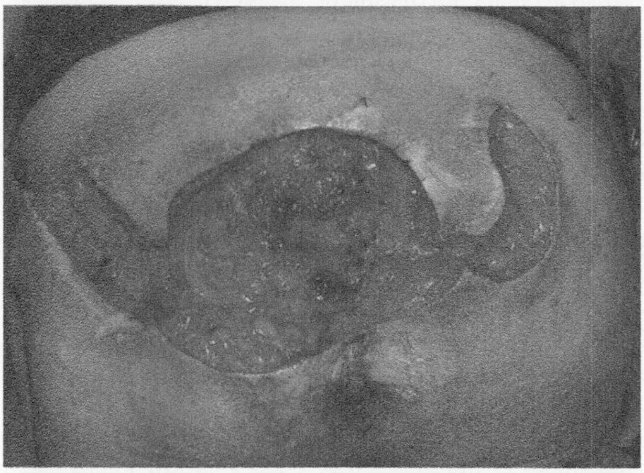

FIGURE 42.12 Clinical case: sacral pressure sore. Harvesting of local cutaneous flap (intraoperative view).

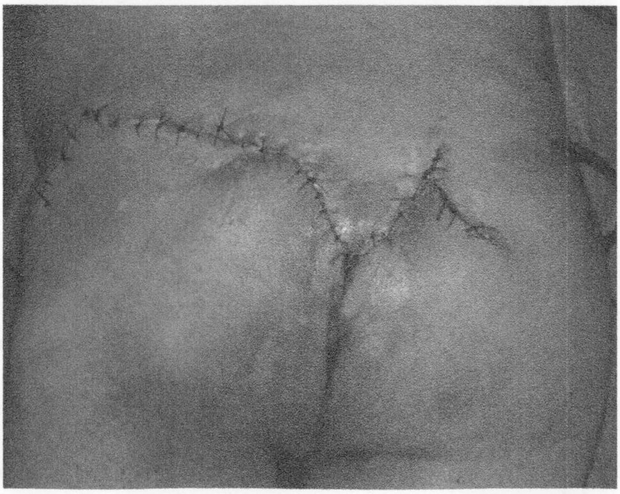

FIGURE 42.13 Clinical case: sacral pressure sore (postoperative view).

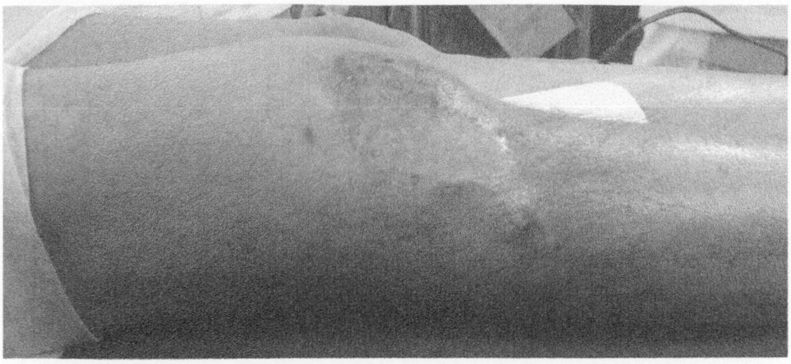

FIGURE 42.14 Clinical case: knee osteomyelitis. Patient previously underwent lateral gastrocnemius flap coverage (preoperative view).

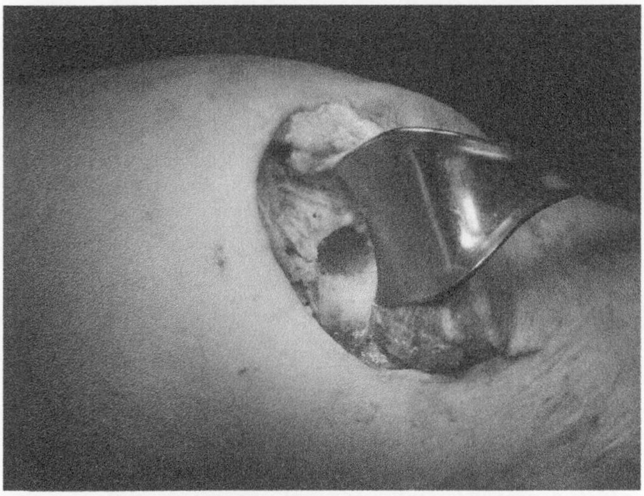

FIGURE 42.15 Clinical case: knee osteomyelitis (intraoperative view).

Despite the benefits deriving from of flap coverage, there are medically compromised patients who may not bear a surgical intervention (Figures 42.14 and 42.15). Nevertheless, surgery is often required for definitive treatment of stage III and IV pressure sores, with high early success rate but variable and not always satisfactory long-term results.[92]

There are many different techniques for the surgical repair of pressure sores, but for years, musculocutaneous flaps have been considered the first choice.[93]

Fasciocutaneous flaps and perforator-based flaps, respectively, described for the first time in 1988[94] and 1993,[95] have recently gained more and more popularity, showing to be a safe and reliable alternative to muscular transposition for pressure sores coverage.

The selection of the surgical technique may depend on different factors such as the type of patients (level of spinal cord injury, ambulatory status, daily habits, educational status, motivational level, co-morbidities, state of local tissues, nutritional status, etc.), the size and location of the ulcer, and whether we are treating it for the first time or it is a recurrent sore.

A musculocutaneous flap may be more appropriate for a large, deep ulcer (ischial and sacral coccygeal); in fact if the loss of subcutaneous tissue beyond the wound periphery is extensive, then it is difficult to obliterate the dead space with a fasciocutaneous flap. It usually finds its indication in cases complicated by osteomyelitis such as trochanteric pressure sores complicated by femoral head osteomyelitis and joint capsule involvement (e.g. vastus lateralis flap acts as a *carrier* for the antibiotic therapy and also obliterates dead spaces). The most popular myocutaneous flap is the gluteus maximus muscle that can be performed as a rotation flap, advancement island flap, or split flap.[96–98]

The main advantage offered by muscular flaps is that they represent good vascularised tissues for local antibiotic delivery. On the other hand, they present several disadvantages: They are invasive, provide a limited arc of rotation, and show an important atrophic degeneration with time, and, if used as primary option, they are not repeatable and, in case of pressure sore relapse, limit the possibility of secondary fasciocutaneous flap mobilisation, due to poor blood supply. Finally, covering pressure sores by muscle is contradictory to normal anatomy. In fact, the sacral area is normally muscular tissue free, and the muscular transposition changes the physiological point contact with abnormal body weight distribution, causing the possible onset of a new ischial pressure sore (Figures 42.16 through 42.20).

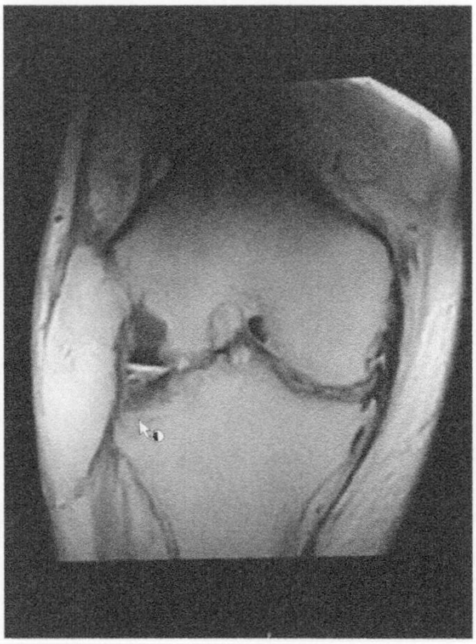

FIGURE 42.16 Knee osteomyelitis. MRI image: presence of bone sequestrum (coronal view).

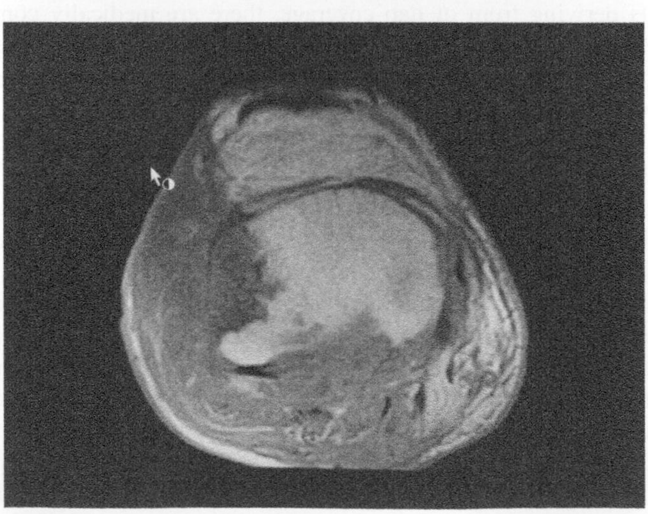

FIGURE 42.17 Knee osteomyelitis: MRI image (axial view).

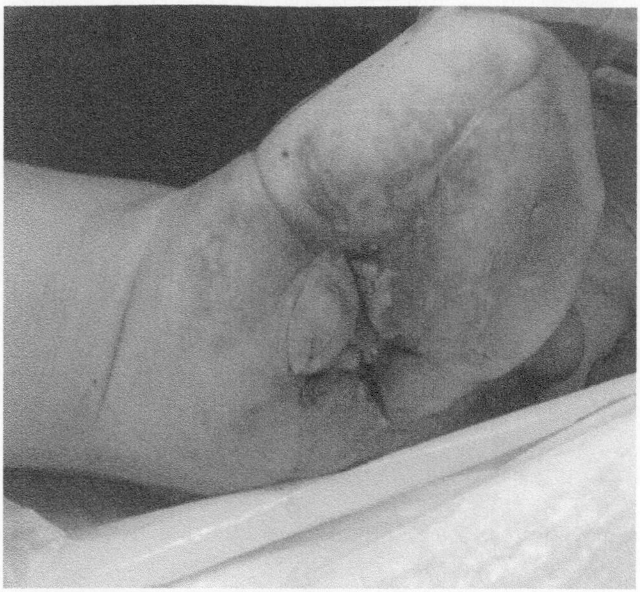

FIGURE 42.18 Clinical case: trochanteric pressure sore with osteomyelitis in paraplegic patient (preoperative view).

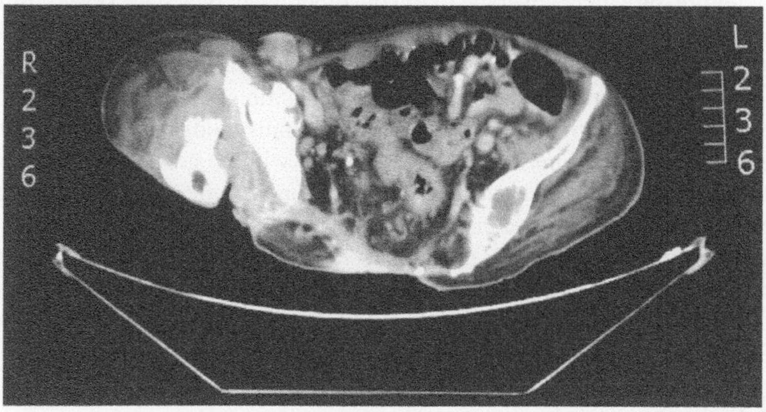

FIGURE 42.19 Trochanteric pressure sore with osteomyelitis in paraplegic patient: TC Image.

For this reason, fasciocutaneous flaps (gluteal rotation, posterior thigh, gluteal perforator, and transverse lumbar sacral for sacrum, ischium, and trochanter coverage) and perforator flaps (superior and inferior gluteal and island inferior gluteal thigh for sacrum, trochanter, and ischium coverage) could play an effective role for covering and filling these kinds of defects especially over pressure-bearing areas. Sameem et al. reviewed the literature for comparing musculocutaneous, fasciocutaneous, and perforator-based flaps for treatment of pressure sores and found no significant difference among these approaches in terms of complication or recurrence rates.[61]

Using fasciocutaneous and perforator-based flaps entails a muscle-/nerve-sparing and poorly invasive procedure, makes easier the simultaneous treatment of multiple lesions with minimal operative blood loss, decreases postoperative pain, shortens hospital stays, and reduces costs.

They were found to be appropriate to cover pressure sore and do not show a greater risk of wound breakdown or flap failure than musculocutaneous. In fact, the effects of constant pressure seem to be heavier on muscular tissues causing remarkable atrophic change and earlier ischaemia and

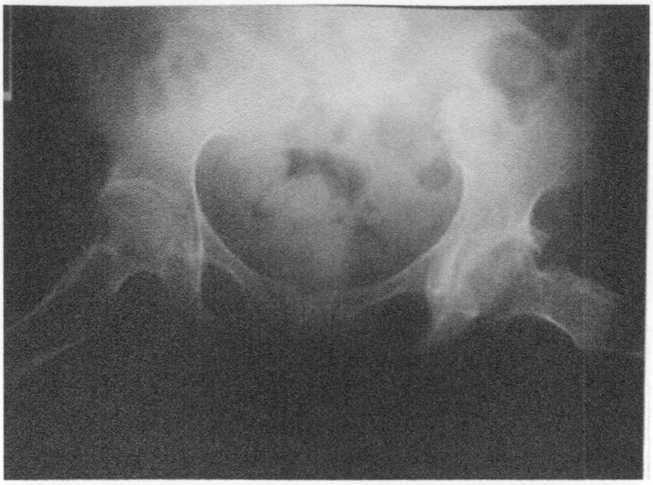

FIGURE 42.20 Osteomyelitis in paraplegic patient: plain RX image. Demineralisation and bone destruction, with inflammatory changes.

necrosis, than in cutaneous layers.[12,13,99] Fasciocutaneous and perforator flaps offer options for both advancement (in particular freestyle pedicled perforator-based flaps that are harvested directly adjacent to sores) and transposition, thanks to their longer pedicle, resulting in increased flexibility and versatility for pressure ulcer coverage.[100] On the other hand, they have several limitations: they are technically more difficult due to the meticulous pedicle dissection and susceptible to venous congestion. A multidisciplinary team plays a key role for a successful outcome. During surgery, a bone culture has to be performed to determine a targeted antibiotic therapy. To avoid excessive tension/pressure on flaps during the postoperative period, an air fluidised therapy bed is mandatory. This device also reduces the importance of nursing care with no need of regular turning on bed. The protocol foresees postoperative physical examination with interventions that include strategies to reduce extrinsic and intrinsic risk factors associated with tissue ischaemia, furthermore monitoring and optimising the patient's nutritional status. Neurological and psychiatric consulting registered neurologic status according to the standards of the American Spinal Injury Association (ASIA)[101] and functional status by the Functional Independence Measure (FIM).[102]

REFERENCES

1. Lipsky BA, Berendt AR, Deery HG et al. Diagnosis and treatment of diabetic foot infections. Infectious Diseases Society of America. *Plast Reconstr Surg* 2006;117(7 Suppl):212S–238S.
2. Bonham P. A critical review of the literature: Part I: Diagnosing osteomyelitis in patients with diabetes and foot ulcers. *J WOCN* 2001;28:73–88.
3. Anderson CA, Roukis TS. The diabetic foot. *Surg Clin N Am* 2007;87:1149–1177.
4. Frykberg RG, Zgonis T, Armstrong DG et al. Diabetic foot disorders: A clinical practice guideline (2006 revision). *J Foot Ankle Surg* 2006;45:S1–S66.
5. Croll SD, Nicholas GG, Osborne MA, Wasser TE, Jones S. Role of magnetic resonance imaging in the diagnosis of osteomyelitis in diabetic foot infections. *J Vasc Surg* 1996;24:266–270.
6. Keenan AM, Tindel NL, Alavi A. Diagnosis of pedal osteomyelitis in diabetic patients using current scintigraphic techniques. *Arch Intern Med* 1989;149:2262–2266.
7. Blume PA, Dey HM, Daley LJ, Arrighi JA, Soufer R, Gorecki GA. Diagnosis of pedal osteomyelitis with Tc-99m HMPAO labeled leukocytes. *J Foot Ankle Surg* 1997;36:120–126, discussion 160.
8. Devillers A, Moisan A, Hennion F, Garin E, Poirier JY, Bourguet P. Contribution of technetium-99m hexamethylpropylene amine oxime labelled leucocyte scintigraphy to the diagnosis of diabetic foot infection. *Eur J Nucl Med* 1998;25:132–138.

9. Fox IM, Zeiger L. Tc-99m-HMPAO leukocyte scintigraphy for the diagnosis of osteomyelitis in diabetic foot infections. *J Foot Ankle Surg* 1993;32:591–594.
10. Newman LG. Imaging techniques in the diabetic foot. *Clin Podiatr Med Surg* 1995;12:75–86.
11. Hughes DK. Nuclear medicine and infection detection: The relative effectiveness of imaging with 111In-Oxine-, 99mTc-HMPAO-, and 99mTc-stannous fluoride colloid-labeled leukocytes and with 67Ga-citrate. *J Nucl Med Technol* 2003;31(4):196–201; quiz 203–204.
12. Gill EA Jr, Stevens DL. Primary sternal osteomyelitis. *West J Med* 1989;151:199–203; Boll KL, Jurik AG. Sternal osteomyelitis in drug addicts. *J Bone Joint Surg Br* 1990;72:328–329; Narchi H. Primary sternal osteomyelitis in children with sickle cell disease. *Pediatr Infect Dis J* 1999;18:940–942.
13. Chen YL, Tsai SH, Hsu KC, Chen CS, Hsu CW. Primary sternal osteomyelitis due to *Peptostreptococcus anaerobius*. *Infection* 2012;40(2):195–197. Epub Aug 17, 2011.
14. Patel NV, Woznick AR, Welsh KS, Bendick PJ, Boura JA, Mucci SJ. Predictors of mortality after muscle flap advancement for deep sternal wound infections. *Plast Reconstr Surg* 2009;123(1):132–138.
15. Klesius AA, Dzemali O, Simon A, Kleine P, Abdel-Rahman U, Herzog C, Wimmer-Greinecker G, Moritz A. Successful treatment of deep sternal infections following open heart surgery by bilateral pectoralis major flaps. *Eur J Cardiothorac Surg* 2004;25(2):218–223.
16. Li AE, Fishman EK. Evaluations of complications after sternotomy using single- and multidetector CT with three-dimensional volume rendering. *AJR Am J Roentgenol* 2003;181:1065–1070.
17. Vogel H, Nagele B, Bleese N. X-Ray findings of the sternum after sternotomy (in German, English abstract). *Rontgen-Blatter* 1982;35:325–330.
18. Restrepo CS, Martinez S, Lemos DF, Washington L, McAdams HP, Vargas D, Lemos JA, Carrillo JA, Diethelm L. Imaging appearances of the sternum and sternoclavicular joints. *Radiographics* 2009;29(3):839–859.
19. Aslam M, Rajesh A, Entwisle J, Jeyapalan K. Pictorial review: MRI of the sternum and sternoclavicular joints. *Br J Radiol* 2002;75:627–634.
20. Turpin S, Lambert R. Role of scintigraphy in musculoskeletal and spinal infection. *Radiol Clin North Am* 2001;39:169–189.
21. Love C, Din AS, Tomas MB, Kalapparambath TP, Palestro CJ. Radionuclide bone imaging: An illustrative review. *Radiographics* 2003;23:341–358.
22. Rosenthall L, Lisbona R, Hernandez M et al. 99mTc-PP and 67Ga imaging following insertion of orthopedic devices. *Radiology* 1979;133:717–721.
23. Schauwecker DS, Park HM, Mock BH et al. Evaluation of complicating osteomyelitis with Tc-99m MDP, In-111 granulocytes, and Ga-67 citrate. *J Nucl Med* 1984;25:849–853.
24. Schauwecker DS. The scintigraphic diagnosis of osteomyelitis. *AJR Am J Roentgenol* 1992;158:9–18.
25. Palestro CJ, Torres MA. Radionuclide imaging in orthopedic infections. *Semin Nucl Med* 1997;27:334–345.
26. Browdie DA, Berustein RV, Agnew K, Damie A, Fischer M, Balz J. Diagnosis of poststernotomy infection: Comparison of three means of assessment. *Ann Thorac Surg* 1991;51:290–292.
27. Bessette PR, Hanson MJ, Czarnecki DJ, Yuilie DL, Rankin JJ. Evaluation of postoperative osteomyelitis of the sternum comparing CT and dual Tc-99m MDP hone and ln-111 WBC SPECT. *Clin Nucl Med* 1993;18:197–202.
28. Jeevanandam V, Smith CR, Rose EA, Malm JR, Hugo NE. Single stage management of sternal wound infections. *J Thorac Cardiovasc Surg* 1990;99:256–263.
29. Schumacher Jr. HB, Mandelbaum I. Continuous antibiotic irrigation in the treatment of infection. *Arch Surg* 1963;86:384–387.
30. Molina JE. Primary closure for infected dehiscence of the sternum. *Ann Thorac Surg* 1993;55:459–463.
31. Levi N, Olsen PS. Primary closure of deep sternal wound infection following open heart surgery: A safe operation? *J Cardiovasc Surg* 2000;41:241–245.
32. Krabatsch T, Fleck E, Hetzer R. Treating poststernotomy mediastinitis by transposition of the greater omentum: Late angiographic findings. *J Card Surg* 1995;10(1):46–51.
33. Lopez-Monjardin H, de-la-Pena-Salcedo A, Mendoza-Munoz M, Lopez-Yanez-de-la-Pena A, Palacio-Lopez E, Lopez-Garcia A. Omentum flap versus pectoralis major flap in the treatment of mediastinitis. *Plast Reconstr Surg* 1998;101(6):1481–1485.
34. Seguin JR, Loisance DY. Omental transposition for closure of median sternotomy following severe mediastinal and vascular infection. *Chest* 1985;88:684–690.
35. Loose R, Birekandt S, Möller F. Deep sternal wound complications after CABG with unilateral and bilateral internal thoracic artery grafts in diabetic patients. *J Thorac Cardiovasc Surg* 2000;48(Suppl 1):48.

36. Castello JR, Centella T, Garro L, Barros J, Oliva E, Sanchez-Olaso A, Epeldegui A. Muscle flap reconstruction for the treatment of major sternal wound infections after cardiac surgery: A 10-year analysis. *Scand J Plast Renonstr Surg Hand Surg* 1999;67(2):462–465.
37. Yasuura K, Okamoto H, Morita S, Ogawa Y, Sawazaki M, Seki A, Masumoto H, Matsuura A, Maseki T, Torii S. Results of omental flap transposition for deep sternal wound infection after cardiovascular surgery. *Ann Surg* 1999;227(3):455–459.
38. Bauer J, Phillips LG. MOC-PSSM CME article: Pressure sores. *Plast Reconstr Surg* 2008 Jan;121(1 Suppl):1–10.
39. Agrawal K, Chauhan N. Pressure ulcers: Back to the basics. *Indian J Plast Surg* 2012;45(2):244–254.
40. EPUAP. 2003. European Pressure Ulcer Advisory Panel. Volume 5, number 2, 2003.
41. Matsui Y, Furue M, Sanada H, Tachibana T, Nakayama T, Sugama J, Furuta K, Tachi M, Tokunaga K, Miyachi Y. Development of the DESIGN-R with an observational study: An absolute evaluation tool for monitoring pressure ulcer wound healing. *Wound Repair Regen* 2011;19(3):309–315.
42. Bass MJ, Phillips LG. Pressure sores. *Curr Probl Surg* 2007;44(2):101–143. Review.
43. Ruan CM, Escobedo E, Harrison S, Goldstein B. Magnetic resonance imaging of nonhealing pressure ulcers and myocutaneous flaps. *Arch Phys Med Rehabil* 1998;79(9):1080–1088.
44. Deficit Reduction Act of 2005, Section 5001. Hospital Quality Improvement, Centers for Medicare and Medicaid Services (CMS). 2005.
45. The National Quality Forum (NQF) on Serious Reportable Events (SRE's) in Healthcare. 2002.
46. Hauptfleisch J, Meagher TM, Hughes RJ, Singh JP, Graham A, López de Heredia L. Interobserver agreement of magnetic resonance imaging signs of osteomyelitis in pelvic pressure ulcers in patients with spinal cord injury. *Arch Phys Med Rehabil* 2013 June;94(6):1107–1111.
47. Larson DL, Gilstrap J, Simonelic K, Carrera GF. Is there a simple, definitive, and cost-effective way to diagnose osteomyelitis in the pressure ulcer patient? *Plast Reconstr Surg* 2011;127(2):670–676.
48. European Pressure Ulcer Advisory Panel and National Pressure Ulcer Advisory Panel. *Prevention and Treatment of Pressure Ulcers: Quick Reference Guide*. Washington, DC: National Pressure Ulcer Advisory Panel. 2009.
49. Yabunaka K, Iizaka S, Nakagami G, Aoi N, Kadono T, Koyanagi H, Uno M, Ohue M, Sanada S, Sanada H. Can ultrasonographic evaluation of subcutaneous fat predict pressure ulceration? *J Wound Care* 2009;18(5):192,194,196.
50. Quintavalle PR, Lyder CH, Mertz PJ, Phillips-Jones C, Dyson M. Use of high-resolution, high-frequency diagnostic ultrasound to investigate the pathogenesis of pressure ulcer development. *Adv Skin Wound Care* 2006;19(9):498–505.
51. Rifai A, Nyman R. Scintigraphy and ultrasonography in differentiating osteomyelitis from bone infarction in sickle cell disease. *Acta Radiol* 1997;38:139.
52. Esposito G, Ziccardi P, Meoli S et al. Multiple CT imaging in pressure sores. *Plast Reconstr Surg* 1994;94:333–342.
53. Burdge DR, Gribble MJ. Histologically proven pressure sore related osteomyelitis in the setting of negative technetium bone scans. *Am J Phys Med Rehabil* 1993;72:386–389.
54. Sugarman B. Infection and pressure sores. *Arch Phys Med Rehabil* 1985;66:177–179.
55. Sugarman B. Pressure sores and underlying bone infection. *Arch Intern Med* 1987;147:553–555.
56. Lewis VL, Bailey MH, Pulawski G, Kind G, Bashioum RW, Hendrix RW. The diagnosis of osteomyelitis in patients with pressure sores. *Plast Reconstr Surg* 1988;81:229–232.
57. Thomhill-James M, Gonzales F, Stewart CA, Kanel GC, Lee GC, Capen DA. Osteomyelitis associated with pressure ulcers. *Arch Phys Med Rehabil* 1986;67:314–318.
58. Huang AB, Schweitzer ME, Hume E, Batte WG. Osteomyelitis of the pelvis/hips in paralyzed patients: Accuracy and clinical utility of MRI. *J Comput Assist Tomogr* 1998;22:437–443.
59. Sammak B, Abd El Bagi M, Al Shahed M et al. Osteomyelitis: A review of currently used imaging techniques. *Eur Radiol* 1999;9:894–900.
60. Daniali LN, Keys K, Katz D, Mathes DW. Effect of preoperative magnetic resonance imaging diagnosis of osteomyelitis on the surgical management and outcomes of pressure ulcers. *Ann Plast Surg* 2011;67:520–525.
61. Greco M, Marchetti F, Tempesta M, Ruggiero M, Marcasciano M, Carlesimo B. Cutaneous flaps in the treatment of 338 pressure sores: a better choice. *Ann Ital Chir*. 2013 Nov–Dec;84(6):655–659.
62. Krause JS, Carter RE, Pickelsimer EE, Wilson D. A prospective study of health and risk of mortality after spinal cord injury. *Arch Phys Med Rehabil* 2008;89:1482–1491.
63. Raghavan P, Raza WA, Ahmed YS, Chamberlain MA. Prevalence of pressure sores in a community sample of spinal injury patients. *Clin Rehabil* 2003;17:879–884.

64. Fuhrer MJ, Garber SL, Rintala DH, Clearman R, Hart KA. Pressure ulcers in community-resident persons with spinal cord injury: Prevalence and risk factors. *Arch Phys Med Rehabil* 1993;74:1172.
65. Grayson ML, Gibbons GW, Balogh K, Levin E, Karchmer AW. Probing to bone in infected pedal ulcers: A clinical sign of underlying osteomyelitis in diabetic patients. *JAMA* 1995;273:721–723.
66. Lipsky BA, Berendt AR, Cornia PB et al. 2012 Infectious Diseases Society of America clinical practice guideline for the diagnosis and treatment of diabetic foot infections. *J Am Podiatr Med Assoc* 2013;103(1):2–7.
67. Darouiche RO, Landon GC, Klima M, Musher DM, Markowski J. Osteomyelitis associated with pressure ulcers. *Arch Intern Med* 1994;154:753–758.
68. Hartemann-Heurtier A, Senneville E. Diabetic foot osteomyelitis. *Diabetes Metab* 2008;34:87–95.
69. Waldvogel FA, Medoff G, Swartz MN. Osteomyelitis: A review of clinical features, therapeutic considerations and unusual aspects. *N Engl J Med* 1970;282:198–206.
70. Santiago Restrepo C, Giménez CR, McCarthy K. Imaging of osteomyelitis and musculoskeletal soft tissue infections: Current concepts. *Rheum Dis Clin North Am* 2003;29(1):89–109. Review.
71. Han H, Lewis VL Jr, Wiedrich TA, Patel PK. The value of Jamshidi core needle bone biopsy in predicting postoperative osteomyelitis in grade IV pressure ulcer patients. *Plast Reconstr Surg* 2002;110(1):118–122.
72. Hendrix RW, Calenoff L, Lederman RB, Nieman HL. Radiology of pressure sores. *Radiology* 1981;138(2):351–356. PubMed PMID: 7455114.
73. Lewis VL Jr, Bailey MH, Pulawski G, Kind G, Bashioum RW, Hendrix RW. The diagnosis of osteomyelitis in patients with pressure sores. *Plast Reconstr Surg* 1988;81(2):229–232.
74. Wrobel JS, Connolly JE. Making the diagnosis of osteomyelitis: The role of prevalence. *J Am Podiatr Med Assoc* 1998;88:337–343.
75. Pineda C, Vargas A, Rodríguez AV. Imaging of osteomyelitis: Current concepts. *Infect Dis Clin North Am* 2006;20(4):789–825. Review.
76. Ram PC, Martinez S, Korobin M et al. CT detection of intraosseous gas: A new sign of osteomyelitis. *AJR Am J Roentgenol* 1981;137:721–723.
77. Bohndorf K. Infection of the appendicular skeleton. *Eur Radiol* 2004;14:E53–E63.
78. Rennert R, Golinko M, Yan A, Flattau A, Tomic-Canic M, Brem H. Developing and evaluating outcomes of an evidence-based protocol for the treatment of osteomyelitis in stage IV pressure ulcers: A literature and wound electronic medical record database review. *Ostomy Wound Manage* 2009;55:42–53.
79. Mahnken AH, Bucker A, Adam G, Gunther RW. MRI of osteomyelitis: Sensitivity and specificity of STIR sequences in comparison with contrast enhanced T1 spin echo sequences. *Rofo* 2000;172:1016–1019.
80. Schmid MR, Hodler J, Vienne P, Binkert CA, Zanetti M. Bone marrow abnormalities of foot and ankle: STIR versus T1-weighted contrast enhanced fat-suppressed spin-echo MR imaging. *Radiology* 2002;224:463–469.
81. Kocher M, Lee B, Dolan M et al. Pediatric orthopedic infections: Early detection and treatment. *Pediatr Ann* 2006;35:112–122.
82. Luchs JS, Hines J, Katz DS. MR imaging of squamous cell carcinoma complicating chronic osteomyelitis of the femur. *Am J Roentgenol* 2002;178:512–513.
83. Flemming D, Murphey M, McCarthy K. Imaging of the foot and ankle: Summary and update. *Curr Opin Orthop* 2005;16:54–59.
84. Bauer J, Phillips LG. MOC-PSSM CME article: Pressure sores. *Plast Reconstr Surg* 2008;121(1 Suppl):1–10. doi: 10.1097/01.prs.0000294671.05159.27. Review.
85. Rubayi S, Chandrasekhar BS. Trunk, abdomen, and pressure sore reconstruction. *Plast Reconstr Surg* 2011;128(3):201e–215e.
86. Peters AM. The use of nuclear medicine in infections. *Br J Radiol* 1998;71:252–261.
87. Merkel KD, Brown ML, Dewanjee MK et al. Comparison of Indium-labeled leukocyte imaging with sequential technetium–gallium scanning in diagnosis of low grade musculoskeletal sepsis. *J Bone Joint Surg Am* 1985;67:465–476.
88. Melkun ET, Lewis VL Jr. Evaluation of (111) indium-labeled autologous leukocyte scintigraphy for the diagnosis of chronic osteomyelitis in patients with grade IV pressure ulcers, as compared with a standard diagnostic protocol. *Ann Plast Surg* 2005;54(6):633–636.
89. Kolindou A, Liu Y, Ozker K et al. In-111 WBC imaging of osteomyelitis in patients with underlying bone scan abnormalities. *Clin Nucl Med* 1996;21:183–191.
90. Larson DL, Hudak KA, Waring WP, Orr MR, Simonelic K. Protocol management of late-stage pressure ulcers: A 5-year retrospective study of 101 consecutive patients with 179 ulcers. *Plast Reconstr Surg* 2012;129(4):897–904.

91. Sameem M, Au M, Wood T, Farrokhyar F, Mahoney J. A systematic review of complication and recurrence rates of musculocutaneous, fasciocutaneous, and perforator-based flaps for treatment of pressure sores. *Plast Reconstr Surg* 2012;130(1):67e–77e. doi: 10.1097/PRS.0b013e318254b19f. Review.
92. Thiessen FE, Andrades P, Blondeel PN, Hamdi M, Roche N, Stillaert F, Van Landuyt K, Monstrey S. Flap surgery for pressure sores: Should the underlying muscle be transferred or not? *J Plast Reconstr Aesthet Surg* 2011;64(1):84–90.
93. Ger R, Levine SA. The management of decubitus ulcers by muscle transposition. An 8-year review. *Plast Reconstr Surg* 1976;58:419–428.
94. Park C, Park BY. Fasciocutaneous V-Y advancement flap for repair of sacral defects. *Ann Plast Surg* 1988;21:23–26.
95. Koshima I, Moriguchi T, Soeda S, Kawata S, Ohta S, Ikeda A. The gluteal perforator-based flap for repair of sacral pressure sores. *Plast Reconstr Surg* 1993;91:678–683.
96. Parkash S, Banerjee S. The total gluteus maximus rotation and other gluteus maximus musculocutaneous flaps in the treatment of pressure ulcers. *Br J Plast Surg* 1986;39:66–71.
97. Rees RS, Reilley AF, Nanney LB, Lynch JB. Sacral pressure sores: Treatment with island gluteus maximus musculocutaneous flaps. *South Med J* 1985;78:1147–1151.
98. Rubayi S, Doyle BS. The gluteus maximus muscle splitting myocutaneous flap for treatment of sacral and coccygeal pressure ulcer. *Plast Reconstr Surg* 1995;96:1366–1371.
99. Nola GT, Vistnes LM. Differential response of skin and muscle in the experimental production of pressure sores. *Plast Reconstr Surg* 1980;66:728e33.
100. Coskunfirat OK, Ozgentas HE. Gluteal perforator flaps for coverage of pressure sores at various locations. *Plast Reconstr Surg* 2004;113:2012–2017.
101. Kirshblum SC, Waring W, Biering-Sorensen F et al. Reference for the 2011 revision of the International Standards for Neurological Classification of Spinal Cord Injury. *J Spinal Cord Med* 2011;34(6):547–554.
102. Young Y, Fan MY, Hebel JR, Boult C. Concurrent validity of administering the functional independence measure (FIM) instrument by interview. *Am J Phys Med Rehabil* 2009;88(9):766–770.

43 Image Guided 3D Printing and Haptic Modelling in Plastic Surgery

Michael P. Chae, David J. Hunter-Smith, and Warren M. Rozen

CONTENTS

43.1 BACKGROUND

Modern imaging techniques have become an essential component of preoperative planning in plastic surgery. In the last decade, computed tomographic angiography (CTA) has demonstrated a reliable and accurate method of characterising a flap in perforator flap surgery for the selection of donor site, flap, perforator, and the optimal mode of dissection (Rozen et al. 2008,b,c). Furthermore, CTA has been shown to minimise donor site morbidity and improve operative outcomes in breast reconstruction (Rozen et al. 2008a). Recently, three-dimensional (3D) and 4D CTA have emerged, producing superior spatial resolution of perforator vessels, their vascular territory, and the dynamic flow characteristics (Colohan et al. 2012, Nie et al. 2013). However, all current imaging modalities are limited by being represented in 2D on a flat surface, like a computer screen or a hard film. A 3D-printed haptic model can provide a tactile feedback to the surgeon and, hence, a superior anatomical representation for surgical planning.

43.2 INTRODUCTION TO 3D PRINTING

3D printing is a form of rapid prototyping (RP) where a physical model is fabricated from 3D design achieved by computer-aided design process or directly from a medical imaging modality, such as computed tomography (CT) and magnetic resonance imaging (MRI) (Goiato et al. 2011).

RP or additive manufacturing has been utilised in industrial design for more than three decades, but it has only come to the fore in medical application in the last decade. Using an appropriate medical imaging software, such as Osirix (Pixmeo, Geneva, Switzerland) and 3D Slicer (Version 4.3, Surgical Planning Laboratory, Boston, MA), routine CT or MRI data can be reconstructed in 3D and manipulated to produce a virtual model of the organ or tissue of interest. This data can be sectioned into ultrathin data slices suitable for 3D printing using a 3D printer software, such as Cube software (Version 2.0.1, 3D Systems, Rock Hill, SC).

For surgeons, RP technologies have demonstrated a significant potential as a visualisation tool that can be an effective addition alongside the conventional imaging methods for preoperative planning and intraoperative surgical guidance. Numerous surgical disciplines have reported the usefulness of RP and its beneficial effect on clinical outcome, such as maxillofacial surgery (Cohen et al. 2009), orthopaedic surgery (Chen et al. 2012), neurosurgery (D'Urso et al. 2000, Wurm et al. 2004), cardiac surgery (Mottl-Link et al. 2008), and ear, nose, throat surgery (Suzuki et al. 2004).

For medical application, stereolithography, selective laser sintering (SLS), and 3D printing are currently the most commonly used RP technologies. Stereolithography is the earliest 3D technology described where a liquid polymer media is placed in a vat for *curing* with laser into an ultraviolet-sensitive solid resin (Hannen 2006, Rozen et al. 2012a,b). The end product must be *cured* in a UV chamber and the support structures, produced at the same time, must be removed manually by hand. Stereolithography is currently considered a *gold standard* for medical RP and can produce models accurate to 0.1 mm (Cohen et al. 2009). Moreover, its efficiency increases as larger products are manufactured and it can reproduce the inner structures accurately and reliably (Ono et al. 1994). The disadvantages are that stereolithography is labour intensive, requires more than a day to produce a large model, and is associated with high costs for materials and maintenance, and, hence, more expensive compared to SLS (Herlin et al. 2011) and 3D printing (Cohen et al. 2009).

SLS describes a process where small particles of thermoplastic, metal, ceramic, or glass powder on a build tray are selectively fused by a high-power laser as dictated by the computer-aided design (Rengier et al. 2010). Once a layer of sintering is completed, the build tray is lowered and then, filled with the particles for solidification by laser beams. The unsintered powders can be removed or brushed away at the end, leaving only the final product. The main advantage of SLS lies in its ability to build without requiring support structures due to the surrounding unsintered powders. In comparison, 3D models by stereolithography and 3D printing necessitate simultaneous fabrication of the support structures for certain designs. Although they can be manually removed, for example, using a surgical needle holder, the aftermath leaves sufficient damage to the surface superficially. Hence, SLS potentially produces smoother models and uses less amount of materials, leading to cost savings. However, SLS is still significantly more expensive than 3D printing (Mottl-Link et al. 2008).

3D printing consists of a number of techniques where the material is ejected from a single nozzle and deposited onto a build tray in a layer-by-layer fashion for the production of a physical model that can be handled afterwards immediately without any curing (Cohen et al. 2009).

43.3 TYPES OF 3D PRINTING

3D printing technology can be primarily divided into fused deposition modelling (FDM) or inkjet modelling. First described by S. Scott Crump two decades ago (US patent: US5121329 A), FDM is the most commonly used technique where melted filament of thermoplastic material is extruded through a single nozzle and solidifies after it is deposited (Cohen et al. 2009, Gerstle et al. 2014). Polylactic acid (PLA) and acrylonitrile–butadiene–styrene (ABS) are the most commonly used materials for FDM in household 3D printers, such as Cube 2 printer (Figure 43.1).

Inkjet 3D printers eject, from a single nozzle, droplets of melted thermoplastic materials for build and wax for support scaffolding. After the deposition of each layer, the surface is smoothed out using a milling head and residual particles are blown away by vacuum. Inkjet technology produces precise models with smooth surfaces, but at a slow speed. This has been recently overcome by

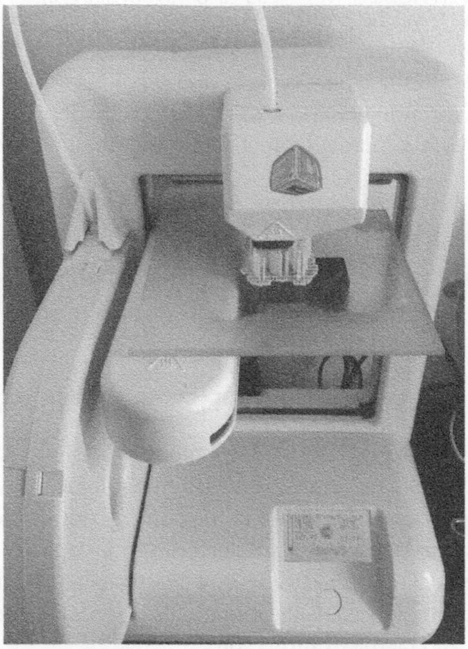

FIGURE 43.1 An office-based 3D printer (Cube 2, 3D Systems, Rock Hill, SC) using FDM technology and fluorescent green-coloured PLA filament.

Multijet printing technology (3D Systems, Rock Hill, SC) and PolyJet technology (Stratasys, Edina, MN) where materials are ejected from multiple nozzles. Unfortunately, with the current technology, only few material options are available for inkjet printing.

43.4 ADVANTAGES AND DISADVANTAGES OF 3D PRINTING

Advantages of 3D printing stem from the haptic models that provide a tactile feedback to the user, in addition to their accurate 3D visualisation of the anatomy. A surgeon can interact hands on with the model and appreciate the potential patient-specific anatomical details and the spatial relationship between certain parts. The tactile quality of the physical model produces superior spatial information than a 3D visualisation or a 2D image (Way and Barner 1997), and they can also be used to improve physician communication with patients. In plastic and reconstructive surgery, this information can be useful in designing free flaps (Chae et al. 2014b). Furthermore, having a solid model in one's hands enables one to simulate complex movements, such as temporomandibular joint (TMJ) movements, that are difficult to replicate using 3D imaginations in a computer software (Chen et al. 2014). Some authors have been able to simulate operative procedures on 3D biomodels (Stoker et al. 1992, Heissler et al. 1998, D'Urso et al. 1999, Mavili et al. 2007). As a result, biomodels have been numerously reported to reduce the length of operation, leading to multiple benefits, such as reduced exposure to general anaesthesia, shortened wound exposure time, and decreased intraoperative blood loss (D'Urso et al. 1999, Guarino et al. 2007, Rozen et al. 2012b).

Recent advancements in 3D printers have enabled the production of quality biomodels in high resolution using materials, such as PLA, that are shown to be light, tough, biocompatible, easy to fabricate, and uniform in quality (Xu et al. 2010). Moreover, 3D printers are faster, cheaper, and are a superior option for manufacturing smaller, more complex models in comparison to stereolithography (Cohen et al. 2009).

The most significant disadvantage of 3D printing is related to cost. Amongst the most well-known brands, the cost of a professional 3D printer ranges between USD 40,000 and 300,000 [unpublished data]. Fortunately, the technology has become more widely available and personal 3D printers can currently be purchased at USD 1300–5000. Despite being faster than stereolithography, 3D printing is still a relatively time-consuming process (Wurm et al. 2004). Furthermore, users relying on a third-party company for 3D printing would have to wait lengthy periods for the delivery. In addition, most of current standard 3D print materials, such as PLA and ABS, are hard and make it difficult to simulate operative procedures like cutting biomodels using a scalpel (Mottl-Link et al. 2008).

43.5 3D PRINTING IN PLASTIC SURGERY

3D printed haptic biomodels can be potentially valuable in plastic surgery by facilitating preoperative planning, education, and individualised prosthesis manufacturing.

43.6 PREOPERATIVE PLANNING: SOFT TISSUE MAPPING

Perforator flap surgery is routinely performed by reconstructive surgeons for the correction of large soft tissue defects and breast reconstructions after oncological resection. CTA is the imaging modality of choice for the selection of donor site, flap, and perforator for free flap transfer, as well as flap and perforator selection for locoregional perforator flap options (Rozen et al. 2008c, 2011). Furthermore, evidences demonstrate that these benefits translate to improved clinical outcomes (Rozen et al. 2008a,b). In addition to CTA, the biomodels can provide an additional layer of clinical information through visual and tactile examination.

Recently, we reported a case where a *reverse model* of an ankle soft tissue defect (Figure 43.2) was 3D printed for preoperative planning (Chae et al. 2014b). CT scan data of the patient's lower limbs was reconstructed into a 3D image using Osirix (Pixmeo, Geneva, Switzerland) and exported in STL (standard tessellation language) file format. Using Magics (Materialise, Leuven, Belgium), a mirror image of the normal contralateral ankle was created (Figure 43.3). This was virtually superimposed onto the pathological ankle, which was then subtracted away, leaving only the *reverse*

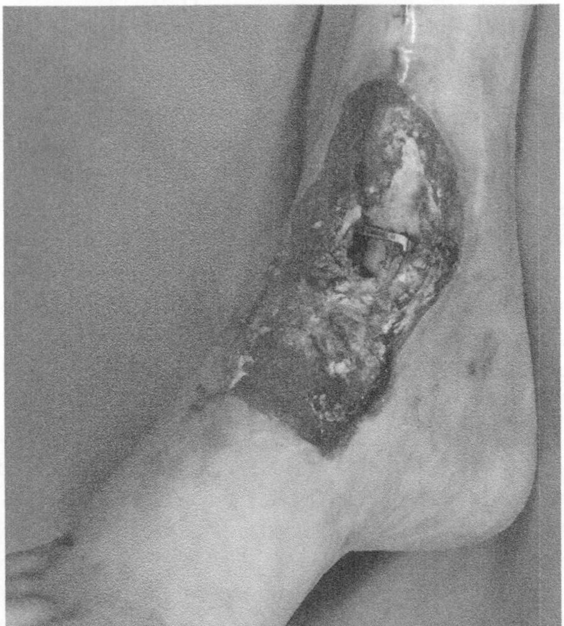

FIGURE 43.2 Photograph of the soft tissue ankle defect. (Reprinted from Chae, M.P. et al., *Microsurgery*, in press. With permission.)

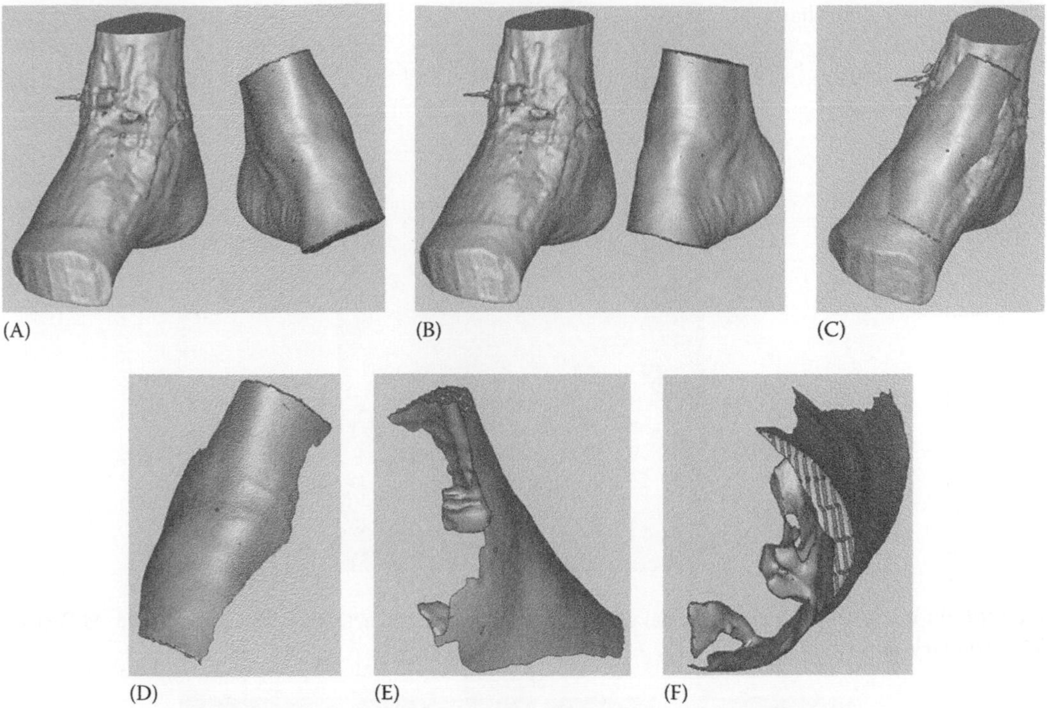

FIGURE 43.3 3D images of the ankle defect and the normal contralateral side are superimposed onto each other and, then, subtracted on Magics software (Materialise, Leuven, Belgium) to create a *reverse image* representing the defect. (Reprinted from Chae, M.P. et al., *Microsurgery*, in press. With permission.)

image representing the defect. 3D image of the donor site (i.e., forearm) was similarly created using Magics. The *reverse image* was placed initially alongside and then, superimposed onto the forearm. From this, spatial information, such as the depth and width of the defect compared to the thickness and width of the forearm respectively, could be gathered. Both the ankle and the defect were preoperatively 3D printed using PLA filament and a Cube 2 printer (3D Systems, Rock Hill, SC) (Figures 43.4 and 43.5). Interestingly, using FDM 3D printer to print the ankle in anatomical position led to the wound defect being filled with support structures. Although they were easily removable, this made the surface appear rough affecting its aesthetics. This could have been prevented by printing the models in an orientation where the defect is pointing up. Of note, the ankle and *reverse model* took 12.5 and 8.5 h, respectively, to print and together, they required approximately 75% of the entire printer cartridge (worth USD 54).

43.7 PREOPERATIVE PLANNING: VASCULAR MAPPING

Using the same technique, we attempted to 3D print perforator anatomy from a CTA data for a deep inferior epigastric artery perforator (DIEP) flap breast reconstruction. The biomodel made the process of appreciating the arterial anatomy and its relationship with bony landmarks was intuitive and useful. One of the major drawbacks was that the model was scaled down significantly in order to fit within the maximum print dimensions on our Cube 2 printer (i.e., 15.6 × 15.6 × 15.6 mm). As 3D printing becomes more widespread, printers able to produce large dimensions may become more affordable. Furthermore, the current technique precluded perforators from deep inferior epigastric artery (DIEA) being printed. Interestingly, the Cube 2 printer can potentially print to a resolution of 200 μm. However, the software 3D Slicer (Surgical Planning Laboratory, Boston, MA) could only 3D reconstruct the DIEA and not its perforators. 3D Slicer is a rapidly evolving open-source software

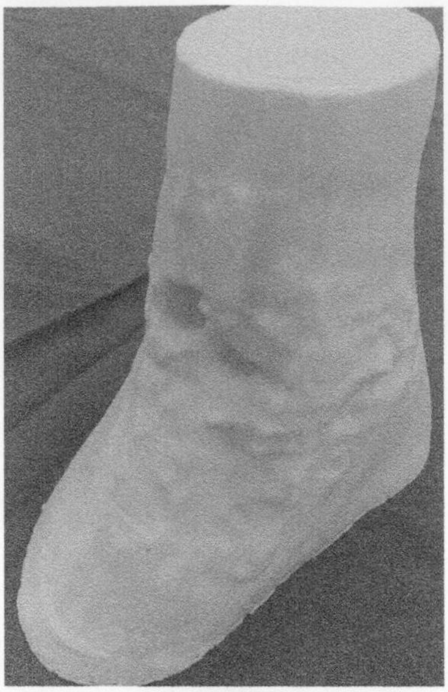

FIGURE 43.4 3D printed haptic model of the soft tissue ankle defect. (Reprinted from Chae, M.P. et al., *Microsurgery*, in press.)

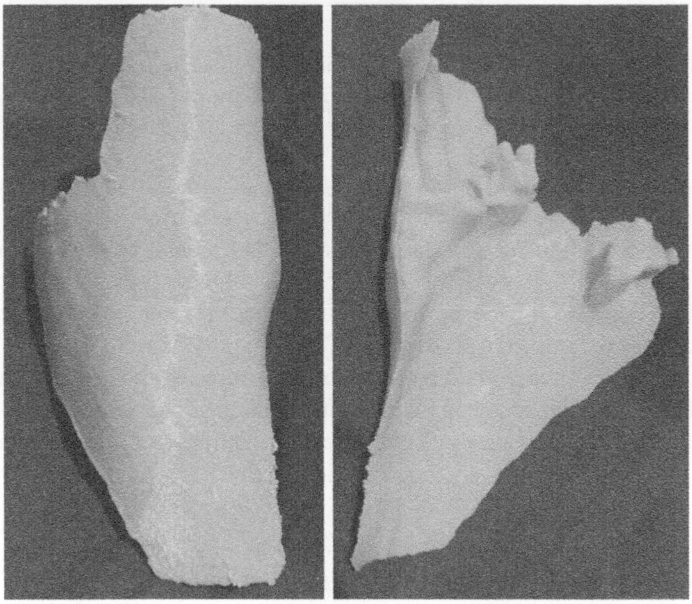

FIGURE 43.5 3D printed haptic model of the ankle defect alongside the *reverse model* representing the defect. (Reprinted from Chae, M.P. et al., *Microsurgery*, in press. With permission.)

platform, and hence, we would expect the software resolution to improve and match the printers soon. Of note, the printing took 42 h and approximately 55% of the entire cartridge. This is due to a significant amount of *noise* detected during the 3D reconstruction process, leading to an excessive amount of support structures being printed. In the future, this can be prevented by installing a *segmentation* technique, such as open-source Vascular Modeling Toolkit (VMTK, Orobix, Bergamo, Italy).

3D printing can be a valuable for volumetric analysis. Volume assessment is an important aspect of preoperative planning for breast reconstructive surgery. Currently, plastic surgeons rely on

2D photography or 3D imaging, such as VECTRA (Canfield Imaging Systems, Fairfield, NJ) and subjective visual assessment. Pitfalls with using 3D photography like VECTRA is the presence of chest wall asymmetry, leading to asymmetrical appearance superficially despite having equal breast volumes. A recent report (Chae et al. 2014a) presented a case of breast asymmetry where Osirix (Pixmeo, Geneva, Switzerland) was used to calculate the volume difference between the breasts, excluding the chest wall, using their routine chest CT data (Figure 43.6). Using the same technique as above, the breasts were 3D printed, illustrating the difference in volume (Figure 43.7). We have subsequently used this same approach and same technology to print soft tissue defects in

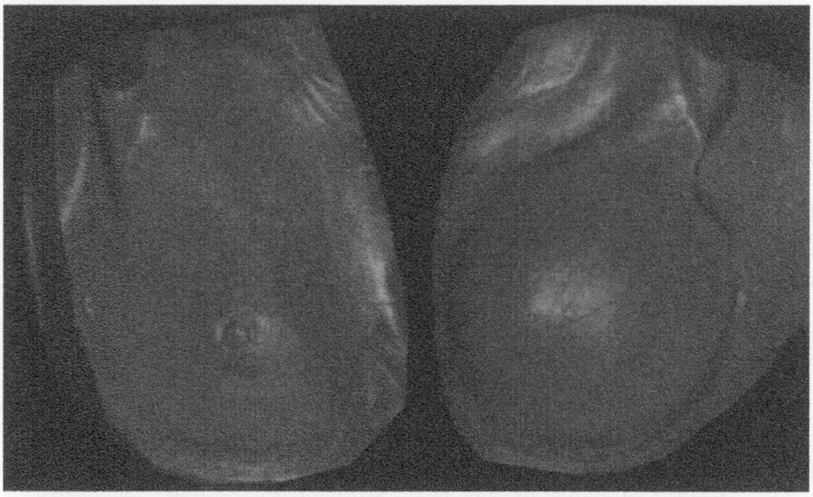

FIGURE 43.6 3D reconstructed CT images of a woman with left breast implant and normal right breast presenting for correction of asymmetry. (Reprinted from Chae, M.P. et al., *Breast Cancer Res. Treat.*, in press. With permission.)

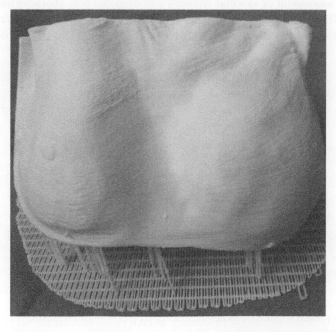

FIGURE 43.7 3D printed breast model of the woman described in Figure 43.6. (Reprinted from Chae, M.P. et al., *Breast Cancer Res. Treat.*, in press. With permission.)

multiple body regions, including the lower limb, gluteal region, lower trunk, breast, and head and neck. These models could not be printed in real-life size due to the printer dimensions. However, the models were printed with anatomical landmarks that facilitated intuitive appreciation of the shape and size of the breasts and the defect. Of note, the breast and the sacral pressure ulcer models took 15 and 12.5 h to print, respectively, and each used up approximately 50% of the printer cartridge.

43.8 PREOPERATIVE PLANNING: BONE MAPPING

3D printing of bony pathology in the hand can be useful for plastic surgeons. Bone 3D printing has been numerously reported in other surgical disciplines, such as maxillofacial surgery (Lee et al. 2007, Cohen et al. 2009, Cao et al. 2010, Herlin et al. 2011, Katsuragi et al. 2011, Chen et al. 2014,), craniofacial surgery (Ono et al. 2000, Ciocca et al. 2010, Lee et al. 2012), and orthopaedic surgery (Hsieh et al. 2010, Gan et al. 2011, Kunz et al. 2013, Kataoka et al. 2013, Minns et al. 2003). Using the same principles as already mentioned, we 3D printed a haptic model of a subluxed first carpometacarpal joint. The spatial relationship between the trapezium and the first metacarpal was easy to appreciate from the biomodel. Moreover, the model could be viewed from various angles in order to determine the method of reduction.

43.9 A NEW EVOLUTION: 4D PRINTING

To our knowledge, we are the first to apply 3D printing to 4D CT technology. Time-resolved CT data acquisition or 4D CT can provide information about spatiotemporal relationship of anatomical structures (Rietzel et al. 2005), such as the position of carpal bones during a hand movement. 4D CT has been developed and used extensively in respiratory medicine to remove lung motion artefact for precise radiotherapy planning and delivery (Reinhardt et al. 2008). 4D CT is performed by oversampling CT data acquisition at each slice and retrospectively reconstructing the data accounting for the chest wall movement during a respiratory cycle. In plastic surgery, 4D CTA has been utilised primarily for the assessment of vascular territory and dynamic flow characteristics of a perforator (Colohan et al. 2012, Nie et al. 2013). Recently, we 3D printed the 4D CT scan data of carpal bones of a patient in various stages of the thumb movement, such as abduction (Figure 43.8). All models

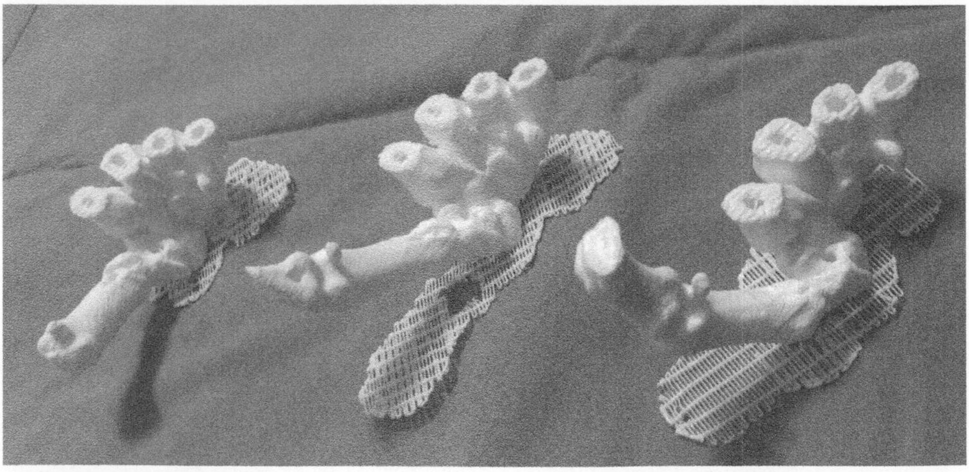

FIGURE 43.8 4D printed haptic models demonstrating progressive abduction (from left to right) of the first carpometacarpal joint.

were printed in real-life size, and each took 2–7 h to print. Encouragingly, the biomodels accurately reproduced the position of carpal bones during each movement and were easier to appreciate than 3D images on a computer screen. A potential challenge associated with this technique is that it relies on the discretion of the clinician reviewing the 4D data to determine which stage scan best represents the transition in carpal bone position during movement.

43.10 EDUCATION

Intuitive, detailed understanding of the anatomical structures and their spatial composition is an important asset of a plastic surgeon before performing an invasive procedure. Through a standard medical training, a surgical aspirant gains procedural experiences via human cadaveric dissections as a medical student and assisting senior surgeons in operating theatres as a resident towards a gradual improvement in competence. To this end, 3D printed haptic models can function as an accurate, tactile, visualisation medium to practice operative procedures on for a surgical trainee. In addition to producing a generic standardised anatomical model, a 3D printer is capable of replicating patient-specific situations. Furthermore, a haptic biomodel can be utilised to simulate an operation before a challenging, complex anatomical and pathological condition. This enables the operator to predict potential intraoperative challenges and postoperative outcomes. Subsequent improvement in the surgeon's ability and confidence leads to potentially superior patient outcomes and reduced risk of complications (Wurm et al. 2004, Knox et al. 2005, Armillotta et al. 2007, Mavili et al. 2007, Sulaiman et al. 2008, Bruyere et al. 2008, Kalejs and von Segesser 2009).

Furthermore, these biomodels can be used to facilitate physician–patient communication during a consultation. Better understanding of the intended procedure and potential outcomes and complications can form an important aspect of informed consent. For patients from non-medical background, an image of CT or MRI can be a foreign experience. In plastic surgery, 3D photography technology, such as VECTRA (Canfield Imaging Systems, Fairfield, NJ), has been utilised primarily in cosmetic procedures. However, evidences demonstrate that a haptic model that enables hands-on interaction may provide a superior, more intuitive understanding of a complex anatomical detail than a 2D or 3D imaging technique (Suzuki et al. 2004, Kim et al. 2008).

43.11 INDIVIDUALISED PROSTHESIS

RP technology, like 3D printing, has facilitated introduction of a more convenient and standardised method of manufacturing a custom prosthesis. Standard 3D printing materials can be sterilised by gas or autoclaving for intraoperative manipulation (Mottl-Link et al. 2008, Herlin et al. 2011, Lee et al. 2012). Currently, commercially available breast implants come in different volumes but in the same shape. To this effect, a 3D printed breast implant customised to account for individual variation in the chest wall anatomy and the desired breast shape and size may lead to a more aesthetic and satisfactory outcome. In the last decade, numerous reports have demonstrated the utility of 3D printed prostheses of the nose (Wu et al. 2008, Ciocca et al. 2010), the ear (Sykes et al. 2004, Subburaj et al. 2007, Karayazgan-Saracoglu et al. 2009), the eyes (Ciocca and Scotti 2013), the face (Tsuji et al. 2004), and hand (De Laurentis and Mavroidis 2002, Gerstle et al. 2014). Most reports indicate their superior aesthetics compared to wax-based prosthetics hand crafted by prosthetists (Sykes et al. 2004, Karayazgan-Saracoglu et al. 2009). Furthermore, they are associated with improved clinical outcome due to a reduction in the length of operation, leading to reduction in complications, such as infection (Eppley 2002, Sammartino et al. 2004).

43.12 FUTURE AND CONCLUSION

In the last decade, RP technologies, especially 3D printing, has introduced the production of haptic biomodels in medicine that can be a valuable addition to the conventional imaging modalities for comprehensive surgical planning, education of surgical trainees and patients, and fabrication of individualised prosthesis. Aided by extensive media exposure in recent times, 3D printing has garnered significant public interest and, hence, the technology is expected to become faster, cheaper, more accurate, more accessible, and easier to use. In plastic surgery, this technology ultimately has a potential to become an essential office-based tool for a surgeon.

ACKNOWLEDGEMENT

The authors would like to acknowledge the support from Prof. Robert T Spychal at Peninsula Health.

REFERENCES

Armillotta, A., Bonhoeffer, P., Dubini, G. et al. 2007. Use of rapid prototyping models in the planning of percutaneous pulmonary valved stent implantation. *Proc Inst Mech Eng H* 221 (4):407–416.

Bruyere, F., Leroux, C., Brunereau, L., and Lermusiaux, P. 2008. Rapid prototyping model for percutaneous nephrolithotomy training. *J Endourol* 22 (1):91–96.

Cao, D., Yu, Z., Chai, G., Liu, J., and Mu, X. 2010. Application of EH compound artificial bone material combined with computerized three-dimensional reconstruction in craniomaxillofacial surgery. *J Craniofac Surg* 21 (2):440–443.

Chae, M. P., Hunter-Smith, D. J., Spychal, R. T., and Rozen, W. M. 2014. 3D volumetric analysis for planning breast reconstructive surgery. *Breast Cancer Res Treat*, in press.

Chae, M. P., Lin, F., Spychal, R. T., Hunter-Smith, D. J., and Rozen, W. M. 3D-printed haptic models for preoperative planning in reconstructive surgery. *Microsurgery*, in press.

Chen, Y., Niu, F., Yu, B. et al. 2014. Three-dimensional preoperative design of distraction osteogenesis for hemifacial microsomia. *J Craniofac Surg* 25 (1):184–188.

Chen, Y. X., Zhang, K., Hao, Y. N., and Hu, Y. C. 2012. Research status and application prospects of digital technology in orthopaedics. *Orthop Surg* 4 (3):131–138.

Ciocca, L., De Crescenzio, F., Fantini, M., and Scotti, R. 2010. Rehabilitation of the nose using CAD/CAM and rapid prototyping technology after ablative surgery of squamous cell carcinoma: A pilot clinical report. *Int J Oral Maxillofac Implants* 25 (4):808–812.

Ciocca, L. and Scotti, R. 2013. Oculo-facial rehabilitation after facial cancer removal: Updated CAD/CAM procedures. A pilot study. *Prosthet Orthot Int*. [Epub ahead of Print].

Cohen, A., Laviv, A., Berman, P., Nashef, R., and Abu-Tair, J. 2009. Mandibular reconstruction using stereolithographic 3-dimensional printing modeling technology. *Oral Surg Oral Med Oral Pathol Oral Radiol Endod* 108 (5):661–666.

Colohan, S., Wong, C., Lakhiani, C. et al. 2012. The free descending branch muscle-sparing latissimus dorsi flap: Vascular anatomy and clinical applications. *Plast Reconstr Surg* 130 (6):776e–787e.

D'Urso, P. S., Barker, T. M., Earwaker, W. J. et al. 1999. Stereolithographic biomodelling in cranio-maxillofacial surgery: A prospective trial. *J Craniomaxillofac Surg* 27 (1):30–37.

D'Urso, P. S., Earwaker, W. J., Barker, T. M. et al. 2000. Custom cranioplasty using stereolithography and acrylic. *Br J Plast Surg* 53 (3):200–204.

De Laurentis, K. J. and Mavroidis, C. 2002. Mechanical design of a shape memory alloy actuated prosthetic hand. *Technol Health Care* 10 (2):91–106.

Eppley, B. L. 2002. Craniofacial reconstruction with computer-generated HTR patient-matched implants: Use in primary bony tumor excision. *J Craniofac Surg* 13 (5):650–657.

Gan, Y., Xu, D., Lu, S., and Ding, J. 2011. Novel patient-specific navigational template for total knee arthroplasty. *Comput Aided Surg* 16 (6):288–297.

Gerstle, T. L., Ibrahim, A. M., Kim, P. S., Lee, B. T., and Lin, S. J. 2014. A plastic surgery application in evolution: Three-dimensional printing. *Plast Reconstr Surg* 133 (2):446–451.

Goiato, M. C., Santos, M. R., Pesqueira, A. A. et al. 2011. Prototyping for surgical and prosthetic treatment. *J Craniofac Surg* 22 (3):914–917.

Guarino, J., Tennyson, S., McCain, G. et al. 2007. Rapid prototyping technology for surgeries of the pediatric spine and pelvis: Benefits analysis. *J Pediatr Orthop* 27 (8):955–960.

Hannen, E. J. 2006. Recreating the original contour in tumor deformed mandibles for plate adapting. *Int J Oral Maxillofac Surg* 35 (2):183–185.

Heissler, E., Fischer, F. S., Bolouri, S. et al. 1998. Custom-made cast titanium implants produced with CAD/CAM for the reconstruction of cranium defects. *Int J Oral Maxillofac Surg* 27 (5):334–338.

Herlin, C., Koppe, M., Beziat, J. L., and Gleizal, A. 2011. Rapid prototyping in craniofacial surgery: Using a positioning guide after zygomatic osteotomy—A case report. *J Craniomaxillofac Surg* 39 (5):376–379.

Hsieh, M. K., Chen, A. C., Cheng, C. Y. et al. 2010. Repositioning osteotomy for intra-articular malunion of distal radius with radiocarpal and/or distal radioulnar joint subluxation. *J Trauma* 69 (2):418–422.

Kalejs, M. and von Segesser, L. K. 2009. Rapid prototyping of compliant human aortic roots for assessment of valved stents. *Interact Cardiovasc Thorac Surg* 8 (2):182–186.

Karayazgan-Saracoglu, B., Gunay, Y., and Atay, A. 2009. Fabrication of an auricular prosthesis using computed tomography and rapid prototyping technique. *J Craniofac Surg* 20 (4):1169–1172.

Kataoka, T., Oka, K., Miyake, J. et al. 2013. 3-Dimensional prebent plate fixation in corrective osteotomy of malunited upper extremity fractures using a real-sized plastic bone model prepared by preoperative computer simulation. *J Hand Surg Am* 38 (5):909–919.

Katsuragi, Y., Kayano, S., Akazawa, S. et al. 2011. Mandible reconstruction using the calcium-sulphate three-dimensional model and rubber stick: A new method, 'mould technique', for more accurate, efficient and simplified fabrication. *J Plast Reconstr Aesthet Surg* 64 (5):614–622.

Kim, M. S., Hansgen, A. R., Wink, O., Quaife, R. A., and Carroll, J. D. 2008. Rapid prototyping: A new tool in understanding and treating structural heart disease. *Circulation* 117 (18):2388–2394.

Knox, K., Kerber, C. W., Singel, S. A., Bailey, M. J., and Imbesi, S. G. 2005. Rapid prototyping to create vascular replicas from CT scan data: Making tools to teach, rehearse, and choose treatment strategies. *Catheter Cardiovasc Interv* 65 (1):47–53.

Kunz, M., Ma, B., Rudan, J. F., Ellis, R. E., and Pichora, D. R. 2013. Image-guided distal radius osteotomy using patient-specific instrument guides. *J Hand Surg Am* 38 (8):1618–1624.

Lee, J. W., Fang, J. J., Chang, L. R., and Yu, C. K. 2007. Mandibular defect reconstruction with the help of mirror imaging coupled with laser stereolithographic modeling technique. *J Formos Med Assoc* 106 (3):244–250.

Lee, S. J., Lee, H. P., Tse, K. M., Cheong, E. C., and Lim, S. P. 2012. Computer-aided design and rapid prototyping-assisted contouring of costal cartilage graft for facial reconstructive surgery. *Craniomaxillofac Trauma Reconstr* 5 (2):75–82.

Mavili, M. E., Canter, H. I., Saglam-Aydinatay, B., Kamaci, S., and Kocadereli, I. 2007. Use of three-dimensional medical modeling methods for precise planning of orthognathic surgery. *J Craniofac Surg* 18 (4):740–747.

Minns, R. J., Bibb, R., Banks, R., and Sutton, R. A. 2003. The use of a reconstructed three-dimensional solid model from CT to aid the surgical management of a total knee arthroplasty: A case study. *Med Eng Phys* 25 (6):523–526.

Mottl-Link, S., Hubler, M., Kuhne, T. et al. 2008. Physical models aiding in complex congenital heart surgery. *Ann Thorac Surg* 86 (1):273–277.

Nie, J. Y., Lu, L. J., Gong, X., Li, Q., and Nie, J. J. 2013. Delineating the vascular territory (perforasome) of a perforator in the lower extremity of the rabbit with four-dimensional computed tomographic angiography. *Plast Reconstr Surg* 131 (3):565–571.

Ono, I., Abe, K., Shiotani, S., and Hirayama, Y. 2000. Producing a full-scale model from computed tomographic data with the rapid prototyping technique using the binder jet method: A comparison with the laser lithography method using a dry skull. *J Craniofac Surg* 11 (6):527–537.

Ono, I., Gunji, H., Suda, K., and Kaneko, F. 1994. Method for preparing an exact-size model using helical volume scan computed tomography. *Plast Reconstr Surg* 93 (7):1363–1371.

Reinhardt, J. M., Ding, K., Cao, K. et al. 2008. Registration-based estimates of local lung tissue expansion compared to xenon CT measures of specific ventilation. *Med Image Anal* 12 (6):752–763.

Rengier, F., Mehndiratta, A., von Tengg-Kobligk, H. et al. 2010. 3D printing based on imaging data: Review of medical applications. *Int J Comput Assist Radiol Surg* 5 (4):335–341.

Rietzel, E., Pan, T., and Chen, G. T. 2005. Four-dimensional computed tomography: Image formation and clinical protocol. *Med Phys* 32 (4):874–889.

Rozen, W. M., Anavekar, N. S., Ashton, M. W. et al. 2008a. Does the preoperative imaging of perforators with CT angiography improve operative outcomes in breast reconstruction? *Microsurgery* 28 (7):516–523.

Rozen, W. M., Ashton, M. W., Grinsell, D. et al. 2008b. Establishing the case for CT angiography in the preoperative imaging of abdominal wall perforators. *Microsurgery* 28 (5):306–313.

Rozen, W. M., Ashton, M. W., Stella, D. L. et al. 2008c. The accuracy of computed tomographic angiography for mapping the perforators of the deep inferior epigastric artery: A blinded, prospective cohort study. *Plast Reconstr Surg* 122 (4):1003–1009.

Rozen, W. M., Chubb, D., Grinsell, D., and Ashton, M. W. 2011. Computed tomographic angiography: Clinical applications. *Clin Plast Surg* 38 (2):229–239.

Rozen, W. M., Ting, J. W., Baillieu, C., and Leong, J. 2012a. Stereolithographic modeling of the deep circumflex iliac artery and its vascular branching: A further advance in computed tomography-guided flap planning. *Plast Reconstr Surg* 130 (2):380e–382e.

Rozen, W. M., Ting, J. W., Leung, M. et al. 2012b. Advancing image-guided surgery in microvascular mandibular reconstruction: Combining bony and vascular imaging with computed tomography-guided stereolithographic bone modeling. *Plast Reconstr Surg* 130 (1):227e–229e.

Sammartino, G., Della Valle, A., Marenzi, G. et al. 2004. Stereolithography in oral implantology: A comparison of surgical guides. *Implant Dent* 13 (2):133–139.

Stoker, N. G., Mankovich, N. J., and Valentino, D. 1992. Stereolithographic models for surgical planning: Preliminary report. *J Oral Maxillofac Surg* 50 (5):466–471.

Subburaj, K., Nair, C., Rajesh, S., Meshram, S. M., and Ravi, B. 2007. Rapid development of auricular prosthesis using CAD and rapid prototyping technologies. *Int J Oral Maxillofac Surg* 36 (10):938–943.

Sulaiman, A., Boussel, L., Taconnet, F. et al. 2008. In vitro non-rigid life-size model of aortic arch aneurysm for endovascular prosthesis assessment. *Eur J Cardiothorac Surg* 33 (1):53–57.

Suzuki, M., Ogawa, Y., Kawano, A. et al. 2004. Rapid prototyping of temporal bone for surgical training and medical education. *Acta Otolaryngol* 124 (4):400–402.

Sykes, L. M., Parrott, A. M., Owen, C. P., and Snaddon, D. R. 2004. Applications of rapid prototyping technology in maxillofacial prosthetics. *Int J Prosthodont* 17 (4):454–459.

Tsuji, M., Noguchi, N., Ihara, K. et al. 2004. Fabrication of a maxillofacial prosthesis using a computer-aided design and manufacturing system. *J Prosthodont* 13 (3):179–183.

Way, T. P. and Barner, K. E. 1997. Automatic visual to tactile translation – Part II: Evaluation of the TACTile image creation system. *IEEE Trans Rehabil Eng* 5 (1):95–105.

Wu, G., Zhou, B., Bi, Y., and Zhao, Y. 2008. Selective laser sintering technology for customized fabrication of facial prostheses. *J Prosthet Dent* 100 (1):56–60.

Wurm, G., Tomancok, B., Pogady, P., Holl, K., and Trenkler, J. 2004. Cerebrovascular stereolithographic biomodeling for aneurysm surgery. Technical note. *J Neurosurg* 100 (1):139–145.

Xu, H., Han, D., Dong, J. S. et al. 2010. Rapid prototyped PGA/PLA scaffolds in the reconstruction of mandibular condyle bone defects. *Int J Med Robot* 6 (1):66–72.

Index

A

B

C

D

E

F

G

H

K

L

M

N

O

P

R

T

U

V

Printed and bound by CPI Group (UK) Ltd, Croydon, CR0 4YY
22/10/2024
01777614-0018